Access Videos, Quizzes, Self Assessments, and More!

Self-study Companion Website resources included with any book.

Access to MyHealthLab, including assignments and eText, sold separately. To purchase access to MyHealthLab, visit www.mypearsonstore.com.

REGISTER NOW!

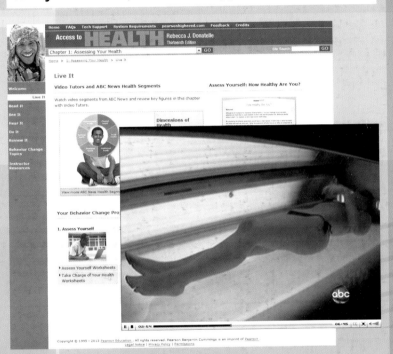

Registration will let you:

- See It! with *ABC News* videos and student behavior change Vlogs.
- Hear It! with MP3 Tutor Sessions and MP3 Case Studies.
- Do It! with essay-question quizzes, Nutritools activities, and web links.
- Live It! with *Assess Yourself* activities, Video Tutors, and other worksheets.

Registration also gives you access to multiple practice quizzes, mobile apps, web links, and more.

www.pearsonhighered.com/donatelle

TO REGISTER

1. Go to www.pearsonhighered.com/donatelle
2. Click on your book cover.
3. Select any chapter from the drop-down menu and click "Go."
4. Click "See It."
5. Click "Register."
6. Follow the on-screen instructions to create your login name and password.

Your Access Code is:

Note: If there is no silver foil covering the access code, it may already have been redeemed, and therefore may no longer be valid. In that case, you can purchase access online using a major credit card or PayPal account. To do so, go to www.pearsonhighered.com/donatelle, click on "Buy Access," and follow the on-screen instructions.

TO LOG IN

1. Go to www.pearsonhighered.com/donatelle
2. Click on your book cover.
3. Select any chapter from the drop-down menu and click "Go."
4. Click "See It" and then click one of the video options.
5. Enter your login name and password.

Hint:
Remember to bookmark the site after you log in.

Technical Support:
http://247pearsoned.custhelp.com

BEHAVIOR CHANGE CONTRACT

Complete the Assess Yourself questionnaire. After reviewing your results and considering the various factors that influence your decisions, choose a health behavior that you would like to change, starting this quarter or semester. Sign the contract at the bottom to affirm your commitment to making a healthy change and ask a friend to witness it.

My behavior change will be:

_____

My long-term goal for this behavior change is:

_____

These are three obstacles to change (things that I am currently doing or situations that contribute to this behavior or make it harder to change):

1. _____
2. _____
3. _____

The strategies I will use to overcome these obstacles are:

1. _____
2. _____
3. _____

Resources I will use to help me change this behavior include:

a friend/partner/relative: _____

a school-based resource: _____

a community-based resource: _____

a book or reputable website: _____

In order to make my goal more attainable, I have devised these short-term goals:

_____   _____   _____
short-term goal   target date   reward

_____   _____   _____
short-term goal   target date   reward

_____   _____   _____
short-term goal   target date   reward

When I make the long-term behavior change described above, my reward will be:

_____   target date: _____

I intend to make the behavior change described above. I will use the strategies and rewards to achieve the goals that will contribute to a healthy behavior change.

Signed: _____   Witness: _____

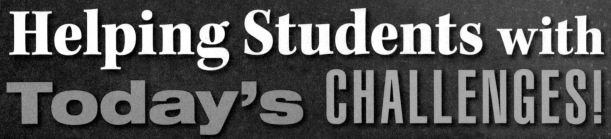

Helping Students with Today's CHALLENGES!

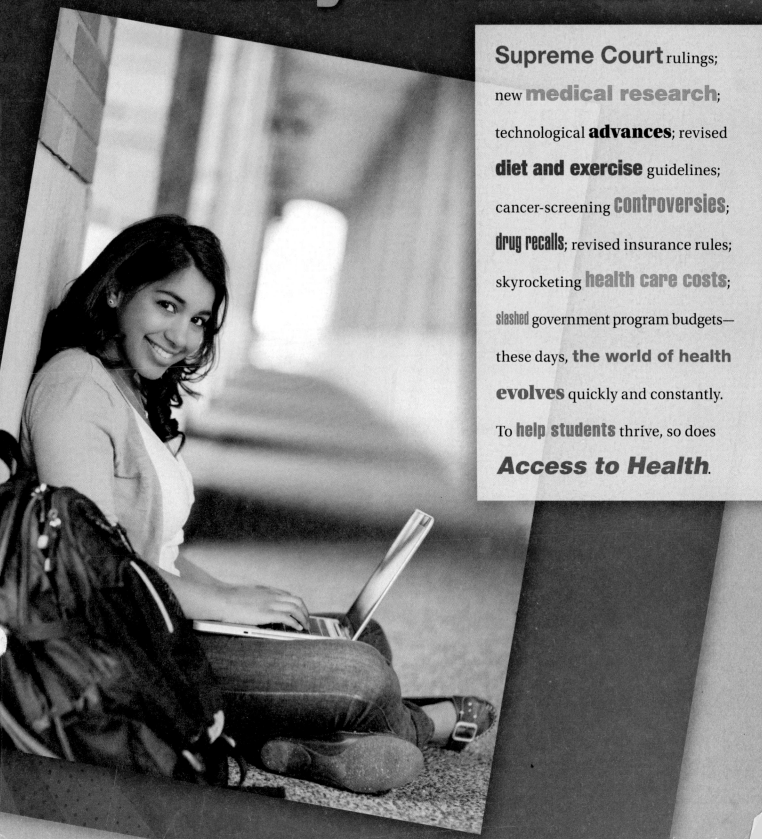

Supreme Court rulings; new **medical research**; technological **advances**; revised **diet and exercise** guidelines; cancer-screening **controversies**; **drug recalls**; revised insurance rules; skyrocketing **health care costs**; slashed government program budgets— these days, **the world of health evolves** quickly and constantly. To **help students** thrive, so does *Access to Health*.

New *Money & Health* Features Help Students Become Savvy Health Consumers

Students Profit from Learning to Have a Healthier Relationship with Money

Read about money-related health topics such as maximizing health care services while minimizing costs, easing the financial stress of college, and understanding how the recent U.S. health care legislation impacts the cost of contraception.

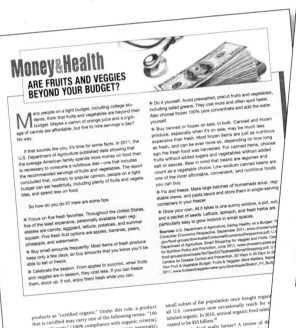

Money&Health
ARE FRUITS AND VEGGIES BEYOND YOUR BUDGET?

Many people on a tight budget, including college students, think that fruits and vegetables are beyond their budget. Maybe a carton of orange juice and a package of carrots are affordable, but five to nine servings a day? No way.

If that sounds like you, it's time for some facts. In 2011, the U.S. Department of Agriculture published data showing that the average American family spends more money on food than is necessary to consume a nutritious diet—one that includes the recommended servings of fruits and vegetables. The report concluded that, contrary to popular opinion, people on a tight budget can eat healthfully, including plenty of fruits and vegetables, and spend less on food.

So how do you do it? Here are some tips:

✱ **Focus on five fresh favorites.** Throughout the United States, five of the least expensive, perennially available fresh vegetables are carrots, eggplant, lettuce, potatoes, and summer squash. Five fresh fruit options are apples, bananas, pears, pineapple, and watermelon.

✱ **Buy small amounts frequently.** Most items of fresh produce keep only a few days, so buy amounts that you know you'll be able to eat or freeze.

✱ **Celebrate the season.** From apples to zucchini, when fruits and veggies are in season, they cost less. If you can freeze them, stock up. If not, enjoy them fresh while you can.

✱ **Do it yourself.** Avoid prewashed, precut fruits and vegetables, including salad greens. They cost more and often spoil faster. Also choose frozen 100% juice concentrate and add the water yourself.

✱ **Buy canned or frozen on sale, in bulk.** Canned and frozen produce, especially when it's on sale, may be much less expensive than fresh. Most frozen items are just as nutritious as fresh, and can be even more so, depending on how long ago the fresh food was harvested. For canned items, choose fruits without added sugars and vegetables without added salt or sauces. Bear in mind that beans are legumes and count as a vegetable choice. Low-sodium canned beans are one of the most affordable, convenient, and nutritious foods you can buy.

✱ **Fix and freeze.** Make large batches of homemade soup, vegetable stews, and pasta sauce and store them in single-serving containers in your freezer.

✱ **Grow your own.** All it takes is one sunny window, a pot, soil, and a packet of seeds. Lettuce, spinach, and fresh herbs are particularly easy to grow indoors in small spaces.

Sources: U.S. Department of Agriculture, *Eating Healthy on a Budget: The Consumer Economics Perspective, September 2011, www.choosemyplate. gov/food-groups/downloads/ConsumerEconomicsPerspective.pdf; U.S. Department of Agriculture, Smart Shopping for Veggies and Fruits, Center for Nutrition Policy and Promotion, June 2011, www.choosemyplate.gov/ food-groups/downloads/TenTips/DGTipsheet9SmartShopping.pdf; U.S. Centers for Disease Control and Prevention, 30 Ways in 30 Days to Stretch Your Fruit & Vegetable Budget, Fruits & Veggies: More Matters, September 2011, www.fruitsandveggiesmatter.gov/downloads/Stretch_FV_Budget.pdf.*

products as "certified organic." Under this rule, a product that is certified may carry one of the following terms: "100 percent Organic" (100% compliance with organic criteria), "Organic" (must contain at least 95% organic materials), "Made with Organic Ingredients" (must contain at least 70% organic ingredients), or "Some Organic Ingredients" (contains less than 70% organic ingredients—usually listed individually). To be labeled with any of the above terms, the foods also must be produced without hormones, antibiotics, or genetic modification. However, reliable monitoring systems to ensure credibility are still under development.

The market for organic foods has been increasing by more than 20 percent per year—five times faster than food sales in general. Where only a small subset of the population once bought organic, all U.S. consumers now occasionally reach for something labeled organic. In 2010, annual organic food sales were estimated to be $25 billion.[41]

Is organic food really better? A review of the studies published over the past 50 years found no substantive difference in nutrient quality of organic versus traditionally grown foods.[42] However, pesticide residues do remain on conventionally grown produce. In 2011, the USDA reported that 3 percent of food samples harvested in 2009 had pesticide residues that exceeded the established tolerance level or for which no tolerance level has been established. The USDA advises that consumers always rinse fruits and vegetables before cooking or consuming them.[43]

USDA ORGANIC
U.S. FDA label for organic foods.

Money&Health
INVESTING IN YOUR PHYSICAL HEALTH! HOW TO SHOP FOR FITNESS FACILITIES, EQUIPMENT, AND CLOTHING

Do you really need to belong to the best gym or have the latest equipment and fashionable clothing to meet your physical fitness goals? The short answer is no. You can achieve your personal goals without joining a fitness center, without buying equipment, and without spending lots of money on the latest fitness fashions. All you need is a good pair of shoes, comfortable clothing to suit the environment you will be physically active in, your own body to use as resistance, and a safe place for activity. However, you may enjoy the experience of going to a wellness center or prefer to buy exercise equipment for your home, and you may need new exercise clothing. Use the following tips to help guide you through this process.

CHOOSING A FACILITY

✱ Visit several facilities before making a decision, if possible during the time when you intend to use them (so you can see how busy or crowded they are at that time).

✱ Determine the location and hours of operation; are these convenient for you?

✱ Consider the exercise classes offered. What is the schedule? Can you try one for free?

✱ Evaluate their equipment. Is it sufficient to cover your training needs (i.e., aerobic exercise machines, resistance-training equipment, including both free weights and machines, mats, and other items to assist with stretching)?

Before you sign on the dotted line, check out the classes, equipment, and personnel a fitness center offers.

✱ Consider the personnel (including training in first aid and CPR), options for working with a personal trainer, and how friendly and approachable they are.

✱ Consider the financial implications. What membership benefits, student rates, or other discounts are available? Steer clear of clubs that pressure you for a long-term commitment and do not offer trial memberships or grace periods that allow you to get a refund.

BUYING EQUIPMENT

✱ Ignore claims that an exercise device provides lasting "no sweat" results in a short time.

✱ Question claims that an exercise device can target or burn fat.

✱ Read the fine print. Advertised results may be based on more than just using this machine; they may also involve caloric restriction.

✱ Be skeptical of testimonials and before-and-after pictures of satisfied customers.

✱ Calculate the total cost by including shipping and handling fees, sales tax, delivery and setup charges, or long-term commitments.

✱ Ask about warranties, guarantees, and return policies.

✱ Try the equipment at a gym, if you can, or borrow it from someone.

✱ Consider how this piece of equipment will fit in your home. Where will you store it? Will you be able to get to it easily?

✱ Check out consumer reviews or online resources for the best product ratings.

BUYING EXERCISE CLOTHING

✱ Choose your exercise clothing based on comfort, not looks. It should be neither too loose nor too tight.

✱ Consider the environment (temperature, humidity, ventilation) when making your selection.

✱ Dress in layers, ensuring that your skin can breathe in the cold (see also the section Exercising in the Cold).

✱ Dress to allow for optimal heat dissipation in hot and humid environments (see also the section Exercising in the Heat).

✱ Choose clothing that helps you to feel good about yourself and the activity you are undertaking.

New *Tech & Health* Features Discuss Social Media, Smart Phone Apps, Gadgets, and Other Tech Advances

Giving Students the Knowledge to Harness Technology to Improve Their Health

Students use technology all the time in their everyday lives. The new *Tech & Health* features address issues such as privacy and safety concerns with social media and Internet addiction. These features also highlight trusted sources of health information online, talk about tech developments that impact health, and give a heads up on useful smartphone applications for diet, fitness, and much more.

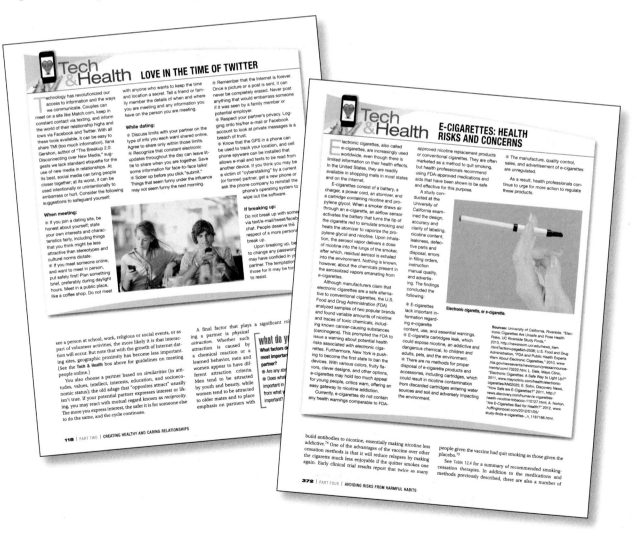

Cutting-Edge Concepts Come Alive through Technology

New: Quick Response (QR) Codes Provide Instant Access to Video Tutors!

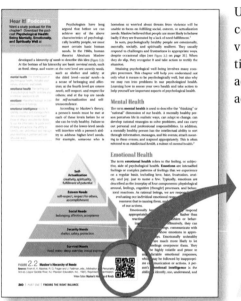

Using a QR code reader app on your smartphone, scan the code and quickly load *Video Tutors* on your device. These videos dynamically use book art and photos along with narration to reinforce key concepts such as reading food labels, the acute stress response, benefits of regular exercise, how drugs act on the brain, and the chain of infection.

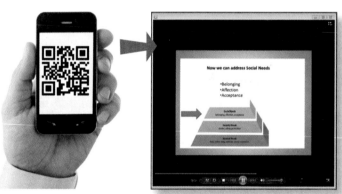

See It!, *Hear It!*, and *Do It!* Boxes Link to Key Online Content

Hear It! boxes reference study podcasts and *See It!* boxes call out *ABC News* videos in all chapters. Now the "Eating for a Healthier You" chapter also contains *Do It!* boxes that reference Pearson *NutriTools* nutrition activities. Content is accessible through the Companion Website or in MyHealthLab. Pre-built, gradable assignments are available through MyHealthLab for the *ABC News* videos.

See It! Videos
Put down that cell phone! Watch **The Multi-Tasking Myth** at www.pearsonhighered.com/donatelle to understand why doing multiple things at once might not be the best idea.

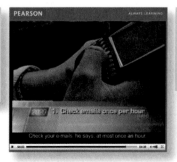

Hear It! Podcasts
Want a study podcast for this chapter? Download the podcast **Personal Fitness: Improving Health through Exercise** at www.pearsonhighered.com/donatelle

Do It! Nutritools
Ever wondered how your favorite meal stacks up, nutrition-wise? Go to the Do It! section of www.pearsonhighered.com/donatelle to complete the **Build a Meal, Build a Salad, Build a Pizza,** and **Build a Sandwich** activities. Put your food choices on a virtual plate and see where it falls on a healthy-eating scale.

So Many Options for You and Your Students

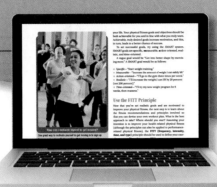

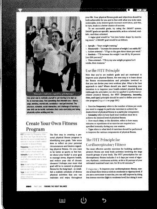

Students today want options when it comes to learning and textbooks. *Access to Health* gives students flexibility, offering a wide range of formats for the book and a large array of online learning resources. Let your students find a version that works best for them!

Access to Health Pearson eText in MyHealthLab

0-321-85956-1/978-0-321-85956-3

Available at no additional charge within MyHealthLab, the eText version of the print book gives students access to the text whenever and wherever they please. Pearson eText pages look just like the printed book, but allow students to click on linked resources such as study podcasts and videos. You can highlight, bookmark, and zoom text. Students who purchase access to MyHealthLab also get access to the eText via the Pearson Apple iPad application.

Access to Health CourseSmart eTextbook

0-321-85964-2/978-0-321-85964-8

CourseSmart eTextbooks are an exciting new choice for students looking to save money. Students can subscribe to content online and save up to 40 percent compared to the print book price. Go to www.coursesmart.com.

Access to Health Books a la Carte

0-321-85965-0/978-0-321-85965-5

Books a la Carte features exactly the same content as *Access to Health* but provides it in a convenient, three-hole-punched, loose-leaf version. Books a la Carte offers a great value for students, costing 35 percent less than a standard new textbook package.

Pearson Custom Library: You Create Your Perfect Text

www.pearsonlearningsolutions.com/custom-library

Access to Health is also available in the Pearson Custom Library, allowing you to create the perfect text for your course. Select the chapters you need in the sequence you want. Delete chapters you opt not to use—your students pay only for what you choose.

MyHealthLab®

http://www.pearsonhighered.com/myhealthlab

The new **MyHealthLab**® from Pearson has been designed and refined with a single purpose in mind: to help educators create that moment of understanding for their students.

The MyHealthLab system helps instructors maximize class time with customizable, easy-to-assign, and automatically graded assignments that motivate students to learn outside of class and arrive prepared for the lecture.

By complementing your teaching with our engaging technology and content, you can be confident your students will arrive at that moment—the moment of true understanding.

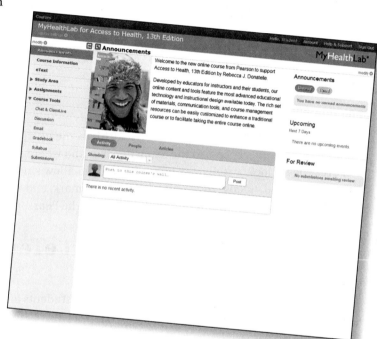

Engaging Experiences

MyHealthLab provides a one-stop spot for accessing a wealth of preloaded content and tools, while giving you the ability to customize your course as much as you'd like.

The fresh, clean layout is pleasing to both new and experienced users.

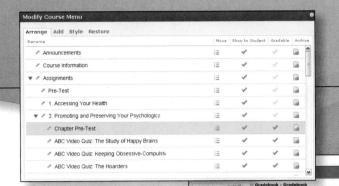

New! Over 150 Pre-Built Assignments

Instructors can lessen their prep time and simplify their lives with preloaded quiz and test questions (specific to the textbook) that they can assign and/or edit, a gradebook that automatically records student results from assigned tests, and the ability to customize the course as much (or as little) as desired.

New! *Video Tutors* and *ABC News* Videos

Video Tutors are 27 brand-new videos that use book figures and photos. These videos are referenced in the textbook with Quick Response (QR) Codes—just scan the code with your phone for quick loading and viewing. Additionally, the book comes with access to over 60 *ABC News* videos that bring personal health topics to life. These are available on the Instructor Resource DVD, MyHealthLab, and the Companion Website.

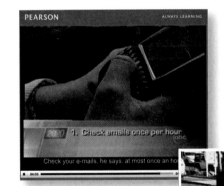

New! Pre- and Post-Evaluations

You can now easily measure before and after results for Student Learning Outcomes. A 50-question exam can be assigned at the start of the course, and again at the end, to effectively measure Student Learning Outcomes.

Dynamic Instructor Supplements for Teaching and Class Preparation

Teaching Tool Box

0-321-85962-6/978-0-321-85962-4

Instructors find a wealth of resources that reinforce key learning from the text and suit virtually any teaching style. The Teaching Tool Box includes the following:

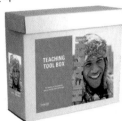

- **New!** Printed *Assess Yourself* Activities self-assessment student supplement
- Instructor Resource DVD
- Printed Test Bank
- Instructor Resource and Support Manual
- User's Quick Guide
- MyLab Instructor Access Card
- *Take Charge* Self-Assessment Worksheets

- *Teaching with Student Learning Outcomes*
- *Teaching with Web 2.0*
- *Great Ideas: Active Ways to Teach Health and Wellness*
- *Behavior Change Log Book and Wellness Journal* student supplement
- *Eat Right! Healthy Eating in College and Beyond* student supplement
- *Live Right! Beating Stress in College and Beyond* student supplement

Instructor Resource DVD

The Instructor Resource DVD contains the Computerized Test Bank, over 60 *ABC News* videos, PowerPoint lecture outlines, PowerPoint step-edit images, clicker questions, quiz-show questions, jpeg files for book figures, tables and selected photos, transparency masters, and Word® files for the Test Bank.

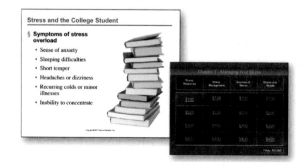

New! Printed *Assess Yourself* Activities

0-321-86014-4/978-0-321-86014-9

Long available online and reporting to the electronic gradebook, these popular behavior-change assessments and activities are now also available as a printed booklet for instructors who prefer to assign traditional, paper homework. (For more details on *Assess Yourself* worksheets, see the inside front cover.)

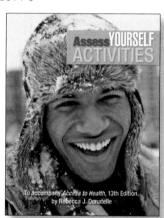

Teaching with Student Learning Outcomes

0-321-80265-9/ 978-0-321-80265-1

This new publication contains essays from 11 instructors who are teaching using student learning outcomes. They share goals in using outcomes, the processes that they follow to develop and refine outcomes, and many tips and suggestions for successfully incorporating outcomes into a personal health course.

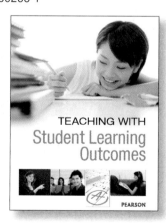

Access to

HEALTH

Thirteenth Edition

Rebecca J. Donatelle

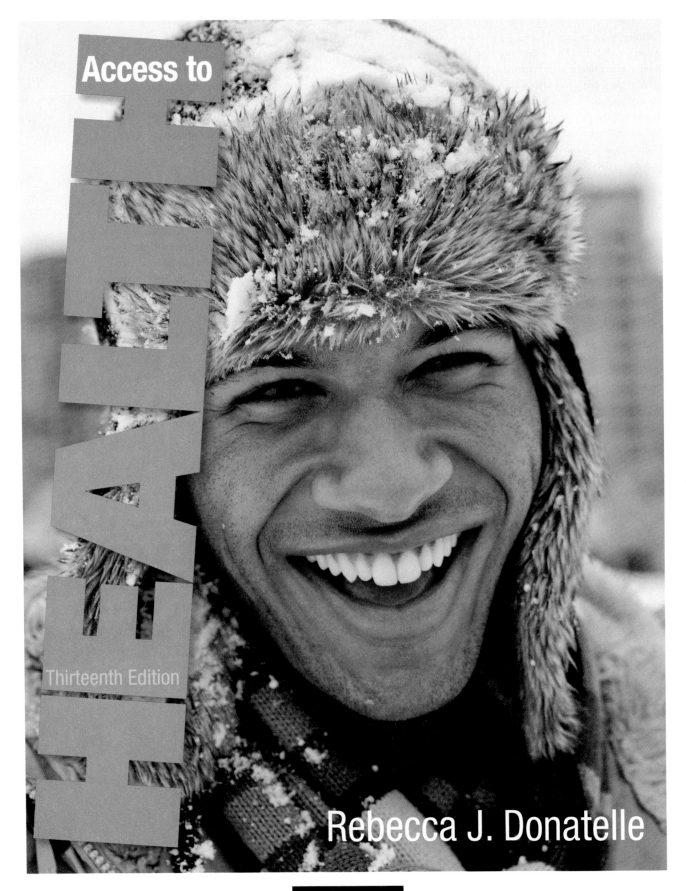

PEARSON

Boston Columbus Indianapolis New York San Francisco Upper Saddle River
Amsterdam Cape Town Dubai London Madrid Milan Munich Paris Montréal Toronto
Delhi Mexico City São Paulo Sydney Hong Kong Seoul Singapore Taipei Tokyo

Executive Editor: Sandra Lindelof

Project Development Editor: Erin Strathmann

Development Editors: Alice Fugate, Tanya Martin

Editorial Manager: Susan Malloy

Editorial Assistant: Briana Verdugo

Managing Editor: Deborah Cogan

Production Project Manager: Megan Power

Production Management: Thistle Hill Publishing Services

Compositor: Nesbitt Graphics

Interior Designer and Cover Designer: Gary Hespenheide

Illustrator: Precision Graphics

Photo Editor: Donna Kalal

Manufacturing Buyer: Stacey Weinberger

Executive Marketing Manager: Neena Bali

Text Printer: Donnelley/Menasha

Cover Printer: Lehigh-Phoenix Color

Cover Photo Credit: Noel Hendrickson/Getty Images

Credits and acknowledgments borrowed from other sources and reproduced, with permission, in this textbook appear on the appropriate page within the text and on page C-1.

Many of the designations used by manufacturers and sellers to distinguish their products are claimed as trademarks. Where those designations appear in this book, and the publisher was aware of a trademark claim, the designations have been printed in initial caps or all caps.

Library of Congress Cataloging-in-Publication Data

Donatelle, Rebecca J., 1950–

 Access to health / Rebecca J. Donatelle, Oregon State University. — Thirteenth edition.

   pages ; cm

 Includes bibliographical references and index.

 ISBN 978-0-321-83202-3 (pbk.) — ISBN 0-321-83202-7 (pbk.)

 1. Health. I. Title.

 RA776.D66 2014

 613—dc23

                      2012032629

ISBN 10: 0321832027 (Student edition)

ISBN 13: 9780321832023 (Student edition)

ISBN 10: 0321859596 (Instructor's Review Copy)

ISBN 13: 9780321859594 (Instructor's Review Copy)

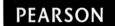

Brief Contents

Contents

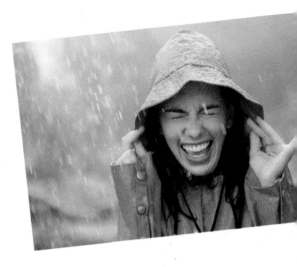

2 Promoting and Preserving Your Psychological Health   28

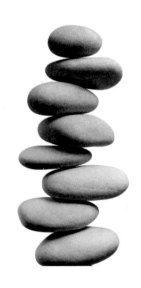

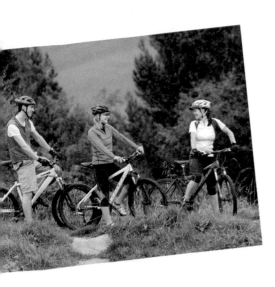

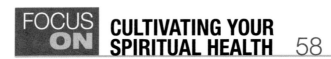

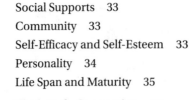 **CULTIVATING YOUR SPIRITUAL HEALTH** 58

3 Managing Stress and Coping with Life's Challenges   70

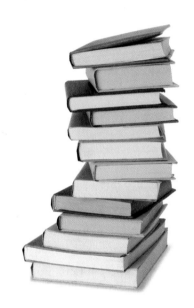

FOCUS ON IMPROVING YOUR SLEEP   98

Part Two: Creating Healthy and Caring Relationships

4 Building Healthy Relationships and Communicating Effectively   112

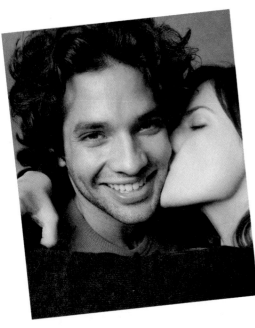

5 Understanding Your Sexuality 136

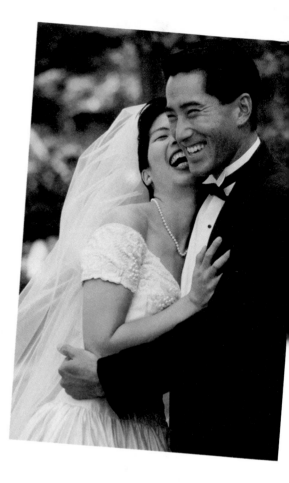

6 Considering Your Reproductive Choices 162

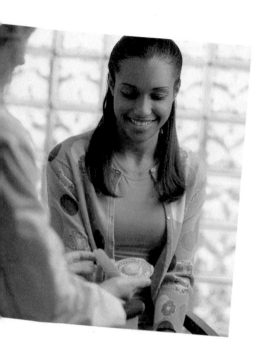

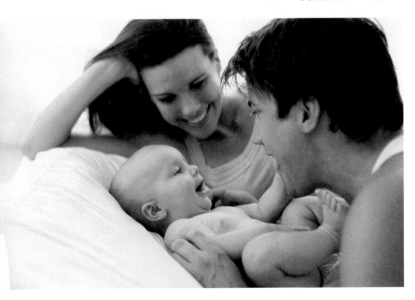

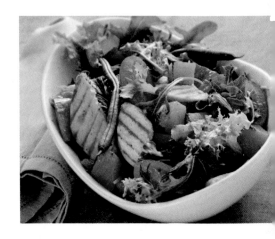

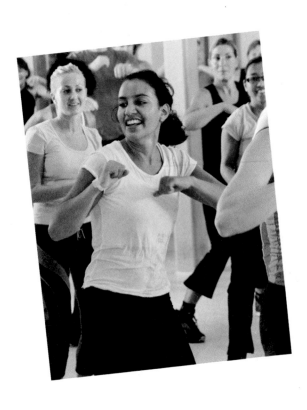

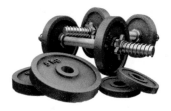

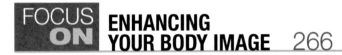

FOCUS ON ENHANCING YOUR BODY IMAGE   266

9 Improving Your Physical Fitness   280

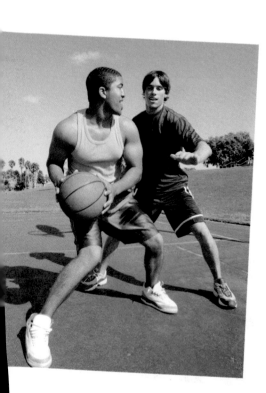

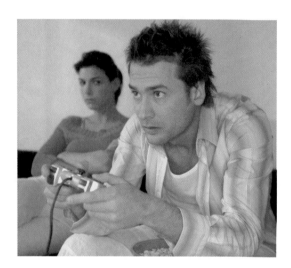

12 Ending Tobacco Use   354

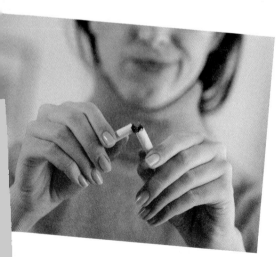

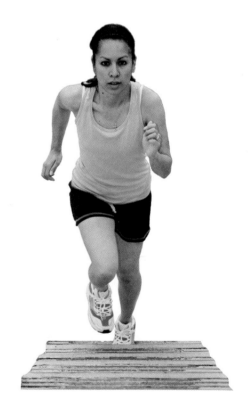

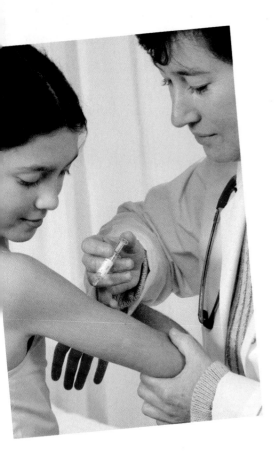

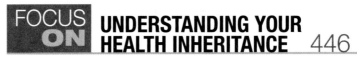

FOCUS ON **UNDERSTANDING YOUR HEALTH INHERITANCE** 446

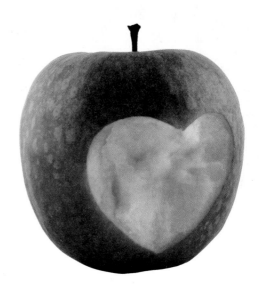

 MINIMIZING YOUR RISK FOR DIABETES 482

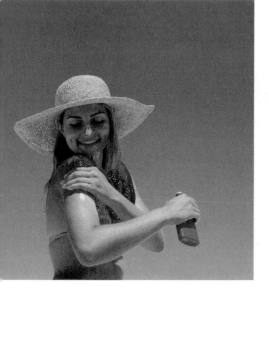

16 Reducing Your Cancer Risk   496

17 Reducing Risks and Coping with Chronic Conditions   522

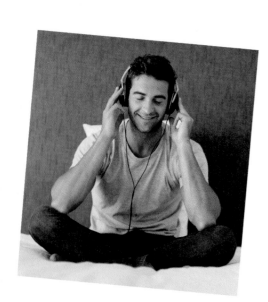

Part Six: Facing Life's Challenges

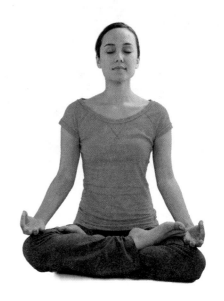

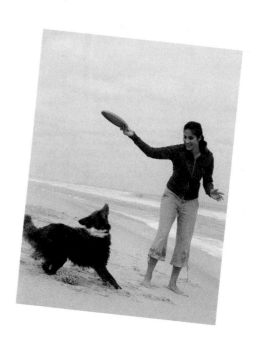

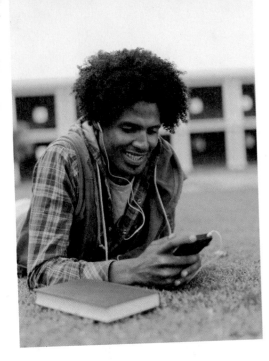

 REDUCING YOUR RISK OF UNINTENTIONAL INJURY   598

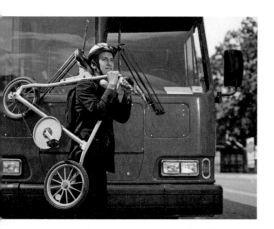

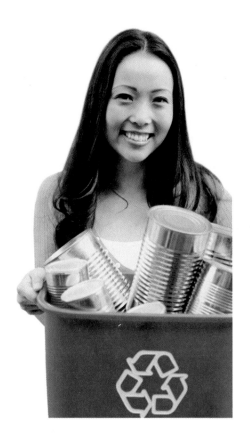

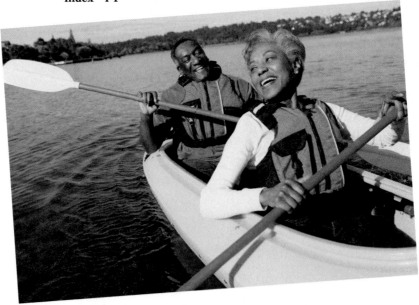

Feature Boxes

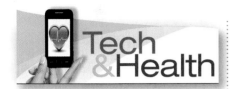

Money&Health

Skills for Behavior Change

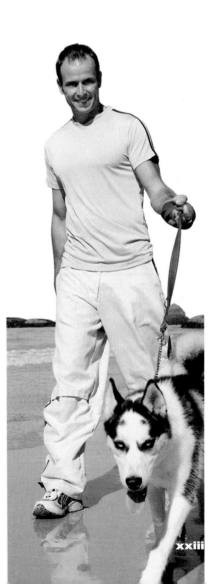

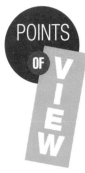

POINTS OF VIEW

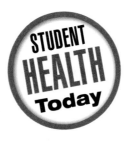

STUDENT HEALTH Today

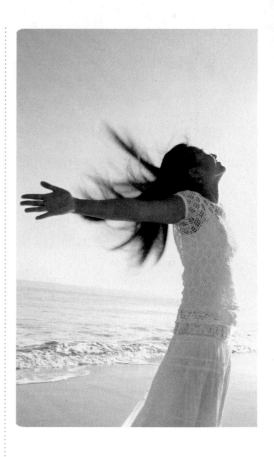

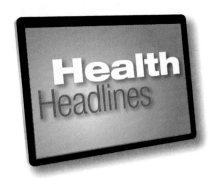

Health In a Diverse World

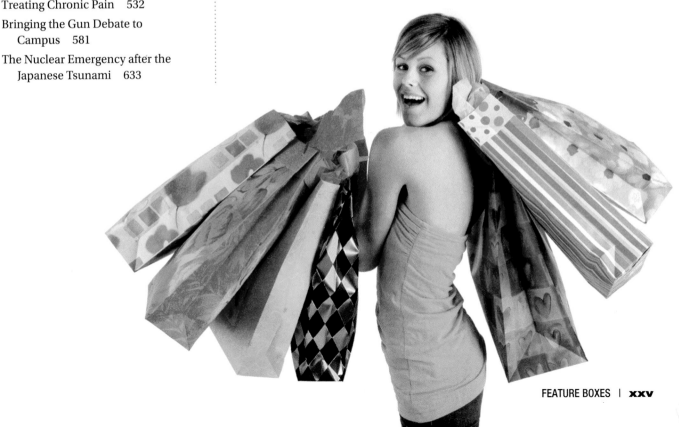

BE HEALTHY, BE GREEN

Online Access to Health

Assess yourself

Go to **www.pearsonhighered.com/donatelle** and select the book you use. Find the chapter you want in the drop down menu, and then you will see the Assess Yourself activities. Printed versions of these same worksheets can be made available to students if instructors so choose.

Video Tutors

Chapter 1: Accessing Your Health
Dimensions of Health

Chapter 4: Building Healthy Relationships and Communicating Effectively
Gender Differences in Communication

Chapter 2: Promoting and Preserving Your Psychological Health
Maslow's Hierarchy of Needs

Chapter 5: Understanding Your Sexuality
Male and Female Sexual Response

Focus On: Cultivating Your Spiritual Health
Facets of Spirituality

Chapter 6: Considering Your Reproductive Choices
Choosing Contraception

Chapter 3: Managing Stress and Coping with Life's Challenges
Body's Stress Response

Chapter 7: Eating for a Healthier You
Understanding Food Labels

Focus On: Improving Your Sleep
Sleep Cycle

Chapter 8: Reaching and Maintaining a Healthy Weight
Obesity Health Effects

 **Focus On:** Enhancing Your Body Image
Body Image Continuum

 **Chapter 13:** Avoiding Drug Misuse and Abuse
Psychoactive Drugs Acting on the Brain

 **Chapter 9:** Improving Your Physical Fitness
Health Benefits of Regular Exercise

 **Chapter 14:** Protecting against Infectious Diseases and Sexually Transmitted Infections
Chain of Infection

 **Chapter 10:** Recognizing and Avoiding Addiction
Addiction Cycle

 **Focus On:** Understanding Your Health Inheritance
Inheritance Pattern of Single-Gene Disorders

 **Chapter 11:** Drinking Alcohol Responsibly
Long- and Short-Term Effects of Alcohol

 **Chapter 15:** Preventing Cardiovascular Disease
Atheroschlerosis and Coronary Artery Disease

 **Chapter 12:** Ending Tobacco Use
Long- and Short-Term Effects of Tobacco

 **Focus On:** Minimizing Your Risk for Diabetes
How Diabetes Develops

Chapter 16: Reducing Your Cancer Risk

Metastasis

Focus On: Reducing Your Risk of Unintentional Injury

Biking Safety

Chapter 17: Reducing Risks and Coping with Chronic Conditions

Lungs During an Asthma Attack

Chapter 20: Preserving and Protecting Your Environment

Enhanced Greenhouse Effect

Chapter 18: Choosing Conventional and Complementary Health Care

CAM: Risks vs. Benefits

Chapter 21: Preparing for Aging, Death, and Dying

Effects of Aging Body

Chapter 19: Preventing Violence and Abuse

Acquaintance Rape on Campus

Preface

In today's world, health is headline news. The issues and information may seem so complex and contradictory that you may wonder how to make sense of it all. What can you do to ensure a life that is healthy and long and to help improve the health of the people around you? Getting healthy and staying healthy can be a challenge, but it is a worthwhile goal, and one that is well within reach for most of us. No matter where your health is now, you can make positive changes for a healthier future, you can help others maintain health, and you can become an agent for healthy change in your community.

My goal in writing *Access to Health,* Thirteenth Edition, is to provide students with just what that title says: access to health information and to their own health potential. This book provides the most scientifically valid information available to help students be smarter in their health decision making, more positively involved in their personal health, and more active as advocates for healthy changes in their communities. Change isn't something that just happens: It takes knowledge, preparation, and effort; therefore, this book places emphasis on empowering students to identify their health risks, create plans for change, and make healthy lifestyle changes part of their daily routines.

Access to Health is designed to help students quickly grasp the information presented and understand its relevance to their own lives and the lives of others. Exciting revisions have been made to the art and design of the book in this new edition, with the purpose of capturing students' interest, engaging them in the subject matter, and helping them to be better prepared for whatever the future holds. In addition, there are six Focus On chapters delving into areas of health that are of practical importance to college students but are not always given sufficient coverage in a personal health text. These Focus On chapters spotlight spiritual health, sleep, body image, health inheritance, diabetes, and unintentional injury.

Looking back from the time when I taught my first Personal Health course as a teaching assistant in graduate school to the completion of this, the Thirteenth Edition of *Access to Health,* I am gratified by the overwhelming success that this text has enjoyed through its many revisions and changes. With each edition of the text, I have listened to the thoughtful suggestions of instructors and students using the book, as well as to the feedback from my own students in keeping the book relevant, interesting, and accessible. I hope that this edition's rich foundation of scientifically valid information, its wealth of technological tools and resources, and its thought-provoking features will stimulate you to share my enthusiasm for personal health and to become actively engaged in behaviors that will lead to better health for all.

New to This Edition

Access to Health, Thirteenth Edition, maintains many features that the text has become known for, while incorporating several major revisions and exciting new features. The most noteworthy changes to the text as a whole include the following:

- **New Tech & Health** This new box category focuses on how technology use can improve our health.
- **New Money & Health** This new box category gives college students tips and information regarding health topics that also relate to the wallet.
- **More Web Tie-Ins with the Book** Now QR codes in the text make it quick and easy to view video tutors on your phone as part of classroom discussion. Boxes throughout also indicate where podcasts, assessments, and the *ABC News* videos can be found online.
- **Changes to the Companion Website include the following:**

  * The **See It** section is SMS-protected and contains *ABC News* videos with assessment questions.
  * The **Hear It** section contains new audio case studies with assessment questions.
  * The **Do It** section contains new exercises and assessments based on the Points of View boxes in the text.
  * The **Live It** section has enhanced navigation and behavior change features, including a new How Healthy Are You? module.
  * **New On the Go** section includes Tweet Your Health, a brand new Twitter-based service that keeps students focused on behavior change.

- **MyHealthLab® updates include the following:**

  * **All of the same sections that appear in the Companion Website now also appear in MyHealthLab,** and the assignments all speak to the grade book. An additional set of review questions is also available for instructor assignment only.
  * **New discussion questions** about controversial health issues make creation and implementation of an online discussion forum easier and more accessible for instructors. The discussion features tie in to the Points of View boxes, *ABC News* videos, and audio case studies.
  * **New Pearson eText** is laid out just like the printed textbook. Students can create notes, highlight text in different colors, create bookmarks, zoom in and out, click hyperlinked words and phrases to view definitions, and view a video or visit a website as they read the text.

Chapter-by-Chapter Revisions

Access to Health, Thirteenth Edition, has been updated line by line to provide students with the most current information and references for further exploration. Portions of chapters have been reorganized to improve the flow of topics, while figures, tables, feature boxes, and photos have all been added, improved on, and updated. The following is a chapter-by-chapter listing of some of the most noteworthy changes, updates, and additions.

Chapter 1: Accessing Your Health
- New **Health Headlines** box explaining the Affordable Care Act and the implications of the recent Supreme Court ruling
- Updated figures and discussion statistics covering health disparities, causes of death, and life expectancy
- New figures on Healthy People 2020 and dimensions of health
- New **Tech & Health** box on finding health news on the Internet
- New **Money & Health** box on maximizing health care and minimizing costs

Chapter 2: Promoting and Preserving Your Psychological Health
- New **Health Headlines** box titled "Overdosing on Self-Esteem"
- Revised figure covering the mental health concerns reported by college students
- Updated mental health statistics related to incidence of schizophrenia, suicide, and other disorders

Focus On: Cultivating Your Spiritual Health
- New **Student Health Today** box on the physiological effects of meditation
- Updated research information about psychological and physical benefits of meditation, prayer, and other spiritual practices

Chapter 3: Managing Stress and Coping with Life's Challenges
- New **Money & Health** box with tips for financially stressed college students
- Revised figure covering what stresses Americans
- New **Tech & Health** box on decreasing tech-related stress
- New studies referenced that explain role of stress in poor immune response and heart disease

Focus On: Improving Your Sleep
- New National Sleep Foundation survey results in discussions about typical amounts of sleep Americans get each night
- Updated table covering sleep difficulties of adults

Chapter 4: Building Healthy Relationships and Communicating Effectively
- New **Tech & Health** box "Love in the Age of Twitter"
- New **Money & Health** box on studies showing that marriage may increase both wealth and health
- **Points of View** box on Defense of Marriage Act updated to reflect political happenings in states over the past few years
- Changed presentation of the figure showing healthy versus unhealthy relationships continuum to enhance readability

Chapter 5: Understanding Your Sexuality
- New **Tech & Health** box on the pleasures and perils of online dating
- New table on types of sexual dysfunction

Chapter 6: Considering Your Reproductive Choices
- New **Money & Health** box on health care reform and ontraceptives
- New **Tech & Health** box covering phone apps for tracking the fertility cycle
- New **Health in a Diverse World** box on how men can be more involved in birth control
- Updated abortion statistics (U.S. and worldwide)
- Revised table on birth control use among college students

Chapter 7: Eating for a Healthier You
- Expanded MyPlate information
- New **Health in a Diverse World** box on global malnutrition
- New **Money & Health** box titled "Are Fruits and Veggies Beyond Your Budget?"
- Expanded information in figure covering foods providing complementary amino acids

Chapter 8: Reaching and Maintaining a Healthy Weight
- Updated discussion and figure on obesity trends in the United States
- New figure in the **Health in a Diverse World** box titled "Globesity"
- New **Health Headlines** box debunking the HCG fad diet
- New **Tech & Health** box on diet-tracking smartphone apps

Focus On: Enhancing Your Body Image
- Updated eating disorder statistics and study references

Chapter 9: Improving Your Physical Fitness
- Revised Figure 9.5 to reflect newer recommendations on maximum heart rate ranges
- Reworked Figure 9.4 (FITT Principle) to improve readability
- New **Money & Health** box on shopping for fitness clothes, equipment, and facilities

Chapter 10: Recognizing and Avoiding Drug Addiction
- New **Tech & Health** box and related figure on technology and Internet addiction
- New **Health Headlines** box on a Parkinson's disease treatment whose side effect can be compulsive gambling
- Revised figure on the cycle of psychological addiction

Chapter 11: Drinking Alcohol Responsibly
- New **Health Headlines** box on global health and alcohol abuse
- New **Tech & Health** box on pitfalls of smartphone programs that estimate blood alcohol levels
- New Figure 11.8 on trends in drunk-driving fatalities
- Updated figures covering college student drinking patterns and negative consequences from drinking

Chapter 12: Ending Tobacco Use
- New **Tech & Health** box on electronic cigarette risks and concerns
- New **Money & Health** box on the cost of quitting versus smoking
- New **Student Health Today** box explaining recent research regarding effectiveness of hypnosis or acupuncture to quit smoking
- Updated Figure 12.1, "Trends in Smoking among U.S. College Students"

Chapter 13: Avoiding Drug Misuse and Abuse
- New **Tech & Health** box on types of drug tests
- New before-and-after type photos showing how methamphetamine use ravages the body

Chapter 14: Protecting against Infectious Diseases and Sexually Transmitted Infections
- New **Tech & Health** box on new cheap and easy tests that help AIDs patients cope in developing nations
- Revised **Health Headlines** box with more information debunking most anti-vaccination rhetoric
- Updated vaccination recommendations table
- HIV/AIDs infection statistics updated and recent treatment developments explained

Focus On: Understanding Your Health Inheritance
- New **Tech & Health** box on at-home genetic test kits

Chapter 15: Preventing Cardiovascular Disease
- New table on heart attack signs and symptoms
- New figure showing prevalence of heart attacks in the United States by state
- Updated figure showing prevalence of cardiovascular disease in Americans
- New figure showing where heart disease and stroke deaths in the U.S. rank among the four most common causes of death
- New **Health Headlines** box on stroke

Focus On: Minimizing Your Risk for Diabetes
- Improved figure on blood glucose levels
- Updated figure and discussion statistics on U.S. incidence of diabetes

Chapter 16: Reducing Your Cancer Risk
- New figure on trends in cancer survival rates
- Updated statistics on estimated new cancer cases and cancer deaths
- Latest recommendations on cancer screenings and tests

Chapter 17: Reducing Risks and Coping with Chronic Conditions
- Updated figures and statistics relating to incidence of asthma, migraines, bronchitis, allergies, back pain, and other chronic conditions

Chapter 18: Choosing Conventional and Complementary Health Care
- New **Money & Health** box on health care spending accounts
- Updated figure covering health care spending by nations
- **Points of View** box rewritten to reflect recent events in the debate over whether the government should facilitate health care
- New figure on main meridian channels

Chapter 19: Preventing Violence and Abuse
- Updated figure showing declining crime rate statistics
- Updated figure on U.S. homicide rates
- Updated figure on child abuse and neglect victims

Focus On: Reducing Your Risk of Unintentional Injury
- New **Points of View** box regarding bans on cell phone use while driving

Chapter 20: Preserving and Protecting Your Environment
- New **Points of View** box and figure on fracking
- New **Money & Health** box on plastic bag bans and taxes
- New **Health Headlines** box on the nuclear emergency in Fukushima, Japan
- New figure on world energy consumption by type of fuel
- Updated statistics and figure on world population growth
- New statics and updated figures on U.S. trash and recycling

Chapter 21: Preparing for Aging, Death, and Dying
- New **Health in a Diverse World** box on keeping fit as we age
- New figure on organ donation
- Updated figure on living arrangements of senior citizens in the United States

Text Features and Learning Aids

Access to Health, Thirteenth Edition, includes the following special features, all of which have been revised and improved upon for this edition:

- **Chapter objectives** summarize the main competencies that students will gain from each chapter and alert students to the key concepts.
- **Chapter opener questions** capture students' attention and engage them in what they will be learning. Questions are repeated and answered in photo legends within the chapter.
- **What Do You Think?** critical thinking questions within the chapter prompt students to reflect on personal and societal issues relating to the material they have just learned.
- **What's Working for You?** features (new to this edition) reinforce healthy behaviors by calling students' attention to positive things they are already doing to promote good health.
- **Why Should I Care?** features (new to this edition) lead students to recognize the relevance of health issues to their own lives in the here and now.
- **Did You Know?** figures call attention to statistics that are relevant to the lives of college students in a fun format.
- **Assess Yourself and Your Plan for Change** boxes are combined in each chapter. Students assess their current health behaviors and are given specific ideas for setting goals and following through on behavior change.
- **Skills for Behavior Change** boxes give students specific strategies for making lasting changes to their health behaviors.
- **Points of View** boxes (new to this edition) present viewpoints on a controversial health issue and ask students **Where Do You Stand?** questions, encouraging students to critically evaluate the information and consider their own opinions.
- **Tech & Health** boxes cover the new technology innovations, from medical tests to calorie-counting smartphone apps, that can help students stay healthy.
- **Student Health Today** boxes offer current data and information about health trends specific to college students, including potential risks and safety issues that affect students' lives.
- **Health Headlines** boxes highlight new discoveries and research, as well as interesting trends in the fields of public and personal health.
- **Health in a Diverse World** boxes expand discussion of health topics to diverse groups within the United States and around the world.
- **Money & Health** boxes cover health topics from the financial perspective, discussing everything from how to lessen money stress during school to how something like a plastic bag tax at the grocery store might impact behavior.
- **Be Healthy, Be Green** boxes offer information on how students can make environmentally responsible health choices.
- A **running glossary** in the margins defines terms where students first encounter them, emphasizing and supporting understanding of material.
- **QR codes and media callout boxes** indicate when podcasts, videos, and assessments are available online for use with the book.
- The sections at the ends of chapters focus on student application: **Summary** wraps up chapter content, **Pop Quiz** multiple-choice questions and **Think about It!** discussion questions encourage students to evaluate and apply new information, **Accessing Your Health on the Internet** and **References** sections offer more opportunities to explore areas of interest.
- The **appendices** at the end of the book include practical information on providing emergency care and a table of nutritive values for selected foods and fast foods.
- A **Behavior Change Contract** for students to fill out is included at the front of the book.

Supplementary Materials

Available with *Access to Health,* Thirteenth Edition, is a comprehensive set of ancillary materials designed to enhance learning and to facilitate teaching.

Student Supplements

- **MyHealthLab** (www.pearsonhighered.com/myhealthlab). Organized by learning areas and a snap to navigate, MyHealthLab is a course management platform that makes it easier than ever to learn about personal health and wellness:

  * **Read It** contains the new Pearson eText, a full-featured electronic book that allows for note creation, highlighting, bookmarking, zooming, and linking to definitions and external sites; chapter objectives to direct student learning; and chapter-specific RSS feeds.
  * **See It** houses 27 brand-new video tutors, brief videos that can be accessed quickly through scanning-related QR codes in chapters. There are also more than 30 *ABC News* videos about important health topics, each 5 to 10 minutes long, and followed by assignable quiz questions.
  * **Hear It** offers MP3 tutor sessions with assignable quizzes to explain the big picture concepts for each chapter and new audio case studies with accompanying essay questions.
  * **Do It** contains activities related directly to the book's Points of View boxes, critical thinking questions, news quizzes, and Web links. This edition also includes seven "nutri-tools" activities in the healthy eating chapter.
  * **Review It** provides an online glossary, flashcards available for mobile phones, and practice quizzes for each chapter.
  * **Live It** is an electronic toolkit to help jump-start behavior change projects. With 30 assessments from the book, additional worksheets, and the new How Healthy

Are You? module, it guides students through planning for change, creating a behavior change contract, journaling and logging their behaviors as they implement change, and preparing a reflection piece to aid in behavior change evaluation.

✳ **On the Go** houses tools to help students study on the go using their mobile devices, including Tweet Your Health, a brand-new Twitter application that sends students reminders about their behavior change project and allows them to track their progress using their mobile phone.

● **Companion Website** (www.pearsonhighered.com/donatelle). Like MyHealthLab, this website is organized by learning areas. Students can study chapter objectives and follow RSS feeds (Read It), view SMS-protected *ABC News* videos on health topics (See It), listen to MP3 clips of main concepts and case studies (Hear It), learn hands-on with critical thinking activities (Do It), take practice quizzes (Review It), access the behavior-change tool kit (Live It), and utilize mobile health-tracking tools (On the Go).

● *Assess Yourself* **Activities:** These behavior-change assessments are available on the book website where they report to the online gradebook when assigned. They are also available as a printed supplement.

● *Take Charge of Your Health!* **Worksheets.** A total of 50 self-assessment exercises are now available. Worksheets are available as a gummed pad and can be packaged at no additional charge with the main text. About half of these worksheets report to the online gradebook.

● *Behavior Change Log Book and Wellness Journal.* This assessment tool helps students track daily exercise and nutritional intake and create a long-term nutrition and fitness prescription plan. It includes Behavior Change Contracts and topics for journal-based activities.

● *Eat Right! Healthy Eating in College and Beyond.* This handy, full-color booklet provides students with practical guidelines, tips, shopper's guides, and recipes that turn healthy eating principles into blueprints for action. Topics include healthy eating in the cafeteria, dorm room, and fast-food restaurants; planning meals on a budget; weight management; vegetarian alternatives; and how alcohol affects health.

● *Live Right! Beating Stress in College and Beyond.* This booklet gives students useful tips for coping with a variety of life's challenges both during college and for the rest of their lives. Topics include sleep, managing finances, time management, coping with academic pressure, relationships, and a closer look at advertised products that promise to make our lives better.

● **Tweet Your Health** (www.tweetyourhealth.com). This Twitter-based app lets students track and keep on online journal of everyday health behaviors via any computer or mobile device.

● **Digital 5-Step Pedometer.** Take strides to better health with this pedometer, which measures steps, distance (miles), activity time, and calories and provides a time clock.

● **MyDietAnalysis** (www.mydietanalysis.com). Powered by ESHA Research, Inc., MyDietAnalysis features a database of nearly 20,000 foods and multiple reports. It allows students to track their diet and activity using up to three profiles and to generate and submit reports electronically.

Instructor Supplements

A full resource package accompanies *Access to Health,* Thirteenth Edition, to assist the instructor with classroom preparation and presentation.

● **MyHealthLab** (www.pearsonhighered.com/myhealthlab). This course managment tool provides a one-stop spot for accessing a wealth of preloaded content and makes paper-free assigning and grading easier than ever. Instructors can electronically assign the self-assessments to students, who can complete them anonymously and still have their work reflected in the grade book. Reports on cumulative class responses allow instructors to better target certain issues in lectures. MyHealthLab contains the Pearson eText, which allows for instructor annotation to be shared with the class; includes over 30 *ABC News* videos; houses assignable chapter-specific quizzes, MP3 tutor sessions, case studies, activities, and flashcards; and provides robust electronic behavior-change tools, including the How Healthy Are You? module and Tweet Your Health.

● **Video Tutors,** *ABC News* **Health and Wellness Lecture Launcher Videos.** Twenty-seven brand-new brief videos accessible via QR codes in the text, plus 60 *ABC News* videos, each 5 to 10 minutes long, help instructors stimulate critical discussion in the classroom. Videos are provided already linked within PowerPoint® lectures and are available separately in large-screen format with optional closed captioning on the Instructor Resource DVD and through MyHealthLab.

● **Instructor Resource DVD.** The Instructor Resource DVD includes 60 new *ABC News* Lecture Launcher videos; clicker questions; Quiz Show questions; PowerPoint® lecture outlines; all illustrations and tables from the text; selected photos; Transparency Masters; as well as Microsoft Word® files for the Instructor Resource and Support Manual and the Test Bank. The DVD also holds the Computerized Test Bank.

● **Teaching Tool Box.** Save hours of valuable planning time with one comprehensive course planning kit. The Teaching Tool Box provides all the prepping and lecture tools an instructor needs: the Course-at-a-Glance Quick Reference Guide; an Instructor Resource DVD including PowerPoint® Lecture Outlines, PRS Clicker Questions, Quiz Show questions, *ABC News* videos, and Transparency Masters; a MyHealthLab access kit; the Instructor Resource and Support Manual to easily find visual assets; *Great Ideas: Active Ways to Teach Health and Wellness*; Printed and Computerized Test Banks—along with helpful student supplements, including the *Take Charge of Your Health!* worksheets, the *Behavior Change Log Book*, *Eat Right!*, and *Live Right!*—all in one convenient package!

● **User's Quick Reference Guide.** This valuable supplement acts as your road map to the Teaching Tool Box and everything it contains, with resources broken down by chapter and page number. The side for instructors provides assets that you can use when preparing for a lecture or while in class. The student side outlines where to find the resources to aid your students in their homework or in-class activities.

● **Instructor Resource and Support Manual.** Easier to use than a typical instructor's manual, this key guide provides a step-by-step visual walk-through of all the resources available to you for preparing your lectures. Also included are tips and strategies for new instructors, sample syllabi, and suggestions for integrating MyHealthLab into your classroom activities and homework assignments.

● **New! Teaching with Student Learning Outcomes.** This feature provides essays from 11 instructors who teach using student learning outcomes. They share goals and suggestions for developing good learning outcomes and give tips and suggestions for how to teach personal health in this manner.

● **New! Teaching with Web 2.0.** From Facebook to Twitter and blogs, students are interacting with technology constantly. This *handbook* gives tips on how to incorporate technology in your course.

● **Test Bank.** The Test Bank incorporates Bloom's Taxonomy, or the Higher Order of Learning, to help instructors create exams that encourage students to think analytically and critically, rather than simply to regurgitate information.

● *Great Ideas! Active Ways to Teach Health & Wellness.* This manual provides ideas for classroom activities related to specific health and wellness topics, as well as suggestions for activities that can be adapted to various topics and class sizes.

● **Course Management.** In addition to MyHealthLab, Blackboard is available. Contact your Benjamin Cummings sales representative for details.

● **Health & Wellness Teaching Community Website** (www.pearsonhighered.com/healthcommunity). This community serves instructors by offering teaching tips and ideas and a forum for peers to talk to one another about health-related issues.

Acknowledgments

It is hard for me to believe that *Access to Health* is in its thirteenth edition! Since its inception, the personal health textbook market has undergone remarkable changes. Whereas the text remains the foundation of information, the ability to communicate with students through the Internet and other media provides textbook authors and publishers entirely new and exciting ways of teaching, sharing information, and covering up-to-the minute health topics in every class. Today's text offers opportunities for student engagement and thought-provoking exercises that help students understand complex issues surrounding health so they can make better decisions related to health care and behaviors. To maximize student learning we sought input from faculty members and experts in technology and e-learning—those who work with students daily and who understand how to engage today's learner with written and visual content.

Producing a text students like to read goes well beyond the written word. In addition to the background research, a small army of publishing professionals take the basic information and make it come alive for the reader. Each step in planning, developing, and marketing a high-quality textbook and supplemental materials requires a tremendous amount of work from many dedicated professionals. I often think how fortunate I have been to work with the many gifted publishing professionals who make up the Pearson family. There have been so many names and faces along the way—people who have worked behind the scenes, in many cases, to make *Access to Health* a resounding success from the first edition to this one. I owe each of them a debt of gratitude, for without their efforts, this book may have languished on the shelves along the way. From this author's perspective, Pearson personnel personify key aspects of what it takes to be successful in the publishing world: (1) skill and competence; (2) drive and motivation; (3) creativity and commitment to excellence; (4) a vibrant, youthful, and enthusiastic approach; and (4) personalities that motivate an author to continually strive to produce market-leading texts.

In particular, I am indebted to Erin Strathmann, who took over the reins of project development editor with this edition of *Access to Health* and never dropped a beat in ensuring that the project kept on schedule and continued to reflect excellent editorial skills. Erin's upbeat manner and encouragement—and her creative insights in improving each chapter—were definite pluses, both for me and for contributors to this edition. A gifted writer herself, she was able to synthesize, refine, and improve sections of the manuscript with a deft stroke of the keyboard—skills that are invaluable in the editorial process. Her background and knowledge about key health issues also helped bring a refreshing new perspective to many of the health topics. In short, Erin did a simply outstanding job, and I am very grateful for her wonderful work ethic, attention to detail, keen eye, skill, and positive approach to the editorial process. Pearson has clearly scored a "hit" by adding Erin to their editorial team! Thank you, Erin!

Further praise and thanks go to the executive editor, Sandra Lindelof, for going the extra mile to ensure that the book has the necessary resources and is "cutting edge" when it comes to both being a leader in the personal health market and using state-of-the-art technology. Sandy's positive attitude, hard work, tenacity, and dedication to the success of the Pearson's team is unparalleled. Sandy keeps a steady finger on the pulse of the personal health market and is quick to suggest strategies to improve a text and meet the needs of instructors. She has been instrumental in the ongoing success of this text. Although she has an extensive and growing list of authors, Sandy "worries the details," and this interest and enthusiasm carries over into all aspects of the published work. Thank you Sandy for all of your efforts on our behalf!

Although these women were key contributors to the finished work, there were many other people who worked on this revision of *Access to Health*. In particular, I would like to thank Production Project Manager Megan Power, who skillfully navigated production pitfalls and handled every detail, every obstacle, with patience, professionalism, and good grace. Thanks also to Angela Williams Urquhart and Andrea Archer at Thistle Hill Publishing Services, who put everything together to make a polished finished product. Gary Hespenheide and his staff at Hespenheide Design worked wonders in giving the book an exciting and fresh new look, both inside and out. Editorial Assistant Briana Verdugo gets major kudos for skillfully overseeing the print supplements package, and Sade McDougal, assistant media producer, once again pulled together an innovative and comprehensive media supplements package. Editorial Manager Susan Malloy deserves special recognition for saving the day on more than one occasion and for being ready and willing to lend a helping hand wherever needed. Additional thanks go to the rest of the team at Pearson, especially Design Manager Marilyn Perry, Photo Team Lead Donna Kalal, Senior Managing Editor Deborah Cogan, and Director of Development Barbara Yien.

The editorial and production teams are critical to a book's success, but I would be remiss if I didn't thank another key group who ultimately help determine a book's success: the textbook representative and sales group and their leader, Senior Marketing Manager Neena Bali. Neena does a superb job of making sure that *Access to Health* gets into instructors' hands and that adopters receive the service they deserve. In keeping with my overall experiences with Pearson, the members of the marketing and sales staff are among the best of the best. I am very lucky to have them working with me on this project and want to extend a special thanks to all of them!

Contributors to the Thirteenth Edition

Many colleagues, students, and staff members have provided the feedback, reviews, extra time, assistance, and encouragement that have helped me meet the rigorous demands of publishing this book over the years. Whether acting as reviewers, generating new ideas, providing expert commentary, or revising chapters, each of these professionals has added his or her skills to our collective endeavor.

I would like to thank other key contributors to chapters in this edition. As always, I would like to give particular thanks to Dr. Patricia Ketcham, who has helped with the *Access to Health* series since its beginnings. As associate director of health promotion in Student Health Services at Oregon State University and with her high level of involvement in national groups focused on college student issues, Dr. Ketcham has provided a current and unique perspective on key campus challenges and the innovative ways in which campuses are coping with problems that invariably arise. Although she has been instrumental in the development and updating of several different chapters over the years, for this edition she focused her attention on Chapter 10, "Recognizing and Avoiding Addiction"; Chapter 11, "Drinking Alcohol Responsibly"; and Chapter 13, "Avoiding Drug Misuse and Abuse."

Dr. Peggy Pederson, Associate Professor and Chair of Health Education at Western Oregon University, used her background in Health Promotion and Health Behavior and her specialization in Human Sexuality to complete a thorough, issues-oriented revision of Chapter 6, "Considering Your Reproductive Choices."

Dr. Tanya Littrell, coauthor of the textbook *Get Fit-Stay Well* and exercise scientist in the Fitness Technology and Physical Education Department at Portland Community College, provided a wealth of knowledge and expertise, as well as an engaging writing style, in revising Chapter 9, "Improving your Physical Fitness."

Dr. Karen Elliot, assistant professor in the Department of Public Health at Oregon State University, has assisted with revisions of several chapters over the last editions of *Access to Health*. In this edition, she utilized her expertise in the health promotion and health behavior areas to provide detailed, cutting-edge information to improve the content and quality of each chapter. Her thoughtful revisions are reflected in Chapter 2, "Promoting and Preserving Your Psychological Health"; "Focus On: Cultivating Your Spiritual Health"; Chapter 12, "Ending Tobacco Use"; and Chapter 21, "Preparing for Aging, Death, and Dying." Dr. Elliot also revised the sexually transmitted infections portion of Chapter 14.

Laura Bonazzoli, development editor and author, provided a thorough and timely revision of Chapter 7, "Eating for a Healthier You." In this chapter, key strategies for dealing with the unique dietary challenges are discussed based on the best available scientific research, and practical tips are provided to help students eat in more healthful ways. Laura Bonazzoli also revised Chapter 1, "Accessing Your Health," Chapter 18, "Choosing Complementary Health Care," as well as the Focus On chapters "Reducing Your Risk of Unintentional Injury" and "Understanding Your Health Inheritance."

Finally, a special thank you to Dr. Susan Dobie, associate professor in the Department of Health, Physical Education and Leisure Sciences at the University of Northern Iowa for her work in revising Chapter 4, "Building Healthy Relationships and Communicating Effectively", and Chapter 6, "Considering Your Reproductive Choices." Her attention to detail, expertise in these areas, and excellent writing style combined to provide a top-notch revision of these important chapters. These contributors were brought on because of their history of working with college students and their vital, enthusiastic approach to student learning. Importantly, they are all experts in subject matter content and have proven academic training and research background in related fields. Thank you to each of you for your help in making this edition of *Access to Health* one of the best yet!

Many thanks are also due to the talented people who contributed to the supplement package: Jennifer Jabson (Boston University), Brenda Moore (Georgia Perimeter College), Karla Rues (Ozarks Technical Community College), and Tanya Martin.

Reviewers for the Thirteenth Edition

With each new edition of *Access to Health*, we have built on the combined expertise of many colleagues throughout the country who are dedicated to the education and healthy behavioral changes of students. I thank the many reviewers of the past 13 edition of *Access to Health* who have made such valuable contributions. I want you, the instructors who have used and reviewed the book over the years, to know that I am grateful for your support and guidance. You are one of most essential resources for knowing how to best stimulate students to learn, grow, and tackle the health challenges that lie ahead of them.

For the Thirteenth Edition, reviewers who have helped us continue this tradition of excellence include:

Louvenia Askew (Southeastern Louisiana University)
J. Ausherman (Cleveland State University)
Claire Belles (Central Piedmont Community College)
Mathew Belles (Central Piedmont Community College)
Leigh Bovard (West Liberty University)
Shannon Carl (Baylor University)
Sarah Collins (St. Vincent's Medical Center)
Pamela Coward (Bristol Community College)
Jennifer Susan Dearden (Morehead State)
Bill Dunscombe (Union County College)
Ari Fisher (Louisiana State University)
Patrick Honey (Middlesex Community College)
Elizabeth Hopkins (Las Positas College)
Grace Lartey (Western Kentucky University)
Susie Myers (Kansas City Kansas Community College)
Lisa O'Leary (Kean University)
Kandice Porter (Kennesaw State University)
Todd Sabato (James Madison University)

Gaynelle Schmieder (Pennsylvania Highlands
    Community College)
John P. Seabolt (University of Kentucky)
Christine Sholtey (Waubonsee Community College)
Debra G. Smith (Ohio University Lancaster)
David Stronck (California State University, East Bay)

Heidi Uperesa (New Mexico State University)
Dr. Patricia Wright (The University of Scranton)
Jodi Zieverink (Central Piedmont Community College)

Many thanks to all,
Rebecca J. Donatelle, PhD

Access to HEALTH

Thirteenth Edition

Rebecca J. Donatelle

1 Accessing Your Health

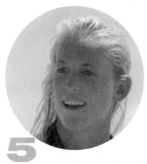

5
What is meant by *quality of life*?

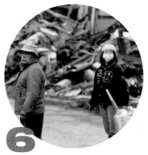

6
Why should I be concerned about health conditions in other places?

18
How can I stay motivated to improve my health habits?

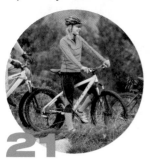

21
How do other people influence my health behaviors?

OBJECTIVES

✳ Describe the immediate and long-term rewards of healthy behaviors and the effects that your health choices may have on others.

✳ Compare and contrast the medical model of health and the public health model, and discuss the six dimensions of health.

✳ Identify several personal factors that influence your health and classify them as modifiable or nonmodifiable.

✳ Explain how aspects of the social and physical environment influence your health.

✳ Discuss the importance of a global perspective on health, and explain how gender, racial, economic, and cultural factors influence health disparities.

✳ Compare and contrast three models of behavior change.

✳ Identify your own current risk behaviors, the factors that influence those behaviors, and the strategies you can use to change them.

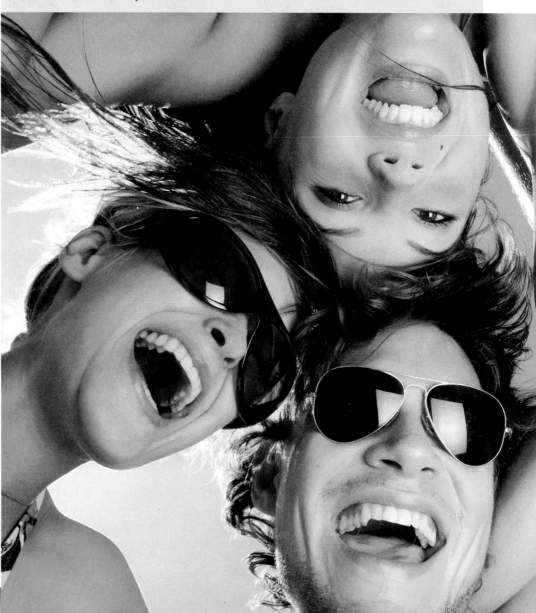

Got health? That may sound like a simple question, but it isn't; health is a process, not something we just "get." People who are healthy in their forties, fifties, sixties, and beyond aren't just lucky or the beneficiaries of hardy genes. In most cases, those who are healthy and thriving in later years set the stage for good health by making it a priority in their early years. You've probably heard from your parents and grandparents that your college years are some of the best of your life. Here the canvas is hung upon which you will paint the story of your life. Whether your story is filled with good health, productive careers, happiness, special relationships, and fulfillment of life goals is largely dependent on the health choices you make—beginning right now.

Why Health, Why Now?

In addition to our desires to improve our health, constant messages via television, the Internet, and magazines remind us of health challenges facing the world, the nation, your community, and your campus. We can't run from these issues, and we can't ignore them. Even health issues occurring in another part of the world affect us. In the twenty-first century your health is connected, not only to the people you directly interact with and the environments where you spend time, but also to people you've never met and to the well-being of the entire planet.

How does what you do today influence you and those around you? Let's take a look at how your actions and inactions matter.

Choose Health Now for Immediate Benefits

Almost everyone knows that overeating leads to weight gain, or that drinking and driving increases the risk of motor vehicle accidents. But other, subtler choices you make every day may be influencing your well-being in ways you're not aware of. For instance, did you know that the amount of sleep you get each night could affect your body weight, your ability to ward off colds, your mood, and your driving? What's more, inadequate sleep is one of the most commonly reported impediments to academic success (Figure 1.1). Another example is smoking: It has many immediate health effects, including fatigue, throat irritation, and breathing problems. And like poor sleep, it increases your vulnerability to colds and other infections.

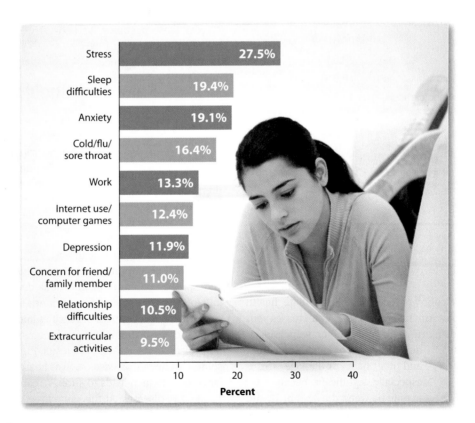

FIGURE 1.1 Top Ten Reported Impediments to Academic Performance—Past 12 Months
In a recent survey by the National College Health Association, students indicated that stress, poor sleep, recurrent minor illnesses, and anxiety, among other things, had prevented them from performing at their academic best.
Source: Data are from American College Health Association, *American College Health Association—National College Health Assessment II (ACHA-NCHA II) Reference Group Data Report, Spring 2011* (Baltimore: ACHA, 2012).

TABLE 1.1 Leading Causes of Death in the United States, 2009, Overall and by Age Group (15 and older)

All Ages	Number of Deaths
Diseases of the heart	595,444
Malignant neoplasms (cancer)	573,855
Chronic lower respiratory diseases	137,789
Cerebrovascular diseases	129,180
Accidents (unintentional injuries)	118,043
Aged 15–24	
Unintentional injuries	12,015
Assault (homicide)	4,651
Suicide	4,559
Malignant neoplasms (cancer)	1,594
Diseases of the heart	984
Aged 25–44	
Unintentional injuries	28,149
Malignant neoplasms	15,389
Diseases of the heart	13,447
Suicide	12,119
Homicide	6,674
Aged 45–64	
Malignant neoplasms (cancer)	159,379
Diseases of the heart	103,812
Unintentional injuries	32,667
Chronic lower respiratory diseases	18,616
Chronic liver disease and cirrhosis	18,348
Aged 65+	
Diseases of the heart	476,519
Malignant neoplasms	396,173
Chronic lower respiratory diseases	117,856
Cerebrovascular diseases	109,764
Alzheimer's disease	82,438

Source: Sherry L. Murphy, Jiaquan Xu, and Kenneth D. Kochanek, "Deaths: Preliminary Data for 2010," *National Vital Statistics Reports* 60, no. 4 (Hyattsville, MD: National Center for Health Statistics, 2012.)

diate benefits. When you're well nourished, fit, rested, and free from the influence of nicotine, alcohol, and other drugs, you're more likely to avoid illness, succeed in school, maintain supportive relationships, participate in meaningful work and community activities, and enjoy your leisure time.

Choose Health Now for Long-Term Rewards

The choices you make today are like seeds: Planting good seeds means you're more likely to enjoy the fruits of good health, including not only a longer life, but also a higher quality of life. In contrast, poor choices increase the likelihood of a shorter life, as well as persistent illness, addiction, and other limitations on quality of life. In other words, successful aging starts now.

Personal Choices Influence Your Life Expectancy According to current **mortality** and death statistics—which reflect the proportion of deaths within a population—the average **life expectancy** at birth in the United States is projected to be 78.5 years for a child born in 2012.[1] In other words, we can expect that American infants born today will live to an average age of over 78 years; much longer than the 47-year life expectancy for people born in the early 1900s. That's because life expectancy 100 years ago was largely determined by our susceptibility to infectious disease. In 1900, over 30 percent of all deaths occurred among children under 5 years old, and the leading cause of death was infection.[2] Even among adults, infectious diseases such as tuberculosis and pneumonia were the leading causes of death, and widespread epidemics of infectious diseases such as cholera and influenza crossed national boundaries to kill millions.

With the development of vaccines and antibiotics, life expectancy increased dramatically as premature deaths from infectious diseases decreased. As a result, the leading cause of death shifted to **chronic diseases** such as heart disease, cerebrovascular disease (which leads to strokes), cancer, and chronic lower respiratory diseases. At the same time, advances in diagnostic technologies, heart and brain surgery, radiation and other cancer treatments, as well as new medications continued the trend of increasing life expectancy into the twenty-first century.

Unfortunately, some researchers question whether this trend of

"Why Should I Care?"

Just as health problems can create challenges for success, improving your health can lead to better academics, career success, increased relationship satisfaction, and more joy in living overall.

Similarly, drinking alcohol reduces your immediate health and your academic performance. It also sharply increases your risk of unintentional injuries—not only motor vehicle accidents, but also falls, drownings, and other harm or damage. This is especially significant because for people between the ages of 15 and 44, unintentional injury—whether related to alcohol use or any other factor—is the leading cause of death (Table 1.1).

It isn't an exaggeration to say that healthy choices have imme-

mortality The proportion of deaths to population.

life expectancy Expected number of years of life remaining at a given age, such as at birth.

chronic disease A disease that typically begins slowly, progresses, and persists, with a variety of signs and symptoms that can be treated but not cured by medication.

increasing life expectancy will continue. In fact, a recent study projects that today's newborns will be the first generation to have a lower life expectancy than that of their parents.[3] One major contributor to future reductions in life expectancy relates to obesity and sedentary lifestyle. A recent study led by researchers from the Harvard School of Public Health and the University of Washington indicates that smoking, high blood pressure, elevated blood glucose, and overweight/obesity currently reduce life expectancy in the United States by 4.9 years in men and 4.1 years in women.[4]

67 & 71

are the *healthy* life expectancy ages of men and women, respectively, in the U.S., while the average total life expectancy ages are 75.7 and 80.6.

Whereas lifestyle choices may be the biggest reason for future declines in life expectancy, health care decisions may also have an impact. For example, a growing number of persons are opting out of vaccinations for their children, while there are increasing threats from resistant pathogens and new strains of diseases. Other individual choices, such as texting while driving or failing to properly dispose of toxic chemicals, also are part of life expectancy projections.

Personal Choices Influence Your *Healthy* Life Expectancy By now you're probably beginning to see how healthful choices, such as watching what you eat, enjoying physical activity, and avoiding smoking and alcohol abuse, increase your life expectancy. But another benefit of these healthful choices is that they increase your **healthy life expectancy;** that is, the number of years of full health you enjoy, without disability, chronic pain, or significant illness.

Another dimension of healthy life expectancy is **health-related quality of life (HRQoL),** a multidimensional concept that includes elements of physical, mental, emotional, and social function. HRQoL goes beyond mortality rates and life expectancy and focuses on the impact health status has on overall quality of life. Closely related to this is *well-being*, which assesses the positive aspects of a person's life, such as positive emotions and life satisfaction.[5]

Choose Health Now to Benefit Others

Our personal health choices don't affect only our own lives. They affect the lives of others, because they contribute to global health or the global burden of disease. For example, we've said that overeating and inadequate physical activity contribute to obesity. But obesity isn't a problem only for the individual. Along with its associated health problems, obesity burdens the U.S. health care system and the U.S. economy overall. *Direct* medical costs, including the costs of diagnosis and treatment, reached as high as $147 billion in 2008, and roughly half of those costs were paid by public programs (Medicaid and Medicare).[6] In addition, obesity costs the public *indirectly*. These indirect costs include reduced tax revenues because of income lost from absenteeism and premature death, increased disability payments because of an inability to remain in the workforce, and increased health insurance rates as claims rise for treatment of obesity itself as well as its associated diseases.

> **healthy life expectancy** Expected number of years of full health remaining at a given age, such as at birth.
>
> **health-related quality of life** Assessment of impact of health status—including elements of physical, mental, emotional, and social function—on overall quality of life.

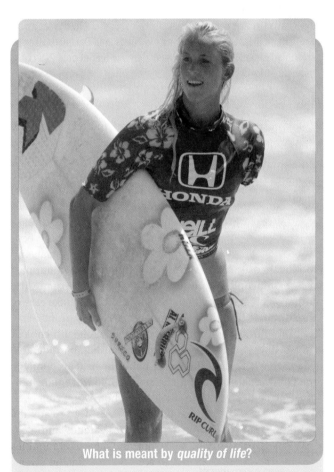

What is meant by *quality of life*?

Health-related *quality of life* refers to a person's or group's perceived physical and mental health over time. Just because a person has an illness or disability doesn't mean his or her quality of life is necessarily low. Hawaiian surfer Bethany Hamilton lost her arm in a shark attack while surfing at age 13, but that hasn't prevented her from achieving her goals and a high quality of life. She returned to surfing just 1 month after the attack and has since traveled around the world competing as a professional surfer.

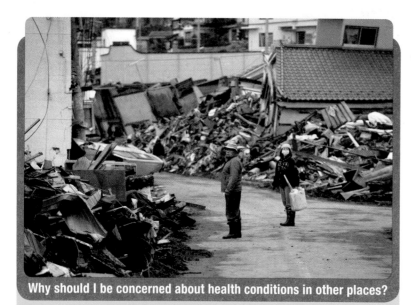

Why should I be concerned about health conditions in other places?

Unhealthy conditions in one location can have far-reaching impacts on the economy and health. When the 2011 earthquake and tsunami in Japan caused devastation in that country, productivity losses were felt as far away as Europe. The natural disaster also damaged the Fukushima Daiichi nuclear power plant, spreading radiation throughout the region and fear of potential nuclear fallout throughout the world.

health The ever-changing process of achieving individual potential in the physical, social, emotional, mental, spiritual, and environmental dimensions.

medical model A view of health in which health status focuses primarily on the individual and a biological or diseased organ perspective.

Direct and indirect costs are also associated with smoking, excessive alcohol consumption, and illegal drug use. All of these choices place an economic burden on our communities and our society as a whole. The disease burden goes beyond pure economics and includes social and emotional costs, such as those on families left without parents or on people who lose loved ones in their prime. The burden on caregivers who personally sacrifice to take care of those disabled by diseases is another part of this problem.

At the root of the concern that individual health choices cost society is an ethical question causing considerable debate: To what extent should the public be held accountable for an individual's unhealthy choices? Should we require individuals to somehow pay for their poor choices? Of course, in some cases, we already do. We tax cigarettes and alcohol, and a few communities are currently taxing sweetened soft drinks, which have been blamed for rising obesity rates.[7] On the other side of the argument are those who argue that smoking and drinking are addictions that require treatment, not punishment, and that obesity is a product of a society

what do you think?

Is obesity always a matter of lacking willpower or discipline?
● Since we tax cigarettes, is it reasonable to tax high-calorie sodas?
● What about taxing prepackaged, high-fat foods?
● Who should decide?
● Would you draw the line?

of excess in which small children learn behaviors early in life that are difficult to break. Should individuals be punished for choices that society influenced and the media promoted? Who is ultimately responsible?

Before you decide where you stand on this issue, hold on: It's not as black and white as it may first appear. That's because seemingly personal choices that influence health are not always entirely within our personal control. We'll explain shortly, but first it's essential to understand what health actually is and which factors we actually may be able to control.

What Is Health?

For some, the word **health** simply means the antithesis of sickness. To others, it means being in good physical shape and able to resist illness. Still others use terms such as *wellness* or *well-being* to include a wide array of factors that seem to lead to positive health status. Why are there all of these variations? In part, the differences are due to an increasingly enlightened way of viewing health that has taken shape over time. As our collective understanding of illness has improved, so has our ability to understand the many nuances of health.

Models of Health

Over the centuries, different ideals—or models—of human health have dominated. Our current model of health has broadened from a focus on the individual physical body to an understanding of health as a reflection not only of ourselves, but also of our communities.

Medical Model Prior to the twentieth century, if you made it to your fiftieth birthday, you were regarded as lucky. Survivors were believed to be of hearty, healthy stock—having what we might refer to today as "good genes." We didn't have the means to delve into factors influencing risks, and as such, cleanliness, good behavior, and a bit of luck were part of the good health formula.

Throughout these years, perceptions of health were dominated by the **medical model,** in which health status focused primarily on the individual and his or her tissues and organs. The surest way to bring about improved health was to cure the individual's disease, either with medication to treat the disease-causing agent or through surgery to remove the diseased body part. Thus, government resources focused on initiatives that led to treatment, rather than prevention, of disease.

Public Health Model Not until the early decades of the 1900s did researchers begin to recognize that entire populations of poor people, particularly those living in certain locations, were victims of environmental factors over which they

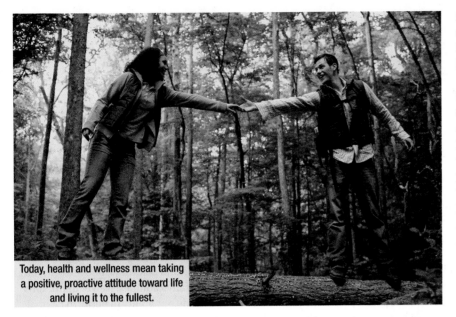

Today, health and wellness mean taking a positive, proactive attitude toward life and living it to the fullest.

had little control: things such as polluted water, air, and food; poor housing; and unsafe work settings. As a result of this new understanding, researchers began to focus on an **ecological or public health model,** which views diseases and other negative health events more as a result of an individual's interaction with his or her social and physical environment.

Recognition of the public health model enabled health officials to move to control contaminants in water, for example, by building adequate sewers, and to control burning and other forms of air pollution. In the early 1900s colleges began offering courses in health and hygiene to teach students about these important factors. And over time, public health officials began to recognize and address many other forces affecting human health, including hazardous work conditions; negative influences in the home and social envi-

ronment; abuse of drugs and alcohol; stress; unsafe behavior; diet; sedentary lifestyle; and cost, quality, and access to health care.

By the 1940s progressive thinkers began calling for policies, programs, and services to improve individual health and that of the population as a whole. In other words, their focus shifted from treatment of individual illness to **disease prevention** by reducing or eliminating the factors that cause illness and injury. For example, childhood vaccination programs reduced the incidence and severity of infectious disease; installation of safety features such as seatbelts and airbags in motor vehicles reduced traffic injuries and fatalities; and laws governing occupational safety reduced injuries to and deaths of American workers. In 1947 at an international conference focusing on global health issues, the World Health Organization (WHO) proposed a new definition of health: "Health is the state of complete physical, mental, and social well-being, not just the absence of disease or infirmity."[8] This new definition definitively rejected the old medical model.

Alongside prevention, the public health model began to emphasize **health promotion,** that is, policies and programs that promote behaviors known to support good health. Health-promotion programs identify healthy people who are engaging in **risk behaviors** (those that increase susceptibility to negative health outcomes) and motivate them to change their actions by changing aspects of the larger environment to increase an individual's chances of success. Numerous policies, individual actions, and public services have worked to improve our overall health status greatly in the past 100 years. (Figure 1.2 lists the ten greatest public health achievements of the twentieth century.)

ecological or public health model A view of health in which diseases and other negative health events are seen as a result of an individual's interaction with his or her social and physical environment.

disease prevention Actions or behaviors designed to keep people from getting sick.

health promotion The combined educational, organizational, procedural, environmental, social, and financial supports that help individuals and groups reduce negative health behaviors and promote positive change.

risk behaviors Actions that increase susceptibility to negative health outcomes.

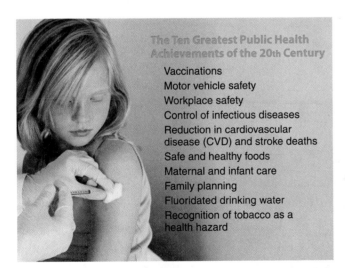

The Ten Greatest Public Health Achievements of the 20th Century

Vaccinations
Motor vehicle safety
Workplace safety
Control of infectious diseases
Reduction in cardiovascular disease (CVD) and stroke deaths
Safe and healthy foods
Maternal and infant care
Family planning
Fluoridated drinking water
Recognition of tobacco as a health hazard

FIGURE 1.2 **The Ten Greatest Public Health Achievements of the Twentieth Century**

Source: Adapted from Centers for Disease Control and Prevention, "Ten Great Public Health Achievements—United States, 1900–1999," *Morbidity and Mortality Weekly Report* 48, no. 12 (April 1999): 241–43.

Wellness and the Dimensions of Health

In 1968, biologist, environmentalist, and philosopher René Dubos proposed an even broader definition of health. In his Pulitzer Prize–winning book, *So Human an Animal*, Dubos defined health as "a quality of life, involving social, emotional, mental, spiritual, and biological fitness on the part of the individual, which results from adaptations to the environment."[9] This concept of adaptability, or the ability to

Irreversible disability and/or death	Chronic illness	Signs of illness	Signs of health/ wellness	Improved health/ wellness	Optimal wellness/ well-being

▲
Neutral
point

FIGURE 1.3 **The Wellness Continuum**

cope successfully with life's ups and downs, became a key element in our overall understanding of health.

Eventually the word **wellness** entered the popular vocabulary. This word further enlarged Dubos's definition of health by recognizing levels—or gradations—of health within each category **(Figure 1.3)**. To achieve *high-level wellness,* a person must move progressively higher on a continuum of positive health indicators. Those who fail to achieve these levels may slip into illness, premature disability, or death.

Today, the words *health* and *wellness* are often used interchangeably to mean the dynamic, ever-changing pro-

wellness The achievement of the highest level of health possible in each of several dimensions.

cess of trying to achieve one's potential in each of six interrelated dimensions **(Figure 1.4)**:

● **Physical health.** This dimension includes characteristics such as body size and shape, sensory acuity and responsiveness, susceptibility to disease and disorders, body functioning, physical fitness, and recuperative abilities. Newer definitions of physical health also include our ability to perform normal *activities of daily living (ADLs),* or those tasks that are necessary to normal existence in society, such as getting up out of a chair, bending over to tie your shoes, or writing a check.

● **Social health.** The ability to have a broad social network and have satisfying interpersonal relationships with friends, family members, and partners is a key part of overall

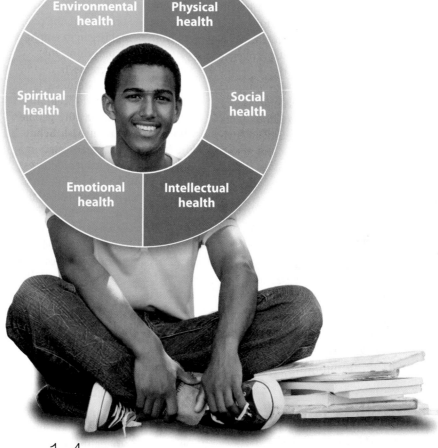

FIGURE 1.4 **The Dimensions of Health**
When all dimensions are balanced and well developed, they support your active, thriving lifestyle.

Video Tutor: Dimensions of Health

wellness. This implies being able to give and receive love and to be nurturing and supportive in social interactions. Successfully interacting and communicating with others, adapting to various social situations, and other daily behaviors are all part of social health.

- **Intellectual health.** The ability to think clearly, reason objectively, analyze critically, and use brainpower effectively to meet life's challenges are all part of this dimension. This includes learning from successes and mistakes and making sound, responsible decisions that consider all aspects of a situation. It also includes having a healthy curiosity about life and an interest in learning new things.
- **Emotional health.** This is the feeling component—being able to express emotions when appropriate, and to control them when not. Self-esteem, self-confidence, self-efficacy, trust, love, and many other emotional reactions and responses are all part of emotional health.
- **Spiritual health.** This dimension involves having a sense of meaning and purpose in your life. This may involve a belief in a supreme being or a specified way of living prescribed by a particular religion. It also may include the ability to understand and express one's purpose in life; to feel a part of a greater spectrum of existence; to experience peace, contentment, and wonder over life's experiences; and to care about and respect all living things.
- **Environmental health.** This dimension entails understanding how the health of the environments in which you live, work, and play can positively or negatively affect you; protecting yourself from hazards in your own environment; and working to preserve, protect, and improve environmental conditions for everyone.

Achieving wellness means attaining the optimal level of well-being for your unique limitations and strengths. For example, a physically disabled person may function at his or her optimal level of performance; enjoy satisfying interpersonal relationships; work to maintain emotional, spiritual, and intellectual health; and have a strong interest in environmental concerns. In contrast, those who spend hours lifting weights to perfect the size and shape of each muscle but pay little attention to their social or emotional health may look healthy but may not maintain a good balance in all dimensions.

Although we often consider physical attractiveness and athletic performance key measures of health, these external trappings reveal very little about a person's overall health. The perspective we need is *holistic*, emphasizing the balanced integration of mind, body, and spirit.

What Influences Your Health?

If you're lucky, aspects of your world conspire to promote your health: Everyone in your family is slender and fit; your mom reminds you when it's time to see the dentist;

there are fresh apples on sale at the neighborhood farmer's market; and a new bike trail opens along the river (and you have a bike!). If you're not so lucky, aspects of your world discourage health: Everyone in your family is overweight and they eat high-fat diets; your peers urge you to keep up with their drinking; there are only cigarettes, alcohol, and junk food for sale at the corner market; and you wouldn't dare walk or ride alongside the river for fear of being mugged. This variety of influences explains why we said earlier that seemingly personal choices aren't totally within an individual's control.

Public health experts refer to the factors that influence health as **determinants of health,** a term the U.S. Surgeon General defines as "the range of personal, social, economic, and environmental factors that influence health status."[10] The Surgeon General's health promotion plan, called *Healthy People,* has been published every 10 years since 1990 with the goal of improving the quality and years of life for all Americans. The overarching goals set out by the newest version, *Healthy People 2020,* are:

> **determinants of health** The range of personal, social, economic, and environmental factors that influence health status.

- Attain high-quality, longer lives free of preventable diseases
- Achieve health equity, eliminate disparities, and improve health of all groups
- Create social and physical environments that promote good health for all
- Promote quality of life, healthy development, and healthy behaviors across all life stages

Healthy People 2020 classifies health determinants into five large groupings: individual behavior, biology and genetics, social factors, policymaking, and health services (Figure 1.5).

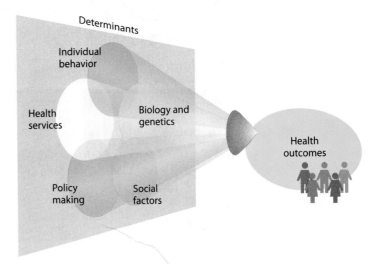

FIGURE 1.5 *Healthy People 2020* **Determinants of Health**
The determinants of health often overlap with one another. Collectively, they impact health of individuals and communities.

Individual Behavior

Individual behaviors can help you attain, maintain, or regain good health, or they can deteriorate your health and promote disease. From birth onward, your behaviors are shaped by a multitude of influences. Fortunately, most behaviors are things you can change, so health experts refer to them as *modifiable determinants*. Modifiable determinants significantly influence your risk for chronic disease. Earlier, we said that chronic diseases are the leading causes of death and disability in the United States; indeed, they are responsible for 7 out of 10 deaths.[11] Incredibly, just four modifiable determinants are responsible for most of the illness and early death related to chronic diseases (Figure 1.6). These are the following:[12]

- **Lack of physical activity.** Physical inactivity and overweight/obesity are each responsible for nearly 1 in 10 deaths in U.S. adults.
- **Poor nutrition.** High dietary salt, low dietary omega-3 fatty acids, and high dietary *trans* fatty acids are the dietary risks with the largest mortality effects.
- **Excessive alcohol consumption.** Alcohol causes 90,000 deaths in adults annually through cardiovascular disease, other medical conditions, traffic accidents, and violence.
- **Tobacco use.** Tobacco smoking and the high blood pressure and cancer it causes are responsible for about 1 in 5 deaths in American adults.

On the flip side, studies show people who exercise regularly, drink alcohol in moderation, eat five daily servings of fruits and vegetables, and don't smoke can add up to 14 extra years to their lives.[13]

Other modifiable determinants include use of vitamins and other supplements, caffeine, over-the-counter medications, and illegal drugs; sexual behaviors and use of contraceptives; sleep habits; and hand washing and other simple infection-control measures.

Biology and Genetics

Biological and genetic determinants are things you can't typically change or modify. Health experts frequently refer to these factors as *nonmodifiable determinants*. They include genetically inherited traits, conditions, and predispositions to diseases such as sickle cell disease, hemophilia, cystic fibrosis, allergies and asthma, cardiovascular disease, diabetes, certain cancers, and other problems. They also refer to certain innate characteristics, such as your age, race, ethnicity, metabolic rate, and body structure. Your gender is a key biological determinant: Women are at risk for low bone density, sexually transmitted infections, autoimmune diseases (in which the immune system attacks the body's own cells), and depression. Your own history of illness and injury also classifies as biology; for instance, if you had a serious knee injury in high school, it may cause pain with walking and exercise, which in turn may predispose you to weight gain.

See It! Videos
What behaviors should you change to live longer? Watch **Months to a Healthier Lifestyle** at
www.pearsonhighered.com/donatelle

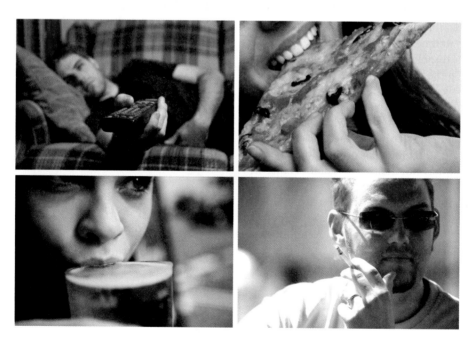

FIGURE 1.6 **Four Leading Causes of Chronic Disease in the United States**
Lack of physical activity, poor nutrition, excessive alcohol consumption, and tobacco use—all modifiable health determinants—are the four most significant factors leading to chronic disease among Americans today.

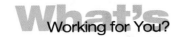
Social Factors

Social factors include both the social and physical conditions in the environment in which people are born or live. Exposure to crime, violence, mass media, technology, and poverty, as well as availability of healthful foods, transportation, living wages, social support, and educational or job opportunities are all examples. Physical conditions include the natural environment; conditions such as good lighting, trees, or benches; the state of buildings—homes, schools, or workplaces; exposure to toxic substances; and the presence of physical barriers, which can challenge people with disabilities.

Economic Factors Among the most powerful of all determinants of health are economic factors: Even in affluent nations such as the United States, people who are in lower socioeconomic brackets have substantially shorter life expectancies and more illnesses than people who are wealthy.[14] Economic disadvantages exert their effects on human health within nearly all domains of life. They include the following:

● Lacking access to quality education from early childhood through adulthood

● Living in poor housing with potential exposure to asbestos, lead, dust mites, rodents and other pests, inadequate sanitation, tap water that's not safe to drink, and high levels of crime

● Being unable to pay for nourishing food, warm clothes, and sturdy shoes; heat and other utilities; medications and medical supplies; transportation; and counseling services, fitness classes, and other wellness measures

● Having insecure employment or being stuck in a low-paying job with few benefits

● Having few assets to fall back on in case of illness or injury

As a student, you're likely to face economic challenges. In a recent survey, 33 percent of college students reported that in the past year their finances had been "very difficult to handle."[15] When you're injured or sick and the money is tight, what can you do to get the best care for the lowest price? Read the **Money & Health** box on page 12 for ideas on maximizing care while minimizing costs.

The Built Environment One part of the physical environment that is getting a fair amount of attention from public health officials these days is the *built environment*. As the name implies, the built environment includes anything created or modified by human beings, from buildings to roads that serve recreation areas and transportation systems to electric transmission lines and communications cables.

Researchers in public health have increasingly been promoting changes to the built environment that can improve the health of community members.[16] For example, Walter Willett of the Harvard School of Public Health proposes that sidewalks and bike lanes be part of every federally funded road project.[17] He asserts that when sidewalks are built in neighborhoods, people are more apt to start walking and slim down. Similarly, when a supermarket selling fresh produce replaces side-by-side fast-food outlets in an inner-city neighborhood, residents' dietary choices improve. Simple changes in community environments can make a difference by enabling you to make better choices.

Pollutants and Infectious Agents Physical conditions also include the quality of the air we breathe, our land, water, and foods. When individuals and communities are exposed to toxins, radiation, irritants, and infectious agents via their environment, they can suffer significant harm.

These effects are not necessarily limited to the local community. With the rise of global travel and commerce, the health status of people in one region can affect the health of people around the world. These environmental determinants are a grim reminder of the need for a proactive international response for disease prevention and climate change.

Policymaking

Public policies and interventions can have a powerful and positive effect on the health of individuals and communities. Examples include policies banning smoking, laws mandating seat belt use in motor vehicles and helmets for bikes and motorcycles, vaccination programs, and public funding for mental health services.[18] For example, in 2009 the

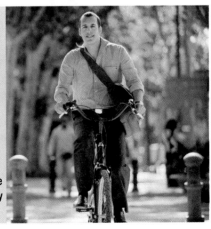

The built environment of your community can promote positive health behaviors. The bike-friendly nature of Amsterdam, Netherlands, with its wide bike paths and major thoroughfares closed to automobile traffic, encourages residents to incorporate healthy physical activity into their daily lives.

Money&Health

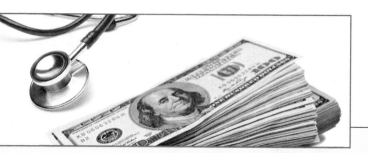

MAXIMIZING CARE WHILE MINIMIZING COSTS

Maybe you're like the 6 percent of college students who reported in a 2010 survey that they had no health care insurance. Or maybe you're on your parents' plan or one sponsored by your college or university, but there's a hefty deductible or co-payment, or the test or medication you need isn't covered. Whatever your situation, following a few strategies will help you get the best care for the lowest cost.

✳ **Preserve your health.** Remember that four behaviors—overeating, failing to exercise, smoking, and abusing alcohol—account for the majority of preventable disease. Your most important cost-sparing strategy is to take care of your health in the first place.

✳ **Avoid unnecessary risks.** Unintentional injuries aren't just the top cause of death in young adults, they're also a primary reason young adults seek emergency care. (For additional information, see Focus On: Reducing Your Risk of Unintentional Injury.)

✳ **Do your research.** If you have health care insurance, read the Summary Plan Description (SPD). This explains what doc-

If you are uninsured or underinsured, ask your doctor for generic prescriptions to save on your costs.

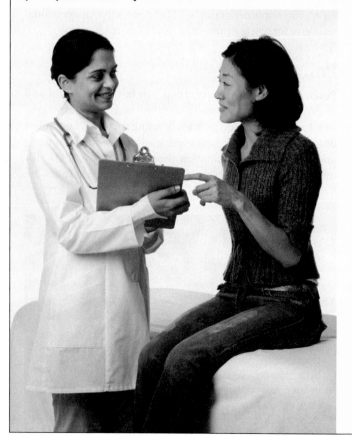

tor, emergency room, and hospital visits are covered and also specifies if vision, dental, or prescription benefits are included. The SPD also outlines any co-payments, annual deductibles, and in- and out-of-network rules for seeing specialists. When you know the answers to these questions, you're less likely to make decisions resulting in large bills.

✳ **Make sure you need health care, not self-care.** The number one reason behind doctor visits is the common cold—for which there's no treatment. For many conditions, rest, nutritious fluids, and the passage of time are the only healers. So think before you spend money on health care you don't need.

✳ **Try the least expensive health care options first.** For instance, your student health center may be able to provide exactly the level of care you need for little or no cost. Or call the nurse hotline available on your insurance plan.

✳ **Go prepared.** When you do visit your doctor, come with a list of symptoms, concerns, and questions. If you think you need a diagnostic test, request it and explain why. If you're sexually active, ask your doctor what tests you should have for sexually transmitted infections, even if you don't have symptoms.

✳ **Ask your doctor to help you get the lowest cost care.** For instance, generic versions of most prescription medications are available, at a cost that may be 50 to 75 percent lower than that of the brand-name drug. So ask the doctor for the generic version of the drug, when possible.

✳ **Use the emergency room (ER) only for emergencies.** Studies show that almost 70 percent of ER visits are not really emergencies at all—and care in an ER can cost ten times as much as the same care in a walk-in clinic.

✳ **When you get a bill from your provider, check it for accuracy.** Medical-bill errors are common, especially duplicated charges and simple typos. Also review the statements you get from your plan to make sure that you received the care described and the right reimbursements.

✳ **Be aware that if your plan denies coverage for a test or treatment your physician says is necessary, you have the right to appeal the decision.** Check your SPD for your plan's appeals process, which typically involves writing a letter explaining your grievance. Copy both your physician and your state insurance commissioner, and keep a copy for your own records.

Sources: American College Health Association. *American College Health Association-National College Health Assessment II: Reference Group Executive Summary Fall 2010.* (Linthicum, MD: American College Health Association, 2011), www.acha.org; U.S. Department of Labor. *Top 10 Ways to Make Your Health Benefits Work for You* (September 29, 2010), www.dol.gov/ebsa/publications/10working4you.html; Aetna. *Six Ways to Save Money With Your Aetna Student Health Benefits,* Aetnastudenthealth.com, www.aetna studenthealth.com/schools/SavingMoneyFlyer.pdf; CalCPA. *How to Minimize Health Care Costs* (2007), American Institute of Certified Public Accountants, www.calcpa.org/Content/25713.aspx.

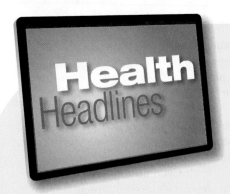

NATIONAL HEALTH CARE REFORM

The United States saw four major political movements supporting national health insurance during the past century, but none had succeeded. The Obama administration put health care reform at the top of its domestic agenda, and on March 23, 2010, the Patient Protection and Affordable Care Act (ACA) became law. The main goal of the ACA is to provide access to health insurance for more than 30 million previously uninsured Americans and also to reform some insurance practices and policies deemed unfair or counter to the public good. The legislation is structured to achieve its goals by expanding Medicaid eligibility to include an additional 17 million people. Although individual states could opt out of the expansion, it is largely funded by federal dollars, which few states are expected to refuse. The law also provides tax credits to small businesses to help them pay for coverage for their employees.

One of the most contentious aspects of the ACA is the so-called individual mandate: All Americans will be required to carry health insurance by 2014 or face an annual (and progressively increasing) fine if they fail to do so. To help Americans find the most affordable plan for their needs, starting in 2014, they will be able to shop for and compare plans in state-based Affordable Insurance Exchanges. ACA supporters say that the individual mandate is necessary to push young, healthy Americans into the insurance pool and thereby dilute the cost of care overall. Opponents argue that compelling individuals to purchase an expensive product such as health insurance is an overreaching by the federal government and violates the Constitution's constraints on federal powers. In June 2012 the U.S. Supreme Court ruled that Congress could enact the ACA under its authority to raise and collect taxes. Some critics immediately charged that a tax levied on an American who refuses to purchase a product or service is not comparable to a general income tax nor a tax incentive, such as for purchasing energy-saving devices for one's home.

Thus, the ACA is likely to face further challenges.

Some reforms are already in effect. These include a provision allowing young adults to stay on their parents' health insurance plan up to age 26 if they do not have access to coverage through an employer. In addition, most employer-based and individual plans are now required to cover preventive services such as blood pressure screenings, certain cancer screenings, vaccinations, prenatal care, well-baby care, smoking-cessation programs, and certain other services with no co-payment or deductible.

Other provisions now in effect ban or place restrictions on certain insurance industry practices such as the following:

✳ Insurers are no longer allowed to deny coverage to children with preexisting conditions, and in 2014, this provision will be expanded to include adults.
✳ Insurers are not allowed to cancel coverage because the insured made an honest mistake on his or her application.
✳ Insurers now have to publicly justify rate hikes.
✳ New health insurance plans cannot impose lifetime coverage limits.

More information and updates on health care reform can be found at www.healthcare.gov.

---

residents of Albert Lea, Minnesota, signed on to an ambitious citywide initiative to improve the health of its residents. It mandated that local restaurants make healthful changes to their menus, that schools ban eating in hallways and selling candy for fundraisers, and that neighborhoods form "walking school buses" to escort kids to school on foot. It also funded changes to the built environment, including laying new sidewalks and digging plots for community gardens. The efforts appeared to pay off with noteworthy improvements in health care claims and other behavioral improvements in less than a year.[19]

Access to Quality Health Services

The health of individuals and communities is also determined by access to quality health care, including not only services for physical and mental health, but also accurate and relevant health information and products such as eye-glasses, medical supplies, and medications. In 2010, more than 27 percent of young Americans (age 18 to 24) lacked health insurance.[20] Individuals without health insurance may delay going to the doctor for regular preventative care. If they are sick, their disease may not be diagnosed until it is advanced, reducing the chance of recovery and leading to higher rates of hospitalization, longer stays, and more costly health care than for those who have insurance and get preventive screenings and prompt treatment.

In addition to the uninsured is the problem of the millions of "underinsured"—those who have some coverage, but not enough. These individuals cannot afford to pay the difference between what their insurance covers and what their providers and medications cost. Therefore, like the uninsured, they tend to delay care or try other cost-saving measures such as taking only half of the prescribed dose of their medications.

health disparities Differences in the incidence, prevalence, mortality, and burden of diseases and other health conditions among specific population groups.

belief Appraisal of the relationship between some object, action, or idea and some attribute of that object, action, or idea.

health belief model (HBM) Model for explaining how beliefs may influence behaviors.

Access to health services is affected by economics, public policies, and health insurance legislation. Early in 2010, President Obama signed into law a set of health care reforms intended to reduce the nation's health care costs while increasing Americans' access to quality care. These reforms, which are being implemented gradually over several years, are meeting significant legal challenges. For details on the new health care legislation, see the accompanying **Health Headlines** box on page 13.

Health Disparities

In recognition of the changing demographics of the U.S. population and the vast differences in health status based on racial or ethnic background, *Healthy People 2020* includes strong language about the importance of reducing these **health disparities.**[21] See the **Health in a Diverse World** box on page 15 for examples of groups that often experience health disparities.

How Can You Improve Your Health Behaviors?

We've just identified many factors critical to your health status. However, you have the most control over factors in just one category: your individual behaviors (or modifiable determinants). Clearly, change is not always easy. Your chances of successfully changing negative habits improve when you identify a behavior that you want to change and then develop a plan for gradual transformation that allows you time to unlearn negative patterns and substitute positive ones. To successfully change a behavior, you need to see change not as a singular *event* but instead as a *process* that requires preparation, has several steps or stages, and takes time to occur.

Models of Behavior Change

Over the years, social scientists and public health researchers have developed a variety of models to reflect this multifaceted process of behavior change. We explore three of those here.

Health Belief Model
We often assume that when rational people realize their behaviors put them at risk, they will change those behaviors and reduce that risk. However, it doesn't work that way for many of us. Consider the number of health professionals who smoke, consume junk food, and act in other unhealthy ways. They surely know better, but their "knowing" is disconnected from their "doing." One classic model of behavior change proposes that our beliefs may help to explain why this occurs.

A **belief** is an appraisal of the relationship between some object, action, or idea (e.g., smoking) and some attribute of that object, action, or idea (e.g., "Smoking is expensive, dirty, and causes cancer" or "Smoking is sociable and relaxing"). Psychologists studying the relationship between beliefs and health behaviors have determined that although beliefs may subtly influence behavior, they may or may not cause people to behave differently. In 1966, psychologist I. Rosenstock developed a classic theory, the **health belief model (HBM),** to show when beliefs affect behavior change.[22] The HBM holds that several factors must support a belief before change is likely:

- **Perceived seriousness of the health problem.** The more serious the perceived effects are, the more likely it is that action will be taken.
- **Perceived susceptibility to the health problem.** What is the likelihood of developing the health problem? People who perceive themselves at high risk are more likely to take preventive action.
- **Cues to action.** A person who is reminded or alerted about a potential health problem is more likely to take action.

People follow the HBM many times every day. Take, for example, smokers. Older smokers are likely to know other smokers who have developed serious heart or lung problems. They are thus more likely to perceive tobacco as a threat to their health than are teenagers who have just begun

See It! Videos
How can you change your habits and stick with it? Watch **New Year's Resolutions** at www.pearsonhighered.com/donatelle

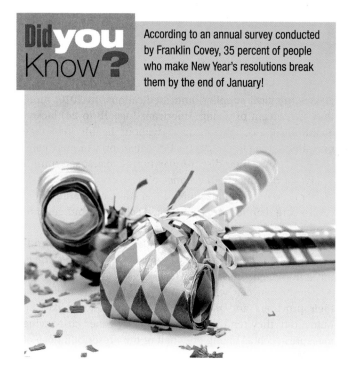

Did you Know?
According to an annual survey conducted by Franklin Covey, 35 percent of people who make New Year's resolutions break them by the end of January!

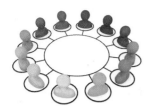

THE CHALLENGE OF HEALTH DISPARITIES

The following factors can affect an individual's ability to attain optimal health:

✱ **Race and ethnicity.** Research indicates dramatic health disparities among people of certain racial and ethnic backgrounds. Socioeconomic differences, stigma based on "minority status," poor access to health care, cultural barriers and beliefs, discrimination, and limited education and employment opportunities can all affect health status.

✱ **Inadequate health insurance.** A large and growing number of people are *uninsured* or *underinsured*. Those without adequate insurance coverage may face high co-payments, high deductibles, or limited care in their area.

✱ **Sex and gender.** At all ages and stages of life, men and women experience major differences in rates of disease and disability. For instance, men smoke more than women, but women who smoke have higher rates of lung disease. And women are ten times more likely than men to contract HIV (which causes AIDS) when having unprotected sex. In contrast, men have much higher

One of the ways public health officials attempt to address the problem of health disparities due to location, poverty, and lack of insurance is to organize Remote Area Medical (RAM) clinics. At a clinic like this, rural families, most with little or no insurance, wait in line for hours to receive free health care from hundreds of professional doctors, nurses, dentists, and other health workers.

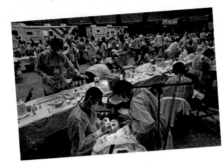

death rates from both unintentional injuries and violence.

✱ **Economics.** One's economic status can influence one's health. For example, persistent poverty may make it difficult to buy healthy food or to afford preventive medical visits or medication. Eco-

nomics also influences access to safe, affordable exercise.

✱ **Geographic location.** Whether you live in an urban or rural area and have access to public transportation or your own vehicle can have a huge impact on what you choose to eat, the amount of physical activity you get, and your ability to visit the doctor or dentist.

✱ **Sexual orientation.** Gay, lesbian, bisexual, or transgender individuals may lack social support, are often denied health benefits due to unrecognized marital status, and face unusually high stress levels and stigmatization by other groups.

✱ **Disability.** Disproportionate numbers of disabled individuals lack access to health care services, social support, and community resources that would enhance their quality of life.

Source: Data from Centers for Disease Control and Prevention, "CDC Health Disparities and Inequalities Report," *Morbidity and Mortality Weekly Report*, Supplement 60 (January 14, 2011): 1–116. www.cdc.gov/mmwr/preview/ind2011_su.html; H. Mead, L. Cartwright-Smith, K. Jones, C. Ramos, K. Woods, and B. Siegel, *Racial and Ethnic Disparities in U.S. Health Care: A Chartbook* (New York: The Commonwealth Fund, March 2008).

smoking. The greater the perceived threat of health problems caused by smoking, the greater the chance a person will quit.

However, many chronic smokers know the risks yet continue to smoke. Why do they miss these cues to action? According to Rosenstock, some people do not believe they are susceptible to a severe problem—they act as though they are immune to it—and are unlikely to change their behavior. They also may feel that the immediate pleasure outweighs the long-range cost.

Social Cognitive Model The **social cognitive model** developed from the work of several researchers over the past several decades, but it is most closely associated with the work of psychologist Albert Bandura. Fundamentally, the model proposes that three factors interact in a reciprocal fashion to promote and motivate change. These are the social environment in which we live, our thoughts or cognition (including our values, perceptions, beliefs, expecta-

tions, and sense of self-efficacy), and our behaviors (**Figure 1.7** on page 16). We change our behavior in part by observing models in our environments—from childhood to the present moment—reflecting on our observations, and regulating ourselves accordingly.

For instance, if as a child we observed our mother successfully quitting smoking, we are more apt to believe we can do it, too. In addition, when we succeed in changing ourselves, we change our thoughts about ourselves, and this in turn may promote further behavior change: After we've successfully quit smoking, we may feel empowered to increase our level of physical activity. Moreover, as we change ourselves, we change our world; in our example, we become a model of successful smoking cessation for others to observe. Thus, we are not just products of our environments, but producers.

social cognitive model Model of behavior change emphasizing the role of social factors and thought processes (cognition) in behavior change.

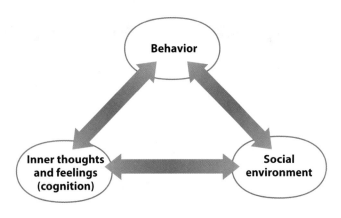

FIGURE 1.7 **Social Cognitive Model**
We constantly change our behavior in response to factors in our social environment and our thoughts and feelings. In a reciprocal fashion, our behaviors change our environments as well as our thoughts and feelings—including our sense of our ability to make positive change.

Transtheoretical Model Why do so many New Year's resolutions fail before Valentine's Day? According to Drs. James Prochaska and Carlos DiClemente, it's because we are going about things in the wrong way; fewer than 20 percent of us are really prepared to take action. After considerable research, Prochaska and DiClemente have concluded that behavior changes usually do not succeed if they start with the change itself. Instead, we must go through a series of stages to adequately prepare ourselves for that eventual change.[23] According to Prochaska and DiClemente's **transtheoretical model** of behavior change (also called the *stages of change model*), our chances of keeping those New Year's resolutions will be greatly enhanced if we have proper reinforcement and help during each of the following stages:

transtheoretical model Model of behavior change that identifies six distinct stages people go through in altering behavior patterns; also called the *stages of change model.*

1. Precontemplation. People in the precontemplation stage have no current intention of changing. They may have tried to change a behavior before and given up, or they may be in denial and unaware of any problem.

2. Contemplation. In this phase, people recognize that they have a problem and begin to contemplate the need to change. Despite this acknowledgment, people can languish in this stage for years, realizing that they have a problem but lacking the time or energy to make the change.

3. Preparation. Most people at this point are close to taking action. They've thought about what they might do and may even have come up with a plan.

4. Action. In this stage, people begin to follow their action plans. Those who have prepared for change appropriately and made a plan of action are more ready for action than those who have given it little thought.

5. Maintenance. During the maintainance stage, a person continues the actions begun in the action stage and works toward making these changes a permanent part of his or her life. In this stage, it is important to be aware of the potential for relapses and to develop strategies for dealing with such challenges.

6. Termination. By this point, the behavior is so ingrained that constant vigilance may be unnecessary. The new behavior has become an essential part of daily living.

We don't necessarily go through these stages sequentially. They may overlap, or we may shuttle back and forth from one to another—say, contemplation to preparation, then back to contemplation—for a while before we become truly committed to making the change. Still, it's useful to recognize "where we are" with a change, so that we can consider the appropriate strategies to move us forward.

Step One: Increase Your Awareness

Before you can decide what you might want to change, you need to learn what researchers know about the behaviors that contribute to and detract from your health. Each chapter in this book provides a foundation of information focused on these factors. Check out the Table of Contents at the front of the book to locate chapters with the information you're looking for.

This is also a good time to take stock of the health determinants in your life: What aspects of your biology and behavior support your health, and which are obstacles to overcome? What elements of your social and physical environment could you tap into to help you change, and what elements might hold you back? Making a list of all of the health determinants that affect you—both positively and negatively—should greatly increase your understanding of what you might want to change, and what you might need to do to make that change happen.

Step Two: Contemplate Change

Now that you've increased your awareness of the behaviors that contribute to wellness in populations, and the specific health determinants affecting you, you may find yourself contemplating change. In this stage, the following strategies may be helpful.

Examine Your Current Health Habits and Patterns Do you routinely stop at Dunkin' Donuts for breakfast? Smoke when you're feeling stressed? Party too much on the weekends? Get to bed way past 2 AM? When considering behavior you may want to change, ask yourself the following:

● How long and how frequently has this been going on?
● How serious are the consequences of the habit or pattern in the short and long term?
● What are some of your reasons for continuing this problematic behavior?
● What kinds of situations trigger the behavior?
● Are other people involved in this behavior? If so, in what way?

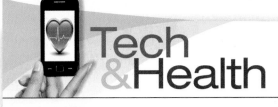

Tech & Health

SURFING FOR THE LATEST IN HEALTH

The Internet can be a wonderful resource for quickly finding answers to your questions, but it can also be a source of much *misinformation.* If you're not careful, you could end up feeling frazzled, confused, and—worst of all—misinformed. To ensure that the sites you visit are reliable and trustworthy, follow these tips.

❋ Look for websites sponsored by an official government agency, a university or college, or a hospital/medical center. Government sites are easily identified by their *.gov* extensions (e.g., the National Institute of Mental Health's website is www.nimh.nih.gov). College and university sites typically have *.edu* extensions (e.g., Johns Hopkins University's website is www.jhu.edu). Hospitals often have an extension of *.org* (e.g., the Mayo Clinic's website is www.mayoclinic.org). Major philanthropic foundations, such as the Robert Wood Johnson Foundation, the Kellogg Foundation, and others, often provide information about selected health topics. In addition, national nonprofit organizations, such as the American Heart Association and the American Cancer Society, are often good, authoritative sources of information. Foundations and nonprofits usually have URLs ending with a *.org* extension.

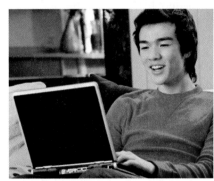

Find reliable health information at your fingertips!

❋ Search for well-established, professionally peer-reviewed journals such as the *New England Journal of Medicine* (http://content.nejm.org) or the *Journal of the American Medical Association (JAMA;* http://jama.ama-assn.org). Although some of these sites require a fee for access, you can often locate concise abstracts and information, such as a weekly table of contents, that can help you conduct a search. Other times, you can pay a basic fee for a certain number of hours of unlimited searching. Your college may have Internet access to these journals that they make available to students for no cost.

❋ Consult the Centers for Disease Control and Prevention (www.cdc.gov) for consumer news, updates, and alerts.

❋ For a global perspective on health issues, visit the World Health Organization (www.who.int/en).

❋ There are many government- and education-based sites that are independently sponsored and reliable. The following is just a sample. We provide more in each chapter as we cover specific topics:

1. Aetna Intelihealth: www.intelihealth.com
2. FamilyDoctor.org: familydoctor.org
3. MedlinePlus: www.nlm.nih.gov/medlineplus
4. Go Ask Alice!: www.goaskalice.columbia.edu
5. WebMD Health: webmd.com

❋ The nonprofit health care accrediting organization Utilization Accreditation Review Commission (URAC; www.urac.org) has devised more than 50 criteria that health sites must satisfy to display its seal. Look for the "URAC Accredited Health Web Site" seal on websites you visit.

❋ And, finally, don't believe everything you read. Cross-check information against reliable sources to see whether facts and figures are consistent. Be especially wary of websites that try to sell you something. When in doubt, check with your own health care provider, health education professor, or state health division website.

As we've explored throughout this chapter, health behaviors involve elements of personal choice, but they are also influenced by other determinants that make them more or less likely. Some are *predisposing factors*—for instance, if your parents smoke, you're 90 percent more likely to start smoking than someone whose parents don't smoke. Some are *enabling factors*—for example, if your peers smoke, you are 80 percent more likely to smoke. Identifying the factors that encourage or discourage a habit is part of contemplating behavior change.

Various *reinforcing factors* can also contribute to your current habits. If you decide to stop smoking, but your family and friends all smoke, you may lose your resolve. In such cases, it can be helpful to employ the social cognitive model and deliberately change aspects of your social environment.

For instance, you could spend more time with nonsmoking friends to give yourself a chance to observe people modeling the positive behavior you want to emulate.

Identify a Target Behavior To clarify your thinking about the various behaviors you might like to target, ask yourself these questions:

● **What do I want?** What is your ultimate goal: To lose weight, exercise more, reduce stress, have a lasting relationship? You need a clear picture of your target outcome.
● **Which change is the greatest priority at this time?** People often decide to change several things at once. Suppose you are gaining unwanted weight. Rather than saying, "I need to

eat less and start exercising," identify one specific behavior that contributes significantly to your greatest problem, and tackle that first.

● **Why is this important to me?** Think through why you want to change. Are you doing it because of your health? To improve your academic performance? To look better? To win someone else's approval? It's best to target a behavior because it's right for you rather than because you think it will help you win others' approval.

Another aspect of targeting is filling in the details. Identifying the specific behavior you would like to change—in contrast to the general problem—will allow you to set clear goals.

Learn More about the Target Behavior Once you've clarified exactly what behavior you'd like to change, you're ready to learn more about that behavior. Again, the information in this textbook will help. In addition, this is a great time to learn how to gain access to accurate and reliable health information on the Internet (see the **Tech & Health** box on page 17).

---
motivation A social, cognitive, and emotional force that directs human behavior.

As you conduct your research, don't limit your focus to the behavior and its effects. Also think about what aspects of your world might pose obstacles to your success, and learn all you can about those. For instance, let's say you decide you want to meditate for 15 minutes a day. You face a big ramp-up just in learning what meditation is, how it's practiced, and what benefits you might expect from it. But in addition, what might pose an obstacle to meditation? Do you think of yourself as hyper? Do you live in a super-noisy dorm? Are you afraid your friends might think meditating is weird? In short, learn everything you can—positive and negative—about your target behavior now, and you'll be better prepared for change.

Assess Your Motivation and Your Readiness to Change On any given morning, many of us get out of bed and resolve to change a given behavior that day. However, most of us soon return to our old behavior patterns.

Wanting to change is an essential prerequisite of the change process, but to achieve change, you need more than desire. You need real **motivation,** which isn't just a feeling, but a social and cognitive force that directs your behavior. To understand what goes into motivation, let's return for

3 to 5

is the number of times most people will attempt to change an unhealthy behavior before succeeding.

a moment to two models of change discussed earlier: the health belief model and the social cognitive model.

Remember that, according to the HBM, your beliefs affect your ability to change. For example, when reaching for another cigarette, smokers sometimes tell themselves, "I'll stop tomorrow," or "They'll have a cure for lung cancer before I get it." These beliefs allow them to continue what they're doing. To put it another way, they dampen motivation. So as you contemplate change, take some time to think about your beliefs and consider whether they are likely to motivate you to achieve lasting change. Ask yourself the following.

Do you believe that your current pattern could lead you to a serious problem? The more severe the consequences are, the more motivated you'll be to change the behavior. For example, smoking can cause cancer, emphysema, and other deadly diseases. The fear of developing those diseases can help you stop smoking. But what if cancer and emphysema were just words to you? In that case, you could study up on these disorders and the tissue destruction, pain, loss of function, and emotional suffering they cause. Doing so might increase your motivation: In Canada, a recent law

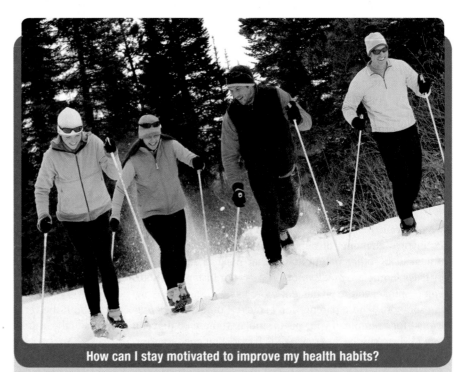

How can I stay motivated to improve my health habits?

Many people find it easiest to stay motivated by planning small incremental changes, working toward a goal, and rewarding themselves along the way. Friends can also help you stay motivated by modeling healthy behaviors, offering support, joining you in your change efforts, and providing reinforcement.

requires that graphic images of gangrenous limbs, diseased organs, and chests sawed open for autopsy cover at least half of cigarette packages. The year after the law took effect, 38 percent of smokers who tried to quit cited the images as a motivating factor.[24]

Do you believe that you are personally likely to experience the consequences of your behavior? For example, losing a loved one to lung cancer could motivate you to work harder to stop smoking. If you really couldn't convince yourself that your behavior will affect you personally, you might ask your health care provider to give you an honest assessment of your risk.

Let's say you're still struggling to perceive the behavior as serious or the consequences as personal. If that's true, try employing the social cognitive model to help change those beliefs. For instance, you could interview people struggling with the consequences of the behavior you want to change. Ask them what their life is like, and if, when they were engaging in the behavior, they believed that it would harm them. Your health care provider may be able to put you in touch with patients who would be happy to support your behavior change plan in this way. And don't ignore the motivating potential of positive role models. Do you know people who have successfully lost weight, stopped drinking, or quit smoking? Hang out with them! Finding ways to stay motivated is a key purpose behind many of the behavior change steps and processes we have been describing throughout this section. The **Skills for Behavior Change** box summarizes some of these tips for maintaining motivation.

Even though motivation is powerful, by itself it's not enough to achieve change. Motivation has to be combined with common sense, commitment, and a realistic understanding of how best to move from point A to point B. *Readiness* is the state of being that precedes behavior change. People who are ready to change possess the knowledge, skills, and external and internal resources that make change possible.[25]

what do you think?

Do you have an internal or an external locus of control?
● Can you think of some friends whom you'd describe as more internally or externally controlled?
● How do people with the different views deal with similar situations?

Maintain Your Motivation

Skills for Behavior Change

❭ **Pick one specific behavior you want to change.** Trying to change too many things at once can be overwhelming.
❭ **Assess the one behavior you wish to change.** Figure out why it is important to change. If it doesn't feel important, then you'll have a hard time finding motivation, and it probably isn't a behavior you should address at this time.
❭ **Set achievable and incremental goals.** By developing both short- and long-term goals, you improve your chances of accomplishing them and staying motivated to move forward.
❭ **Give yourself rewards.** Create a list of things you would find rewarding and plan for giving yourself specific rewards once you reach specific goals.
❭ **Avoid or anticipate barriers and temptation.** By controlling or eliminating the environmental cues that provoke the behavior you want to change, you'll make it easier for yourself to succeed at lasting change.
❭ **Remind yourself why you are trying to change.** Prepare a list of benefits you'll realize from making this change, both now and down the road. You can also prepare a list of the risks you face if you don't make this change. Post the lists where you will see them daily.
❭ **Enlist the help and support of others.** Other people can be major motivators for positive change—either as role models, a cheering squad, or partners in change. Let the people you care about know about your plans for change and ask them for help.
❭ **Don't be discouraged by lapses.** Everyone experiences temporary setbacks, and a brief lapse doesn't mean the entire cause is lost. Reexamine your plan, look for new strategies to motivate you, set some new short-term goals, and get right back on the horse.

Develop Self-Efficacy

Self-efficacy—an individual's belief that he or she is capable of achieving certain goals or of performing at a level that may influence events in life—is one of the most important factors that influences our health status. Prior success will lead to expectations of success in the future. In general, people who exhibit high self-efficacy are confident that they can succeed, and they approach challenges with a positive attitude. In turn, they may be more motivated to change and more likely to succeed.

Conversely, someone with low self-efficacy or with self-doubts may give up easily or never even try to change a behavior. These people tend to shy away from difficult challenges. They may have failed before, and when the going gets tough, they are more likely to give up or revert to old patterns of behavior.

If you suspect you have low self-efficacy, the contemplation stage is a great time to get to work developing it! A technique of cognitive-behavioral therapy called *cognitive restructuring* can help. (See Chapter 3 for information on cognitive restructuring.) Find out more by visiting your campus student counseling services.

self-efficacy Belief in one's ability to perform a task successfully.

Cultivate an Internal Locus of Control

The conviction that you have the power and ability to change is a powerful motivator. Individuals who feel they have limited control over their lives often find it more difficult to initiate positive changes.[26] If they believe that someone or something else controls a situation or that they dare not act in a particular way because of peer repercussions, they may become easily frustrated and give up. People with these characteristics have an *external* **locus of control.** In contrast, people who have a stronger *internal* locus of control believe that they have power over their own actions. They are more driven by their own thoughts and are more likely to state their opinions and be true to their own beliefs.

Having an internal or external locus of control can vary according to circumstance. For instance, someone who finds out that diabetes runs in his family may resign himself to facing the disease one day instead of taking an active role in modifying his lifestyle to minimize his risk of developing diabetes. On this front, he would be demonstrating an external locus of control. However, the same individual might exhibit an internal locus of control when resisting a friend's pressure to smoke.

Step Three: Prepare for Change

You've contemplated change for long enough! Now it's time to set a realistic goal, anticipate barriers, reach out to others, and commit. Here's how.

Set a Realistic Goal
A realistic goal is one that you truly can achieve within the circumstances of your life right now. Knowing that your goal is attainable increases your motivation. This, in turn, leads to a better chance of success and to a greater sense of self-efficacy—which can motivate you to succeed even more.

Use the SMART System
Unsuccessful goals are vague and open-ended: for instance, "Get into shape by exercising more." In contrast, successful goals are SMART—specific, measurable, action-oriented, realistic, and time-oriented. Examples of SMART goals are:

- **S**pecific. "Attend a Tuesday/Thursday aerobics class at the YMCA."
- **M**easurable. "Reduce my alcohol intake on Saturday nights from three drinks to two."
- **A**ction-oriented. "Volunteer at the animal shelter on Friday afternoons."
- **R**ealistic. "Increase my daily walk from 15 to 20 minutes."
- **T**ime-oriented. "Stay in my strength-training class for the full 10-week session, then reassess."

Use Shaping
A stepwise process of making a series of small changes known as **shaping** can help you achieve your goal. Suppose you want to start jogging 3 miles every other day, but right now you get tired and winded after half a mile. Shaping would dictate a process of slow, progressive steps, such as walking 1 hour every other day at a slow, relaxed pace for the first week; walking for an hour every other day, but at a faster pace that covers more distance the second week; and speeding up to a slow run the third week.

Regardless of the change you plan, remember that current habits didn't develop overnight, and they won't change overnight, either. Start changes slowly to avoid hurting yourself or causing undue stress. Keep the steps of your program small. Be flexible and willing to change the original plan if it proves too uncomfortable, and master one step before moving on to the rest.

Anticipate Barriers to Change
Recognizing possible stumbling blocks in advance will help you prepare fully for change. Various social determinants, aspects of the built environment, or lack of adequate health care can inhibit change. In addition to negative determinants, a few general barriers to change include the following:

- **Overambitious goals.** Remember the advice to set realistic goals? Even with the strongest motivation, overambitious goals can derail change. Habits are best changed one small step at a time.
- **Self-defeating beliefs and attitudes.** As the health belief model explains, believing you're too young, fit, or lucky to worry about the consequences of your behavior can keep you from making a solid commitment to change. Likewise, thinking you are helpless to change your habits can also undermine efforts.
- **Failing to accurately assess your current state of wellness.** You might assume that you will be able to walk 2 miles to campus each morning, for example, only to discover that you're aching and winded after only a mile. Failing to make sure that the planned change is realistic for *you* can be a barrier that leaves you with weakened motivation and commitment.
- **Lack of support and guidance.** If you want to cut down on your drinking, peers who drink heavily may be powerful barriers to that change. To succeed, you need to recognize and limit interactions with people in your life who might oppose your decision to change.
- **Emotions that sabotage your efforts and sap your will.** Sometimes the best laid plans go awry because you're having a bad day or are fighting with someone. Emotional reactions to life's challenges aren't inherently

To reach your behavior change goals, you need to take things one step at a time.

bad. However, they can sabotage your efforts to change by distracting you and draining your reserves. Seek help for more severe psychological problems, and recognize that you may need to focus on those issues before you can effect significant change in other aspects of your health.

Enlist Others as Change Agents The social cognitive model recognizes the importance of our social contacts in successful change. Most of us are highly influenced by the approval or disapproval (real or imagined) of close friends, family members, and other social and cultural groups. In addition, watching others successfully change their behavior can give you ideas and encouragement for your own change. This **modeling,** or learning from role models, is a key component of the social cognitive model of change. Observing a friend who is a good conversationalist, for example, can help you improve your communication skills.

Family Members From the time of your birth, your parents and other family members have given you strong cues about which actions are and are not socially acceptable. Your family also influenced your food choices, your religious beliefs, your political beliefs, and many of your other values and actions. Strong and positive family units provide care, trust, and protection; are dedicated to the healthful development of all family members; and work to reduce problems. When the loving family unit does not exist or when it does not provide for basic human needs, many young people have great difficulties.

Friends Just as your family influences your actions during your childhood, your friends and significant others influence your behaviors as you grow older. Most of us desire to fit the "norm" and avoid hassles in our daily interactions with others. If you deviate from the expected actions, you may suffer ostracism, strange looks, and other negative social consequences. But if your friends offer encouragement, or even express interest in joining with you in the behavior change, you are more likely to remain motivated. Thus, cultivating and maintaining close friends who share your personal values can greatly affect your behaviors.

Professionals You may want to enlist support from professionals such as your health instructor, PE instructor, coach, health care provider, academic adviser, or minister. As appropriate, consider the counseling services offered on campus, as well as community services such as smoking cessation programs, Alcoholics Anonymous support groups, and your local YMCA.

Sign a Contract It's time to get it in writing! A formal *behavior change contract* serves many powerful purposes. It functions as a promise to yourself, as a public declaration of intent, as an organized plan that lays out start and end dates and daily actions, as a listing of barriers you may encounter, as a place to brainstorm strategies to overcome barriers, as a list of sources of support, and as a reminder of the benefits of sticking with the program. Writing a behavior change contract will help you clarify your goals and make a commitment to change. Fill out the Behavior Change Contract at the beginning of this book to help you set a goal, anticipate obstacles, and create strategies to overcome those obstacles. Figure 1.8 on page 22 shows an example of a completed contract.

modeling Learning specific behaviors by watching others perform them.
imagined rehearsal Practicing, through mental imagery, to become better able to perform an event in actuality.

Step Four: Take Action to Change

It's time to put your plan into action! Behavior change strategies include visualization, countering, controlling the situation, changing your self-talk, rewarding yourself, and journaling. The options don't stop here, but these are a good place to start.

Visualize New Behavior Mental practice can transform unhealthy behaviors into healthy ones. Athletes and others often use a technique known as **imagined rehearsal** to reach their goals. Careful mental and verbal rehearsal of how you intend to act will help you anticipate problems and greatly improve the likelihood of success.

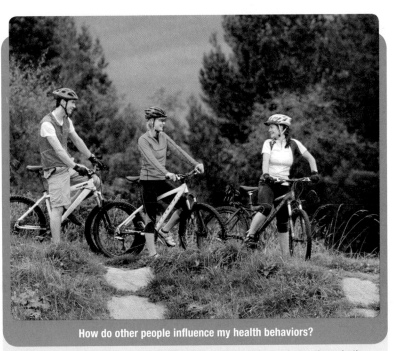

How do other people influence my health behaviors?

The people in your life can play a huge role—both positive and negative—in the health choices you make. The behaviors of those around you can predispose you to certain health habits, at the same time enabling and reinforcing them. Seeking out the support and encouragement of friends who have similar goals and interests will strengthen your commitment to develop and maintain positive health behaviors.

Behavior Change Contract

My behavior change will be:
To snack less on junk food and more on healthy foods.

My long-term goal for this behavior change is:
Eat junk food snacks no more than once a week

These are three obstacles to change (things that I am currently doing or situations that contribute to this behavior or make it harder to change):
1. The grocery store is closed by the time I come home from school
2. I get hungry between classes, and the vending machines only carry candy bars.
3. It's easier to order pizza or other snacks than to make a snack at home.

The strategies I will use to overcome these obstacles are:
1. I'll leave early for school once a week so I can stock up on healthy snacks in the morning.
2. I'll bring a piece of fruit or other healthy snack to eat between classes.
3. I'll learn some easy recipes for snacks to make at home.

Resources I will use to help me change this behavior include:
a friend/partner/relative: my roommates: I'll ask them to buy healthier snacks instead of chips when they do the shopping.
a school-based resource: The dining hall: I'll ask the manager to provide healthy foods we can take to eat between classes.
a community-based resource: The library: I'll check out some cookbooks to find easy snack ideas
a book or reputable website: The USDA nutrient database at www.ars.usda.gov: I'll use this site to make sure the foods I select are healthy choices.

In order to make my goal more attainable, I have devised these short-term goals:
short-term goal Eat a healthy snack 3 times per week   target date September 15   reward new CD
short-term goal Learn to make a healthy snack   target date October 15   reward concert tickets
short-term goal Eat a healthy snack 5 times per week   target date November 15   reward new shoes

When I make the long-term behavior change described above, my reward will be:
ski lift tickets for winter break   target date: December 15

I intend to make the behavior change described above. I will use the strategies and rewards to achieve the goals that will contribute to a healthy behavior change.

Signed: Elizabeth King   Witness: Susan Bauer

FIGURE 1.8 Example of a Completed Behavior Change Contract
A blank version is included in the front of the book for you to fill out.

Learn to "Counter" Countering means substituting a desired behavior for an undesirable one. If you want to stop eating junk food, for example, compile a list of substitute foods and places to get them and have this ready before your mouth starts to water at the smell of a burger and fries.

Control the Situation Sometimes, the right setting or the right group of people will positively influence your behaviors. Any behavior has both antecedents and consequences. *Antecedents* are the events or aspects of the situation that come beforehand; these cue or stimulate a person to act in certain ways. Antecedents can be physical events, thoughts, emotions, or the actions of other people. *Consequences*—the results of behavior—affect whether a person will repeat that action. Consequences can also consist of physical events, thoughts, emotions, or the actions of other people. A diary noting your undesirable behaviors and identifying the settings in which they occur can be useful in helping you determine the antecedents and consequences involved. Once you have recognized the antecedents of a given behavior, you can employ **situational inducement** to modify those that are working against you. By carefully considering which settings will help and which will hurt your effort to change, and by seeking the first and avoiding the second, you will improve your chances for change. Similarly, identifying substitute antecedents that can support a more positive result gives you a strategy for controlling the situation.

Change Your Self-Talk The way you think to yourself, known as **self-talk,** can also play a role in modifying health-related behaviors. It can reflect your feelings of *self-efficacy,* discussed earlier in this chapter. When we don't feel self-efficacious, it's tempting to engage in negative self-talk, which can sabotage our best intentions. In the **Skills for Behavior Change** box on the next page are some suggested strategies for changing self-talk.

Use Rational, Positive Statements The rational-emotive form of cognitive therapy, or self-directed behavior change, is based on the premise that there is a close connection between what people say to themselves and how they feel. According to psychologist Albert Ellis, most emotional problems and related behaviors stem from irrational statements that people make to themselves when events in their lives are different from what they would like them to be.[27]

For example, suppose that after doing poorly on a test you say to yourself, "I can't believe I flunked that easy exam. I'm

countering Substituting a desired behavior for an undesirable one.
situational inducement Attempt to influence a behavior through situations and occasions that are structured to exert control over that behavior.
self-talk The customary manner of thinking and talking to yourself, which can affect your self-image.

so stupid." Now change this irrational self-talk into rational, positive statements about what is really going on: "I really didn't study enough for that exam. I'm certainly not stupid; I just need to prepare better for the next test." Such self-talk will help you recover quickly from disappointment and take positive steps to correct the situation.

Practice Blocking and Stopping By purposefully blocking or stopping negative thoughts, a person can concentrate on taking positive steps toward behavior change. For example, suppose you are preoccupied with your ex-partner, who has recently left you for someone else. By refusing to dwell on negative images and forcing yourself to focus elsewhere, you can avoid wasting energy, time, and emotional resources and move on to positive change.

Reward Yourself Another way to promote positive behavior change is to reward yourself for it. This is called **positive reinforcement.** Each of us is motivated by different reinforcers.

Most positive reinforcers can be classified under five headings: consumable, activity, manipulative, possessional, and social:

- *Consumable reinforcers* are edible items, such as your favorite fruit or snack mix.
- *Activity reinforcers* are opportunities to do something enjoyable, such as going on a hike or taking a trip.
- *Manipulative reinforcers* are incentives such as getting a lower rent in exchange for mowing the lawn or the promise of a better grade for doing an extra-credit project.
- *Possessional reinforcers* are tangible rewards, such as a new electronic gadget or sports car.
- *Social reinforcers* are signs of appreciation, approval, or love, such as loving looks, affectionate hugs, and praise.

The difficulty with employing positive reinforcement often lies in determining which incentive will be most effective. Your reinforcers may initially come from others (extrinsic rewards), but as you see positive changes in yourself, you will begin to reward and reinforce yourself (intrinsic rewards). Keep in mind that reinforcers should immediately follow a behavior, but beware of overkill. If you reward yourself with a movie every time you go jogging, this reinforcer will soon lose its power. It would be better to give yourself this reward after, say, a full week of adherence to your jogging program.

<what do you think?>
what do you think?
What type of reinforcers would most likely get you to change a behavior: money, praise, or recognition from someone?
- Why would it motivate you?
- Can you think of options to reinforce behavior changes?

Skills for Behavior Change

Challenge the Thoughts That Sabotage Change

Are any of the following thought patterns and beliefs holding you back? Try these strategies to combat self sabotage:

❭ **"I don't have enough time!"** Chart your hourly activities for 1 day. What are your highest priorities and what can you eliminate? Plan to make time for a healthy change next week.

❭ **"I'm too stressed!"** Assess your major stressors right now. List those you can control and those you can change or avoid. Then identify two things you enjoy that can help you reduce stress now.

❭ **"I'm worried about what others may think."** Ask yourself how much others influence your decisions about drinking, sex, eating habits, and the like. What is most important to you? What actions can you take to act in line with these values?

❭ **"I don't think I can do it."** Just because you haven't done something before doesn't mean you can't do it now. To develop some confidence, take baby steps and break tasks into small segments of time.

❭ **"I can't break this habit!"** Habits are difficult to break, but not impossible. What triggers your behavior? List ways you can avoid these triggers. Ask for support from friends and family.

Journal Writing personal experiences, interpretations and results in a journal, notebook, or online in a blog is an important skill for behavior change. You can log your daily activities, monitor your progress, record how you feel about it, and note ideas for improvement.

Let's Get Started!

After you acquire the skills to support successful behavior change, you're ready to apply those skills to your target behavior. Create a behavior change contract incorporating the goals and skills we've discussed, and place it where you will see it every day and where you can refer to it as you work through the chapters in this text. Consider it a visual reminder that change doesn't "just happen." Reviewing your contract helps you to stay alert to potential problems, to be aware of your alternatives, to maintain a firm sense of your values, and to stick to your goals under pressure.

positive reinforcement Presenting something positive following a behavior that is being reinforced.

How Healthy Are You?

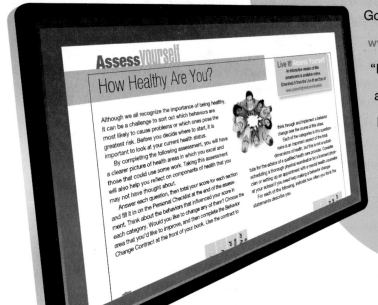

Assess yourself

How Healthy Are You?

Although we all recognize the importance of being healthy, it can be a challenge to sort out which behaviors are most likely to cause problems or which ones pose the greatest risk. Before you decide where to start, it is important to look at your current health status.

By completing the following assessment, you will have a clearer picture of health areas in which you excel and those that could use some work. Taking this assessment will also help you reflect on components of health that you may not have thought about.

Answer each question, then total your score for each section and fill it in on the Personal Checklist at the end of the assessment. Think about the behaviors that influenced your score in each category. Would you like to change any of them? Choose the area that you'd like to improve, and then complete the Behavior Change Contract at the front of your book. Use the contract to

Go online to the **Live It!** section of **www.pearsonhigherd.com/donatelle** to take the "How Healthy Are You?" assessment. If the assessment shows areas of your life that could be improved, then try the strategies listed in the **YOUR PLAN FOR CHANGE** box.*

*If your instructor so chooses, Assess Yourself Activities are available as a printed supplement or as assignable homework online at www.pearsonhighered.com/myhealthlab.

MyHealthLab®

YOUR PLAN FOR CHANGE

Once you've gone online and used the **Assess yourself** activity to gauge your total health status, you may see various dimensions where you could improve your health.

Today, you can:

○ Evaluate your behavior and identify patterns and specific things you are doing.

○ Select one pattern of behavior that you want to change.

○ Fill out the Behavior Change Contract at the front of your book. Be sure to include your long- and short-term goals for change, the rewards you'll give yourself for reaching these goals, the potential obstacles along the way, and the strategies for overcoming these obstacles. For each goal, list the small steps and specific actions that you will take.

Within the next 2 weeks, you can:

○ Start a journal and begin charting your progress toward your behavior change goal.

○ Tell a friend or family member about your behavior change goal, and ask them to support you along the way.

○ Reward yourself for reaching your short-term goals, and reevaluate your plan if you find they are too ambitious.

By the end of the semester, you can:

○ Review your journal entries and consider how successful you have been in following your plan. What helped you be successful? What made change more difficult? What will you do differently next week?

○ Revise your plan as needed: Are the goals attainable? Are the rewards satisfying? Do you have enough support and motivation?

Summary

* Choosing good health has immediate benefits, such as reducing the risk of injury and illnesses and improving academic performance; long-term rewards, such as disease prevention, longevity, and improved quality of life; and societal and global benefits, such as reducing the global disease burden.

* For the U.S. population as a whole, the leading causes of death are heart disease, cancer, and chronic lower respiratory diseases. In the 15- to 24-year-old age group, the leading causes are unintentional injuries, homicide, and suicide.

* The average life expectancy at birth in the United States is 78.3 years. This has increased greatly over the past century; however, unhealthy behaviors related to chronic disease may prevent further increases in total life expectancy and cause a reduction in *healthy* life expectancy.

* The definition of *health* has changed over time. The medical model focused on treating disease, whereas the current ecological or public health model focuses on factors contributing to health, disease prevention, and health promotion.

* Health can be seen as existing on a continuum and encompassing the dynamic process of fulfilling one's potential in the physical, social, emotional, spiritual, intellectual, and environmental dimensions of life. Wellness means achieving the highest level of health possible in each of the health dimensions.

* Health is influenced by factors called *determinants*. The Surgeon General's health promotion plan, *Healthy People,* classifies determinants as individual behavior, biology and genetics, social factors, policymaking, and health services. Disparities in health among different groups contribute to increased risks.

* Models of behavior change include the health belief model, the social cognitive model, and the transtheoretical (stages of change) model. A person can increase the chance of successfully changing a health-related behavior by viewing change as a process containing several steps and components.

* When contemplating a behavior change, it is helpful to examine current habits, learn about a target behavior, and assess motivation and readiness to change. When preparing to change, it is helpful to set realistic and incremental goals that employ shaping, anticipate barriers to change, enlist the help and support of others, and sign a behavior change contract. When taking action to change, it is helpful to visualize new behavior, practice countering, control the situation, change self-talk, reward oneself, and keep a log, blog, or journal.

Pop Quiz

1. What statistic is used to describe the number of deaths from heart disease this year?
   a. Morbidity
   b. Mortality
   c. Incidence
   d. Prevalence

2. Your ability to perform everyday tasks, such as walking up the stairs or tying your shoes, is an example of
   a. improved quality of life.
   b. healthy life expectancy.
   c. health promotion.
   d. activities of daily living.

3. Janice describes herself as confident and trusting, and she displays both high self-esteem and high self-efficacy. The dimension of health this relates to is the
   a. social dimension.
   b. emotional dimension.
   c. spiritual dimension.
   d. intellectual dimension.

4. *Healthy People 2020* is a(n)
   a. blueprint for health actions designed to improve health in the United States.
   b. projection for life expectancy rates in the United States in the year 2020.
   c. international plan for achieving health priorities for the environment in the year 2020.
   d. set of specific goals that states must achieve in order to receive federal funding for health care.

5. Because Craig's parents smoked, he is 90 percent more likely to start smoking than someone whose parents didn't. This is an example of what factor influencing behavior change?
   a. Circumstantial factor
   b. Enabling factor
   c. Reinforcing factor
   d. Predisposing factor

6. Suppose you want to lose 20 pounds. To reach your goal, you take small steps. You start by joining a support group and counting calories. After 2 weeks, you begin an exercise program and gradually build up to your desired fitness level. What behavior change strategy are you using?
   a. Shaping
   b. Visualization
   c. Modeling
   d. Reinforcement

7. After Kirk and Tammy pay their bills, they reward themselves by watching TV together. The type of positive reinforcement that motivates them to pay their bills is a(n)
   a. activity reinforcer.
   b. consumable reinforcer.
   c. manipulative reinforcer.
   d. possessional reinforcer.

8. Jake is exhibiting *self-efficacy* when he
   a. believes that he can and will be able to bench-press 125 pounds in his specified time frame.
   b. is doubtful that his bad shoulder will heal enough to bench-press the weight he is hoping for.
   c. claims he is not good enough to do any physical exercise that will ever allow him to bench-press 125 pounds.
   d. does not possess personal control over this situation.

9. The setting events for a behavior that cue or stimulate a person to act in certain ways are called
   a. antecedents.
   b. frequency of events.
   c. consequences.
   d. cues to action.

10. What strategy for change is advised for an individual in the preparation stage of change?
    a. Seeking out recommended readings
    b. Finding creative ways to maintain positive behaviors
    c. Setting realistic goals
    d. Publicly stating the desire for change

Answers to these questions can be found on page A-1.

Think about It!

1. How are the words *health* and *wellness* similar? What, if any, are important distinctions between these terms? What is health promotion? Disease prevention?
2. How healthy is the U.S. population today? Are we doing better or worse in terms of health status than we have done previously? What factors influence today's disparities in health?
3. What are some of the health disparities existing in the United States today? Why do you think these differences exist? What policies do you think would most effectively address or eliminate health disparities?
4. What is the health belief model? How may this model be working when a young woman decides to smoke her first cigarette? Her last cigarette?
5. Using the transtheoretical model, discuss what you might do (in stages) to help a friend stop smoking. Why is it important that a person be ready to change before trying to change?

Accessing Your Health on the Internet

The following websites explore further topics and issues related to personal health. For links to the websites below, visit the Companion Website for *Access to Health,* 13th Edition, at www.pearsonhighered.com/donatelle.

1. *CDC Wonder.* This is a clearinghouse for comprehensive information from the Centers for Disease Control and Prevention (CDC), including special reports, guidelines, and access to national health data. http://wonder.cdc.gov
2. *MayoClinic.com.* This reputable resource for specific information about health topics, diseases, and treatment options is provided by the staff of the Mayo Clinic. It is easy to navigate and is consumer friendly. www.mayoclinic.com
3. *National Center for Health Statistics.* This is an outstanding place to start for information about health status in the United States. It contains links to key reports; national survey information; and information on mortality by age, race, gender, geographic location, and other important data. www.cdc.gov/nchs
4. *National Health Information Center.* This is an excellent resource for consumer information about health. www.health.gov/nhic
5. *World Health Organization.* This resource for global health information provides information on the current state of health around the world, such as illness and disease statistics, trends, and illness outbreak alerts. www.who.int/en

References

1. The World Factbook—Country Comparisons: Life Expectancy at Birth—2012 Estimates," CIA, June 1, 2012. https://www.cia.gov/library/publications/the-world-factbook/rankorder/2102rank.html.
2. Centers for Disease Control and Prevention, "Achievements in Public Health, 1900–1999: Control of Infectious Diseases," *Morbidity and Mortality Weekly Report* 48, no. 29 (1999): 621–29, www.cdc.gov/mmwr/preview/mmwrhtml/mm4829a1.htm.
3. S. J. Olshansky et al., "A Potential Decline in Life Expectancy in the United States in the 21st Century," *New England Journal of Medicine* 352, no. 11 (2005): 1138–45.
4. G. Danaei et al., "The Promise of Prevention: The Effects of Four Preventable Risk Factors on National Life Expectancy and Life Expectancy Disparities by Race and County in the United States," *PLoS Medicine* 7, no. 3 (2010): e1000248, www.plosmedicine.org/article/info%3Adoi%2F10.1371%2Fjournal.pmed.1000248.
5. U.S. Department of Health and Human Services, *Healthy People 2020,* www.healthypeople.gov/2020/about/QoL.WBabout.aspx.
6. E. A. Finkelstein et al., "Annual Medical Spending Attributable to Obesity: Payer- and Service-Specific Estimates," *Health Affairs* 28, no. 5 (2009): w822–31.
7. M. Bittman, "Soda: A Sin We Sip Instead of Smoke?" *New York Times,* February 12, 2010, www.nytimes.com/2010/02/14/weekinreview/14bittman.html.
8. World Health Organization (WHO), "Constitution of the World Health Organization," *Chronicles of the World Health Organization* (Geneva: WHO, 1947), www.who.int/governance/eb/constitution/en/index.html.
9. R. Dubos, *So Human an Animal: How We Are Shaped by Surroundings and Events* (New York: Scribner, 1968), 15.
10. U.S. Department of Health and Human Services, *Healthy People 2020* (Washington, DC: U.S. Government Printing Office, 2011), www.healthypeople.gov/2020/about/DOHAbout.aspx.

11. Centers for Disease Control and Prevention, Chronic Disease and Health Promotion, *Chronic Disease Overview*, December 17, 2009, www.cdc.gov/chronicdisease/overview/index.htm#2.

12. G. Danaei et al., "The Preventable Causes of Death in the United States: Comparative Risk Assessment of Dietary, Lifestyle, and Metabolic Risk Factors," *PLoS Medicine* 6, no. 4 (2009): e1000058, www.plosmedicine.org/article/info:doi/10.1371/journal.pmed.1000058; Centers for Disease Control and Prevention, *Chronic Disease Overview*, 2009.

13. K-T. Khaw et al., "Combined Impact of Health Behaviours and Mortality in Men and Women: The EPIC-Norfolk Prospective Population Study." *PLoS Medicine* 5, no. 1 (2008): e12, doi:10.1371/journal.pmed.0050012.

14. U.S. Department of Health and Human Services, *Healthy People 2020*, 2011.

15. American College Health Association, *American College Health Association-National College Health Assessment II: Reference Group Executive Summary Fall 2010* (Linthicum, MD: American College Health Association, 2011), www.acha.org.

16. H. Gagnon, S. Tessier, and J. Cote, et al., "Psychosocial Factors and Beliefs Related to Intentions to Not Binge Drink Among Young Adults," *Alcohol and Alcoholism*, 2012. May, 02. Doi 10.1093/alcalc/ags049; J. Macy, S. Middlestadt, L. Kolbe, et al., "Applying the Theory of Planned Behavior to Explore the Relationship Between Smoke-Free Air Laws and Quitting Intention," *Health Education and Behavior*, 2012.39(1):27–34.

17. W. C. Willett and A. Underwood, "Crimes of the Heart," *Newsweek*, February 5, 2010, www.newsweek.com/id/233006.

18. U.S. Department of Health and Human Services, *Healthy People 2010*, 2011.

19. W. C. Willett and A. Underwood, "Crimes of the Heart," 2010.

20. K. Sebelius, Affordable Care Act in Action: Fewer Uninsured Young Adults in America (2011, September 13). U.S. Department of Health and Human Services. www.healthcare.gov/blog/2011/09/fewer_uninsured091311.html.

21. National Institutes of Health, *National Institutes of Health (NIH) Strategic Research Plan and Budget to Reduce and Ultimately Eliminate Health Disparities: Volume 1, Fiscal Years 2002–2006* (Bethesda, MD: National Institutes of Health, May 12, 2006), http://ncmhd.nih.gov/our_programs/strategic/pubs/VolumeI_031003EDrev.pdf.

22. I. Rosenstock, "Historical Origins of the Health Belief Model," *Health Education Monographs* 2, no. 4 (1974): 328–35.

23. J. O. Prochaska and C. C. DiClemente, "Stages and Processes of Self-Change of Smoking: Toward an Integrative Model of Change," *Journal of Consulting and Clinical Psychology* 51 (1983): 390–95.

24. W. C. Willett and A. Underwood, "Crimes of the Heart," 2010.

25. M. Hesse, "The Readiness Ruler as a Measure of Readiness to Change Polydrug Use in Drug Abusers," *Journal of Harm Reduction* 3, no. 3 (2006): 1477–81; M. Cismaru, "Using Protection Motivation Theory to Increase the Persuasiveness of Public Service Communications," The Saskatchewan Institute of Public Policy, Public Policy Series paper no. 40 (February 2006); E. A. Fallon, S. Wilcox, and M. Laken, "Health Care Provider Advice for African American Adults Not Meeting Health Behavior Recommendations," *Preventing Chronic Disease* 3, no. 2 (2006): A45; M. R. Chacko et al., "New Sexual Partners and Readiness to Seek Screening for Chlamydia and Gonorrhea: Predictors among Minority Young Women," *Sexually Transmitted Infections* 82 (2006): 75–79.

26. H. Gagnon, S. Tessier, and J. Cote, et al., "Psychosocial Factors and Beliefs Related to Intentions to Not Binge Drink Among Young Adults," *Alcohol and Alcoholism*, 2012. May, 02. Doi 10.1093/alcalc/ags049; J. Macy, S. Middlestadt, L. Kolbe, et al., "Applying the Theory of Planned Behavior to Explore the Relationship Between Smoke-Free Air Laws and Quitting Intention," *Health Education and Behavior*, 2012.39(1):27–34.

27. A. Ellis and M. Benard, *Clinical Application of Rational Emotive Therapy* (New York: Plenum, 1985).

Promoting and Preserving Your Psychological Health

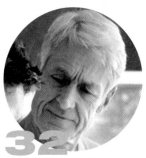

32

How do others influence my psychological well-being?

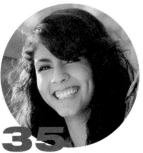

35

Is laughter really the best medicine?

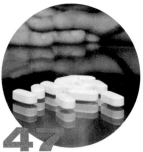

47

What should I do if someone I know is suicidal?

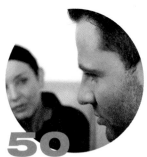

50

How can I choose the right therapist for me?

OBJECTIVES

✱ Define each of the four components of psychological health, and identify the basic traits shared by psychologically healthy people.

✱ Learn what factors affect your psychological health; discuss the positive steps you can take to enhance psychological well-being.

✱ Identify psychological disorders, such as mood disorders, anxiety disorders, personality disorders, and schizophrenia, and explain their causes and treatments.

✱ Discuss warning signs of suicide and actions that can be taken to help a suicidal individual.

✱ Explain the different types of treatments and mental health professionals, and examine how they can play a role in managing mental health disorders.

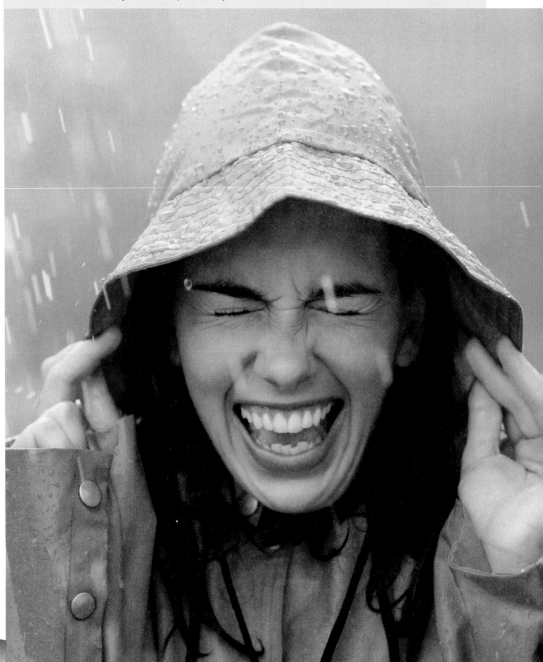

Although the vast majority of students describe their college years as among the best of their lives, many also find the pressure of grades, financial concerns, relationship problems, and the struggle to find themselves to be extraordinarily difficult. Psychological distress caused by relationship issues, family issues, academic competition, and adjusting to college life is rampant today. Experts believe that the anxiety-inducing campus environment is a major contributor to poor health decisions such as high levels of alcohol consumption and, in turn, to health problems that ultimately affect academic success and success in life.

Fortunately, humans possess resiliency, a trait that enables us to cope, adapt, and thrive, regardless of life's challenges. How we feel and think about ourselves, those around us, and our environment can tell us a lot about our psychological health.

What Is Psychological Health?

Psychological health is the sum of how we think, feel, relate, and exist in our day-to-day lives. Our thoughts, perceptions, emotions, motivations, interpersonal relationships, and behaviors are a product of our experiences and the skills we have developed along the way to meet life's challenges. **Psychological health** includes mental, emotional, social, and spiritual dimensions (Figure 2.1).

Most experts identify several basic elements shared by psychologically healthy people:

- **They feel good about themselves.** They are not typically overwhelmed by fear, love, anger, jealousy, guilt, or worry. They know who they are, have a realistic sense of their capabilities, and respect themselves even though they realize they aren't perfect.
- **They feel comfortable with other people, respect others, and have compassion.** They enjoy satisfying and lasting personal relationships and do not take advantage of others or allow others to take advantage of them. They recognize that there are others whose needs are greater than their own and take responsibility for their fellow human beings. They can give love, consider others' interests, take time to help others, and respect personal differences.
- **They control tension and anxiety.** They recognize the underlying causes and symptoms of stress and anxiety in their lives and consciously avoid irrational thoughts, hostility, excessive excuse making, and blaming others for their problems. They use resources and learn skills to control reactions to stressful situations.
- **They meet the demands of life.** They try to solve problems as they arise, accept responsibility, and plan ahead. They set realistic goals, think for themselves, and make independent decisions. Acknowledging that change is inevitable, they welcome new experiences.

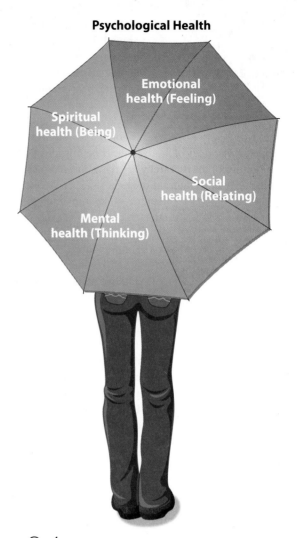

Psychological Health

Emotional health (Feeling)

Spiritual health (Being)

Social health (Relating)

Mental health (Thinking)

FIGURE 2.1 **Psychological Health**
Psychological health is a complex interaction of the mental, emotional, social, and spiritual dimensions of health. Possessing strength and resiliency in these dimensions can maintain your overall well-being and help you weather the storms of life.

- **They curb hate and guilt.** They acknowledge and combat tendencies to respond with anger, thoughtlessness, selfishness, vengefulness, or feelings of inadequacy. They do not try to knock others aside to get ahead, but rather reach out to help others.
- **They maintain a positive outlook.** They approach each day with a presumption that things will go well. They look to the future with enthusiasm rather than dread. Fun and making time for themselves are integral parts of their lives.
- **They value diversity.** They do not feel threatened by those of a different race, gender, religion, sexual orientation, ethnicity, or political party. They are nonjudgmental and do not force their beliefs and values on others.
- **They appreciate and respect nature.** They take time to enjoy their surroundings, are conscious of their place in the universe, and act responsibly to preserve their environment.

psychological health The mental, emotional, social, and spiritual dimensions of health.

Psychologists have long argued that before we can achieve any of the above characteristics of psychologically healthy people, we must meet certain basic human needs. In the 1960s, human theorist Abraham Maslow developed a *hierarchy of needs* to describe this idea (Figure 2.2): At the bottom of his hierarchy are basic *survival needs,* such as food, sleep, and water; at the next level are *security needs,* such as shelter and safety; at the third level—*social needs*—is a sense of belonging and affection; at the fourth level are *esteem needs,* self-respect, and respect for others; and at the top are needs for *self-actualization* and self-transcendence.

According to Maslow's theory, a person's needs must be met at each of these levels before he or she can be truly healthy. Failure to meet one of the lower-level needs will interfere with a person's ability to address higher-level needs. For example, someone who is homeless or worried about threats from violence will be unable to focus on fulfilling social, esteem, or actualization needs. Maslow believed that people are more likely to behave badly if they are frustrated by a lack of need fulfillment.[1]

In sum, psychologically healthy people are emotionally, mentally, socially, and spiritually resilient. They usually respond to challenges and frustrations in appropriate ways, despite occasional slips (see Figure 2.3 on page 31). When they do slip, they recognize it and take action to rectify the situation.

Attaining psychological well-being involves many complex processes. This chapter will help you understand not only what it means to be psychologically well, but also why we may run into problems in our psychological health. Learning how to assess your own health and take action to help yourself are important aspects of psychological health.

Mental Health

The term **mental health** is used to describe the "thinking" or "rational" dimension of our health. A mentally healthy person perceives life in realistic ways, can adapt to change, can develop rational strategies to solve problems, and can carry out personal and professional responsibilities. In addition, a mentally healthy person has the intellectual ability to sort through information, messages, and life events; attach meaning to these events; and respond appropriately. This is often referred to as *intellectual health,* a subset of mental health.[2]

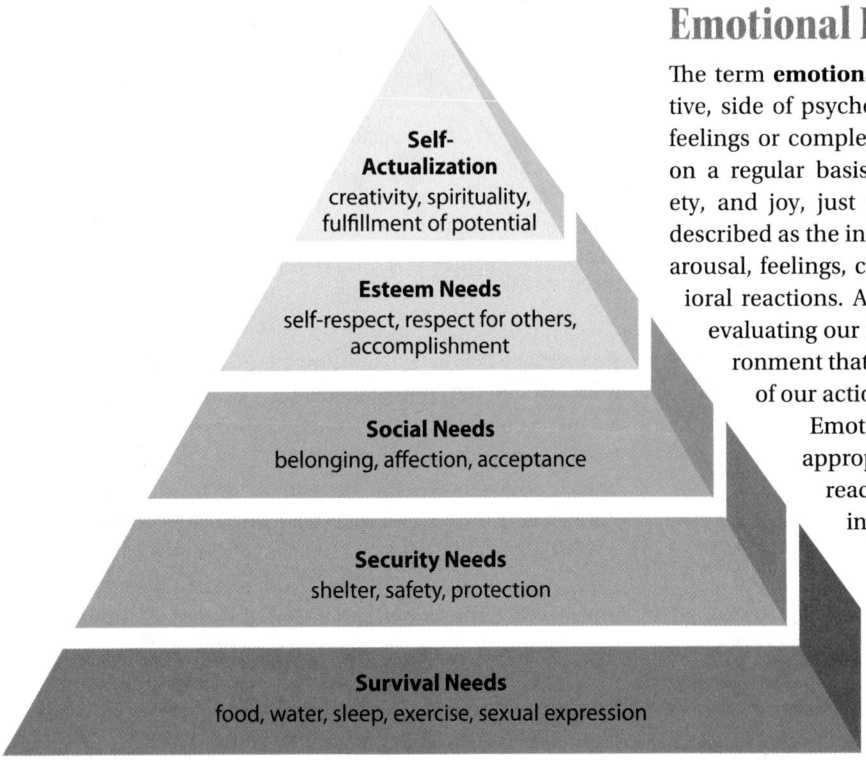

Emotional Health

The term **emotional health** refers to the feeling, or subjective, side of psychological health. **Emotions** are intensified feelings or complex patterns of feelings that we experience on a regular basis, including love, hate, frustration, anxiety, and joy, just to name a few. Typically, emotions are described as the interplay of four components: physiological arousal, feelings, cognitive (thought) processes, and behavioral reactions. As rational beings, we are responsible for evaluating our individual emotional responses, the environment that is causing them, and the appropriateness of our actions.

Emotionally healthy people usually respond appropriately to upsetting events. Rather than reacting in an extreme fashion or behaving inconsistently or offensively, they can express their feelings, communicate with others, and show emotions in appropriate ways. Emotionally unhealthy people are much more likely to let their feelings overpower them. They may be highly volatile and prone to unpredictable emotional responses, which may be followed by inappropriate communication or actions. A person's **emotional intelligence** is the ability to identify, use, understand, and

---

mental health The thinking part of psychological health; includes your values, attitudes, and beliefs.

emotional health The feeling part of psychological health; includes your emotional reactions to life.

emotions Intensified feelings or complex patterns of feelings.

emotional intelligence Ability to identify, monitor, and manage one's own emotions and to understand those of others; includes the ability to use the information to guide one's thinking and actions The ability to identify, use, understand and manage your emotions in positive and constructive ways.

Self-Actualization
creativity, spirituality, fulfillment of potential

Esteem Needs
self-respect, respect for others, accomplishment

Social Needs
belonging, affection, acceptance

Security Needs
shelter, safety, protection

Survival Needs
food, water, sleep, exercise, sexual expression

FIGURE 2.2 **Maslow's Hierarchy of Needs**

Source: From A. H. Maslow. R. D. Frager and J. Fadiman, eds., *Motivation and Personality,* 3rd ed. (Upper Saddle River, NJ: Pearson Education, Inc., 1987). Reprinted by permission.

Video Tutor: Maslow's Hierarchy of Needs

No zest for life; pessimistic/cynical most of the time; spiritually down	Shows poorer coping than most, often overwhelmed by circumstances	Works to improve in all areas, recognizes strengths and weaknesses	Possesses zest for life; spiritually healthy and intellectually thriving
Laughs, but usually at others, has little fun	Has regular relationship problems, finds that others often disappoint	Healthy relationships with family and friends, capable of giving and receiving love and affection	High energy, resilient, enjoys challenges, focused
Has serious bouts of depression, "down" and tired much of time; has suicidal thoughts	Tends to be cynical/critical of others; tends to have negative/critical friends	Has strong social support, may need to work on improving social skills but usually no major problems	Realistic sense of self and others, sound coping skills, open-minded
A "challenge" to be around, socially isolated	Lacks focus much of the time, hard to keep intellectual acuity sharp	Has occasional emotional "dips", but overall good mental/emotional adaptors	Adapts to change easily, sensitive to others and environment
Experiences many illnesses, headaches, aches/pains, gets colds/infections easily	Quick to anger, sense of humor and fun evident less often		Has strong social support and healthy relationships with family and friends

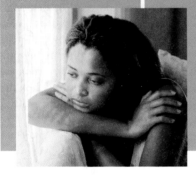
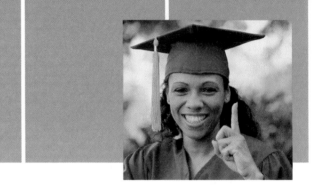

FIGURE 2.3 **Characteristics of Psychologically Healthy and Unhealthy People**
Where do you fall on this continuum?

manage one's emotions in positive and constructive ways. It is about recognizing your own emotional state and the emotional states of others. Emotional intelligence consists of four core abilities: self-awareness, self-management, relationship management, and social awareness. Developing or increasing your emotional intelligence can help you build strong relationships, succeed at work, and achieve your goals.[3]

Emotional health also affects social and intellectual health. People who feel hostile, withdrawn, or moody may become socially isolated.[4] Because they are not much fun to be around, their friends may avoid them at the very time they are most in need of emotional support. For students, a more immediate concern is the impact of emotional trauma on academic performance. Have you ever tried to study for an exam after a fight with a friend or family member? Emotional turmoil may seriously affect your ability to think, reason, and act rationally.

Social Health

Social health includes your interactions with others on an individual and group basis, your ability to use social resources and support in times of need, and your ability to adapt to a variety of social situations. Socially healthy individuals enjoy a wide range of interactions with family, friends, and acquaintances and are able to have healthy interactions with an intimate partner. Typically, socially healthy individuals can listen, express themselves, form healthy attachments, act in socially acceptable and responsible ways, and find the best fit for themselves in society. Numerous studies have documented the importance of positive relationships with family members, friends, and significant others in overall well-being and longevity.[5]

Social bonds reflect the level of closeness and attachment that we develop with individuals and are the very foundation of human life. They provide intimacy, feelings of belonging, opportunities for giving and receiving nurturance, reassurance of one's worth, assistance and guidance, and advice. Social bonds take multiple forms, the most common of which are social support and community engagements.

social health Aspect of psychological health that includes interactions with others, ability to use social supports, and ability to adapt to various situations.

social bonds Degree and nature of interpersonal contacts.

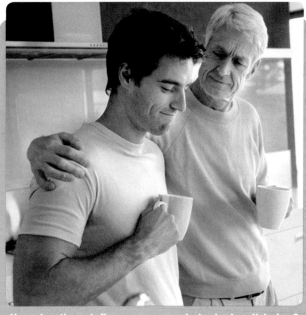

How do others influence my psychological well-being?

Your outlook on life is determined in part by your social and cultural surroundings, and the positive or negative nature of your social bonds can strongly affect your sense of well-being. In particular, your family members shape your psychological health. As you were growing up, they modeled behaviors and skills that helped you develop cognitively and socially. Their love and support can give you a sense of self-worth and encourage you to treat others with compassion and care.

social support Network of people and services with whom you share ties and from whom you get support.

spiritual health Aspect of psychological health that relates to having a sense of meaning and purpose to one's life, as well as a feeling of connection with others and with nature.

dysfunctional families Families in which there is violence; physical, emotional, or sexual abuse; parental discord; or other negative family interactions.

The concept of **social support** is more complex than many people realize. In general, it refers to the people and services with whom we interact and share social connections. These ties can provide *tangible support,* such as babysitting services or money to help pay the bills, or *intangible support,* such as encouraging you to share intimate thoughts. Sometimes, support can be felt as perceiving that someone would be there for us in a crisis. Generally, the closer and the higher the quality of the social bond, the more likely a person is to ask for and receive social support. For example, if your car broke down on a dark country road in the middle of the night, whom could you call for help and know that the person would do everything possible to get there? Common descriptions of strong social support include the following:[6]

- Being cared for and loved, with shared intimacy
- Being esteemed and valued; having a sense of self-worth
- Sharing companionship, communication, and mutual obligations with others; having a sense of belonging

- Having "informational" support—access to information, advice, community services, and guidance from others

Social health also reflects the way we react to others. (Look for more information about interpersonal relationships in **Chapter 4.**)

Spiritual Health

It is possible to be mentally, emotionally, and socially healthy and still not achieve optimal psychological well-being. What is missing? For many people, the difficult-to-describe element that gives purpose to life is the spiritual dimension.

The term *spirituality* is broader in meaning than religion and is defined as an individual's sense of purpose and meaning in life; it goes beyond material values.[7] Spirituality may be practiced in many ways, including through religion; however, religion does not have to be part of a spiritual person's life. **Spiritual health** refers to the sense of belonging to something greater than the purely physical or personal dimensions of existence. For some, this unifying force is nature; for others, it is a feeling of connection to other people; for still others, the unifying force is a god or other higher power.

(**Focus On: Cultivating Your Spiritual Health**, which begins on page 58, will help you explore your spiritual health in more detail and better understand the role spirituality plays in your overall psychological health.)

Factors That Influence Psychological Health

Psychological health is the product of many influences throughout our lives. It can be influenced by multiple factors, including family, social supports, and the community in which you live. Your psychological health is also shaped by your sense of self-efficacy and self-esteem, your personality, and your developmental stage.

The Family

Families have a significant influence on psychological development. Healthy families model and help develop the cognitive and social skills necessary to solve problems, express emotions in socially acceptable ways, manage stress, and develop a sense of self-worth and purpose. Children raised in healthy, nurturing homes are more likely to become well-adjusted, productive adults. In adulthood, family support is one of the best predictors of health and happiness.[8] Children brought up in **dysfunctional families**—in which there is violence; distrust; anger; dietary deprivation; drug abuse; parental discord; or sexual, physical, or emotional abuse—may have a harder time adapting to life and may run an increased risk of psychological problems. In dysfunctional families, love, security, and unconditional trust may be so lacking that children become psychologically damaged. Yet not all people raised in dysfunctional families become psychologically unhealthy, and not all people from healthy environments become well adjusted.

Social Supports

Our initial social support may be provided by family members, but as we grow and develop, the support of peers and friends becomes more and more important. We rely on friends to help us figure out who we are and what we want to do with our lives. A recent study of college students clearly demonstrated that the availability of social support (a sense of belonging) predicted overall well-being.[9] We often check in with friends to bounce ideas off them to see if they think we are being logical or smart or practical or fair. Having people in our lives who provide positive support and who we can trust and rely on is important to our psychological health.

Community

The communities we live in can have a positive impact on our psychological health through collective actions. For example, neighbors may join together to get rid of trash on the street, participate in a neighborhood watch to keep children safe, help each other with home repairs, or organize a community picnic. Religious institutions, schools, clinics, and local businesses can also engage in efforts that demonstrate support and caring for community members. Likewise, you are a part of a campus community. That community can support and care for your psychological health by creating a safe environment to explore and develop your mental, emotional, social, and spiritual dimensions.

what do you think?

What are some ways in which people in your community work together toward a common goal?
● What type of groundwork must be established before this type of working together can occur?
● What factors can get in the way of collaboration and cooperation?

Self-Efficacy and Self-Esteem

During our formative years, successes and failures in school, athletics, friendships, intimate relationships, our jobs, and every other aspect of life subtly shape our beliefs about our personal worth and abilities. These beliefs in turn become internal influences on our psychological health.

Self-efficacy describes a person's belief about whether he or she can successfully engage in and execute a specific behavior. **Self-esteem** refers to one's realistic sense of self-respect or self-worth. People with high levels of self-efficacy and self-esteem tend to express a positive outlook on life.

Self-esteem results from the relationships we have with our parents and family growing up; with friends as we grow older; with our significant others as we form intimate relationships;

and with our teachers, coworkers, and others throughout our lives. How can you build your self-esteem? The **Skills for Behavior Change** box below suggests small things you can do every day that can make a difference in how you feel about yourself, and the **Health Headlines** box on page 34 discusses the downside of having too much self-esteem.

Learned Helplessness versus Learned Optimism Psychologist Martin Seligman proposed that people who continually experience failure may develop a pattern of response known as **learned helplessness** in which they give up and fail to take action to help themselves. Seligman ascribes this response in part to society's tendency toward *victimology*—blaming one's problems on other people and circumstances.[10] Although viewing ourselves as victims may make us feel better temporarily, it does not address the underlying causes of a problem. Ultimately, it can erode

self-efficacy Describes a person's belief about whether he or she can successfully engage in and execute a specific behavior.

self-esteem Refers to one's realistic sense of self-respect or self-worth.

learned helplessness Pattern of responding to situations by giving up because of repeated failure in the past.

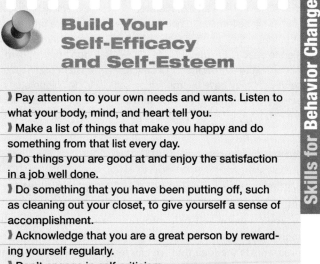

Build Your Self-Efficacy and Self-Esteem

❭ Pay attention to your own needs and wants. Listen to what your body, mind, and heart tell you.
❭ Make a list of things that make you happy and do something from that list every day.
❭ Do things you are good at and enjoy the satisfaction in a job well done.
❭ Do something that you have been putting off, such as cleaning out your closet, to give yourself a sense of accomplishment.
❭ Acknowledge that you are a great person by rewarding yourself regularly.
❭ Don't engage in self-criticism.
❭ Write down the good things about yourself and practice affirmations.
❭ Spend time with people who make you feel good about yourself. Avoid people who treat you poorly or make you feel bad about yourself.
❭ Take time to reflect on your achievements, friends, or special memories.
❭ Take advantage of any opportunity to learn something new.
❭ Do something nice for another person. There is no greater way to feel better about yourself than to help someone else. (This applies to helping or protecting animals, too!)

Skills for Behavior Change

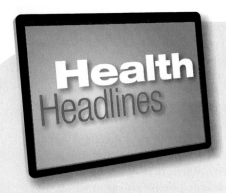

OVERDOSING ON SELF-ESTEEM?

Since the late 1960s, fostering self-esteem in children was seen as key to keeping them away from drugs and violence and to ensuring well-adjusted lives. While it's true people tend to thrive when praised for hard work and accomplishments, society is now questioning the downside of over-praising and the handing out of so many ribbons just for showing up. There is a point at which *healthy self-esteem* hits the slippery slope of vanity and narcissism, leading some to have an exaggerated investment in self-image, a need for constant compliments, and a sense of feeling entitled to special treatment in life.

According to a growing list of critics, Generation Y may have overdosed on self-esteem by growing up in an environment where nobody fails and everyone is gifted.

Dr. Jean Twenge, author of *Generation Me: Why Today's Young Americans are More Confident, Assertive, Entitled and More Miserable Than Ever*, discusses a study of over 16,000 college students who took the Narcissistic Personality Inventory between 1982 and 2006. In 1982, only a third of the students scored above average on narcissism on the test, but in 2006 over 65 percent did. Some point to the look-at-me-all-the-time dynamics of Twitter, Facebook, and YouTube as enforcing narcissism. Psychologists theorize people who judge self-worth by the number of followers for their Twitter feed may have a distorted perspective on what it takes to maintain healthy relationships in real life. The problem is that being special and important in a virtual world, where status is measured by the number of Facebook friends or video hits, doesn't translate into automatic success at work or in higher education.

In fact, preliminary research points indicate people who never fail and have extremely high levels of self-esteem might be more prone to anger, aggression, and other negative behaviors when others don't praise them or meet their needs for instant gratification. A recent University of Michigan study sounded an interesting new alarm about just how important self-esteem may be to the self-esteem generation. Although the sample size was small, students reported liking and wanting moments that boost their self-esteem more than having sex, eating a favorite food, drinking, or nearly all other pleasurable events!

Psychologists continue to support the idea that self-esteem is important for positive growth and development. However, knowing what the criteria are for healthy self-esteem remains somewhat illusive. More research is needed to examine potential risks of too much self-esteem and the best ways to deal with it once it occurs.

Sources: "Narcissistic and Entitled to Everything—Does Gen Y Have Too Much Self-Esteem?" Aspen Educational Group, Accessed February 11, 2012, www.aspeneducation.com/article-entitlement.html; J. M. Twenge et al., "Egos Inflating Over Time: A Cross Temporal Meta-analysis of the Narcissistic Personality Inventory," *Journal of Personality* 76, no. 4 (2008): 875–902; L. Martin, "Twitter and YouTube: Unexpected Consequences of the Self-Esteem Movement?" PsychCentral.com, Accessed February 9, 2012, from http://pro.psychocentral.com/2011/twitter-and-youtube-unexpected-consequences-of-the-self-esteem-movement/00545.html; M. Wei, K. Yu-Hsin Liao, T. Ku, and P. Shaffer, "Attachment, Self Compassion, Empathy, and Subjective Well-Being among College Students and Community Adults," *Journal of Personality*, 79, no. 1(2011):191–221; B. J. Bushman, S. J. Moeller, and J. Crocker, "Sweets, Sex, or Self-Esteem? Comparing the Value of Self-Esteem Boosts with Other Pleasant Rewards," *Journal of Personality* (2011), DOI: 10.1111/j.1467-6494.2011.00712.

self-efficacy by making us feel that we cannot do anything to improve the situation.

Today, many self-help programs use elements of Seligman's principle of **learned optimism.** The basis for these programs is the idea that we can teach ourselves to be optimistic. By changing our self-talk, examining our reactions, and blocking negative thoughts, we can "unlearn" negative thought processes that have become habitual. Some programs practice positive affirmations with clients, teaching them the sometimes difficult task of acknowledging positive things about themselves. Often we are our own worst critics, and learning to be kinder to ourselves is difficult.

learned optimism Teaching oneself to think positively.

Personality

Your personality is the unique mix of characteristics that distinguish you from others. Heredity, environment, culture, and experience influence how each person develops. Personality determines how we react to the challenges of life, interpret our feelings, and resolve conflicts.

75%

of Americans are extroverted, as measured by the Myers–Briggs Type Indicator personality test.

Most recent schools of psychological theory promote the idea that we have the power to understand our behavior and to change it, thus molding our own personalities. Although this is more difficult if social environments are inhospitable, there may be opportunities for making positive changes. One way to examine personality is by looking at traits that are associated with psychological health. In general, the following personality traits are often related to psychological well-being:[11]

- **Extroversion**—the ability to adapt to a social situation and demonstrate assertiveness as well as power or interpersonal involvement
- **Agreeableness**—the ability to conform, be likable, and demonstrate friendly compliance and love
- **Openness to experience**—the willingness to demonstrate curiosity and independence (also referred to as inquiring intellect)
- **Emotional stability**—the ability to maintain emotional control
- **Conscientiousness**—the qualities of being dependable and demonstrating self-control, discipline, and a need to achieve
- **Resiliency**—the ability to adapt to change and stressful events in healthy and flexible ways

Life Span and Maturity

Although our temperaments are largely determined by genetics, as we age, we learn to control the volatile emotions of youth and channel our feelings in more acceptable ways. The college years mark a critical transition period as young adults move away from families and establish themselves as independent adults. This transition is easier for those who have successfully accomplished earlier developmental tasks such as learning how to solve problems, make and evaluate decisions, define and adhere to personal values, and establish both casual and intimate relationships. Graduating from college can also be another transition for many into adulthood and further independence. Anticipating an adjustment period and creating new patterns typically ensures an easier transition. Developing a schedule and accessing alumni resources and campus resources for new graduates can be helpful with adjusting and developing autonomy after graduation.[12] People who have not fulfilled these earlier tasks may find their lives interrupted by recurrent crises left over from earlier stages. For example, if they did not learn to trust others in childhood, they may have difficulty establishing intimate relationships as adults.

The Mind–Body Connection

Can negative emotions make us physically ill? Can positive emotions help us stay

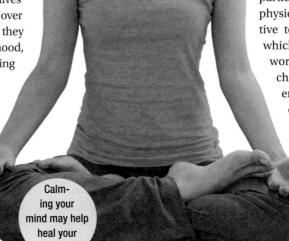

Calming your mind may help heal your body.

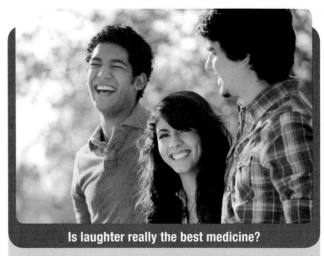

Is laughter really the best medicine?

Research is inconclusive regarding whether laughing actually improves your health, but we've all experienced the sense of well-being that a good laugh can bring. Regardless of whether it actually increases blood flow, boosts immune response, lowers blood sugar levels, or facilitates better sleep, there is no doubting that sharing laughter and fun with others can strengthen social ties and bring joy to your everyday life.

well? Researchers are exploring the interaction between emotions and health, especially in conditions of uncontrolled, persistent stress. In fact, the NCCAM and other organizations are investing more and more dollars in large research projects designed to explore the link between mind and body. At the core of the mind–body connection is **psychoneuroimmunology (PNI),** the study of the interactions of behavioral, neural, and endocrine functions and the functioning of the body's immune system.

psychoneuroimmunology (PNI)
The study of the interactions of behavioral, neural, and endocrine functions and the functioning of the body's immune system.

One area of study that appears to be particularly promising in enhancing physical health is *happiness*—a collective term for several positive states in which individuals actively embrace the world around them.[13] In examining the characteristics of happy people, scientists have found that this emotion can have a profound impact on the body. Happiness, or related mental states such as hopefulness, optimism, and contentment, appears to reduce the risk or limit the severity of cardiovascular disease, pulmonary disease, diabetes, hypertension, colds, and other infections. Laughter can promote

Using Positive Psychology to Enhance Your Happiness

Implement the following strategies to enhance happiness and employ a more positive outlook:

❯ **Check yourself.** Throughout the day, stop and evaluate what you're thinking. If you find that your thoughts are mainly negative, try to find a way to put a positive spin on them.

❯ **Use your sense of humor.** Give yourself permission to smile or laugh, especially during difficult times. Seek humor in everyday happenings. When you can laugh at life, you feel less stressed.

❯ **Follow a healthy lifestyle.** Exercise at least three times a week to positively affect mood and reduce stress. Follow a healthy diet to fuel your mind and body. And learn to manage stress.

❯ **Surround yourself with positive people.** Make sure those in your life are positive, supportive people you can depend on to give helpful advice and feedback. Negative people, those who believe they have no power over their lives, may increase your stress level and may make you doubt your ability to manage stress in healthy ways.

❯ **Practice positive self-talk.** Start by following one simple rule: Don't say anything to yourself that you wouldn't say to anyone else. Be gentle and encouraging with yourself. If a negative thought enters your mind, evaluate it rationally and respond with affirmations of what is good about yourself.

Source: Abridged from MayoClinic.com, "Positive Thinking: Reduce Stress by Eliminating Negative Self-talk," 2011, www.mayoclinic.com/health/positive-thinking/SR00009/NSECTIONGROUP=2.

increases in heart and respiration rates and can reduce levels of stress hormones in much the same way as light exercise can. For this reason, it has been promoted as a possible risk reducer for people with hypertension and other forms of cardiovascular disease.[14]

Subjective well-being is that uplifting feeling of inner peace or an overall "feel-good" state, which includes happiness. Subjective well-being is defined by three central components: satisfaction with present life, relative presence of positive emotions, and relative absence of negative emotions.[15] You do not have to be happy all the time to achieve overall subjective well-being. Everyone experiences disappointments, unhappiness, and times when life seems unfair. However, people with a high level of subjective well-being are typically resilient, are able to look on

subjective well-being An uplifting feeling of inner peace.

the positive side and get back on track fairly quickly, and are less likely to fall into despair over setbacks.

Scientists suggest that some people may be biologically predisposed to happiness. One study of 2,574 Americans showed that variants of a gene actually influenced how satisfied or dissatisfied people were with their lives and their overall levels of happiness. This marks an advance toward explaining why some people seem naturally happier than others. However, researchers are careful to point out that happiness is only partly influenced by genetics.[16] Other psychologists suggest that we can develop happiness by practicing positive psychological actions.[17] The **Skills for Behavior Change** box provides some suggestions for things you can do to incorporate positive psychology principles into your own life.

Strategies to Enhance Psychological Health

As we have seen, psychological health involves four dimensions. Attaining self-fulfillment is a lifelong, conscious process that involves enhancing each of these components. Strategies include building self-efficacy and self-esteem, understanding and controlling emotions, maintaining support networks, and learning to solve problems and make decisions. In addition to the advice in this chapter, see Chapter 3 for tips on managing stress and other tools for enhancing your psychological health.

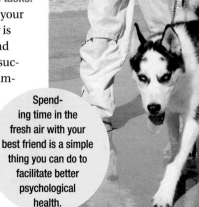

Spending time in the fresh air with your best friend is a simple thing you can do to facilitate better psychological health.

● **Develop a support system.** One of the best ways to promote self-esteem is through a support system of peers and others who share your values. Members of your support system can help you feel good about yourself and force you to take an honest look at your actions and choices. Keeping in contact with old friends and family members can provide a foundation of unconditional love that will help you through life's transitions.

● **Complete required tasks.** A good way to boost your sense of self-efficacy is to learn new skills and develop a history of success. Most college campuses provide study groups and learning centers that can help you manage time, develop study skills, and prepare for tests.

- **Form realistic expectations.** If you expect perfect grades, a steady stream of Saturday-night dates, and the perfect job, you may be setting yourself up for failure. Assess your current resources and the direction in which you are heading. Set small, incremental goals that you can actually meet.
- **Make time for you.** Taking time to enjoy yourself is another way to boost your self-esteem and psychological health. View a new activity as something to look forward to and an opportunity to have fun. Anticipate and focus on the fun things that you have to look forward to each day.
- **Maintain physical health.** Regular exercise fosters a sense of well-being. More and more research supports the role of exercise and good nutrition in improved mental health.
- **Examine problems and seek help when necessary.** Knowing when to seek help from friends, family, or professionals is an important factor in boosting self-esteem. Sometimes you can handle life's problems alone; at other times, you need assistance.
- **Get adequate sleep.** Getting enough sleep on a daily basis is a key factor in physical and psychological health. Not only do our bodies need to rest to conserve energy for daily activities, but we also need to restore supplies of many of the neurotransmitters that we use up during our waking hours. (For more information on the importance of sleep, see Focus On: Improving Your Sleep beginning on page 98.)

"Why Should I Care?"

Mental health problems can affect people of any age and have a huge impact on the kind of life you lead—including your success in academics, career, and relationships, as well as your general ability to function and enjoy life. Also, mental health concerns are so prevalent among college students that it is possible your roommate or a friend could have a problem and may need your help and support.

cal relatives with a mental illness; malnutrition or exposure to viruses while in the womb; stressful life situations, such as financial problems, a loved one's death, or a divorce; chronic medical conditions, such as cancer; combat; taking psychoactive drugs during adolescence; childhood abuse or neglect; and lack of friendships or healthy relationships.[19] As with physical disease, mental illnesses can range from mild to severe and can exact a heavy toll on quality of life, both for people with the illnesses and those who come in contact with them.

Mental disorders are common in the United States and worldwide. The basis for diagnosing mental disorders in the United States is the *Diagnostic and Statistical Manual of Mental Disorders,* Fourth Edition, Text Revision (*DSM-IV-TR*). An estimated 26.2 percent of Americans aged 18 and older—about 1 in 4 adults—suffer from a diagnosable mental disorder in a given year, and nearly half of them have more than one mental illness at the same time.[20] This translates to 57.7 million people. Out of these, about 6 percent, or 1 in 17, suffer from a serious mental illness requiring close monitoring, residential care in many instances, and medication. Mental disorders are the leading cause of disability in the United States and Canada for people aged 15 to 44.[21]

57.7 million

U.S. adults suffer from a diagnosable mental disorder in any given year.

When Psychological Health Deteriorates

Sometimes circumstances overwhelm us to such a degree that we need help to get back on track to healthful living. Stress, abusive relationships, anxiety, loneliness, financial upheavals, and other traumatic events can derail our coping resources. Chemical imbalances, drug interactions, trauma, neurological disruptions, and other physical problems also may contribute to mental health problems.

Mental illnesses are disorders that disrupt thinking, feeling, moods, and behaviors, and cause varying degrees of impaired functioning in daily living. They are believed to be caused by a variety of biochemical, genetic, and environmental factors.[18] Risk factors for developing or triggering mental illness include the following: having other biologi-

Mental Health Threats to College Students

Mental health problems are common among college students and they appear to be increasing in number and severity.[22] The most recent National College Health Assessment survey found that approximately 1 in 3 undergraduates reported "feeling so depressed it was difficult to function" at least once in the past year. Just over 6 percent of students reported "seriously considering attempting suicide" in the past year.[23] In another study based on a sample of over 3,000 students, approximately 41 percent of students met the criteria for moderate to severe depression.[24] Although these data may appear alarming, it is important to note that increases in help-seeking behavior rather than actual increases in overall prevalence of disorders may be contributing to these trends.

mental illnesses Disorders that disrupt thinking, feeling, moods, and behaviors, and that impair daily functioning.

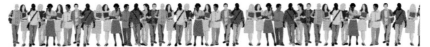

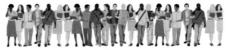

Felt overwhelmed by all they needed to do 86.3%

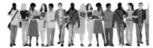

Felt things were hopeless 45.1%

Felt so depressed that it was difficult to function 31.1%

Seriously considered suicide 6.4%

Intentionally injured themselves 5.2%

 = 2%

Attempted suicide 1.1%

FIGURE 2.4 **Mental Health Concerns of American College Students, Past 12 Months**
Source: Data from American College Health Association, *American College Health Association–National College Health Assessment II (ACHA-NCHA II): Reference Group Data Report Spring 2011* (Baltimore: American College Health Association, 2012).

---

chronic mood disorder Experience of persistent emotional states, such as sadness, despair, and hopelessness.

major depression Severe depressive disorder with physical effects such as sleep disturbance and exhaustion, and mental effects such as the inability to concentrate; also called *clinical depression*.

Although there are many types of mental illnesses, we will focus here on those disorders that are most common among college students: mood disorders, anxiety disorders, personality disorders, and schizophrenia (see the **Health Headlines** box on page 39 for information on another growing mental health concern among young adults, attention-deficit/hyperactivity disorder). For information about other disorders, consult the websites listed at the end of this chapter or ask your instructor for local resources. Figure 2.4 shows the mental health concerns of American college students.

Mood Disorders

Chronic mood disorders are disorders that affect how you feel, such as persistent sadness or feelings of euphoria. They include major depression, dysthymic disorder, bipolar disorder, and seasonal affective disorder. In any given year, approximately 10 percent of Americans aged 18 or older suffer from a mood disorder.[25]

Major Depression

Sometimes life throws us down the proverbial stairs. We experience loss, pain, disappointment, or frustration, and we can be left feeling beaten and bruised. How do we know if these emotions are really signs of a **major depression**? Major or clinical depression is not the same as having a bad day or feeling down after a negative experience. It is also not something that can be willed or wished away, or ignored for the sake of "growing a thicker skin." Major depression is the most common mood disorder, affecting approximately 14.8 million American adults, or about 7 percent of the U.S. population.[26] These numbers likely do not reflect all those who suffer from depression because many are misdiagnosed or underdiagnosed.

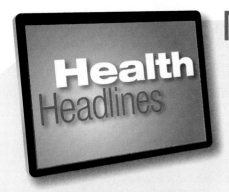

WHEN ADULTS HAVE ADHD

Attention-deficit/hyperactivity disorder (ADHD) is a common neurobehavioral condition that affects 5 to 8 percent of school-aged children. In as many as 60 percent of cases, symptoms persist into adulthood. In any given year, 4.1 percent of adults are identified as having ADHD.

People with ADHD are hyperactive or distracted most of the time. Even when they try to concentrate, they find it hard to pay attention. They have a hard time organizing things, listening to instructions, remembering details, and controlling their behavior. As a result, people with ADHD often have problems getting along with other people.

ADULT ADHD MYTHS AND FACTS

Myth: ADHD is just a lack of willpower. Persons with ADHD focus well on things that interest them; they could focus on any other tasks if they really wanted to.
Fact: ADHD looks very much like a willpower issue, but it isn't. It's essentially a chemical problem in the management systems of the brain.
Myth: Everybody has the symptoms of ADHD, and anyone with adequate intelligence can overcome these difficulties.
Fact: ADHD affects persons of all levels of intelligence. Although everyone sometimes is prone to distraction or impulsivity, only those with chronic impairments from ADHD symptoms warrant an ADHD diagnosis.
Myth: Someone can't have ADHD and also have depression, anxiety, or other psychiatric problems.

Fact: A person with ADHD is six times more likely to have another psychiatric or learning disorder. Attention-deficit/hyperactivity disorder usually overlaps with other disorders.
Myth: Unless you have been diagnosed with ADHD as a child, you can't have it as an adult.
Fact: Many adults struggle all their lives with unrecognized ADHD. They haven't received help because they assumed that their chronic difficulties, like depression or anxiety, were caused by other impairments that did not respond to treatment.

EFFECTS OF ADULT ADHD

Left untreated, ADHD can disrupt everything from careers to relationships and financial stability. Although most of us sometimes have challenges in these areas, the persistent chaos and disorganization of ADHD can make managing the problems worse and worse. Some key areas of disruption might include:

✱ **Health.** Impulsivity and trouble with organization can lead to problems with health, such as compulsive eating, alcohol or drug abuse, or forgetting to take medication for a chronic condition.
✱ **Work and finances.** Difficulty concentrating, completing tasks, listening, and relating to others can lead to trouble at work. Managing finances also may be a concern. You may find yourself struggling to pay bills, losing paperwork, missing deadlines, or spending impulsively, resulting in debt.
✱ **Relationships.** You might wonder why loved ones constantly nag you to tidy up, get organized, and take care of business. Or if your loved one has ADHD, you might be hurt that he or she doesn't seem to listen to you, blurts out hurtful things, and leaves you responsible for the bulk of organizing and planning.

GET EDUCATED ABOUT ADHD

If you suspect that you or someone close to you has ADHD, learn as much as you can about adult ADHD and treatment options. Children and Adults with

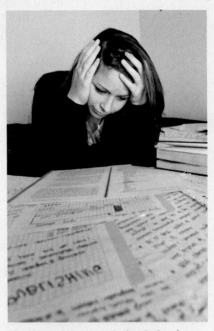

Disorder and chaos can be headaches for us all, but ADHD sufferers may find them insurmountable obstacles.

Attention-Deficit Hyperactivity Disorder (CHADD) is a good source of information and support (www.chadd.org). Adult ADHD can be a challenge to diagnose, as there is no simple test for it and it often occurs concurrently with other conditions, such as depression or anxiety disorders. To ensure that you receive the best treatment, secure a diagnosis and treatment plan from a qualified professional with experience in ADHD.

Sources: Centers for Disease Control and Prevention, "Attention-Deficit Hyperactivity Disorder," updated December 2011, www.cdc.gov/ncbddd/adhd; Helpguide.org, "Adult ADD/ADHD: Signs, Symptoms, Effects, and Treatment," updated December 2011, www.helpguide.org/mental/adhd_add_adult_symptoms.htm; National Institute of Mental Health, "The Numbers Count," 2010, www.nimh.nih.gov/health/publications/the-numbers-count-mental-disorders-in-america/index.shtml; H. R. Searight, J. M. Burke, and F. Rottnek, "Adult ADHD: Evaluation and Treatment in Family Medicine," *American Family Physician* 62, no. 9 (2000): 2091–92; T. Brown, *Attention Deficit Disorder: The Unfocused Mind in Children and Adults* (New Haven, CT: Yale University Press, 2005).

dysthymic disorder (dysthymia)
Type of depression that is milder and harder to recognize than major depression; chronic; and often characterized by fatigue, pessimism, or a short temper.

bipolar disorder Form of mood disorder characterized by alternating mania and depression; also called *manic depression.*

Major depression is characterized by a combination of symptoms that interfere with work, study, sleep, appetite, relationships, and enjoyment of life. Symptoms can last for weeks, months, or years and vary in intensity.[27] Sadness and despair are the main symptoms of depression. Other common signs include:

- Sadness and despair
- Loss of motivation or interest in pleasurable activities
- Preoccupation with failures and inadequacies; concern over what others are thinking
- Difficulty concentrating; indecisiveness; memory lapses
- Loss of sex drive or interest in close interactions with others
- Fatigue and loss of energy; slow reactions
- Sleeping too much or too little; insomnia
- Feeling agitated, worthless, or hopeless
- Withdrawal from friends and family
- Diminished or increased appetite
- Significant weight loss or weight gain
- Recurring thoughts that life isn't worth living; thoughts of death or suicide

The **Health in a Diverse World** box on page 41 discusses in the differences in depression prevalence across different ages, genders, and ethnicities.

Depression in College Students

Mental health problems, particularly depression, have gained increased recognition as major obstacles to success and healthy adjustment. Students who have weak communication skills, who find that college isn't what they expected, or who find that people they've known seem different often have difficulties. Stressors such as anxiety over relationships, pressure to get good grades and win social acceptance, abuse of alcohol and other drugs, poor diet, and lack of sleep can create a toxic cocktail that can overwhelm even the most resilient students. In its most recent survey, the American College Health Association found that the number of students who reported "having been diagnosed with depression" was approximately 10 percent.[28]

Being far from home without the security of family and friends can exacerbate problems. International students are particularly vulnerable to depression and other mental health concerns.

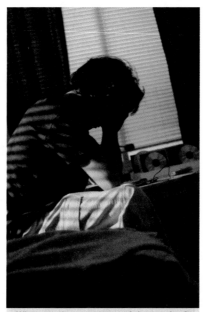

What are the symptoms of depression? There is more to depression than simply feeling blue. When a person is clinically depressed, he or she finds it difficult to function, sometimes struggling just to get out of bed in the morning or to follow a conversation.

Most campuses have counseling centers and other services available; however, many students do not use them because of persistent stigma about seeing a counselor. The **Student Health Today** box on page 42 describes some of the strategies colleges are adopting to address mental health concerns.

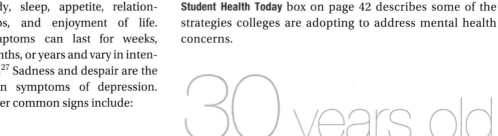

30 years old
is the median age of onset for mood disorders.

Dysthymic Disorder

Many people suffer from **dysthymic disorder (dysthymia),** a less severe syndrome of chronic mild depression. Dysthymia can be harder to recognize than major depression. Dysthymic individuals may appear to function all right, but they may lack energy or may fatigue easily; be short-tempered, overly pessimistic, and ornery; or just not feel quite up to par without having any significant, overt symptoms. People with dysthymia may cycle into major depression over time. For a diagnosis, symptoms must persist for at least 2 years in adults (1 year in children). This disorder affects approximately 1.5 percent of the U.S. population aged 18 and older in a given year, or about 3.3 million American adults.[29]

Bipolar Disorder

People with **bipolar disorder** (also called *manic depression*) often have severe mood swings, ranging from extreme highs (mania) to extreme lows (depression). Sometimes these swings are dramatic and rapid; other times they are slow and gradual. When in the manic phase, people may be overactive, talkative, and have tons of energy; in the depressed phase, they may experience some or all of the symptoms of major depression.

Although the cause of bipolar disorder is unknown, biological, genetic, and environmental factors, such as drug abuse and stressful or psychologically traumatic events, seem to be involved in triggering episodes. Once diagnosed, persons with bipolar disorder have several counseling and pharmaceutical options, and most will be able to live a healthy, functional life while being treated. Bipolar disorder affects 5.7 million U.S. adults, representing 2.6 percent of the population.[30]

DEPRESSION ACROSS GENDER, AGE, AND ETHNICITY

Although depression may affect persons of every age, gender, and ethnicity, it does not always manifest itself in the same way across all populations.

DEPRESSION AND GENDER

Women are almost twice as likely as men to experience depression. Hormonal changes may be one factor. Women also face various stressors related to multiple responsibilities—work, child rearing, single parenthood, household work, and caring for elderly parents— at rates that are higher than those of men. Researchers have observed gender differences in coping strategies (responses to certain events or stimuli) and have proposed that some women's strategies make them more vulnerable to depression. Typically, men try to distract themselves from a depressed mood, whereas women focus on it. If focusing obsessively on negative feelings intensifies these feelings, women who do this may predispose themselves to depression.

Depression in men is often masked by alcohol or drug abuse, or by the socially acceptable habit of working excessively long hours. Typically, depressed men present not as hopeless and helpless, but as irritable, angry, and discouraged—often personifying a "tough guy" image. Men are less likely to admit they are depressed, and doctors are less likely to suspect it, based on what men report during doctor's visits.

Depression can affect men's physical health differently than it can women's health. Although depression is associated with an increased risk of coronary heart disease in both men and women, it is also associated with a higher risk of death by heart disease in men. Men are also more likely to act on suicidal feelings, and they are usually more successful at suicide; suicide rates among depressed men are four times those among depressed women.

Regardless of gender, age or ethnicity, none of us is immune to depression.

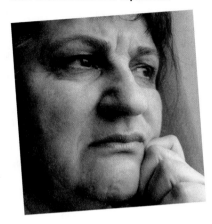

DEPRESSION AND AGE

Today, depression in children is increasingly reported, with 1 in 10 children between ages 6 and 12 experiencing persistent feelings of sadness, the hallmark of depression. Depressed children may pretend to be sick, refuse to go to school or have a sudden drop in school performance, sleep excessively, engage in self-mutilation, abuse drugs or alcohol, feel misunderstood, or attempt suicide.

Before adolescence, girls and boys experience depression at about the same rate, but by adolescence and young adulthood, girls experience depression more than boys do. This may be due to biological and hormonal changes; girls' struggles with self-esteem and perceptions of success and approval; and an increase in girls' exposure to traumas that may contribute to depression, such as childhood sexual abuse.

As adults reach their middle and older years, most are emotionally stable and lead active and satisfying lives. However, when depression does occur, it is often undiagnosed or untreated, particularly in people in lower income groups or who lack access to community resources or

medications. Depression is considered the most common mental disorder of people aged 65 and older. Older adults may be less likely to discuss feelings of sadness, loss, helplessness, or other symptoms, or they may attribute their depression to aging.

DEPRESSION AND RACE/ ETHNICITY

Rates of depression among Latino, African American, and Asian American/ Pacific Islander populations are difficult to determine, as members of these groups may have difficulty accessing mental health services because of economic barriers, social and cultural differences, language barriers, and lack of culturally competent providers. Data from the 2008 U.S. National Health and Wellness Survey indicated that when whites report depression symptoms to a health care provider, they are much more likely to be officially diagnosed with depression. Seventy-six percent of whites with reported depressive symptoms were officially diagnosed versus 58.7 percent of African Americans, 62.7 percent of Latinos, and 47.4 percent of Asian Americans.

Sources: National Institute of Mental Health (NIMH), *Women and Depression: Discovering Hope,* revised 2011, NIH Publication no. 09-4779. Available from www.nimh.nih.gov/health/ publications/women-and-depression-discovering-hope/index.shtml; NIMH, "Depression and Men," 2009, www.nimh.nih.gov/health/topics/depression/ men-and-depression/depression-in-men.shtml; American Psychiatric Association (APA), Healthy Minds. Healthy Lives. "Children," 2010, www .healthyminds.org/More-Info-For/Children.aspx; APA, Healthy Minds. Healthy Lives. "Seniors," 2011, www.healthyminds.org/More-Info-For/ Seniors.aspx; H. Kannan, S. Bolge, and S. Wagner, "Depression: Ethnic Differences in Prevalence, Diagnosis, and Symptoms" (Princeton, NJ: Consumer Health Sciences, 2009), Poster presented at the International Society of Pharmacoeconomics and Outcomes Research (ISPOR) 14th Annual International Meeting, May 2009, www .chsinternational.com/Resources/2009_05_20_ ISPOR_Poster_no3_Depression-Ethnicity.pdf.

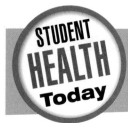

Mental Health Problems on Campus: Universities Respond

According to the latest National College Health Assessment Survey, nearly 33 percent of female students and 27 percent of male students throughout the country reported that they had felt too depressed to function at least once during the past year. At the same time, 49 percent of college women and 38 percent of college men felt hopeless one or more times, and another 6 percent of college women and 6 percent of college men had seriously considered suicide. Universities are enacting a range of policies to help these students, including the following:

- Student leave is a growing trend on campuses. For example, New York University, Texas A&M, and Cornell University have established various forms of a mandatory 6-month or 1-year leave of absence for students who seem to be at highest risk for mental health problems.
- Some institutions, such as the University of Illinois at Urbana-Champaign, mandate counseling for students who are suicidal, requiring a minimum of four therapy sessions following a suicide attempt.

- Increasing numbers of institutions offer time-management workshops, massage and stress management sessions during examinations, and workshops on relationships, coping with loss and grief, and other challenges.
- Classes on stress management, coping, relaxation, meditation, yoga, and other mental health strategies are increasingly common, either as electives or as part of a professional curriculum.
- Most campus health services now include counseling centers with 24/7 access. Students are encouraged to use them, and increased advertising in new-student orientation sessions lets students know what kind of help is available.
- Many universities offer extensive first-year orientations at the beginning of each academic year. Students engage in group activities, such as camping trips and special seminars, to get to know one another in social settings. Professors, upperclassmen, and others offer special assistance and lead discussion groups to help incom-

First-year orientation programs are one strategy universities have adopted to help students transition into college life and to address potential mental health concerns.

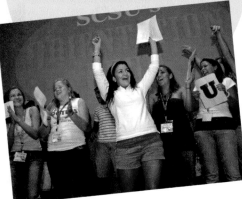

ing students adjust to life away from home and to foster awareness of the wide range of resources available when students can't handle multiple pressures.

Source: J. Feirman, "The New College Drop-Out," *Psychology Today* 38, no. 3 (2005): 38–39; American College Health Association, *American College Health Association–National College Health Assessment II (ACHA–NCHA II): Reference Group Data Spring 2011* (Baltimore: American College Health Association, 2012).

Seasonal Affective Disorder

Another form of depression, **seasonal affective disorder (SAD),** strikes during the winter months and is associated with reduced exposure to sunlight. People with SAD suffer from irritability, apathy, carbohydrate craving and weight gain, increased sleep time, and general sadness. Several factors are implicated in SAD development, including disruption in the body's circadian rhythms and changes in levels of the hormone melatonin and the brain chemical serotonin.[31]

The most beneficial treatment for SAD is light therapy, which exposes patients to lamps that simulate sunlight. Eighty percent of patients experience relief from their symptoms within 4 days. Other treatments for SAD include diet change (such as eating more complex carbohydrates), increased exercise, stress-management techniques, sleep

seasonal affective disorder (SAD)
Type of depression that occurs in the winter months, when sunlight levels are low.

restriction (limiting the number of hours slept in a 24-hour period), psychotherapy, and prescription medications.

What Causes Mood Disorders?

Mood disorders are caused by the interaction between multiple factors, including biological differences, hormones, inherited traits, life events, and early childhood trauma.[32] The biology of mood disorders is related to individual levels of brain chemicals called *neurotransmitters*. Several types of depression, including bipolar disorder, appear to have a genetic component. Depression can also be triggered by a serious loss, difficult relationships, financial problems, and pressure to succeed. Early childhood trauma, such as loss of a parent, may cause permanent changes in the brain, making one more prone to depression. Changes in the body's physical health can be accompanied by mental changes, particularly depression. Stroke, heart attack, cancer, Parkinson's disease, chronic pain, type 2 diabetes, certain medications, alcohol, hormonal disorders, and a wide range of other afflictions can cause a person to become depressed, frustrated, or angry. When this happens, recovery is often more difficult. A person who feels exhausted and defeated may lack the will to fight illness and do what is necessary to optimize recovery.

Anxiety Disorders

Anxiety disorders include generalized anxiety disorder, panic disorders, phobic disorders, obsessive-compulsive disorder, and post-traumatic stress disorder. They are characterized by persistent feelings of threat and worry. Consider John Madden, former head coach of the Oakland Raiders, who outfitted his own bus and, for many years, drove every weekend across the country to serve as commentator for NFL games. Why this exhausting driving schedule? Madden is terrified of getting on a plane.

Anxiety disorders are the number one mental health problem in the United States, affecting more than 18 percent of all adults.[33] Anxiety is also a leading mental health problem among adolescents, affecting 25.1 percent of Americans aged 13 to 18. Among U.S. undergraduates, approximately 11 percent report being diagnosed with or treated for anxiety in the past year.[34]

Did you Know?

About 1 in 3 people with panic disorder develops agoraphobia, a condition in which the person becomes afraid of being in any place or situation—such as a crowd or a wide-open space—where escape might be difficult in the event of a panic attack.

Costs associated with an overly anxious U.S. populace are growing rapidly; conservative estimates cite nearly $50 billion a year spent in medical costs and workplace losses.[35]

Generalized Anxiety Disorder

One common form of anxiety disorder, **generalized anxiety disorder (GAD),** is severe enough to interfere significantly with daily life. Generally, the person with GAD is a consummate worrier who develops a debilitating level of anxiety. To be diagnosed with GAD, one must exhibit at least three of the following symptoms for more days than not during a 6-month period: restlessness or feeling keyed up or on edge; being easily fatigued; difficulty concentrating or mind going blank; irritability; muscle tension; sleep disturbances.[36] Generalized anxiety disorder often runs in families, but it is readily treatable.

Panic Disorders

Panic disorders are characterized by the occurrence of **panic attacks,** an acute anxiety reaction that brings on an intense physical reaction. You may dismiss the feelings as the jitters from too much stress, or the reaction may be so severe that you fear you will have a heart attack and die. Approximately 4.7 percent of Americans aged 18 and older experience panic attacks, usually in early adulthood.[37] Panic attacks and disorders are increasing in incidence, particularly among young women.

Although highly treatable, panic attacks may become debilitating and destructive, particularly if they happen often and cause the person to avoid going out in public or interacting with others. A panic attack typically starts abruptly, peaks within 10 minutes, lasts about 30 minutes, and leaves the person tired and drained.[38] Symptoms include increased respiration, chills, hot flashes, shortness of breath, stomach cramps, chest pain, difficulty swallowing, and a sense of doom or impending death.

Although researchers aren't sure what causes panic attacks, heredity, stress, and certain biochemical factors may play a role. Your chances of having a panic attack increase if a close relative has them. Some researchers believe that people who suffer panic attacks are experiencing an overreactive fight-or-flight physical response. (See **Chapter 3.**)

Phobic Disorders

Phobias, or phobic disorders, involve a persistent and irrational fear of a specific object, activity, or situation, often out of proportion to the circumstances. Phobias result in a compelling

anxiety disorders Mental illness characterized by persistent feelings of threat and worry in coping with everyday problems.

generalized anxiety disorder (GAD) A constant sense of worry that may cause restlessness, difficulty in concentrating, tension, and other symptoms.

panic attack Severe anxiety reaction in which a particular situation, often for unknown reasons, causes terror.

phobia Deep and persistent fear of a specific object, activity, or situation that results in a compelling desire to avoid the source of the fear.

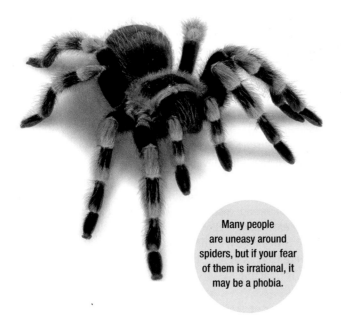

Many people are uneasy around spiders, but if your fear of them is irrational, it may be a phobia.

Post-Traumatic Stress Disorder

People who have served in combat or have experienced or witnessed a natural disaster, serious accident, violent assault, terrorist incident, or other traumatic life event may develop **post-traumatic stress disorder (PTSD).** The lifetime risk of PTSD is nearly 7 percent in the United States, with rates as high as 30 percent in strife-torn regions of the world. Combat soldiers have high rates of PTSD, ranging from 17 percent of those who fought in Iraq and Afghanistan to more than 30 percent of those who returned from Vietnam.[42]

Symptoms of PTSD include:

- Dissociation, or perceived detachment of the mind from the emotional state or even the body
- Intrusive recollections of the traumatic event, such as flashbacks, nightmares, and recurrent thoughts or images
- Acute anxiety or nervousness, in which the person is hyperaroused, may cry easily, or experiences mood swings
- Insomnia and difficulty concentrating
- Intense physiological reactions, such as shaking or nausea, when something reminds the person of the traumatic event

Although these symptoms may be appropriate as initial responses to traumatic events, PTSD may be diagnosed if a person experiences them for at least 1 month following the traumatic event. In some cases, symptoms don't appear until months or even years later.

What Causes Anxiety Disorders?

Because anxiety disorders vary in complexity and degree, scientists have yet to find clear reasons why one person develops them and another doesn't. The following factors are often cited as possible causes:[43]

- **Biology.** Some scientists trace the origin of anxiety to the brain and its functioning. Using sophisticated positron-emission tomography (PET) scans, scientists can analyze areas of the brain that react during anxiety-producing events. Families appear to display similar brain and physiological reactivity, so we may inherit tendencies toward anxiety disorders.
- **Environment.** Anxiety can be a learned response. Although genetic tendencies may exist, experiencing a repeated pattern of reaction to certain situations programs the brain to respond in a certain way. For example, if your mother screamed whenever a large spider crept into view or if other anxiety-raising events occurred frequently, you might be predisposed to react with anxiety to similar events later in life.
- **Social and cultural roles.** Cultural and social roles also may be a factor in risks for anxiety. Because men and women are taught to assume different roles (such as man as protector, woman as victim), women may find it more acceptable to scream, tremble, or otherwise express extreme anxiety. Men, in contrast, may have learned to repress anxious feelings rather than act on them.

desire to avoid the source of the fear. About 9 percent of American adults suffer from specific phobias, such as fear of spiders, snakes, or public speaking.[39]

Another 15 million of American adults suffer from **social phobia,** also called *social anxiety disorder*.[40] Social phobia is an anxiety disorder characterized by the persistent fear and avoidance of social situations. Essentially, the person dreads these situations for fear of being humiliated, embarrassed, or even looked at. These disorders vary in scope. Some cause difficulty only in specific situations, such as getting up in front of the class to give a report. In extreme cases, a person avoids all contact with others.

Obsessive-Compulsive Disorder

People who feel compelled to perform rituals over and over again; who are fearful of dirt or contamination; who have an unnatural concern about order, symmetry, and exactness; or who have persistent intrusive thoughts that they can't shake may be suffering from **obsessive-compulsive disorder (OCD).** Approximately 2 million Americans aged 18 and over (1 percent) have OCD.[41] Not to be confused with being a perfectionist, a person with OCD often knows the behaviors are irrational, yet is powerless to stop them. According to the *DSM-IV-TR,* for a person to be diagnosed with OCD, the obsessions must consume more than 1 hour per day and interfere with normal social or life activities. Although the exact cause is unknown, genetics, biological abnormalities, learned behaviors, and environmental factors have all been considered. Obsessive-compulsive disorder usually begins in adolescence or early adulthood; the median age of onset is 19.

social phobia Phobia characterized by fear and avoidance of social situations; also called *social anxiety disorder.*

obsessive-compulsive disorder (OCD) Form of anxiety disorder characterized by recurrent, unwanted thoughts and repetitive behaviors.

post-traumatic stress disorder (PTSD) Collection of symptoms that may occur as a delayed response to a traumatic event or series of events.

Personality Disorders

According to the *DSM-IV-TR,* a **personality disorder** is an "enduring pattern of inner experience and behavior that deviates markedly from the expectation of the individual's culture and is pervasive and inflexible."[44] It is estimated that 10 percent of adults in the United States have some form of personality disorder as defined by the *DSM-IV-TR.*[45] People who live, work, or are in relationships with individuals suffering from personality disorders often find interactions with them to be challenging and destructive.

One common type of personality disorder is *paranoid personality disorder,* which involves pervasive, unfounded suspicion and mistrust of other people, irrational jealousy, and secretiveness. Persons with this illness have delusions of being persecuted by everyone, from family members and loved ones to the government.

Narcissistic personality disorders involve an exaggerated sense of self-importance and self-absorption. Persons with narcissistic personalities are preoccupied with fantasies of how wonderful they are. Typically, they are overly needy and demanding and believe that they are "entitled" to nothing but the best.

Borderline personality disorder (BPD) is characterized by impulsiveness and risky behaviors such as gambling sprees, unsafe sex, use of illicit drugs, and daredevil driving.[46] Sufferers have unstable moods and can experience erratic mood swings. Other characteristics include reality distortion and the tendency to see things in only black-and-white terms. In addition, 70 to 80 percent of persons diagnosed with BPD engage in **self-injury,** in which they deliberately mutilate or harm their own body—such as by cutting or burning—as a way to cope with their emotions.[47] For more about self-injury, see the **Student Health Today** box on page 46.

Schizophrenia

Perhaps the most frightening psychological disorder is **schizophrenia,** which affects about 1 percent of the U.S. population.[48] Schizophrenia is characterized by alterations of the senses (including auditory and visual hallucinations); the inability to sort and process incoming stimuli and make appropriate responses; an altered sense of self; and radical changes in emotions, movements, and behaviors. Typical symptoms of schizophrenia include fluctuating courses of delusional behavior, hallucinations, incoherent and rambling speech, inability to think logically, erratic movement, odd gesturing, and difficulty with normal activities of daily living.[49] Such individuals are often regarded as odd or dangerous, and viewed that way, they have difficulties in social interactions and may withdraw.

For decades, scientists believed that schizophrenia was an environmentally provoked form of madness. They blamed abnormal family interactions or early childhood traumas.

In the mid-1980s, magnetic resonance imaging (MRI) and PET scans began allowing scientists to study brain function more closely; based on that knowledge, schizophrenia was found to be a biological disease of the brain. The brain damage occurs early in life, possibly as early as the second trimester of fetal development. Fetal exposure to toxic substances, infections, or medications has been studied as a possible risk, and hereditary links are being explored. Symptoms usually appear in men in their late teens and twenties and in women in their late twenties and early thirties.[50]

Even though environmental theories of the causes of schizophrenia have been discarded in favor of biological ones, a stigma remains attached to the disease. Families of people with schizophrenia frequently experience anger and guilt. They often need information, family counseling, and advice on how to meet the schizophrenic person's needs for shelter, medical care, vocational training, and social interaction.

At present, schizophrenia is treatable but not curable. Treatments usually include some combination of hospitalization, medication, and psychotherapy. Supportive psychotherapy, as opposed to psychoanalysis, can help the patient acquire skills for living in society. With proper medication, public understanding, support of loved ones, and access to therapy, many schizophrenics lead normal lives. Without these forms of assistance and treatment, they may have great difficulty.

personality disorder Mental disorder characterized by inflexible patterns of thought and beliefs that lead to socially distressing behavior.

self-injury Intentionally causing injury to one's own body in an attempt to cope with overwhelming negative emotions; also called *self-mutilation, self-harm,* or *nonsuicidal self-injury* (NSSI).

schizophrenia Mental illness with biological origins characterized by irrational behavior, severe alterations of the senses, and often an inability to function in society.

| Patient with schizophrenia off all medication | Patient with schizophrenia on medication |

These brain images reveal a significant reduction in brain activity in a person with untreated schizophrenia. Yellow and red identify areas of greatest activity, and blue signifies reduced activity.

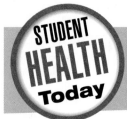

STUDENT HEALTH Today

CUTTING THROUGH THE PAIN

When some people are unable to deal with the pain, pressure, or stress they experience in everyday life, they may resort to self-harm in an effort to cope. *Self-injury,* also termed *self-mutilation, self-harm,* or *nonsuicidal self-injury* (NSSI), is the act of deliberately harming one's body in an attempt to cope with overwhelming negative emotions. Self-injury is an attempt at coping; it is not an attempt at suicide.

The most common method of self-harm is cutting (with razors, glass, knives, or other sharp objects). Other methods include burning, bruising, excessive nail biting, breaking bones, pulling out hair, and embedding sharp objects under the skin. Seventy-five percent of those who harm themselves do so in more than one way.

Researchers estimate that between 2 and 8 million Americans have engaged in self-harm at some point in their lives, and the prevalence of NSSI in college students is reported between 17 and 38 percent. Many people who harm themselves suffer from larger mental health conditions and have experienced sexual, physical, or emotional abuse as children or adults. Self-harm is also commonly associated with mental illnesses such as borderline personality disorder, depression, anxiety disorders, substance abuse disorders, post-traumatic stress disorder, and eating disorders.

Signs of self-injury include multiple scars, current cuts and abrasions, and implausible explanations for wounds and ongoing injuries. A self-injurer may attempt to conceal scars and injuries by wearing long sleeves and pants. Other symptoms can include difficulty handling anger, social withdrawal, sensitivity to rejection, or body alienation. If you or someone you know is engaging in self-injury, seek professional help. Treatment is challenging; not only must the self-injurious behavior be stopped, but the sufferer must also learn to recognize and manage the feelings that triggered the behavior.

If you are a recovering cutter, some of the following steps may be part of your treatment:

1. Start by being aware of feelings and situations that trigger your urge to cut.
2. Identify a plan of what you can do instead of cutting when you feel the urge.
3. Create a list of alternatives, including:

✱ Things that might distract you
✱ Things that might soothe and calm you
✱ Things that might help you express the pain and deep emotion
✱ Things that might help release physical tension and distress
✱ Things that might help you feel supported and connected
✱ Things that might substitute for the cutting sensation

For more information, try these resources: American Self-Harm Information Clearinghouse, www.selfinjury.org; S.A.F.E. Alternatives, www.selfinjury.com; and Self-Injury Support, www.sisupport.org.

Previously, self-injury was thought to be more common in females, but recent research indicates that rates are generally the same for men and women.

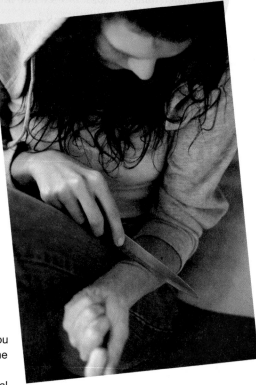

Sources: J. Bennett, "Why She Cuts," *Newsweek* Web Exclusive, December 29, 2008, www .newsweek.com/id/177135; M. J. Prinstein, "Introduction to the Special Section on Suicide and Nonsuicidal Self-Injury: A Review of Unique Challenges and Important Directions for Self-Injury Science," *Journal of Consulting and Clinical Psychology* 76, no. 1 (2008): 1–8; Mayo Clinic Staff, MayoClinic.com, "Self-Injury/ Cutting," August 2010, www.mayoclinic.com/ health/self-injury/DS00775.

Suicide: Giving Up on Life

Each year there are more than 34,000 reported suicides in the United States.[51] Experts estimate that there may actually be closer to 100,000 cases; the discrepancy is due to the difficulty in determining the cause of many suspicious deaths.

More lives are lost to suicide than to any other cause except cancer and cardiovascular disease. It is the third leading cause of death for 15- to 24-year-olds and the fifth leading cause of death for 5- to 14-year-olds.[52]

College students are more likely than the general population to attempt suicide; it is the second leading cause of death

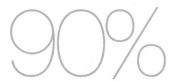

90%

of people who kill themselves have a diagnosable mental disorder, most commonly a depressive disorder or a substance abuse disorder.

on college campuses. The pressures, disappointments, challenges, and changes of the college environment are believed to be partially responsible for the emotional turmoil that can lead a young person to contemplate suicide. However, young adults who do not attend college but who are searching for direction in careers, relationships, and other areas are also at risk. Risk factors include a family history of suicide, previous suicide attempts, excessive drug and alcohol use, prolonged depression, financial difficulties, serious illness in oneself or a loved one, and loss of a loved one through death or rejection.

Recent studies indicate that suicide is the seventh leading cause of death for men and the fifteenth leading cause of death for women.[53] Whether they are more likely to attempt suicide or are more often successful, nearly four times as many men die by suicide than women. Firearms, suffocation, and poison are the most common methods of suicide. Men are almost twice as likely as women to commit suicide with firearms, whereas women are almost three times as likely as men to commit suicide by poisoning.[54]

Warning Signs of Suicide

In most cases, suicide does not occur unpredictably. In fact, 75 to 80 percent of people who commit suicide give an indication of their intentions, though the warnings are not always recognized.[55] Anyone who expresses a desire to kill himself or herself or who has made an attempt is at risk. Common signs that a person may be contemplating suicide include:

- Recent loss and a seeming inability to let go of grief
- History of depression
- Change in personality, such as sadness, withdrawal, irritability, anxiety, tiredness, indecisiveness, apathy
- Change in behavior, such as inability to concentrate, loss of interest in classes or work, unexplained demonstration of happiness following a period of depression
- Sexual dysfunction (such as impotence) or diminished sexual interest
- Expressions of self-hatred and excessive risk-taking, or an "I don't care what happens to me" attitude
- Change in sleep patterns and/or eating habits
- A direct statement about committing suicide, such as "I might as well end it all"
- An indirect statement, such as "You won't have to worry about me anymore"
- Final preparations such as writing a will, giving away prized possessions, or writing revealing letters
- Preoccupation with themes of death
- Marked changes in personal appearance[56]

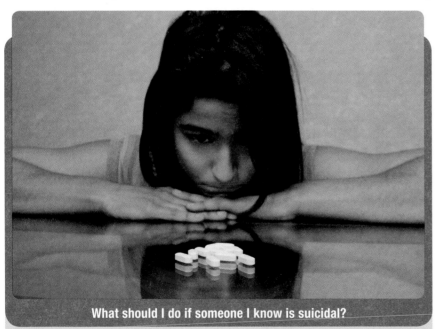

What should I do if someone I know is suicidal?

If you notice warning signs of suicide in someone, take action. Suicidal people urgently need professional assistance; your willingness to talk to the person about depression and suicide in a nonjudgmental way can be the encouragement he or she needs to seek help. Remember: Always take thoughts of or plans for suicide seriously; a life may depend on it.

Preventing Suicide

Most people who attempt suicide really want to live but see death as the only way out of an intolerable situation. Crisis counselors and suicide hotlines may help temporarily, but the best way to prevent suicide is to get rid of conditions and substances that may precipitate attempts, including alcohol, drugs, loneliness, isolation, and access to guns.

If someone you know threatens suicide or displays warning signs, get involved—ask questions and seek help. Specific actions you can take include:

- **Monitor the warning signals.** Keep an eye on the person or see that someone else is present. Don't leave him or her alone.
- **Take threats seriously.** Don't brush them off as "just talk."

Money&Health
LOW-COST TREATMENT OPTIONS FOR MENTAL HEALTH CONDITIONS

Mental health disorders are treatable, yet people don't always seek help. Often the cost of therapy and prescription drugs is a major barrier, since many otherwise comprehensive insurance plans may not cover the cost of mental health services. If you are on a tight budget and struggle with depression, anxiety, or other mental health issues, it's always a good idea to speak with your family physician about low-cost treatment resources in your region and state. Here is a roundup of possible treatment options one can pursue, along with tips on easing the expense:

THERAPY

Cognitive behavioral therapy (CBT) can cost $100 or more per hour. However, some therapists or clinics offer therapy on a sliding scale, which means the fee fluctuates based on income. Ask about a sliding scale or other payment options when you call or visit for a consultation. Federally funded health centers can also be a good resource for those without health insurance or with a limited budget. Many of these centers include mental health services, and they also have sliding scales for payment. Finally, some colleges and universities offer low-cost therapy for mental health problems. Call the psychology, psychiatry, or behavioral health department and inquire about sessions with graduate students, who are supervised and can provide services at a lower cost as they gain counseling experience. Keep in mind that these sessions aren't always open to the public; some departments may limit them to students of that college or university.

PRESCRIPTION DRUGS

Medication can help reduce symptoms of certain mental health disorders, including anxiety and depression, but for people without health insurance drugs can be very expensive. Most pharmaceutical companies offer patient-assistance programs for uninsured patients. These programs provide prescribed medication at little to no cost. It's also a good idea to ask your doctor if a generic (non-brand-name) drug might work for you as well as a brand-name drug. The cost different between generic and brand-name drugs can be substantial. You can also see if your doctor might have medication samples he or she could give you for free.

Note that if you are considering medication, it must be prescribed and monitored by your physician. Do not adjust the dosage or frequency or stop taking it abruptly, even if cost is a factor, without first discussing it with your doctor.

Sources: ADAA, Low Cost Treatment, 2011, www.adaa.org/finding-help/treatment/low-cost-treatment; Partnership for Prescription Assistance, 2011, Patient Frequently Asked Questions, www.pparx.org/en/patient_faqs; J. Grohol, 2011, "Finding Low-Cost Psychotherapy," PsychCentral, Accessed January 25, 2012, from http://psychcentral.com/lib/2007/finding-low-cost-psychotherapy/.

- **Let the person know how much you care.** State that you are there to help.
- **Listen.** Try not to discredit or be shocked by what the person says. Empathize, sympathize, and keep the person talking.
- **Ask directly,** "Are you thinking of hurting or killing yourself?"
- **Do not belittle the person's feelings.** Don't tell the person that he or she doesn't really mean it or couldn't succeed at suicide. To some, these comments offer the challenge of proving you wrong.
- **Help the person think about alternatives to suicide.** Offer to go for help along with the person. Call your local suicide hotline, and use all available community and campus resources.
- **Tell the person's spouse, partner, parents, siblings, or counselor.** Do not keep your suspicions to yourself. Don't let a suicidal friend talk you into keeping your discussions confidential. If your friend succeeds in a suicide attempt, you may find that others will question your decision, and you may blame yourself.[57]

Seeking Professional Help

A physical ailment will readily send most of us to the nearest health professional, but many people view seeking professional help for psychological problems as an admission of personal failure. However, increasing numbers of Americans are turning to mental health professionals, and nearly 1 in 5 seeks such help. Researchers view breakdowns in support systems, high societal expectations, and dysfunctional families as three major reasons why more people are asking for assistance than ever before.

Consider seeking help if:

- You feel that you need help or feel out of control.
- You experience wild mood swings or inappropriate emotional responses to normal stimuli.
- Your fears or feelings of guilt frequently distract your attention.
- You begin to withdraw from others.
- You have hallucinations.

POINTS OF VIEW

Self-Help Books:
BENEFICIAL OR BALONEY?

Self-help books abound, and they cover everything from losing weight to having a better sex life to improving your golf swing to managing your finances. These books, and the programs, seminars, DVDs, and other products that support them, offer accessible, relatively inexpensive guidance to individuals hoping to bring about positive change in their lives. But are these books really helpful, or are they a marketing scam, taking money from innocent consumers without providing any real service?

Arguments in Favor of Self-help Books
○ Self-help books can provide another perspective on a problem, helping the reader become "unstuck."
○ Some self-help books are directive and practical enough to help people change their lives for the better.
○ They can provide useful information and can point people to concrete resources.
○ They provide a private way for people to find information about problems that they may have difficulty discussing.
○ Using a self-help book to read up on a condition or disease may help a person empathize more with another struggling person.
○ Self-help books are generally inexpensive compared with many other kinds of help, such as psychological counseling.

Arguments against Self-help Books
○ Books can't make you change—real change has to come from within an individual.
○ These books often make claims of an outcome that seem too good to be true.
○ Merely reading a self-help book may give a person a false sense of solving a problem without actually dealing with the problem.
○ Self-help books encourage self-diagnosis of health problems, which carries many risks.
○ Anyone can write a self-help book—you don't have to be a professional to be published and the book doesn't have to be based on scientific evidence.
○ When it comes to your health, it's worth it to find qualified health care providers who can help you, even if doing so costs more than a book.

Where Do You Stand?
○ Do you think self-help books tend to be helpful or harmful? In which situations do you think a self-help book is most likely to be valuable?
○ Would you use a self-help book if you felt you had a problem? If so, how would you determine what book to use?
○ Do you know anyone who has used one? Did it help? How?
○ Suppose your cousin was looking for a self-help book. What advice would you give her?

- You feel inadequate or worthless or that life is not worth living.
- Your daily life seems to be nothing but a series of repeated crises.
- You are considering suicide.
- You turn to drugs or alcohol to escape your problems.

Low-cost or free support groups are available to help with all types of issues, including recovery from substance abuse, eating disorders, and other addictions; dealing with health conditions such as diabetes or cancer; and addressing other challenges, such as managing stress, overcoming fear of public speaking, becoming more physically fit, or losing weight. See the **Money & Health** box on page 48 for tips on how to get good mental health care on a tight budget. You may find certain self-help books useful, as well, but be cautious in your selection (see the **Points of View** box).

Mental Illness Stigma

Stigmas are negative perceptions about groups of people or about a certain situation or condition. Common stigmas about people with mental illness are that they are dangerous, irresponsible, require constant care, or that they "just need to get over it." Derogatory terms such as *nut job*, *wacko*, *crazy*, *insane*, *madman*, *bonkers*, and *demented* are still commonly used to describe persons with mental illness. In truth, very few people who suffer with a mental illness are dangerous. Most live independently, go to school, hold jobs, and are productive members of society. A mental illness is like any other chronic disease. You can't just decide to "get over it."

The stigma of mental illness often leads to feelings of shame, guilt, loss of self-esteem, and a sense of isolation and hopelessness. Many people who have successfully managed their mental illness report that the stigma they faced was more disabling at times than the illness itself.[58] The stigma may cause people who are struggling with a mental illness to delay seeking treatment or avoid care that could dramatically improve their symptoms and quality of life.

College student Alison Malmon founded the group Active Minds after her older brother, Brian, committed suicide. Brian had suffered from mental illness for several years, but had concealed his symptoms from everyone close to him. Today there are over 270 Active Mind chapters on college campuses across the country, working to end the stigma of mental illness and to encourage those at risk to seek help.[59]

stigma Negative perception about a group of people or a certain situation or condition.

Getting Evaluated for Treatment

If you are considering treatment for a psychological problem, schedule a complete evaluation first. Consult a credentialed health professional for a thorough examination, which should include three parts:

1. *A physical checkup*, which will rule out thyroid disorders, viral infections, and anemia—all of which can result in depressive-like symptoms—and a neurological check of coordination, reflexes, and balance to rule out brain disorders

2. *A psychiatric history*, which will trace the course of the apparent disorder, genetic or family factors, and any past treatments

3. *A mental status examination*, which will assess thoughts, speaking processes, and memory, and will include an in-depth interview with tests for other psychiatric symptoms.

Once physical factors have been ruled out, you may decide to consult a professional who specializes in psychological health.

Mental Health Professionals

Several types of mental health professionals are available; Table 2.1 on the next page provides information on the most common types of practitioners. When choosing a therapist, it is important to verify that he or she has the appropriate training. But the most important factor is whether you feel you can work with him or her. A qualified mental health professional should be willing to answer all your questions during an initial consultation. Questions to ask the therapist and yourself include:

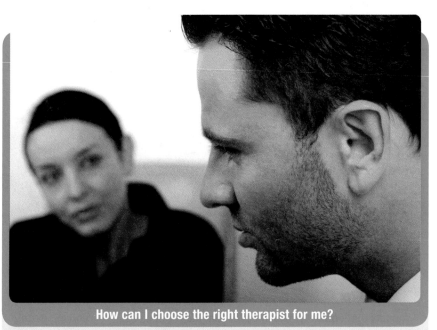

How can I choose the right therapist for me?

The choice of therapist is very individual—seeing a mental health professional is a form of relationship, and as in any relationship, it is important to establish a connection. Depending on your concerns, you may need to find someone with a particular specialty or degree, but regardless, you'll want to be comfortable with the therapist you choose. Schedule an initial interview with more than one professional and ask a lot of questions. Trust your instincts and don't settle for someone who doesn't "feel right." Remember that your mental health is important; you deserve to find the best possible help and support.

- **Can you interview the therapist before starting treatment?** An initial meeting will help you determine whether this person will be a good fit for you.
- **Do you like the therapist as a person?** Can you talk to him or her comfortably?
- **Is the therapist watching the clock or easily distracted?** You should be the main focus of the session.
- **Does the therapist demonstrate professionalism?** Be concerned if your therapist is frequently late or breaks appointments, suggests social interactions outside therapy sessions, talks inappropriately about himself or herself, has questionable billing practices, or resists releasing you from therapy.
- **Will the therapist help you set your own goals and timetables?** A good professional should evaluate your general situation and help you set small goals to work on between sessions.

Remember, in most states, the use of the title *therapist* or *counselor* is unregulated. Check credentials and make your choice carefully.

What to Expect in Therapy

Before making an appointment, call for information and to briefly explain your needs. Ask about office hours, policies and procedures, fees, and insurance participation. The first trip to a therapist can be difficult. Most of us have misconceptions about what therapy is and what it can do. The first visit serves as a sizing-up between you and the therapist. If you decide that this professional is not for you, you will at least have learned how to present your problem and what qualities you need in a therapist.

Arrive on time, wear comfortable clothing, and expect your visit to last about an hour. The therapist will record your history and details about the problem that has brought you to therapy. Answer honestly and do not be embarrassed to acknowledge your feelings. It is critical to the success of your treatment that you trust the therapist enough to be open and honest.

Do not expect the therapist to tell you what to do or how to behave. The responsibility for improved behavior lies with

TABLE 2.1   **Mental Health Professionals**

What Are They Called?	What Kind of Training Do They Have?	What Kind of Therapy Do They Do?	Professional Association
Psychiatrist	Medical doctor (MD) degree, followed by 4 years of specialized mental health training	As a licensed MD, a psychiatrist can prescribe medications and may have admitting privileges at a local hospital.	American Psychiatric Association www.psych.org
Psychologist	Doctoral (PhD) degree in counseling or clinical psychology, followed by several years of supervised practice to earn license	Psychologists are trained in various types of therapy, including cognitive and behavior therapy. May be trained in certain specialties, such as family counseling or sexual counseling.	American Psychological Association www.apa.org
Clinical/psychiatric social worker	Master's degree in social work (MSW) followed by 2 years of experience in a clinical setting to earn license	Social workers may be trained in certain specialties, such as substance abuse counseling or child counseling.	National Association of Social Workers www.socialworkers.org
Counselor	Master's degree in counseling, psychology, educational psychology, or related human service; generally must complete at least 2 years of supervised practice to obtain a license	Many counselors are trained to provide individual and group therapy. They often specialize in one type of counseling, such as family, marital, relationship, children, or substance abuse.	American Counseling Association www.counseling.org
Psychoanalyst	Postgraduate degree in psychology or psychiatry (PhD or MD), followed by 8 to 10 years of training in psychoanalysis, which includes undergoing analysis themselves	Psychoanalysis is based on the theories of Freud and his successors. It focuses on patterns of thinking and behavior and the recall of early traumas that have blocked personal growth. Treatment is intensive, lasting 5 to 10 years, with 3 or 4 sessions per week.	American Psychoanalytic Association www.apsa.org
Licensed marriage and family therapist (LMFT)	Master's or doctoral degree in psychology, social work, or counseling, specializing in family and interpersonal dynamics; generally must complete at least 2 years of supervised practice to obtain a license	LMFTs treat individuals or families in the context of family relationships. Treatment is typically brief (20 sessions or fewer) and focused on finding solutions to specific relational problems.	American Association for Marriage and Family Therapy www.aamft.org

Antidepressants	Used to treat depression, panic disorders, anxiety disorders	
Selective serotonin-reuptake inhibitors (SSRIs)	*Examples:* fluoxetine (Prozac), paroxetine (Paxil, Seroxat), escitalopram (Lexapro, Esipram), citalopram (Celexa), and sertraline (Zoloft)	The current standard drug treatment for depression; also frequently prescribed for anxiety disorders
Noradrenergic and specific serotonergic antidepressants (NaSSAs)	*Examples:* mirtazapine (Avanza, Zispin, Remeron)	Reportedly has fewer sexual dysfunction side effects than do SSRIs
Serotonin-norepinephrine reuptake inhibitors (SNRIs)	*Examples:* venlafaxine (Effexor), duloxetine (Cymbalta)	Also sometimes prescribed for ADHD
Norepinephrine-dopamine reuptake inhibitors (NDRIs)	*Examples:* bupropion (Wellbutrin, Zyban)	Also used in smoking cessation; fewer weight gain or sexual dysfunction side effects than SSRIs
Tricyclic antidepressants (TCAs)	*Examples:* imipramine, amitriptyline, nortriptyline, and desipramine	Negative side effects; usually used as a 2nd or 3rd line of treatment when other medications prove ineffective
Monoamine oxidase inhibitors (MAOIs)	*Examples:* phenelzine (Nardil), tranylcypromine (Parnate), and isocarboxazid (Marplan)	Dangerous interactions with many other drugs and substances in food; generally no longer prescribed
Anxiolytics (antianxiety drugs)	Used to treat anxiety disorders, including OCD, GAD, panic disorders, phobias, PTSD	
Benzodiazepines	*Examples:* lorazepam (Ativan), clonazepam (Klonopin), alprazolam (Xanax), diazepam (Valium)	Short-term relief, sometimes taken on an as-needed basis; dangerous interactions with alcohol; possible to develop tolerance or dependence
Serotonin 1A agonists	*Examples:* buspirone (BuSpar)	Longer-term relief; must be taken for at least 2 weeks to achieve antianxiety effects
Mood stabilizers	Used to treat bipolar disorder, schizophrenia	
Lithium	*Examples:* lithium carbonate	Drug most commonly used to treat bipolar disorder; blood levels must be closely monitored to determine proper dosage and avoid toxic effects
Anticonvulsants	*Examples:* valproic acid (Depakene), divalproex sodium (Depakote), sodium valproate (Depacon)	Used more frequently for acute mania than for long-term maintenance of bipolar disorder
Antipsychotics (neuroleptics)	Used to treat schizophrenia, mania, bipolar disorder	
Atypical antipsychotics	*Examples:* clozapine (Clozaril), risperidone (Risperdal)	First line of treatment for schizophrenia; fewer adverse effects than earlier antipsychotics
First-generation antipsychotics	*Examples:* haloperidol (Haldol), chlorpromazine (Thorazine)	Earliest forms of antipsychotics; unpleasant side effects such as tremor and muscle stiffness
Stimulants	Used to treat ADHD, narcolepsy	
Methylphenidate	Brand names: Ritalin, Metadate, Concerta	Can lead to tolerance and dependence; frequently abused for both performance enhancement and recreational use
Amphetamines	*Examples:* amphetamine (Adderall), dextroamphetamine (Dexedrine, Dextrostat), pemoline (Cylert)	Can lead to tolerance and dependence; frequently abused for both performance enhancement and recreational use

Source: Data from National Institute of Mental Health, Mental Health Medications, "Alphabetical List of Medications," 2011, www.nimh.nih.gov/health/publications/mental-health-medications/alphabetical-list-of-medications.shtml.

you. If after your first visit (or even after several visits), you feel you cannot work with this person, say so. You have the right to find a therapist with whom you feel comfortable.

Treatment Models Many different types of counseling exist, including psychodynamic therapy, interpersonal therapy, and cognitive behavioral therapy.

Psychodynamic therapy focuses on the psychological roots of emotional suffering. This type of therapy involves self-reflection, self-examination, and the use of the relationship between therapist and patient as a window into problematic relationship patterns in the patient's life. Its goal is not only to alleviate the most obvious symptoms, but also to help people lead healthier lives.[60]

Interpersonal therapy focuses on social roles and relationships. The patient works with a therapist to evaluate specific problem areas in the patient's life, such as conflicts with family and friends or significant life changes or transition. While past experiences help inform the process, interpersonal therapy focuses mainly on improving relationships in the present.[61]

Treatment for mental disorders can include various cognitive behavioral therapies. *Cognitive therapy* focuses on the impact of thoughts and ideas on feelings and behavior. It helps a person to look at life rationally and correct habitually pessimistic or faulty thinking patterns. *Behavioral therapy,* as the name implies, focuses on what we do. Behavior therapy uses the concepts of stimulus, response, and reinforcement to alter behavior patterns. With cognitive behavioral therapy, you work with a mental health counselor (psychotherapist) in a structured way, attending a limited number of sessions to become aware of inaccurate or negative thinking. Cognitive behavioral therapy allows you to view challenging situations more clearly and respond to them in a more effective and positive way. Cognitive behavioral therapy can be a very helpful tool in treating mental anxiety or depression.[62]

Pharmacological Treatment

Treatment for some conditions combines cognitive behavioral therapies with medication prescribed by the patient's physician or by a psychiatrist. Table 2.2 on page 52 includes information about the major classes of medications used to treat the most common mental illnesses. These drugs require a doctor's prescription and have been approved by the U.S. Food and Drug Administration (FDA). These medications are not, however, without side effects and risks. For example, the FDA proposed new warnings for antidepressant medications, including a labeling change that warns about increased risks of suicidal thinking and behavior in young adults aged 18 to 24 during initial treatment.[63]

Potency, dosage, and side effects of drugs can vary greatly. It is vital to talk to your health care provider and completely understand the risks and benefits of any prescribed medication. Likewise, your doctor needs to be notified as soon as possible of any adverse effects you may experience. With some drug therapies, such as antidepressants, you may not feel the therapeutic effects for several weeks, so patience is important. Finally, be sure to follow your doctor's recommendations for beginning or ending a course of any medication.

How Psychologically Healthy Are You?

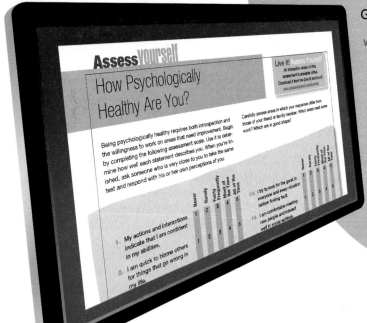

Go online to the **Live It!** section of

www.pearsonhighered.com/donatelle

to take the "How Psychologically Healthy Are You?" assessment.* For areas where you determine that you need to change your behaviors, follow the tips found in the **YOUR PLAN FOR CHANGE** box.

*If your instructor so chooses, Assess Yourself Activities are available as a printed supplement or as assignable homework online at www.pearsonhighered.com/myhealthlab.

MyHealthLab®

YOUR PLAN FOR CHANGE

The **Assess yourself** activity "How Psychologically Health Are You?" gives you the chance to look at various aspects of your psychological health and compare your self-assessment with a friend's perceptions. Once you have considered these results, you can take steps to change behaviors that may be detrimental.

Today, you can:

○ Evaluate your behavior and identify patterns and specific things you are doing that negatively affect your psychological health. What can you change now? What can you change in the near future?

○ Start a journal and note erratic or extreme changes in your mood. Look

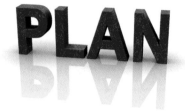

for trends and think about ways you can change your behavior to address them.

○ Make a list of the things that bring you joy—friends, family, activities, entertainment, nature. Commit yourself to making more room for these joy-givers in your life.

Within the next 2 weeks, you can:

○ Visit your campus health center and find out about counseling services they offer. If you are feeling overwhelmed, depressed, or anxious, make an appointment with a counselor.

○ Pay attention to negative thoughts that pop up throughout the day. Note times when you find yourself undermining your abilities and notice when you

project negative attitudes. Bringing your awareness to these thoughts gives you an opportunity to stop and reevaluate them.

By the end of the semester, you can:

○ Make a commitment to an ongoing therapeutic practice aimed at improving your psychological health. Depending on your current situation, this could mean anything from seeing a counselor or joining a support group to practicing meditation or attending religious services.

○ Volunteer regularly with a local organization you care about. Focus your energy and gain satisfaction by helping to improve others' lives or the environment.

Summary

* Psychological health is a complex phenomenon involving mental, emotional, social, and spiritual dimensions.
* Many factors influence psychological health, including life experiences, family, the environment, other people, self-esteem, self-efficacy, and personality.
* The mind–body connection is an important link in overall health and well-being. Positive psychology emphasizes happiness as a key factor in determining overall reaction to life's challenges.
* Developing self-esteem and self-efficacy, making healthy connections, having a positive outlook on life, and maintaining physical health are key to enhancing psychological health.
* College life is a high-risk time for developing disorders such as depression or anxiety because of high stress levels, pressures for grades, and financial problems, among others.
* Mood disorders include major depression, dysthymic disorder, bipolar disorder, and seasonal affective disorder. Anxiety disorders include generalized anxiety disorder, panic disorders, phobic disorders, obsessive-compulsive disorder, and post-traumatic stress disorder. Personality disorders include paranoid, narcissistic, and borderline personality disorders.
* Schizophrenia is a disorder once believed to result from environmental causes. Brain function studies have now shown that it is instead a biological disease of the brain.
* Suicide is a result of negative psychological reactions to life. People intending to commit suicide often give warning signs of their intentions. Such people can often be helped.
* Mental health professionals include psychiatrists, psychoanalysts, psychologists, social workers, and counselors. Many therapy methods exist, including interpersonal, psychodynamic, and cognitive behavioral therapy.

Pop Quiz

1. A person with high self-esteem
   a. possesses feelings of self-respect and self-worth.
   b. believes he or she can successfully engage in a specific behavior.
   c. believes external influences shape one's psychological health.
   d. has a high altruistic capacity.

2. All of the following traits have been identified as characterizing psychologically healthy people *except*
   a. conscientiousness.
   b. introversion.
   c. openness to experience.
   d. agreeableness.

3. Subjective well-being includes all of the following components *except*
   a. psychological hardiness.
   b. satisfaction with present life.
   c. relative presence of positive emotions.
   d. relative absence of negative emotions.

4. People who have experienced repeated failures at the same task may eventually give up and quit trying altogether. This pattern of behavior is termed
   a. post-traumatic stress disorder.
   b. learned helplessness.
   c. self-efficacy.
   d. introversion.

5. The term that most accurately refers to the feeling or subjective side of psychological health is
   a. social health.
   b. mental health.
   c. emotional health.
   d. spiritual health.

6. Which statement below is *false*?
   a. One in four adults in the United States suffers from a diagnosable mental disorder in a given year.
   b. Mental disorders are the leading cause of disability in the United States.
   c. Dysthymia is an example of an anxiety disorder.
   d. Bipolar disorder can also be referred to as manic depression.

7. This disorder is characterized by a need to perform rituals over and over again; fear of dirt or contamination; or an unnatural concern with order, symmetry, and exactness.
   a. Personality disorder
   b. Obsessive-compulsive disorder
   c. Phobic disorder
   d. Post-traumatic stress disorder

8. What is the number one mental health problem in the United States?
   a. Depression
   b. Anxiety disorders
   c. Alcohol dependence
   d. Schizophrenia

9. Every winter, Stan suffers from irritability, apathy, weight gain, and sadness. He most likely has
   a. panic disorder.
   b. generalized anxiety disorder.
   c. seasonal affective disorder.
   d. chronic mood disorder.

10. A person with a PhD in counseling psychology and training in various types of therapy is a
    a. psychiatrist.
    b. psychologist.
    c. social worker.
    d. psychoanalyst.

Answers to these questions can be found on page A-1.

Think about It!

1. What is psychological health? What indicates that you are or are not psychologically healthy? Why might the college environment provide a challenge to psychological health?

2. Discuss the factors that influence your overall level of psychological health. Which factors can you change? Which ones may be more difficult to change?

3. Which psychological dimensions do you need to work on? Which are most important to you, and why? What actions can you take today?

4. What are the warning signs of suicide? What are the symptoms of major depression? Why are some groups of people more vulnerable to suicide and depression than others? What would you do if you heard a friend say to no one in particular that he was going to "do the world a favor and end it all"?

5. Describe the various types of mental health professionals and types of therapies. If you felt depressed about breaking off a long-term relationship, which professional and which therapy do you think would be most beneficial to you?

Accessing Your **Health** on the Internet

The following websites explore further topics related to psychological health. For links to the websites below, visit the Companion Website for *Access to Health*, 13th Edition, at www.pearsonhighered.com/donatelle.

1. *American Foundation for Suicide Prevention.* Provides resources for suicide prevention and support for family and friends of those who have committed suicide. www.afsp.org

2. *American Psychological Association Help Center.* Includes information on psychology at work, the mind–body connection, understanding depression, psychological

responses to war, and other topics. www.apa.org/helpcenter/wellness/index.aspx

3. *National Alliance on Mental Illness.* Support and advocacy organization of families and friends of people with severe mental illnesses. www.nami.org

4. *National Institute of Mental Health (NIMH).* Provides an overview of mental health information and new research. www.nimh.nih.gov

5. *Mental Health America.* Works to promote mental health through advocacy, education, research, and services. www.nmha.org

6. *Helpguide.* Resources for improving mental and emotional health as well as specific information on topics such as self-injury, sleep, depressive disorders, and anxiety disorders. www.helpguide.org

7. *Active Minds.* Campus education and advocacy organization formed to combat the stigma of mental illness, encourage students who need help to seek it early, and prevent tragedies related to untreated mental illness. www.activeminds.org

References

1. A. H. Maslow, *Motivation and Personality,* 2nd ed. (New York: Harper and Row, 1970).

2. U.S. Department of Health and Human Services, *Mental Health: A Report of the Surgeon General—Executive Summary* (Rockville, MD: U.S. Department of Health and Human Services, Substance Abuse and Mental Health Services Administration, National Institute of Mental Health, 1999), Available at www.surgeongeneral .gov/library/mentalhealth/summary.html.

3. Helpguide.org, Emotional Intelligence, Accessed January 2012, http://helpguide .org/mental/eq5_raising_emotional_ intelligence.htm.

4. Helpguide.org, Improving Emotional Health, Strategies and Tips for Good Mental Health, 2011, http://helpguide .org/mental/ mental_emotional_health.htm.

5. Mayo Clinic, "Social Support: Tap this Tool to Combat Stress," 2010, www .mayoclinic.com/health/social-support/ SR000033; M. Umberson and J. Montez, "Social Relationships and Health," *Journal of Health and Social Behavior* 51, no. 1, Supplement (2010):S54–S66;

J. Holt-Lunstad, T. B. Smith, and J. B. Layton, "Social Relationships and Mortality Risk: A Meta-analytic Review," *PLoS Medicine* 7, no. 7 (2010): e1000316, DOI: 10.1371/journal.pmed.1000316; T. Inagaki and N. Eisenberger, "Neural Correlates of Giving Support to a Loved One," *Psychosomatic Medicine* (2011): DOI: 10.1097/PSY.0b013e3182359335; T. Antonucci, K. Birditt, and N. Webster, "Social Relations and Mortality: A More Nuanced Approach," *Journal of Health Psychology* 15, no. 5 (2010): 649–59, DOI: 10.1177/1359105310368189.

6. K. Karren et al., *Mind/Body Health,* 4th ed. (San Francisco: Benjamin Cummings, 2010).

7. Dowshen, S., "How Can Spirituality Affect Your Family's Health?" 2011, http:// kidshealth.org/parent/emotions/feelings/ spirituality.html#; National Center for Cultural Competence, Georgetown University. Definitions and Discussion of Spirituality and Religion. 2011, http:// nccc.georgetown.edu/body_mind_spirit/ definitions_spirituality_religion.html.

8. C. Carter, *Raising Happiness: 10 Simple Steps for More Joyful Kids and Happier Parents* (New York: Ballantine Publishing, 2010).

9. J. Mattanah, J. Ayers, B. Brand, and L. Brooks, "A Social Support Intervention to Ease the College Transition: Exploring Main Effects and Moderators," *Journal of College Student Development* 51, no. 1 (2010): 93–108.

10. M. Seligman and C. Peterson, "Learned Helplessness," in *International Encyclopedia for the Social and Behavioral Sciences,* vol. 13, ed. N. Smelser (New York: Elsevier, 2002), 8583–866.

11. M. Seligman, *Learned Optimism: How to Change Your Mind and Your Life* (New York: Free Press, 1998); J. H. Martin, *Motivation Processes and Performance: The Role of Global and Facet Personality,* PhD dissertation, University of North Carolina at Chapel Hill, 2002.

12. R. Curtis. "Post-Graduation Advising: Needed More Now Than Ever," *The Mentor,* Penn State's Division of Undergraduate Studies, January 13, 2010, http://dus.psu.edu/mentor/old/ articles/100113rc.htm.

13. S. Rimer, Harvard School of Public Health, "The Biology of Emotion—And What It May Teach Us about Helping People to Live Longer," 2012, www.hsph .harvard.edu/news/hphr/chronic- disease-prevention/happiness-stress- heart-disease/.

14. Ibid.; M. Miller and W. F. Fry, "The Effect of Mirthful Laughter on the Human Cardiovascular System," *Medical Hypotheses*

73, no. 5 (2009): 636–39; S. Horowitz, "The Effect of Positive Emotions on Health: Hope and Humor," *Alternative and Complementary Therapies* 15, no. 4 (2009): 196–202.

15. R. I. Dunbar et al., "Social Laughter Is Correlated with an Elevated Pain Threshold," *Proceedings of the Royal Society,* September 14, 2011, DOI: 10.1098/rspb.2011.1373.

16. De Neve, J. "Functional Polymorphism (*5-HTTLPR*) in the Serotonin Transporter Gene Is Associated with Subjective Well-being: Evidence from a U.S. Nationally Representative Sample," *Journal of Human Genetics* 56 (2011):456–459, DOI: 10.1038/jhg.2011.39.

17. C. Carter, "Raising Happiness," 2010;. R. I. Dunbar, "Social Laughter," 2011;

18. Mayo Clinic Staff, MayoClinic.com, "Mental Illness: Causes," September 2010, www.mayoclinic.com/health/mental-illness/DS01104/DSECTION=causes.

19. Ibid.

20. National Institute of Mental Health, Report of the National Advisory Mental Health Council's Workgroup, *From Discovery to Cure: Accelerating the Development of New and Personalized Interventions for Mental Illnesses,* August 2010, www.nimh.nih.gov/about/advisory-boards-and groups/namhc/reports/fromdiscoverytocure.pdf.

21. Ibid.

22. J. Hunt and D. Eisenberg, "Mental Health Problems and Help-Seeking Behavior among College Students," *Journal of Adolescent Health* 46, no. 1 (2010): 3–10.

23. American College Health Association, *American College Health Association–National College Health Assessment II (ACHA–NCHA II): Reference Group Data Report Spring 2011* (Baltimore: American College Health Association, 2012), Available at www.acha-ncha .org/reports_ACHA-NCHAII.html.

24. American Psychological Association, "College Students Exhibiting More Severe Mental Illness, Study Finds," *ScienceDaily,* August 12, 2010, www.sciencedaily.com/releases/2010/08/100812111053.htm.

25. National Institute of Mental Health, "Mood Disorders," Updated February 2011, http://report.nih.gov/NIHfactsheets/ViewFactSheet.aspx?csid=48&key=M#M.

26. National Institutes of Mental Health, "The Numbers Count: Mental Disorders in America," 2009, www.nimh.nih.gov/health/publications/the-numbers-count-mental-disorcers-in-america.shtml.

27. National Institute of Mental Health, "Depression," Revised 2011, www.nimh .nih.gov/publicat/depression.cfm.

28. American College Health Association, *ACHA–NCHA II: Reference Group Data Report Spring 2011,* 2012.

29. National Institute of Mental Health, "The Numbers Count," 2009.

30. Ibid.

31. American Psychiatric Association, Healthy Minds. Healthy Lives. "Seasonal Affective Disorder," 2011, www.healthyminds.org/Main-Topic/Seasonal-Affective-Disorder.aspx.

32. Mayo Clinic Staff, MayoClinic.com, "Depression: Causes," 2010, www .mayoclinic.com/health/depression/DS00175/DSECTION=causes.

33. National Institute of Mental Health, "The Numbers Count," 2009.

34. American College Health Association, *ACHA–NCHA II: Reference Group Data Report Spring 2011,* 2012.

35. M. Jacofsky et al., MentalHelp.net, "Understanding Anxiety and Anxiety Disorders Introduction," Updated June 2010, www.mentalhelp.net/poc/view_doc .php?type=doc&id=38463&cn=1.

36. National Institute of Mental Health, "Generalized Anxiety Disorder, GAD," Reviewed July 7, 2009, www.nimh.nih .gov/health/publications/anxiety-disorders/generalized-anxiety-disorder-gad.shtml.

37. National Institute of Mental Health, "The Numbers Count," 2009.

38. Mayo Clinic Staff, MayoClinic.com, "Panic Attacks and Panic Disorder: Symptoms," 2010, www.mayoclinic .com/health/panic-attacks/DS00338/DSECTION=symptoms.

39. National Institute of Mental Health, "The Numbers Count," 2009.

40. Ibid.

41. Ibid.

42. J. Gradus, United States Department of Veterans Affairs. National Center for PTSD, Epidemiology of PTSD. Updated December 2011, www.ptsd.va.gov/professional/pages/epidemiological-facts-ptsd.asp.

43. National Institute of Mental Health, "Generalized Anxiety Disorder, GAD," 2009.

44. Allpsych, Personality Disorders, 2011, http://allpsych.com/disorders/personality/index.html.

45. About Recovery, 2010, Personality Disorders. http://aboutrecovery.com/addictions-mental-health/personality-disorder.htm.

46. Mayo Clinic Staff, MayoClinic.com, "Borderline Personality Disorder," 2010, www.mayoclinic.com/health/borderline-personality-disorder/DS00442.

47. J. Cole, "Facts," BPDWORLD, 2010, www .bpdworld.org/demo-category/106-facts.

48. National Institute of Mental Health, "The Numbers Count," 2009.

49. National Institute of Mental Health, "Schizophrenia," Reviewed March 2010, www.nimh.nih.gov/health/topics/schizophrenia/index.shtml.

50. Ibid.

51. National Institute of Mental Health, "Suicide in the U.S.: Statistics and Prevention," NIH Publication no. 06-4594, Reviewed September 2010, www.nimh.nih.gov/health/publications/suicide-in-the-us-statistics-and-prevention/index.shtml.

52. J. Xu et al., "Deaths: Final Data for 2007," *National Vital Statistics Reports* 58, no. 19 (Hyattsville, MD: National Center for Health Statistics, 2010).

53. National Institute of Mental Health, "Suicide in the U.S.: Statistics and Prevention," 2010.

54. Ibid.

55. Crisis Link, "Suicide Myths (Adult)," 2009, www.crisislink.org/resources/suicide/suicide_myths_adult.html.

56. NIH, "Suicide in the U.S," 2010.

57. American Association of Suicidology, "Understanding and Helping the Suicidal Individual," January 2012, www .suicidology.org/web/guest/how-can-you-help.

58. Mayo Clinic Staff, MayoClinic.com, "Mental Health: Overcoming the Stigma of Mental Illness," 2011, www.mayoclinic .com/health/mental-health/MH00076; Mental Health America, Stigma: Building Awareness and Understanding, 2012, www.nmha.org/go/action/stigma-watch.

59. Active Minds: Changing the Conversation about Mental Health, "About Us: FAQ," Accessed January 2012, www.activeminds .org/index.php?option=com_content&task=view&id=40&Itemid=109.

60. APA, 2010. Psychodynamic Psychotherapy Brings Lasting Benefits through Self-Knowledge, 2010, www.apa.org/news/press/releases/2010/01/psychodynamic-therapy.aspx

61. CRC Health Group, Interpersonal Therapy What Is It?, 2011, www .crchealth.com/types-of-therapy/what-is-interpersonal-therapy/.

62. Mayo Clinic, Cognitive Behavioral Therapy, 2010, www.mayoclinic .com/health/cognitive-behavioral-therapy/MY00194.

63. U.S. Food and Drug Administration, "Understanding Antidepressant Medications," 2009, www.fda.gov/ForConsumers/ConsumerUpdates/ucm095980.htm.

Cultivating Your Spiritual Health

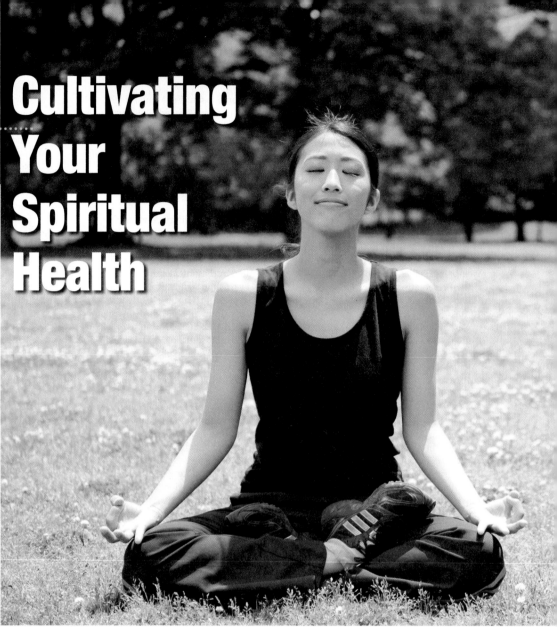

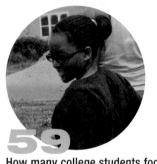

59 How many college students focus on their spiritual health?

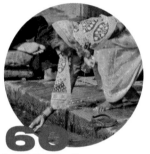

60 Is spirituality the same as religion?

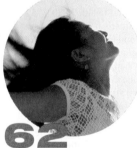

62 Does spirituality influence health?

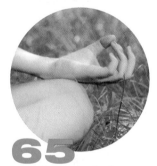

65 Is meditation boring?

Lia's favorite spot on campus is the secluded Japanese garden on the south side of the library. Whether she's feeling stressed about exams or is mulling over an important decision, a few minutes alone in the garden always seem to help. Sometimes she sits quietly and watches the birds come and go. Sometimes she gets out her camera and photographs particularly brilliant blossoms. Often she simply rests, eyes closed, feeling the sun's warmth on her face, and lets her thoughts turn to gratitude for her health, her loving family, and her opportunity to study. However she spends it, her "garden break" leaves Lia feeling refreshed and refocused, with greater confidence in her ability to tackle the challenges of her day.

Lia's desire to find a sense of purpose, meaning, and harmony in her life is shared by a majority of American college students. According to UCLA's Higher Education Research Institute (HERI), undergraduates show significant growth in a wide spectrum of spiritual and ethical considerations.[1] Data from more than 24,450 students at 111 colleges and universities (taken as they entered college in the fall of 2005 and again as they prepared for their senior

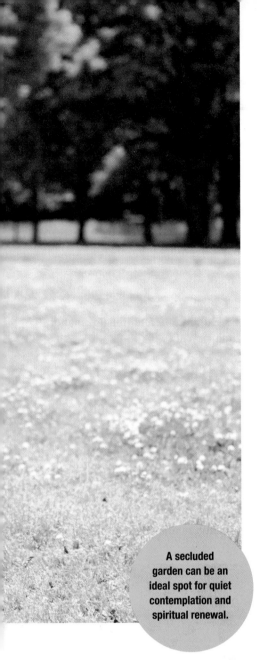

76%

of college students say they are "searching for meaning and purpose in life."

Hear It! Podcasts

Want a study podcast for this chapter text? Download the podcast **Psychological Health: Being Mentally, Emotionally, and Spiritually Well** at www.pearsonhighered.com/donatelle.

A secluded garden can be an ideal spot for quiet contemplation and spiritual renewal.

and cultures. Students also reported high levels of satisfaction with, and recognition of the importance of, expressing diverse beliefs on their campus.

Spiritual health is one of six key dimensions of health (see **Figure 1.4** on page 8 in **Chapter 1**). Lia's sense of wonder and respect for the natural world, her gratitude for the good things in her life, and her belief in a "universal spirit" suggest that spiritual health is an important focus of her daily life, bringing her greater awareness and serenity. If you're feeling as if you could use a little more of these qualities in your own life, read on: This chapter will help you explore ways to enhance your spiritual focus.

What Is Spirituality?

From one day to the next, many of us attempt to satisfy our needs for belonging and self-esteem by acquiring material possessions. But at some point we come to realize that new gadgets, clothes, or concert tickets don't necessarily make us happy or improve our sense of self-worth. That's when many of us begin to contemplate another side of ourselves: our spirituality.

But what is spirituality? It isn't easy to define. Although part of the universal human experience, it's highly personal, and involves feelings and senses

year in 2009) found that interest in the following goals increased during the college years:

- Integrating spirituality into my life
- Developing a meaningful philosophy of life
- Helping others who are in difficulty
- Influencing social values

Also, researchers found that, compared with college first-year students, juniors and seniors were more interested in participating in community action programs and expressed more desire to understand other countries

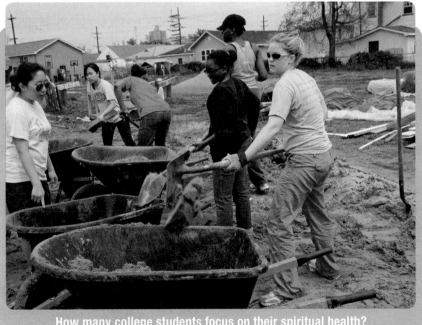

How many college students focus on their spiritual health?

Spiritual and ethical concerns are important to most American college students. For example, more than 80 percent of college seniors desire to become a more loving person. One of the ways students express their spirituality is by working to reduce suffering in the world; many contribute their time and skills to volunteer organizations, as these students are doing by working to build homes for Habitat for Humanity.

that are often intangible. As such, it tends to defy the boundaries that strict definitions would impose. Let's begin by exploring its root, *spirit,* which in many cultures refers to *breath,* or the force that animates life. When you're "inspired," your energy flows. You're not held back by doubts about the purpose or meaning of your work and life. Indeed, many definitions of spirituality incorporate this sense of transcendence. For example, the National Cancer Institute defines **spirituality** as an individual's sense of peace, purpose, and connection to others, and beliefs about the meaning of life.[2] Similarly, Harold G. Koenig, MD, one of the foremost researchers of spirituality and health, defines *spirituality* as the personal quest for understanding answers to ultimate questions about life, about meaning, and about our relationship with the sacred or transcendent.[3] The sacred or transcendent could be a higher power, or it could relate to our relationship with nature or forces we cannot explain.

Religion and Spirituality Are Distinct Concepts

Spirituality may or may not lead to participation in organized **religion,** that is, a system of beliefs, practices, rituals, and symbols designed to facilitate closeness to the sacred or transcendent.[4] Although spirituality and religion share some common elements, they are not the same thing. Most Americans consider spirituality to be important in their lives, but not necessarily in the form of religion: A recent national survey revealed that 73 percent of Americans 30 years and older believe in God, but not all of these respondents identified themselves as being affiliated with a particular religion.[5] Thus, it's clear that religion does not

T A B L E	
1	**Characteristics Distinguishing Religion and Spirituality**

Religion	Spirituality
Community focused	Individualistic
Observable, measurable, objective	Less measurable, more subjective
Formal, orthodox, organized	Less formal, less orthodox, less systematic
Behavior-oriented, outward practices	Emotionally oriented, inwardly directed
Authoritarian in terms of behaviors	Not authoritarian, little accountability
Doctrine separating good from evil	Unifying, not doctrine oriented

Source: National Center for Complementary and Alternative Medicine (NCCAM), "Prayer and Spirituality in Health: Ancient Practices, Modern Science," *CAM at the NIH* 12, no. 1 (2005): 1–4.

have to be part of a spiritual person's life. Table 1 identifies some characteristics that can help you distinguish between religion and spirituality.

Another finding of the same survey was that 74 percent of Americans affiliated with a religious tradition agreed that other religions are also valid.[6] Perhaps this is because all major religions express a belief in a unifying spiritual concept, a oneness with a greater power. It seems that a majority of Americans recognize and respect this underlying unity of spiritual ideas expressed in different religious and spiritual practices.

Spirituality Integrates Three Facets

Brian Luke Seaward, a professor at the University of Northern Colorado and author of several books on spirituality and mind–body healing, identifies three facets of human existence that together constitute the core of human spirituality: relationships, values, and

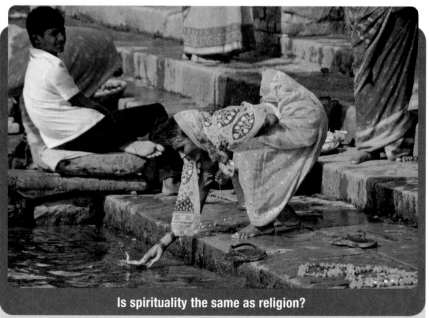

Is spirituality the same as religion?

Spirituality and religion are not the same. Many people find that religious practices, for example, attending services or making offerings—such as the flowers these Hindus are preparing to place in the sacred Ganges River—help them to focus on their spirituality. However, religion does not have to be part of a spiritual person's life.

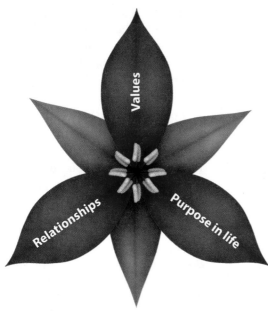

FIGURE 1 **Three Facets of Spirituality**
Most of us are prompted to explore our spirituality because of questions relating to our relationships, values, and purpose in life. At the same time, these three facets together constitute spiritual well-being.

Video Tutor: Facets of Spirituality

purpose in life (**Figure 1**).[7] Questions arising in these three domains prompt many of us to look for spiritual answers. At the same time, spiritual well-being is characterized by healthy relationships, strong personal values, and a sense that we have a meaningful purpose in life.

Relationships Have you ever wondered if someone you were attracted to is really right for you? Or, conversely, if you should break off a long-term relationship? Have you ever wished you had more friends, or that you were a better friend to yourself? Have you ever tried to make a connection with some sort of Presence or Higher Self? For many people, such questions and yearnings are natural triggers for spiritual growth: As we contemplate whom we should choose as a life partner or how to mend a quarrel with a friend, we begin to foster our own inner wisdom. At the same time, healthy relationships are a sign of spiritual well-being. When we treat ourselves and others with respect, honesty, integrity, and love, we are manifesting our spiritual health.

Values Our personal **values** are our principles—not only the things we say we care about, but also the things that cause us to behave the way we do. For instance, if you value honesty, then you are not likely to call in sick for work when you intend to spend the day at the beach. In other words, our value system is the set of fundamental rules by which we conduct our lives. It's what we stand for. When we attempt to clarify our values, and then to live according to those values, we're engaging in spiritual work. Spiritual health is characterized by a strong personal value system.

Meaningful Purpose in Life What career do you plan to pursue? Do you hope to marry? Do you plan to have or adopt children? What things will make you feel happy and "complete"? How do these choices reflect what you hold as your purpose in life? At the end of your days, what would you want people to say about how you've lived your life and what your life has meant to others? Contemplating these questions fosters spiritual growth. People who are spiritually healthy are able to articulate their purpose and to make choices that manifest that purpose. In thinking about your own purpose, avoid the temptation to get too ambitious, as in, "I'm here to eradicate world hunger!" Instead, try to articulate what you see as your unique contribution to the world—something you can actually do, starting now.

Spiritual Intelligence Is an Inner Wisdom

Our relationships, values, and sense of purpose together contribute to our overall **spiritual intelligence (SI).** This term was introduced by physicist and philosopher Danah Zohar, who defined it as "an ability to access higher meanings, values, abiding pur-

values Principles that influence our thoughts and emotions and guide the choices we make in our lives.

spiritual intelligence (SI) The ability to access higher meanings, values, abiding purposes, and unconscious aspects of the self, a characteristic that helps us find a moral and ethical path to guide us through life.

poses, and unconscious aspects of the self."[8] Zohar includes qualities such as the ability to think outside the box, humility, and an access to energies that come from a source beyond the ego in her definition of *spiritual intelligence,* explaining that SI helps us use meanings, values, and purposes to live richer and more creative lives.

Since Zohar's introduction of SI, dozens of clerics, psychologists, and even business consultants have expanded on the definition. For example, Rabbi Yaacov Kravitz of the Center for Spiritual Intelligence explains that SI helps us find a moral and ethical path to help guide us through life.[9] SI also helps us in the search for meaning and purpose. Would you like to find out your own spiritual IQ? See the **Assess Yourself** activity at www.pearsonhighered.com/myhealthlab.

The Benefits of Spiritual Health

Since 2002 our understanding of the importance of the mind–body connection to human health and wellness has been increasing and that importance has been documented by a broad range of large-scale surveys.[10]

Physical Benefits

The emerging science of mind–body medicine is a research focus of the National Center for Complementary and Alternative Medicine (NCCAM) and an important objective of the organization's 2011–2015 Strategic Plan. One aspect being studied is the association between spiritual health and general health. The NCCAM cites evidence that mind–body practices can have a positive influence on health and suggests that the connection may

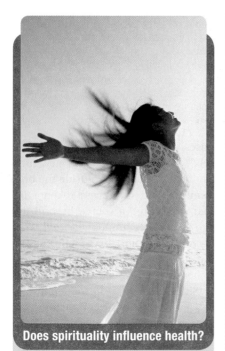

Does spirituality influence health?

Spirituality is widely acknowledged to have a positive impact on health and wellness. Benefits range from reductions in overall morbidity and mortality to improved abilities to cope with illness and stress.

be due to improved immune function.[11] Increasing numbers of studies are showing that certain spiritual practices can affect the mind, body, and behavior in ways that have potential to treat many health problems and promote healthy behavior. Ongoing research is investigating the role spirituality plays in treating insomnia, substance abuse, specific pain conditions, irritable bowel syndrome, obesity, and more.[12]

Some researchers believe that a key to understanding the improved health and longer life of spiritually healthy people is their greater self-control and mindfulness training. People who are more spiritually healthy and incorporate mind–body practices may have an increased capacity to engage in healthy behaviors and reduce the likelihood of overeating, smoking, and abusing alcohol and other drugs. They may also be better able to cope with stress on a daily basis.[13]

When we do get sick, the National Cancer Institute (NCI) contends that spiritual or religious well-being may help restore health and improve quality of life as follows:

- Decreasing anxiety, depression, anger, discomfort, and feelings of isolation
- Decreasing alcohol and drug abuse
- Decreasing blood pressure and the risk of heart disease
- Increasing the person's ability to cope with the effects of illness and with medical treatments
- Increasing feelings of hope and optimism, freedom from regret, satisfaction with life, and inner peace[14]

Several studies show an association between spiritual health and a person's ability to cope with a variety of physical illnesses as well as with cancer.[15] For example, a study of cardiac patients showed a benefit related to spiritual health and mind–body techniques.[16] Researchers have also looked into the overall association between spiritual practices and mortality, and a review of over a decade of research studies indicated that individuals who incorporate spiritual practices regularly have a significant reduction in mortality and risk of cardiovascular events.[17]

Psychological Benefits

Current research also suggests that spiritual health contributes to psychological health. For instance, the NCI and independent studies have found that spirituality reduces levels of anxiety and depression.[18] And certain spiritual practices, such as yoga, deep meditation, and other mindfulness practices, can have positive physiological effects on the body.[19]

People who have found a spiritual community also benefit from increased social support. For instance, participation in religious services, charitable organizations, and social gatherings can help members avoid isolation. At such gatherings, clerics and others may offer spiritual support in regard to challenges that members may be facing. A community may include retired members who offer child care for working parents, meals for those with disabilities, or transportation to medical appointments. All such measures can contribute to members' overall feelings of security and belonging.

Stress Reduction Benefits

The NCI cites stress reduction as one probable mechanism among spiritually healthy people for improved health and longevity and for better coping with illness.[20] In addition, several small studies support the contention that positive religious practices support effective stress management.[21] And a recent study suggests that increasing mindfulness through meditation reduces stress levels not only in people with physical and mental disorders, but also in healthy people as well.[22]

What Can You Do to Focus on Your Spiritual Health?

Cultivating your spiritual side takes just as much work as becoming physically fit or improving your diet. Here, we introduce some ways to develop your spiritual health by training your body, expanding your mind, tuning in, and reaching out.

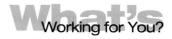
What's Working for You?

Maybe you're already focusing on enhancing your spiritual health. Do you incorporate any of the following behaviors into your daily life?

- ☐ I practice yoga.
- ☐ I meditate.
- ☐ I do volunteer work.
- ☐ I maintain healthy relationships.

Train Your Body

For thousands of years, in regions throughout the world, seekers have cultivated transcendence through physical means. One of the foremost examples is the practice of various forms of **yoga.** Although in the West we think of yoga as involving controlled breathing and physical postures, traditional forms also emphasize meditation, chanting, and other practices that are believed to cultivate unity with the *Atman,* or Absolute.

If you are interested in exploring yoga, sign up for a class on campus, at your local YMCA, or at a yoga center. Choose a form that seems right to you: Some, such as *hatha yoga,* focus on developing flexibility, deep breathing, and tranquility, whereas others, such as *ashtanga yoga,* are fast-paced and demanding and thus more appropriate for developing physical fitness than spiritual health. (See **Chapter 3** and **Chapter 9** for more on various styles of yoga.) For your first class, dress comfortably in fabrics that are somewhat close-fitting but that allow movement so when you bend at the waist or lift your leg, you won't feel constricted or exposed. No shoes or socks are worn. Some facilities provide yoga mats, or you may be asked to bring your own. The instructor will likely begin the class with a series of gentle warm-up poses and then add more challenging poses with coordinated breathing to align, stretch, and invigorate each body region. Classes usually conclude with several minutes of relaxation and deep breathing.

Training your body to improve your spiritual health doesn't necessarily require you to engage in a formal practice such as yoga. By energizing your body and sharpening your mental focus, jogging, biking, aerobics, dance, or any other exercise you do regularly can contribute to your spiritual health. The Eastern meditative movement practices of tai chi or qigong can also increase physical activity and mental focus. Both have been shown to have beneficial effects on bone health, cardiopulmonary fitness, balance, and quality of life. To transform exercise into a spiritual workout, begin by acknowledging gratitude for your body and its abilities, and throughout the session, maintain mindfulness of your breathing. (We'll say more about mindful breathing in the later discussion on meditation.)

You can also cultivate spirituality through fully engaging your body's senses. In fact, you can think of vision, hearing, taste, smell, and touch as five portals to spiritual health. Viewing an engaging piece of art or listening to beautiful music can calm the mind and

yoga System of physical and mental training involving controlled breathing, physical postures *(asanas)*, meditation, chanting, and other practices believed to cultivate unity with the *Atman,* or Absolute.

senses—smelling freshly cut grass, listening to the birds, and photographing the flowers.

The flip side of cultivating your senses is depriving them! Closing your eyes and sitting in silence removes the distraction of visual and auditory stimuli, helping you to focus within. To take advantage of silence, turn off your cell phone and take a long, solitary walk. You might even spend a weekend at one of the many retreat centers throughout the United States. To find one, see the listings at www.SpiritSite.com.

Expand Your Mind

For many people, psychological counseling is a first step toward improving their spiritual health. Therapy helps you let go of past hurts, accept your limitations, manage stress and anger, reduce anxiety and depression, and take control of your life—all steps toward spiritual growth. If you've never engaged in therapy, making the first appointment can feel daunting. Your campus health department can usually help by providing a referral.

Another practical way to expand your mind is to study the sacred texts of the world's major religions and spiritual practices. Many find guidance in the writings of great spiritual teachers. Libraries and bookstores are filled with volumes that explore the diverse approaches humans take to achieving spiritual fulfillment.

Finally, you can expand your awareness of different spiritual practices by exploring on-campus meditation or service-oriented groups, taking classes in spiritual or religious subjects, attending meetings

15.8 million

U.S. adults practice yoga, according to a recent survey by *Yoga Journal.*

soothe the spirit. A key reason that Lia, in our opening story, finds sustenance in nature is that she fully engages her

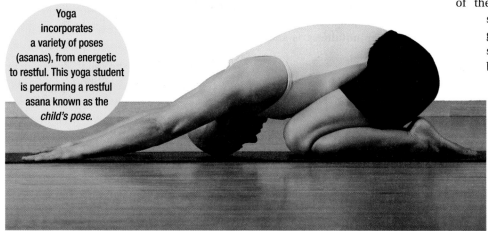

Yoga incorporates a variety of poses (asanas), from energetic to restful. This yoga student is performing a restful asana known as the *child's pose.*

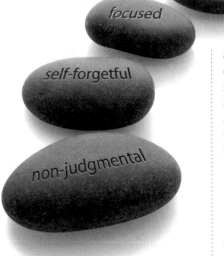

FIGURE 2 Qualities of Mindfulness

or services of area churches, attending public lectures, and checking out the websites of various spiritual and religious organizations. In each case, you can evaluate the messages and ideas you encounter and decide which practices or beliefs hold meaning for you.

contemplation Practice of concentrating the mind on a spiritual or ethical question or subject, a view of the natural world, or an icon or other image representative of divinity.

mindfulness Practice of purposeful, nonjudgmental observation in which we are fully present in the moment.

Tune in to Yourself and Your Surroundings

Focusing on your spiritual health has been likened to tuning in on a radio: Inner wisdom is perpetually available to us, but if we fail to tune our "receiver," we won't be able to hear it through all the "static" of daily life. Fortunately, four ancient practices still in use today can help you tune in. These are contemplation (studying), mindfulness (observing), meditation (emptying), and prayer (communing with the Divine).

Contemplation

If you were to look up the word *contemplation* in a dictionary, you'd find that it means a study of something—whether a candle flame or a theory of quantum mechanics. In the domain of spirituality, **contemplation** refers to concentrating the mind on a spiritual or ethical question or subject, a view of the natural world, or an icon or other image representative of divinity. For instance, a Zen Buddhist might contemplate a riddle, called a *koan,* such as, what is the sound of one hand clapping? A Sufi might contemplate the 99 names of God. A Roman Catholic might contemplate an image of the Virgin Mary. Spiritual people with no religious affiliation might contemplate the natural world, a favorite poem, or an ethical question such as, what is the origin of evil? Most religious and spiritual traditions advocate engaging in the contemplation of gratitude, forgiveness, and unconditional love.

When practicing contemplation, it can be helpful to keep a journal to record any insights that arise, and journaling itself can be a form of contemplation. For example, you might want to make a list of 20 things in your life you are grateful for or write a poem of forgiveness for yourself or a loved one. You might also use your journal to record inspirational quotations that you encounter in your readings. Journaling can fill a larger role in spiritual health and development by providing a sense of overall calmness.

Mindfulness

Mindfulness A practice of focused, nonjudgmental observation, **mindfulness** is the ability to be fully present in the moment (Figure 2). If you have ever been immersed in a moment, experiencing it completely with all your senses, this is mindfulness. You could be watching a sunset, listening to a great pianist, or even perfecting your golf swing. In any case, mindfulness is an awareness of present-moment reality—a holistic sensation of being totally involved in the moment rather than focused on some worry or being on "autopilot."[23]

So how do you practice mindfulness? The range of opportunities is as infinite as the moments of our lives. Living mindfully means to allow ourselves to become more deeply and completely aware of what we are sensing in each moment.[24] For instance, the next time you are going to eat an orange, pay attention! What does it feel like to pierce the skin with your thumbnail? Do you smell the scent of the orange as you peel it? What does the rind really look like? How do the drops of juice splatter as you pull apart the segments? What does it taste like, and how does the taste change from the first bite to the last?

Pursuing almost any endeavor that requires close concentration can help you develop mindfulness. Think of physical and mental challenges, such as a competitive diver leaping from the board or a physician attempting a difficult diagnosis. Or consider creative and performing arts such as sculpting, painting, writing, dancing, or playing a musical instrument. Even household activities such as cooking or cleaning can foster mindfulness—as long as you pay attention while you do them!

Even the most mundane activities—such as peeling and eating an orange—can have spiritual value if done mindfully.

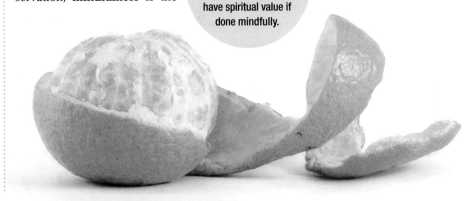

In this era of global environmental concerns, we can also cultivate mindfulness by paying attention to how our choices affect our world. This doesn't only mean recycling soda cans and taking the subway instead of driving. Those are easy examples. Instead, mindfulness of our environment calls on us to examine our values and behaviors as we share our Earth every moment of each day.

Meditation **Meditation** is a practice of emptying the mind, of cultivating stillness. Although the precise details vary with different schools of meditation, the fundamental task is the same: to quiet the mind's noise (referred to as "chatter," "static," or "monkey mind").

Why would you want to cultivate stillness? For thousands of years, human beings of different cultures and traditions have found that achieving periods of meditative stillness each day enhances their spiritual health. Today, researchers are beginning to discover why. The NCCAM reports that by using brain-scanning techniques, researchers found that experienced meditators show a significantly increased level of *empathy,* the ability to understand and share another person's experience.[25] Similarly, a recent study found that meditation increased the capacity for forgiveness among college students.[26] And there are other benefits, too. Studies suggest that meditation improves the brain's ability to process information; reduces stress, anxiety, and depression; improves concentration; and decreases blood pressure.[27] For more on what happens to the body during meditation, see the **Student Health Today** box on page 66.

what do you think?

Why do you think mindfulness practices are gaining more recognition?

● What are benefits of mindfulness?
● In today's fast-paced, multitasking world, do you think it is challenging to practice mindfulness on a regular basis?

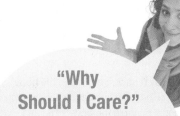

"Why Should I Care?"

Practicing meditation can improve concentration and your brain's ability to process information; it can also reduce stress, anxiety, and depression, all important factors when trying to manage your classes and handle daily demands.

So how do you meditate? Detailed instructions are beyond the scope of this text, but most teachers suggest beginning by sitting in a quiet place with low lighting where you won't be interrupted. Many advocate assuming a "full lotus" position, with legs bent fully at the knees, each ankle over the opposite knee. However, this position can be painful for beginners and those with poor flexibility or joint pain. Thus, you may want to assume a modified lotus position, with your legs simply crossed in front of you. Lying down is not recommended because you may fall asleep. Rest your hands on your knees, palms upward. Beginners usually find it easier to meditate with the eyes closed.

Once you're in position, it's time to start emptying your mind. The various schools of meditation teach different methods to achieve this. For example:

● **Mantra meditation.** Focus on a *mantra,* a single word such as *Om, Amen, Love,* or *God* and repeat this word silently. When a distracting thought arises, simply set it aside. It may help to imagine the thought as a leaf, and visualize placing it on a gently flowing stream that carries it away. Do not fault yourself for becoming distracted. Simply notice the thought, release it, and return to your mantra.
● **Breath meditation.** Count each breath: Pay attention to each inhalation, the brief pause that follows, and

the exhalation. Together, these equal one breath. When you have counted ten breaths, return to one. As with mantra meditation, as distractions arise, release them and return to the breath.
● **Color meditation.** When your eyes are closed, you may perceive a field of color, such as a deep, restful blue. Focus on this color. Treat distractions as in other forms of meditation.
● **Candle meditation.** With your eyes open, focus on the flame of a candle. Allow your eyes to soften as you meditate on this object. Treat distractions as in other forms of meditation.

After several minutes of meditation, and with practice, you may come to experience a sensation sometimes described as "dropping down," in which you feel yourself release into the meditation. In this state, which can be likened to a wakeful sleep, distracting thoughts are far less likely to arise, and yet you may receive surprising insights.

meditation Practice of emptying the mind of thought.

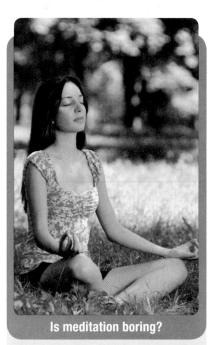

Is meditation boring?

Once you get the hang of it, meditation is anything but boring. As expert Jon Kabat-Zinn notes, "[When] you pay attention to boredom, it gets unbelievably interesting."

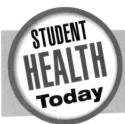

WHAT DOES MEDITATION DO TO THE BODY AND MIND?

The contemplative state of meditation has long been praised as a method of attaining peace and centeredness in life. Research suggests it can also be as good for the body as it is for the psyche. For example, one study found African Americans with coronary artery disease who took part in transcendental meditation had a 43% reduction in risk for mortality from myocardial infarction and stroke compared to a similar group who did not meditate. How can a spiritual practice related to thinking be good for the body?

While people have meditated for spiritual reasons for generations, the exact physiological processes still remain only partially understood. One theory suggests medita-tion works by reducing activity in the body's sympathetic nervous system, which, among other things, controls the body's "fight or flight" stress response. When under stress the body reacts by raising heart rate, increasing breaths, and constricting blood vessels. Over the long run, too much stress can lead to both increased wear and tear on the body and a harried, exhausted outlook on life. By practicing deep, calm contemplation, people who meditate seem to promote parasympathetic nervous system activity, which leads to slower breathing, lower blood pressure, and easier digestion, along with the long-touted spiritual benefits.

Finally, evidence suggests that meditating changes the brain itself. Some studies indicate people that meditate have increased gray and white matter, as well as more gyrification, or folds in the brain, than nonmeditators.

Sources: R. Schneider, S. Nidich, J. M. Kotchen, T. Kotchen, C. Grim, M. Rainforth, C. G. King, and J. Salerno, "Effects of Stress Reduction on Clini-cal Events in African Americans With Coronary Heart Disease: A Randomized Controlled Trial," *Circulation* (2009), 120: S461; "Meditation: An Introduction," National Center for Complemen-tary and Alternative Medicine, *National Institutes of Health,* 2010, http://nccam.nih.gov/health/meditation/overview.htm; E. Luders, F. Kurth, E. A. Mayer, A. W. Toga, K. L. Narr, and C. Gaser, "The Unique Brain Anatomy of Meditation Practition-ers: Alterations in Cortical Gyrification. *Frontiers in Human Neuroscience,* 6:34 (2012), DOI: 10.3389/fnhum.2012.00034.

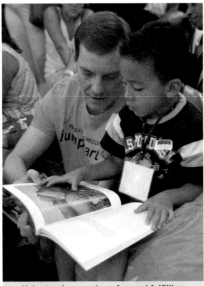

Volunteering can be a fun and fulfilling way to broaden your experience, connect with your community, and focus on your spiritual health.

prayer Communication with a transcendent Presence.

altruism Giving of oneself out of genuine concern for others.

Initially, try meditating for just 10 to 20 minutes, once or twice a day. In time, you can increase your sessions to 30 minutes or more. As you meditate for longer periods, you will likely find yourself feeling more rested and less stressed, and you may begin to experi-ence the increased levels of empathy recorded among expert meditators.

Prayer In **prayer,** rather than empty-ing the mind, an individual focuses the mind in communica-tion with a transcend-ent Presence. Spiritual traditions throughout the world distinguish several forms that this communication can take. For many, prayer offers a sense of com-fort, a sense that we are not alone. It can be the means of express-ing concern for others, for admission of trans-gressions, for seeking forgiveness, and for renewing hope and purpose. Focusing on the things we are grateful for can move people to look to the future with hope and give them the strength to get through the most challenging times.

Reach Out to Others

Altruism, the giving of oneself out of genuine concern for others, is a key aspect of a spiritually healthy lifestyle.

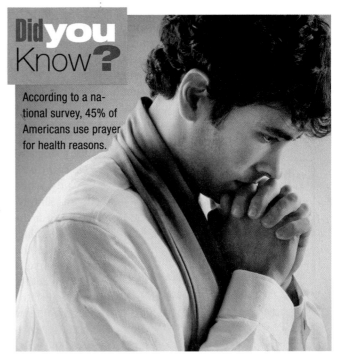

Did you Know?

According to a na-tional survey, 45% of Americans use prayer for health reasons.

39% of Americans meditate at least once a week.

Volunteering to help others, choosing to work for a nonprofit organization, donating money or other resources to a food bank or other program—even spending an afternoon picking up litter in your neighborhood—all of these are ways to serve others and simultaneously enhance your own spiritual and overall health. Researchers have referred to the benefits of volunteering as a "helpers high," or a distinct physical sensation associated with helping. About half of participants in one study reported that they feel stronger and more energetic after helping others; many also reported feeling calmer and less depressed, with increased feelings of self-worth.[28]

Community service can also take the form of **environmental steward-ship,** which the Environmental Protection Agency (EPA) defines as the responsibility for environmental quality shared by all those whose actions affect the environment. Responsibility manifests in action. Simple actions such as reducing and recycling packaging, turning off lights, making sure the heat or air-conditioning maintains an ecofriendly temperature, using energy-efficient lightbulbs and appliances, and taking shorter showers can make a difference.

Finding Your Spiritual Side through Service

Recognizing that we are all part of a greater system and that we have responsibilities to and for others is a key part of spiritual growth. Volunteering your time and energy is a great way to connect with others and help make the world a better place while improving your own health. Here are a few ideas:

〉 Offer to help elderly neighbors by providing lawn care or helping with simple household repairs.

〉 Volunteer with Meals on Wheels, a local soup kitchen, food bank, or other program that helps neighbors obtain adequate food.

〉 Organize or participate in an after-school or summertime activity for neighborhood children.

〉 Participate in a highway, beach, or neighborhood cleanup; restoration of park trails and waterways; or other environmental preservation projects.

〉 Volunteer at the local humane society walking dogs, caring for cats, helping with cleaning, or raising money for shelter programs.

〉 Apply to become a Big Brother or Big Sister and mentor a child who may face significant challenges or have poor role models.

〉 Join an organization working on a cause such as global warming or hunger, or start one yourself. Check out these inspiring examples: Students Against Global Apathy (SAGA) was founded by a University of Alberta student to confront global poverty and injustice; Students for the Environment (S4E) was founded by students at the University of Delaware to focus on local, national, and global environmental issues. The National Student Campaign Against Hunger and Homelessness is a project of student-level Public Interest Research Groups.

〉 Spend time volunteering in a neighborhood challenged by poverty, low literacy levels, or a natural disaster. Or volunteer with an organization such as Habitat for Humanity to build homes or provide other aid to developing communities.

To find out more information on service, the following are some online resources:

Ties community service to learning for K–12 through college: www.servicelearning.org
Locates service opportunities: www.volunteermatch.org
Lists overseas volunteer opportunities: www.projects-abroad.org
Oriented toward students: www.dosomething.org
Competition for money for service projects: www.truehero.org

For more strategies to enhance your spiritual health by reaching out to others, refer to the **Skills for Behavior Change** box.

environmental stewardship Responsibility for environmental quality shared by all those whose actions affect the environment.

Assess Yourself

What's Your Spiritual IQ?

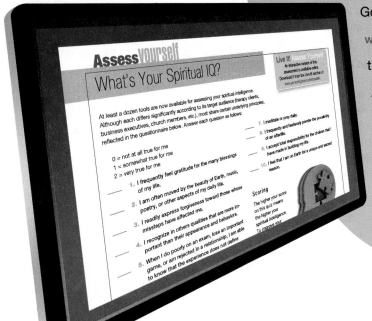

Assess Yourself
What's Your Spiritual IQ?

At least a dozen tools are now available for assessing your spiritual intelligence. Although each differs significantly according to its target audience (therapy clients, business executives, church members, etc.), most share certain underlying principles, reflected in the questionnaire below. Answer each question as follows:

0 = not at all true for me
1 = somewhat true for me
2 = very true for me

1. I frequently feel gratitude for the many blessings of my life.
2. I am often moved by the beauty of Earth, music, poetry, or other aspects of my daily life.
3. I readily express forgiveness toward those whose missteps have affected me.
4. I recognize in others qualities that are more important than their appearance and behaviors.
5. When I do poorly on an exam, lose an important game, or am rejected in a relationship, I am able to know that the experience does not define me.
6. I meditate or pray daily.
7. I frequently and fearlessly ponder the possibility of an afterlife.
8. I accept total responsibility for the choices that I have made in building my life.
9. I feel that I am on Earth for a unique and sacred reason.

Scoring
The higher your score on this quiz means the higher your spiritual intelligence. To improve your

Go online to the **Live It!** section of www.pearsonhighered.com/donatelle to take the "What's Your Spiritual IQ?" assessment.* Afterwards, you can formulate a plan to further develop your spirituality by following the steps outlined in the **YOUR PLAN FOR CHANGE** box.

*If your instructor so chooses, Assess Yourself Activities are available as a printed supplement or as assignable homework online at www.pearsonhighered.com/myhealthlab.

MyHealthLab®

YOUR PLAN FOR CHANGE

The **Assess Yourself** activity gives you the chance to evaluate your spiritual intelligence, and the text introduced you to some practices used successfully by millions over many generations to enhance their spiritual health. If you are interested in further cultivating your spirituality, consider some of the small but significant steps listed below to start on your journey.

Today, you can:

○ Find a quiet spot, turn off your cell phone, close your eyes, and contemplate, meditate, or pray for 10 minutes. Or spend 10 minutes in quiet mindfulness of your surroundings.

○ In a journal or on your computer, compile a list of things you are grateful for. Today, list at least ten things. Include people, pets, talents and abilities, achievements, places, foods . . . whatever comes to mind!

Within the next 2 weeks, you can:

○ Explore the options on campus for beginning psychotherapy, joining a spiritual or religious group, or volunteering with an organization working for positive change.

○ Think of a person in your life with whom you have experienced conflict. Spend a few minutes contemplating forgiveness toward this person and then write a letter or e-mail apologizing for any offense and offering your forgiveness in return. Wait a day or two before deciding whether you are truly ready to send the message.

By the end of the semester, you can:

○ Develop a list of several spiritual texts you would like to read during your break.

○ Begin exploring options for volunteer work that would serve others and have meaning for you.

References

1. A. Asten, H. Asten, and J. Lindholm, *Cultivating the Spirit: How College Can Enhance Students' Inner Lives* (San Francisco: Jossey-Bass, 2010).

2. National Cancer Institute, "General Information on Spirituality," Modified August 2011, www.cancer.gov/cancertopics/pdq/supportivecare/spirituality/Patient/page1.

3. H. G. Koenig, *Medicine, Religion and Health* (West Conshohocken, PA: Templeton Foundation Press, 2008).

4. Ibid.

5. Pew Forum, "Religion Among the Millenials," 2010, www.pewforum.org/Age/Religion-Among-the-Millennials.aspx

6. Ibid.

7. B. L. Seaward, *Managing Stress: Principles and Strategies for Health and Well Being*, 7th ed. (Sudbury, MA: Jones and Bartlett, 2012).

8. DanahZohar.com, "Learn the Qs," Accessed January 2012, http://dzohar.com/?page_id=622.

9. Center for Spiritual Intelligence, What Is SI?, 2008, http://spiritualintelligence.com/?page_id=7.

10. National Institutes of Health, National Center for Complementary and Alternative Medicine, "Exploring the Science of Complementary and Alternative Medicine: Third Strategic Plan: 2011–2015,": NIH Publication No. 11-7643, D458, February 2011, http://nccam.nih.gov/about/plans/2011/objective1.htm.

11. Ibid.

12. Ibid.

13. M. E. McCullough and B. L. B. Willoughby, "Religion, Self-Regulation, and Self-Control: Associations, Explanations, and Implications," *Psychological Bulletin* 135, no. 1 (2009): 69–93.

14. National Cancer Institute (NCI), "Spirituality in Cancer Care," August 2011, www.cancer.gov/cancertopics.pqd/supportivecare/spirituality/patient.

15. C. Lysne, and A. Wachholtz, "Pain, Spirituality and Meaning Making: What Can We Learn from the Literature?" *Religions*, no. 2 (2011): 1–16, DOI:10.3390/rel2010001; H. Koenig and A. Bussing, "Spiritual Needs of Patients with Chronic Diseases." *Religions* 1, no. 1 (2010): 18–27.

16. ClinicalTrials.gov, "Mind–Body Interventions in Cardiac Patients," Retrieved 2011, http://clinicaltrials.gov/ct2/show/NCT01270568.

17. G. Lucchetti, A. Lucchetti, and H. Koenig, "Impact of Spirituality/Religiosity on Mortality: Comparison with Other Health Interventions," *The Journal of Science and Healing* 7, no. 4 (2011): 234–38.

18. National Cancer Institute (NCI), "Spirituality in Cancer Care," August 2011, www.cancer.gov/cancertopics/pdq/supportivecare/spirituality/patient.

19. M. Javnbakht, R. Hejazi Kenari, and M. Ghasemi, "Effects of Yoga on Depression and Anxiety of Women," *Complementary Therapies in Clinical Practice* 15, no. 2 (2009); V. Conn, "The Power of Being Present: The Value of Mindfulness Interventions in Improving Health and Well-Being," *Western Journal of Nursing Research* 33 (2011): 993–95; Y. Matchim, J. Armer, and B. Stewart, "Breast Cancer Survivors Benefit from Practicing Mindfulness-Based Stress Reduction," *Western Journal of Nursing Research* 33, no. 8 (2011): 996–1016, first published on October 18, 2010.

20. Cancer Institute (NCI), "Spirituality in Cancer Care," Modified August 2011, www.cancer.gov/cancertopics/pdq/supportivecare/spirituality/patient; NCCAM, "Prayer and Spirituality in Health," 2005; NCI, "Spirituality in Cancer Care," 2009.

21. G. G. Ano and E. B. Vasconcelles, "Religious Coping and Psychological Adjustment to Stress: A Meta-Analysis," *Journal of Clinical Psychology* 61, no. 4 (2005): 461–80; U. Winter et al., "The Psychological Outcome of Religious Coping with Stressful Life Events in a Swiss Sample of Church Attendees," *Psychotherapy and Psychosomatics* 78, no. 4 (2009): 240–44; G. Lucchetti, "Impact of Spirituality/Religiosity," 2011 Y. Matchim, "Breast Cancer Survivors Benefit," 2011.

22. A. Chiesa and A. Serretti, "Mindfulness-Based Stress Reduction for Stress Management in Healthy People: A Review and Meta-Analysis," *Journal of Alternative and Complementary Medicine* 15, no. (2009): 593–600. G. Lucchetti, "Impact of Spirituality/Religiosity," 2011; Y. Matchim, "Breast Cancer Survivors Benefit," 2011.

23. G. Lucchetti, "Impact of Spirituality/Religiosity," 2011; Y. Matchim, "Breast Cancer Survivors Benefit," 2011.

24. D. Oman, S. Shapiro, C. Thoreson, T. Plante, and T. Flinders, "Meditation Lowers Stress and Supports Forgiveness among College Students: A Randomized Controlled Trial," *Journal of American College Health* 56, no. 5 (2008): 425–31.

25. National Center for Complementary and Alternative Medicine (NCCAM), "Research Spotlight: Meditation May Increase Empathy," Modified March 2011, http://nccam.nih.gov/research/results/spotlight/060608.htm.

26. D. Oman, "Meditation Lowers Stress and Supports Forgiveness," 2008.

27. NCCAM, "Research Spotlight," 2011; A. Chiesa and A. Serretti, "Mindfulness-Based Stress Reduction for Stress Management in Healthy People," 2009; N. Y. Winbush, C. R. Gross, and M. J. Kreitzer, "The Effects of Mindfulness-Based Stress Reduction on Sleep Disturbance: A Systematic Review," *EXPLORE: The Journal of Science and Healing* 3, no. 6 (2007): 585–91; N. E. Morone et al., "'I Felt Like a New Person.' The Effects of Mindfulness Meditation on Older Adults with Chronic Pain: Qualitative Narrative Analysis of Diary Entries," *Journal of Pain*, no. 9 (2008): 841–48. Y. Matchim, "Breast Cancer Survivors Benefit," 2011.

28. C. Carter, *Raising Happiness: 10 Simple Steps for More Joyful Kids and Happier Parents* (New York: Ballantine Publishing, 2010); R. I. Dunbar et al., "Social Laughter Is Correlated with an Elevated Pain Threshold," *Proceedings of the Royal Society,* September 14, 2011, DOI: 10.1098/rspb.2011.1373.39%

3

Managing Stress and Coping with Life's Challenges

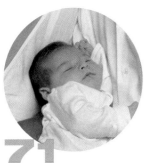

71 Isn't some stress healthy?

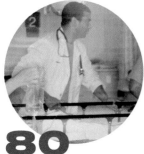

80 Who is most prone to stress?

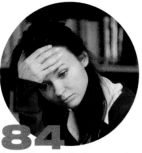

84 Are college students more stressed out than other groups?

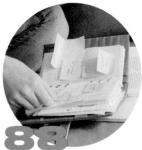

88 How can I manage my time more effectively?

OBJECTIVES

✳ Define stress and examine its potential impact on health, relationships, and success in college.

✳ Explain the phases of the general adaptation syndrome and the physiological changes that occur during them.

✳ Examine the physical, emotional, and social health risks that may occur with chronic stress.

✳ Discuss sources of stress and examine the unique stressors that affect college students.

✳ Explore stress-management techniques and ways to enrich your life with positive experiences and attitudes.

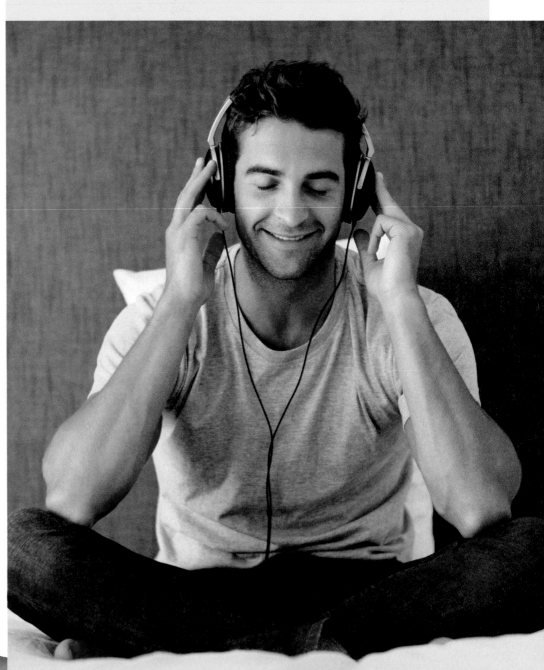

Rising tuition, roommates who bug you, dating anxiety, pressure to get good grades, money, and future career worries—they all lead up to STRESS! In today's fast-paced, 24/7 connected world, stress can cause us to feel overwhelmed. It can also push us to improve performance, bring excitement, and leave us exhilarated. While we work, play, socialize, and sleep, stress affects us in myriad ways, many of which we may not even notice.

According to a recent American Psychological Association poll, chronic stress that interferes with our ability to function normally over an extended period is becoming a public health crisis.[1] Nearly 75 percent of American adults reported experiencing unhealthy levels of stress in the last month and struggled to implement changes they believed would decrease stress and improve their lives.[2] Nearly half of American adults (44%) believe that their stress has increased over the past 5 years, affecting their personal and professional lives. As Norman B. Anderson, chief executive officer of the American Psychological Association said, "America is at a critical crossroads when it comes to stress and our health."[3]

The exact toll stress exerts on us during a lifetime of overload is unknown, but we know stress is a significant health hazard. It can rob the body of needed nutrients, damage the cardiovascular system, raise blood pressure, increase our risks for cancer and diabetes, and dampen the immune system's defenses. In addition, it can drain our emotional reserves and contribute to depression, anxiety, fatigue, and irritability, impacting relationships with friends, family, and coworkers. Importantly, research indicates that stress can take a major toll on kids, with over one third of children reporting they had suffered a stress-related health problem in the last month, such as headaches, stomachaches, difficulty sleeping, or other illnesses. Stress seems to be a particular threat to youth who are overweight. The higher the stress, the greater the chances of overeating, sleeping too much, and too much television, which in turn contributes to weight gain and more stress.

40%
of deaths in the United States are related wholly or in part to stress.

Is too much stress an inevitable negative part of life? Fortunately, the answer is no. We can learn to anticipate and recognize our personal stressors and develop skills to reduce or better manage those stressors we cannot avoid. First, we must understand what stress is and what effects it has on the body.

What Is Stress?

Most current definitions state that **stress** is the mental and physical response and adaptation by our bodies to the real or perceived changes and challenges in our lives. A **stressor** is any real or perceived physical, social, or psychological event or stimulus that causes our bodies to react or respond.[4] Several factors influence one's response to stressors including *characteristics of the stressor* (Can you control it? Is it predictable? Does it occur

stress A series of physiological responses and adaptations in response to a real or imagined threat to one's well-being.

stressor A physical, social, or psychological event or condition that upsets homeostasis and produces a stress response.

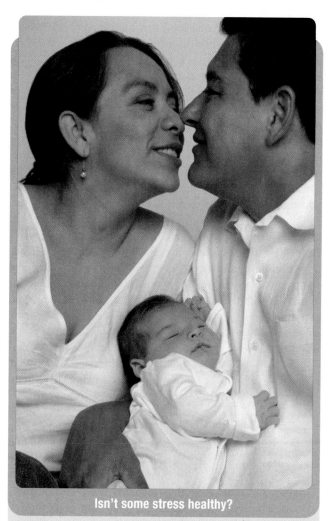

Isn't some stress healthy?

Absolutely! Stress isn't necessarily bad for you: Although events that cause prolonged *distress*, such as a natural disaster, can undermine your health, events that cause *eustress*, such as the birth of a child, can have positive effects on your growth and well-being. People usually live their lives to the fullest when they experience a moderate level of stress—just enough to keep them challenged and motivated—and deal with that stress in a productive manner. Just as too much stress can be detrimental to your health, too little stress leaves you stagnant and unfulfilled.

often?); *biological factors* (e.g., your age or gender); and *past experiences* (e.g., things that have happened to you, their consequences, and how you responded). Stressors may be tangible, such as a failing grade on a test, or intangible, such as the angst associated with meeting your significant other's parents for the first time. Importantly, stress is in the eye of the beholder: Each person's unique combination of heredity, life experiences, personality, and ability to cope influences how the person perceives an event and what meaning he or she attaches to it. What "stresses out" one person may not even bother the next person.

Generally, positive stress is called **eustress.** Eustress presents the opportunity for personal growth and satisfaction and can actually improve health. It can energize you, motivate you, and raise you up when you are down. Getting married or winning a major competition can give rise to the pleasurable rush associated with eustress. **Distress,** or negative stress, is caused by events that result in debilitative tension and strain, such as financial problems, the death of a loved one, academic difficulties, and the breakup of a relationship. In general, the most common manifestation of stress, **acute stress,** comes from demands and pressures of the recent past and anticipated demands and pressures of the near future.[5] Usually acute stress is intense, flares quickly, and disappears quickly without permanent damage to your health. Seeing someone you have a crush on could cause your heart to race and your muscles to tense while you appear cool, calm, and collected on the outside. The positive reaction to acute stress is that you rise to the occasion and put your most charming self forward. In contrast, anticipating a class presentation could cause shaking hands, nausea, headache, cramping, or diarrhea, along with a galloping heartbeat. When you finally make the presentation, the results are hurt by the stress: Your voice shakes horribly and you forget what you were going to say. Another form of stress is *episodic acute stress,* which describes the state of *regularly* reacting with wild, acute stress to various situations. Individuals experiencing episodic acute stress may complain about all they have to do and focus on negative events that may or may not come about. These "awfulizers" are often reactive and anxious, but their thoughts and behaviors can be so engrained that to them they seem normal. Others may regularly react with episodic outbursts that are over-the-top "chirpy" or happy, happy, happy, and they may not realize this is also a stress reaction. While types of acute stress can cause physical and emotional reactions, they may or may not result in negative physical or emotional outcomes. In contrast, **chronic stress** can linger indefinitely and wreak silent havoc on your body systems. Watching a loved one slowly lose a battle with cancer or heart disease can cause family members to have prolonged physiological stress responses while caring for the person and watching his or her suffering. Upon a loved one's eventual death, survivors may struggle to balance the need to process emotions such as anger, grief, loneliness, and guilt, while focusing to stay caught up in classes and with everyday life.[6] Sleep deprivation during times of emotional upset may result in more negative reactions to stressors.

eustress Stress that presents opportunities for personal growth; positive stress.

distress Stress that can have a detrimental effect on health; negative stress.

acute stress The short-term physiological response to an immediate perceived threat.

chronic stress An ongoing state of physiological arousal in response to ongoing or numerous perceived threats.

homeostasis A balanced physiological state in which all the body's systems function smoothly.

adaptive response Form of adjustment in which the body attempts to restore homeostasis.

general adaptation syndrome (GAS) The pattern followed in the physiological response to stress, consisting of the alarm, resistance, and exhaustion phases.

Body Responses to Stress

The body's physiological responses evolved to protect humans from harm. Thousands of years ago, if your ancestors didn't respond by fighting or fleeing, they might have been eaten by a saber-toothed tiger or killed by a marauding enemy clan. Today, when we face real or perceived threats, these same physiological responses are usually larger in scale than needed for the situation at hand, so our instinctual reactions must be contained or repressed. Continually having to "stuff" our reactions rather than letting them run their course can harm our health over time.

The General Adaptation Syndrome

When stress levels are low, the body is often in a state of **homeostasis:** All body systems are operating smoothly to maintain equilibrium. Stressors trigger a "crisis-mode" physiological response, after which the body attempts to return to homeostasis by means of an **adaptive response.** First characterized by Hans Selye in 1936, the internal fight to restore homeostasis in the face of a stressor is known as the **general adaptation syndrome (GAS)** (Figure 3.1). The GAS has three distinct phases: alarm, resistance, and exhaustion.[7]

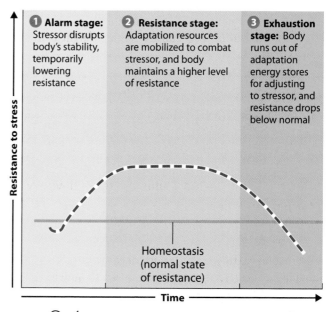

FIGURE 3.1 The General Adaptation Syndrome (GAS)
The GAS describes how we cope with prolonged stress.

Regardless of whether you are experiencing distress or eustress, similar physiological changes occur. The GAS can occur in varying degrees of intensity or time periods. Response to similar stressors varies among people. How an individual reacts depends on perceptions, learned responses, emotional and physiological health, and coping mechanisms.

Alarm Phase Suppose you are walking home after a night class on a dimly lit campus. You hear someone cough behind you and sense them approaching rapidly. You walk faster, only to hear the quickened footsteps of the other person. Your senses become increasingly alert, breathing quickens, heart races, and you begin to perspire. In desperation you stop, rip off your backpack, and prepare to fling it at your would-be attacker to defend yourself. You turn around and let out a blood-curdling yell. To your surprise, the person behind you is a classmate: She has been trying to stay close to you out of her own anxiety about walking alone in the dark. She screams and backs off the sidewalk, and you both stare at each other in startled embarrassment and burst into nervous laughter. You have just experienced the alarm phase of the GAS. Also known as the **fight-or-flight response,** this physiological reaction is one of our most basic, innate survival instincts.[8] (See Figure 3.2.)

When the mind perceives a real or imaginary stressor, the cerebral cortex, the region of the brain that interprets the nature of an event, triggers an **autonomic nervous system (ANS)** response that prepares the body for action. The ANS

fight-or-flight response Physiological arousal response in which the body prepares to combat or escape a real or perceived threat.

autonomic nervous system (ANS) The portion of the central nervous system regulating body functions that a person does not normally consciously control.

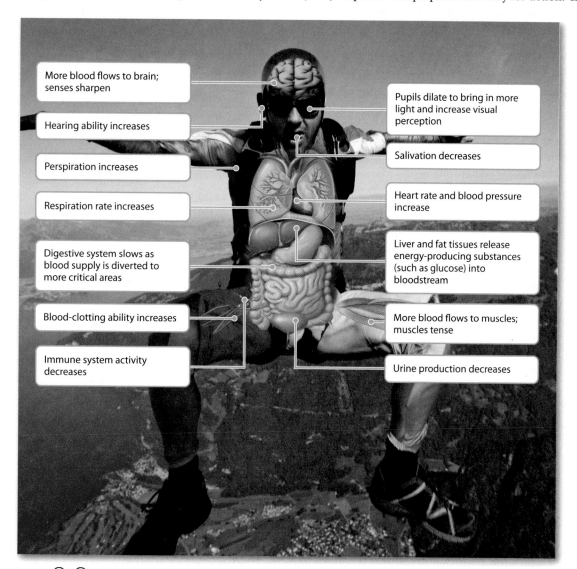

- More blood flows to brain; senses sharpen
- Hearing ability increases
- Perspiration increases
- Respiration rate increases
- Digestive system slows as blood supply is diverted to more critical areas
- Blood-clotting ability increases
- Immune system activity decreases
- Pupils dilate to bring in more light and increase visual perception
- Salivation decreases
- Heart rate and blood pressure increase
- Liver and fat tissues release energy-producing substances (such as glucose) into bloodstream
- More blood flows to muscles; muscles tense
- Urine production decreases

FIGURE 3.2 **The Body's Acute Stress Response**
Exposure to stress of any kind causes a complex series of involuntary physiological responses.

Video Tutor: Body's Stress Respose

is the portion of the central nervous system regulating body functions that we do not normally consciously control, such as heart and glandular functions and breathing.

The ANS has two branches: sympathetic and parasympathetic. The **sympathetic nervous system** energizes the body for fight or flight by signaling the release of several stress hormones. The **parasympathetic nervous system** functions to slow all the systems stimulated by the stress response—in effect, it counteracts the actions of the sympathetic branch.

The responses of the sympathetic nervous system to stress involve a series of biochemical exchanges between different parts of the body. The brain's **hypothalamus** functions as the control center of the sympathetic nervous system and determines the overall reaction to stressors. When the hypothalamus perceives that extra energy is needed to fight a stressor, it stimulates the adrenal glands, located near the top of the kidneys, to release the hormone **epinephrine,** also called *adrenaline*. Epinephrine causes more blood to be pumped with each beat of the heart, dilates the airways in the lungs to increase oxygen intake, increases the breathing rate, stimulates the liver to release more glucose (which fuels muscular exertion), and dilates the pupils to improve visual sensitivity. The body is then poised to act immediately.

In addition to the fight-or-flight response, the alarm phase can also trigger a longer-term reaction to stress. The hypothalamus uses chemical messages to trigger the pituitary gland within the brain to release a powerful hormone, *adrenocorticotropic hormone (ACTH)*. ACTH signals the adrenal glands to release **cortisol,** a hormone that makes stored nutrients more readily available to meet energy demands. Finally, other parts of the brain and body release endorphins, which relieve pain that a stressor may cause.

Resistance Phase In the resistance phase of the GAS, the body tries to return to homeostasis by resisting the alarm responses. However, because some perceived stressor still exists, the body does not achieve complete calm or rest. Instead, the body stays activated or aroused at a level that causes a higher metabolic rate in some organ tissues. For example, if a loved one develops an aggressive form of cancer, you may be wild with grief or anxiety after hearing the diagnosis and all of your systems may respond in the alarm phase. As you get used to the diagnosis, you calm down somewhat, but your body does not return completely to rest. The organs and systems of resistance are working overtime.

Exhaustion Phase A prolonged effort to adapt to the stress response leads to **allostatic load,** or exhaustive wear and tear on the body. In the exhaustion phase of the GAS, the physical and emotional energy used to fight a stressor has been depleted. You may feel tired or drained. As the body adjusts to chronic unresolved stress, the adrenal glands continue to release cortisol, which remains in the bloodstream for longer periods of time as a result of slower metabolic responsiveness. Over time, cortisol can reduce **immunocompetence,** or the ability of the immune system to respond to attack.[9]

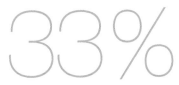

33%

of college students report their finances have been very difficult to handle during the past year.

Life Effects of Stress

Much has been written about the negative effects of stress, but researchers have only recently begun to untangle the complex web of physiological and emotional responses that can take a toll on a person's physical, intellectual, and emotional well-being. Stress is often described as a "disease of prolonged arousal" that leads to a cascade of negative health effects. The longer you are chronically stressed, the more likely will be the negative health effects. Nearly all body systems become potential targets, and the long-term effects may be devastating. Some warning symptoms of prolonged stress are shown in **Figure 3.3** on page 75.

Physical Effects of Stress

The higher the levels of stress you experience, the greater the likelihood of damage to your physical health.[10] Studies have shown that 40 percent of deaths and 70 percent of diseases in the United States are related, in whole or in part, to stress.[11] The list of ailments related to chronic stress includes such problems as heart disease, diabetes, cancer, headaches, ulcers, low back pain, depression, and the common cold. Increases in rates of suicide, mental illness, homicide, and domestic violence across the United States are additional symptoms of a nation under stress.

Stress and Cardiovascular Disease Perhaps the most studied and documented health consequence of unresolved stress is cardiovascular disease (CVD). Research on this topic demonstrates the impact of chronic stress on heart rate, blood pressure, heart attack, and stroke.[12] The largest

sympathetic nervous system Branch of the autonomic nervous system responsible for stress arousal.

parasympathetic nervous system Branch of the autonomic nervous system responsible for slowing systems stimulated by the stress response.

hypothalamus A structure in the brain that controls the sympathetic nervous system and directs the stress response.

epinephrine Also called *adrenaline*, a hormone that stimulates body systems in response to stress.

cortisol Hormone released by the adrenal glands that makes stored nutrients more readily available to meet energy demands.

allostatic load Wear and tear on the body caused by prolonged or excessive stress responses.

immunocompetence The ability of the immune system to respond to attack.

epidemiological study to date, the IN-TERHEART Study, with almost 30,000 participants in 52 countries, identified stress as one of the key modifiable risk factors for heart attack.[13]

Historically, the increased risk of CVD from chronic stress has been linked to increased arterial plaque buildup due to elevated cholesterol, hardening of the arteries, alterations in heart rhythm, increased and fluctuating blood pressures, and difficulties in cardiovascular responsiveness due to all of the above.[14] In the past two decades, research into the relationship between stress and CVD contributors has shown direct links between the incidence and progression of CVD and stressors such as job strain, caregiving, bereavement, and natural disasters.[15] (For more information about CVD, see **Chapter 15.**)

Stress and Weight Gain If you think that when you are extremely stressed, you tend to eat more and gain weight, you didn't imagine it. Higher stress levels may increase cortisol levels in the bloodstream. Because cortisol contributes to increased hunger and seems to activate fat-storing enzymes, people who are stressed may get a double whammy of risks from higher-circulating cortisol levels. Animal and human studies, including those in which subjects suffer from post-traumatic stress, seem to support the theory that cortisol plays a role in laying down extra belly fat and increasing eating behaviors.[16]

Stress and Alcohol Dependence New research from Scripps Research Institute has found a specific stress hormone, the corticotropin-releasing factor (CRF), is key to the development and maintenance of alcohol dependence in animals. CRF is a natural

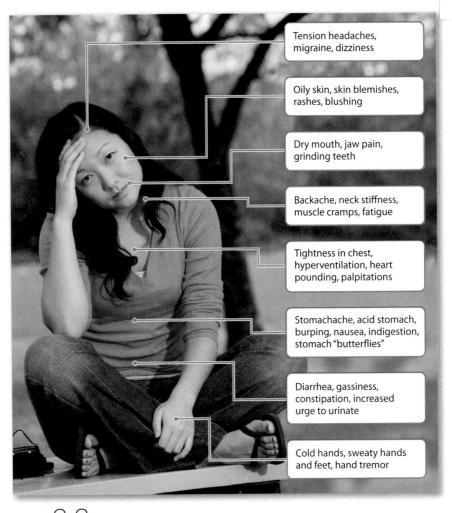

FIGURE 3.3 **Common Physical Symptoms of Stress**
Sometimes you may not even notice how stressed you are until your body starts sending you signals. Do you frequently experience any of these physical symptoms of stress?

Tension headaches, migraine, dizziness

Oily skin, skin blemishes, rashes, blushing

Dry mouth, jaw pain, grinding teeth

Backache, neck stiffness, muscle cramps, fatigue

Tightness in chest, hyperventilation, heart pounding, palpitations

Stomachache, acid stomach, burping, nausea, indigestion, stomach "butterflies"

Diarrhea, gassiness, constipation, increased urge to urinate

Cold hands, sweaty hands and feet, hand tremor

substance involved in the body's stress response, stimulating the secretion of various stress hormones.[17] If found to be true in humans as well as animals, new avenues for tackling both alcohol and stress problems may open up. Stay tuned on this topic!

Stress and Hair Loss Too much stress can lead to thinning hair, and even baldness, in men and women. The most common type of stress-induced hair loss is *telogen effluvium*. Often seen in individuals who have suffered a death in the family, had a difficult pregnancy, or experienced severe weight loss, this condition pushes colonies of hair to go into a resting phase. Over time (usually a few months), simply washing or combing the hair may cause clumps of it to fall out. A similar stress-related condition known as *alopecia areata* occurs when stress triggers white blood cells to attack and destroy hair follicles, usually in patches. If stress is prolonged, varying degrees of baldness may occur.[18]

Losing hair? Maybe you need to de-stress!

Stress and Diabetes Controlling stress levels is critical for preventing development of type 2 diabetes, as well as for successful short- and long-term diabetes management.[19] People under lots of stress often don't get enough sleep, don't eat well, and may drink or take other drugs to help them get through a stressful time. All of these behaviors can alter blood sugar levels and promote development of diabetes. Stress hormones may affect blood glucose levels directly. (For full information on diabetes and lifestyle variables that may contribute to it, see Focus On: Minimizing Your Risk for Diabetes.)

Stress and Digestive Problems Digestive disorders are physical conditions whose causes are often unknown. It is widely assumed that an underlying illness, pathogen, injury, or inflammation is already present when stress triggers nausea, vomiting, stomach cramps and related gut pain, or diarrhea. Although stress doesn't directly cause these symptoms, it is clearly related and may actually make your risk of having symptoms even worse.[20] For example, people with depression or anxiety are more susceptible to irritable bowel syndrome, probably because stress stimulates colon spasms via the nervous system. Some relaxation techniques, such as progressive muscle relaxation, meditation, and guided imagery (discussed later in this chapter) may be helpful in coping with stressors that make your digestive problems worse. These techniques promote relaxation by reducing the activity of the sympathetic nervous system, leading to decreases in heart rate, blood pressure, and other stress responses. Some earlier research also has indicated that relaxation may reduce gastrointestinal reactivity and decrease risks of gastrointestinal flare-ups.[21] More research is necessary to examine why this may be the case in some individuals and not in others.

Stress and Impaired Immunity A growing area of scientific investigation known as *psychoneuroimmunology (PNI)* analyzes the intricate relationship between the mind's response to stress and the immune system's ability to function effectively. (See more on PNI in **Chapter 2.**) Several recent reviews of research linking stress to

adverse health consequences suggest that too much stress over a long period can negatively affect various aspects of the cellular immune response, increasing risks for upper respiratory infections and certain chronic conditions, increasing adverse birth outcomes and fetal development, and exacerbating problems for children and adults suffering from post-traumatic stress.[22] How long do you have to be stressed to suffer from impaired immunity? A look at the research yields evidence of impaired immunity from the initial stress to as long as 6 months later following acute stressors such as arguments, public speaking, and academic examinations.[23] More prolonged stressors, such as socioeconomic disparities and prolonged economic uncertainty, devastating life events such as the loss of a spouse, exposure to a natural disaster, war, caregiving, or living with a chronic disease or handicap, also have been shown to impair the natural immune response among various populations over time.[24]

Stress and Libido Although we might think that a lack of interest in sex occurs only in older people and that young people enjoy constant, regular sex, too much stress can throw a big wrench in your sex life at any age and stage of life.

Intellectual Effects of Stress

In a recent national survey of college students, more than half of the respondents said that they had felt overwhelmed by all that they had to do within the past 2 weeks, with a similar number reporting they felt exhausted. Nearly 43 percent of students said they had experienced a larger than average amount of stress during the past year. Not surprisingly, these same students rated stress as their number one impediment to academic performance, followed by lack of sleep.[25] Stress can play a huge role in whether students

Prolonged stress can compromise the immune system, leaving you vulnerable to infection. If you spend exam week in a state of high stress, sleeping too little and worrying a lot, chances are you will reduce your body's ability to fight off cold and flu viruses.

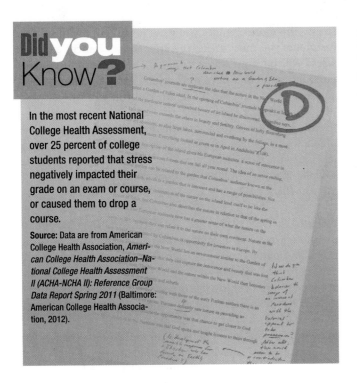
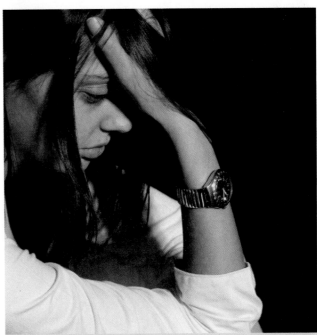

Stress and depression have complicated interconnections based on emotional, physiological, and biochemical processes. Prolonged stress can trigger depression in susceptible people, and prior periods of depression can leave individuals more susceptible to stress.

stay in school, get good grades, and succeed on their career path. It can also wreak havoc on students' ability to concentrate, remember key information for exams, and understand and retain complex information.

Stress, Memory, and Concentration Although the exact reasons stress can affect grades are complex, the mystery of how and why stress affects memory and concentration in humans is slowly unraveling. Animal studies have provided compelling indicators of how chronic exposure to glucocorticoids—stress hormones released from the adrenal cortex—are believed to affect cognitive functioning and overall mental health. In humans, acute stress has been shown to impair short-term memory, particularly verbal memory.[26] Exciting new studies have linked prolonged exposure to cortisol (a key stress hormone) to actual shrinking of the hippocampus, the brain's major memory center. In rats that were chronically stressed, the decision-making regions of the brain actually shriveled, whereas brain sectors responsible for habitual behaviors that didn't rely on memory increased.[27]

"Why Should I Care?"

Exposure to academic stress is associated with increased upper respiratory tract infections among students. Take time to de-stress, and you might avoid a bad cold.

Psychological Effects of Stress

Stress may be one of the single greatest contributors to mental disability and emotional dysfunction in industrialized nations. Studies have shown that the rates of mental disorders, particularly depression and anxiety, are associated with various environmental stressors from childhood through adulthood, including abuse, marital and relationship conflict, poverty, and other stressful life events.[28] In particular, stressful life events and inadequate sources of social support can contribute to mental disorders among people aged 15 to 24 more than among other age groups. Researchers suggest that as individuals move from adolescence into adulthood, they face increased stressors of all kinds, particularly those related to work, finances, school, lack of social support, loneliness, and problems in relationships, which may challenge their mental health.[29]

What Causes Stress?

On any given day, we all experience eustress and distress, usually from a wide range of obvious and not-so-obvious sources. Several studies in recent years have examined sources of stress among various populations in the United States and globally. One of the most comprehensive is conducted annually by the American Psychological Association; the 2010 survey found that concerns over money, work, the economy, family responsibilities, and relationships were major sources of stress among American adults (Figure 3.4, see page 78).[30] Those who were obese or perceived themselves to have health issues reported the most stress. College students, in particular, face stressors that come from internal sources, as well as external pressures to succeed in a competitive environment that is often geographically far from the support of family and lifelong friends. Awareness of the sources of stress can do much to help you develop a plan to avoid, prevent, and control the things that cause you stress.

Psychosocial Stressors

Psychosocial stressors refer to the factors in our daily routines and in our social and physical environments that cause us to experience stress. Key psychosocial stressors include adjustment to change, hassles, interpersonal relationships, academic and career pressures, frustrations and conflicts, overload, and stressful environments.

Adjustment to Change Any time change occurs in your normal routine, whether good or bad, you experience stress. The more changes you experience and the more adjustments you must make, the greater the chances are that stress will have an impact on your health. Unfortunately, although your first days on campus can be exciting, they can also be among the most stressful you will face in your life. Moving away from home, trying to fit in and make new friends from diverse backgrounds, adjusting to a new schedule, learning to live with strangers in housing that is often lacking in the comforts of home: All of these things can cause sleeplessness and anxiety and keep your body in a continual fight-or-flight mode.

Hassles: The Little Things That Bug You Some psychologists have proposed that little stressors, frustrations, and petty annoyances, known collectively as *hassles,* can be just as stressful as the major life changes.[31] Put another way, these cumulative hassles add up, taxing the physiological systems of the body and putting what is sometimes referred to as an *allostatic load* on the body that can result in health issues. Listening to classmates who talk too much during lecture, having to hear someone airing their dirty laundry on a loud cell phone call, not finding parking on campus, and a host of other bothersome situations can push your buttons and result in frustration, anger, and fight-or-flight responses.[32] For many people, the fast pace of technology creates new hassles and adds to their stress. See the **Tech & Health** box on the next page for more on technostress.

The Toll of Relationships Let's face it, relationships can trigger some of the biggest fight-or-flight reactions of all time. Remember that wild, exhilarating feeling of new love? You couldn't focus or sleep, and you didn't get much work done while thinking about your *new* love interest. Likewise, remember the breakups? Again, you couldn't focus, couldn't sleep, and didn't get much done while thinking about your *former* love interest. Love relationships are the ones we often think of first, but friends, family members, and coworkers can be the sources of overwhelming struggles, just as they can be sources of strength and support. The same can be said of other relationships, too. Coworker interactions and relationships can have their challenges; they can make us strive to be the best that we can be and give us hope for the future, keep us motivated to work harder and help build confidence and self-esteem, or they can diminish our self-esteem and leave us reeling from a destructive interaction. A recent comparison of nearly 80 studies of stress and work provides strong evidence that work situations with high demands, little control, and coworkers who are difficult

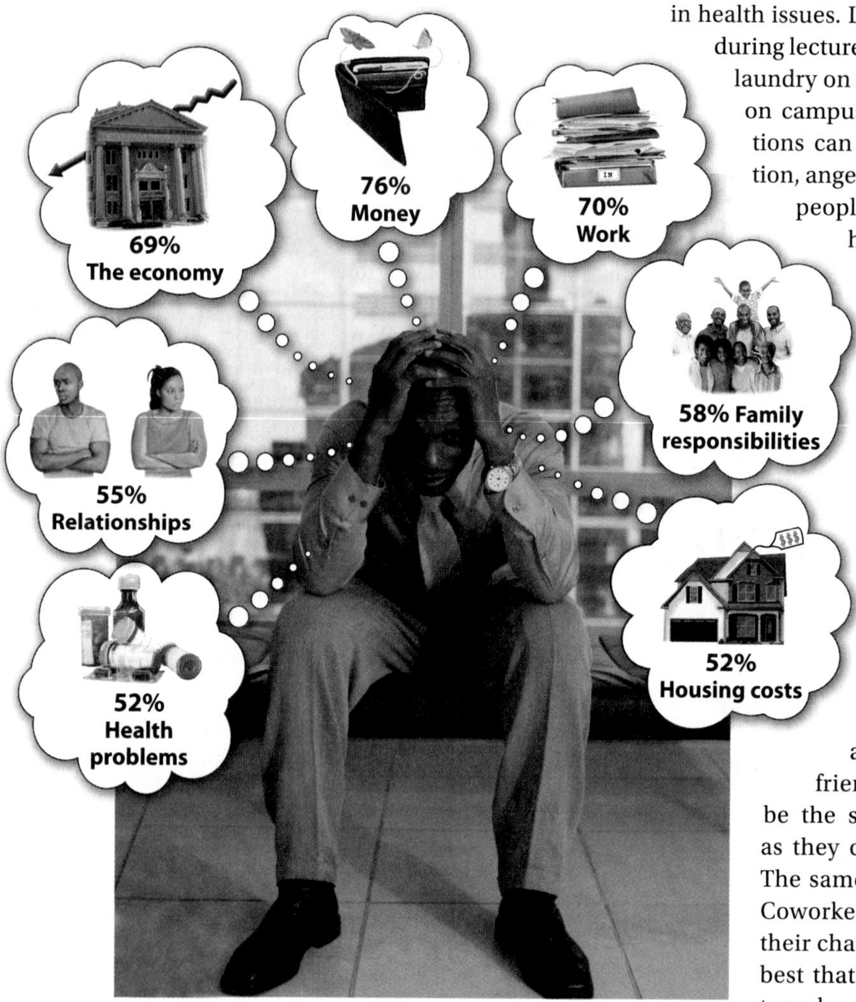

FIGURE 3.4 **What Do We Say Stresses Us?**
The annual *Stress in America* survey indicates American adults are increasingly experiencing money, work, and housing concerns as major sources of stress in their lives.

Source: Data are from the American Psychological Association, *2011 Stress in America, Key Findings,* 2012, www.apa.org/news/press/releases/stress/national-report.pdf.

69% The economy

76% Money

70% Work

58% Family responsibilities

55% Relationships

52% Housing costs

52% Health problems

Tech & Health
TAMING TECHNOSTRESS

Are you "twittered out"? Is all that texting causing your thumbs to seize up in protest? If so, you're not alone. Like millions of others, you may find that all of the pressure for contact is stressing you out! Known as *technostress,* this bombardment is defined as stress created by a dependence on technology and the constant state of connection, which can include a perceived obligation to respond, chat, or tweet.

There is much good that comes from all that technological wizardry. For some folks, however, technomania can become obsessive—when people would rather hang out online talking to strangers than study, talk to friends, socialize in person, or generally connect in the real world. Although technology can allow us to multitask, work on the go, and communicate in new and different ways, there are some clear downsides to all of that "virtual" interaction.

✳ **Social distress.** Authors Michell Weil and Larry Rosen describe *technosis,* a very real syndrome in which people become so immersed in technology that they risk losing their own identity. Worrying about checking your voice mail, constantly switching to e-mail or Facebook to see who has left a message

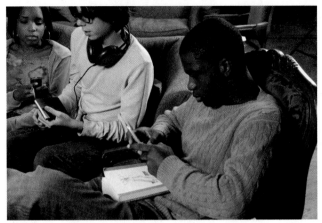
Technology may keep you in touch, but it can also add to your stress and take you away from real-world interactions.

or is online, perpetually posting to Twitter, and so on can keep you distracted and take important minutes or hours from your day.

✳ **Technology dependency.** Increasing research supports the concept that being "wired" 24/7 while studying, working, out with friends, driving, and in just about every other imaginable place can lead to mental overload, neglect of personal needs and activities, time pressures, guilt, physical symptoms, and economic problems. Couple that with frustrations when wireless connections fail or phones are lost, and stress levels can soar.

To avoid technosis and to prevent technostress, set time limits on your

technology usage and make sure that you devote at least as much time to face-to-face interactions with people you care about as a means of cultivating and nurturing your relationships. Screen your contacts, especially when you are in public or engaged in face-to-face communication with someone. You don't always need to answer your phone or respond to a text or e-mail immediately.

Leave your devices at home or turn them off when you are out with others or on vacation. If you can't leave your PDA, laptop, or cell phone at home—or turned off—when you are out with others, or on vacation, then there is a problem. Tune in to your surroundings, your loved ones and friends, your job, and your classes by shutting off your devices.

Sources: Insurance Institute for Highway Safety, Highway Loss Data Division. "Cellphone and Texting Laws," February 2012, www.iihs.org/laws/cellphonelaws.aspx; National Safety Council, "National Safety Council Estimates That at Least 1.6 Million Crashes Are Caused Each Year by Drivers Using Cell Phones and Texting," press release, January 12, 2010, www.nsc.org/Pages/NSCestimates16millioncrashescausedbydriversusingcellphonesandtexting.aspx; Governors Highway Safety Association, "Cell Phone and Texting Laws," 2010, www.ghsa.org/html/stateinfo/laws/cellphone_laws.html.

---

to get along with increase the likelihood of employee complaints about gastrointenstional ailments and sleep difficulties. Competition for rewards and systems that favor certain classes of employees or pit workers against one another are among the most stressful job situations.[33]

Academic and Financial Pressure

It isn't surprising that today's college and university students face mind-boggling amounts of pressure competing for grades, athletic positions, internships, and jobs. Challenging classes can be tough enough, but many students also work at least part-time to pay the bills. Today's economic downturn can have

major effects on college students and make distant dreams even harder to realize. When economic conditions become strained, the effects on people with limited resources (particularly students) can be significant. Increasing reports of mental health problems on college campuses may be one of the results of too much stress.

Frustrations and Conflicts

Whenever there is a disparity between our goals (what we hope to obtain in life) and our behaviors (actions that may or may not lead to these goals), frustration can occur. For example, you realize that you must get good grades in college to enter graduate school, which is your ultimate goal. If you know you should be getting good grades, but are having too much fun with friends when you should be studying, these inconsistencies between your goals and your behavior can cause significant stress.

Conflicts occur when we are forced to decide among competing motives, impulses, desires, and behaviors or when we are forced to face pressures of demands that are incompatible with our own values and sense of importance. College students who are away from their families for the first time may face a variety of conflicts among parental values, their own beliefs, and the beliefs of others who are very different from themselves.

Overload We've all experienced times in our lives when the demands of work, responsibilities, deadlines, and relationships all seem to be pulling us underwater with a 200-pound weight tied to our feet.

overload A condition in which a person feels overly pressured by demands.

background distressors Environmental stressors of which people are often unaware.

Overload occurs when, try as we might, there are not nearly enough hours in the day to do what we are required to do, and our physical, mental, and emotional reserves are not sufficient to deal with all we have on our plate. Students suffering from overload may experience depression, sleeplessness, mood swings, frustration, anxiety, or a host of other symptoms. Binge drinking; high consumption of junk foods; and fighting with friends, family, and coworkers can all add fuel to the overload fire. Unrelenting stress and overload can lead to a state of physical and mental exhaustion known as *burnout*.

Stressful Environments For many students, where they live and the environment around them cause significant levels of stress. Perhaps you cannot afford safe, healthy housing, or a bad roommate constantly makes life uncomfortable, or loud neighbors keep you up at night. Noise, pressure of people in crowded living situations, and uncertainties over food and whether you have a place to sleep can keep even the most resilient person on edge.

Although rare, natural disasters can devastate countries, cities, and communities, leaving individuals fighting for their very survival. Tsunamis, floods, earthquakes, hurricanes, tornadoes, and other disasters wreak havoc on our lives, causing extreme levels of environmentally induced stress. In the aftermath of disasters, events can spiral out of control, leaving food, water, and other resources vulnerable indefinitely. Imagine waking up to find that your family is missing, your home is wiped out, you have no cell phone or communication methods,

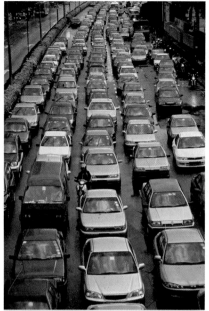

Traffic jams and noise pollution are examples of the daily hassles and frustrations that can add up and jeopardize our health.

your city and university are in shambles, and all you have are the clothes on your back! This type of stress would make that little spat you had with your roommate seem pretty insignificant in comparison. Often as damaging as one-time disasters are **background distressors** in the environment, such as noise, air, and water pollution; allergy-aggravating pollen and dust; and environmental tobacco smoke. As with other challenges, our bodies respond to environmental distressors with the GAS. People who cannot escape background distressors may exist in a constant resistance phase.

Bias and Discrimination Racial and ethnic diversity of students, faculty members, and staff enriches everyone's educational experience on campus. It also challenges us to examine our personal attitudes, beliefs, and biases. Students come to campus from vastly different backgrounds and with very different life experiences. Often, those perceived as dissimilar may become

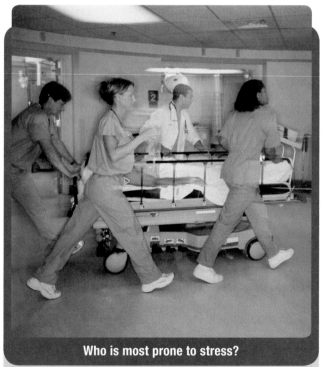

Who is most prone to stress?

Everyone experiences stress in his or her life, but some people have personalities and attitudes that leave them more susceptible, whereas others have careers or life circumstances that impose greater external pressures on them. Individuals such as doctors and nurses face long work hours and a high-stakes work environment, making them especially prone to stress, overload, and burnout.

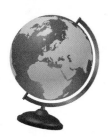

INTERNATIONAL STUDENT STRESS

International students experience unique adjustment issues such as language barriers, cultural barriers, and a lack of social support. Academic stress may pose a particular problem for the more than 670,000 international students who have left support networks of family and friends in their native countries to study in the United States. Accumulating evidence suggests seeking emotional support from others is one effective way to cope with stressful and upsetting situations. Yet, many international students feel ashamed to struggle and fear seeking support is a sign of weakness that calls inappropriate attention to both the individual and the respective ethnic group. This reluctance, coupled with cultural conflicts and other stressors, can lead international students to suffer significantly more stress-related illnesses than their American counterparts. Even if

Language barriers, cultural conflicts, racial prejudices, and a reluctance to seek social support all contribute to a significantly higher rate of stress-related illnesses among international students studying in the United States.

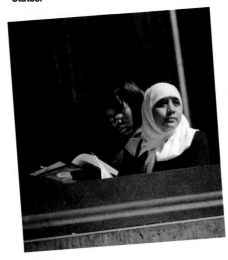

we can't solve the many problems international students encounter, there are things we can do to make one person's life (or maybe two or three persons' lives) a little less stressful: Share companionship and communication, and lend a helping hand. To paraphrase a popular Hindu proverb: "Help thy neighbor's boat across and thine own boat will also reach the shore."

Sources: S. Sumer, "International Students' Psychological and Sociocultural Adaptation in the United States," doctoral dissertation, Georgia State University, 2009, http://digitalarchive .gsu.edu/cps_diss/34; Institute of International Education, "Record Numbers of International Students in U.S. Higher Education," press release, November 16, 2009, http://opendoors .iienetwork.org/?p=150649; S. T. Mortenson, "Cultural Differences and Similarities in Seeking Social Support as a Response to Academic Failure: A Comparison of American and Chinese College Students," *Communication Education* 55, no. 2 (2006): 127–46.

victims of subtle and not-so-subtle forms of bigotry, insensitivity, harassment, or hostility, or they may simply be ignored. Whether real or perceived, race, ethnicity, religious affiliation, age, sexual orientation, or other "differences"—whether in viewpoints, appearance, behaviors, or backgrounds—may hang like a dark cloud over these students.[34] See the **Health in a Diverse World** box above for more on stress and international students.

Evidence of the health effects of excessive stress in minority groups abounds. For example, African Americans suffer higher rates of hypertension, CVD, and most cancers than do whites.[35] Although poverty and socioeconomic status have been blamed for much of the spike in hypertension rates for African Americans and other marginalized groups, this chronic, physically debilitating stress may reflect real and perceived effects of institutional racism rather than individual/interpersonal poverty and perceived racism. More research is necessary to show direct associations between racism, stress, and hypertension; however, it is important to realized that all types of

"isms" may influence stress-related hypertension and make it more difficult for those affected to engage in healthy lifestyle behaviors.[36]

Internal Stressors

Although stress can come from the environment and other external sources, it can result from internal factors as well. Internal stressors such as negative appraisal, low self-esteem, and low self-efficacy can cause unsettling thoughts or feelings and can ultimately affect your health.[37] It is important to address and manage these internal stressors.

Appraisal and Stress Throughout life, we encounter many different types of demands and potential stressors—

> ## what do you think?
> **Do you get stressed out by things in your home or school environment?**
> ● Which environmental stressors bug you the most?
> ● When you encounter these environmental stressors, what actions do you take, if any?

See It! Videos

Put down that cell phone! Watch **The Multi-Tasking Myth** at www.pearsonhighered.com/donatelle to understand why doing multiple things at once might not be the best idea.

some biological, some psychological, and others sociological. In any case, it is our appraisal of these demands, not the demands themselves, that results in our experiencing stress. **Appraisal** is defined as the interpretation and evaluation of information provided to the brain by the senses. As new information becomes available, appraisal helps us recognize stressors, evaluate them on the basis of past experiences and emotions, and decide whether or not we have the ability to cope. When you feel that the stressors of life are overwhelming and you lack control, you are more likely to feel strain and distress.

appraisal The interpretation and evaluation of information provided to the brain by the senses.

suicidal ideation A desire to die and thoughts about suicide.

hostility The cognitive, affective, and behavioral tendencies toward anger and cynicism.

Self-Esteem and Self-Efficacy As we learned in Chapters 1 and 2, *self-esteem* refers to how you feel about yourself. Self-esteem varies; it can and does continually change.[38] When you feel good about yourself, you are less likely to respond to or interpret an event as stressful and more likely to be able to cope when you are stressed.[39] Of particular concern, research with high school and college students has found that low self-esteem and stressful life events significantly predict **suicidal ideation,** a desire to die and thoughts about suicide. On a more positive note, research has also indicated that it is possible to increase an individual's ability to cope with stress by increasing self-esteem.[40] (In **Chapter 2** we discussed several ways to develop and maintain self-esteem.)

Self-efficacy, also introduced in earlier chapters, is another important factor in the ability to cope with life's challenges. Self-efficacy refers to belief or confidence in one's skills and performance abilities.[41] Self-efficacy is considered one of the most important personality traits that influences psychological and physiological stress responses.[42] Developing self-efficacy is also vital to coping with and overcoming academic pressures and worries. For example, by learning to handle anxiety around testing situations, you improve your chances of performing well; the more you feel yourself capable to handle testing situations, the greater will be your sense of academic self-efficacy. For tips on how to deal with test-taking anxiety and build your testing self-efficacy, see the Skills for Behavior Change box.

Type A and Type B Personalities It should come as no surprise to you that personality can have an impact on whether you are happy and socially well-adjusted or sad and socially isolated. However, your personality may affect more than just your social interactions: It may be a critical factor in your stress level, as well as in your risk for CVD, cancer, and other chronic and infectious diseases.

In 1974, physicians Meyer Friedman and Ray Rosenman published a book indicating that Type A individuals had a greatly increased risk of heart disease.[43] *Type A* personalities are defined as hard-driving, competitive, time-driven perfectionists. In contrast, *Type B* personalities are described as being relaxed, noncompetitive, and more tolerant of others.

Today, most researchers recognize that none of us will be wholly Type A or Type B all of the time. We might exhibit either type as we respond to the various challenges of our daily lives. In addition, recent research indicates that not all Type A people experience negative health consequences; in fact, some hard-driving individuals seem to thrive on their supercharged lifestyles. Only those Type A individuals who exhibit a "toxic core"; have disproportionate amounts of anger; are distrustful of others; and have a cynical, glass-half-empty approach to life—a set of characteristics referred to as **hostility**—are at increased risk for heart disease. Relationships fraught with problems may not just be unpleasant happenings in life. In fact, a recent study has shown that couples who have marital discord—who are often in turmoil and are angry and hostile toward each other—have a significantly higher risk of early coronary heart disease.[44]

Type C and Type D Personalities In addition to CVD risks, personality types have been linked to increased risk for a variety of illnesses, ranging from asthma to cancer. *Type C* personality is one such type. Typically, Type C people are stoic and tend to deny feelings. They have a tendency to conform to the wishes of others (or to be "pleasers"), a lack of assertiveness, and an inclination toward feelings of helplessness or hopelessness. Possibly as a result of these characteristics, research indicates they are more susceptible to illnesses such as asthma, multiple sclerosis, autoimmune disorders, and cancer.[45] They are the "nice" guys and gals who really do finish last when it comes to their health.

A more recently identified personality type is *Type D* (distressed), which is characterized by a tendency toward excessive negative worry, irritability, gloom, and social inhibition. Several recent studies have shown that Type D people may be up to eight times more likely to die of a heart attack or sudden cardiac death.[46]

Psychological Hardiness and Resilience According to psychologist Susanne Kobasa, **psychological hardiness** was the key to reducing self-imposed stress associated with Type A behavior. Psychologically hardy people were characterized by *control, commitment,* and willingness to *embrace challenge.*[47] People with a sense of *control* are able to accept responsibility for their behaviors and work to change situations they discover to be debilitating. People with a sense of *commitment* have healthy self-esteem and know their purpose in life. Those who embrace *challenge* see change as a stimulating opportunity for personal growth. Today, the concept of hardiness has evolved to include a person's overall ability to cope with stress and adversity.[48]

Today, it is more common for people to think of this general hardiness concept in terms of **psychological resilience.** This resilience is the process of adapting well in the face of adversity, trauma, tragedy, threats, or significant sources of stress, such as family and relationship problems, serious health problems, or workplace and financial stressors. Essentially, it refers to our ability to "bounce back" from difficult experiences, thrive in the face of adversity, or function at higher levels than expected under stressful situations. Resilient individuals are able to interact more effectively with potentially negative environments as a result of "protective factors" such as strong support networks of family, friends, and healthy communities. The concept of resilience has been studied extensively and appears to be a key indicator of good psychological and social development.[49]

Managing Stress in College

College students thrive under a certain amount of stress, but excessive stress can leave them overwhelmed and unable to cope. Recent studies of college students indicate that the emotional health self-rating of first-year college students is at an all-time low. At the same time, increased percentages report feeling overwhelmed much of the time. These same students report more emotional reactivity in the form of anger, hostility, frustration, and a greater sense of being out of control.[50] Sophomores and juniors reported fewer problems with these issues, and seniors reported the fewest problems. This may indicate students' progressive emotional growth through experience, maturity, increased awareness of support services, and more social connections.[51]

Students generally report using health-enhancing methods to combat stress, but research has found that students sometimes resort to health-compromising activities to escape the stress and anxiety of college.[52] Numerous researchers have found stress among young adults to be correlated to unhealthy behaviors such as substance abuse, lack of physical activity, poor psychological and physical health, lack of social problem solving, depression, and infrequent use of social support networks.[53] Being on your own in college may pose challenges, but it also lets you take control of and responsibility for your life, to evaluate your unique situation, and to take steps that fit your schedule and lifestyle to reduce negative stressors in your life. Although you can't eliminate all life stressors, you can train yourself to recognize the events that cause stress and to anticipate your reactions to them. **Coping** is the act of managing events or conditions to lessen the physical or psychological effects of excess stress.[54] One of the most effective ways to combat stressors is to build coping strategies and skills, known collectively as *stress-management techniques,* such as the ones discussed in the following sections.

How daunting that pile of books and homework is all depends on your own appraisal of it.

psychological hardiness A personality trait characterized by control, commitment, and the embrace of challenge.

psychological resilience The process of adapting well in the face of adversity, trauma, tragedy, threats, or significant sources of stress, such as family and relationship problems, serious health problems, or workplace and financial stressors.

coping Managing events or conditions to lessen the physical or psychological effects of excess stress.

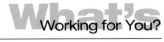

Working for You?

Maybe you're already on your way to a less-stressed life. Below is a list of some things you can do to cope with stress. Which of these are you already incorporating into your life?

☐ I listen to relaxing music.
☐ I exercise regularly.
☐ I get 8 hours of sleep each night.
☐ I practice deep breathing.

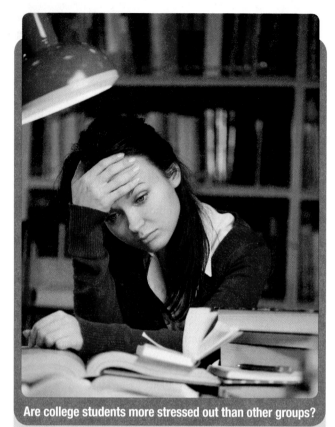

Are college students more stressed out than other groups?

Studies suggest yes—the combination of new environment, peer and parent pressures, and juggling the demands of work, school, and a social life likely contribute to this phenomenon.

Practice Mental Work to Reduce Stress

Stress management isn't something that just happens. It calls for getting a handle on what is going on in your life, taking a careful look at yourself, and coming up with a personal plan of action. Because your perceptions are often part of the problem, assessing your "self-talk," beliefs, and actions are good first steps. Why are you so stressed? How much of it is due to perception rather than reality? What's a realistic plan of action for you? Think about your situation and map out a strategy for change. The tools in this section will help you.

stress inoculation Stress-management technique in which a person consciously tries to prepare ahead of time for potential stressors.

cognitive restructuring The modification of thoughts, ideas, and beliefs that contribute to stress.

Assess Your Stressors and Solve Problems Assessing what is really going on in your life is an important first step to solving problems and reducing stress. Here's how:

- Make a list of the major things that you are worried about right now.
- Examine the causes of the problems and worries.
- Consider how big each problem is. What are the consequences of doing nothing versus taking action?

- List your options, including ones that you may not like very much.
- Outline an action plan, and then *act*. Remember that even little things can sometimes make a big difference and that you shouldn't expect immediate results.
- After you act, evaluate. How did you do? Do you need to change your actions to achieve a better outcome next time? How?

One useful way of coping with your stressors, once you have identified them, is to consciously anticipate and prepare for specific stressors, a technique known as **stress inoculation.** For example, suppose that speaking in front of a class scares you. Practice in front of friends or in front of a video camera to banish panic and prevent your freezing up on the day of the presentation. The assumption is that by dealing with smaller fears, you develop resistance, so that larger fears do not seem so overwhelming.

Change How You Think and Talk to Yourself
As noted earlier, our appraisal of people and situations is what makes these things stressful, not the people or situations themselves. Several types of negative self-talk exist, but among the most common are *pessimism,* or focusing on the negative; *perfectionism,* or expecting superhuman standards; *"should-ing,"* or reprimanding yourself for items that you should have done; *blaming* yourself or others for circumstances and events; and *dichotomous thinking,* in which everything is either black or white (good or bad) instead of gradated.[55] To combat negative self-talk, we must first become aware of it, then stop it, and finally replace the negative thoughts with positive ones—a process referred to as **cognitive restructuring.** Once you realize that some of your thoughts may be irrational or overreactive, interrupt this self-talk by saying "Stop" (under your breath or out loud) and make a conscious effort to think positively. If you can learn to view stressors in a positive light, you can reduce your stress levels without having to remove the stressors. See the **Skills for Behavior Change** box below for other suggestions of ways to rethink your thinking habits.

Rethink Your Thinking Habits

Break the worry habit. The following suggestions can slow the worry drain:

❱ Create a "worry period" when you can journal or fret out loud. After that move on.
❱ Focus on what is going right, deemphasize what's going wrong
❱ Learn to accept what you cannot change.
❱ Seek help from a friend, counselor, or family member if your worries seem out of control

Skills for Behavior Change

Developing a Support Network

As you plan a stress-management program, remember the importance of social networks and social bonds. Friendships are an important aspect of inoculating yourself against harmful stressors. Studies of college students have demonstrated the importance of social support in *buffering* individuals from the effects of stress.[56] It isn't necessary to have a large number of friends. However, different friends often serve different needs, so having more than one is usually beneficial.

Find Supportive People Family members and friends are often a steady base of support when the pressures of life seem overwhelming. But if friends or family are unavailable or if your friends tend to bring you down rather than build you up, most colleges and universities offer counseling services at no cost for short-term crises. Clergy, instructors, and residence hall supervisors also may be excellent resources. If university services are unavailable, or if you are concerned about confidentiality, most communities offer low-cost counseling through mental health clinics.

Invest in Your Loved Ones Imagine if you had absolutely no one you could call when you were in financial trouble or if a loved one died and no one called you. Many people find that they've spent so much of their time pushing ahead in careers or self-improvement that they are alone at the worst times of their lives. As our lives get busy and obligations become overwhelming, we often don't make time for the very people who are most important to us: our friends, family, and other loved ones. In order to have a healthy social support network, we have to invest time and energy. Healthy social connections don't just happen by virtue of location or bloodlines. Cultivate and nurture the relationships that matter: those built on trust, mutual acceptance and understanding, honesty, and genuine caring. In addition, treating others

empathically provides them with a measure of emotional security and reduces *their* anxiety. If you want others to be there for you to help you cope with life's stressors, you need to be there for them.

Cultivating Your Spiritual Side

One of the most important factors in reducing overall stress in your life is taking the time and making the commitment to cultivate your spiritual side: finding your purpose in life and living your days more fully. Spiritual health and spiritual practices can be vital components of your support system, often linking you to a community of like-minded individuals and giving you perspective on the things that truly matter in your life. (For specific information on the various aspects of spirituality and how it can affect your overall health, see Focus On: Cultivating Your Spiritual Health beginning on page 58.)

Managing Emotional Responses

Have you ever gotten all worked up about something only to find that your perceptions were totally wrong? We often get upset not by realities, but by our faulty perceptions. Social networking sites and e-mails are often perfect places for reading meaning into things that are said and perceiving issues that don't exist. Eyeball-to-eyeball interactions, where body language, voice intonation, and opportunities for clarification are present, are much better than cryptic texts or e-mails for interpreting true meanings.

Stress management requires that you examine the validity of a stressor and your emotional responses to interactions with others using all of the available visual and sensory clues. Learning to tell the difference between normal emotions and emotions based on irrational beliefs or expressed and interpreted in an over-the-top manner can help you stop the emotion or express it in a healthy and appropriate way.

Fight the Anger Urge Anger usually results when we feel we have lost control of a situation or are frustrated by a situation that we can do little about. Major sources of anger include (1) perceived *threats* to self or others we care about; (2) *reactions to injustice* such as unfair actions, policies, or behaviors; (3) *fear,* which leads to negative responses; (4) *faulty emotional reasoning,* or misinterpretation of normal events; (5) *low frustration tolerance,* often fueled by stress, drugs, lack of sleep, and other factors; (6) *unreasonable expectations* about ourselves and others; and (7) *people rating,* or applying derogatory ratings to others.

Each of us learned by this point in our lives that there are three main approaches

Spending time communicating and socializing can be an important part of building a support network and reducing your stress level.

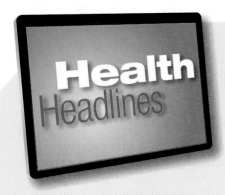

Health Headlines

FIND HAPPINESS AND REDUCE STRESS

Don't we all just want to be happy? In the past few decades, a field of research called *positive psychology* has emerged to study how people can become happier Some psychologists found that people who are generally more optimistic or happier have fewer mental and physical health problems. If happiness and optimism are keys to health and stress reduction, how can *you* find them?

✳ **Set realistic goals.** Psychologist Alice Donner says that striving for a 100 percent dose of contentment and perfection is unrealistic. She suggests that managing your *expectations* is a key. Decide what is realistic for you and work to get to that place.

✳ **Remember that money doesn't buy happiness.** In fact, too much focus on the acquisition of things rather than on relationships and connections may be a major cause of discontent. Also, people who have to pay for a lot of material things tend to work longer hours, vacation less,

and in general not take time for themselves.

✳ **Lose yourself in the moment.** Finding your flow, a state of effortless concentration and enjoyment, should be a daily goal. What is it that energizes you, makes time fly by, and causes you to concentrate fully on the present? The more often you find and follow that, the happier you'll be.

✳ **Count your blessings.** Although we all can find time to be critical and complain, focusing on our many positive attributes and being thankful for all the good things in our lives should become a daily ritual. For some, this might include daily journaling, a time when they can contemplate all of the good things about their day. Telling your parents how much you appreciate them, telling your friends that they enrich your life, and bringing a smile to someone's face—even if you don't know them—are all important.

✳ **Make changes and reinvigorate.** For example, try new recipes, find new ways of exercising, plan a fun outing with someone you enjoy once a month, find a new place on campus to study, plan a trip somewhere different in the next 6 months, learn a new skill, or help someone by volunteering your time.

✳ **Forgive and forget.** Rather than ruminating over some slight or indiscretion, try to understand what may have caused someone to act toward you in a hurtful manner, and then move on.

✳ **Remember to prioritize you.** Your own happiness is as important as that of others in your life. Limit the time you spend with people who bring you down. Instead, find time for breaks, fun interludes, and time alone.

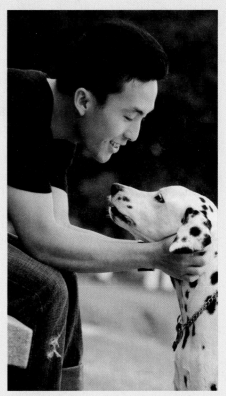

Don't forget to make time for joy and beauty in your life.

Sources: R. Kobau, M Seligman, and C. Peterson, et al, "Mental Health Promotion in Public Health: Perspectives and Strategies from Positive Psychology," *American Journal of Public Health* 101, no. 8 (2011): e1–e9; S. Algoe, B. Fredrickson, and L. Barbara, "Emotional Fitness and the Movement of Affective Science from Lab to Field," *American Psychologist* 66, no. 1 (2011): 35–42; M. E. P. Seligman, *Authentic Happiness: Using the New Positive Psychology to Realize Your Potential for Lasting Fulfillment* (New York: Free Press/Simon & Schuster, 2002).

to dealing with anger: expressing it, suppressing it, or calming it. You may be surprised to find out that expressing your anger is probably the healthiest thing to do in the long run, if you express anger in an assertive rather than an aggressive way. However, it's a natural reaction to want to respond aggressively, and that is what we must learn to keep at bay. To accomplish this, there are several strategies you can use.[57]

● **Identify your anger style.** Do you express anger passively or actively? Do you hold anger in, or do you explode? Do you throw the phone, smash things, or scream at others?

● **Learn to recognize patterns in your anger responses and how to de-escalate them.** For 1 week, keep track of everything that angers you or keeps you stewing. What thoughts or feelings lead up to your boiling point? Keep a journal and listen to your anger. Try to change your self-talk. Explore how you can interrupt patterns of anger, such as counting to 10, getting a drink of water, or taking some deep breaths.

● **Find the right words to de-escalate conflict.** Recent research has shown that when couples are angry and fight, using words that suggest thoughtfulness can reduce conflict.[58]

Words such as *think, because, reason, why* demonstrate more consideration for your partner and the issues under fire, as well as a more rational approach.

● **Plan ahead.** Explore options to minimize your exposure to anger-provoking situations such as traffic jams.

● **Vent to your friends.** Find a few close friends in whom you can confide or to whom you can vent your frustration. Allow them to listen and perhaps provide insight or another perspective that your anger has blinded you to. Don't wear down your supporter with continual rants.

● **Develop realistic expectations of yourself and others.** Anger is often the result of unmet expectations, frustrations, resentments, and impatience. Are your expectations of yourself and others realistic? Try talking with those involved about your feelings at a time when you are calm.

● **Turn complaints into requests.** When frustrated or angry with someone, try reworking the problem into a request. Instead of screaming and pounding on the wall because your neighbors' blaring music woke you up at 2 A.M., talk with them. Try to reach an agreement that works for everyone.

● **Leave past anger in the past.** Learn to resolve issues that have caused pain, frustration, or stress. If necessary, seek the counsel of a professional to make that happen.

Learn to Laugh, Be Joyful, and Cry

Have you ever noticed that you feel better after a belly laugh or a good cry? Adages such as "laughter is the best medicine" and "smile and the world smiles with you" didn't just evolve out of the blue. Humans have long recognized that smiling, laughing, singing, dancing, and other actions can elevate our moods, relieve stress, make us feel good, and help us improve our relationships. Learning to laugh at your own silly actions and taking yourself less seriously is a good starting place. Crying can have similar positive physiological effects in relieving tension. Several research articles have indicated that laughter and joy may increase endorphin levels, increase oxygen levels in the blood, decrease stress levels, relieve pain, enhance productivity, and reduce risks of chronic disease; however, the evidence for *long-term* effects on immune functioning and protective effects for chronic diseases is only just starting to be understood.[59] For ideas on how to find more joy and laughter in your daily life, see the **Health Headlines** box on the previous page.

Taking Physical Action

Physical activities can complement the emotional and mental strategies of stress management.

Exercise Regularly The human stress response is intended to end in physical activity, yet we live in a world where we usually aren't able to fight or flee. Exercise "burns off" existing stress hormones by directing them toward their intended metabolic function.[60] Exercise can also help combat stress by raising levels of endorphins—mood-elevating, painkilling hormones—in the bloodstream, increasing energy, reducing hostility, and improving mental alertness. (For more information on the beneficial effects of exercise, see **Chapter 9.**)

Get Enough Sleep Adequate amounts of sleep allow you to refresh your vital energy, cope with multiple stressors more effectively, and be productive when you need to be. In fact, sleep is one of the biggest stress busters of them all. (These benefits and others are discussed in much more depth in Focus On: Improving Your Sleep beginning on page 98.)

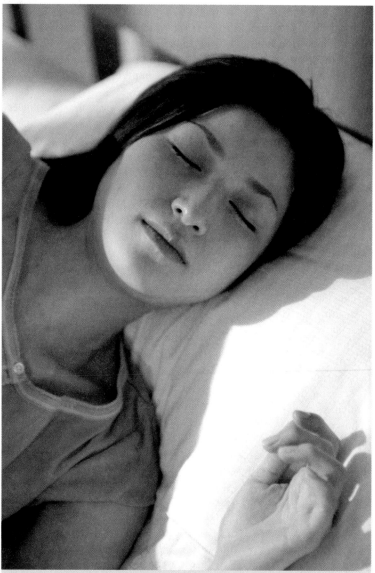

Taking care of your physical health—through quality sleep, sufficient exercise, and healthful nutrition—is a crucial component of stress management.

Learn to Relax Like exercise, relaxation can help you cope with stressful feelings, preserve your energy, and refocus your energies. Once you have learned simple relaxation techniques, you can use them at any time—before a difficult exam, for example. As your body relaxes, your heart rate slows, your blood pressure and metabolic rate decrease, and many other body-calming effects occur, all of which allow you to channel energy appropriately. We discuss specific relaxation techniques later in the chapter.

Eat Healthfully Whether foods can calm us and nourish our psyches is a controversial question. High-potency supplements that are supposed to boost resistance against stress-related ailments are nothing more than gimmicks. However, it is clear that eating a balanced, healthy diet will help provide the stamina you need to get through problems and will stress-proof you in ways that are not fully understood. It is also known that undereating, overeating, and eating the wrong kinds of foods can create distress in the body. In particular, avoid **sympathomimetics,** foods that produce (or mimic) stresslike responses, such as caffeine. (For more information about the benefits of sound nutrition, see **Chapter 7.**)

Managing Your Time

Ever go to a party when an exam was looming? Have you put off writing a paper until the night before it was due? We all **procrastinate,** or voluntarily delay doing some task despite expecting to be worse off for the delay. Procrastination results in academic difficulties, financial problems, relationship problems, and a multitude of stress-related ailments.

How can you avoid the procrastination bug? According to psychologist Peter Gollwitzer and colleagues, setting clear "implementation intentions," a series of goals to be accomplished toward a specific end, is key.[61] You could decide to work on your paper at least 2 hours per day for the next week as a way of ensuring that you'll complete it by the due date. By making a clear plan of action with set deadlines and rewarding yourself for meeting these deadlines, you can motivate yourself toward project completion. Another strategy is to get started early and set a personal end date that is well ahead of the class due date.

Learning to manage your time better overall is key to reducing stress. Keep a journal for 1 week to become aware of how you spend your time. Write down your activities every day—everything from going to class to doing your laundry to texting your friends—and the amount of time you spend doing each. Once you have kept track for several days, you can assess your activities. Are you completing the tasks you need to do on a daily basis? Are there any activities you can stop doing or that you would like to do more frequently? Use the following time-management tips in your stress-management program:

● **Do one thing at a time.** Don't try to watch television, wash clothes, and write your term paper all at once. Stay focused.

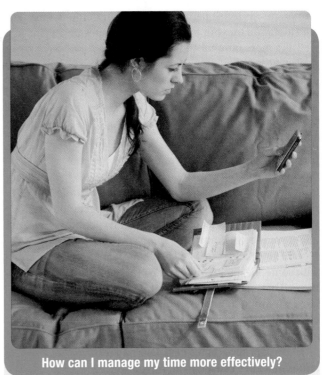

How can I manage my time more effectively?

Learning to manage your time means recognizing that there are only 24 hours in a day and you can't do everything. Instead, you need to prioritize your "to do's" and set realistic time limits. You also need to identify the things that cause you to waste time and find ways to avoid them. Establishing routines and using a calendar or other planning device to keep track of schedules and tasks can help you implement an effective time-management plan.

● **Clean off your desk.** Go through the things on your desk, toss unnecessary papers, and put into folders the papers for tasks that you must do. Read your mail, recycle what you don't need, and file what you will need later.

● **Prioritize your tasks.** Make a daily "to do" list and stick to it. Categorize the things you must do today, the things that you must do but not immediately, and the things that it would be nice to do. Consider the "nice to do" items only if you finish the others or if they include something fun.

● **Find a clean, comfortable place to work, and avoid interruptions.** When you have a project that requires total concentration, schedule uninterrupted time. Don't answer the phone; close your door and post a "Do Not Disturb" sign; or go to a quiet room in the library or student union where no one will find you.

● **Reward yourself for work completed.** Did you finish a task on your list? Then do something nice for yourself. Rest breaks give you time to yourself to help you recharge and refresh your energy levels.

● **Work when you're at your best.** If you're a morning person, study and write papers in the morning, and take breaks when you start to slow down.

● **Break overwhelming tasks into small pieces, and allocate** a certain amount of time to each. If you are floundering on a task, move on and come back to it when you're refreshed.

- **Remember that time is precious.** Many people learn to value their time only when they face a terminal illness. Try to value each day. Time spent not enjoying life is a tremendous waste! If you have trouble saying no to people and projects that steal your time, see the **Skills for Behavior Change** box for some suggestions.

Consider Downshifting

Today's lifestyles are hectic and pressure packed, and stress often comes from trying to keep up. Many people are questioning whether "having it all" is worth it, and they are taking a step back and simplifying their lives. This trend has been labeled *downshifting,* or *voluntary simplicity.* Moving from a large urban area to a smaller town, leaving a high-paying and high-stress job for one that makes you happy, and a host of other changes in lifestyle typify downshifting.

Downshifting involves a fundamental alteration in values and honest introspection about what is important in life. It means cutting down on shopping habits, buying only what you need to get by, and living within modest means. When you contemplate any form of downshift or perhaps even start your career this way, it's important to move slowly and consider the following:

- **Plan for health care costs.** Make sure that you budget for health insurance and basic preventive health services if you're not covered under your parents' plan. Understand your coverage. This should be a top priority.
- **Determine your ultimate goal.** What is most important to you, and what will you need to reach that goal? What can you do without?

Learn to Say No and Mean It!

Is your calendar always so full you barely have time to breathe? Are you unable to say no to other people? When you're asked to do something you don't really want to do, practice the following tips to avoid overcommitment:

❯ **Be sympathetic, but firm.** Explain that although you think it's a great cause or idea, you just can't take on one more project right now. Don't waver if they persist in pressuring you.

❯ **Don't say you want to think about it and will get back to them.** This only leads to more forceful requests later.

❯ **Don't give in to guilt.** Stick to your guns. Remember you don't owe anyone your time.

❯ **Even if something sounds good, avoid spontaneous "yes" responses to new projects.** Make a rule that you will take at least a day to think about committing your time.

❯ **Schedule time for yourself first.** If you don't have time for the things you love to do, stop and prioritize your activities. Don't let time get sucked up doing things you don't want to do.

- **Make both short- and long-term plans for simplifying your life.** Set up your plans in doable steps, and work slowly toward each step.
- **Complete a financial inventory.** How much money will you need to do the things you want to do? Will you live alone or share costs with roommates? Do you need a car, or can you rely on public transportation? Pay off your debt, and get used to paying with cash. If you don't have the cash, don't buy.
- **Select the right career.** Look for work that you enjoy and that isn't necessarily driven by salary. Can you be happy taking a lower-paying job if it is less stressful?
- **Consider options for saving money.** Downshifting doesn't mean you renounce money; it means you choose not to let money dictate your life. Saving is still important. If you're just getting started, you need to prepare for emergencies and for future plans.

Relaxation Techniques for Stress Management

Relaxation is the body's natural antidote to stress. Techniques to reduce stress have been practiced

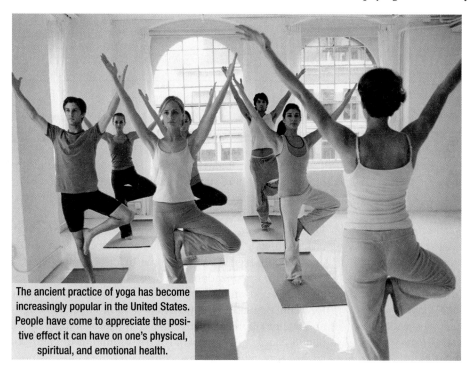

The ancient practice of yoga has become increasingly popular in the United States. People have come to appreciate the positive effect it can have on one's physical, spiritual, and emotional health.

Money&Health

TIPS FOR WHEN FINANCIAL STRESS HITS HARD IN COLLEGE

Financial stress has always been an issue for college students, who often find themselves responsible for money and expenses for the first time. But today's students may also face anxiety over parents becoming tapped out by bills due to unemployment or the loss of a family home. For those who count on parents as a financial "safety net," these situations can be very stressful. Government spending cuts and resulting increases in tuition and fees, coupled with less financial aid, all compound financial stress.

In recent studies, nearly two thirds of students indicated they have "some" or "major" concerns regarding their ability to pay for education. Many worry they may have to drop out. Anxiety rates, depression, and substance abuse are at all-time highs on many campuses, and worries over finances surface as a major issue in students' abilities to do well in school. Trouble sleeping, digestive problems, unexplained weight gain or loss, inability to enjoy regular activities, severe anxiety or panic attacks are all stress-induced symptoms.

No one is completely immune from potential problems in hard economic times. But the following tips can help students cope better with the parts of the financial stress equation they do have control over.

✻ **Develop a realistic budget.** What are your monthly expenses and how much money do you earn? If your parents can't help you, do you have another family member or friend who could help you out? Think about where you spend your money, what you really need, and what you could do without. Necessities first, then wants.

✻ **Pay bills immediately and consider electronic banking.** Late fees and other penalties deplete bank accounts. Sign up for an online account to pay bills quickly and easily. If possible, set up your bills for automatic payment. If you don't have the money to pay the minimum, call your creditors and try to make payment arrangements or pay a smaller amount.

✻ **Use cash instead of credit cards.** Paying for your purchases in cash means you can't spend beyond what you have. Also, most people find handing dollars to a cashier feels more "real" than using a credit card, which makes them think twice before spending.

✻ **Don't take getting into debt lightly.** Some things, like college tuition, may require you to go into debt. Look first to low-interest loans rather than credit cards. Debt should be a last-resort option for most spending. If you want that latest smart phone or an expensive spring break trip, it's better to save up than to put it on a credit card.

✻ **Be willing to make hard choices.** Even in good economic times everyone must learn to live within their means. Embracing this mindset in college will help you cope better with financial stress throughout life. If you feel frustrated or down because of financial stress, remind yourself that possessions are not as important as your education, friendships, or family. Focus on your strengths rather than your possessions as a measure of who you are and what you value in life.

Sources: J. H. Pryor et al., *The American Freshman: National Norms Fall 2010. 2011;* American College Health Association, *American College Health Association–National College Health Assessment II (ACHA-NCHA II): Reference Group Data Report Spring 2011* (Baltimore: American College Health Association, 2012).

---

for centuries and offer opportunities for calming your nervous energy and coping with life's challenges. Some common techniques include yoga, qigong, tai chi, deep breathing, meditation, visualization, progressive muscle relaxation, massage therapy, biofeedback, and hypnosis.

Yoga Yoga is an ancient practice that combines meditation, stretching, and breathing exercises designed to relax, refresh, and rejuvenate. It began about 5,000 years ago in India and has been evolving ever since. Although exact numbers are difficult to obtain, it is estimated that nearly 15 million people in the United States practice one or more of the many versions of yoga today.[62]

Classical yoga is the ancestor of nearly all modern forms of yoga. Breathing, poses, and verbal mantras are often part of classical yoga. Of the many branches of classical yoga, *Hatha yoga* is the most well known because it is the most body focused. This style

of yoga involves the practice of breath control and *asanas*—held postures and choreographed movements that enhance strength and flexibility. (Several other, more athletic, forms of yoga are discussed in Chapter 9.) Recent research shows increased evidence of benefits of Hatha yoga in reducing inflammation, boosting mood, and reducing stress among those who practice regularly.[63]

Qigong *Qigong* (pronounced "chee-kong") is one of the fastest-growing and most widely accepted forms of mind-body health exercises. Even some of the country's largest health care organizations, such as Kaiser Permanente, include this relaxation technique in their system, particularly for people suffering from chronic pain or stress. Qigong is an ancient Chinese practice that involves becoming aware of and learning to control qi (or *chi,* pronounced "chee") or vital energy in your body. According to Chinese medicine, a

what do you think?

Who are your role models?
● Are they constantly "on the go" or more relaxed?
● Would you characterize them as stressed out?
● Could you follow their lead without becoming stressed out yourself?

complex system of internal pathways called *meridians* carry *qi* throughout your body. If your *qi* becomes stagnant or blocked, you'll feel sluggish or powerless. Qigong incorporates a series of flowing movements, breath techniques, mental visualization exercises, and vocalizations of healing sounds designed to restore balance and integrate and refresh the mind and body.

Tai Chi *Tai chi* (pronounced "ty-chee") is sometimes described as "meditation in motion." Originally developed in China as a form of self-defense, this graceful form of exercise has existed for about 2,000 years. Tai chi is noncompetitive and self-paced. To do tai chi, you perform a defined series of postures or movements in a slow, graceful manner. Each movement or posture flows into the next without pause. Tai chi has been widely practiced in China for centuries and is now becoming increasingly popular around the world, both

as a basic exercise program and as a complement to other health care methods. Health benefits include stress reduction, greater balance, and increased flexibility.

Diaphragmatic or Deep Breathing Typically, we breathe using only the upper chest and thoracic region rather than involving the abdominal region. Simply stated, diaphragmatic breathing is deep breathing that maximally fills the lungs by involving the movement of the diaphragm and lower abdomen. This technique is commonly used in yoga exercises and in other meditative practices. (Try the diaphragmatic breathing exercise in **Figure 3.5** right now and see whether you feel more relaxed!)

Meditation There are many different forms of **meditation.** Most involve sitting quietly for 15 or 20 minutes, focusing on a particular word or symbol, and controlling breathing. Practiced by Eastern religions for centuries, meditation is believed to be an important form of introspection and personal renewal. In stress management, it can calm the body and quiet the mind, creating a sense of peace. A recent study found that one form of meditation, transcendental meditation, helped college students decrease stress and

> **meditation** A relaxation technique that involves deep breathing and concentration.

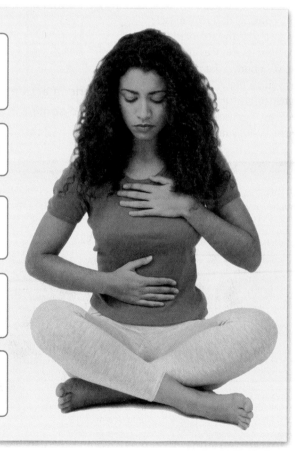

① Assume a natural, comfortable position either sitting up straight with your head, neck, and shoulders relaxed, or lying on your back with your knees bent and your head supported. Close your eyes and loosen binding clothes.

② In order to feel your abdomen moving as you breathe, place one hand on your upper chest and the other just below your rib cage.

③ Breathe in slowly and deeply through your nose. Feel your stomach expanding into your hand. The hand on your chest should move as little as possible.

④ Exhale slowly through your mouth. Feel the fall of your stomach away from your hand. Again, the hand on your chest should move as little as possible.

⑤ Concentrate on the act of breathing. Shut out external noise. Focus on inhaling and exhaling, the route the air is following, and the rise and fall of your stomach.

FIGURE 3.5 **Diaphragmatic Breathing**
This exercise will help you learn to breathe deeply as a way to relieve stress. Practice this for 5 to 10 minutes several times a day, and soon diaphragmatic breathing will become natural for you.

increase coping ability, particularly among those at risk for hypertension.[64] (Meditation and other aspects of spiritual health are discussed in detail in Focus On: Cultivating Your Spiritual Health beginning on page 58.) Meditation can be performed alone or in a group. Many colleges and universities offer classes on how to meditate. Check with your campus Wellness Center.

Visualization

Often it is our own thoughts and imagination that provoke distress by conjuring up worst-case scenarios. Our imagination, however, can also be tapped to reduce stress.

> **visualization** The creation of mental images to promote relaxation.
>
> **biofeedback** A technique using a machine to self-monitor physical responses to stress.
>
> **hypnosis** A trancelike state that allows people to become unusually responsive to suggestion.

In **visualization,** you create mental scenes using your imagination. The choice of mental images is unlimited, but natural settings such as ocean beaches and mountain lakes are often used because they represent stress-free environments. Recalling physical senses of sight, sound, smell, taste, and touch can replace stressful stimuli with peaceful or pleasurable thoughts. Try to make your visualization as real and detailed as possible: Think of all the tiny sounds you might hear, how the air feels about you, and who you are with. The fuller and more nuanced the world you create, the greater the effect.

Progressive Muscle Relaxation

Progressive muscle relaxation involves systematically contracting and relaxing different muscle groups in your body. The standard pattern is to begin with the feet and work your way up your body, contracting and releasing as you go (Figure 3.6). The process is designed to teach awareness of the different feelings of muscle tension and muscle release. With practice, you can quickly identify tension in your body when you are facing stressful situations and consciously release that tension to calm yourself.

Massage Therapy If you have ever had someone massage your stiff neck or aching feet, you know that massage is an excellent way to relax. Techniques vary from deep-tissue massage to the gentler acupressure. Although research on the effectiveness of massage as a stress reducer is in its infancy, a new study indicates that Swedish massage may in fact have a beneficial effect on hormones known to regulate blood pressure and reduce inflammation, as well as invoke a general relaxation response in the body.[65] (**Chapter 18** provides more information about the benefits of massage as well as other body-based methods such as acupressure and shiatsu.)

Biofeedback **Biofeedback** is a technique in which a person learns to control body functions, such as heart rate, body temperature, and breathing rate, with conscious mind control. Using machines as simple as stress dots that change color with body temperature variation to sophisticated electrical sensors, individuals learn to listen to their bodies and make necessary adjustments, such as relaxing certain muscles or changing breathing or concentration, to slow heart rate and relax. Eventually, individuals develop the ability to recognize and lower stress responses without using the machines, and then it can be practiced anywhere.

Hypnosis **Hypnosis** requires a person to focus on one thought, object, or voice, thereby freeing the right hemisphere of the brain to become more active. The person then becomes unusually responsive to suggestion. Whether self-induced or induced by someone else, hypnosis can reduce certain types of stress.

9.4%

of American adults report having practiced some form of meditation in the past 12 months.

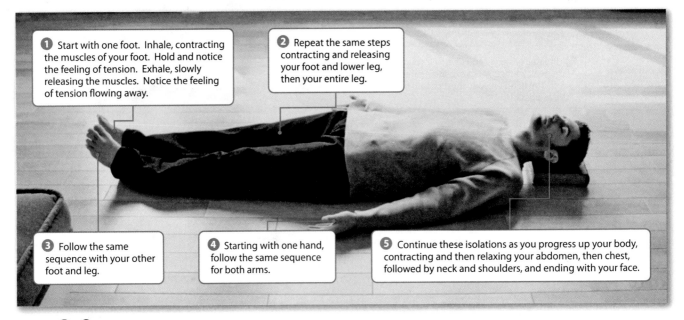

❶ Start with one foot. Inhale, contracting the muscles of your foot. Hold and notice the feeling of tension. Exhale, slowly releasing the muscles. Notice the feeling of tension flowing away.

❷ Repeat the same steps contracting and releasing your foot and lower leg, then your entire leg.

❸ Follow the same sequence with your other foot and leg.

❹ Starting with one hand, follow the same sequence for both arms.

❺ Continue these isolations as you progress up your body, contracting and then relaxing your abdomen, then chest, followed by neck and shoulders, and ending with your face.

FIGURE 3.6 **Progressive Muscle Relaxation**
Sit or lie down in a comfortable position and follow the steps described to increase your awareness of tension in your body.

Assess Yourself

How Stressed Are You?

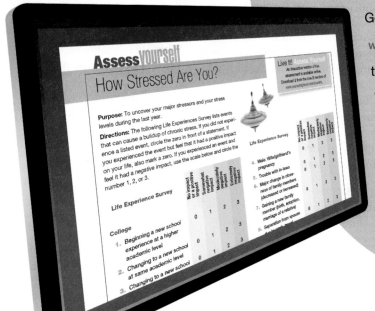

Go online to the **Live It!** section of www.pearson.highered.com/donatelle to take the "How Stressed Are You?" assessment.*

Then try the stress-reducing strategies listed in the **YOUR PLAN FOR CHANGE** box.

*If your instructor so chooses, Assess Yourself Activities are available as a printed supplement or as assignable homework online at www.pearsonhighered.com/myhealthlab.

MyHealthLab®

YOUR PLAN FOR CHANGE

Use the **Assess Yourself** activity "How Stressed Are You?" to rate your stress level. If it is higher than desired, use these tips to reduce stress.

Today, you can:

◯ Practice one new stress-management technique. For example, you could spend 10 minutes doing a deep-breathing exercise or find a good spot on campus to meditate.

◯ Buy a journal and write down stressful events or symptoms of stress that you experience. Try to focus on intense emotional experiences and explore how they affect you.

Within the next 2 weeks, you can:

◯ Attend a class or workshop in yoga, tai chi, qigong, meditation, or some other stress-relieving activity. Look for beginner classes offered on campus or in your community.

◯ Make a list of the papers, projects, and tests that you have over the coming semester and create a schedule for them. Break projects and term papers into small, manageable tasks, and try to be realistic about how much time you'll need to get these tasks done.

By the end of the semester, you can:

◯ Keep track of the money you spend and where it goes. Establish a budget, and follow it for at least a month.

◯ Find some form of exercise you can do regularly. You may consider joining a gym or just arranging regular "walk dates" or pickup basketball games with your friends. Try to exercise at least 30 minutes every day. See Chapter 9 for more information about physical fitness.

Summary

* Stress is always part of life. *Eustress* refers to stress associated with positive events; *distress* is stress associated with negative events.

* The alarm, resistance, and exhaustion phases of the general adaptation syndrome (GAS) involve physiological responses to both real and imagined stressors and cause complex hormonal reactions.

* Undue stress for extended periods of time can compromise the immune system. Stress has been linked to numerous health problems, including cardiovascular disease (CVD), weight gain, hair loss, diabetes, digestive problems, increased susceptibility to infectious diseases, and diminished libido. Psychoneuroimmunology is the study of stress and the immune response.

* Stress can have negative impacts on your intellectual and psychological health, including impaired memory, poor concentration, depression, anxiety, and other disorders.

* Psychosocial factors that impact stress include change, hassles, relationships, pressure, conflict, overload, and environmental stressors. Discrimination or bias may cause unusually high stress. Some sources are internal and are related to appraisal, self-esteem, self-efficacy, personality, and psychological hardiness.

* College can be especially stressful. Managing stress begins with learning coping skills. Managing emotional responses, taking mental or physical action, downshifting, managing finances and time, or learning relaxation techniques will help you cope in the long run.

Pop Quiz

1. Even though Andre experienced stress when he graduated from college and moved to a new city, he viewed these changes as an opportunity for growth. What is Andre's stress called?
    a. Strain
    b. Distress
    c. Eustress
    d. Adaptive response

2. The branch of the autonomic nervous system that is responsible for energizing the body for either fight or flight and for triggering many other stress responses is the
    a. central nervous system.
    b. parasympathetic nervous system.
    c. sympathetic nervous system.
    d. endocrine system.

3. During what phase of the general adaptation syndrome has the physical and psychological energy used to fight the stressor been depleted?
    a. Alarm phase
    b. Resistance phase
    c. Endurance phase
    d. Exhaustion phase

4. A state of physical and mental exhaustion caused by excessive stress is called
    a. conflict.
    b. overload.
    c. hassles.
    d. burnout.

5. Losing your keys is an example of what psychosocial source of stress?
    a. Pressure
    b. Inconsistent behaviors
    c. Hassles
    d. Conflict

6. After 5 years of 70-hour work-weeks, Tom decided to leave his high-paying, high-stress law firm and lead a simpler lifestyle. What is this trend called?
    a. Adaptation
    b. Conflict resolution
    c. Burnout reduction
    d. Downshifting

7. Which of the following test-taking techniques is *not* recommended to reduce test-taking stress?
    a. Plan ahead and study over a period of time for the test.
    b. Take regular breaks to refresh the overstimulated brain.
    c. Do all your studying the night before the exam so it is fresh in your mind.
    d. Practice by using other classmates' sample test questions.

8. Which of the following is *not* an example of a time-management technique?
    a. Scheduling one's time with a calendar or day planner
    b. Identifying time robbers
    c. Procrastinating completion of homework assignments
    d. Developing a game plan

9. Which of the following is an example of a chronic stressor?
    a. Giving a talk in public
    b. Meeting a big project deadline
    c. Having a permanent disability
    d. Dealing with the death of a family member or close friend

10. In which stage of the general adaptation syndrome does the fight-or-flight response occur?
    a. Exhaustion stage
    b. Alarm stage
    c. Resistance stage
    d. Response stage

Answers to these questions can be found on page A-1.

Think about It!

1. Describe the general adaptation syndrome phases and the body's response to stress. Does stress lead to more irritability or emotionality, or does emotionality lead to stress? Provide examples.

2. What are some of the health risks from chronic stress? How does the study of psychoneuroimmunology link stress and illness?

3. Why are the college years often high-stress? What factors increase stress risks? What actions manage your stressors?

4. How does anger affect the body? Discuss the steps you can take to manage your own anger and help your friends control theirs.

5. How much do you procrastinate? What can you do to reduce it?

Accessing Your Health on the Internet

These websites explore personal health topics and issues. For live links, visit the Companion Website for *Access to Health*, 13th Edition, at www.pearsonhighered.com/donatelle.

1. *American College Counseling Association.* This organization for college counselors has useful links and articles. www.collegecounseling.org
2. *American College Health Association.* This site provides information and data from the National College Health Assessment survey. www.acha.org
3. *American Psychological Association.* Here you can find current information and research on stress and stress-related conditions. www.apa.org/topics/stress/index.aspx
4. *Higher Education Research Institute.* This organization provides annual surveys of first-year and senior college students that cover academic, financial, and health-related issues and problems. www.heri.ucla.edu
5. *National Institute of Occupational Safety and Health, Stress at Work.* This site has resources on workplace stress. www.cdc.gov/niosh/topics/stress
6. *National Institute of Mental Health.* This comprehensive site from the National Institutes of Health is a resource for information on all aspects of mental health, including the effects of stress. www.nimh.nih.gov

References

1. American Psychological Association, "Stressed in America," *Monitor on Psychology* 42, no. 1 (2011): 60, www.apa.org/monitor/2011/01/stressed-america.aspx.
2. American Psychological Association, "APA Survey Raises Concern about Health Impact of Stress on Children and Families," press release, November 9, 2010, www.apa.org/news/press/releases/2010/11/stress-in-america.aspx.
3. American Psychological Association, "Stressed in America," 2011.
4. K. Glanz and M. Schwartz, "Stress, Coping and Health Behavior," in *Health Behavior and Health Education: Theory, Research and Practice,* 4th ed., eds.
K. Glanz, B. Rimer, and K. Viswanath (San Francisco: Jossey Bass, 2002), 210–36.
5. American Psychological Association, "Stress: The Different Kinds of Stress," Accessed 2011, www.apa.org/help-center/stress-kinds.aspx.
6. B. L. Seaward, *Managing Stress: Principles and Strategies for Health and Well-Being.* 7th ed. (Sudbury, MA: Jones and Bartlett, 2012), 8.
7. H. Selye, *Stress without Distress* (New York: Lippincott, Williams & Wilkins, 1974), 28–29.
8. W. B. Cannon, *The Wisdom of the Body* (New York: Norton, 1932).
9. B.S. McEwen and P. Tucker. "Critical Biological Pathways for Chronic Psychosocial Stress and Research Opportunities to Advance the Consideration of Stress in Chemical Risk Assessment," *American Journal of Public Health* 101, no. 1, Supplement (2011): S131–39; R. Juster, B. McEwen, and S. Lupien, "Allostatic Load Biomarkers of Chronic Stress and Impact on Health and Cognition," *Neuroscience and Biobehavioral Research,* 35, no. 1 (2010): 2–16.
10. P. Thoits, "Stress and Health: Major Findings and Policy Implications," *Journal of Health and Social Behavior,* no. 51 (2010): 554–55, DOI: 10.1177/0022146510383499.
11. A. Mokdad et al., "Actual Causes of Death in the United States, 2000," *Journal of the American Medical Association* 291 (2004): 1238–45.
12. E. Backe, A.Seidler, U. Latza, K. Rossnagel, and B. Schumann. "The Role of Psychosocial Stress at Work for the Development of Cardiovascular Disease: A Systematic Review," *International Archives of Occupational and Environmental Health* 85, no. 1 (2011): 67–79; A. Steptoe, A. Rosengren, and P. Hjemdahl. "Stress and Cardiovascular Disease: Introduction to Cardiovascular Disease," "Stress and Adaptation (2012): 1–14; J. Bremner et al., "Stress and Health: Effects of a Cognitive Stress Challenge on Myocardial Perfusion and Plasma Cortisol in Coronary Heart Disease Patients with Depression" (San Francisco: John Wiley & Sons, 2009); F. Sparrenberger et al., "Does Psychological Stress Cause Hypertension? A Systematic Review of Observational Studies," *Journal of Human Hypertension* 23 (2009): 12–19.
13. S. Yusef et al., "Effect of Potentially Modifiable Risk Factors Associated with Myocardial Infarction in 52 Countries (The INTERHEART Study): Case-Control Study," *Lancet* 364, no. 9438 (2004): 937–52.
14. Marshall, G., "The Adverse Effects of Psychological Stress on Immunoregulatory Balance: Applications to Human Inflammatory Disease." *Immunology and Allergy Clinics of North America* 31, no. 1 (2011): 133–40; J. Dimsdale, "Psychological Stress and Cardiovascular Disease," *Journal of the American College of Cardiology* 51 (2008): 1237–46.
15. B. Aggarwart, M. Liao, A. Christian, and L. Mosca, "Influence of Care-Giving on Lifestyle and Psychosocial Risk Factors among Family Members of Patients Hospitalized with Cardiovascular Disease," *Journal of General Internal Medicine* 24, no. 1 (2009): 1497–1525; F. Sparrenberger et al., "Does Psychological Stress Cause Hypertension?" 2009; M. Kivimäki et al., "Socioeconomic Position, Psychosocial Work Environment, and Cerebrovascular Disease among Women: The Finnish Public Sector Study," *International Journal of Epidemiology* (January 20, 2009); A. M. Hansen, A. D. Larsen, R. Rugulies, A. H. Garde, and L. E. Knudsen, "A Review of the Effect of the Psychosocial Working Environment on Physiological Changes in Blood and Urine," *Basic Clinical Pharmacology and Toxicology* 105, (2009): 73–83; T. Theorell, "Evaluating Life Events and Chronic Stressors in Relation to Health: Stressors and Health in Clinical Work," in *The Psychosomatic Assessment Strategies to Improve Clinical Practice. Advanced Psychosomatic Medicine,* eds. G. Fava, N. Sonina, and T. Wise, 32 (2012): 58–71.
16. K. Scott, S. Melhorn, and R. Sakai. "Effects of Chronic Social Stress on Obesity," *Current Obesity Reports Online First,* Accessed January 12, 2012, DOI: 10.1007/s13679-011-0006-3; V. Vicennati et al. "Cortisol, Energy Intake, and Food Frequency in Overweight/Obese Women," *Nutrition* 27, no. 6 (2011): 677–80; E. Lambert and G. Lambert., "Stress and Its Role in Sympathetic Nervous System Activation in Hypertension and the Metabolic Syndrome," *Current Hypertension Reports* 13, no. 3 (2011): 244–48; S. Pagota et al. "Association of Post-Traumatic Stress Disorder and Obesity in a Nationally Representative Sample," *Obesity* 20, no. 1 (2012): 200–205; V. Vicennati et al., "Stress-Related Development of Obesity and Cortisol in Women," *Obesity* 17, no. 19 (2009): 1678–83.
17. N. Ribertim et al. "Corticotropin Releasing Factor-Induced Amygdala Gamma Aminobutyric Acid Release Plays a Key Role in Alcohol Dependence," *Biological Psychiatry* 67, no. 9 (2010): 831–39[0].
18. D. K. Hall-Flavin, "Stress and Hair Loss: Are They Related?" Mayo Clinic.com, 2010, www.mayoclinic.com/health/stress-and-hair-loss/AN01442.
19. American Diabetes Association, "How Stress Affects Diabetes," 2011, www.diabetes.org/living-with-diabetes/complications/stress.html; H. Soo, "Stress Management Training in Diabetes Mellitus," *Journal of Health Psychology* 14, no. 7 (2009): 933–43; A. Pandy et al, "Alternative Therapies Useful in the Management of Diabetes: A Systematic Review,"

Journal of Bioallied Science 3, no. 4 (2011): 504–12.

20. C. Bernstein, "Quality of Life in Chronic Immune-Mediated Inflammatory Diseases," *The Journal of Rheumatology Supplement* 88, (2011): 62–65; Mayo Clinic Staff, "Stress: Constant Stress Puts Your Health at Risk," Mayo Foundation for Medical Education and Research, 2010, www.mayclinic.com/;print/stress/SR00001/METHOD=print; National Digestive Diseases Information Clearinghouse (NDDIC), "What I need to know about Irritable Bowel Syndrome," December, 2011.

21. S. Margolis. "Digestive Disorders White Paper–2011," *Johns Hopkins Health Alerts Relaxation*, 2011, www.johnshopkinshealthalerts.com/; C. Fang et al., "Enhanced Psychosocial Well-Being Following Participation in a Mindfulness-Based Stress Reduction Program Is Associated with Increased Natural Killer Cell Activity," *Journal of Alternative and Complementary Medicine* 16, no. 5 (2010): 531–36.

22. G. Miller, E. Chen, and K. Parker, "Psychological Stress in Childhood and Susceptibility to the Chronic Disease of Aging: Moving Toward a Model of Behavioral and Biological Mechanisms," *Psychological Bulletin* 137, no. 6 (2011): 959–97, DOI: 10.1037/a0024768; L. Christian, "Psychoneuroimmunology in Pregnancy: Immune Pathways Linking Stress with Maternal Health, Adverse Birth Outcomes and Fetal Development," *Neuroscience and Biobehavioral Reviews* 36, no. 1 (2012): 350–61, DOI: 10.1016/j.neubiorev.2011.07.005; A. Pedersen, R. Zachariae, and D. Bovbjerb, "Influence of Psychological Stress on Upper Respiratory Infection: A Meta-Analysis of Prospective Studies," *Psychosomatic Medicine* 7 (2010): 823–32; J. Walburn et al., "Psychological Stress and Wound Healing in Humans: A Systematic Review and Meta-Analysis," *Journal of Psychosomatic Research* 67, no. 3 (2009): 253–71.

23. G. Miller, N. Rohleder, and S. Cole, "Chronic Interpersonal Stress Predicts Activation of Pro- and Anti-Inflammatory Signaling 6 Months Later," *Psychosomatic Medicine* 71, no. 1 (2009): 57–62; T. Pace and C. Helm, "A Short Review on the Psychoneuroimmunology of Posttraumatic Stress Disorder: From Risk Factors to Medical Comorbidities," *Brain, Behavior and Immunity* 25, no. 1 (2011): 6–13[0].

24. M. Kondo, N., "Socioeconomic Disparities and Health: Impacts and Pathways," *Journal of Epidemiology* 22, no. 1 (2012): 2–6; [0]T. Theorell, "Evaluating Life Events and Chronic Stressors in Relation to Health: Stressors and Health in Clinical Work," *Advances in Psychosomatic Medicine* 32 (2012): 58–71; J. Gouln and J. Kiecolt-Glaser, "The Impact of Psychological Stress on Wound Healing: Methods and Mecha-

nisms," *Immunology and Allergy Clinics of North America* 31, no. 1 (2011): 81–93.

25. American College Health Association (ACHA), *American College Health Association–National College Health Assessment II (ACHA-NCHA II): Reference Group Data Report Spring, 2011* (Baltimore: American College Health Association, 2012).

26. M. Marin et al., "Chronic Stress, Cognitive Functioning and Mental Health." *Neurobiology of Learning and Memory* 96, no. 4 (2011): 583–95; L. Schwabe, T. Wolf, and M. Oitzi, "Memory Formation under Stress: Quantity and Quality," *Neuroscience and Biobehavioral Reviews* 34, no. 4 (2009): 584–91.

27. E. Dias-Ferreira et al., "Chronic Stress Causes Frontostriatal Reorganization and Affects Decision-Making," *Science* 325, no. 5940 (2009): 621–25; D. de Quervan et al., "Glucocorticoids and the Regulation of Memory in Health and Disease," *Frontiers in Neuroendocrinology* 30, no. 3 (2009): 358–70.

28. J. Fox, L. Halpern, J. Ryan, and K. Lowe, "Stressful Life Events and the Tripartite Model: Relations to Anxiety and Depression in Adolescent Females," *Journal of Adolescence* 33, no. 1 (2010): 43–54; J. Boardman and K. Alexander, "Stress Trajectories, Health Behaviors, and the Mental Health of Black and White Young Adults," *Social Science and Medicine* 72, no. 10 (2011): 1659–66; K. Scott et al., "Association of Childhood Adversities and Early-Onset Mental Disorders with Adult-Onset Chronic Physical Conditions," *Archives of General Psychiatry* 68, no. 8 (2011): 833–44.

29. J. Hunt and D. Eisenbe, "Mental Health Problems and Help Seeking Behaviors among College Students-Review Article," *Journal of Adolescent Health* 46, no. 1 (2010): 3–10; C. Segrin and S. Passalacqua, "Functions of Loneliness, Social Support, Health Behaviors, and Stress in Association with Poor Health," *Health Communication* 25, no. 4 (2010): 312.

30. American Psychological Association, *Stress in America Annual Survey. 2010. Key Findings,* 2011, www.apa.org/news/press/releases/stress/national-report.pdf.

31. R. Lazarus, "The Trivialization of Distress," in *Preventing Health Risk Behaviors and Promoting Coping with Illness,* eds. J. Rosen and L. Solomon (Hanover, NH: University Press of New England, 1985), 279–98.

32. D. Hellhammer, A. Stone, J. Hellhammer, and J. Broderick, "Measuring Stress," *Encyclopedia of Behavioral Neurosciences* 2 (2010): 186–91.

33. A. Nixon et al., "Can Work Make You Sick? A Meta-Analysis of the Relationships between Job Stressors and Physical Symptoms," *Work and Stress,* no. 1 (2011): 1–22.

34. A. Pieterse, R. Carter, S. Evans, and R. Walter, "An Exploratory Examination of the Associations among Racial and Ethnic Discrimina-

tion, Racial Climate, and Trauma-Related Symptoms in a College Student Population," *Journal of Counseling Psychology* 57, no. 3 (2010): 255–63; A. McAleavey, L. Castonguay, and B. Locke, "Sexual Orientation Minorities in College Counseling: Prevalence, Distress, and Symptom Profiles," *Journal of College Counseling* 14, no. 2 (2011): 127–42; M. Wei et al. *Journal of Counseling Psychology* 57, no. 4 (2010): 411–22.

35. Z. Djuric et al., "Biomarkers of Psychological Stress in Health Disparities Research," *The Open Biomarkers Journal* 1 (2008): 7–19; J. Watson, H. Logan, and S. Tomar, "The Influence of Active Coping and Perceived Stress on Health Disparities in a Multi-Ethnic Low Income Sample," *BMC Public Health* 8 (2008): 41; D. Iwamoto, L, Kenji, and W. Ming, "The Impact of Racial Identity, Ethnic Identity, Asian Values and Race-Related Stress on Asian Americans and Asian International College Students' Psychological Well-Being," *Journal of Counseling Psychology* 57, no. 1 (2010): 79–91.

36. E. Brondolo et al. "Racism and Hypertension: A Review of the Empirical Evidence and Implications for Clinical Practice," *American Journal of Hypertension* 24, no. 5 (2011): 518–24; F. Fuchs, "Editorial: Why Do Black Americans Have Higher Prevalence of Hypertension?" Hypertension 57 (2011): 370–80; N. Buchanan et al., "Unique and Joint Effects of Sexual and Racial Harassment on College Students' Well-Being," *Basic and Applied Social Psychology* 31, no. 3 (2009): 267–85.

37. D. Stang, "Calming Down: An Introduction to Stress and Stress Solutions," HealthVideo.com, Accessed November 2010, www.healthvideo.com/article.php?id=1174.

38. K. Karren, L. Smith, B. Hafen, and K. Frandren, Mind/Body Health: The Effects of Attitudes, Emotions, and Relationships. 4th ed. (San Francisco: Benjamin Cummings, 2010).

39. B. L. Seaward, *Managing Stress,* 2012.

40. Brown, K., *Predictors of Suicide Ideation and the Moderating Effects of Suicide Attitudes,* masters thesis, University of Ohio, 2011, http://etd.ohiolink.edu/view.cgi?acc_num=tolego1301765761; J. Gomez, R. Miranda, and L Polanco, "Acculturative Stress, Perceived Discrimination and Vulnerability to Suicide Attempts among Emerging Adults," *Journal of Youth and Adolescence* 40, no. 11 (2011): 1465–76.

41. K. Glanz, B. Rimer, and F. Levis, eds., *Health Behavior and Health Education: Theory, Research, and Practice.* 4th ed. (San Francisco: Jossey-Bass, 2008).

42. B. L.Seaward, *Managing Stress: Principles and Strategies for Health and Well-Being,* 2012.

43. M. Friedman and R. H. Rosenman, Type *A Behavior and Your Heart* (New York: Knopf, 1974).

44. M. Whooley and J. Wong, "Hostility and Cardiovascular Disease," *Journal of the American Collage of Cardiology* 58 (2011): 1228–30; J. Newman et al. "Observed Hostility and the Risk of Incident Ischemic Heart Disease: A Perspective Population Study from the 1995 Canadian Nova Scotia Health Survey," *Journal of the American Collage of Cardiology* 58 (2011): 1222–28; T. Smith., B. Uchino, B. Berg, and P. Florscheim, "Marital discord and Coronary Artery Disease: A Comparison of Behaviorally Defined Discrete Groups," *Journal of Consulting and Clinical Psychology* 80, no. 1 (2012): 87–92.

45. M. Jawer and M. Micozzi, *The Spiritual Anatomy of Emotion: How Feelings Link the Brain, the Body, and the Sixth Sense* (Rochester, VT: Park Street Press, 2009).

46. J. Denollet, "Prognostic Value of Type D Personality Compared with Depressive Symptoms," *Archives of Internal Medicine* 168, no. 4 (2008): 431–35; L. Williams et al., "Type D Personality Mechanisms of Effect: The Role of Health-Related Behavior and Social Support," *Journal of Psychosomatic Research* 64, no. 1 (2008): 63–68; H. Versteeg, V. Spek, and S. Pedersen, "Type D Personality and Health Status in Cardiovascular Disease Populations: A Meta-Analysis of Prospective Studies," *European Journal of Cardiovascular Prevention and Rehabilitation* (2011), DOI: 10.1177/1741826711425338.

47. S. Kobasa, "Stressful Life Events, Personality, and Health: An Inquiry into Hardiness," *Journal of Personality and Social Psychology* 37 (1979): 1–11.

48. C. D. Schetter and C. Dolbier, "Resilience in the Context of Chronic Stress and Health in Adults," *Social and Personality Psychology Compass* 5 (2011): 634–52, DOI: 10.1111/j.1751-9004.2011.00379.x.

49. The American Psychological Association Help Center, "What Is Resilience?" 2012. www.apa.org/helpcenter/road-resilience.aspx#; F. Castro and K. Murray, "Cultural Adaptations and Resilience: Controversies, Issues and Emerging Models," in *Handbook of Adult Resilience,* eds. J. Reich, A. Zautra, and J. Hall (New York: Guilford Press., 2010), 375–403; B. J. Crowley, B. Hayslip, and J. Hobdy, "Psychological Hardiness and Adjustment to Life Events in Adulthood," *Journal of Adult Development* 10 (2003): 237–48; S. R. Maddi, "The Story of Hardiness: Twenty Years of Theorizing, Research, and Practice," *Consulting Psychology Journal: Practice and Research* 54 (2002): 173–86.

50. J. H. Pryor et al., *The American Freshman: National Norms Fall 2009* (Los Angeles: Higher Education Research Institute, 2010), Available at www.heri.ucla.edu/publications-brp.php; J. Pryer, "The Changing First-Year Student: Challenges for 2011. Higher Education Research Institute of UCLA-Freshman Survey 2010." Presented at AAC&U 2011 Annual Meeting (San Francisco, CA).

51. J. Pryer, "The Changing First-Year Student," 2011.

52. H. Morrell, L. Cohen, and D. McChargue, "Depression Vulnerability Predicts Cigarette Smoking among College Students: Gender and Negative Reinforcement Expectancies as Contributing Factors," *Addictive Behavior* 35(2010): 607–11; J. Cranford, S. Nolen-Hoeksema, and R. Zucker, "Alcohol Involvement as a Function of Co-occurring Alcohol Use Disorders and Major Depressive Episode: Evidence from the National Epidemiologic Survey on Alcohol and Related Conditions," *Drug and Alcohol Dependence* 117, no. 3 (2011): 145–51; C. L. Broman, "Stress, Race, and Substance Use in College," *College Student Journal* 39, no. 2 (2005): 340–52; D. Kariv, D. Heilman, and T. Heilman, "Task-Oriented versus Emotion-Oriented Coping Strategies: The Case of College Students," *College Student Journal* 39, no. 1 (2005): 72–84; K. M. Kieffer et al., "Test and Study Worry and Emotionality in the Prediction of College Students' Reasons for Drinking: An Exploratory Investigation," *Journal of Alcohol and Drug Education* 50, no. 1 (2006): 57–81.

53. J. Boardman and K. Alexander, "Stress Trajectories, Health Behaviors and the Mental Health of Black and White Young Adults," *Social Science and Medicine* 72, no. 10 (2011): 1659–66; M. Cerda and V. Johnson-Lawrence, "Lifetime Income Patterns and Alcohol Consumption: Investigating the Association between Long and Short Term Income Trajectories and Drinking," *Social Science and Medicine* 73, no. 8 (2011): 1178–85; E. Avant., J. Davis, and C. Cranston, "Posttraumatic Stress Symptom Clusters, Trauma History, and Substance Use among College Students," *Journal of Aggression, Maltreatment and Trauma* 20, no. 5 (2011): 539–55; M. Terlecki, J. Buckner, M. Larimer, and A. Copeland, "The Role of Social Anxiety in a Brief Alcohol Intervention for Heavy-Drinking College Students," *Journal of Cognitive Psychotherapy* 25, no. 1 (2011): 7–21.

54. B. L. Seaward, Managing *Stress: Principles and Strategies for Health and Well-Being.* 7th ed. (New York: Barnes and Noble, 2012).

55. Ibid.

56. P. Thoits, "Mechanisms Linking Social Ties and Support to Physical and Mental Health," *Journal of Health and Social Behavior* 52, no. 2 (2011): 145–61; B. Lake and E. Oreheck, "Relational Regulation Theory: A New Approach to Explain the Link between Perceived Social Support and Mental Health," *Psychological Review* 118, no. 3 (2011): 482–95; M. Neely et al., "Self Kindness When Facing Stress: The Role of Compassion, Self Regulation and Support in College Students' Well Being," *Motivation and Emotion* 33 (2009): 88–97; J. Ruthig et al., "Perceived Academic Control: Mediating the Effects of Optimism and Social Support on College Students' Psychological Health," *Social Psychology of Education* 12, no. 7 (2009): 233–49.

57. B. L. Seaward, *Managing Stress,* 2012.

58. J. Graham et al., "Cognitive Word Use during Marital Conflict and Increases in Pro-inflammatory Cytokines," *Health Psychology* 28, no. 5 (2009): 621–30.

59. G. Colom, C. Alcover, C. Sanchez-Curto, and J. Zarate-Osuna, "Study of the Effect of Positive Humour as a Variable That Reduces Stress. Relationship of Humour with Personality and Performance Variables," *Psychology in Spain* 15, no. 1 (2011): 9–21; E. Garland et al., "Upward Spirals of Positive Emotions Counter Downward Spirals of Negativity. Insights from the Broaden-and-Build Theory and Affects of Neuroscience on the Treatment of Emotion Dysfunctions and Psychopathology," *Clinical Psychology Review* 30, no. 7, (2010): 549–64.

60. L. Poole et al., "Associations of Objectively Measured Physical Activity with Daily Mood Ratings and Psychophysiological Stress Responses in Women," *Psychophysiology* 48 (2011): 1165–72; DOI: 10.1111/j.1469-8986.2011.01184.x; D. A. Girdano, D. E. Dusek, and G. S. Everly, *Controlling Stress and Tension.* 9th ed. (San Francisco: Benjamin Cummings, 2012), 375.

61. P. Gollwitzer and P. Sheeran, "Implementation Intentions," 2009, National Cancer Institute, http://cancercontrol.cancer.gov/brp/constructs/implementation_intentions/goal_intent_attain.pdf.

62. A. Grant, "Yoga Teaching Increasingly Popular as Second Career," *U.S. News and World Report,* Money, 2012, http://money.usnews.com/money/careers/articles/2011/04/26/yoga-teaching-increasingly-popular-as-second-career.

63. J. Kiecolt-Glaser et al., "Stress, Inflammation, and Yoga Practice," *Psychosomatic Medicine* 72, no. 2 (2010): 113–21.

64. S. Nidich et al., "A Randomized Controlled Trial on the Effects of Transcendental Meditation Program on Blood Pressure, Psychological Distress, and Coping in Young Adults," *American Journal of Hypertension* 22, no. 12 (2009): 1326–31.

65. M. Rapaport, P. Schettler, and C. Bresee, "A Preliminary Study of the Effects of a Single Session of Swedish Massage on Hypothalamic-Pituitary-Adrenal and Immune Function in Normal Individuals," *The Journal of Alternative and Complementary Medicine* 16, no. 10 (2010): 1–10.

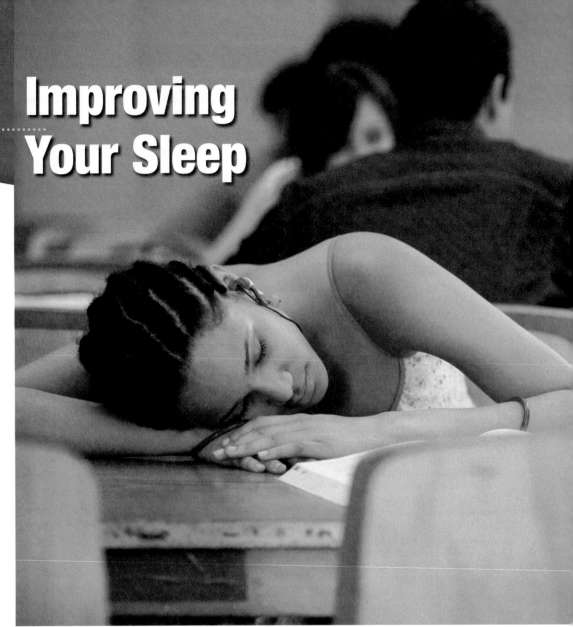

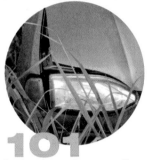

101

Is sleepiness dangerous?

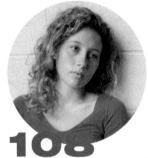

104

Why do caffeinated drinks keep me awake?

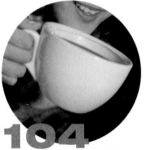

106

Are sleep disorders common?

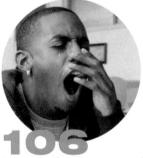

108

What should I do if I can't fall asleep?

Josh knew he wasn't ready for tomorrow's physics exam, but he went to his roommate's basketball game anyway. It was past 11 PM when he finally hit the books. To keep himself awake he drank an energy drink and then a cup of coffee as he plowed through the text, his notes, and the online study guide. Just before 4 AM he fell into bed exhausted. But instead of sleeping, his mind kept racing. *Dynamics, inertia, action,* and *reaction* tumbled around with disjointed memories of all the stressful situations he'd been through in the past few days: losing his cell phone, the argument with his dad. . . .

He glanced at the clock: It was 5:30 AM, and the exam was in 3 hours.

You can probably predict what happened—Josh failed the test.

All people need **sleep,** which is clinically defined as a readily reversible state of reduced responsiveness to, and interaction with, the environment.[1] New evidence links inadequate sleep with a variety of health problems Americans have struggled with for decades, including weight gain, high blood pressure, depression, lowered immunity, and other ailments. Seventy-six percent of Americans want to improve the quantity and quality of the sleep

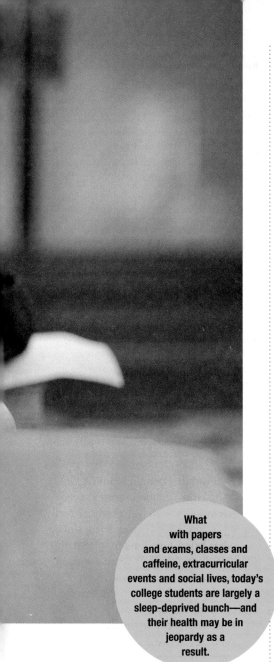

What with papers and exams, classes and caffeine, extracurricular events and social lives, today's college students are largely a sleep-deprived bunch—and their health may be in jeopardy as a result.

owls" who are still awake in the wee hours of the morning yet must get up early—resulting in regular sleep deficiency."[4] In fact, several major studies indicate that younger Americans, particularly those between the ages of 18 and 24, and those over the age of 65 are most likely to fall asleep unintentionally during the day, suffering from a condition known as **excessive daytime sleepiness**, or EDS.[5] Whether due to sleep deficiency or one of the growing list of sleep disorders, between 15 to 30 percent of students report that they fall asleep in class on a regular basis. Those students who carry full course loads and struggle to sleep are significantly more likely to perform worse on academic tests, use more alcohol, and experience higher rates of depression.

44%

of college students say they don't feel rested most days of the week.

One factor commonly implicated in reduced sleep time among college students is the Internet and its 24-hour access to online games, social networks, videos, and news. Unfortunately, the statistics don't improve much for working adults. A recent *Sleep in America* poll from the National Sleep Foundation (NSF) found over 35 percent of adults reported getting less than 7 hours of sleep per day.[6] These sleepy workers are more likely to have on-the-job accidents, perform poorly, and have motor vehicle accidents when commuting. In a recent survey, over 30 percent of workers reported falling asleep or being barely awake in the past month while at work and/or driving drowsy. Shift workers are particularly susceptible to sleep-related problems.[7] When there just aren't enough hours in the day, what typically gets shortchanged is sleep. Because Americans are managing to function with less sleep, you might

they get. Globally, sleep deprivation affects the quality of life of 45 percent of the world's population.[2] In a recent survey from the American College Health Association (ACHA), only about 11 percent of students reported getting enough sleep to feel well rested in the morning 6 or more days a week. Over 60 percent of students said they felt tired or sleepy for 3 or more days in the past week.[3] It's widely acknowledged that college students are among the most sleep-deprived age group in the United States, with nearly 60 percent of those in the 18- to 29-year-old age group describing themselves as "night

sleep A readily reversible state of reduced responsiveness to, and interaction with, the environment.

excessive daytime sleepiness(EDS): disorder characterized by unusual patterns of falling asleep during normal waking hours

conclude that sufficient sleep isn't all that necessary. In fact, getting an adequate amount of sleep is much more important than most people realize. Let's look at the benefits of sleep and find out what happens when you don't get enough.

Why Do You Need to Sleep?

Sleep serves at least two biological purposes: (1) It conserves body energy. When you sleep, your core body temperature and the rate at which you burn calories drop. This leaves you with more energy to perform activities throughout your waking hours. (2) It restores you both physically and mentally. For example, certain reparative chemicals are released while you sleep. And there is some evidence, discussed shortly, that during sleep the brain is cleared of daily minutiae, learning is synthesized, and memories are consolidated. In short, getting enough sleep to feel ready to meet daily challenges is essential.

Sleep Maintains Your Physical Health

Sleep has beneficial effects on most body systems. That's why, when you consistently don't get a good night's rest, your body doesn't function as well, and you become more vulnerable to a wide variety of health problems.[8] Researchers are only just beginning to explore the physical benefits of sleep. Here is a brief summary of what we've learned so far.

● **Sleep helps maintain your immune system.** The common cold, strep throat, flu, mononucleosis, cold sores, and a variety of other ailments are more common when your immune system is depressed. And that's more likely to happen if you're not getting enough sleep. For instance, one recent study found that poor sleep quality and shorter sleep duration increased susceptibility to the common cold.[9] Another study reports that sleep disruption, particularly when circadian rhythms are disturbed repeatedly, disrupts overall immune function.[10]

- **Sleep helps reduce your risk for cardiovascular disease.** Several studies have indicated that high blood pressure is more common in people who get fewer than 7 hours of sleep a night.[11] In addition, two separate studies found that poor sleep quality or reduced sleep time increased the levels of a substance called C-reactive protein (CRP) in the blood, which is a risk factor for heart disease.[12] A study of more than 93,000 women also suggested that sleep duration of 6 or fewer hours a night increases the risk of stroke.[13]

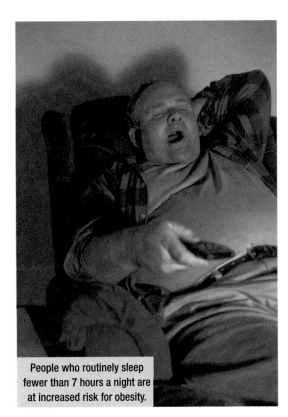

People who routinely sleep fewer than 7 hours a night are at increased risk for obesity.

- **Sleep contributes to a healthy metabolism.** Chemical reactions in your body's cells break down food and synthesize compounds that the body needs. The sum of all these reactions is called *metabolism*. Several recent studies suggest sleep contributes to healthy metabolism and possibly a healthy body weight. Those who sleep less tend to eat more, particularly high-fat, high-protein foods, and exercise less than those who get adequate amounts of sleep.[14] There is evidence that sleep deficiencies, and particularly sleep disorders such as sleep apnea, can increase the risk of *type 2 diabetes*, a disorder of glucose metabolism.[15]

Sleep Affects Your Ability to Function

The evidence is compelling. Shortchange your sleep and you could be sabotaging your health, your job, your relationships, your grades and increasing your risks for accidents. If you drive while drowsy, you could endanger your life and the lives of others. Let's look at what research reveals about how sleep helps you to function.

- **Sleep contributes to neurological functioning.** Restricting sleep can cause a wide range of neurological problems, including lapses of attention, slowed or poor memory, reduced cognitive ability, and a tendency for your thinking to get "stuck in a rut."[16] Your ability not only to remember facts, but also to integrate those facts, make meaningful generalizations about them, and consolidate what you've learned into lasting memories requires adequate sleep time.[17] College students who pull all-nighters, as well as students who are short sleepers, have significantly lower overall grade-point averages compared with classmates who get adequate sleep.[18]

- **Sleep improves motor tasks.** Sleep also has a restorative effect on motor function, or the ability to perform tasks such as shooting a basket, playing a musical instrument, or driving a car. Motor function is affected by sleep throughout the life span.[19] Some researchers contend that a night without sleep impairs your motor skills and reaction time as much as if you were driving drunk.[20] As Americans have become more and more sleep-deprived, the incidence of drowsy driving and so-called fall-asleep crashes has become a national concern. The NSF reports that nearly one third of Americans admit to having fallen asleep at the wheel in the past year, with more than 55 percent saying they had driven while drowsy. It is estimated that over 1,500 Americans die in fatigue-related crashes annually.[21]

Sleep Promotes Your Psychosocial Health

It is believed that certain brain regions, including the cerebral cortex (your "master mind"), only get essential rest during sleep. Metabolism may slow, but other brain functions may actually increase during sleep.[22] Adequate sleep serves as a form of restorative cyclical pattern in which hormones are secreted, and the body has time to balance essential processes, repair systems, and conserve energy. When sleep cycles are disrupted, these repair/restore cycles are also disrupted. Irritability after a sleepless night may in part be due to disruptions in essential brain functions.

In addition, you're more likely to feel stressed-out, worried, or sad when you're sleep deprived. The relationship between sleep and stress is highly complex: Stress can cause or contribute to sleep problems, and sleep problems can cause or increase your level of stress! The same is true of clinical psychiatric conditions such as depression and anxiety disorders: Reduced or poor-quality sleep can trigger these disorders, but it's also a common symptom resulting from them. Nondepressed individuals who suffer from chronic insomnia have over twice the risk of developing depression.[23]

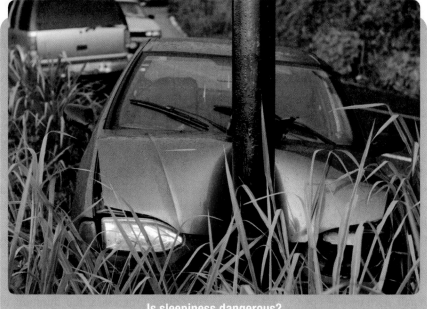

Is sleepiness dangerous?

Lack of sleep impairs your reflexes, cognitive functioning, and motor skills, all of which you need to ride a bike or operate a car safely. The National Sleep Foundation estimates that 100,000 sleep-related auto accidents, resulting in more than 1,500 deaths, occur in the United States every year. If you have difficulty falling asleep, it may be that noises, lights, interruptions, or persistent worries are keeping you awake. Use ear plugs or a white noise machine to block out noise, wear an eye shade to block out light, and turn off your phone and computer.

circadian rhythm The 24-hour cycle by which you are accustomed to going to sleep, waking up, and performing habitual behaviors.

hormone A "chemical messenger" that is released from one of the body's endocrine glands and travels in the bloodstream to another site where it helps to regulate body functions.

REM sleep A period of sleep characterized by brain-wave activity similar to that seen in wakefulness; rapid eye movement and dreaming occur during REM sleep.

non-REM (NREM) sleep A period of restful sleep dominated by slow brain waves; during non-REM sleep, rapid eye movement is rare.

What Goes on When You Sleep?

If you've ever taken a flight that crossed two or more time zones, you've probably experienced *jet lag,* a feeling that your body's "internal clock" is out of sync with the hours of daylight and darkness at your destination. Jet lag happens because the new day/night pattern disrupts the 24-hour cycle by which you are accustomed to going to sleep, waking up, and performing habitual behaviors throughout your day. This cycle, known as your **circadian rhythm,** is regulated in part by a tiny gland in your brain called the *pineal body:* It releases a **hormone** called *melatonin* that induces drowsiness.

You can fight the effects of melatonin for hours—even days!—especially if, like Josh in our opening story, you load up on caffeine. But all mammals will eventually succumb to sleep. Humans should spend roughly one third of our lives asleep. Sleep researchers generally distinguish between two primary sleep states. During **REM sleep,** rapid eye movement occurs, brain wave activity appears similar to being awake, and dreams occur. **Non-REM (NREM) sleep,** in contrast, is the period of restful sleep with slowed brain activity that does *not* include rapid eye movement. During the night, you alternate between periods of NREM and REM sleep, repeating one full cycle about once every 90 minutes.[24] Overall, you spend about 75 percent of each night in NREM sleep and 25 percent in REM **(Figure 1).**

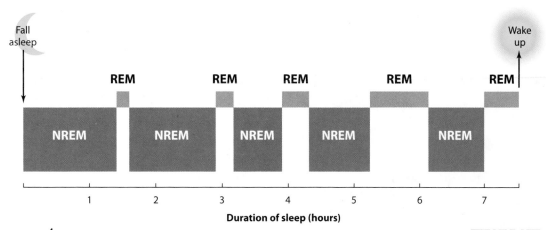

FIGURE 1 The Nightly Sleep Cycle
As the number of hours you sleep increases, your brain spends more and more time in REM sleep. Thus, sleeping for too few hours could mean you're depriving yourself primarily of needed REM sleep.

Video Tutor: Sleep Cycle

Non-REM Sleep Is Restorative

During non-REM sleep, the body rests. Movement can occur, for instance, to shift your position in bed, but muscle tension is reduced. Both your body temperature and your energy use drop; sensation is dulled; and your brain waves, heart rate, and breathing slow. In contrast, digestive processes speed up, and your body stores nutrients. During NREM sleep, you do not typically dream. Four distinct stages of NREM sleep have been distinguished by their characteristic brain-wave patterns.

Stage 1. Your eyes may be open or closed, but essentially, you're drifting off. Stage 1 lasts only a few minutes, and it is the lightest stage of sleep from which you are most easily awakened. This is the transition between wakefulness and sleep in which the brain produces *theta waves,* which are slow brain waves. Many experience a sudden feeling of falling in this stage, which may cause a quick, jerky muscular reaction.

Stage 2. This stage is slightly deeper than stage 1 and lasts 5 to 15 minutes. Your eyes are closed, eye and body movements gradually cease, and you disengage from your environment.

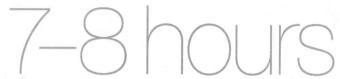

7–8 hours
is the sleep period associated with optimal health.

Stage 3. NREM sleep is also called *slow-wave sleep*, because during stages 3 and 4, a sleeper's brain generates slow, large-amplitude delta waves as shown on an electroencephalogram (EEG). Your blood pressure drops, your heart rate and respiration slow considerably, and you enter deep sleep.

Stage 4. This is the deepest stage of sleep. Human growth hormone is released and signals your body to repair worn tissues. Speech and movement are rare during this stage, but can and do sometimes occur. For example, sleepwalking typically occurs during the first stage 4 period of the night. You've probably heard that it's difficult to awaken a sleepwalker, and that's true of anyone in stage 4 sleep.

REM Sleep Energizes

Dreaming takes place primarily during REM sleep. On an EEG, a REM sleeper's brain-wave activity is almost indistinguishable from that of someone who is wide awake, and the brain's energy use is higher than that of a person who is performing a difficult math problem![25] Your muscles are paralyzed during REM sleep: You may dream that you're rock climbing, but your body is incapable of movement. Almost the only exceptions are your respiratory muscles, which allow you to breathe, and the tiny muscles of your eyes, which move your eyes rapidly as if you were following the scenario of your dream. This rapid eye movement gives REM sleep its name.

During REM sleep, your brain processes the ex-periences you've had and consolidates the information you've learned during the day. A growing chorus of researchers have theorized that if you are deprived of REM sleep, you may well have declines in cognitive function, particularly memory.[26] As the night progresses, the duration of NREM sleep declines and you spend more time in REM. That's why a full night's sleep is important for getting adequate REM cycles.

How Much Sleep Do You Need?

Researchers find that most people need between 7 and 8 hours of sleep per day, on average.[27] But sleep needs vary from person to person, and your gender, health, and lifestyle will also affect how much rest your body demands. It is worth noting that sleep patterns change over the life span, with newborns needing 16 to 18 sleeping hours daily and teens and younger adults needing 8 to 9 hours per night, slightly more than the adult average. Women need more sleep than men overall. It is a myth to think that people need less sleep as they grow older, though older adults may experience sleep difficulties that result in fewer hours of rest per night due to health conditions, pain, and the need to use the bathroom more frequently.[28]

Research has consistently shown that sleep really is the "great elixir" and that sleep deprivation and disorders contribute significantly to premature death and disability from a variety of causes. In general, those who get adequate amounts of sleep live longer and enjoy more quality days than those who don't.[29]

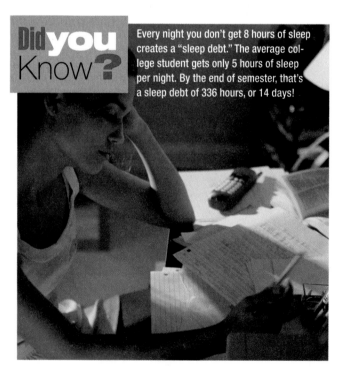

Did you Know? Every night you don't get 8 hours of sleep creates a "sleep debt." The average college student gets only 5 hours of sleep per night. By the end of semester, that's a sleep debt of 336 hours, or 14 days!

Sleep Need Includes Baseline Plus Debt

Pay attention to how you feel after different amounts of sleep, and aim for the duration that feels best for you.[30] In addition to your body's physiological need, consider your current **sleep debt.** That's the total number of hours of missed sleep you're carrying around with you, either because you got up before you were fully rested or because your sleep was interrupted. Let's say that last week you managed just 5 hours of sleep a night, Monday through Thursday. Even if you get 7 to 8 hours a night Friday through Sunday, that unresolved sleep debt of 8 to 12 hours will still leave you tired and groggy when you start the week again. That means you need *more than* 8 hours a night for the next several nights to "catch up."

The good news is that you *can* catch up if you go about it sensibly. Getting 5 hours of sleep a night all semester long, then sleeping 48 hours the first weekend you're home on break won't restore your functioning, and it's likely to disrupt your circadian rhythm. Instead, whittle away at that sleep debt by sleeping 9 hours a night throughout your break—then start the new term resolved to sleep 7 to 8 hours a night.

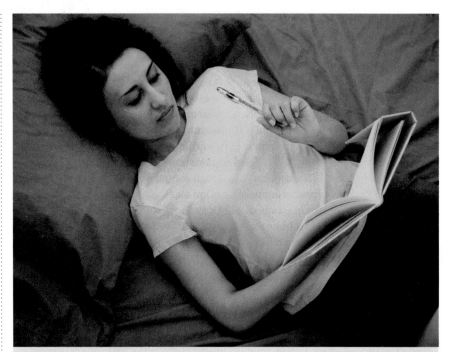

If a worry keeps you awake, jot it down in a journal. You'll be better prepared to handle it in the morning after a good night's sleep.

what do you think?

Do you find it difficult to get 7 or 8 hours of sleep each night?
● Do you think you are able to catch up on sleep you miss?
● Have you noticed any negative consequences in your own life when you get too little sleep?

Do Naps Count?

Speaking of catching up, do naps count? Although naps can't entirely cancel out a significant sleep debt, they can improve your mood, alertness, and performance. A nap may also improve immune functioning and help ward off infections.[31]

It's best to nap in the early to mid-afternoon, when the pineal body in your brain releases a small amount of melatonin and your body experiences a natural dip in its circadian rhythm. Never nap in the late afternoon, as it could interfere with your ability to fall asleep that night. Keep your naps short, because a nap of more than 30 minutes can leave you in a state of **sleep inertia,** which is characterized by cognitive impairment, grogginess, and a disoriented feeling. If you find that your nap makes you feel a bit nauseated or ill, napping might not be right for you.

How to Get a Good Night's Sleep

Do you need a jolt of caffeine to get started in the morning? Do you find it hard to stay awake in class? Have you ever nodded off behind the wheel? These are all signs of inadequate or poor quality sleep. To find out whether you're sleep deprived, go online to www.pearsonhighered.com/donatelle and take the **Assess Yourself** questionnaire.

To Promote Restful Sleep, Try These Tips

The following tips can help you get a more restful night's sleep.

● **Let there be light.** Throughout the day, stay in sync with your circadian rhythm by spending time in the sunlight. If you live in an area where the sun seldom shines for weeks at a time, invest in special light-emitting diode (LED) lighting designed to mimic the sun's rays. Exposure to natural light outdoors is most beneficial, but opening the shades indoors and, on overcast days, turning on room lights can also help keep you alert.
● **Stay active.** It's hard to feel sleepy if you've been sedentary all day, so get plenty of physical activity during the day. Resist the temptation to postpone

sleep debt The difference between the number of hours of sleep an individual needed in a given time period and the number of hours he or she actually slept.

sleep inertia A state characterized by cognitive impairment, grogginess, and disorientation that is experienced upon rising from short sleep or an overly long nap.

exercise until you're sleeping better. Start gently, but start now, because regular exercise can help you maintain regular sleep habits.

● **Sleep tight.** Don't let a pancake pillow, scratchy or pilled sheets, or a threadbare blanket keep you from sleeping soundly. If your mattress is uncomfortable and you can't replace it, try putting a foam mattress overlay on top of it.

● **Create a sleep "cave."** Take a lesson from bats, bears, and burrowing animals! As bedtime approaches, keep your bedroom quiet, cool, and dark. Start by turning off your computer and cell phone. If you live in an apartment or dorm where there's noise outside or in the halls, wear ear plugs or get an electronic device that produces "white noise" such as the sound of gentle rain. Turn down the thermostat or, on hot nights, run an electric fan. Install room-darkening shades

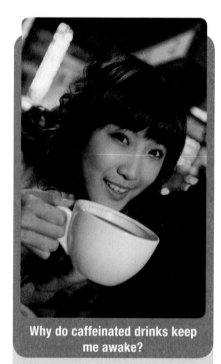

Why do caffeinated drinks keep me awake?

After-dinner coffee? Not unless it's decaf. Caffeine promotes alertness by blocking the neurotransmitter adenosine in your brain—a useful thing when you are studying, but a potential problem when you are trying to sleep. Your body needs 6 hours to process half of the caffeine you drink (and another 6 to process half of what remains, and so on). So coffee at 8 PM means you won't be sleeping soundly until well after midnight.

or curtains or wear an eye mask if necessary to block outside light.

● **Condition yourself into better sleep.** Go to bed and get up at the same time each day. Establish a bedtime ritual that signals to your body that it's time for sleep. For instance, listen to a quiet song, take a warm shower, or read something that lets you quietly wind down. Practice relaxation strategies such as deep breathing.

● **Make your bedroom a mental escape.** Don't stew about things you can't fix right now. Clear your mind of worries and frustrations. Breathe deeply. Focus on listening to your body unwind.

● **Get rid of technology in the bedroom.** Make a rule: No TV, texting, or chatting online after a certain time. If you can't sleep, don't surf the net or check out your Facebook page.

● **Forget about it!** You aren't going to solve your problems or the world's problems during your sleep time. Consciously make a rule that when the problems of the day "intrude" into your sleep time, that you are going to "change the subject or hit your mind's "PAUSE" or "STOP button," focusing on something different that is pleasant and relaxing.

● **Don't toss and turn.** If you're not asleep after 20 minutes, get up. Turn on a low light, and read something relaxing, not stimulating, or listen to some gentle music. Once you feel sleepy, go back to bed.

Problematic Sleep Behaviors to Avoid

Maybe you're already doing most of the actions suggested above, and you still can't sleep. If so, perhaps it's time to learn what *not* to do:

● Don't nap in the late afternoon or evening, and don't nap for longer than 30 minutes.

● Don't engage in strenuous exercise within several hours of bedtime. Activity speeds up your metabolism and makes it harder to fall asleep.

● Don't read, study, watch TV, use your laptop, talk on the phone, eat, or smoke in bed. In fact, don't smoke at all: Besides promoting cancer and heart disease, smoking is known to disturb your sleep.

● Don't try to sleep if you're starving or stuffed. Allow at least 3 hours between your evening meal and bedtime, and if you feel hungry before bed, have a light snack.

● Don't drink coffee, energy drinks, or anything else that contains caffeine within several hours of bedtime. Once you consume caffeine, which is a powerful stimulant, it takes your body about 6 hours to clear just *half* of it from your system.[32]

● Don't drink alcohol within several hours of bedtime. Although initially it can make you drowsy, it interferes with your natural sleep stages and can cause you to awaken in the middle of the night, unable to get back to sleep.

● Don't drink large amounts of any liquid before bed, to prevent having to get up in the night to use the bathroom.

● Avoid sleeping pills and nighttime pain medications unless they have been prescribed by your health care provider. Over-the-counter sleeping aids can interfere with your brain's natural progression through the healthy stages of sleep. You may also experience "payback" later when you try to stop using the drug and your sleep challenges return, at a level worse than they were before you started the medication.

● Don't get triggered. Remember the earlier advice about turning off your cell phone as you begin to prepare for bed? One reason is to avoid those late-night phone calls that can end up in arguments, disappointments, and other emotional stressors. If something—or someone—does trigger you shortly before bed, journal about it briefly, then promise yourself that you'll make time the next day to explore your feelings.

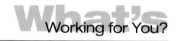

What's Working for You?

Maybe you're already practicing ways to get a better night's sleep. Which of the following sleep-promoting behaviors are you already incorporating into your life?

☐ I exercise regularly.

☐ I turn off my computer at night.

☐ I drink only caffeine-free beverages late in the day.

☐ I make sure not to nap late in the day.

What Do You Do If You're Still Not Sleeping Well?

Fewer than 5 percent of college students are diagnosed and in treatment for sleep disorders.[33] However, the Centers for Disease Control and Prevention estimates that sleeplessness has hit epidemic levels in the United States, causing millions of people to have difficulty performing everyday tasks (Table 1). If you're following the advice in this chapter and you still aren't sleeping well, visit your health care provider; you may be one of the estimated 50 to 70 million Americans who have a clinical sleep disorder.[34]

TABLE 1

Self-Reported Sleep-Related Difficulties among Adults 20 Years Old and Older

Difficulty	Percentage of Adults
Concentrating on things	23.2%
Remembering things	18.2%
Working on hobbies	13.3%
Driving or taking public transportation	11.3%
Taking care of financial affairs	10.5%
Performing employed or volunteer work	8.6%

Source: Centers for Disease Control and Prevention, "Insufficient Sleep Is a Public Health Epidemic," Accessed October 5, 2011, www.cdc.gov/features/dsSleep/.

In a large study of college students, approximately 27 percent of students were at risk for a sleep disorder, with narcolepsy and insomnia being the most common problems. To aid in diagnosis, you will probably be asked to keep a sleep diary like the one in Figure 2. You may also be referred to

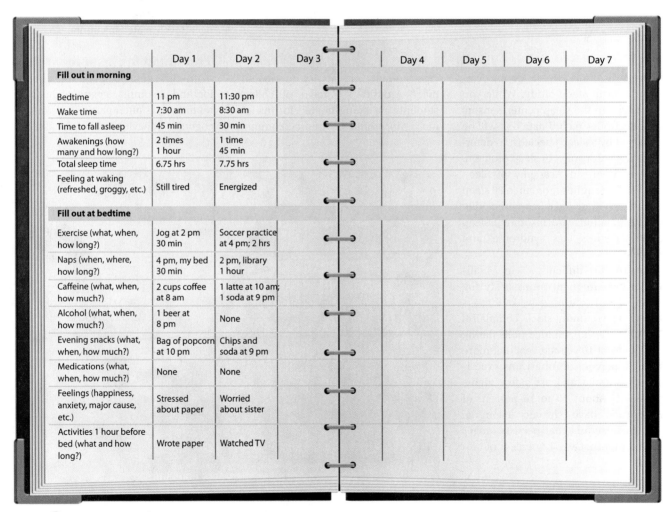

	Day 1	Day 2	Day 3	Day 4	Day 5	Day 6	Day 7
Fill out in morning							
Bedtime	11 pm	11:30 pm					
Wake time	7:30 am	8:30 am					
Time to fall asleep	45 min	30 min					
Awakenings (how many and how long?)	2 times 1 hour	1 time 45 min					
Total sleep time	6.75 hrs	7.75 hrs					
Feeling at waking (refreshed, groggy, etc.)	Still tired	Energized					
Fill out at bedtime							
Exercise (what, when, how long?)	Jog at 2 pm 30 min	Soccer practice at 4 pm; 2 hrs					
Naps (when, where, how long?)	4 pm, my bed 30 min	2 pm, library 1 hour					
Caffeine (what, when, how much?)	2 cups coffee at 8 am	1 latte at 10 am; 1 soda at 9 pm					
Alcohol (what, when, how much?)	1 beer at 8 pm	None					
Evening snacks (what, when, how much?)	Bag of popcorn at 10 pm	Chips and soda at 9 pm					
Medications (what, when, how much?)	None	None					
Feelings (happiness, anxiety, major cause, etc.)	Stressed about paper	Worried about sister					
Activities 1 hour before bed (what and how long?)	Wrote paper	Watched TV					

FIGURE 2 Sample Sleep Diary
Using a sleep diary such as this one can help you and your health care provider discover behavioral factors that might be contributing to your sleep problem.

Beat Jet Lag

Insomnia, fatigue, stomachache, and headache: These are symptoms of jet lag and not a great way to spend a vacation. In general, the more time zones you cross, the worse the jet lag will be. Here's how to avoid or reduce jet lag:

❭ Begin the trip rested (preexisting sleep deprivation intensifies jet lag).
❭ Schedule a daytime flight.
❭ Reset your watch as soon as you depart.
❭ Avoid alcohol and caffeine while traveling.
❭ Eat small meals at the appropriate mealtime for your destination.
❭ A few days before going west, go to bed and wake up 1 hour later each day.
❭ Once in the west, seek morning light and avoid afternoon light.
❭ A few days before going east, go to bed and wake up 1 hour earlier each day.
❭ Once in the east, seek evening light and avoid morning light.
❭ If you take an overnight flight, avoid sleeping too much on the day of your arrival. You'll find it hard to fight the fatigue, but sleeping during the day will make it harder for you to adjust to your new time zone's schedule.

a sleep disorders center for an overnight clinical **sleep study.** While you are asleep in the sleep center, sensors and electrodes record data that will be reviewed by a sleep specialist to determine the nature of your sleep problem.

The American Academy of Sleep Medicine identifies more than 80 sleep disorders. The most common disorders in adults are insomnia, sleep apnea, restless legs syndrome, and narcolepsy.

Insomnia—difficulty in falling asleep, frequent arousals during sleep, or early morning awakening—is the most common sleep complaint. Annual *Sleep in America* polls dating back at least 10 years reveal that more than 50 percent of Americans experience insomnia at least a few nights a week.[35] About 10 to 15 percent of Americans have chronic insomnia, that is, insomnia that persists longer than a month. Over 12 percent of college students are at risk for insomnia.[36] Around 3 percent of college students are being treated for insomnia.[37] Insomnia is more common among women than men, and its prevalence increases with age.

Insomnia Symptoms and Causes Symptoms of insomnia include difficulty falling asleep, waking up frequently during the night, difficulty returning to sleep, waking up too early in the morning, unrefreshing sleep, daytime sleepiness, and irritability. Sometimes insomnia is related to stress and worry. In other cases it may be related to disruptions to the body's circadian rhythms, which may occur with travel across time zones, shift work, and other major schedule changes. Insomnia can also occur as a side effect from taking medications for heart disease, depression, asthma, thyroid disease, high blood pressure, and allergies. Untreated insomnia can be associated with increased illness or morbidity. See the **Skills for Behavior Change** box on ways to beat travel-related insomnia.

Treatment for Insomnia Because of the close connection between behavior and insomnia, cognitive behavioral therapy is often part of treatment. A cognitive behavioral therapist assists a

sleep study A clinical assessment of sleep in which the patient is monitored while spending the night in a sleep disorders center.

insomnia A disorder characterized by difficulty in falling asleep quickly, frequent arousals during sleep, or early morning awakening.

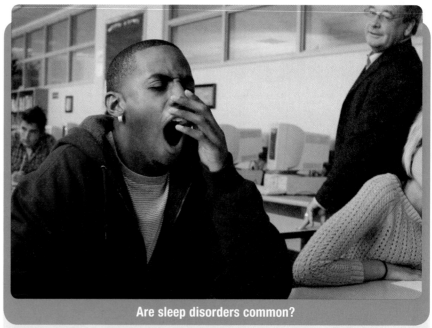

Are sleep disorders common?

From insomnia to narcolepsy, sleep disorders are more common than you might think. There are more than 80 different clinical sleep disorders, and it is estimated that 50 to 70 million Americans—children and adults—suffer from one. Many aren't even aware of their disorder, and many others never seek treatment.

patient in identifying thought and behavioral patterns that contribute to the inability to fall asleep. Once these patterns are recognized, the patient practices new habits that produce positive change.

In some cases of insomnia, *hypnotic* or *sedative* medications may be prescribed. These drugs induce sleep, and some may help relieve anxiety. However, some have undesirable side effects ranging from daytime sleepiness and hallucinations to sleepwalking and other strange nighttime behaviors. Some actually promote anxiety or depression. Many sedatives are also addictive and can lead to tolerance and dependence. Antidepressants are also commonly prescribed for insomnia.

Relaxation techniques, including yoga and meditation, can be especially helpful in preparing the body to sleep. Exercise, done early in the day, can also be helpful in reducing stress and promoting deeper sleep.

Sleep Apnea

Sleep apnea is a disorder in which breathing is briefly and repeatedly interrupted during sleep.[38] *Apnea* refers to a breathing pause that lasts at least 10 seconds. During that time, the chest may rise and fall, but little or no air may be exchanged, or the person may actually not breathe until the brain triggers a gasping inhalation. Sleep apnea affects more than 18 million Americans, or 1 in every 15 people.[39]

Causes and Symptoms of Sleep Apnea There are two major types of sleep apnea: central and obstructive. *Central sleep apnea* occurs when the brain fails to tell the respiratory muscles to initiate breathing. Consumption of alcohol, certain illegal drugs, and certain medications can contribute to central sleep apnea.

Obstructive sleep apnea (OSA), the more common form, occurs when air cannot move in and out of a person's nose or mouth, even though the body tries to breathe. Typically, OSA occurs when a person's throat muscles and tongue relax during sleep and block

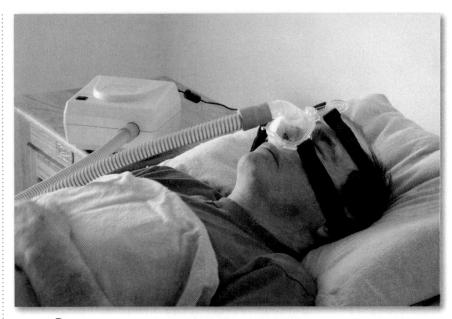

FIGURE 3 **Continuous Positive Airway Pressure (CPAP) Device**
People with sleep apnea can get a better night's sleep by wearing a CPAP device. A gentle stream of air flows continuously into the nose through the tube connected to the mask. This steady stream of air keeps the sleeper's airway open.

the airways, causing snorting, snoring, and gagging These sounds occur because falling oxygen saturation levels in the blood stimulate the body's autonomic nervous system to trigger inhalation, often via a sudden gasp of breath. This response may wake the person, preventing deep sleep and causing the person to wake in the morning feeling tired and unwell.

People who are overweight often have sagging throat tissue, which puts them at higher risk for sleep

"Why Should I Care?"

If you experience persistent trouble sleeping, it's worth your time to see a doctor. Not only can sleep disorders by themselves be threatening to your health, but the fact that they deprive you of quality sleep can also lead to a host of other problems, including academic difficulties, high blood pressure, and chronic stress.

sleep apnea A disorder in which breathing is briefly and repeatedly interrupted during sleep.

apnea. More serious risks of OSA include chronic high blood pressure, irregular heartbeats, heart attack, and stroke. Apnea-associated sleeplessness may also increase the risk of type 2 diabetes, immune system deficiencies, and a host of other problems.[40]

Treatment for Sleep Apnea The most commonly prescribed therapy for OSA is continuous positive airway pressure (CPAP), which consists of an airflow device, long tube, and mask (see Figure 3). People with sleep apnea wear this mask during sleep, and air is forced into the nose to keep the airway open.

Other methods for treating OSA include dental appliances, which reposition the lower jaw and tongue, and surgery to remove tissue in the upper airway. In general, these approaches are most helpful for mild disease or heavy snoring. Lifestyle changes, which may include losing weight, avoiding alcohol, and quitting smoking, are often effective ways of reducing symptoms of OSA.

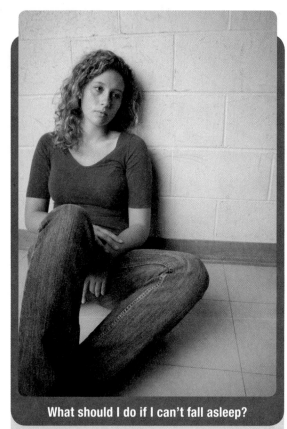

What should I do if I can't fall asleep?

If you can't fall asleep, noises, lights, or persistent worries could be keeping you awake. Try ear plugs or white noise machines to block out sounds, an eye shade to block out light, and keep phones and other devices away from the bedroom to cut down on sleep interruptions. Try to avoid dwelling on worries at bedtime—make it a habit to deal with them in the morning.

Restless Legs Syndrome

Restless legs syndrome (RLS) is a neurological disorder characterized by unpleasant sensations in the legs when at rest combined with an uncontrollable urge to move in an effort to relieve these feelings. These sensations range in severity from uncomfortable to irritating to painful. Some researchers estimate

restless legs syndrome (RLS) A neurological disorder characterized by an overwhelming urge to move the legs when they are at rest.

narcolepsy Excessive, intrusive sleepiness.

that RLS affects as many as 12 million Americans, whereas others think it may be even more common but is underdiagnosed or misdiagnosed.[41]

Symptoms and Causes of RLS Restless legs syndrome sensations are often described as burning, creeping, or tugging, or like insects crawling inside the legs. Moving the legs relieves the discomfort. In general, the symptoms are more pronounced at night. Lying down or trying to relax activates the symptoms, so people with RLS often have difficulty falling and staying asleep.

In most cases, the cause of RLS is unknown. A family history of the condition is seen in approximately 50 percent of cases, suggesting a genetic form of the disorder. People with familial RLS tend to be younger when symptoms start and have a slower progression of the condition. In other cases, RLS appears to be related to other conditions including Parkinson's disease, kidney failure, diabetes, peripheral neuropathy, and anemia. Pregnancy or hormonal changes can worsen symptoms.[42]

Treatment of RLS If there is an underlying condition, treatment of that condition may provide relief. Other treatment options include prescribed medications, decreasing tobacco and alcohol use, and applying heat to the legs. For some people relaxation techniques or stretching exercises can alleviate symptoms.

Narcolepsy

Narcolepsy is a neurological disorder caused by the brain's inability to properly regulate sleep—wake cycles. The result of this disorder is excessive, intrusive sleepiness and daytime sleep attacks. Narcolepsy occurs in about 1 of every 3,000 people and affects men and women equally. Narcolepsy is not rare, but it is an underrecognized and underdiagnosed condition.[43]

Symptoms and Causes of Narcolepsy Narcolepsy is characterized by overwhelming and uncontrollable sleepiness during the day. Narcoleptics are prone to falling asleep at inappropriate times and places—in class, at work, while driving or eating, or even mid-conversation. These sleep attacks can last from a few seconds to several minutes. Other symptoms include *cataplexy* (the sudden loss of voluntary muscle tone, often triggered by emotional stimuli), hallucinations during sleep onset or upon awakening, and brief episodes of paralysis during sleep—wake transitions.

In most cases narcolepsy appears to be caused by a deficiency in the brain of hypocretin, a chemical that plays a role in sleep regulation. There may be a genetic basis for the disorder.[44] Other factors can contribute to the development of narcolepsy, including having another sleep disorder, using certain medications, or having a mental disorder or substance abuse disorder.

Treatment for Narcolepsy Narcolepsy is commonly treated with medications. Stimulants are often prescribed to improve alertness, and antidepressants may be prescribed to treat cataplexy, hallucinations, and sleep paralysis. Behavioral therapy can also help narcoleptics cope with their condition. Some lifestyle changes, such as scheduling brief naps during the day or not eating heavy meals, may also be helpful.

Assess Yourself

Are You Sleeping Well?

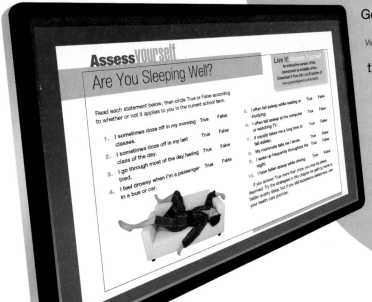

Go online to the **Live It!** section of

www.pearsonhighered.com/donatelle to take

the "Are You Sleeping Well?" assessment.*

If you learn you are sleep deprived,

then try the strategies listed in the

YOUR PLAN FOR CHANGE box.

*If your instructor so chooses, Assess Yourself Activities are available as a printed supplement or as assignable homework online at www.pearsonhighered.com/myhealthlab.

MyHealthLab®

YOUR PLAN FOR CHANGE

Now that you have considered how sleep deprived you may be by filling out the **Assess Yourself** activity, you can take steps to improve your sleep, starting tonight.

Today, you can:
○ Evaluate your behaviors and identify things you're doing that get in the way of a good night's sleep. Develop a plan. What can you do differently starting today?

○ Write a list of personal Dos and Don'ts. For instance: Do turn off your cell phone after 11 PM. Don't drink anything with caffeine after 3 PM.

Within the next 2 weeks, you can:
○ Keep a sleep diary, noting not only how many hours of sleep you get each night, but also how you feel and how you function the next day.

○ Arrange your room to promote restful sleep. Remember the "cave": Keep it quiet, cool, dark, and comfortable.

○ Visit your campus health center and ask for more information about getting a good night's sleep.

By the end of the semester, you can:
○ Establish a regular sleep schedule. Get in the habit of going to bed and waking up at the same time, even on weekends.

○ Create a ritual, such as stretching, meditation, reading something light, or listening to music, that you follow each night to help your body ease from the activity of the day into restful sleep.

○ If you are still having difficulty sleeping and feel you may have a sleep disorder or an underlying health problem disrupting your sleep, contact your health care provider.

References

1. M. F. Bear, B.W. Connors, and M. A. Paradiso, *Neuroscience*, 3rd. ed. (Philadelphia: Lippincott, Williams & Wilkins, 2007), 594.

2. National Sleep Foundation, "National Consumer Research Institute Predicts Top Five Health Trends for 2012," 2012, www.sleepfoundation.org/alert/national-consumer-research-institute-predicts.

3. American College Health Association, *American College Health Association–National College Health Assessment II (ACHA–NCHA II): Reference Group Data Report Spring, 2011* (Baltimore: American College Health Association, 2012), Available at www.achancha.org/reports_ACHA-NCHAII.html.

4. J. Gaultney, "The Prevalence of Sleep Disorders in College Students: Impact on Academic Performance," *Journal of American College Health* 59, no. 2 (2010): 91–97; H. Lund, B. Reider, A. Whitling, and J. Prichard, "Sleep Predictors of Disturbed Sleep in a Large Population of College Students," *Journal of Adolescent Health* 46, no. 2 (2010): 124–32; D. Taylor and A. Bramoweth, "Patterns and Consequences of Inadequate Sleep in College Students: Substance Abuse and Motor Vehicle Accidents," *Journal of Adolescent Health* 46, no. 6 (2010): 610–12; Central Michigan University, "College Student Sleep Patterns Could Be Detrimental," ScienceDaily May 13, 2008, Accessed January 16, 2012., www.sciencedaily.com/releases/2008/05/080512145824.htm.

5. L. R. McKnight-Eily et al., "Unhealthy Sleep-Related Behaviors–2009," *Morbidity and Mortality Weekly* 60, no. 8 (2011): 233–38; National Sleep Foundation Annual Survey, 2011, Accessed January 15, 2012, www.sleepfoundation.org/article/press-release/annual-sleep-america-poll-exploring-connections-communications-technology-use; J. Gaultney, "The Prevalence of Sleep Disorders in College Students: Impact on Academic Performance," *Journal of American College Health* 59, no. 2 (2010): 91–97.

6. L. Swanson et al., "Sleep Disorders and Work Performance: Findings from the 2008 National Sleep Foundation Sleep in American," *Journal of Sleep Research* 20, no. 3 (2011): 487–94, DOI: 10.1111/j.1365-2869.2010.00890; National Sleep Foundation, "Longer Work Days Leave Americans Nodding Off on the Job," press release, March 3, 2008, Accessed January 17, 2012.

7. F. Cappuccio et al., "Sleep Duration and All-Cause Mortality: A Systematic Review and Meta-Analysis of Prospective Studies," *Sleep* 33, no. 5 (2010): 585–92.

8. Ibid.

9. S. Cohen et al., "Sleep Habits and Susceptibility to the Common Cold," *Archives of Internal Medicine* 169, no. 1 (2009): 62–67.

10. T. Bollinger, A. Bollinger, H. Oster, and W. Scolbach, "Sleep, Immunity and Circadian Clocks: A Mechanistic Model," *Gerontology* 56, no. 6 (2010): 574–80. DOI: 10.1159/000281827.

11. R. Lanfranchi, F. Prince, D. Filipini, and J. Carrier, "Sleep Deprivation Increases Blood Pressure in Healthy Normotensive Elderly and Attenuates the Blood Pressure Response to Orthostatic Challenges," *Sleep* 34, no. 3 (2010): 335–39; F. Cappucio, D. Cooper, and D. Lanfranco, "Sleep Duration Predicts Cardiovascular Outcomes: A Systematic Review and Meta-Analysis of Prospective Studies," *European Heart Journal,* first published online February 7, 2011. DOI: 10.1093/eurheart.

12. S. R. Patel et al., "Sleep Duration and Biomarkers of Inflammation," *Sleep* 32, no. 2 (2009): 200–204; M. L. Okun, M. Coussons-Read, and M. Hall, "Disturbed Sleep Is Associated with Increased C-Reactive Protein in Young Women," *Brain, Behavior, and Immunity* 23, no. 3 (2009): 351–54.

13. J-C. Chen et al., "Sleep Duration and Risk of Ischemic Stroke in Postmenopausal Women," *Stroke* 30, no. 12 (2008): 3185–92.

14. L. Nielson, T. Danielson, and A. Serensen, "Short Sleep Duration as a Possible Cause of Obesity: Critical Analysis of the Epidemiological Evidence," *Obesity Reviews* 12, no. 2 (2011): 78–92; M. P. St-Onge et al., "Short Sleep Duration Increases Energy Intakes But Does Not Change Energy Expenditure in Normal-Weight Individuals," *American Journal of Clinical Nutrition* 94 (2011): 2410–416, first published online June 29, 2011, DOI:10.3945/ajcn.111.013904; National Sleep Foundation, "Obesity and Sleep," Accessed January 17, 2012, www.sleepfoundation.org/article/sleep-topics/obesity-and-sleep.

15. National Sleep Foundation, "Sleep Apnea and Diabetes," 2010, Accessed January, 2012, http://www.sleepfoundation.org/alert/sleep-apnea-and-diabetes.

16. National Institutes of Health, "Information about Sleep," 2011, http://science.education.nih.gov/supplements/nih3/sleep/guide/info-sleep.htm; C. Peri and M. Smith, "What Lack of Sleep Does to Your Mind," WebMD, Accessed January 20, 2012, www.webmd.com/sleep-disorders/excessive-sleepiness-10/emotions-cognitive.

17. E. Fortier-Brochu, S. Beauliew-Bonneau, H. Ivers, and C. Morin, "Insomnia and Daytime Cognitive Performance: A Meta-Analysis," *Sleep Medicine Reviews* (2011), DOI: 10-1016/j.smrv.2011.03.008; J. M. Ellenbogen, J. C. Hulbert, Y. Jiang, and R. Stickgold, "The Sleeping Brain's Influence on Verbal Memory: Boosting Resistance to Interference," *PLoS ONE* 4, no. 1 (2009): e4117.

18. A. Gomes, J. Tavares, and M. Azevedo. "Sleep and Academic Performance in Undergraduates: A Multi-Measure, Multi-Predictor Approach." *Chronobiology* 28, no. 9 (2011): 786–801, DOI:10.3109/07420528.2011.606518; V. Thatcher, "University Students and the 'All-Nighter': Correlates and Patterns of Students' Engagement in a Single Night of Total Sleep Deprivation," *Behavioral Sleep Medicine* 6, no. 1 (2008): 16–31.

19. M. Tucker, S McKinley, and R. Stickgold, "Sleep Optimizes Motor Skill in Older Adults," *Journal of the American Geriatrics Society* 59, no. 4 (2011): 603–609; B. R. Sheth, D. Janvelyan, and M. Khan, "Practice Makes Imperfect: Restorative Effects of Sleep on Motor Learning," *PLoS ONE* 3, no. 9 (2008): e3190.

20. D. Taylor and A. Bramoweth, "Patterns and Consequences of Inadequate Sleep in College Students: Substance Abuse and Motor Vehicle Accidents" *Journal of Adolescent Health* 46. no. 6 (2010): 610–12.

21. National Sleep Foundation, "Drowsy Driving Prevention Week, Sleep in America Poll–November, 2011. Facts about Drowsy Driving," 2012, http://drowsydriving.org/2010/11/drowsy-driving-prevention-week%C2%AE-highlights-prevalent-and-preventable-accidents/.

22. National Institutes of Health (NIH), "Teacher's Guide–Information about Sleep," Accessed January, 2012, http://science.education.nih.gov/supplements/nih3/sleep/guide/info-sleep.htm.

23. H. Oster, "Does Late Sleep Promote Depression?" *Expert Reviews of Endocrinology and Metabolism* 7, no. 1, (2012): 27–29, www.expert-reviews.com/doi/abs/10.1586/eem.11.80; C. Baglioni et al., "Insomnia as a Predictor of depression: A Meta-Analytic Evaluation of Longitudinal Epidemiological Studies," *Journal of Affective Disorders* 135, no. 1 (2011): 10–19; A. Gregory et al., "The Direction of Longitudinal Associations between Sleep Problems and Depression Symptoms:

A Study of Twins Aged 8 and 10 Years," *Sleep* 32, no. 2 (2009): 189–99.

24. Bear et al., *Neuroscience*, 596.

25. NIH, "Teacher's Guide–Information About Sleep."

26. M. Kopasz et al. "Sleep and Memory in Healthy children and Adolescents–A Critical Review," *Sleep Medicine Reviews* 14, no. 3 (2010): 167–77; M. Fantini et al., "Longitudinal Study of Cognitive Function in Idiopathic REM Sleep Behavior Disorder," *Sleep* 34, no. 5 (2011): 619–25, www.ncbi.nlm.nih.gov/pmc/articles/PMC3079941/.

27. F. Cappucino et al. "Sleep Duration and All-Cause Mortality: Systematic Review," Sleep 33, no. 5 (2010): 585–92; F. Cappucino, L. D'Elia, P. Strazzullo, and M. Miller, "Quantity and Quality of Sleep and Incidence of Type 2 Diabetes: A Systematic Review and Meta-Analysis," *Diabetes Care* 33, no. 2 (2009): 414–20.

28. NIH, "Teacher's Guide-Sleep-Information about Sleep."

29. N. Marshall et al., "Sleep Apnea as an Independent Risk Factor for All-Cause Mortality: The Busselton Health Study," *Sleep* 31, no. 6 (2008): 1079–85; F. Capuccio et al., "Sleep Duration Predicts Cardiovascular Outcomes: A Systematic Review and Meta-Analysis of Prospective Studies," *European Heart Journal* 32, no. 12 (2011): 1484–92; A. Tamakoshi et al., "Multiple Roles and All-Cause Mortality: The Japan Collaborative Cohort Study," *European Journal of Public Health,* January, 2012, DOI: 10.1093/erpub/ckr194; E. Kronhom et al., "Self-Reported Sleep Duration, All-Cause Mortality, Cardiovascular Mortality and Morbidity in

Finland," *Sleep Medicine* 12, no. 3 (2011): 215–21; F. Cappucino et al. "Sleep Duration and All-Cause Mortality," 2010; F. Cappucino, L. D'Elia, P. Strazzullo, and M. Miller, "Quantity and Quality of Sleep and Incidence of Type 2 Diabetes: A Systematic Review and Meta-Analysis," *Diabetes Care* 33, no. 2 (2009): 414–20.

30. National Sleep Foundation, " How Much Sleep Do We Really Need?," 2011, www.sleepfoundation.org/article/how-sleep-works/how-much-sleep-do-we-really-need.

31. National Sleep Foundation, "Napping," 2011, www.sleepfoundation.org/article/sleep-topics/napping; National Sleep Foundation, "Drowsy Driving—Is There a Perfect Time to Take a Nap?," Accessed January 19, 2012; B. Faraut et al., "Benefits of Napping and an Extended Duration of Recovery Sleep on Alertness and Immune Cells After Acute Sleep Restriction," *Brain, Behavior and Immunity* 25, no. 1 (2011): 18–24.

32. National Sleep Foundation, "Caffeine and Sleep," 2011, www.sleepfoundation.org/article/sleep-topics/caffeine-and-sleep.

33. American College Health Association, *American College Health Association–National College Health Assessment II (ACHA–NCHA II): Reference Group Data Report Spring 2011* (Baltimore: American College Health Association, 2012), Available at www.achancha.org/reports_ACHA-NCHAII.html.

34. Centers for Disease Control and Prevention, "Unhealthy Sleep-Related Behaviors—12 States, 2009," *Morbidity and Mortality Weekly* 60, no. 8 (2011): 233–38.

35. National Sleep Foundation, "Can't Sleep? What to Know about Insomnia," 2009, www.sleepfoundation.org/article/sleep-related-problems/insomnia-and-sleep.

36. J. Gaultney, "The Prevalence of Sleep Disorders in College Students: Impact on Academic Performance," *Journal of American College Health* 59, no. 2 (2010): 91–97.

37. American College Health Association, *American College Health Association–National College Health Assessment II (ACHA–NCHA II): Reference Group Data Report Spring 2011* (Baltimore: American College Health Association, 2012), Available at www.achancha.org/reports_ACHA-NCHAII.html.

38. National Sleep Foundation, "Obstructive Sleep Apnea and Sleep," 2011, Accessed January 18, 2012, www.sleepfoundation.org/article/sleep-related-problems/obstructive-sleep-apnea-and-sleep.

39. Sleep Disorders Guide, "Sleep Apnea Statistics," Accessed January 18, 2012, www.sleepdisordersguide.com/sleepapnea/sleep-apnea-statistics.html.

40. National Sleep Foundation, "Obstructive Sleep Apnea and Sleep," Accessed January 18, 2012.

41. National Institute of Neurological Disorders and Stroke, "Restless Legs Syndrome Fact Sheet," updated November 20,2011, www.ninds.nih.gov/disorders/restless_legs/detail_restless_legs.htm.

42. Ibid.

43. National Institute of Neurological Disorders and Stroke, "Narcolepsy Fact Sheet," updated December 28, 2011, ninds.nih.gov/disorders/narcolepsy/detail_narcolepsy.htm.

44. National Sleep Foundation, 2012.

Building Healthy Relationships and Communicating Effectively

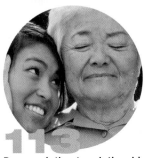

113
Does an intimate relationship have to be sexual?

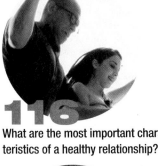

116
What are the most important characteristics of a healthy relationship?

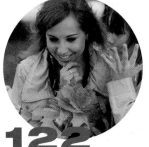

122
How can I communicate better?

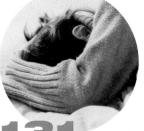

131
How do I cope with a bad breakup?

OBJECTIVES

✱ Identify the characteristics of successful relationships, including how to maintain them and overcome common barriers.

✱ Discuss ways to improve communication skills and interpersonal interactions.

✱ Examine what determines the success of an intimate relationship and how to cope when a relationship has problems.

✱ Examine relationship factors that affect life decisions, such as whether to have children.

✱ Discuss when and why relationships end and how to cope when they do.

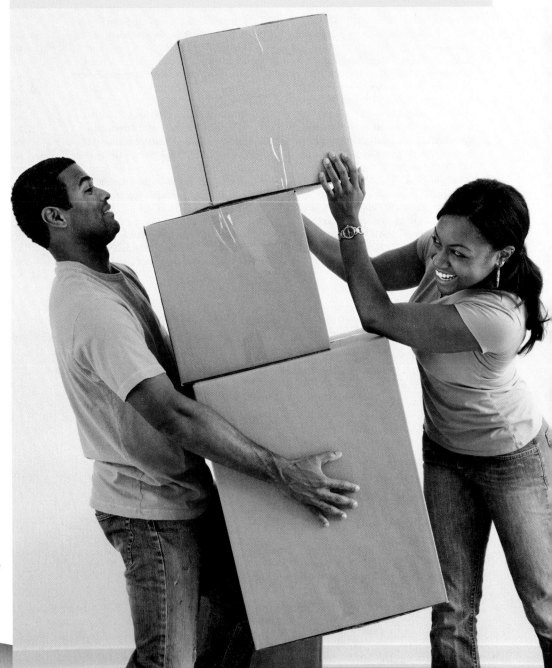

Humans are social beings—we have a basic need to belong and to feel loved, accepted, and wanted. We can't live without interacting with others in some way. The ability to relate well and to give and receive love and support are essential components of a productive and healthy life.

We build networks of supportive friends, significant others, family members, and others who play important roles in helping us meet life's challenges. Numerous studies have shown that having supportive interpersonal relationships is beneficial to health.[1]

All relationships involve a degree of risk. However, only by taking these risks can we grow and truly experience all that life has to offer. In this chapter, we examine healthy relationships and the communication skills necessary to create and maintain them. Expressing ourselves well and knowing how to understand others are vitally important skills. These abilities lay the groundwork for healthy relationships, which are significant factors in overall health.

Intimate Relationships

We can define **intimate relationships** in terms of four characteristics: *behavioral interdependence, need fulfillment, emotional attachment,* and *emotional availability.* Each of these characteristics may be related to interactions with family, close friends, and romantic partners.

Behavioral interdependence refers to the mutual impact that people have on each other as their lives intertwine. What one person does influences what the other person wants to do and can do. Behavioral interdependence may become stronger over time to the point that each person would feel a great void if the other were gone.

Intimate relationships also fulfill psychological needs and thus are a means of *need fulfillment.* Through relationships with others, we fulfill our needs for:

- **Intimacy**—someone with whom we can share our feelings freely.
- **Social integration**—someone with whom we can share worries and concerns.
- **Nurturance**—someone we can take care of and who will take care of us.
- **Assistance**—someone to help us in times of need.
- **Affirmation**—someone who will reassure us of our own worth and tell us that we matter.

In mutually rewarding intimate relationships, partners and friends meet each other's needs. They disclose feelings, share confidences, and provide support and reassurance. Each person comes away feeling better for the interaction and validated by the other person.

In addition to behavioral interdependence and need fulfillment, intimate relationships involve strong bonds of *emotional attachment,* or feelings of love. When we hear the word *intimacy,* we often think of a sexual relationship. Although sex can play an important role in emotional attachment, a relationship can be very intimate without being sexual. Two people can be emotionally intimate (share feelings) or spiritually intimate (share spiritual beliefs and meanings), or they can be intimate friends.

Emotional availability, the ability to give to and receive emotionally from others without fear of being hurt or rejected, is the fourth characteristic of intimate relationships. At times, all of us may limit our emotional availability. For example, after a painful breakup, we may decide not to jump into another relationship immediately, or we may decide to talk about it with only one or two close friends. Holding back can offer time for introspection and healing and for considering the lessons learned. Some people who have experienced intense trauma find it difficult to ever be fully available emotionally. This limits their ability to experience intimate relationships.

> **intimate relationships** Relationships with family members, friends, and romantic partners, characterized by behavioral interdependence, need fulfillment, emotional attachment, and emotional availability.

Relating to Yourself

You have probably heard the idea that you must love and care for yourself before you can love someone else. Ultimately, the most important relationship in your life is the

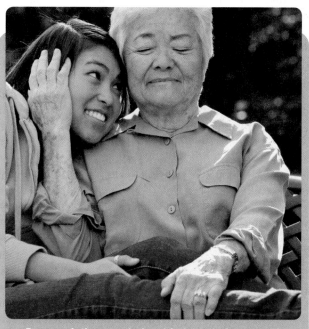

Does an intimate relationship have to be sexual?

We may be accustomed to hearing "intimacy" used to describe romantic or sexual relationships, but intimate relationships can take many forms. The emotional bonds that characterize intimate relationships often span the generations and help individuals gain insight and understanding into each other's worlds.

CHAPTER 4 | BUILDING HEALTHY RELATIONSHIPS AND COMMUNICATING EFFECTIVELY | **113**

one you have with yourself. But how do you learn to value and accept who you are? People with high self-esteem show respect for themselves by remaining true to their values and beliefs. They feel worthy of success in love, relationships, and life in general.

Two personal qualities that are especially important to any good relationship are *accountability* and *self-nurturance.* **Accountability** means that you recognize that you are responsible for your own decisions, choices, and actions. You don't hold others responsible for positive or negative experiences. **Self-nurturance,** which goes hand in hand with accountability, means developing individual potential through a balanced and realistic appreciation of self-worth and ability. To make good choices in life, a person must balance many physical and emotional needs, including sleeping, eating, exercising, working, relaxing, and socializing. When the balance is disrupted, as it will inevitably be at times, self-nurturing people are patient with themselves and try to put things back on course. It is a lifelong process to learn to live in a balanced and healthy way. Individuals who are on a path of accountability and self-nurturance have a much better chance of achieving this balance and maintaining satisfying relationships with others.

Self-Esteem and Self-Acceptance Important factors that affect your ability to nurture yourself and maintain healthy relationships with others include the way you define yourself (*self-concept*) and the way you evaluate yourself (*self-esteem*). Your self-concept is like a mental mirror that reflects how you view your physical features, emotional states, talents, likes and dislikes, values, and roles. A person might define herself as an activist, mother, honor student, athlete, or musician. How you feel about yourself or evaluate yourself constitutes your self-esteem. You might consider yourself an excellent student, a horrible singer, a great lover, or a "10" in terms of appearance. Taken together, such judgments indicate your level of self-esteem or self-evaluation.

Your perception and acceptance of yourself influences your relationship choices. If you feel unattractive, insecure, or inferior to others, you may choose not to interact with other people or to avoid social events. Or you may unconsciously seek out individuals who confirm your negative view of yourself by treating you poorly. Conversely, if you are secure about your unique characteristics and talents, that positive self-concept will make it easier to form relationships with people who support and nurture you and to interact with a variety of people in a healthy, balanced way.

accountability Accepting responsibility for personal decisions, choices, and actions.

self-nurturance Developing individual potential through a balanced and realistic appreciation of self-worth and ability.

family of origin People present in the household during a child's first years of life—usually parents and siblings.

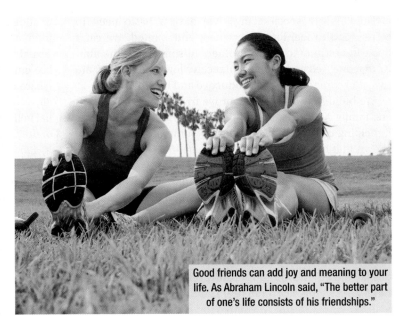

Good friends can add joy and meaning to your life. As Abraham Lincoln said, "The better part of one's life consists of his friendships."

Family Relationships

A family is a recognizable group of people with roles, tasks, boundaries, and personalities whose central focus is to protect, care for, love, and socialize with one another. Because the family is a dynamic institution that changes as society changes, the definition of *family* changes over time. Who are members of today's families? Historically, most families have been made up of people related by blood, marriage or long-term committed relationships, or adoption. Yet today, many other groups of people are recognized and function as family units. Although there is no "best" family type, we do know that a healthy family's key roles and tasks are to nurture and support. Healthy families foster a sense of security and feelings of belonging that are central to growth and development.

During the childhood years, families provide our most significant relationships. It is from our **family of origin,** the people present in our household during our first years of life, that we initially learn about feelings, problem solving, love, intimacy, and gender roles. We learn to negotiate relationships and have opportunities to communicate effectively, develop attitudes and values, and explore spiritual belief systems. It is not uncommon when we establish relationships outside the family to rely on these initial experiences and on skills modeled by our family of origin.

what do you think?

What values about relationships did you learn from your family?
● Did your family foster open, caring communication?
● Were they demonstrative in showing their love and feelings for others?
● How do you think they influenced you in your relationships today?

Friendships Friendships are often the first relationships we form outside of our immediate families, and they can be some of life's most stable and enduring relationships.

<div>

</div>

<table>
<tr><td>

</td></tr>
</table>

<div class="what-do-you-think">

what do you think?

What characteristics keep your friendship intact?

● What do you gain from the friendship?

● What does your friend gain?

</div>

Establishing and maintaining strong friendships may be a good predictor of your success in establishing love relationships, as each requires shared interests and values, mutual acceptance, trust, understanding, respect, and levels of confiding. Healthy friendships involve[2]:

● Understanding the roles and boundaries within the friendship.

● Communicating needs, expectations, limitations, and affections.

● Having a sense of equity in which confidences are shared and both participants contribute fairly and equally to maintaining the friendship.

● Consistently trying to give as much as one gets from the relationship.[3]

Developing meaningful friendships is more than merely "friending" someone on Facebook. Getting to know someone well requires time, effort, and commitment. But the effort is worth it: a good friend can be a trustworthy companion, someone who respects your strengths as well as your weaknesses, someone who can share your joys and your sorrows, and someone you can count on for support.

Romantic Relationships

Most people choose at some point to enter into an intimate romantic and sexual relationship with another person. Romantic relationships typically include all the characteristics of friendship as well as the following characteristics related to passion and caring:

● **Fascination.** Lovers tend to pay attention to the other person even when they should be involved in other activities. They are preoccupied with the other and want to think about, talk to, and be with the other.

● **Exclusiveness.** Lovers have a special relationship that usually precludes having the same kind of relationship with a third party. The love relationship often takes priority over all others.

● **Sexual desire.** Lovers desire physical intimacy and want to touch, hold, and engage in sexual activities with the other.

● **Giving the utmost.** Lovers care enough to give the utmost when the other is in need, sometimes to the point of extreme sacrifice.

● **Being a champion or advocate.** Lovers actively champion each other's interests and attempt to ensure that the other succeeds.

Theories of Love What is love? For centuries, love has been the theme of paintings, sculpture, novels, poems, and plays (and in the modern era, movies). There is no single definition of *love,* and the word may mean different things to different people, depending on cultural values, age, gender, and situation. Although we may not know how to put our feelings into words, we all know it when the "lightning bolt" of love strikes.

Several theories related to how and why love develops have been proposed. In his classic Triangular Theory of Love, psychologist Robert Sternberg proposes the following three key components to loving relationships (Figure 4.1):[4]

● **Intimacy.** The emotional component, which involves closeness, sharing, and mutual support.

● **Passion.** The motivational component, which includes lust, attraction, and sexual arousal.

● **Commitment.** The cognitive component, which includes the decision to be open to love in the short term and the commitment to the relationship in the long term.

The quality of love relationships is reflected by the level of intimacy, passion, and commitment each person

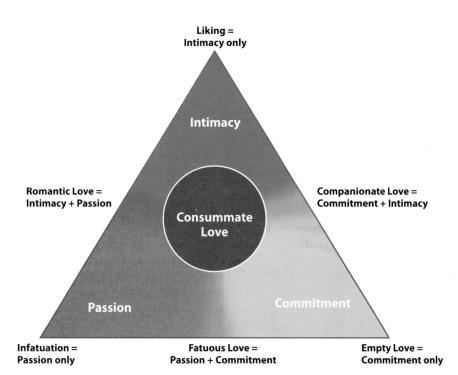

FIGURE 4.1 Sternberg's Triangular Theory of Love
According to Sternberg's model, three elements—intimacy, passion, and commitment—existing alone or in combination, form different types of love. The most complete, ideal type of love in the model is consummate love, which combines balanced amounts of all three elements.

brings to the relationship over time. Sternberg suggests that relationships that include two or more of those components are more likely to endure than those that include only one. He uses the term **consummate love** to describe a combination of intimacy, passion, and commitment—an ideal and deep form of love that is, unfortunately, rare.

Quite different from Sternberg's approach, are theories of love and attraction based on brain circuitry and chemistry. Anthropologist Helen Fisher, among others, hypothesizes that attraction and falling in love follow a fairly predictable pattern based on (1) *imprinting,* in which our evolutionary patterns, genetic predispositions, and past experiences trigger a romantic reaction; (2) *attraction,* in which neurochemicals produce feelings of euphoria and elation; (3) *attachment,* in which endorphins (natural opiates) cause lovers to feel peaceful, secure, and calm; and (4) *production of a cuddle chemical,* in which the brain secretes the hormone oxytocin, stimulating sensations during lovemaking and eliciting feelings of satisfaction and attachment.[5]

According to Fisher's theory, lovers who claim to be swept away by passion may not be far from the truth. A love-smitten person's endocrine system secretes chemical substances such as dopamine, norepinephrine, and phenylethylamine (PEA), which are chemical cousins of amphetamines.[6] Attraction may in fact be a "natural high"; however, this passion "buzz" loses effectiveness over time as the body builds up a tolerance. Fisher speculates that some people become attraction junkies, seeking out the intoxication of new love much as a drug user seeks a chemical high. Fisher also suggests that the significant drop in PEA levels over a 3- to 4-year period leads to the "4-year itch" that manifests in peaking fourth-year divorce rates present in more than 60 cultures. Romances that last beyond the 4-year mark are influenced by endorphins that give lovers a sense of security, peace, and calm.[7]

Strategies for Success in Relationships

Our definition of success in a relationship is often based on whether a couple stays together and remains close over the years. Learning to communicate, respecting each other, and sharing a genuine fondness are crucial. Many social scientists agree that the happiest committed relationships are flexible enough to allow the partners to grow throughout their lives.

How can you increase the odds that a romantic relationship will succeed? Most relationships start with great optimism and true caring. So why do so many run into trouble? One contributing factor is the myth of living "happily ever after" once the right person is found. The myth doesn't account for the fact that healthy relationships don't just happen; they require certain attributes and continued effort.

consummate love A combination of intimacy, compassion, and commitment.

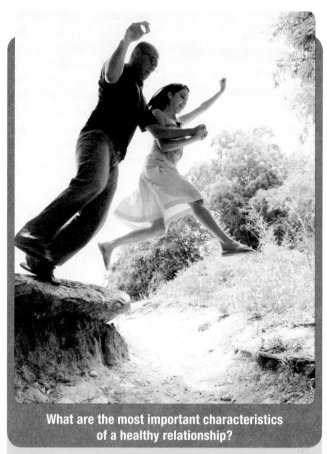

What are the most important characteristics of a healthy relationship?

Healthy relationships can come in all shapes and sizes, but they do have some characteristics in common, including communication, caring, respect, and support. One of the most important components of a strong relationship is trust, which is made up of predictability, dependability, and faith.

Characteristics of Healthy Relationships

Satisfying and stable relationships are based on good communication, intimacy, friendship, and other factors. A key ingredient is trust, the degree to which each partner feels he or she can rely on the integrity of the other. Without trust, intimacy will not develop, and the relationship will likely fail. With time, relationships that lack trust can build it, but that requires opening one's self to others, which carries the risk of hurt or rejection. Trust includes three fundamental elements:

● **Predictability**—the ability to predict your partner's behavior based on past actions.
● **Dependability**—the ability to rely on your partner to emotionally support you in all situations, particularly those in which you feel threatened or hurt.
● **Faith**—your belief in your partner having positive intentions and behavior.

What does a healthy relationship look and feel like? Characteristics of healthy and unhealthy relationships are contrasted in Figure 4.2. Answering some basic questions can also help you determine if a relationship is working.

● Do you love and care for yourself to the same extent that you did before the relationship? Can you be yourself in the relationship?

● Is there genuine caring and goodwill? Do you share interests, values, and opinions? Is there mutual respect for differences?

● Is there mutual encouragement? Are you there for each other and do you support each other unconditionally?

● Do you trust each other? Are you honest with each other? Can you comfortably express your feelings, opinions, and needs?

● Is there room in your relationship for growth as you both evolve and mature?

Relationships are nurtured by consistent communication, actions, and self-reflection. Poor communication can weaken bonds and create mistrust. We all need to reflect periodically on how we typically relate to others through our words and actions. Have we been honest, direct, and fair in our conversations? Have we listened to others' thoughts, wants, and needs? Have we behaved in ways consistent with our words, values, and beliefs?

Choosing a Romantic Partner

Choosing a partner is influenced by more than just chemical and psychological processes. Another factor is *proximity*, or being in the same place at the same time. The more often you

In an unhealthy relationship...	In a healthy relationship...
You care for and focus on another person only and neglect yourself or you focus only on yourself and neglect the other person.	You both love and take care of yourselves before and while in a relationship
One of you feels pressure to change to meet the other person's standards and is afraid to disagree or voice ideas.	You respect each other's individuality, embrace your differences, and allow each other to "be yourselves."
One of you has to justify what you do, where you go, and whom you see.	You both do things with friends and family and have activities independent of each other.
One of you makes all the decisions and controls everything without listening to the other's input.	You discuss things with each other, allow for differences of opinion, and compromise equally.
One of you feels unheard and is unable to communicate what you want.	You express and listen to each other's feelings, needs, and desires.
You lie to each other and find yourself making excuses for the other person.	You both trust and are honest with yourselves and with each other.
You don't have any personal space and have to share everything with the other person.	You respect each other's need for privacy.
Your partner keeps his or her sexual history a secret or hides a sexually transmitted infection from you, or you do not disclose your history to your partner.	You share sexual histories and information about sexual health with each other.
One of you is scared of asking the other to use protection or has refused the other's requests for safer sex.	You both practice safer sex methods.
One of you has forced or coerced the other to have sex.	You both respect sexual boundaries and are able to say no to sex.
One of you yells and hits, shoves, or throws things at the other in an argument.	You resolve conflicts in a rational, peaceful, and mutually agreed upon way.
You feel stifled, trapped, and stagnant. You are unable to escape the pressures of the relationship.	You both have room for positive growth, and you both learn more about each other as you develop and mature.

FIGURE 4.2 **Healthy versus Unhealthy Relationships**
Source: Advocates for Youth, Washington, DC, 2006, www.advocatesforyouth.org. Copyright © 2000. Used with permission.

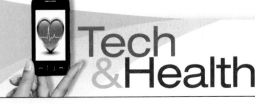

Tech & Health

LOVE IN THE TIME OF TWITTER

Technology has revolutionized our access to information and the ways we communicate. Couples can meet on a site like Match.com, keep in constant contact via texting, and inform the world of their relationship highs and lows via Facebook and Twitter. With all these tools available, it can be easy to share TMI (too much information). Ilana Gershon, author of "The Breakup 2.0: Disconnecting over New Media," suggests we lack standard etiquette for the use of new media in relationships. At its best, social media can bring people closer together; at its worst, it can be used intentionally or unintentionally to embarrass or hurt. Consider the following suggestions to safeguard yourself:

When meeting:

✳ If you join a dating site, be honest about yourself; state your own interests and characteristics fairly, including things that you think might be less attractive than stereotypes and cultural norms dictate.
✳ If you meet someone online, and want to meet in person, put safety first! Plan something brief, preferably during daylight hours. Meet in a public place, like a coffee shop. Do not meet

with anyone who wants to keep the time and location a secret. Tell a friend or family member the details of when and where you are meeting and any information you have on the person you are meeting.

While dating:

✳ Discuss limits with your partner on the type of info you each want shared online. Agree to share only within those limits.
✳ Recognize that constant electronic updates throughout the day can leave little to share when you are together. Save some information for face-to-face talks!
✳ Sober up before you click "submit." Things that seem funny under the influence may not seem funny the next morning.

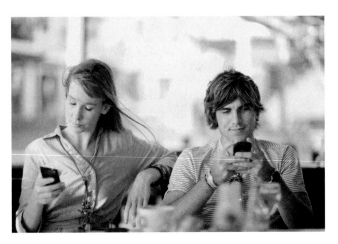

✳ Remember that the Internet is forever. Once a picture or a post is sent, it can never be completely erased. Never post anything that would embarrass someone if it was seen by a family member or potential employer.
✳ Respect your partner's privacy. Logging onto his/her e-mail or Facebook account to look at private messages is a breach of trust.
✳ Know that the GPS in a phone can be used to track your location, and cell phone spyware can be installed that allows e-mail and texts to be read from another device. If you think you may be a victim of "cyberstalking" by a current (or former) partner, get a new phone or ask the phone company to reinstall the phone's operating system to wipe out the software.

If breaking up:

Do not break up with someone via text/e-mail/tweet/facebook/chat. People deserve the respect of a more personal break up.

Upon breaking up, be sure to change any passwords you may have confided in your partner. The temptation to use those for ill may be too strong to resist.

---

see a person at school, work, religious or social events, or as part of volunteer activities, the more likely it is that interaction will occur. But note that with the growth of Internet dating sites, geographic proximity has become less important. (See the **Tech & Health** box above for guidelines on meeting people online.)

You also choose a partner based on *similarities* (in attitudes, values, intellect, interests, education, and socioeconomic status); the old adage that "opposites attract" usually isn't true. If your potential partner expresses interest or liking, you may react with mutual regard known as *reciprocity*. The more you express interest, the safer it is for someone else to do the same, and the cycle continues.

A final factor that plays a significant role in selecting a partner is *physical attraction*. Whether such attraction is caused by a chemical reaction or a learned behavior, men and women appear to have different attraction criteria. Men tend to be attracted by youth and beauty, while women tend to be attracted to older mates and to place emphasis on partners with

what do you think?

What factors do you consider most important in a potential partner?
● Are any absolute musts?
● Does what you believe to be important in a relationship differ from what your parents feel is important?

good financial prospects and who appear to be dependable and industrious. Attraction is a complex notion and influenced by social, biological, and cultural factors.[8]

Communicating: A Key to Good Relationships

From the moment of birth, we struggle to be understood. We flail our arms, cry, scream, smile, frown, and make sounds and gestures to attract attention or to communicate what we want or need. By adulthood, each of us has developed a unique way of communicating with others via gestures, words, expressions, and body language. No two people communicate exactly the same way or have the same need for connecting with others.

Different cultures have different ways of expressing feelings and using body language. Members of some cultures gesture broadly; others maintain a closed body posture. Some are offended by direct eye contact; others welcome a steady gaze. Men and women also tend to have different styles of communication that are largely dictated by culture and socialization (see the **Student Health Today** box on page 120).

Although people differ in the way they communicate, this doesn't mean that one gender, culture, or group is better at communication than another. We have to be willing to accept differences and work to keep communication lines open and fluid. Remaining interested, actively engaged in the interaction, and open and willing to exchange ideas and thoughts are all things that we can typically learn with practice. By understanding how to deliver and interpret information, we can enhance our relationships. Three aspects of strong communications skills are sharing information through self-disclosure, becoming a better listener, and understanding nonverbal communication.

Learning Appropriate Self-Disclosure

Sharing personal information with others is called **self-disclosure.** If you are willing to share personal information with others, they will likely share personal information with you. If you want to learn more about someone, you usually have to be willing to share some of your personal background and interests with that person, as well. Self-disclosure is not only storytelling or sharing secrets; it is also revealing how you are reacting to the present situation and giving any information about the past that is relevant to the other person's understanding of your current reactions.

Self-disclosure can be a double-edged sword, for there is risk in divulging personal insights and feelings. If you sense that sharing feelings and personal thoughts will result in a closer relationship, you will likely take such a risk. But if you believe that the disclosure may result in rejection or alienation, you may not open up so easily. If the confidentiality of previously shared information has been violated, you may hesitate to be as open in the future. However, the risk in not disclosing yourself to others is that you will lack intimacy in relationships. Psychologist Carl Rogers stressed the importance of understanding yourself and others through self-disclosure. He believed that weak relationships were characterized by inhibited self-disclosure.[9]

self-disclosure Sharing personal feelings or information with others.

If self-disclosure is a key element in creating healthy communication, but fear is a barrier to that process, what can we do? The following suggestions can help:

- **Get to know yourself.** Remember that your *self* includes your feelings, beliefs, thoughts, and concerns. The more you know about yourself, the more likely you will be able to share yourself with others.
- **Become more accepting of yourself.** No one is perfect or has to be.
- **Be willing to talk about sex.** The U.S. culture puts many taboos on discussions of sex, so it's no wonder we find it hard to disclose our sexual past to those with whom we are intimate. However, with today's triple threat of unintended pregnancy, sexually transmitted infections, and HIV/AIDS, there has never been a more important time to discuss sexual history with a partner.
- **Choose a safe context for self-disclosure.** When and where you make such disclosures and to whom may greatly influence the response you receive. Choose a setting in which you feel safe to let yourself be known.
- **Be thoughtful about self-disclosure via social media.** Self-disclosure can be an effective method of building intimacy with another person, but not with large groups. Sharing too much personal information via Facebook or Twitter may cause you to feel vulnerable or embarrassed later (see the **Tech & Health** box on the previous page for more on social media and relationships).

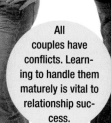

All couples have conflicts. Learning to handle them maturely is vital to relationship success.

Becoming a Better Listener

Listening is a vital part of interpersonal communication; it allows us to share feelings, express concerns, communicate wants and needs, and let our thoughts and opinions be known. Improving listening skills will enhance our relationships, improve our grasp of information, and allow us to interpret more

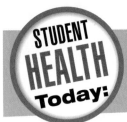

HE SAYS/SHE SAYS

There are some gender-specific communication patterns and behaviors that are obvious to the casual observer (see graphic). However, according to Dr. Cynthia Burggraf Torppa at Ohio State University, the bigger difference is the way in which men and women interpret or process the same message. She indicates that that women are more sensitive to interpersonal meanings "between the lines" and men are more sensitive to subtle messages about status. Recognizing these differences and how they make us unique is a good first step in avoiding unnecessary frustrations and miscommunications.

Sources: C. Burggraf Torppa, Family and Consumer Sciences, Ohio State University Extension, "Gender Issues: Communication Differences in Interpersonal Relationships," 2010, http://ohioline.osu.edu/flm02/pdf/fs04.pdf; J. Wood, *Gendered Lives: Communication, Gender, and Culture.* 8th ed. (Belmont, CA: Cengage, 2008); M. L. Knapp and A. L. Vangelisti, *Interpersonal Communication and Human Relationships.* 6th ed. (Boston: Allyn & Bacon, 2008).

Video Tutor: Gender Differences in Communication

Women

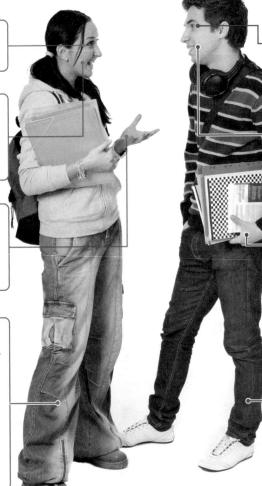

FACIAL EXPRESSIONS
• Smile and nod more often
• Maintain better eye contact

SPEECH PATTERNS
• Higher pitched, softer voices
• Use approximately 5 speech tones
• May sound more emotional
• Make more tentative statements
• Interrupt less often

BODY LANGUAGE
• Take up less space
• Gesture toward the body
• Lean forward when listening
• More gentle when touching others
• More feedback via body language

BEHAVIORAL DIFFERENCES
• More emotional approach
• Express intimate feelings more readily
• Tendency to hold grudges
• Give more compliments
• Gossip more
• More likely to ask for help
• Tend to take rejection more personally
• Apologize more frequently
• Talk is primarily a means of rapport, establishing connections, and negotiating relationships

Men

FACIAL EXPRESSIONS
• Frown more often
• Often avoid eye contact

SPEECH PATTERNS
• Lower pitched, louder voices
• Use approximately 3 speech tones
• May sound more abrupt
• Make more direct statements
• More likely to interrupt

BODY LANGUAGE
• Occupy more space
• Gesture away from the body
• Lean back when listening
• More forceful gestures
• Less feedback via body language

BEHAVIORAL DIFFERENCES
• More inclined to be analytical
• Have more difficulty in expressing intimate feelings
• Hold fewer grudges
• Give fewer compliments
• Gossip less
• Less likely to ask for help
• Tend to take rejection less personally
• Apologize less often
• Talk is primarily a means of preserving independence and negotiating and maintaining status

effectively what others say. We listen best when (1) we believe that the message is somehow important and relevant to us; (2) the speaker holds our attention through humor, dramatic effect, use of the media, or other techniques; and (3) we are in the mood to listen (free of distractions and worries).

When we listen effectively, we try to understand what people are thinking and feeling from their perspective. We not only hear the words, we try to understand what is really being said. How many times have you been caught pretending to listen when you were not? Sometimes this tuned-out behavior is due to lack of sleep, stress, being preoccupied, having too much to drink, or being under the influence of drugs. Other times it's because the speaker is a "motor mouth" who talks for the sake of talking or because you find the speaker or the subject boring. Some of the most common listening difficulties are things that we can work to improve. See the **Skills for Behavior Change** box for suggestions on improving your listening skills.

The Three Basic Listening Modes There are three main ways in which we listen:

- **Competitive, or combative, listening** happens when we are more interested in promoting our own point of view than in understanding or exploring someone else's.
- **Passive, or attentive, listening** occurs when we are genuinely interested in hearing and understanding the other person's point of view. This type of listening encourages further discussion.
- **Active, or reflective, listening** is the single most useful and important listening skill. In active listening, we genuinely want to understand what the other person is thinking and feeling. We are active in confirming our understanding by restating or paraphrasing the speaker's message before we respond. This feedback process is what distinguishes active listening and makes it effective.

Using Nonverbal Communication

Understanding what someone is saying often involves much more than listening and speaking. Often, what is not actually said may speak louder than any words could. Rolling the eyes, looking at the floor or ceiling rather than maintaining eye contact, body movements and hand gestures—all these nonverbal clues influence the way we interpret messages. **Nonverbal communication** includes all unwritten and unspoken messages, both intentional and unintentional. Ideally, our nonverbal communication matches and supports our verbal communication, but this is not always the case. Research shows that when verbal and nonverbal communication doesn't match, we are more likely to believe the nonverbal cues.[10] This is one reason it is important to be aware of the nonverbal cues we use regularly and to understand how others might interpret them.

Nonverbal communication can include the following:[11]

- **Touch.** This can be a handshake, a warm hug, a hand on the shoulder, or a kiss on the cheek.
- **Gestures.** These can include gestures that replace words, such as a thumbs-up or a wave hello or good-bye, or movements that augment verbal communication, such as indicating with your hands how big the fish was that got away. Gestures can also be rude, such as glancing at one's watch to indicate a wish to escape or rolling one's eyes to indicate disdain for what has been said.

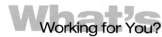
☐ Maybe you already communicate well. Below is a list of some things you can do to improve communication. Which of these are you already incorporating into your life?

☐ I listen actively—I actively try to understand what my friend or partner is saying.

☐ I let people finish what they are saying before I offer my thoughts.

☐ I tell my friends when I am upset and work to resolve problems with them.

☐ When the right time comes, I discuss my intimate thoughts and feelings with my partner.

- **Interpersonal space.** This is the amount of physical space that separates two people. Getting too close can be offensive.
- **Body language.** This includes movements such as folding your arms across your chest, indicating defensiveness, or leaning forward in your chair to show interest.
- **Tone of voice.** This refers not to what you say, but how you say it—including the pitch and volume of your voice and speed of your speech.
- **Facial expressions.** These signal moods and emotions, such as smiling when you are happy.

nonverbal communication Unwritten and unspoken messages, both intentional and unintentional.

Learning to Really Listen

Skills for Behavior Change

To become a better listener, try practicing the following skills on a daily basis:

❭ To avoid distractions, turn off the TV and put your phone away.

❭ Be present in the moment. Good listeners participate and acknowledge what the other person is saying through nonverbal cues such as nodding or smiling and asking questions at appropriate times.

❭ Show empathy and sympathy appropriately.

❭ Ask for clarification. If you aren't sure what the speaker means, say that you don't completely understand or paraphrase what you think you heard.

❭ Control that deadly desire to interrupt. Try taking a deep breath for 2 seconds, then hold your breath for another second, and really listen to what is being said as you slowly exhale.

❭ Avoid snap judgments based on what other people look like or a few statements they have made.

❭ Resist the temptation to "set the other person straight."

❭ Focus on the speaker. Hold back the temptation to launch into a story of your own experience in a similar situation.

conflict Emotional state that arises when opinions differ or the behavior of one person interferes with the behavior of another.

conflict resolution Concerted effort by all parties to constructively resolve points of contention.

Facial expressions are believed to have near universal meaning; however, most other body language is culturally specific. A gesture of agreement in one culture can be offensive in another. To communicate as effectively as possible, it is important to recognize and use appropriate nonverbal cues that support and help clarify your verbal messages. Awareness and practice of your verbal and nonverbal communication will also enhance your skills in interpreting others' messages.

Managing Conflict through Communication

A **conflict** is an emotional state that arises when the behavior of one person interferes with that of another. Conflict is inevitable whenever people live or work together. Not all conflict is bad; in fact, airing feelings and coming to some form of resolution over differences can sometimes strengthen relationships. **Conflict resolution** and successful conflict management form a systematic approach to resolving differences fairly and constructively, rather than allowing them to fester. The goal of conflict resolution is to solve differences peacefully and creatively.

Prolonged conflict can destroy relationships unless the parties agree to resolve points of contention constructively. As two people learn to negotiate and compromise on their differences, the number and intensity of conflicts should diminish. Conflict resolution can therefore be a growth process as people learn to recognize problems and find solutions based on past experience.

Here are some strategies for conflict resolution:

1. **Identify the problem or issue.** Talk with each other to clarify exactly what the conflict or problem is. Try to understand both sides of the problem. In this first stage, you must say what you want and listen to what the other person wants. Focus on using "I" messages and avoid using blaming "you" messages. Be an active listener—repeat what the other person has said and ask questions for clarification. See the **Skills for Behavior Change** box on the next page for some guidelines on how to express difficult feelings.

2. **Generate several possible solutions.** Base your search for solutions on the goals and interests identified in the first step. Come up with several different alternatives, and avoid evaluating any of them until you have finished brainstorming.

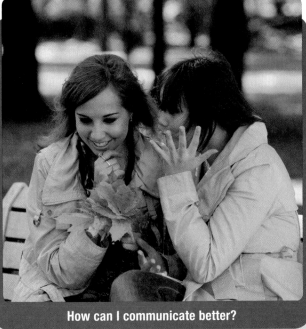

How can I communicate better?

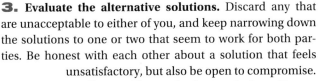

One way to communicate better is to pay attention to your body language. Researchers have found that 93 percent of communication effectiveness is determined by nonverbal cues. Laughing, smiling, and gesturing all help convey meaning and assure your partner that you are actively engaged in the conversation.

3. **Evaluate the alternative solutions.** Discard any that are unacceptable to either of you, and keep narrowing down the solutions to one or two that seem to work for both parties. Be honest with each other about a solution that feels unsatisfactory, but also be open to compromise.

4. **Decide on the best solution.** Choose an alternative that is acceptable to both parties. You both need to be committed to the decision for this solution to be effective.

5. **Implement the solution.** Discuss how the decision will be carried out. Establish who is responsible to do what and when. The solution stands a better chance of working if you agree on how it will be implemented.

6. **Follow up.** Evaluate whether the solution is working. Check in with the other person to see how he or she feels about it. Are you satisfied with the way the solution is working out? If something is not working as planned, or if circumstances have changed, discuss revising the plan. Remember that

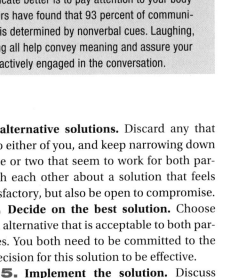

"Why Should I Care?"

Learning how to communicate effectively isn't just some touchy-feely notion—it's actually vitally important. Unless you decide to be a hermit, there is hardly a career or life path you might choose that won't require communicating and cooperating with others. Develop good communication skills now, and you'll be poised for success.

what do you think?

How well do you manage conflict in your personal relationships?
● What could you improve about the way you resolve conflicts?

Communicating When Emotions Run High

How many times have you struggled to find just the right words in an emotionally charged situation? The following guidelines can help you express your feelings more effectively:

❭ Try to be specific rather than general about how you feel.

❭ When expressing anger or irritation, first describe the specific behavior you don't like, then your feelings.

❭ If you have mixed feelings, say so; express each feeling, and explain what each is about.

❭ Use "I" messages, rather than "you" statements that can cast blame. By using "I" messages, the speaker takes responsibility for communicating his or her own feelings, thoughts, and beliefs.

❭ Avoid making judgmental statements, lecturing, or projecting superiority.

❭ During a heated conflict, pause before responding and consider the possible impact of your comment. Wait to discuss a problem if you can't remain calm.

❭ Keep an open mind, and use qualifying statements to invite others to state their opinions.

❭ When you ask for feedback, be prepared for an honest answer.

❭ Be careful when trying to communicate or interpret emotionally charged messages via e-mail or text. It can be hard to interpret their intended meaning without the nonverbal support of tone of voice and body language.

both parties must agree to any changes to the plan, as they did the original idea.

Committed Relationships

Commitment in a relationship means that one intends to act over time in a way that perpetuates the well-being of the other person, oneself, and the relationship. Polls show that the majority of Americans—as many as 95 percent—strive to develop a committed relationship,[12] even though many have difficulty maintaining them. These relationships can take several forms, including partnerships, cohabitation, and marriage.

Marriage

In many societies, traditional committed relationships take the form of marriage. In the United States, marriage means entering into a legal agreement that includes shared finances, property, and responsibility for raising children. Many Americans also view marriage as a religious sacrament that emphasizes certain rights and obligations for each spouse.

Historically, close to 90 percent of Americans married at least once during their lifetime, and at any given time, close to 60 percent of U.S. adults are married (Figure 4.3). However, in recent years Americans have become less likely to marry. Since 1960, annual marriages of adult men and women have steadily declined.[13] This decrease may be due to several factors, including delay of first marriages, an increase in cohabitation, and a small decrease in the number of divorced persons who remarry. In 1960, the median age for first marriage was 23 years for men and 20 years for women; by 2010, the median age of first marriage had risen to 28 years for men and 26 years for women.[14] Many Americans believe that marriage involves **monogamy,** or exclusive sexual involvement with one partner. In fact, the lifetime pattern for many Americans appears to be **serial monogamy,** which means that a person has a monogamous sexual relationship with one partner before moving on to another monogamous relationship. Some couples choose an **open relationship** (or open marriage), in which the partners agree that there may be sexual involvement outside their relationship.

Marriage is socially sanctioned and highly celebrated in American culture, so there are numerous

monogamy Exclusive sexual involvement with one partner.

serial monogamy Series of monogamous sexual relationships.

open relationship Relationship in which partners agree that sexual involvement can occur outside the relationship.

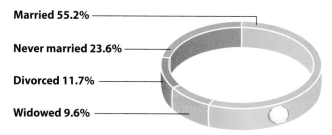

Women

Married 55.2%
Never married 23.6%
Divorced 11.7%
Widowed 9.6%

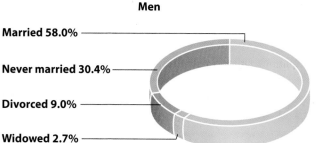

Men

Married 58.0%
Never married 30.4%
Divorced 9.0%
Widowed 2.7%

FIGURE 4.3 Marital Status of the U.S. Population by Sex
Source: U.S. Census Bureau, *Statistical Abstract,* Table 57, "Marital Status of the Population by Sex and Age: 2010," 2012, www.census.gov/compendia/statab/2012/tables/12s0057.pdf.

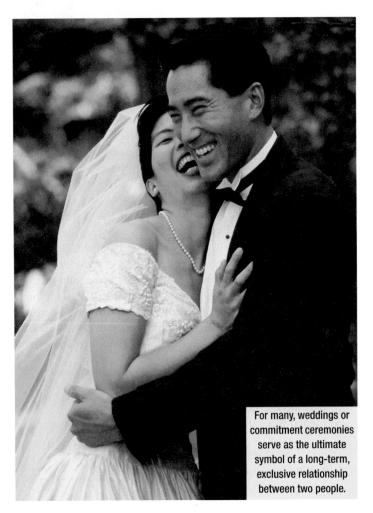

For many, weddings or commitment ceremonies serve as the ultimate symbol of a long-term, exclusive relationship between two people.

incentives for couples to formalize their relationship in this way. A healthy marriage provides emotional support by combining the benefits of friendship and a loving committed relationship. A happy marriage also provides stability for both the couple and for those involved in their lives. Considerable research indicates that married people live longer, feel happier, remain mentally alert longer, and suffer fewer physical and mental health problems.[15] Couples in healthy marriages have less stress, which in turn contributes to better overall health. A healthy marriage contributes to lower stress levels in three important ways: improved personal behaviors, expanded support networks, and financial stability.

cohabitation Intimate partners living together without being married.
common-law marriage Cohabitation lasting a designated period of time (usually 7 years) that is considered legally binding in some states.

Married adults are about half as likely to be smokers as are single, divorced, or separated adults.[16] They are also less likely to be heavy drinkers or to engage in risky sexual behavior.[17] The one negative health indicator for married people is body weight. Married adults, particularly men, weigh more than single adults.[18] Marriage additionally provides the opportunity for strong integration into a network of family and friends to provide assistance and help couples cope when stressors inevitably arise. Finally, marriage is strongly related to economic well-being, which can impact both health status and stress levels.[19] See the **Money & Health** box on page 125 for more on how marriage contributes to financial health.

Cohabitation

Cohabitation is defined as a relationship in which two unmarried people with an intimate connection live together in the same household. For a variety of reasons, increasing numbers of Americans are choosing cohabitation. In some states, cohabitation that lasts a designated number of years (usually 7) legally constitutes a **common-law marriage** for purposes of purchasing real estate and sharing other financial obligations.

Cohabitation can offer many of the same benefits as marriage: love, sex, companionship, and the opportunity to know a partner better over time. In addition to emotional and physical benefits, some people may live together for practical reasons, such as the opportunity to share bills and housing costs. Over the past 20 years, there has been a large increase in the number of persons who have cohabited. In fact, cohabitation is increasingly the first coresidential partnership formed by young adults.[20]

Until recently, many people thought that cohabitation before marriage was likely to lead to the ultimate breakup of the marriage. However, according to a report from the National Center for Health Statistics, cohabitation isn't a clear predictor of marriage success or failure. In a group of 13,000 men and women aged 15 to 44, 71 percent of men who were engaged when they moved in with their fiancée were still married to the same woman after 10 years. For men who didn't cohabit before getting married, the success rate dropped slightly, to 69 percent. Sixty-five percent of cohabiting engaged women were still married after 10 years, compared to 66 percent of women who waited until after marriage to move in with their husband.[21]

While cohabitation can serve as a prelude to marriage, for some people, it is an alternative to marriage. Cohabitation is more common among those of lower socioeconomic status, those who are less religious, people who have been divorced, and those who have experienced parental divorce or high levels of parental conflict during childhood. Although cohabitation has its advantages, it also has some drawbacks. Perhaps the greatest disadvantage is the lack of societal validation for the relationship, especially if the couple subsequently has children. Many cohabitants must deal with pressures from parents and friends, difficulties in obtaining insurance and tax benefits, and legal issues over property.

Gay and Lesbian Partnerships

Whether they are gay or straight, male or female, most adults want inti-

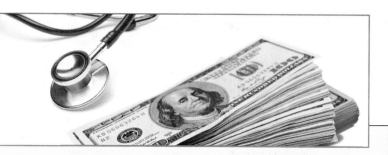

Money&Health
FOR RICHER OR FOR POORER?

If you want to retire rich, stay married! Jay Zagorsky, an Ohio State University researcher, found that a person who gets married and stays married accumulates almost twice as much personal wealth as a person who gets divorced or never marries. Using the National Longitudinal Survey of Youth, Zagorsky followed 9,055 people for 15 years, finding that married people accumulated 77 percent more wealth than divorced people.

This accumulation of wealth is attributed to a number of factors. It is cheaper to run one household of two than two households of one. Married people share items and buy them in larger quantities, which usually cost loss. Additionally, because of task sharing, they are able to

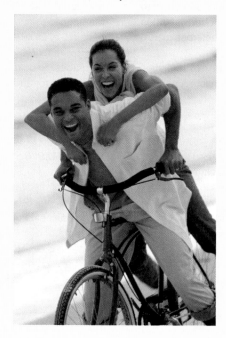

Studies indicate married people may experience higher levels of health and wealth than their unmarried counterparts.

produce more in the same time as a couple than they could individually. For example, if one does laundry and the other vacuums, in the same time they have accomplished two tasks.

Married people behave differently; they work harder, and thus advance further in their jobs, and they save more money. They are more likely to own homes and stocks. Long term wealth and stability are one more reason to invest in a healthy relationship, as according to Zagorsky, "Divorce is as crushing to finances, as it is to emotions."

Sources: J. Zagorsky, "Marriage and Divorce's Impact on Wealth," *Journal of Sociology* 41 (2005): 406–24; Associated Press, "Study: Marriage Builds Wealth and Divorce Destroy It," *USA Today*, January 18, 2006.

mate, committed relationships. Lesbians and gay men seek the same things in primary relationships that heterosexual partners do: love, friendship, communication, validation, companionship, and a sense of stability. The 2010 American Community Survey identified an estimated 646,464 same-sex couples in the United States, 20 percent of whom are legally married.[22]

In addition to the same challenges to successful relationships faced by heterosexual couples, such as effective communication and conflict resolution, lesbian and gay couples often face discrimination and difficulties dealing with social, legal, and religious doctrines. For lesbian and gay couples, obtaining the same level of "marriage benefits," such as tax deductions, power-of-attorney rights, partner health insurance, child custody rights, and other rights, continues to be a challenge. In 1996, the U.S. Congress reaffirmed tax advantages for married couples and effectively blocked cohabitating couples—both homosexual and heterosexual—from these benefits through the Defense of Marriage Act (DOMA). The purpose of DOMA was to normalize heterosexual mar-

riage on a federal level and to permit each state to decide whether or not to recognize same-sex unions. See the **Points of View** box on page 126 for more on this topic.

At the time of this writing in 2012, New York, Massachusetts, Connecticut, Iowa, New Hampshire, Vermont, and the District of Columbia are the only states or districts to grant same-sex couples full marriage equality. The governors of Washington and Maryland have signed legislation making same-sex marriage legal, but the laws are not yet in effect. Nine other states have broad relationship-recognition laws that extend to same-sex couples all, or nearly all, the state rights and responsibilities of married heterosexual couples, whether labeled "civil unions" or "domestic partnerships." More limited rights and protections for same-sex couples are legislated in five additional states.[23] Worldwide, the number of countries that have legalized same-sex marriages or that approve civil unions or registered domestic partnerships for same-sex couples continues to grow. In 2000, the Netherlands was the first country to legalize same sex marriage. Today, seven countries now allow marriage, ten grant broad

The Defense of Marriage Act:
FOR BETTER OR FOR WORSE?

The federal Defense of Marriage Act (DOMA) is a law defining *marriage* as a legal union exclusively between one man and one woman and establishing that no state must recognize the relationship between persons of the same sex as a marriage, even if the relationship is considered a marriage in another state. Thus, DOMA denies gay couples the federal protections and benefits that apply to heterosexual couples. In addition, it says that federal statutes, regulations, and rulings applicable to married heterosexuals do not apply to married people of the same sex.

Before DOMA was enacted, federal law deferred to states in defining marriage. At the time DOMA was enacted, same-sex couples were not allowed to marry in any U.S. state. Since then, eight states and the District of Columbia have recognized equal marriage rights for same-sex couples, and thousands of couples have married. Two of those state laws were later overturned (California and Maine), but California still honors the marriages that took place while the law was in effect. Two additional states (Washington and Maryland) have passed gay marriage legislation that has not yet taken effect. However, because of DOMA, the federal government does not recognize or provide federal legal protections for any of these same-sex marriages. Should DOMA be repealed? Here are some of the arguments for and against the law.

Arguments to Keep DOMA

○ Marriage is largely a religious institution, and most religious groups are opposed to the idea of same-sex marriage.

○ Civil unions and domestic partnerships offer same-sex couples many of the same protections and rights as marriage, so allowing same-sex couples to marry is unnecessary.

○ Allowing same-sex couples to marry would undermine the institution of marriage itself.

Arguments to Repeal DOMA

○ The U.S. Constitution is supposed to guarantee equal rights for all U.S. citizens. Having unequal marriage rights is a form of discrimination.

○ Civil unions and domestic partnerships do not offer all of the benefits of marriage, and they vary greatly from state to state.

○ The U.S. Constitution requires each state to give "full faith and credit" to the laws of other states, including states' obligations to honor marriages validated in other states and districts.

Where Do You Stand?

○ Do you think all legally married couples should be treated equally under the law? Do you think states should be able to make their own determinations about who can legally marry?

○ Are you aware of the rights, responsibilities, and protections

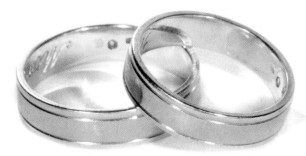

granted to married couples by the federal government?

○ What person(s) or institution(s) should define marriage?

○ Do you think DOMA should be repealed? Why or why not?

---

relationship-recognition laws, and seven offer some protections to same-sex couples.[24]

Staying Single

Increasing numbers of adults of all ages are electing to marry later or to remain single. In 2009, 54.4 percent of women aged 20 to 34 had never been married. Likewise, men in this age group postponed marriage in increasing numbers, with 64.4 percent remaining unmarried in 2009.[25]

Singles clubs, social outings arranged by communities and religious groups, extended family environments, and many social services support the single lifestyle. Many singles live rich, rewarding lives and maintain a large network of close friends and family. Although sexual intimacy may

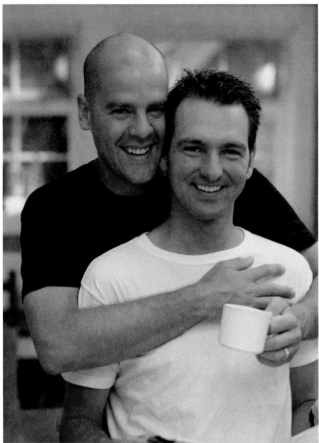

Most adults want to form committed, lasting relationships regardless of their sexual orientation.

Changing patterns in family life affect the environment in which children are raised. In modern society, it is not always clear which partner will adjust his or her work schedule to provide the primary care of children. Nearly half a million children each year become part of a blended family when their parents remarry; remarriage creates a new family of stepparents and stepsiblings.[26] In addition, you might be among the increasing numbers of individuals choosing to have children in a family structure other than a heterosexual marriage. Single women or lesbian couples can choose adoption or alternative insemination as a way to create a family. Single men or gay couples can choose to adopt or obtain the services of a surrogate mother. According to the U.S. Census Bureau, in 2009 over 26 percent of all children under age 18 were living in families headed by a man or woman raising a child alone, reflecting a growing trend in America.[27] Regardless of the structure of the family, certain factors remain important to the well-being of the unit: consistency, communication, affection, and mutual respect. Good parenting does not necessarily come naturally. Many people parent as they were parented (see Table 4.1). This strategy may or may not follow sound child-rearing principles. Establishing a positive, respectful parenting style sets the stage for healthy family growth and development.

Finally, as a potential parent you must consider the financial implications of deciding to have a child. It is estimated that a family with a child born in 2010 can expect to spend an average of $226,920 for food, clothing, shelter, education, and other necessities for the child over the first 17 years of life. Keep in mind that these numbers do not include the cost of childbearing or the major expense of a college education.[28]

Compared to 1975, when only 39 percent of women with children under the age of 5 worked outside the home, nearly 64 percent of mothers with young children work outside the home today.[29] Most families rely on a network of day care workers, family members, friends, grandparents, neighbors, and nannies to provide child care. Child care can be a major financial strain on families. In 2010, the average annual cost for full-time care of an infant in a child care center ranged

or may not be present, the intimacy achieved through other interactions with loved ones is a key aspect of the single lifestyle.

Choosing Whether to Have Children

If you decide to raise children, your relationship with your partner will change. Resources of time, energy, and money are split many ways, and you will no longer be able to give each other undivided attention. Babies and young children do not time their requests for food, sleep, and care for the convenience of adults. Therefore, if your own basic needs for security, love, and purpose are already met, you will be better parents. Any stresses existing in your relationship will be further accentuated when parenting is added to your responsibilities. Having a child does not save a bad relationship—in fact, it seems only to compound the problems that already exist. A child cannot and should not be expected to provide the parents with self-esteem and security.

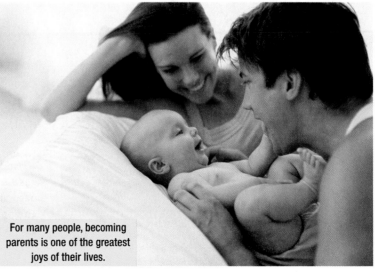

For many people, becoming parents is one of the greatest joys of their lives.

TABLE
4.1 | **Common Parenting Styles**

Authoritarian "Giving orders"	Parents use a set of rules that are clear and unbending. Obedience is highly valued and rewarded. Misbehavior is punished. Children may behave for a reward or out of fear of punishment. Children are not encouraged to think for themselves or to question those in authority.
Permissive "Giving in"	Parents take a hands-off approach. Children are allowed great freedom with few boundaries, minimal guidance, and little discipline. Without limits and expectations, children often struggle with impulse control, poor choices, and insecurity, and have trouble taking responsibility for their actions.
Assertive–Democratic "Giving choices"	Parents have clear expectations for children, clarify issues, and give reasons for limits. Children are given lots of practice in making choices and are guided to see the consequences of their decisions. Encouragement and acknowledgment of good behavior form the focal point of this style. Misbehavior is handled with an appropriate consequence or by problem solving with the child.

Source: S. Dinwiddie, *Effective Parenting Styles: Why Yesterday's Models Won't Work Today.* Accessed January 12, 2009, www.kidsource.com/better.world.press/ parenting.html. Copyright © Sue Dinwiddie. Used with permission.

from $4,650 in Mississippi to $18,200 a year in Washington D.C.[30]

Given that 49 percent of pregnancies in the United States are unintended,[31] some people become parents without a lot of forethought. Some children are born into a relationship that was supposed to last and didn't. This does not mean it is impossible to do a good job of parenting. Children are amazingly resilient and forgiving if parents show respect and communicate about household activities that affect their lives. Even children who grow up in households full of conflict can feel loved and respected if their parents treat them fairly. This means that parents must take responsibility for their

own emotions and make it clear to children that they are not the reason for conflict.

When Relationships Falter

Breakdowns in relationships usually begin with a change in communication, however subtle. Either partner may stop listening and cease to be emotionally present for the other. In turn, the other feels ignored, unappreciated, or unwanted. Unresolved conflicts increase, and unresolved anger can cause problems in sexual relations, which can further increase communication difficulties.

When a couple who previously enjoyed spending time together find themselves continually in the company of others, spending time apart, or preferring to stay home alone, it may be a sign that the relationship is in trouble. Of course, the need for individual privacy is not a cause for worry—it's essential to health. If, however, a partner decides to change the amount and quality of time spent together without the input or understanding of the other, it may be a sign of hidden problems.

Did you Know?

An estimated 65,500 adopted children in the United States are being raised by a gay or lesbian parent—that's more than 4 percent of U.S. adopted children.

Source: Data from G. Gates, L. M. V. Badgett, J. E. Macomber, and K. Chambers, *Adoption and Foster Care by Gay and Lesbian Parents in the United States,* The Urban Institute and the Charles R. Williams Institute on Sexual Orientation Law and Public Policy, March 2007.

95%

of single Americans under the age of 30 report they would like to marry someday.

College students, particularly those who are socially isolated and far from family and hometown friends, may be particularly vulnerable to staying in unhealthy relationships. They may become emotionally dependent on a partner for everything from eating meals to recreation and study time. Mutual obligations, such as shared rental, financial, or transportation arrangements, and sometimes, child care, can

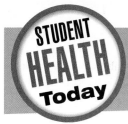

STUDENT HEALTH Today

Recognizing a Potential Abuser

Is the new love in your life really what he or she appears to be? In the beginning, your new love interest may seem like the perfect catch. He or she appears to be sensitive, gentle, caring, respectful, considerate—all the things you've been looking for. Early on, it can be hard to tell what someone is really like because he or she is trying to make a good impression. To avoid getting into a long-term relationship with an abuser, watch carefully and trust your instincts. Ask others about the person's family background, friends, and relationship history. All are important indicators of a person's emotional stability. Be immediately wary if your partner demonstrates any of the following red flags:

✳ Gets extremely angry and swears at you or others.
✳ Regularly makes fun of you or puts you down.
✳ Takes too much control. In a healthy relationship, partners share decision making.

✳ Displays excessive jealousy. Someone who is constantly jealous may lack the self-esteem to have a healthy relationship.
✳ Tries to shut out people you want to see, and wants to spend more and more time alone with you.
✳ Expresses continual negativity. Sulks, angers easily, throws tantrums when things don't go his or her way.
✳ Pushes you verbally or physically to be intimate or have unwanted sex.
✳ Damages your property in fits of anger.
✳ Verbally or physically threatens you.
✳ Verbally or physically harms children or animals.
✳ Is often in trouble or fighting with someone.

The list above is not exhaustive, and there are degrees of seriousness for each. However, if someone you are involved

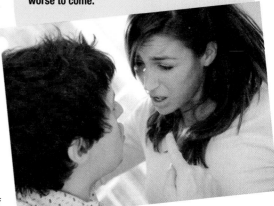

Verbal and physical threats are never part of a healthy relationship—and they may be signs of worse to come.

with displays any sign of physical anger or pushes, shoves, slaps, restrains, or threatens you, it's time to walk away. The National Domestic Violence Hotline offers phone support 24/7 to those who need help recognizing or escaping abuse. Call 1-800-799-SAFE (7233) or visit their website: www.thehotline.org.

---

complicate a decision to end a bad relationship. It's also easy to mistake sexual advances for physical attraction or love. Without a network of friends and supporters to talk with, to obtain validation for feelings, or to share concerns, a student can feel stuck in a relationship that is headed nowhere.

Honesty and verbal affection are usually positive aspects of a relationship. In a troubled relationship, however, they can be used to cover up irresponsible or hurtful behavior. Saying "at least I was honest" is not an acceptable substitute for acting in a trustworthy way, and claiming "but I really do love you" is not a license for being inconsiderate or rude. Relationships that are lacking in mutual respect and consideration can become physically or emotionally abusive; see the **Student Health Today** box describing some warning signs.

Confronting Couples Issues

Couples seeking a long-term relationship must confront a number of issues that can either enhance or diminish their chances of success. These issues can involve power sharing, gender roles, and communication about unmet expectations.

Jealousy **Jealousy** is a negative reaction evoked by a real or imagined relationship involving one's partner and a third person. Contrary to what many people believe, jealousy is not a sign of intense devotion. Instead, jealousy often indicates underlying problems, such as insecurity or possessiveness, which may prove to be a significant barrier to a healthy relationship. Often, jealousy is rooted in a past relationship in which an individual experienced deception and loss. Other causes of jealousy typically include:

jealousy Aversive reaction evoked by a real or imagined relationship involving a person's partner and a third person.

● **Overdependence on the relationship.** People who have few social ties and who rely exclusively on their partner tend to be overly fearful of losing them.
● **Severity of the threat.** People may feel uneasy if someone with stunning good looks and a great personality appears to be interested in his or her partner.
● **High value on sexual exclusivity.** People who believe that sexual exclusivity is a crucial indicator of love are more likely to become jealous.

● **Low self-esteem.** People who think poorly of themselves are more likely to fear that someone else will gain their partner's affection.

● **Fear of losing control.** Some people need to feel in control of every situation. Feeling that they may be losing control over a partner can cause jealousy.

In both men and women, jealousy is related to believing it would be difficult to find another relationship if the current one ends. For men, jealousy is positively correlated with the degree to which the man's self-esteem is affected by his partner's judgments. Although a certain amount of jealousy can be expected in any loving relationship, it doesn't have to threaten the relationship as long as partners communicate openly about it.[32]

Changing Gender Roles Throughout history, women and men have taken on various roles in relationships. In colonial America, gender roles were determined by tradition, and each task within a family unit held equal importance. Our modern society has very few gender-specific roles. Both women and men work, care for children, drive, run businesses, manage family finances, and perform equally well in the tasks of daily living. Rather than taking on traditional female and male roles, many couples find it makes more sense to divide tasks on the basis of schedule, convenience, and preference. However, the division is rarely equal. Even when women work full-time, they tend to bear heavy family and household responsibilities. Today, many working women juggle the responsibilities of being a partner, mother, and a full-time professional and find their never-ending duties to be stressful, frustrating, and overwhelming. According to the Bureau of Labor Statistics, in 2010, on an average day, only 20 percent of men engaged in housework, compared to 49 percent of women; on the days men did engage in household ac-

power Ability to make and implement decisions.

tivities, they spent 30 minutes less completing them.[33] Over time, if couples are unable to communicate how they feel about the division of household responsibilities and arrive at an equitable solution, the relationship is likely to suffer.

Sharing Power **Power** can be defined as the ability to make and implement decisions. Powerful people know what they want and have the ability to attain it. In traditional relationships, men were the wage-earners and consequently, had decision-making power. Women exerted much influence, but ultimately, they needed a man's income for survival. As increasing numbers of women have entered the workforce and generated their own financial resources, the power dynamics between women and men have shifted considerably. The increase in the divorce rate in the past century was partly due to working women gaining the ability to support themselves by choice rather than remaining in difficult or abusive relationships solely for financial reasons.

In successful relationships, partners share responsibilities, power, and control. Even when both partners are financially equal, power in other areas may be an issue. If one partner always has the final say in deciding social plans, for example, the unequal distribution of power in that area may affect the quality of the relationship.

Unmet Expectations We all have expectations—how we will spend our time and our money, how we will express love and intimacy, and how we will grow together as a couple. Expectations are an extension of our values, beliefs, hopes, and dreams for the future. When communicated and agreed upon, these expectations help relationships thrive. If we are unable to communicate our expectations, we set ourselves up for disappointment and hurt. Partners in healthy relationships can communicate wants and needs and have honest discussions when things aren't going as expected or as planned.

When and Why Relationships End

Often we hear in the news that 50 percent of American marriages end in divorce. This number is based on the annual marriage rate compared with the annual divorce rate. This is misleading, because in any given year, the people who are divorcing are not the same as those who are marrying.

The preferred method to determine the divorce rate is to calculate how many people who have ever married subsequently divorce. Using this calculation, the divorce rate in the United States has never exceeded 41 percent.[34] Although this number is still high, the U.S. divorce rate has declined from previous decades. This decrease may be related to an

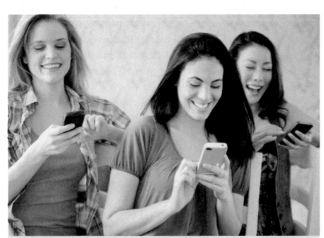

There's more to good communication than just sending a lot of texts.

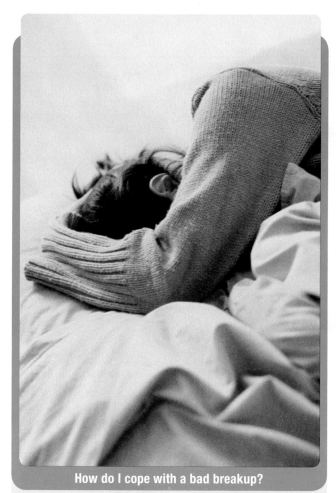

How do I cope with a bad breakup?

It may feel as if there is no end to the sorrow, anger, and guilt that often accompany a difficult breakup, but time is a miraculous healer. Acknowledging your feelings, finding healthful ways to express them, spending time with friends, and allowing yourself to take as much time as you need to heal are all helpful in dealing with the end of a romantic relationship.

increase in the age at which persons first marry and also a higher level of education among those who are marrying—as both contribute to marital stability.[35]

The risk of divorce is lower for educated people marrying for the first time and lower still for people who wait to marry until at least their mid-twenties, who haven't lived with multiple partners prior to marriage, or who are strongly religious and marry someone of the same faith.[36] The divorce rate represents only a portion of the actual number of failed relationships. Many people never go through a legal divorce process so they are not counted in these statistics. Cohabitants and unmarried partners who raise children, own homes together, and exhibit all the outward appearances of marriage without the license are also not included.

Why do relationships end? There are many reasons, including illness, financial concerns, and career problems. Other breakups arise from unmet expectations. Many people enter a relationship with certain expectations about how they and their partner will behave. Failure to communicate these beliefs can lead to resentment and disappointment. Differences in sexual needs may also contribute to the demise of a relationship. Under stress, communication and cooperation between partners can break down. Conflict, negative interactions, and a general lack of respect between partners can erode even the most loving relationship.

Coping with Failed Relationships

No relationship comes with a guarantee. Losing a love is as much a part of life as falling in love. That being said, uncoupling can be very painful. Whenever we risk getting close to another, we also risk being hurt if things don't work out. Remember that knowing, understanding, and feeling good about oneself before entering a relationship is very important. Consider the following tips for coping with a failed relationship:[37]

- **Recognize and acknowledge your feelings.** These may include grief, loneliness, rejection, anger, guilt, relief, or sadness. Seek professional help and support if needed.
- **Find healthful ways to express your emotions, rather than turning them inward.** Go for a walk, talk to friends, listen to music, work out at the gym, volunteer with a community organization, or write in a journal.
- **Spend time with current friends, or reconnect with old friends.** Get reacquainted with yourself, what you enjoy doing, and the people whose company you enjoy.
- **Don't rush into a "rebound" relationship.** You need time to resolve your experience rather than escape from it. You can't be trusting and intimate in a new relationship if you are still working on getting over a past relationship.

Assess yourself

How Well Do You Communicate?

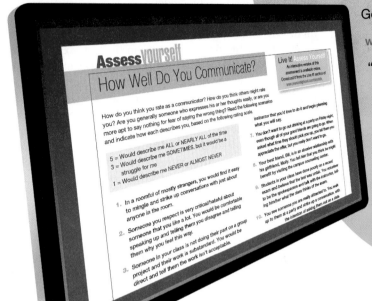

Go online to the **Live It!** section of www.pearsonhighered.com to take the "How Well Do You Communicate?" assessment.*

Use the steps outlined in the **YOUR PLAN FOR CHANGE** box to improve your communication skills.

*If your instructor so chooses, Assess Yourself Activities are available as a printed supplement or as assignable homework online at www.pearsonhighered.com/myhealthlab.

MyHealthLab®

YOUR PLAN FOR CHANGE

The **Assess yourself** activity "How Well Do You Communicate?" is available at www.pearsonhighered.com/myhealthlab. This activity gives you the chance to look at how you communicate. After completing the activity and considering your responses, you can take steps toward becoming a better communicator and improving your relationships.

Today, you can:

○ Call a friend you haven't talked to in a while or arrange a coffee date with a new acquaintance you'd like to get to know better.

○ Start a journal and keep track of communication and relationship issues that arise. Look for trends and think about ways you can change your behavior to address them.

Within the next 2 weeks, you can:

○ Spend some time letting the people you care about know how important they are to you.

○ If there is someone with whom you have a conflict, arrange a time to talk about the issues. Be sure to meet in a neutral setting away from distractions.

By the end of the semester, you can:

○ Practice being an active listener.

○ Take note of your nonverbal communication. Work on maintaining eye contact and using positive body language and facial expressions.

Summary

* Characteristics of intimate relationships include behavioral interdependence, need fulfillment, emotional attachment, and emotional availability. These influence how we interact with others and the types of intimate relationships we form. Family, friends, and partners provide the most common opportunities for intimacy. Each relationship may include healthy and unhealthy characteristics that can affect daily functioning.

* There are many strategies for building better relationships. Examining one's own behaviors to determine what to change and how to change is an important ingredient of success. Characteristics of successful relationships include good communication, intimacy, friendship, and trust.

* To improve our communication skills, we need to address factors that include appropriate self-disclosure, listening effectively, conveying and interpreting nonverbal communication, and managing and resolving conflicts.

* For most people, commitment is an important piece of a successful relationship. Types of committed relationships include marriage, cohabitation, and gay and lesbian partnerships (which can involve either marriage or cohabitation). Success in committed relationships requires understanding the elements of a good relationship.

* Life decisions such as whether to marry or have children require serious consideration. Remaining single is more common than ever before. Most single people lead healthy, happy, and well-adjusted lives. Having children can also be part of a rewarding, productive life as long as parents make the decision with full awareness and acceptance of the demands and responsibilities of parenting.

* Factors that can cause relationship problems include breakdowns in communication, erosion of mutual respect, jealousy, differences over gender roles, power struggles, and unmet expectations. Before relationships fail, warning signs often appear. By recognizing these signs and taking action to change behaviors, partners may save and enhance their relationship.

Pop Quiz

1. Intimate relationships fulfill our psychological need for someone to listen to our worries and concerns. This is known as our need for
   a. dependence.
   b. social integration.
   c. enjoyment.
   d. spontaneity.

2. Lovers tend to pay attention to their significant other even when they should be involved in other activities. This is called
   a. inclusion.
   b. exclusivity.
   c. fascination.
   d. authentic intimacy.

3. All of the following are typical causes of jealousy *except*
   a. overdependence on the relationship.
   b. low self-esteem.
   c. a past relationship that involved deception.
   d. belief that relationships can easily be replaced.

4. According to anthropologist Helen Fisher, attraction and falling in love follow a pattern based on
   a. lust, attraction, and attachment.
   b. intimacy, passion, and commitment.
   c. imprinting, attraction, attachment, and the production of a cuddle chemical.
   d. fascination, exclusiveness, sexual desire, giving the utmost, and being a champion.

5. The goal of conflict resolution is to
   a. constructively resolve points of contention.
   b. declare a winner and a loser.
   c. ensure that couples argue as little as possible.
   d. set a time limit on discussion of difficult issues.

6. Terms such as *behavioral interdependence, need fulfillment,* and *emotional availability* describe which type of relationship?
   a. dysfunctional
   b. sexual
   c. intimate
   d. behavioral

7. Predictability, dependability, and faith are three fundamental elements of
   a. trust.
   b. friendship.
   c. attraction.
   d. attachment.

8. *Competitive listening* refers to
   a. attentive listening to what the other person is saying.
   b. paraphrasing what the other person is communicating to you.
   c. allowing the speaker to complete a thought before asking questions.
   d. a desire to promote your own point of view.

9. One of the most important ways to express difficult feelings is to
   a. be specific rather than general about how you feel.
   b. express anger and resentment so the other person feels your heartache.
   c. point your finger at the other person.
   d. blame the other person for the difficulty you are experiencing.

10. One important factor in choosing a partner is *proximity,* which refers to
    a. smutual regard.
    b. attitudes and values.
    c. physical attraction.
    d. being in the same place at the same time.

Answers to these questions can be found on page A-1.

Think about It!

1. What are the characteristics of intimate relationships? What are behavioral interdependence, need fulfillment, emotional attachment, and emotional availability, and why is each important in relationship development?
2. What problems can form barriers to intimacy? What actions can you take to reduce or remove these barriers?
3. What are common elements of good relationships? What are some warning signs of trouble? What actions can you take to improve your own interpersonal relationships?
4. What is nonverbal communication, and why is it important to develop skills in this area? Give examples of some things you do to communicate without words.
5. How can you tell the difference between a love relationship and one that is based primarily on attraction? What characteristics do love relationships share?
6. Name some common misconceptions about people who choose to remain single and about couples who choose not to have children. Do you want to have children? Why or why not? What characteristics show that a couple is ready to have children?

Accessing Your Health on the Internet

The following websites explore further topics and issues related to personal health. For links to the websites below, visit the Companion Website for *Access to Health,* 13th Edition, at
www.pearsonhighered.com/donatelle.

1. *Relationship Growth Online.* This site provides information, quizzes, games, advice, and links to more information on how to build better relationships. www.relationshipweb.com
2. *Gay and Lesbian Couples National Network.* This is a link to a network for same-sex couples and singles, with resources about gay and lesbian issues. http://couples-national.org
3. *The Gottman Institute.* This organization helps couples directly and provides training to therapists. The website includes research information, self-help tips for relationship building, and a relationship quiz. www.gottman.com
4. *National Center for Health Statistics.* This division of the Centers for Disease Control and Prevention has up-to-date statistics on trends in marriage, divorce, and cohabitation. www.cdc.gov/nchs
5. *The Conflict Resolution Information Source.* This site provides information, news, research, and links to resources for resolving conflicts in interpersonal relationships, marriages, families, organizations, and more. www.crinfo.org
6. *The Hotline.* This site provides information about domestic violence, including how to recognize abuse and how to get help in your local area. www.thehotline.org

References

1. J. Holt-Lunstad, T. Smith, and J. Layton, "Social Relationships and Mortality Risk: A Meta-Analytic Review," *PLoS Medicine* 7, no.7 (2010); J. Snelgrove, P. Hynek, and M. Stafford, "A Multi-Level Analysis of Social Capital and Self-Rated Health: Evidence from the British Household Panel Survey," *Social Science and Medicine* 68, no. 11 (2009): 1993–2001; S. Braithwaite, R. Delevi, and F. Fincham, "Romantic Relationships and the Physical and Mental Health of College Students," *Personal Relationships* 17, no. 1 (2010): 1–12; E. Cornwell and L. Waite, "Social Disconnectedness, Perceived Isolation, and Health among Older Adults," *Journal of Health and Social Behavior,* 50, no.11 (2009): 31–48.
2. D. Akst, "America: Land of Loners?" *The Wilson Quarterly,* Summer 2010, www.wilsonquarterly.com/article.cfm?aid=1631.
3. Ibid.
4. R. Sternberg, "A Triangular Theory of Love," *Psychological Review* 93, (1986): 119–35.
5. H. Fisher, *Why We Love* (New York: Henry Holt, 2004); H. Fisher, A. Aron, D. Mashek, H. Li, and L. L. Brown, "Defining the Brain System of Lust, Romantic Attraction, and Attachment," *Archives of Sexual Behavior* 31, no. 5 (2002): 413–19.
6. Ibid.
7. Ibid.
8. S. A. Rathus, J. Nevid, and L. Fichner-Rathus, *Human Sexuality in a World of Diversity.* 8th ed. (Boston: Allyn & Bacon, 2010).
9. C. R. Rogers, "Interpersonal Relationship: The Core of Guidance" in *Person to Person: The Problem of Being Human,* eds. C. R. Rogers and B. Stevens (Lafayette, CA: Real People Press, 1967).
10. J. Wood, *Interpersonal Communication: Everyday Encounters* (Belmont, CA: Cengage, 2010).
11. R. S. Miller, D. Perlman, and S. S. Brehm, *Intimate Relationships.* 4th ed. (New York: McGraw-Hill, 2007), 150–56.
12. D. Bohon, "Pew Study Shows U.S. Marriages at an All-time Low," December 16, 2011, http://thenewamerican.com/culture/family/10222-pew-study-shows-us-marriages-at-an-all-time-low.
13. The National Marriage Project, University of Virginia, *The State of Our Unions: Marriage in America, 2009: Money & Marriage* (Charlottesville, VA: National Marriage Project and the Institute for American Values, 2009), www.stateofourunions.org.
14. U.S. Census Bureau, "U.S. Census Bureau Reports Men and Women Wait Longer to Marry," November 10, 2010, www.census.gov/newsroom/releases/archives/families_households/cb10-174.html.
15. K. McCoy, "Can Marriage Help You Live Longer?" HealthLibrary, EBSCO Publishing, April 2010, http://healthlibrary.epnet.com/GetContent

.aspx?token=af362d97-4f80-4453-a175-02cc6220a387&chunkiid=43793.

16. C. A. Schoenborn, "Marital Status and Health: United States, 1999–2002," *Advance Data from Vital and Health Statistics,* no. 351, DHHS Publication No. 2005-1250 (Hyattsville, MD: National Center for Health Statistics, 2004), www.cdc.gov/nchs/products/ad.htm.

17. Ibid.

18. Ibid.

19. S. Steiner, "Marrying for Richer Rather Than Poorer," February 11, 2011, www.foxbusiness.com/personal-finance/2011/02/04/marrying-richer-poorer/.

20. P. Y. Goodwin, W. D. Mosher, and A. Chandra," Marriage and Cohabitation in the United States: A Statistical Portrait Based on Cycle 6 (2002) of the National Survey of Family Growth, National Center for Health Statistics," *Vital Health Statistics* 23, no. 28 (2010), www.cdc.gov/nchs/nsfg/nsfg_products.htm.

21. Ibid.

22. U.S. Census Bureau, "Census Bureau Releases Estimates of Same-Sex Married Couples," September 27, 2011, www.census.gov/newsroom/releases/archives/2010_census/cb11-cn181.html.

23. National Gay and Lesbian Task Force, "Relationship Recognition Map for Same-Sex Couples in the U.S.," June 2011, www.thetaskforce.org/reports_and_research/relationship_recognition.

24. D. Masci, H. Lozana-Bielat, M. Ralston, and E. Podrebarac, "Gay Marriage Around the World," July 9, 2009, www.pewforum.org/Gay-Marriage-and-Homosexuality/Gay-Marriage-Around-the-World.aspx.

25. U.S. Census Bureau, "2008 American Community Survey, Marital Status," table S1210, 2008, http://factfinder.census.gov/servlet/DatasetMainPageServlet?_program=ACS&_submenuId=datasets_3&_lang=en&_ts=.

26. U.S. Census Bureau, Housing and Household Economic Statistics Division, Fertility & Family Statistics Branch, "America's Families and Living Arrangements: 2009," 2010, www.census.gov/population/www/socdemo/hh-fam/cps2009.html.

27. Ibid.

28. M. Lino, *Expenditures on Children by Families, 2010* (Alexandria, VA: U.S. Department of Agriculture, Center for Nutrition Policy and Promotion, 2011), www.cnpp.usda.gov/ExpendituresonChildrenbyFamilies.htm.

29. U.S. Bureau of Labor Statistics, "Women in the Labor Force: A Databook, 2010 Edition," 2010, http://data.bls.gov/cps/wlf-databook2010.htm.

30. National Association of Child Care Resource and Referral Agencies, Parents and the High Cost of Child Care, 2011 Report," August 2011, www.naccrra.org/sites/default/files/default_site_pages/2011/cost_report_2011_full_report_0.pdf.

31. L. Finer and M. Zolna, "Unintended Pregnancy in the United State: Incidence and Disparities, 2006," *Contraception* 5, (2011): 478–85.

32. M. Gatzeva and A. Paik, "Emotional and Physical Satisfaction in Noncohabiting, Cohabiting, and Marital Relationships: The Importance of Jealous Conflict," *Journal of Sex Research* 25, (2009): 1–14; D. Nannini and L. Mayers, "Jealousy in Sexual and Emotional Infidelity: An Alternative to the Evolutionary Explanation," *Journal of Sex Research* 37, no. 2 (2000): 117–22.

33. United States Department of Labor, Bureau of Labor Statistics, "American Time Use Survey Summary," June 22, 2011, www.bls.gov/news.release/atus.nr0.htm.

34. D. Hurley, "Divorce Rate: It's Not as High as You Think," *New York Times,* April 19, 2005.

35. The National Marriage Project, University of Virginia, *The State of Our Unions: Marriage in America, 2009: Money & Marriage,* 2009.

36. D. Popenoe and B. D. Whitehead, "Ten Important Research Findings on Marriage and Choosing a Marriage Partner," 2004, www.virginia.edu/marriageproject/tenthingsseries.html.

37. G.F. Kelly, *Sexuality Today,* 2006.

5
Understanding Your Sexuality

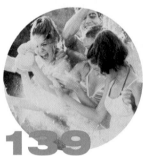

139
What influences sexual identity besides biology?

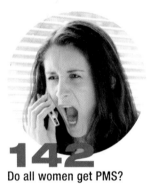

142
Do all women get PMS?

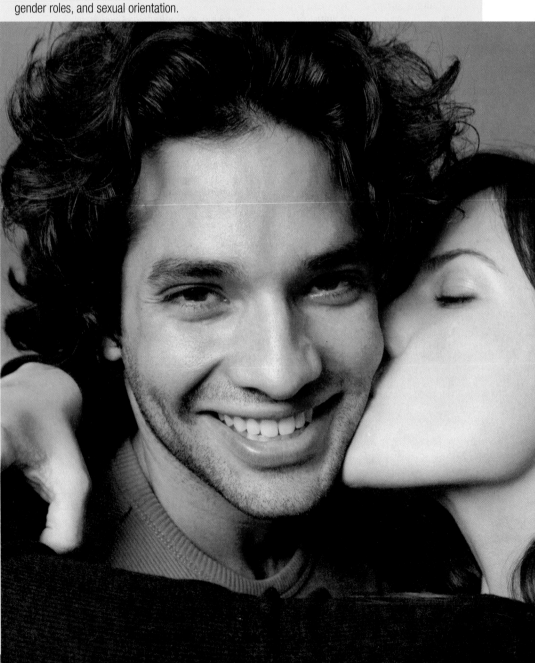

OBJECTIVES

✳ Identify the primary structures of male and female sexual anatomy and explain the functions of each.

✳ Discuss the stages of the human sexual response and what factors may influence these.

✳ Define *sexual identity* and discuss its major components, including biology, gender identity, gender roles, and sexual orientation.

✳ Discuss the options available for the expression of one's sexuality.

✳ Classify sexual dysfunctions, describe major disorders, and discuss treatment options.

✳ Examine the effects of various drugs on sexual behavior.

148
What is "normal" sexual behavior?

155
Are sexual disorders more physical or more psychological?

How do you see yourself as a sexual person? Do you identify yourself as gay or straight? Are you comfortable in your own skin? Do you know enough about sexual anatomy and physiology to maximize your sexual pleasure and control your fertility? Human sexuality is complex and involves physical health, personal values, interpersonal relationships, cultural traditions, social norms, new technologies, current research findings, and changing political agendas. **Sexuality** is much more than sexual feelings or intercourse. Rather, it includes all the thoughts, feelings, and behaviors associated with being male or female, experiencing attraction, being in love, and being in relationships that include sexual intimacy. Elements of sexuality include:

- **Sensuality.** Awareness and feelings about your body and others' bodies, especially that of your sexual partner. Sensuality enables us to feel good about how our bodies look and feel and to enjoy the pleasure they can give to us and others.
- **Intimacy.** The ability to have a positive, close relationship with another human being.
- **Sexual identity.** One's sense of oneself as a sexual being, including gender identity.
- **Sexual health and reproduction.** Attitudes and behaviors related to the health of the sexual organs, the ability to have children, and the health consequences of sexual behavior.
- **Sexualization.** The use of sexuality to influence or manipulate others in ways that may be harmful or exploitative.

Our sexuality is central to who we are as humans. In this chapter, we will focus on sexual identity and aspects of sexual health, reproduction, and sexual behaviors. Having a comprehensive understanding of your sexuality will help you make responsible and satisfying decisions about your life and your interpersonal relationships.

Your Sexual Identity: More than Biology

Sexual identity, the recognition and acknowledgment of oneself as a sexual being, is determined by a complex interaction of genetic, physiological, environmental, and social factors. The beginning of sexual identity occurs at conception with the combining of chromosomes that determine sex. All eggs carry an X chromosome; sperm may carry either an X or a Y chromosome. If a sperm carrying an X chromosome fertilizes an egg, the resulting combination of sex chromosomes (XX) produces a female. If a sperm carrying a Y chromosome fertilizes an egg, the XY combination produces a male.

Sometimes chromosomes are added, lost, or rearranged in this process and the sex of the offspring is not clear, a condition known as **intersexuality.** *Disorders of sexual development* (*DSDs*) is a less confusing term that has been recommended to refer to intersex conditions, which may occur as often as 1 in 1,500 live births (see the **Health in a Diverse World** box on page 138).[1]

The genetic instructions included in the sex chromosomes lead to the development of male and female **gonads** (reproductive organs) at about the eighth week of fetal life. Once the male gonads (testes) and the female gonads (ovaries) develop, they play a key role in all future sexual development because the gonads are responsible for the production of sex hormones. The primary female sex hormones are estrogen and progesterone. The primary male sex hormone is testosterone. The release of testosterone in a maturing fetus signals the development of a penis and other male genitals. If no testosterone is produced, female genitals form.

At the time of **puberty,** sex hormones again play major roles in development. Hormones released by the **pituitary gland,** called gonadotropins, stimulate the testes and ovaries to make appropriate sex hormones. Increased estrogen production in females and testosterone production in males leads to the development of **secondary sex characteristics.** Male secondary sex characteristics include deepening of the voice, development of facial and body hair, and growth of the skeleton and musculature. Female characteristics include growth of the breasts, widening of the hips, and the development of pubic and underarm hair.

Thus far, we have described sexual identity only in terms of a person's biological status as a male or female. Another important component of our sexual identity is gender. **Gender** refers to characteristics and actions typically associated with men or women (masculine or feminine) as defined by the culture in which one lives. Our sense of masculine and feminine traits is largely a result of **socialization** during our childhood. **Gender roles** are the behaviors and activities we use to express masculinity or femininity in ways that conform to society's expectations. For example, children may learn to play with dolls or toy trucks based on how parents influence their actions. For some, gender roles can be very confining when they lead to stereotyping. Bounds established by **gender-role stereotypes** can make it difficult to express one's true sexual identity. Men are traditionally

sexuality Thoughts, feelings, and behaviors associated with being male or female, experiencing attraction, being in love, and being in relationships that include sexual intimacy.

sexual identity Recognition of oneself as a sexual being; a composite of biological sex characteristics, gender identity, gender roles, and sexual orientation.

intersexuality Not exhibiting exclusively male or female sex characteristics.

gonads Reproductive organs that produce germ cells and sex hormones. In males, the testes, and in females, the ovaries).

puberty Period of sexual maturation.

pituitary gland Endocrine gland that controls the release of hormones from the gonads.

secondary sex characteristics Characteristics associated with sex but not directly related to reproduction, such as vocal pitch, body hair, and location of fat deposits.

gender Characteristics and actions associated with being feminine or masculine as defined by the society in which one lives.

socialization Process by which a society communicates behavioral expectations to its members.

gender roles Expression of maleness or femaleness in everyday life.

gender-role stereotypes Generalizations concerning how men and women should express themselves and the characteristics each possesses.

See It! Videos
What's it like to change your gender in society? Watch **Gender Transition** at www.pearsonhighered.com/donatelle.

DISORDERS OF SEXUAL DEVELOPMENT

The South African middle-distance runner Caster Semenya is one of the fastest women around today. But after she won the gold medal in the 800-meter race at the 2009 World Championships, she was required to undergo gender testing and was subsequently barred from competition. Officials at the International Association of Athletics Federations (IAAF) wanted to determine whether Semenya has a disorder of sexual development (DSD; also called intersexuality) resulting in testosterone levels that give her an unfair athletic advantage over other female competitors. In July 2010, the IAAF announced that Semenya was again eligible to compete. The decision of the IAAF council was the culmination of an 18-month-long review by an expert working group that has studied issues relating to the participation of female athletes with hyperandrogenism, a condition involving overproduction of male sex hormones. The ruling by the IAAF states a female with hyperandrogenism who is recognized as a female in law will be eligible to compete in women's competition in athletics provided that she has androgen levels below the male range (measured by reference to testosterone levels in serum) or, if she has androgen

Many people considered it an invasion of privacy when World Champion runner Caster Semenya was required to submit to gender testing before being allowed to return to competition.

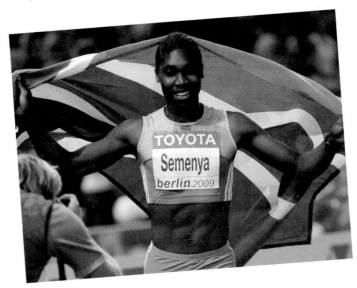

levels within the male range, she also has an androgen resistance such that she derives no competitive advantage from such levels.

The details of Semenya's test results and whether she received medical treatment to regain her eligibility remain confidential; however, Semenya's case highlights the challenges facing athletes and others with both male and female characteristics. People with DSDs are born with various levels of male and female biological characteristics, ranging from different chromosomal arrangements to altered hormone production to variation in primary and secondary sex characteristics. While most people are born with either XX or XY chromosomes, some are born with XXY or XO chromosomes (where O signifies a missing or

damaged chromosome). In some people, gonads do not develop fully into ovaries or testicles, although there may be no external signs to indicate this, and in others, external genitalia may be ambiguous.

Many, but not all, DSDs require some degree of medical intervention, whether hormonal or surgical, to ensure a person's physical health. It is also necessary to "assign" a gender to all children as early as possible to ensure their psychological health. If this assignment is later found to be inconsistent with the child's own sense of gender, he or she may choose to adopt a different gender identity. Most people born with DSDs today are allowed to grow up, establish their own gender identity, and choose as adults whether to have additional surgeries to alter any sexual tissues they feel that are incongruent with their gender. To find out more about DSDs, visit the website of Accord Alliance at www.accordalliance.org.

Sources: A. Kessel, "Caster Semenya May Return to Track This Month after IAAF Clearance," *The Guardian,* July 6, 2010, www.guardian.co.uk/sport/2010/jul/06/caster-semenya-iaaf-clearance; "Consensus Statement on Management of Intersex Disorders," *Pediatrics* 118 (2006): e488–e500; "IAFF Approves New Rules on Hyperandrogenism," *The Guardian,* April 12, 2011, www.guardian.co.uk/sport/2011/apr/12/iaaf-athletics-rules-hyperandrogenism-caster-semenya.

Sexual Orientation

Sexual orientation refers to a person's enduring emotional, romantic, or sexual attraction to others. You may be primarily attracted to members of the opposite sex (**heterosexual**), the same sex (**homosexual**), or both sexes (**bisexual**). Many homosexuals prefer the terms **gay,** queer, or **lesbian** to describe their sexual orientation. *Gay* and *queer* can apply to both men and women, but *lesbian* refers specifically to women.

Gay and bisexual people are often targets of **sexual prejudice.** Sexual prejudice refers to negative attitudes and hostile actions directed at members of a particular social group. Hate crimes, discrimination, and hostility toward sexual minorities are evidence of ongoing sexual prejudice.[2] Recent data from the Department of Justice indicated that bias regarding sexual orientation was the motivation for approximately 18.5 percent of all hate crimes reported.[3]

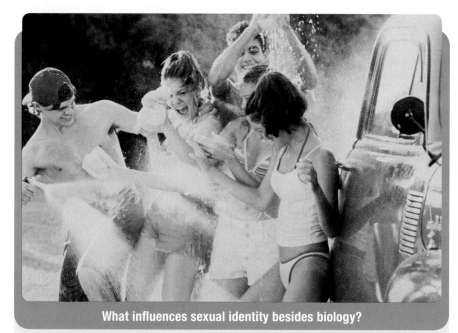

What influences sexual identity besides biology?

How you perceive yourself as a sexual being is influenced by socialization and personal experience. Your understanding of gender roles, your contact with people of various gender identities or sexual orientations, and your own degree of emotional maturity can all affect your sense of sexual identity.

expected to be independent, aggressive, logical, and always in control of their emotions. Women are traditionally expected to be passive, nurturing, intuitive, sensitive, and emotional. **Androgyny** refers to the combination of traditional masculine and feminine traits in a single person. Androgynous people do not always follow traditional gender roles but instead choose behaviors based on a given situation.

Whereas gender roles are an expression of cultural expectations for behavior, **gender identity** refers to a person's sense or awareness of being masculine or feminine. A person's gender identity does not always match his or her biological sex: This is called being **transgendered.** There is a broad spectrum of expression among transgendered persons that reflects the degree of dissatisfaction they have with their sexual anatomy. Some transgendered persons are very comfortable with their bodies and are content simply to dress and live as the other gender. *Transvestism,* also referred to as cross-dressing, is the term used to describe the practice of wearing the clothing of the opposite sex. Most transvestites are male, heterosexual, and married.

At the other end of the spectrum are **transsexuals,** who feel extremely trapped in their bodies and may opt for therapeutic interventions, such as sex reassignment surgery. In short, a transsexual wears clothes of the opposite sex because those clothes are associated with the gender they identify with, whereas a cross-dresser wears clothes of the opposite sex because those clothes are associated with the opposite gender.

Most researchers today agree that sexual orientation is best understood using a model that incorporates biological, psychological, and socioenvironmental factors. Biological explanations focus on research into genetics, hormones, and differences in brain anatomy. Psychological and socioenvironmental explanations examine parent–child interactions, sex roles, and early sexual and interpersonal interactions. Collectively, this growing body of research suggests that the origins of homosexuality, like heterosexuality, are complex.[4] To diminish the complexity of sexual orientation to "a choice" is a clear misrepresentation of current research. Homosexuals do not "choose" their sexual orientation any more than heterosexuals do.

Researcher Fritz Klein developed a questionnaire that not only looks at who you are attracted to and actually have sex with, but also considers factors such as those individuals you feel close to

androgyny Combination of traditional masculine and feminine traits in a single person.

gender identity Personal sense or awareness of being masculine or feminine, a male or a female.

transgendered Having a gender identity that does not match one's biological sex.

transsexual Person who is psychologically of one sex but physically of the other.

sexual orientation A person's enduring emotional, romantic, or sexual attraction to other persons.

heterosexual Experiencing primary attraction to and preference for sexual activity with people of the opposite sex.

homosexual Experiencing primary attraction to and preference for sexual activity with people of the same sex.

bisexual Experiencing attraction to and preference for sexual activity with people of both sexes.

gay Sexual orientation involving primary attraction to people of the same sex.

lesbian Sexual orientation involving attraction of women to other women.

sexual prejudice Negative attitudes and hostile actions directed at those with a different sexual orientation.

See It! Videos

Is there a gay gene? How do you feel about same-sex couples expressing affection in public? Watch **Gay Gene** and **Homophobia** at www.pearsonhighered.com/donatelle.

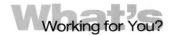
Maybe you're already quite comfortable with your own sexual orientation and that of the people around you. Which of these attitudes and behaviors describe you?

☐ I'm comfortable with my sexual orientation.

☐ I'm trying to become more understanding of those with a sexual orientation different from mine by talking with people who have a different orientation.

☐ I have friends and family members with sexual orientations that differ from my own, and I am comfortable relating to them.

☐ I've attended meetings of the lesbian, gay, bisexual, and transgendered (LGBT) group on my campus to better understand what the challenges are.

☐ I'm already "out," and to get support I've joined the LGBT group on campus.

emotionally, who you enjoy socializing with, and in which "community" you feel most comfortable. This questionnaire is available as the **Assess Yourself** activity "What Are Your Sexual Attitudes and Preferences?" at www.pearsonhighered.com/myhealthlab. After completing the questionnaire, you may realize that there are not just three sexual orientations (homosexual, heterosexual, or bisexual), but indeed a whole range of complex, interacting, and fluid factors that influence your sexuality over time.

Sexual Anatomy and Physiology

Understanding the functions of the male and female reproductive systems will help you derive pleasure and satisfaction from your sexual relationships, be sensitive to your partner's wants and needs, and make responsible choices regarding your own sexual health.

Female Sexual Anatomy and Physiology

The female reproductive system includes two major groups of structures, the external genitals and the internal organs (**Figure 5.1**). The external female genitals are collectively known as the **vulva** and include all structures that are outwardly visible, specifically the mons pubis, the labia minora and majora, the clitoris, the urethral and vaginal openings, and

the vestibule of the vagina and its glands. The **mons pubis** is a pad of fatty tissue covering and protecting the pubic bone; after the onset of puberty, it becomes covered with coarse hair. The **labia majora** are folds of skin and erectile tissue that enclose the urethral and vaginal openings; the **labia minora,** or inner lips, are folds of mucous membrane found just inside the labia majora.

The **clitoris** is located at the upper end of the labia minora and beneath the mons pubis, and its only known function is to provide sexual pleasure. Directly below the clitoris is the **urethral opening** through which urine is expelled from the body. Below the urethral opening is the vaginal opening. In some women, the vaginal opening is covered by a thin membrane called the **hymen.** It is a myth that an intact hymen is proof of virginity, as the hymen can be stretched or torn by physical activity and is not present in all women.

The **perineum** is the area of smooth tissue found between the vulva and the anus. Although not technically part of the external genitalia, the tissue in this area has many nerve endings and is sensitive to touch; it can play a part in sexual excitement.

vulva External female genitalia.

mons pubis Fatty tissue covering the pubic bone in females; in physically mature women, the mons is covered with coarse hair.

labia majora "Outer lips," or folds of tissue covering the female sexual organs.

labia minora "Inner lips," or folds of tissue just inside the labia majora.

clitoris Pea-sized nodule of tissue located at the top of the labia minora; central to sexual arousal in women.

urethral opening Opening through which urine is expelled.

hymen In some women, a thin tissue covering the vaginal opening.

perineum Tissue that forms the "floor" of the pelvic region.

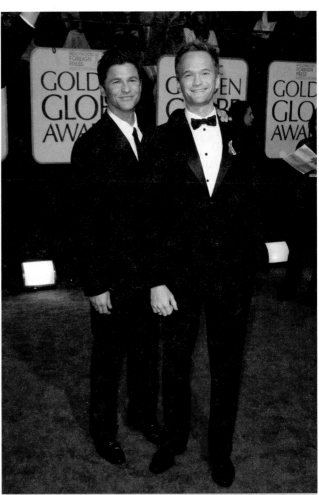

The presence of gay and lesbian celebrities in the media contributes to the increasing acceptance of gay relationships in everyday life. Actor Neil Patrick Harris and his partner David Burtka are an openly gay couple who are parents to twins born via surrogate in October 2010. They announced their engagement after New York state legalized gay marriage in 2011.

External Anatomy

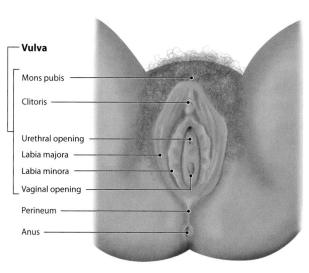

Vulva

- Mons pubis
- Clitoris
- Urethral opening
- Labia majora
- Labia minora
- Vaginal opening
- Perineum
- Anus

Internal Organs

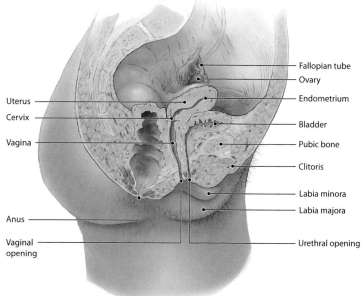

- Fallopian tube
- Ovary
- Endometrium
- Bladder
- Pubic bone
- Clitoris
- Labia minora
- Labia majora
- Urethral opening
- Uterus
- Cervix
- Vagina
- Anus
- Vaginal opening

FIGURE 5.1 **Female Sexual Anatomy**

The internal female genitals include the vagina, uterus, fallopian tubes, and ovaries. The **vagina** is a muscular, tube-shaped organ that serves as a passageway from the uterus to the outside of the body. This passage allows menstrual flow to exit from the uterus during a woman's monthly cycle, receives the penis during intercourse, and serves as the birth canal during childbirth. The **uterus (womb)** is a hollow, muscular, pear-shaped organ. Hormones acting on the inner lining of the uterus (the **endometrium**), either prepare the uterus for implantation and development of a fertilized egg or signal that no fertilization has taken place, in which case the endometrium deteriorates and becomes menstrual flow.

The lower end of the uterus, the **cervix,** extends downward into the vagina. The **ovaries,** almond-sized organs suspended on either side of the uterus, have two main functions: producing hormones (estrogen, progesterone, and small amounts of testosterone) and serving as the reservoir for immature eggs. All the eggs a woman will ever have are present in her ovaries at birth. Eggs mature and are released from the ovaries in response to hormone levels. Extending from the upper end of the uterus are two thin, flexible tubes called the **fallopian tubes** (also known as oviducts). The fallopian tubes, which do not actually touch the ovaries, capture eggs as they are released from the ovaries

during ovulation, and they are the site where sperm and egg meet and fertilization takes place. The fallopian tubes then serve as the passageway to the uterus, where the fertilized egg becomes implanted and development continues.

The Onset of Puberty and the Menstrual Cycle
With the onset of puberty, the female reproductive system matures, and the development of secondary sex characteristics transforms young girls into young women. The first sign of puberty is the beginning of breast development, which generally occurs around age 11. The pituitary gland, the **hypothalamus,** and the ovaries all secrete hormones that act as chemical messengers. Working in a feedback system, hormonal levels in the bloodstream act as the trigger mechanism for release of more or different hormones.

Around age 9½ to 11½, the hypothalamus receives the message to begin secreting *gonadotropin-releasing hormone* (*GnRH*). The release of GnRH in turn signals the pituitary gland to release hormones called *gonadotropins.* Two gonadotropins, *follicle-stimulating*

"Why Should I Care?"

It is more difficult to please a partner sexually or to describe to a partner how to please you if you don't understand basic sexual anatomy. For example, the clitoris in females is very responsive to touch and when stimulated often leads to orgasm. The urethral opening located nearby is not.

vagina Muscular, tube-shaped organ in females that serves as a passageway connecting the vulva to the uterus.

uterus (womb) Hollow, pear-shaped muscular organ whose function is to contain a developing fetus.

endometrium Soft, spongy matter that makes up the uterine lining.

cervix Lower end of the uterus that opens into the vagina.

ovaries Almond-sized organs that house developing eggs and produce hormones.

fallopian tubes Tubes that extend from near the ovaries to the uterus; site of fertilization and passageway for fertilized eggs.

hypothalamus Area of the brain located near the pituitary gland; works in conjunction with the pituitary gland to control reproductive functions.

estrogens Hormones secreted by the ovaries that control the menstrual cycle.

progesterone Hormone secreted by the ovaries; helps the endometrium develop and helps maintain pregnancy.

menarche The first menstrual period.

ovarian follicles Areas within the ovary in which individual eggs develop.

graafian follicle Mature ovarian follicle that contains a fully developed egg (ovum).

ovum Single mature egg cell.

ovulation The point of the menstrual cycle at which a mature egg ruptures through the ovarian wall.

corpus luteum Cells that form from the remains of the graafian follicle following ovulation; it secretes estrogen and progesterone during the second half of the menstrual cycle.

hormone (*FSH*) and *luteinizing hormone* (*LH*), signal the ovaries to start producing **estrogens** and **progesterone.** Estrogens regulate the menstrual cycle, and increased estrogen levels assist in the development of female secondary sex characteristics. Progesterone helps the endometrium develop in preparation for nourishing a fertilized egg and helps maintain pregnancy. The normal age range for the onset of the first menstrual period, or **menarche,** is 9 to 17 years, with the average age being 11½ to 13½ years. Body fat heavily influences the onset of puberty, and increasing rates of obesity in children may account for the fact that girls in the United States and other developed countries seem to be reaching puberty much earlier than they used to.[5] Very thin girls, such as young athletes, tend to start menstruating later.

The average menstrual cycle lasts 28 days and consists of three phases: the proliferative phase, the secretory phase, and the menstrual phase (**Figure 5.2**). The *proliferative phase* begins with the end of menstruation. During this time, the endometrium develops or "proliferates." How does this process work? By the end of menstruation, the hypothalamus senses very low levels of estrogen and progesterone in the blood. In response, it increases its secretions of GnRH, which in turn triggers the pituitary gland to release FSH. When FSH reaches the ovaries, it signals several **ovarian follicles** to begin maturing. Normally, only one of the follicles, the **graafian follicle,** reaches full maturity in the days preceding ovulation. While the follicles mature, they begin producing estrogen, which in turn signals the endometrial lining of the uterus to proliferate. If fertilization occurs, the endometrium will become a nesting place for the developing embryo. High estrogen levels signal the pituitary to slow down FSH production and increase release of LH. Under the influence of LH, the ovarian follicle ruptures and releases a mature **ovum** (plural: *ova*), a single mature egg cell, near a fallopian tube (around day 14). This is the process of **ovulation.** The other ripening follicles degenerate and are reabsorbed by the body. Occa-

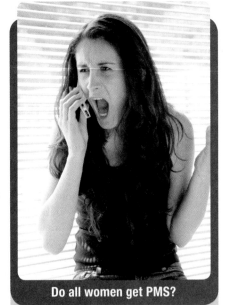

Do all women get PMS?

About 75 percent of menstruating women experience some PMS symptoms every month, but for most women these symptoms are mild and short-lived. Stress reduction, regular exercise, and a healthy diet are all good strategies for coping with PMS symptoms, which can include irritability and moodiness, fatigue, bloating, breast tenderness, and food cravings.

Surface of endometrium is sloughed off; bleeding occurs

Estrogens increase

Egg develops and endometrium proliferates

Menstrual phase

Proliferative phase

Ovulation occurs

Estrogens and progesterone decrease suddenly

Secretory phase

Endometrium thickens; secretion and blood supply increase; follicle manufactures progesterone

FIGURE 5.2 The Three Phases of the Menstrual Cycle

Source: Rathus et al., *Human Sexuality in a World of Diversity*, 6th Ed., © 2009. Figure "The Three Phases of the Menstrual Cycle," © 2005 Allyn & Bacon. Reproduced with permission of Pearson Education, Inc.

sionally, two ova mature and are released during ovulation. If both are fertilized, fraternal (nonidentical) twins develop. Identical twins develop when one fertilized ovum (called a *zygote*) divides into two separate zygotes.

The phase following ovulation is called the *secretory phase*. The ruptured graafian follicle, which has remained in the ovary, is transformed into the **corpus luteum** and begins secreting large amounts of estrogen and progesterone. These hormone secretions peak around day 20 or 21 of the average cycle and cause the endometrium to thicken. If fertilization and implantation take place, cells surrounding the developing embryo release a hormone called *human chorionic gonadotropin* (*HCG*), increasing estrogen and progesterone secretions that maintain the endometrium and signal the pituitary gland not to start a new menstrual cycle. If no implantation occurs, the hypothalamus responds by signaling the pituitary to stop producing FSH and LH, thus peaking the levels of progesterone in the blood. The corpus luteum begins to decompose, leading to rapid declines in estrogen and progesterone levels. These hormones are needed to sustain the lining of the uterus. Without them, the endometrium is sloughed off in the menstrual flow, and this begins the *menstrual phase*. The low estrogen levels of the menstrual phase signal the hypothalamus to release GnRH, which acts on

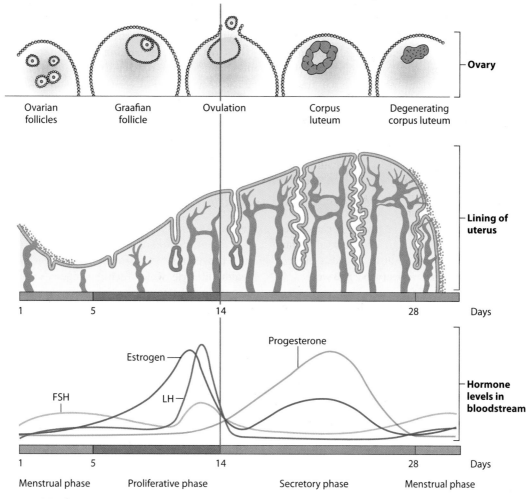

Ovary
Ovarian follicles — Graafian follicle — Ovulation — Corpus luteum — Degenerating corpus luteum

Lining of uterus

Days: 1 5 14 28

Estrogen — Progesterone — FSH — LH

Hormone levels in bloodstream

Days: 1 5 14 28

Menstrual phase — Proliferative phase — Secretory phase — Menstrual phase

FIGURE 5.3 **Hormonal Control and Phases of the Menstrual Cycle**

the pituitary to secrete FSH, and the cycle (shown in Figure 5.3) begins again.

Menstrual Problems **Premenstrual syndrome (PMS)** is a term used for a collection of physical, emotional, and behavioral symptoms that many women experience 7 to 14 days prior to their menstrual period. The most common symptoms are tender breasts, bloating, food cravings, fatigue, irritability, and depression. It is estimated that 75 percent of menstruating women experience some signs and symptoms of PMS each month.[6] For the majority of women, these disappear as their period begins, but for a small subset of women (3 to 5 percent), their symptoms are severe enough to affect their daily routines and activities to the point of being disabling. This severe form of PMS has its own psychiatric designation, **premenstrual dysphoric disorder (PMDD),** with symptoms that include severe depression, hopelessness, anger, anxiety, low self-esteem, difficulty concentrating, irritability, and tension.

There are several natural approaches to managing PMS that can also help PMDD. These strategies include eating more carbohydrates (whole grains, fruits, and vegetables), reducing caffeine and salt intake, exercising regularly, and taking measures to reduce stress.[7] Recent investigation into methods of controlling severe emotional swings has led to the use of antidepressants for treating PMDD, primarily selective serotonin reuptake inhibitors (SSRIs; e.g., Prozac, Paxil, and Zoloft).

Dysmenorrhea is a medical term for menstrual cramps, the pain or discomfort in the lower abdomen that many women experience just before or during menstruation. Along with cramps, some women experience nausea and vomiting, loose stools, sweating, and dizziness. Menstrual cramps can be classified as primary or secondary dysmenorrhea. Primary dysmenorrhea doesn't involve any physical abnormality and usually begins 6 months to a year after a woman's first period, while secondary dysmenorrhea has an underlying physical cause such as endometriosis or uterine fibroids.[8] If you experience primary dysmenorrhea, you can reduce your discomfort

premenstrual syndrome (PMS) Mood changes and physical symptoms that occur in some women 1 to 2 weeks prior to menstruation.

premenstrual dysphoric disorder (PMDD) Group of symptoms similar to but more severe than PMS, including severe mood disturbances.

dysmenorrhea Condition of pain or discomfort in the lower abdomen just before or during menstruation.

by using over-the-counter nonsteroidal anti-inflammatory drugs (NSAIDs) such as aspirin, ibuprofen (Advil or Motrin), or naproxen (Aleve). Other self-care strategies, such as soaking in a hot bath or using a heating pad on your abdomen, may also ease your cramps. For severe cramping, your health care provider may recommend a low-dose oral contraceptive to prevent ovulation, which in turn may reduce the production of prostaglandins and therefore the severity of your cramps. Managing secondary dysmenorrhea involves treating the underlying cause.

Toxic shock syndrome (*TSS*), although rare, is still something women should be aware of. It is caused by a bacterial infection facilitated by tampon or diaphragm use (see Chapters 6). Symptoms occur during one's period or a few days afterward and are sometimes hard to recognize because they mimic the flu. They include sudden high fever, vomiting, diarrhea, dizziness, fainting, or a rash that looks like sunburn. Proper treatment usually assures recovery in 2 to 3 weeks.

Menopause Just as menarche signals the beginning of a woman's potential reproductive years, **menopause**—the permanent cessation of menstruation—signals the end. *Perimenopause* refers to the 4 to 6 years preceding menopause when hormonal changes take place and menstrual cycles and flow can become irregular. Menopause generally occurs between the ages of 45 and 55, with the average being age 51 among U.S. women. Menopausal changes result in decreased estrogen levels, which may produce troublesome symptoms in some women. Decreased vaginal lubrication, hot flashes, night sweats, headaches, dizziness, and joint pain have been associated with the onset of menopause.

menopause Permanent cessation of menstruation, generally occurs between the ages of 45 and 55.

hormone replacement therapy (menopausal hormone therapy) Use of synthetic estrogens and progesterone to compensate for hormonal changes in a woman's body during menopause.

Synthetic forms of estrogen and progesterone have long been prescribed as **hormone replacement therapy** to relieve menopausal symptoms and reduce the risk of heart disease and osteoporosis. (The National Institutes of Health prefers the term **menopausal hormone therapy,** because hormone therapy is not a replacement and does not restore the physiology of youth.) However, recent studies, including results from the Women's Health Initiative (WHI), suggest that hormone therapy using synthetic hormones may actually do more harm than good. In fact, the WHI terminated this research ahead of schedule due to concerns about participants' increased risk of breast cancer, heart attack, stroke, blood clots, and other health problems.[9] All women need to discuss the risks and benefits of menopausal hormone therapy with their health care provider to make an informed decision. Adopting a healthy lifestyle, which includes regular exercise, a balanced diet, and adequate calcium intake, can also help protect postmenopausal women from heart disease and osteoporosis.

Male Sexual Anatomy and Physiology

The structures of the male reproductive system are divided into external and internal genitals (Figure 5.4). The external genitals are the penis and the scrotum. The internal male genitals include the testes, epididymides, vasa deferentia, ejaculatory ducts, urethra, and other structures—the seminal vesicles, the prostate gland, and the Cowper's glands—that secrete components that, with sperm, make up semen. These three structures are sometimes referred to as the *accessory glands*.

External Anatomy

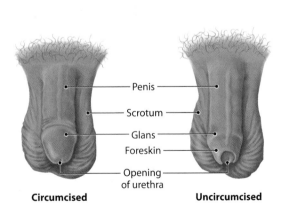

Circumcised   Uncircumcised

Internal Organs

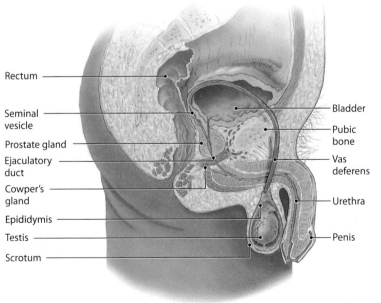

FIGURE 5.4 **Male Sexual Anatomy**

Circumcision:
RISK VERSUS BENEFIT

Circumcision, the surgical removal of the foreskin from the penis, can be a controversial issue for parents. They must balance personal, cultural, and health issues in deciding whether to circumcise a son.

Although circumcision rates are on the decline in the United States, 32 percent of all newborn boys are still circumcised each year. Here are some of the arguments against and for circumcision.

Arguments against Circumcision

○ It is a surgical procedure that may cause pain to the infant, and there are potential complications such as bleeding, infection, improper healing, or cutting the foreskin too long or too short.

○ Families may feel the foreskin is needed for identity reasons, sexual pleasure, or other reasons linked to religion or culture.

○ Much of the research on the relationship between circumcision and sexually transmitted infections was done in developing countries and may not be indicative of outcomes in developed nations.

○ Men lose a degree of sexual pleasure and stimulation when the foreskin is removed. Many unique nerve endings—found only in the foreskin—are lost forever.

Arguments for Circumcision

○ Circumcised males have a lower risk of penile cancer.

○ Circumcised males have a lower risk of urinary tract infections during their first year, easier genital hygiene, and a lower risk of foreskin infections.

○ Circumcision has been shown to have a protective effect against human immunodeficiency virus (HIV), herpes simplex virus 2 (HSV-2), and human papillomavirus (HPV) transmission in males.

○ Families may have religious or cultural reasons for wishing to circumcise their sons (in the Jewish faith, for example, circumcision is performed in a ceremony called a bris, and it represents the covenant God made with the patriarch Abraham).

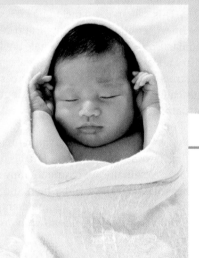

Where Do You Stand?

○ If you had a son, what decision would you make regarding circumcising him?

○ What factors—religious, cultural, aesthetic, or health-related—would have the most influence on your decision?

○ If you are male, does your circumcised or uncircumcised status affect your opinion?

Sources: R.C. Rabin, "Steep Drop Seen in Circumcisions in US," *The New York Times,* August 16, 2010, www.nytimes.com/2010/08/17/health/research/17circ .html?ref=health; A. A. R. Tobian, R. H. Gray, and T. C. Quinn, "Male Circumcision for the Prevention of Acquisition and Transmission of Sexually Transmitted Infections: The Case for Neonatal Circumcision," *Archives of Pediatrics & Adolescent Medicine* 164 (2010): 78–84; M. Moreno, "Advice for Patients: Male Circumcision," *Archives of Pediatrics & Adolescent Medicine* 164, no. 1 (2010): 104; Centers for Disease Control and Prevention, "Male Circumcision and Risk for HIV Transmission and Other Health Conditions: Implications for the United States, Centers for Disease Control and Prevention," Updated February 2008, www.cdc.gov/hiv/resources/factsheets/circumcision.htm; Mayo Clinic Staff, "Circumcision (Male): Why It's Done," February 2010, www.mayoclinic.com/health/circumcision/MY01023/DSECTION=why-its-done.

The **penis** is the organ that deposits sperm in the vagina during intercourse. The urethra, which passes through the center of the penis, acts as the passageway for both semen and urine to exit the body. During sexual arousal, the spongy tissue in the penis becomes filled with blood, making the organ stiff (erect). Further sexual excitement leads to **ejaculation,** a series of rapid, spasmodic contractions that propel semen out of the penis.

Debate continues over the practice of *circumcision,* the surgical removal of a fold of skin covering the end of the penis, known as the *foreskin.* Most circumcisions are performed for religious or cultural reasons or because of hygiene concerns. However, recent research supports the claim that circumcision yields medical benefits, including decreased risk of urinary tract infections in the first year, decreased risk of penile cancer (although cancer of the penis is very rare), and decreased risk of sexual transmission of human papillomavirus (HPV) and human immunodeficiency virus (HIV).[10] See the **Points of View** box on the previous page for a discussion of the controversy surrounding circumcision.

Situated behind the penis is a sac called the **scrotum.** The scrotum protects the testes and helps control their internal temperature, which is vital to proper sperm production. The **testes** (singular: *testis*) manufacture sperm and **testosterone,** the hormone responsible for the development of male secondary sex characteristics.

The development of sperm is referred to as **spermatogenesis.** Like the maturation of eggs in the female, this process is governed by the pituitary gland. Follicle-stimulating hormone (FSH) is secreted into the bloodstream to stimulate the testes to manufacture sperm. Immature sperm are released into a comma-shaped structure on the back of each testis called the **epididymis** (plural: *epididymides*), where they ripen and reach full maturity.

Each epididymis contains coiled tubules that gradually straighten out to become the **vas deferens** (plural: *vasa deferentia*). These make up the tubular transportation system whose sole function is to store and move sperm. Along the way, the **seminal vesicles** provide sperm with nutrients and other fluids that compose **semen.**

The vasa deferentia eventually connect each epididymis to the **ejaculatory ducts,** which pass through the prostate gland and empty into the urethra. The **prostate gland** contributes more fluids to the semen, including chemicals that help the sperm fertilize an ovum and neutralize the acidic environment of the vagina to make it more conducive to sperm motility (ability to move) and potency (potential for fertilization). Just below the prostate gland are two pea-shaped nodules called the **Cowper's glands.** The Cowper's glands secrete a preejaculate fluid that lubricates the urethra and neutralizes any acid that may remain in the urethra after urination. Urine and semen do not come into contact with each other. During ejaculation of semen, a small valve closes off the tube to the urinary bladder.

Andropause Testosterone levels in men vary greatly, and in general, older men have lower testosterone levels than do younger men. Men, however, do not experience a rapid hormone decline in middle age that affects their reproductive capacity as women do during menopause. Instead, men typically experience a gradual decline in testosterone levels throughout adulthood, about 1 percent a year on average after the age of 30.[11] Many doctors use the term *andropause* to describe age-related hormone changes in men. Some men with lower testosterone levels do not experience signs and symptoms. Those who do may experience the following:

- **Changes in sexual function.** These may include reduced sexual desire, fewer spontaneous erections—such as during sleep—and infertility. Testes may become smaller, as well.
- **Changes in sleep patterns.** Low testosterone may cause insomnia or other sleep disturbances.
- **Physical changes.** Various physical changes may occur, including increased body fat, reduced muscle bulk and strength, and decreased bone density. Abnormal enlargement of the male breasts (gynecomastia) and hair loss are possible.
- **Emotional changes.** Low testosterone levels may contribute to a decrease in motivation or self-confidence, cause sadness or depression, or interfere with concentration or memory.[12]

Treatment is available for age-related low testosterone levels, but it is not without controversy. For some men, testosterone therapy relieves the symptoms. For others, especially older men, the benefits aren't clear. And there are risks; testosterone therapy may increase the risk of prostate cancer or other health problems.

Human Sexual Response

Psychological traits greatly influence sexual response and sexual desire. Thus, you may find a sexual relationship with one partner vastly different from experiences with other partners. Sexual response is a physiological process that generally follows a pattern that can be roughly divided into four stages: excitement/arousal, plateau, orgasm, and resolution (Figure 5.5). Researchers agree that each individual has a personal response pattern that may or may not conform to these phases.

penis Male sexual organ that releases sperm into the vagina.

ejaculation Propulsion of semen from the penis.

scrotum External sac of tissue that encloses the testes.

testes Male sex organs that manufacture sperm and produce hormones.

testosterone Male sex hormone manufactured in the testes.

spermatogenesis The development of sperm.

epididymis Duct system atop the testis where sperm mature.

vas deferens Tube that transports sperm from the epididymis to the ejaculatory duct.

seminal vesicles Glandular ducts that secrete nutrients for the semen.

semen Fluid containing sperm and nutrients that increase sperm viability and neutralize vaginal acid.

ejaculatory duct Tube formed by the junction of the seminal vesicle and the vas deferens that carries semen to the urethra.

prostate gland Gland that secretes nutrients and neutralizing fluids into the semen.

Cowper's glands Glands that secrete a preejaculate fluid that lubricates the urethra and neutralizes any acid remaining in the urethra after urination.

Regardless of the type of sexual activity (stimulation by a partner or self-stimulation), the response stages are the same.

During the first stage, *excitement/arousal,* **vasocongestion** (increased blood flow that causes swelling in the genitals) stimulates male and female genital responses. The vagina begins to lubricate, and the penis becomes partially erect. Both sexes may exhibit a "sex flush" or light blush all over their bodies. Excitement/arousal can be generated through fantasy or by touching parts of the body, kissing, viewing erotic images, or reading erotic literature.

During the *plateau phase,* the initial responses intensify. Voluntary and involuntary muscle tensions increase. A woman's nipples become erect, as does a man's penis. The penis secretes a few drops of preejaculatory fluid, which may contain sperm.

During the *orgasmic phase,* vasocongestion and muscle tensions reach their peak, and rhythmic contractions occur through the genital regions. In women, these contractions are centered in the uterus, outer vagina, and anal sphincter. In men, the

vasocongestion Engorgement of the genital organs with blood.

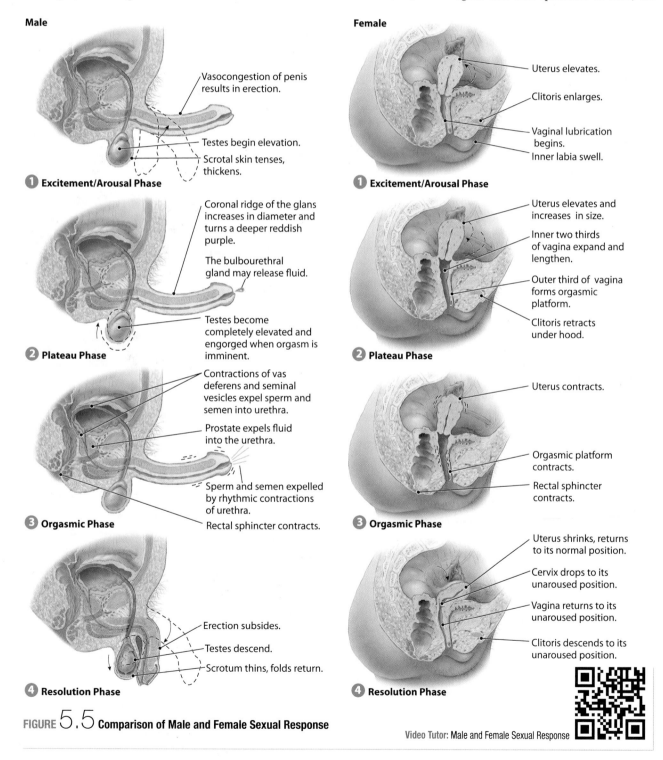

Male

Vasocongestion of penis results in erection.

1 Excitement/Arousal Phase
- Vasocongestion of penis results in erection.
- Testes begin elevation.
- Scrotal skin tenses, thickens.

2 Plateau Phase
- Coronal ridge of the glans increases in diameter and turns a deeper reddish purple.
- The bulbourethral gland may release fluid.
- Testes become completely elevated and engorged when orgasm is imminent.

3 Orgasmic Phase
- Contractions of vas deferens and seminal vesicles expel sperm and semen into urethra.
- Prostate expels fluid into the urethra.
- Sperm and semen expelled by rhythmic contractions of urethra.
- Rectal sphincter contracts.

4 Resolution Phase
- Erection subsides.
- Testes descend.
- Scrotum thins, folds return.

Female

1 Excitement/Arousal Phase
- Uterus elevates.
- Clitoris enlarges.
- Vaginal lubrication begins.
- Inner labia swell.

2 Plateau Phase
- Uterus elevates and increases in size.
- Inner two thirds of vagina expand and lengthen.
- Outer third of vagina forms orgasmic platform.
- Clitoris retracts under hood.

3 Orgasmic Phase
- Uterus contracts.
- Orgasmic platform contracts.
- Rectal sphincter contracts.

4 Resolution Phase
- Uterus shrinks, returns to its normal position.
- Cervix drops to its unaroused position.
- Vagina returns to its unaroused position.
- Clitoris descends to its unaroused position.

FIGURE 5.5 **Comparison of Male and Female Sexual Response**

Video Tutor: Male and Female Sexual Response

Why do we place so much importance on orgasm?
● Can sexual pleasure and satisfaction be achieved without orgasm?
● What is the role of desire in sexual response?

contractions occur in two stages. First, contractions within the prostate gland begin propelling semen through the urethra. In the second stage, the muscles of the pelvic floor, urethra, and anal sphincter contract. Semen usually, but not always, is ejaculated from the penis. In both sexes, spasms in other major muscle groups also occur, particularly in the buttocks and abdomen. Feet and hands may also contract, and facial features often contort.

Muscle tension and congested blood subside in the *resolution phase* as the genital organs return to their pre-arousal states. Both sexes usually experience deep feelings of well-being and profound relaxation. Many women can experience multiple orgasms during the orgasmic phase. Some men experience a refractory period, during which their systems are incapable of subsequent arousal. This refractory period may last from a few minutes to several hours and tends to lengthen with age.

Men and women experience the same stages in the sexual response cycle; however, the length of time spent in any one stage varies. Thus, one partner may be in the plateau phase while the other is in the excitement or orgasmic phase. Such variations in response rates are entirely normal. Some couples believe that simultaneous orgasm is desirable for sexual satisfaction. Although simultaneous orgasm is pleasant, so are orgasms achieved at different times.

Sexual pleasure and satisfaction are also possible without orgasm or even intercourse. Expressing sexual feelings for another person involves many pleasurable activities, of which intercourse and orgasm may be only a part.

Sexual Responses among Older Adults

Older adults are commonly stereotyped as being incapable of or uninterested in sexual relations. The truth is, though we do experience some physical changes as we age, they generally do not cause us to stop enjoying sex.

In women, the most significant physical changes follow menopause. Skin becomes less elastic; most internal sexual organs, including the uterus and cervix, shrink somewhat; the vaginal walls become thinner; and vaginal lubrication during sexual arousal may decrease. The resulting increased friction during penetration can be painful, and the use of artificial lubricants usually resolves this problem. Women who remain sexually active as they age report fewer problems with age-related changes in sexual functioning.

Although men do not experience menopause, their bodies also change as a result of the aging process. They require more direct and prolonged stimulation to achieve an erection, and erections become less firm. They are slower to reach orgasm, and their refractory periods are longer. Older men also experience a decrease in the intensity of ejaculation. Semen seeps out during ejaculation rather than being forcefully expelled as is typical in younger men.

The majority of healthy older men and women enjoy a regular and satisfying sex life. Among the advantages experienced by adults at this stage of life are a level of comfort with and appreciation of their body as well as no longer needing contraception (although protection from sexually transmitted infections (STIs) is still necessary if there are new or multiple partners).

Expressing Your Sexuality

Finding healthy ways to express your sexuality is an important part of sexual maturity. Many avenues of sexual expression are available.

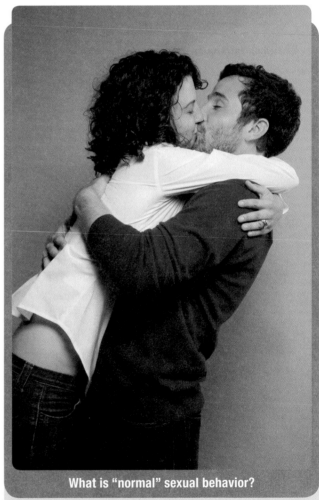

What is "normal" sexual behavior?

As with any other human behavior, the idea of "normal" sexual behavior varies from person to person and from society to society, usually along a spectrum of perceived acceptability or appropriateness. For example, in most modern cultures kissing is a common way to express affection; however, societies have different standards—and individuals have different comfort levels—for the circumstances in which a full-on smack on the lips is considered appropriate.

Sexual Behavior: What Is "Normal"?

How do we know which sexual behaviors are considered normal? What or whose criteria should we use? These are not easy questions.

Every society sets standards and attempts to regulate sexual behavior. Boundaries arise that distinguish good from bad, acceptable from unacceptable, and result in criteria used to establish what is viewed as normal or abnormal. Some of the common standards for sexual behavior in Western culture today include the following:[13]

- **The coital standard.** Penile–vaginal intercourse (coitus) is viewed as the ultimate sex act.
- **The orgasmic standard.** Sexual interaction should lead to orgasm.
- **The two-person standard.** Sex is an activity to be experienced by two people.
- **The romantic standard.** Sex should be related to love.
- **The safer-sex standard.** If we choose to be sexually active, we should act to prevent unintended pregnancy or disease transmission.

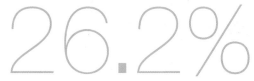

26.2%

of college students report having had more than one sex partner in the past 12 months.

These are not laws or rules, but rather are rather social scripts that have been adopted over time. Sexual standards often shift through the years, and many people choose not to follow them. Rather than making blanket judgments about normal versus abnormal, we might ask the following questions:[14]

- Is a sexual behavior healthy and fulfilling for a particular person?
- Is it safe?
- Does it involve the exploitation of others?
- Does it take place between responsible, consenting adults?

In this way, we can view behavior along a continuum that takes into account many individual factors. As you read about the options for sexual expression in the pages ahead, use these questions to explore your feelings about what is normal for you.

Options for Sexual Expression

The range of human sexual expression is virtually infinite. What you find enjoyable may not be an option for someone else (see the **Health in a Diverse World** box on page 150 for a discussion of sexuality and disability). The ways you choose to meet your sexual needs today may be very different from what they were 2 weeks ago or will be 2 years from now. Accepting yourself as a sexual person with individual desires and preferences is the first step in achieving sexual satisfaction. Are you curious about your peers' sexual behavior? Then check out the **Student Health Today** box on page 151 and the **Tech & Health** box on technology and dating on page 153.

celibacy State of not engaging in sexual activity.

autoerotic behaviors Sexual self-stimulation.

sexual fantasies Sexually arousing thoughts and dreams.

masturbation Self-stimulation of genitals.

erogenous zones Areas of the body that, when touched, lead to sexual arousal.

Celibacy **Celibacy** is abstention from sexual activities with others. Some people choose celibacy for religious or moral reasons. Others may be celibate for a period of time due to illness, the breakup of a long-term relationship, or lack of an acceptable partner. For some, celibacy is a lonely, agonizing state, but others find it an opportunity for introspection, values assessment, and personal growth.

Autoerotic Behaviors **Autoerotic behaviors** involve self-stimulation. The two most common are sexual fantasy and masturbation.

Sexual fantasies are sexually arousing thoughts and dreams. Fantasies may reflect real-life experiences, forbidden desires, or the opportunity to practice new or anticipated sexual experiences. The fact that you fantasize about a particular sexual experience does not necessarily mean that you want to, or have to, act out that experience. Sexual fantasies are just that—fantasy.

Masturbation is self-stimulation of the genitals. Although many people are uncomfortable discussing masturbation, it is a common sexual practice across the life span. Masturbation is a natural pleasure-seeking behavior in infants and children. It is a valuable and important means for adolescents, as well as adults, to explore sexual feelings and responsiveness. In one survey of college students, 48 percent of women and 92 percent of men reported that they have masturbated.[15]

Kissing and Erotic Touching Kissing and erotic touching are two very common forms of nonverbal sexual communication. Both men and women have **erogenous zones,** areas of the body that when touched lead to sexual arousal. Erogenous zones may include genital and nongenital areas, such as the earlobes, mouth, breasts, and inner thighs. Almost any area of the body can be conditioned to respond erotically to touch. Spending time with your partner to explore and learn about his or her erogenous areas is another pleasurable, safe, and satisfying means of sexual expression.

Manual Stimulation Both men and women can be sexually aroused and achieve orgasm through manual stimulation of the genitals by a partner. For many women, orgasm is more likely to be achieved through manual stimulation than through intercourse. *Sex toys* include a wide variety of

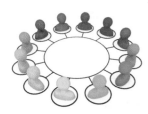

SEXUALITY AND DISABILITY

Many of us tend to think of disabled people as asexual. It may be difficult to understand what sex would be like as or with a disabled person, but disabled people are not asexual, and it is possible for a disabled person to have a sex life. A major challenge for those who are single is meeting others who are interested in a romantic or sexual relationship. There are many hurdles to overcome, including cultural standards of beauty and perfection and our preconceptions about what disabled people can and can't do sexually.

Disabled people may be born with a disability or may have become disabled as a child or later in life. These distinctions are significant; for people who became disabled after they became sexually active, there may be the expectation of performing sexually the way they used to. Coming to terms with a change in sexual performance due to disability can be a difficult process.

The challenges a disabled person faces with respect to having a satisfying sexual relationship include both physical and psychological difficulties. Being disabled means that a person has certain limitations in physical function. That can mean many things, and the disability may or may not directly affect sexual function. For example, someone who is deaf is legally disabled, but sexually functional. A person who is paralyzed from the neck down may still be able to have an orgasm, in spite of being unable to move.

Some people have disabilities that have minimal impact on their ability to pursue social connections. A person who has lost a limb, for example, is often still able to take part in social—and perhaps athletic—activities to the same extent as most able-bodied people. Other disabilities can even foster certain social connections—for example, many deaf individuals consider themselves part of

Whether able-bodied or disabled, we are all sexual beings deserving of intimacy and fulfilling sexual relationships.

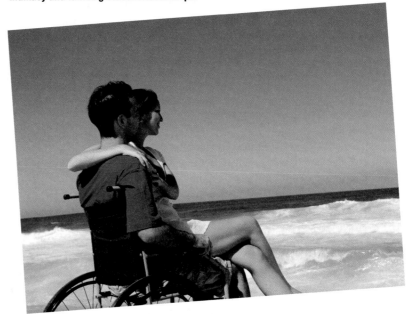

a vibrant culture that provides rich social interaction and support.

On the other hand, some disabilities can be very socially isolating. For example, a single person who is paralyzed has obstacles to overcome in finding a romantic or sexual partner. Help may be needed for travel, and the number of people the person meets will be limited by how often he or she can get out socially. Help may be needed with various tasks of daily life. He or she may not be able to move to touch and arouse a partner. The psychological challenges for disabled people in finding a romantic or sexual partner can also be significant and may include overcoming anger, dealing with the feeling that their sexual drives are not legitimate, and overcoming feelings that they don't measure up in the estimation of other people.

For anyone with a disability, counseling or therapy to deal with sexuality issues can help. Cognitive therapy and

sex therapy—the treatment of sexual dysfunction, lack of sexual confidence, and other sexual problems—may help, or the person may want to see a certified sex surrogate. Surrogates offer therapeutic exercises to help the patient. These may include relaxation techniques, intimate communication, social skills, and sexual touching. One or a combination of these methods may help disabled people who want to explore the sexual side of their life. Resources such as the National Sexuality Resource Center (http://nsrc.sfsu.edu/issues/sex-and-disability) can help those who want more information about sexuality and disability.

Each disabled person is unique, and it's important to consider his or her specific challenges, problems, and feelings involved in addressing his or her sexuality.

Sources: www.christopherreeve.org/site/ c.mtKZKgMWKwG/b.4453431/k.A0C5/ Sexuality_for_Men.htm

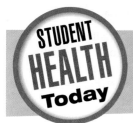

SEX ON CAMPUS

College students often think that everyone is having more sex than they are and with numerous partners. These perceptions may cause self-consciousness about a lack of sexual activity or encourage increased promiscuity in order to "measure up." In reality, students' opinions and attitudes about sex, relationships, and contraception vary greatly. Results from a recent national survey of college students might surprise you:

* Approximately 74 percent of college students reported having had 0 to 1 sexual partners within the past school year.
* Forty-five percent reported having had oral sex one or more times in the past 30 days.
* Almost 50 percent reported having had vaginal intercourse one or more times in the past 30 days.

Are you the only one on your campus not living the life of the typical reality TV hottie? Probably not. You may think everyone else is having more sex with more partners than you are, but generally speaking, the actual numbers don't measure up to college students' perceptions.

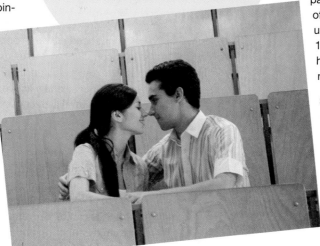

* Five percent reported having anal intercourse one or more times in the past 30 days.
* Of college females who had vaginal intercourse within the past school year, 1.7 percent of reported experiencing an unintentional pregnancy, and 1.9 percent of males reported having gotten someone pregnant unintentionally.

Source: American College Health Association, *American College Health Association—National College Health Assessment II (ACHA-NCHA II) Reference Group Data Report Spring 2011* (Baltimore: American College Health Association, 2012).

---

objects that can be used for sexual stimulation alone or with a partner. Vibrators and dildos are two common types of toys and can be found in a variety of shapes, styles, and sizes. Sex toys can be used both to enhance the sexual experience and also as therapeutic devices to help with issues such as orgasmic difficulty and erectile dysfunction. For women who may not reach orgasm through intercourse, they can provide another option for sexual satisfaction. (Note that toys must be cleaned after each use.)

Working for You?

Maybe you already make healthful, responsible, and satisfying decisions about your sex life. Which of these behaviors are you already practicing?

☐ I've chosen to be celibate—with so many other obligations and pressures in my life, this choice makes sense to me right now.

☐ I'm in a monogamous sexual relationship. We're not ready to start a family, so we're using birth control.

☐ My partner doesn't want to have sex—he says he's not ready. We still manage to show each other our love by kissing and touching.

College Health Assessment (NCHA), 44.9 percent of college students reported having oral sex in the past month.[16] For some people, oral sex is not an option because of moral or religious beliefs. Remember, HIV and other STIs can be transmitted via unprotected oral–genital sex just as they can through intercourse. Use of an appropriate barrier device is strongly recommended if either partner's health status is in question.

cunnilingus Oral stimulation of a woman's genitals.

fellatio Oral stimulation of a man's genitals.

vaginal intercourse Insertion of the penis into the vagina.

Vaginal Intercourse The term *intercourse* generally refers to **vaginal intercourse** (*coitus,* or insertion of the penis into the vagina), which is the most frequently practiced form of sexual expression. In the latest NCHA survey, more than 49.7 percent of college students reported having vaginal intercourse in the past month.[17] Coitus can involve a variety of positions, including the missionary position (man on top facing the woman), woman on top, side by side, or man behind (rear entry). Many partners enjoy experimenting with different positions. Knowledge of yourself and your body, along with your ability to communicate effectively, will play a large part in determining the enjoyment and meaning of intercourse for you and your partner. Whatever your circumstances, you should practice safer sex to avoid disease and unintended pregnancy.

Oral–Genital Stimulation **Cunnilingus** refers to oral stimulation of a woman's genitals and **fellatio** to oral stimulation of a man's genitals. Many partners find oral stimulation intensely pleasurable. In the most recent National

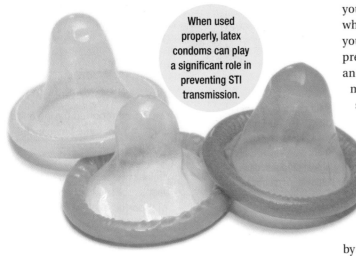

When used properly, latex condoms can play a significant role in preventing STI transmission.

Anal Intercourse The anal area is highly sensitive to touch, and some couples find pleasure in stimulation of this area. **Anal intercourse** is insertion of the penis into the anus. Research indicates that 5 percent of college-aged men and women have had anal sex in the past month.[18] Stimulation of the anus by mouth, fingers, or sex toys is also practiced. As with all forms of sexual expression, anal stimulation or intercourse is not for everyone. If you do enjoy this form of sexual expression, remember to use condoms and/or dental dams to avoid transmitting disease. Also, anything inserted into the anus should not then be directly inserted into the vagina, because bacteria commonly found in the anus can cause vaginal infections.

56.8%

of college students report using a contraceptive the last time they had vaginal intercourse.

Responsible and Satisfying Sexual Behavior

Healthy sexuality doesn't happen by chance. It is a product of assimilating information and building skills, of exploring values and beliefs, and of making responsible and informed choices. Healthy and responsible sexuality includes the following:

- **Good communication as the foundation.** Open and honest communication with your partner is the basis for establishing respect, trust, and intimacy. Do you communicate with your partner in caring and respectful ways? Can you share your thoughts and emotions freely with your partner? Do you talk about being sexually active and what that means? Can you share your sexual history with your partner? Do you discuss contraception and disease prevention? Are you able to communicate what you like and don't like? These are all components of the open communication that is necessary for healthy, responsible sexuality.

  - **Acknowledging that you are a sexual person.** People who can see and accept themselves as sexual beings are more likely to make informed decisions and take responsible actions. If you see yourself as a potentially sexual person, you will plan ahead for contraception and disease prevention. If you are comfortable being a sexually active person, you will not need or want your sexual experiences to be clouded by alcohol or other drug use. If you choose not to be sexually active, you do so consciously, as a personal decision. Even if you are not sexually active, it is important to acknowledge that sex is a natural aspect of everyone's life and to recognize that you are in charge of your own decisions about your sexuality.

- **Understanding sexual structures and their functions.** If you understand how your body works, sexual pleasure and response will not be mysterious events. You will be able to pleasure yourself and communicate to your partner how best to pleasure you. You will understand how pregnancy and STIs can be prevented. You will be able to recognize sexual dysfunction and take responsible actions to address the problem.

- **Accepting and embracing your gender identity and your sexual orientation.** "Being comfortable in your own skin" is an old saying that is particularly relevant when it comes to sexuality. It is difficult to feel sexually satisfied if you are conflicted about your gender identity or sexual orientation. You should explore and address questions and feelings you may have about either your gender identity or your sexual orientation. Good communication skills, acknowledging that you are a sexual person, and understanding your sexual structures and their functions will allow you to complete this task.

See the **Skills for Behavior Change** box on page 154 for tips on taking steps toward healthy sexuality.

Variant Sexual Behavior

Although attitudes toward sexuality have changed substantially, some behaviors are still considered to be outside the norm. People who study sexuality prefer to use the neutral term **variant sexual behavior** to describe less common sexual behaviors, for example:

- **Group sex.** Sexual activity involving more than two people. Participants in group sex run a higher risk of exposure to HIV and other STIs than that associated with a sexual encounter with only one partner.
- **Swinging.** Also known as partner-swapping.

anal intercourse Insertion of the penis into the anus.

variant sexual behavior A sexual behavior that is not commonly practiced.

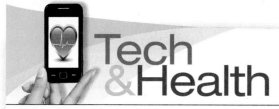

Tech & Health

THE PLEASURES AND PERILS OF TECHNOLOGY AND DATING

More than ever before, people can instantaneously connect with potential love interests, flirt with partners, or stay in touch with that special someone, all with the click of a send button. But along with that instant gratification comes several dangers. Top among them are meeting unscrupulous strangers through online dating sites and sending a suggestive message, photo, or video that makes its way into the hands of people it wasn't intended for.

Internet Dating Safety

In April 2011, a Los Angeles entertainment executive filed a lawsuit against Match.com after being sexually assaulted by a man she met on the site. In a statement released by her attorney, she said "This horrific ordeal completely blindsided me because I had considered myself savvy about online dating safety. Things quickly turned into a nightmare, beyond my control." After the assault, the woman performed an Internet search that revealed that her date had been convicted of several counts of sexual battery in the past. Her lawsuit is not seeking monetary damages, but rather is asking that no new members be allowed to join Match.com until the site enacts a policy of screening members' names against public sex offender registries.

This case highlights the fact that the people you meet on dating sites could be potentially dangerous and you should treat them as complete strangers, even after chatting for hours online. Internet dating sites don't perform screening checks of their users, and you have no real means of knowing the person is who he or she claims to be. Just as you would do with any stranger you meet at a café or bar, use common sense and always meet up in a public place when getting to know someone. (For a review of social networking safety tips, see the **Student Health Today** box on page 151.)

Sexting

Most people realize that "sexting," or sending sexual texts, photos, or videos on your cell phone, has the potential for loss of privacy and embarrassment. However, some still do it. Why? According to some students, sexting is a way for couples to express their feelings even if they are apart; for others, sexting is considered a "safe" way to be sexual, where you don't run the risk of unintended pregnancy or infection with a sexually transmitted disease. In one survey, 4 percent of cell phone–owning 12- to 17-year-olds have texted nude or nearly nude photos of themselves to someone else, and 15 percent of phone-owning 12- to 17-year-olds have received sexually suggestive images as texts. It is not uncommon for such explicit images to get passed from one person to another, beyond the intended recipient. When that happens, the person who sent the text is open to a variety of consequences, including getting dropped by friends, being bullied, receiving unwanted sexual come-ons, or even facing violence. The effects can lead to emotional and social isolation or other problems, or even have negative impacts on one's self-esteem and self-concept. While it's easy to send a "sext" without thinking too much about it, it's also easy for the recipient to pass it on. So before you pick up that phone, think carefully about what could happen if your explicit text gets around.

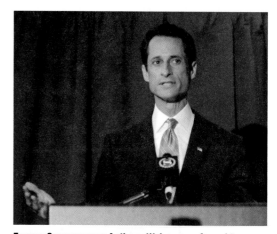

Former Congressman Anthony Weiner was forced to resign after he posted lewd photos of himself on Twitter and admitted to sexting with several women.

Sources: A. Zavis, "Woman Sues Online Dating Site over Alleged Sexual Assault," *Los Angeles Times: L.A. Now*, April 13, 2011; "What They're Saying about Sexting," *New York Times*, March 26, 2011; A. Lenhart, "Teens and Sexting," Pew Internet & American Life Project, Pew Research Center, December 15, 2009; SafetyWeb.com, "Sexting 101—Guide for Parents," February 14, 2010.

Taking Steps toward Healthy Sexuality

Healthy and responsible sexuality means having information and skills, exploring values and beliefs, and making responsible and informed choices. The following tips can help:

❭ Give some thought to your own sexuality. Do you choose to be sexually active now, or are you more comfortable waiting?

❭ Get to know your body and how you respond sexually to make communicating easier and sex better.

❭ If you have a partner now, sit down and talk about your sexual relationship. Are you both comfortable and satisfied with all aspects of the relationship? Discuss what you like and don't like.

❭ Explore and address any questions and feelings you may have about your gender identity or your sexual orientation.

● **Fetishism.** Using inanimate objects to heighten sexual arousal. Objects of fetishes often enhance one of the senses, such as silky clothing or lingerie, food with pleasant smells, or fancy shoes.

Some variant sexual behaviors can be harmful to the individual, to others, or to both. Some of the following activities are illegal in certain states:

● **Exhibitionism.** Exposing one's genitals to strangers in public places. Most exhibitionists are seeking a reaction of shock or fear. Exhibitionism is a minor felony in most states.

● **Voyeurism.** Observing other people for sexual gratification. Most voyeurs are men who attempt to watch women undressing or bathing. Voyeurism is an invasion of privacy and is illegal in most states.

● **Sadomasochism.** Sexual activities in which gratification is received by inflicting pain (verbal or physical abuse) on a partner or by being the object of such infliction. A sadist is a person who enjoys inflicting pain, and a masochist enjoys experiencing pain. These activities are legal when they involve consenting partners.

● **Pedophilia.** Sexual activity or attraction between an adult and a child. Any sexual activity involving a minor, including possession of child pornography, is illegal.

● **Autoerotic asphyxiation.** The practice of reducing or eliminating oxygen to the brain, usually by tying a cord around one's neck while masturbating to orgasm. Tragically, some individuals accidentally strangle themselves.

---

sexual dysfunction Problems associated with achieving sexual satisfaction.

sexual performance anxiety Sexual difficulties caused by anticipating some sort of problem with the sex act.

libido Sexual drive or desire.

inhibited sexual desire Lack of sexual appetite or lack of interest and pleasure in sexual activity.

TABLE
5.1
Types of Sexual Dysfunction

	Description
Desire Disorders	
Inhibited sexual desire	When a person is not interested in sexual activity
Sexual aversion disorder	When a person experiences phobias (fears) or anxiety about sexual contact
Arousal Disorders	
Erectile dysfunction	When a man cannot achieve or maintain an erection
Female sexual arousal disorder	When a woman cannot stay sexually aroused
Orgasmic Disorders	
Premature ejaculation	When a man reaches orgasm rapidly or prematurely
Delayed ejaculation	When a man has difficulty reaching orgasm despite normal desire and stimulation
Female orgasmic disorder	When a woman can't have an orgasm or has difficulty or delay in reaching orgasm
Pain Disorders	
Dyspareunia	When there is pain during or after sex
Vaginismus	When the vaginal muscles contract so forcefully that penetration cannot occur

Sexual Dysfunction

Research indicates that **sexual dysfunction,** the term used to describe problems that can hinder sexual functioning, is quite common. Sexual dysfunction can be divided into four categories: desire disorders, arousal disorders, orgasmic disorders, and pain disorders. (See Table 5.1.) All can be treated successfully.

Both men and women can experience **sexual performance anxiety** when they anticipate some sort of problem in the sex act. A man may become anxious and unable to maintain an erection (an arousal disorder), or he may experience premature ejaculation (an orgasmic disorder). A woman may be unable to achieve orgasm or to allow penetration because of the involuntary contraction of vaginal muscles. Both can overcome performance anxiety by learning to focus on immediate sensations and pleasures rather than on orgasm.

Sexual Desire Disorders

Libido is a person's sexual drive or desire. The most frequent reason people seek out a sex therapist is **inhibited sexual desire.**[19]

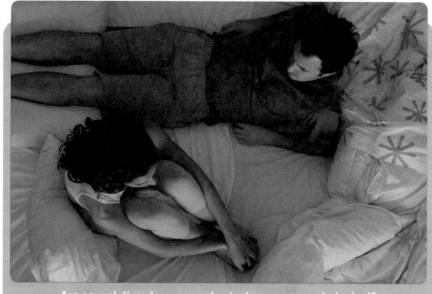

Are sexual disorders more physical or more psychological?

Sexual disorders can have both physical and psychological roots and can occur as a result of stress, fatigue, depression, or anxiety. They frequently have a physiological origin, such as overall poor health, chronic disease, or the use of alcohol or drugs. Arousal disorders and pain disorders are often strongly related to physical conditions and risk factors, but they may be exacerbated by stress and mental health problems. Interpersonal problems, including lack of trust and communication between partners, also contribute significantly to the development of sexual dysfunctions.

diabetes. These, in turn, affect blood flow. The most common sexual arousal disorder is **erectile dysfunction (ED)**—difficulty in achieving or maintaining an erection sufficient for intercourse. At some time in his life, every man experiences erectile dysfunction. Risk factors that can contribute to ED include certain medical conditions, treatments, and medications; using tobacco; being overweight; injuries; psychological conditions; drug and alcohol use; and prolonged bicycling.[21] Some 30 million men in the United States, half of them under age 65, suffer from ED. The condition generally becomes more of a problem as men age, affecting 1 in 4 men over the age of 65.[22] The first line of treatment for arousal disorders is lifestyle change. The FDA has approved several drugs, such as Viagra (sildenafil citrate), Levitra (vardenafil hydrochloride), and Cialis (tadalafil) to treat ED. These drugs work by relaxing the smooth muscle cells in the penis, allowing for increased blood flow to the erectile tissues. The best prevention for ED is to maintain overall physical and mental health.

Inhibited sexual desire is a lack of interest and pleasure in sexual activity. A low sex drive (decreased libido) may be caused by hormonal imbalances in women or by low testosterone in both men and women. Fatigue, stress, and common conditions such as depression and anxiety can cause decreased libido. Antidepressant medications (e.g., Prozac, Zoloft, Paxil) are well known for reducing sexual desire in both men and women.[20] **Sexual aversion disorder** is another type of desire dysfunction, characterized by sexual phobias (unreasonable fears) and anxiety about sexual contact. The psychological stress related to a punitive upbringing, a rigid religious background, or a history of physical or sexual abuse may be sources of desire disorders.

Sexual Arousal Disorders

The majority of arousal disorders are caused by lifestyle issues that increase the risk of high cholesterol, hypertension, and chronic diseases such as cardiovascular disease and

50%
of the 30 million American men with erectile dysfunction are under age 65.

Orgasmic Disorders

Premature ejaculation (also known as *early ejaculation*)—ejaculation that occurs prior to or very soon after the insertion of the penis into the vagina—affects up to 50 percent of men at some time in their lives. Treatment first involves a physical examination to rule out organic causes. If the cause is not physiological, therapy is available to help a man learn how to control the timing of his ejaculation. **Delayed ejaculation** is persistent difficulty in reaching orgasm despite normal desire and stimulation. Fatigue, stress, performance pressure, and alcohol use can all contribute to orgasmic disorders in men.

In a woman, the inability to achieve orgasm is called **female orgasmic disorder.** A woman with this disorder often learns to fake orgasm to avoid embarrassment or to preserve her partner's ego. Contributing factors include a conservative upbringing, performance anxiety, lack of trust, relationship issues, and difficulty seeing oneself as a sexual being. Again, the first step in treatment is a physical exam

sexual aversion disorder Desire dysfunction characterized by sexual phobias and anxiety about sexual contact.

erectile dysfunction (ED) Difficulty in achieving or maintaining an erection sufficient for intercourse.

premature ejaculation Ejaculation that occurs prior to or almost immediately following penile penetration of the vagina; also known as *early ejaculation.*

delayed ejaculation Persistent difficulty in reaching orgasm despite normal desire and stimulation.

female orgasmic disorder A woman's inability to achieve orgasm.

dyspareunia Pain experienced by women during intercourse.

vaginismus State in which the vaginal muscles contract so forcefully that penetration cannot occur.

to rule out organic causes. Often the problem is solved by simple self-exploration to learn more about what forms of stimulation are arousing enough to produce orgasm. Through masturbation, a woman can learn how her body responds to various types of touch. Once she has become orgasmic through masturbation, she can then learn to communicate her needs to her partner.

Sexual Pain Disorders

Two common disorders in this category are dyspareunia and vaginismus. **Dyspareunia** is pain experienced by a woman during intercourse that may be caused by conditions such as endometriosis, uterine tumors, chlamydia, gonorrhea, or urinary tract infections. Childbirth trauma and insufficient lubrication during intercourse may also cause discomfort. Dyspareunia can also be psychological in origin. **Vaginismus** is the involuntary contraction of vaginal muscles, making penile insertion painful or impossible. Most cases of vaginismus are related to fear of intercourse or unresolved sexual conflicts. As with other sexual problems, these disorders can be treated, with good results.

Seeking Help for Sexual Dysfunction

Sexual dysfunctions are most common in the early adult years, with the majority of people seeking care for these conditions during their late twenties and into their thirties. The incidence of dysfunction increases again during the perimenopause and postmenopause years in women and in older age for both men and women.[23] Many treatment models can help people with sexual dysfunction. It is important not to be afraid to talk to a sex educator, counselor, or medical professional. If you are looking for a qualified sex educator, therapist, or counselor, the American Association of Sex Educators, Counselors, and Therapists (AASECT) can help. AASECT has been in the forefront of establishing criteria for certifying sex therapists. Lists of certified professionals and clinics can be obtained by visiting the AASECT website: www.aasect.org.

what do you think?

Why do we find it so difficult to discuss sexual dysfunction?

● Do you think it is more difficult for men than for women? Or vice versa?

Drugs and Sex

Because psychoactive drugs affect the body's overall physiological functioning, it is only logical that they affect sexual behavior. Promises of increased pleasure make drugs very tempting to people seeking greater sexual satisfaction. But if drugs are necessary to increase sexual feelings, it is likely that

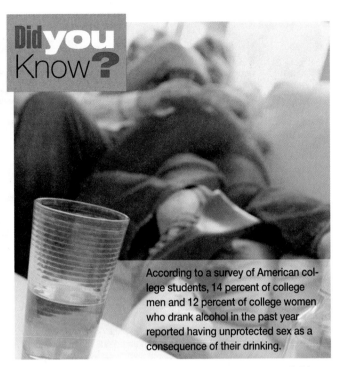

Did you Know?

According to a survey of American college students, 14 percent of college men and 12 percent of college women who drank alcohol in the past year reported having unprotected sex as a consequence of their drinking.

Source: Data from American College Health Association, *American College Health Association—National College Health Assessment II (ACHA-NCHA II) Reference Group Data Report Spring 2011* (Baltimore: American College Health Association, 2012).

partners are being dishonest about their feelings for each other. Good sex should not depend on chemical substances. Alcohol is notorious for reducing inhibitions and promoting feelings of well-being and desirability. At the same time, alcohol inhibits sexual response; thus, the mind may be willing, but not the body. When drugs become central to sexual activities, they inevitably damage the relationship. Perhaps the most common danger associated with the use of drugs during sex is the tendency to blame alcohol or drugs for negative behavior or unsafe or undesired sexual activity.

An increasing number of young men have begun experimenting with the recreational use of drugs intended to treat erectile dysfunction. These drugs work by relaxing the smooth muscle cells in the penis, allowing for increased blood flow to erectile tissues. Young men who take this type of medication are hoping to increase their sexual stamina or counteract performance anxiety or the effects of alcohol or other drugs. However, these drugs probably have only a placebo effect in men with normal erections, and combining them with other drugs, such as ketamine, amyl nitrate, or methamphetamine can lead to potentially fatal drug interactions. In particular, when combined with amyl nitrate, these drugs can lead to a sudden drop in blood pressure and possible cardiac arrest.[24]

"Date rape" drugs have been a growing concern in recent decades. (See more on them discussed in detail in chapters text covering drugs and violence—**Chapters 13** and **19,** respectively.) They have become prevalent on college campuses, where they are often used in combination with alcohol. These drugs are often introduced to unsuspecting women through alcoholic drinks to render them unconscious and vulnerable to rape. This problem is so serious that the U.S. Congress passed the Drug-Induced Rape Prevention and Punishment Act of 1996 to increase federal penalties for using drugs to facilitate sexual assault.

The Sex Industry

Throughout history, sex has been a prominent theme in art, literature, and the media. But when do depictions of the human body and human sexual behaviors cross the line from art to pornography, from story to exploitation, from

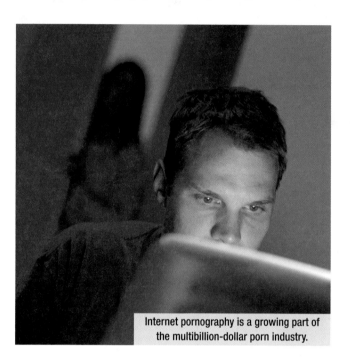

Internet pornography is a growing part of the multibillion-dollar porn industry.

sales tool to public perversion? These are difficult distinctions to make. Two particularly controversial aspects of the sex industry are pornography and prostitution.

pornography Visual or literary depictions of sexual activity intended to be sexually arousing.

prostitution Practice of engaging in sexual acts for money.

Pornography refers to any visual or literary depictions of sexual activity intended to be sexually arousing. An Internet tracking firm recently reported that pornographic websites make up 12 percent (4.2 million) of total websites and that over 40 percent of Internet users in the United States visit adult sites each month.[25] The pornography industry—which includes the Internet, video sales and rentals, cable, pay-per-view, phone sex, exotic dance clubs, computer games, and magazines—generates revenues of $13.33 billion annually in the United States, $2.8 billion of which is from online sources.[26] Clearly, pornography is a booming industry supported by millions of consumers. Why, then, is it so controversial? The fear many people have is that viewing pornographic materials leads to negative attitudes toward women, sexual aggression, and sexual violence. Current evidence suggests that pornography does not lead to sexual violence or predatory behavior in normal, healthy adults, but in those individuals who have preexisting negative attitudes toward women, this may be a legitimate concern.[27]

Prostitution, the practice of engaging in sexual acts for money, is a widespread industry around the world. Estimating the revenue generated by the U.S. prostitution industry is difficult, as most activity is illegal. Several countries have legalized prostitution, but in the United States it is legal only in selected counties in the state of Nevada. Illegal sex workers often struggle with substance abuse, sexual violence, and STIs. Countries that have legalized prostitution have made progress in regulating the industry and reducing these risks.

What Are Your Sexual Attitudes?

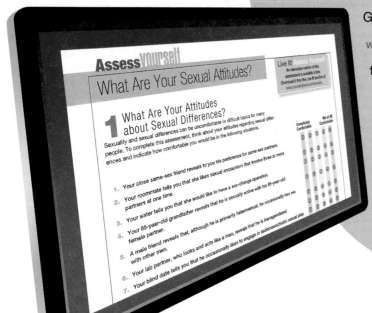

Go online to the **Live It!** section of

www.pearsonhighered.com/donatelle to take

the "What Are Your Sexual Attitudes?"

assessment.* If you want to change any of

your attitudes or opinions, you can use the

plan outlined in the

YOUR PLAN FOR CHANGE box.

*If your instructor so chooses, Assess Yourself Activities are available as a printed supplement or as assignable homework online at www.pearsonhighered.com/myhealthlab.

MyHealthLab®

YOUR PLAN FOR CHANGE

If you were surprised or unhappy with any of your responses to the **Assess yourself** activity, consider ways to change the attitudes you want to work on.

Today, you can:

○ Develop a plan. Review your responses to the questionnaire and think about attitudes you would like to change. Evaluate your behavior and identify patterns and specific things you are doing. What can you change now? What can you change in the near future?

○ Start a journal in which you explore your feelings and beliefs about sexuality. This could simply be a place for you to jot down questions or thoughts as they arise or to set long-term goals and examine your values and behaviors.

Within the next 2 weeks, you can:

○ Establish a time to sit down with the person with whom you are having a sexual relationship and have an honest and open discussion about sex. Before the discussion, think about what you would like to talk about and how you will bring it up. Are there sexual issues between you that need to be addressed? Are both you and your partner satisfied with the nature of your sexual relationship?

○ Take steps to be more responsible about your sexuality. If you have had unprotected sex, make an appointment to be tested for STIs. If you have found yourself without contraception, stop by a drugstore and purchase several packages of condoms. If you feel your sexual decision making is sometimes impaired by drugs or alcohol, set goals to limit and control your use of these substances.

By the end of the semester, you can:

○ Develop a greater understanding of and tolerance for people with different sexual values and lifestyles. Learn about different viewpoints by doing research, attending meetings on campus, or getting to know sexually diverse people.

○ Expand your sense of gender identity. Consider taking a class or workshop in an activity or subject area that you traditionally associate with the opposite gender. Volunteer with a group that focuses on issues relating to the opposite gender.

Summary

* The major structures of female sexual anatomy include the mons pubis, labia minora and majora, clitoris, vagina, uterus, cervix, fallopian tubes, and ovaries. The major structures of male sexual anatomy are the penis, scrotum, testes, epididymides, vasa deferentia, ejaculatory ducts, urethra, and the accessory glands (seminal vesicles, prostate gland, and Cowper's glands).

* Physiologically, both males and females experience four stages of sexual response: excitement/arousal, plateau, orgasm, and resolution.

* *Sexual identity* is determined by the interaction of genetic, physiological, and environmental factors. Biological sex, gender identity, gender roles, and sexual orientation are all blended into our sexual identity.

* *Sexual orientation* refers to a person's enduring emotional, romantic, or sexual attraction to others. Gay, lesbian, and bisexual persons are repeatedly the targets of sexual prejudice. *Sexual prejudice* refers to negative attitudes and hostile actions directed at members of a particular social group.

* People can express themselves sexually in a variety of ways, including celibacy, autoerotic behaviors, kissing and erotic touch, manual stimulation, oral–genital stimulation, vaginal intercourse, and anal intercourse. Variant sexual behaviors are those that are less common. Some variant sexual behaviors are potentially harmful to others and are therefore illegal in some states.

* Sexual dysfunctions can be categorized into four classes: desire disorders, arousal disorders, orgasmic disorders, and pain disorders. Stress, relationship issues, lack of exercise, smoking, alcohol and drug use, and other lifestyle choices can lead to sexual dysfunction.

* Sex is a multibillion-dollar industry in the United States and throughout the world. Pornography and prostitution are two aspects of the sex industry that have varying degrees of legality in different countries. Prostitution is legal in selected counties in Nevada.

* Responsible and satisfying sexuality involves good communication, acknowledging yourself as a sexual being, understanding sexual structures and functions, and accepting your gender identity and sexual orientation.

Pop Quiz

1. Your personal inner sense of maleness or femaleness is known as your
   a. sexual identity.
   b. sexual orientation.
   c. gender identity.
   d. gender.

2. Intimacy is which type of romantic feeling?
   a. Romantic love
   b. Sensual feelings
   c. Empty commitment love
   d. Mutual feelings of emotional closeness

3. The most sensitive part of the female genital region is the
   a. mons pubis.
   b. vagina.
   c. clitoris.
   d. labia.

4. When a woman is ovulating,
   a. she has released an egg.
   b. she is experiencing menstrual bleeding.
   c. an egg has been fertilized and she is pregnant.
   d. None of the above

5. Which of the following is *not* true about a woman's menstrual cycle?
   a. All women will experience premenstrual syndrome (PMS).
   b. Estrogen levels drop during ovulation.
   c. The hypothalamus monitors the hormone levels in the blood.
   d. The endometrium becomes engorged with blood and causes bleeding if the ovum is not fertilized.

6. A condition in which a woman experiences pain when menstruating is known as
   a. premenstrual syndrome.
   b. dysmenorrhea.
   c. premenstrual dysphoric disorder.
   d. amenorrhea.

7. What is the role of testosterone in the male reproductive system?
   a. It is used to produce sperm for reproduction.
   b. It is the hormone that stimulates development of secondary male sex characteristics.
   c. It allows the penis to harden during sexual arousal.
   d. It secretes the seminal fluid preceding ejaculation.

8. The preejaculate fluid that sometimes is seen before a man ejaculates comes from which structure of the male reproductive system?
   a. Prostate gland
   b. Cowper's glands
   c. Vas deferens
   d. Testicles

9. Individuals who are sexually attracted to both men and women are identified as
   a. heterosexual.
   b. bisexual.
   c. homosexual.
   d. intersex.

10. Fellatio is the oral stimulation of the
    a. male genitals.
    b. female genitals.
    c. anal region.
    d. mouth and tongue.

Answers to these questions can be found on page A-1.

Think about It!

1. How have gender roles changed over your lifetime? Do you view the changes as positive for both men and women?
2. Have you ever discussed with your friends what it was like going through puberty? Did you understand what was happening to you physically and emotionally and why?
3. What criteria do you use to determine "normal" sexual behavior? What criteria should we use to determine healthy sexual practices?
4. If scientists are able to establish the combination of factors that interact to produce homosexual, heterosexual, or bisexual orientation, will that put an end to prejudice against gays? Why or why not?
5. How can we remove the stigma that surrounds sexual dysfunction so that individuals feel more comfortable seeking help? Are men and women affected differently by sexual dysfunction?
6. Have you ever viewed pornography? What prompted you to do this? How did you feel about the experience?

Accessing Your Health on the Internet

The following websites explore further topics and issues related to personal health. For links to the websites below, visit the Companion Website for *Access to Health*, 13th Edition, at www.pearsonhighered.com/donatelle.

1. *American Association of Sex Educators, Counselors, and Therapists (AASECT).* AASECT is a professional organization that provides standards of practice for treatment of sexual issues and disorders. www.aasect.org
2. *SmarterSex.org.* This site, created by the peer education group BACCHUS network, presents student-friendly information on sexual health targeted at 18- to 24-year-olds. www.smartersex.org
3. *Go Ask Alice.* Columbia University Health Services provides this interactive question-and-answer resource. "Alice" is available to answer questions about any health-related issues, including relationships, nutrition and diet, exercise, drugs, sex, alcohol, and stress. www.goaskalice.columbia.edu
4. *Sexuality Information and Education Council of the United States (SIECUS).* SIECUS provides information, guidelines, and materials for advancement of healthy and proper sex education. www.siecus.org
5. *Advocates for Youth.* Here, you can find current news, policy updates, research, and other resources about the sexual health of and choices particular to high school and college-aged students. www.advocatesforyouth.org

References

1. Consortium on the Management of Disorders of Sexual Development, *Handbook for Parents* (Rohnert Park, CA: Intersex Society of North America, 2006), Available at at http://dsdguidelines.org.
2. D. A. Hope, ed., "Sexual stigma and sexual prejudice in the United States: A conceptual framework," in *Contemporary Perspectives on Lesbian, Gay and Bisexual Identities: The 54th Nebraska Symposium on Motivation.* (New York: Springer), 65–111.
3. Federal Bureau of Investigation, "Hate Crime Statistics, 2009," Accessed November 2010, www2.fbi.gov/ucr/hc2009/incidents.html.
4. W. J. Jenkins, "Can Anyone Tell Me Why I'm Gay? What Research Suggests Regarding the Origins of Sexual Orientation," *North American Journal of Psychology* 12, no. 2 (2010): 279–96.
5. S. E. Anderson, G. E. Dallal, and A. Must, "Relative Weight and Race Influence Average Age at Menarche: Results from Two Nationally Representative Surveys of U.S. Girls Studied 25 Years Apart," *Pediatrics* 111, no. 4 (2003): 844–50; H. Baer, G. Colditz, W. Willett, and J. Dorgan, "Adiposity and Sex Hormones in Girls," *Cancer Epidemiology Biomarkers Preview* 16, no. 9 (2007): 1880–88; L. Shi, S. Wudy, A. Buyken, M. Hartmann, and T. Remer, "Body Fat and Animal Protein Intakes Are Associated with Adrenal Androgen Secretion in Children," *American Journal of Clinical Nutrition* 90, no. 5 (2009): 1321–28; K. K. Ong et al., "Infancy Weight Gain Predicts Childhood Body Fat and Age at Menarche in Girls," *Journal of Clinical Endocrinology & Metabolism,* no. 94 (2009): 1527–32.
6. Mayo Clinic Staff, "Premenstrual Syndrome (PMS)," 2009, www.mayoclinic.com/health/premenstrual-syndrome/DS00134.
7. Mayo Clinic Staff, "Premenstrual Dysphoric Disorder (PMDD)," 2010, www.mayoclinic.com/health/pmdd/AN01372.
8. Mayo Clinic Staff, "Menstrual Cramps," 2007, www.mayoclinic.com/Health/Menstrual-Cramps/Ds00506.
9. National Institutes of Health, *Facts about Menopausal Hormone Therapy* (NIH Publication no. 05-5200: 2005), Available at www.nhlbi.nih.gov/health/women/pht_facts.htm; NHLBI, "WHI Follow-Up Study Confirms Risk of Long-Term Combination Hormone Therapy Outweigh Benefits for Postmenopausal Women," news release, March 4, 2008, public.nhlbi.nih.gov/newsroom/home/GetPressRelease.aspx?id=2554; NHLBI, "WHI Study Data Confirm Short-term Health Disease Risks of Combination Hormone Therapy for Postmenopausal Women," news release, February 15, 2010, www.nih.gov/news/health/feb2010/nhlbi-15.htm.
10. N. Siegfried et al., "HIV and Male Circumcision—A Systematic Review with the Assessment of Quality of Studies," *The Lancet–Infectious Diseases* 5, no. 3 (2005): 165–73; A. Bertran et al., "Randomized, Controlled Intervention Trial of Male Circumcision for Reduction of HIV Transmission Risk: The ANRS 1265 Trial," *PLoS Medicine* 2, no. 11 (2005): 1112–22; B. G. Williams et al., "The Potential Impact of Male Circumcision on HIV in Sub-Saharan Africa," *PLoS Medicine* 3, no. 7 (2006): e262; B. P. Homeier,

"Circumcision," Paper presented at KidsHealth for Parents, Nemours Foundation (January 2005), Available at kidshealth.org/parent/system/surgical/circumcision.html; Mayo Clinic Staff, "Circumcision (Male): Why It's Done," February 2010, www.mayoclinic.com/health/circumcision/MY01023/DSECTION=why-its-done.

11. Mayo Clinic Staff, "Male Menopause: Myth or Reality?" June 25, 2009, www.mayoclinic.com/health/male-menopause/MC00058.

12. Ibid.

13. G. F. Kelly, "Sexual Individuality and Sexual Values," in *Sexuality Today: The Human Perspective*. 9th ed. (New York: McGraw-Hill, 2008).

14. Ibid.

15. J. A. Higgins, J. Trussell, N. B. Moore, and J. K. Davidson, "Young Adult Sexual Health: Current and Prior Sexual Behaviours among Non-Hispanic White U.S. College Students," *Sexual Health* 7, no. 1 (2010): 35–43.

16. American College Health Association, *American College Health Association–National College Health Assessment II (ACHA-NCHA II) Reference Group Data Report Spring 2011* (Baltimore: American College Health Association, 2012), Available at www.acha-ncha.org/reports_ACHA-NCHAII.html.

17. Ibid.

18. Ibid.

19. G. F. Kelly, "Sexual Individuality and Sexual Values," 2008.

20. Medline Plus, "Sexual Problems Overview: Medline Plus," Updated May 2010, www.nlm.nih.gov/medlineplus/ency/article/001951.htm.

21. Mayo Clinic Staff, "Erectile Dysfunction," January 2010, www.mayoclinic.com/health/erectile-dysfunction/DS00162.

22. National Kidney and Urological Diseases Information Clearinghouse, "Erectile Dysfunction," 2009, http://kidney.niddk.nih.gov/kudiseases/pubs/impotence/index.htm.

23. Medline Plus, "Sexual Problems Overview: Medline Plus," Updated May 2010.

24. K. M. Smith and F. Romanelli, "Recreational Use and Misuse of Phosphodiesterase 5 Inhibitors," *Journal of the American Pharmacists Association* 45, no. 1 (2005): 63–75; R. Kloner, "Erectile Dysfunction and Hypertension," *International Journal of Impotence Research* 19, no. 3 (2007): 296–302.

25. J. Ropelato, "Internet Pornography Statistics," TopTenREVIEWS, Inc., Accessed June 2010, www.internet-filter-review.toptenreviews.com/internet-pornography-statistics.html.

26. Ibid.

27. B. Paul, "Predicting Internet Pornography Use and Arousal: The Role of Individual Difference Variables," *Journal of Sex Research* 46, no. 4 (2009): 344–57; D. Kingston, N. Malamuth, P. Fedoroff, and W. Marchall, "The Importance of Individual Differences in Pornography Use: Theoretical Perspectives and Implications for Treating Sexual Offenders," *Journal of Sex Research* 46, no. 2/3 (2009): 216–32; B. A. Wilson et al., "Predicting Responses to Sexually Aggressive Stories: The Role of Consent, Interest in Sexual Aggression, and Overall Sexual Interest," *Journal of Sex Research* 39, no. 4 (2002): 275–83; M. T. Whitty and W. A. Fisher, "The Sexy Side of the Internet: An Examination of Sexual Activities and Materials in Cyberspace," in *Psychological Aspects of Cyberspace: Theory, Research, Applications,* ed. A. Barak (Cambridge, UK: Cambridge University Press, 2008), 185–208; A. McKee, "The Relationship between Attitudes towards Women, Consumption of Pornography, and Other Demographic Variables in a Survey of 1,023 Consumers of Pornography," *International Journal of Sexual Health* 19 (2007): 31–45.

6 Considering Your Reproductive Choices

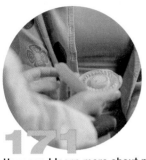
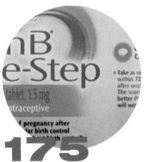
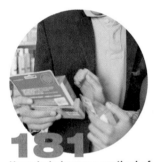

OBJECTIVES

✳ Compare the different types of contraceptive methods and their effectiveness in preventing pregnancy and sexually transmitted infections.

✳ Summarize the legal decisions surrounding abortion and the various types of abortion procedures.

✳ Discuss key issues to consider when planning a pregnancy.

✳ Explain the importance of prenatal care and the physical and emotional aspects of pregnancy.

✳ Describe the basic stages of childbirth and the methods and complications that can arise during labor and delivery.

✳ Review primary causes of and possible solutions to infertility.

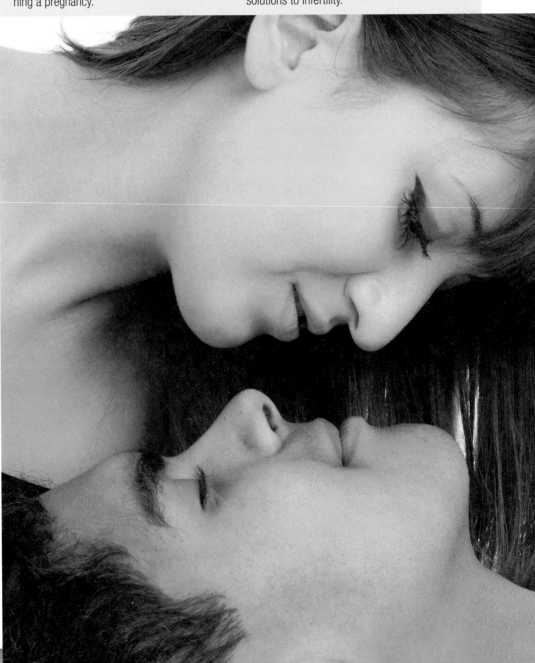

Today, we not only understand the intimate details of reproduction, but also possess technologies that can control or enhance our **fertility.** Along with information and technological advances comes choice, which goes hand in hand with responsibility. As adults, choosing whether and when to have children is one of our greatest responsibilities. Children transform people's lives. They require a lifelong personal commitment of love and nurturing. Before having children, ask yourself: Are you physically, emotionally, and financially prepared to care for another human being right now?

One measure of maturity is the ability to discuss reproduction and birth control with your sexual partner before engaging in sexual activity. Men often assume that their partners are taking care of birth control. Women sometimes feel that broaching the topic implies that they are promiscuous. Both may feel that bringing up the subject interferes with romance and spontaneity.

Too often, no one brings up the topic, and unprotected sex is the result. In a recent survey, only 57 percent of college students (59% of college women and 53% of college men) reported having used a method of contraception the last time they had sexual intercourse.[1] The sad result is too many unintended pregnancies and sexually transmitted infections. In fact, 51 percent of pregnancies in the United States are unintended. So, if you're thinking about becoming sexually active, or you already are but are not using birth control, make time to see your doctor or visit a local family planning clinic to discuss getting contraceptives. Discussing the topic with your health care provider or your sexual partner will be easier and less embarrassing if you understand human reproduction and contraception and honestly consider your attitudes toward these matters. This chapter provides important information for you to think about as you contemplate your own sexual and reproductive choices.

Basic Principles of Birth Control

Video Tutor:
Choosing
Contraception

The term **birth control** (also called **contraception**) refers to methods of preventing conception. **Conception** occurs when a sperm fertilizes an egg. This usually takes place in a woman's fallopian tube. The following conditions are necessary for conception:

1. A viable egg. A sexually mature woman will release one egg (sometimes more) from one of her two ovaries once every 28 days, on average. Eggs remain viable for 24 to 36 hours after their release from the ovary into the fallopian tube.

2. A viable sperm. Each ejaculation contains between 200 and 500 million sperm cells. Once sperm reach the fallopian tubes, they survive an average of 48 to 72 hours—and can survive up to a week.

3. Access to the egg by the sperm. To reach the egg, sperm must travel up the vagina, through the cervical opening into the uterus, and from there to the fallopian tubes.

Birth control methods prevent conception by interfering with one of these three conditions. Different methods offer varying degrees of control over when and whether pregnancy occurs.

Society has searched for a simple, infallible, and risk-free way to prevent pregnancy since people first associated sexual activity with pregnancy. Outside of abstinence, we have not yet found one.

To evaluate the effectiveness of a particular contraceptive method, you must be familiar with two concepts: perfect-use failure rate and typical-use failure rate. **Perfect-use failure rate** refers to the number of pregnancies that are likely to occur in the first year of use (per 100 users of the method) if the method is used absolutely perfectly—without any error. The **typical-use failure rate** refers to the number of pregnancies that are likely to occur in the first year of use with typical use—that is, with the normal number of errors, memory lapses, and incorrect or incomplete use. The typical-use information is much more practical in helping people make informed decisions about contraceptive methods.

Present methods of contraception fall into several categories. **Barrier methods** block the egg and sperm from joining. **Hormonal methods** introduce synthetic hormones into the woman's system that prevent ovulation, thicken cervical mucus, or prevent a fertilized egg from implanting. Surgical methods can prevent pregnancy permanently. Other methods may involve temporary or permanent abstinence or planning intercourse in accordance with fertility patterns. Table 6.1 lists the

fertility A person's ability to reproduce.
contraception (birth control) Methods of preventing conception.
conception Fertilization of an ovum by a sperm.
perfect-use failure rate The number of pregnancies (per 100 users) likely to occur in the first year of use of a particular birth control method if the method is used consistently and correctly.
typical-use failure rate The number of pregnancies (per 100 users) likely to occur in the first year of use of a particular birth control method if the method's use is not consistent or always correct.
barrier method Contraceptive methods that block the meeting of egg and sperm by means of a physical barrier (such as condom, diaphragm, or cervical cap);a chemical barrier (such as spermicide); or both.
hormonal methods Contraceptive methods that introduce synthetic hormones into a woman's system to prevent ovulation, thicken cervical mucus, or prevent a fertilized egg from implanting.

TABLE 6.1 | **Top Reported Means of Contraception Sexually Active College Students or Their Partner Used the Last Time They Had Intercourse**

Method	Male	Female	Total
Male condom	66.3%	60.4%	62.3%
Birth control pills (monthly or extended cycle)	61.5%	60.2%	60.6%
Withdrawal	25.1%	27.4%	26.6%
Fertility awareness (calendar, mucus, basal body temperature)	4.9%	6.0%	5.6%
Spermicide (foam, jelly, cream)	5.8%	3.5%	4.3%
Intrauterine device	4.6%	5.0%	4.9%
Cervical ring	4.7%	5.0%	4.9%

Note: Survey respondents could select more than one method.
Source: Data from American College Health Association, *American College Health Association—National College Health Assessment II: Reference Group Data Spring 2011* (Baltimore: American College Health Association, 2012).

most popular forms of contraception among sexually active college students.

Some contraceptive methods can also protect, to some degree, against **sexually transmitted infections (STIs).** This is an important factor to consider in choosing a contraceptive. Table 6.2 on page 165 summarizes the effectiveness, STI protection, frequency of use, and costs of various methods.

Barrier Methods

Barrier methods work on the simple principle of preventing sperm from ever reaching the egg by use of a physical or chemical barrier during intercourse. Some barrier methods prevent semen from having any contact with the woman's body, and others prevent sperm from going past the cervix. In addition, many barrier methods contain or are used in combination with a substance that kills sperm.

Male Condom

The **male condom** is a thin sheath designed to cover the erect penis and catch semen before it enters the vagina. Most male condoms are made of latex, although condoms made of polyurethane or lambskin also are available. Condoms come in a wide variety of styles and may be purchased in pharmacies, supermarkets, some public bathrooms, and many health clinics. A new condom must be used for each act of vaginal, oral, or anal intercourse.

A condom must be rolled onto the penis before the penis touches the vagina, and it must be held in place when removing the penis from the vagina after ejaculation (see Figure 6.1). Condoms come with or without **spermicide** and

sexually transmitted infections (STIs) Infectious diseases caused by pathogens transmitted through some form of sexual contact.

male condom Single-use sheath of thin latex or other material designed to fit over an erect penis and to catch semen upon ejaculation.

spermicide Substance designed to kill sperm.

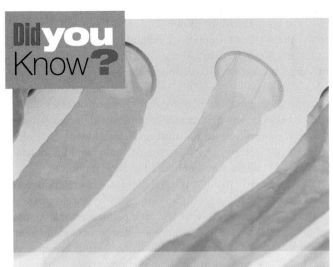

Condoms have been protecting people for millennia. The ancient Egyptians used linen sheaths and animal intestines as condoms as early as 1200 BC. The oldest evidence of condom use in Europe comes from cave paintings at the Grotte des Combarelles in France, dating from AD 100–200.

with or without lubrication. If desired, users can lubricate their own condoms with contraceptive foams, creams, and jellies or other water-based lubricants. Never use products such as baby oil, cold cream, petroleum jelly, vaginal yeast infection medications, or body lotion with a condom. These products contain mineral oil and will cause the latex to disintegrate.

Condoms are less effective and more likely to break during intercourse if they are old or improperly stored. To maintain effectiveness, store them in a cool place (not in a wallet or glove compartment), and inspect them for small tears before use. Lightly squeeze the package before opening to feel that air is trapped inside and the package has not been punctured. Discard all condoms that have passed their expiration date.

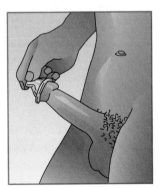

❶ Pinch the air out of the top half-inch of the condom to allow room for semen.

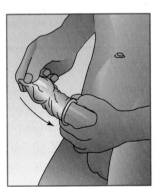

❷ Holding the tip of the condom with one hand, use the other hand to unroll it onto the penis.

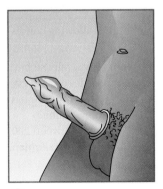

❸ Unroll the condom all the way to the base of the penis, smoothing out any air bubbles.

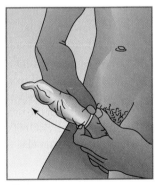

❹ After ejaculation, hold the condom around the base until the penis is totally withdrawn to avoid spilling any semen.

FIGURE 6.1 **How to Use a Male Condom**

TABLE 6.2 Contraceptive Effectiveness, STI Protection, Frequency of Use, and Costs

Method	Failure Rate		STI Protection	Frequency of Use	Cost
	Typical Use	Perfect Use			
Continuous abstinence	0	0	Yes	N/A	None
Implanon	0.05	0.05	No	Inserted every 3 years	$400–$800/exam, device, and insertion; $75–$250 for removal
Male sterilization	0.15	0.1	No	Done once	$350–$1,000/interview, counseling, examination, operation, and follow-up sperm count
Female sterilization	0.5	0.5	No	Done once	$1,500–$6,000/interview, counseling, examination, operation, and follow-up
IUD (intrauterine device)					
ParaGard (copper T)	0.8	0.6	No	Inserted every 10 years	$175–$500/exam, insertion, and follow-up visit
Mirena	0.2	0.2	No	Inserted every 5 years	$500–$1,000/exam, insertion, and follow-up visit
Depo-Provera	3	0.3	No	Injected every 12 weeks	$30–$75/3-month injection; $35–$175 for initial exam; $20–$40 for further visits to clinician for shots
Oral contraceptives (combined pill and progestin-only pill)	8	0.3	No	Take daily	$15–$50 monthly pill pack at drugstores, often less at clinics; check for family planning programs in your student health center, $35–$175 for initial exam
Ortho Evra patch	8	0.3	No	Applied weekly	$15–$70/month at drugstores; often less at clinics, $35–$175 for initial exam
NuvaRing	8	0.3	No	Inserted every 4 weeks	$15–$70/month at drugstores, often less at clinics; $35–$175 for initial exam
Cervical cap (FemCap) (with spermicidal cream or jelly)					
Women who have never given birth	14	4	Some	Used every time	$60–$75 for cap; $50–$200 for initial exam; $8–$17/supplies of spermicide jelly or cream
Women who have given birth	32	No data	Some	Used every time	
Male condom (without spermicides)	15	2	Some	Used every time	$1.00 and up/condom—some family planning or student health centers give them away or charge very little. Available in drugstores, family planning clinics, some supermarkets, and from vending machines
Diaphragm (with spermicidal cream or jelly)	16	6	Some	Used every time	$15–$75 for diaphragm; $50–$200 for initial exam; $8–$17/supplies of spermicide jelly or cream
Today sponge					
Women who have never given birth	16	9	No	Used every time	$9.00–$15/package of three sponges. Available at family planning centers, drugstores, online, and in some supermarkets
Women who have given birth	32	20	No	Used every time	
Female condom (without spermicides)	21	5	Some	Used every time	$4/condom. Available at family planning centers, drugstores, and in some supermarkets
Fertility awareness–based methods	25	12	No	Followed every month	$10–$12 for temperature kits. Charts and classes often free in health centers and churches
Withdrawal	27	4	No	Used every time	None
Spermicides (foams, creams, gels, vaginal suppositories, and vaginal film)	29	18	No	Used every time	$8/applicator kits of foam and gel ($4–$8 refills). Film and suppositories are priced similarly. Available at family planning clinics, drugstores, and some supermarkets
No method	85	85	No	N/A	None
Emergency contraceptive pill	Treatment initiated within 72–120 hours after unprotected intercourse reduces the risk of pregnancy by 75%–89% (with no protection against STIs). Costs depend on what services are needed: $39–$60/Plan B–One Step, available OTC to women 18 and older; $20–$50/one pack of combination pills; $50–$70/two packs of progestin-only pills; $35–$150/visit with health care provider; $10–$20/pregnancy test; ella $77–$97/in addition to visit with health care provider				

Note: "Failure Rate" refers to the number of unintended pregnancies per 100 women during the first year of use. "Typical Use" refers to failure rates for men and women whose use is not consistent or always correct. "Perfect Use" refers to failure rates for those whose use is consistent and always correct.

Some family planning clinics charge for services and supplies on a sliding scale according to income.

Sources: Adapted from R. Hatcher et al., *Contraceptive Technology*, 19th rev. ed. Copyright © 2007 Contraceptive Technology Communications, Inc. Reprinted by permission of Ardent Media, LLC.; Planned Parenthood, Birth Control, 2011, www.plannedparenthood.org/health-topics/birth-control-4211.htm.

Advantages When used consistently and correctly, condoms can be up to 98 percent effective. The condom is the only temporary means of birth control available for men, and latex and polyurethane condoms are the only barriers that effectively prevent the spread of some STIs and HIV. ("Skin" condoms, made from lamb intestines, are not effective against STIs.) Many people choose condoms because they are inexpensive and readily available without a prescription, and their use is limited to times of sexual activity, with no negative health effects. Some men find condoms help them stay erect longer or help prevent premature ejaculation.

Disadvantages The easy availability of condoms is accompanied by considerable potential for user error; as a result, the typical use effectiveness of condoms in preventing pregnancy is around 85 percent. Improper use of a condom can lead to breakage, leakage, or slipping, potentially exposing the users to STI transmission or an unintended pregnancy. Even when used perfectly, a condom doesn't protect against STIs that may have external areas of infection (e.g., herpes). For some people, a condom ruins the spontaneity of sex because stopping to put it on may break the mood. Others report that the condom decreases sensation. These inconveniences and perceptions contribute to improper use or avoidance of condoms altogether. Partners who put on a condom as part of foreplay are generally more successful with this form of birth control. As a new condom is required for each act of intercourse, some users find it difficult to be sure to have a condom available when needed.

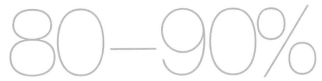

80–90%

is the reduction in risk of STI transmission provided by latex condoms, according to several research studies.

Female Condom

The **female condom** is a single-use, soft, loose-fitting polyurethane sheath meant for internal vaginal use. It is designed as one unit with two flexible rings. One ring lies inside the sheath and serves as an insertion mechanism and internal anchor. The other ring remains outside the vagina once the device is inserted and protects the labia and the base of the penis from infection. Figure 6.2 shows the proper use of the female condom.

female condom Single-use polyurethane sheath for internal use during vaginal or anal intercourse to catch semen upon ejaculation.

Advantages Used consistently and correctly, female condoms can be up to 95 percent effective. They

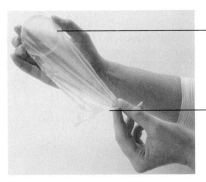

Inner ring is used for insertion and to help hold the sheath in place during intercourse.

Outer ring covers the area around the opening of the vagina.

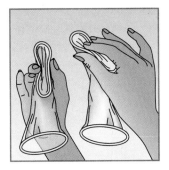

❶ Grasp the flexible inner ring at the closed end of the condom, and squeeze it between your thumb and second or middle finger so it becomes long and narrow.

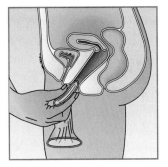

❷ Choose a comfortable position for insertion: squatting, with one leg raised, or sitting or lying down. While squeezing the ring, insert the closed end of the condom into your vagina.

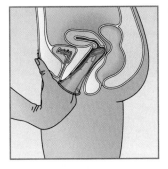

❸ Placing your index finger inside of the condom, gently push the inner ring up as far as it will go. Be sure the sheath is not twisted. The outer ring should remain outside of the vagina.

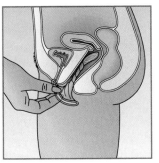

❹ During intercourse, be sure that the penis is not entering on the side, between the sheath and the vaginal wall. When removing the condom, twist the outer ring so that no semen leaks out.

FIGURE 6.2 **How to Use a Female Condom**

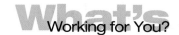
Maybe you are already sexually active and practicing safer sex. Which of the following behaviors are you already incorporating into your life?

☐ I keep a package of condoms handy—I don't want to get caught unprepared.

☐ I made an appointment with my doctor to discuss a more reliable form of birth control.

☐ I've decided I'm not ready to have sex, so I'm choosing to abstain at this point in my life.

☐ My partner and I have agreed to use a condom every time we have sex. Even though it can be awkward to discuss, it's a relief to talk it over!

also can prevent the spread of HIV and other STIs, including those that can be transmitted by external genital contact. The female condom can be inserted up to 8 hours in advance, so its use doesn't have to interrupt lovemaking. Some women choose to use the female condom because it gives them more personal control over pregnancy prevention and STI protection or because they cannot rely on their partner to use a male condom. Because the polyurethane is thin and pliable, there is less loss of sensation with the female condom than there is with the latex male condom. The female condom is relatively inexpensive, readily available without a prescription, and causes no negative health effects.

Disadvantages As with the male condom, there is potential for user error with the female condom, including possible breaking, slipping, or leaking, all of which could lead to STI transmission or an unintended pregnancy. Because of the potential problems, the typical use effectiveness of the female condom is 79 percent. Some people dislike using the female condom because they feel it is disruptive, noisy, odd looking, or difficult to use. Some women have reported external or vaginal irritation from using the female condom. As with the male condom, a new condom is required for each act of intercourse, so users may not always have one available when needed. The female condom can be used effectively for anal sex, but it is difficult to use in this manner and increases the likelihood of rectal bleeding, which increases the risk of contracting HIV. Therefore, it's better to use the male condom for anal sex.

Jellies, Creams, Foams, Suppositories, and Film

Like condoms, some other barrier methods—jellies, creams, foams, suppositories, and film—do not require a prescription. They are referred to as spermicides—substances designed to kill sperm. The active ingredient in most of them is nonoxynol-9 (N-9).

Jellies and creams are packaged in tubes, and foams are available in aerosol cans. All have applicators designed for insertion into the vagina. They must be inserted far enough to cover the cervix, thus providing both a chemical barrier that kills sperm and a physical barrier that stops sperm from continuing toward an egg.

Suppositories are waxy capsules that are inserted deep into the vagina, where they melt. They must be inserted 10 to 20 minutes before intercourse to have time to melt, but no longer than 1 hour prior to intercourse, or they lose their effectiveness. An additional suppository or other spermicide must be inserted for each subsequent act of intercourse.

Vaginal contraceptive film is another method of spermicide delivery. A thin film infused with spermicidal gel is inserted into the vagina so that it covers the cervix. The film dissolves into a spermicidal gel that is effective for up to 3 hours. As with other spermicides, a new film must be inserted for each act of intercourse.

Advantages Spermicides are most effective when used in conjunction with another barrier method (condom, diaphragm, etc.); used alone they offer only 71 percent (typical use) to 82 percent (perfect use) effectiveness at preventing pregnancy. Like condoms, spermicides are simple to use, inexpensive, do not require a prescription or pelvic examination, and are readily available. They are simple to use, and their use is limited to the time of sexual activity.

Disadvantages Spermicides can be messy and must be reapplied for each act of intercourse. Some people experience irritation or allergic reactions to spermicides, and recent studies indicate that while spermicides containing N-9 are effective at preventing pregnancy, they are not effective in preventing transmission of HIV. In fact, frequent (more than once a day) use of N-9 spermicides has been shown to cause irritation and breaks in the mucous layer or skin of the genital tract, creating a point of entry for viruses and bacteria that cause disease.[2] Spermicides containing N-9 have also been associated with increased risk of urinary tract infection. New spermicides without N-9, such as Contragel, are beginning to enter the market.

Diaphragm with Spermicidal Jelly or Cream

Invented in the mid-nineteenth century, the **diaphragm** was the first widely used birth control method for women. The device is a soft, shallow cup made of thin latex rubber. Its flexible, rubber-coated ring is designed to fit snugly behind the pubic bone in front of the cervix and over the back of the cervix on the other side so it blocks access to the uterus. Diaphragms must be used with spermicidal cream or jelly, which is applied to the inside of the diaphragm before it is inserted, up to 6 hours before intercourse. The diaphragm holds the spermicide in

diaphragm Latex, cup-shaped device designed to cover the cervix and block access to the uterus; should always be used with spermicide.

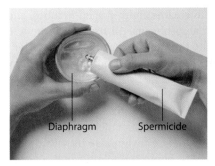
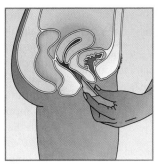
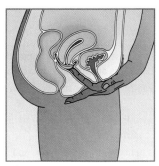

1 Place spermicidal jelly or cream inside the diaphragm and all around the rim.

2 Fold the diaphragm in half and insert dome-side down (spermicide-side up) into the vagina, pushing it along the back wall as far as it will go.

3 Position the diaphragm with the cervix completely covered and the front rim tucked up against your pubic bone; you should be able to feel your cervix through the rubber dome.

FIGURE 6.3 **Proper Use and Placement of a Diaphragm**

place, creating a physical and chemical barrier against sperm (Figure 6.3). Diaphragms are manufactured in different sizes and must be fitted to the woman by a trained practitioner, who should make sure the user knows how to insert her diaphragm correctly before leaving the practitioner's office.

Advantages If used consistently and correctly, diaphragms can be 94 percent effective in preventing pregnancy. When used with spermicidal jelly or cream, the diaphragm also offers some protection against gonorrhea and possibly chlamydia and human papillomavirus (HPV). After the initial prescription and fitting, the only ongoing expense involved with diaphragm use is spermicide. Because the diaphragm can be inserted up to 6 hours in advance and be used for multiple acts of intercourse, some users may find it less disruptive than other barrier methods.

cervical caps Small cup made of latex or silicone that is designed to fit snugly over the entire cervix; should always be used with spermicide.

Disadvantages Although the diaphragm can be left in place for multiple acts of intercourse, additional spermicide must be applied each time, and the diaphragm must then stay in place for 6 to 8 hours after intercourse to allow the chemical to kill any sperm remaining in the vagina. Some women find inserting the device can be awkward. When inserted incorrectly, diaphragms are much less effective. It is also possible for a diaphragm to slip out of place, be difficult to remove, or require refitting by a physician (e.g., following a pregnancy or a significant weight gain or loss).

Cervical Cap with Spermicidal Jelly or Cream

One of the oldest methods used to prevent pregnancy, early **cervical caps** were made from beeswax, silver, or copper. The currently available FemCap is a clear silicone cup that

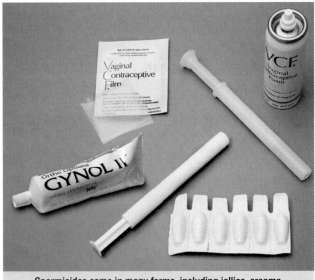

Spermicides come in many forms, including jellies, creams, films, foam, and suppositories.

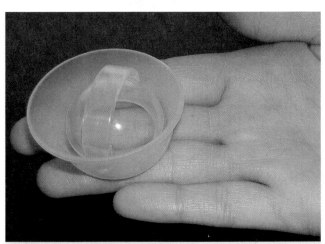

FemCap is used in conjunction with spermicide and is positioned to cover the cervix. It is shaped like a sailor's cap and has a loop to aid in removal.

fits snugly over the entire cervix. It comes in three sizes and must be fitted by a practitioner. The FemCap is designed for use with spermicidal jelly or cream. It is held in place by suction created during application and works by blocking sperm from the uterus.

Advantages Cervical caps can be reasonably effective (up to 86%) with typical use. They also may offer some protection against transmission of gonorrhea and possibly chlamydia and HPV. They are relatively inexpensive, as the only ongoing cost is for the spermicide.

The FemCap can be inserted up to 6 hours prior to intercourse. The device must be left in place for 6 to 8 hours afterward, but after that time period, can be removed, cleaned, and reinserted immediately. Because the FemCap is made of surgical-grade silicone, it is a suitable alternative for people who are allergic to latex.

Disadvantages The FemCap is somewhat more difficult to insert than a diaphragm because of its smaller size. Like a diaphragm, it requires an initial fitting and may require subsequent refitting if a woman's cervix size changes (e.g., after giving birth). Because the FemCap can become dislodged during intercourse by heavy thrusting or certain sexual positions, placement must be monitored. The device cannot be used during the menstrual period or for longer than 48 hours because of the risk of **toxic shock syndrome (TSS).** Some women report unpleasant vaginal odors after use.

Contraceptive Sponge

The **contraceptive sponge** is made of polyurethane foam and contains nonoxynol-9 (sold in the United States as the Today Sponge). Prior to insertion, the sponge must be moistened with water to activate the spermicide. It is then folded and inserted deep into the vagina, where it fits over the cervix and creates a barrier against sperm.

Advantages The sponge is fairly effective (91% perfect use; 84% typical use) when used consistently and correctly. A main advantage of the sponge is convenience, because it does not require a trip to the doctor for fitting. Protection begins immediately on insertion and lasts for up to 24 hours. There is no need to reapply spermicide or insert a new sponge for any subsequent acts of intercourse within the same 24-hour period; it must be left in place for at least 6 hours after the last intercourse. Like the diaphragm and cervical cap, the sponge offers limited protection from some STIs.

Disadvantages The sponge is less effective for women who have previously given birth (80% perfect use; 68% typical use). Allergic reactions, such as irritation of the vagina, are more common with the sponge than with other barrier methods. Should the vaginal lining become irritated, the risk of yeast infections and other STIs may increase. Some cases of TSS have been reported in women using the sponge; the same precautions should be taken as with the diaphragm and cervical cap. Some women find the sponge difficult or messy to remove.

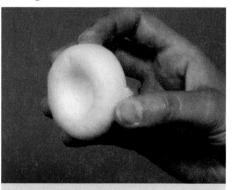

The Today sponge is a barrier method with spermicide that is most effective when used in conjunction with male condoms.

toxic shock syndrome (TSS) Potentially life-threatening disease that occurs when specific bacterial toxins multiply and spread to the bloodstream, most commonly through improper use of tampons or diaphragms.

contraceptive sponge Contraceptive device, made of polyurethane foam and containing nonoxynol-9, that fits over the cervix to create a barrier against sperm.

oral contraceptives Pills containing synthetic hormones that prevent ovulation by regulating hormones.

Hormonal Methods

The term *hormonal contraception* refers to birth control that contains synthetic estrogen and/or progestin. These ingredients are similar to the hormones estrogen and progesterone, which a woman's ovaries produce naturally for the process of ovulation and the menstrual cycle. In recent years, hormonal contraception has become available in a variety of forms (transdermal, injection, and oral). All forms require a prescription from a health care provider.

Hormonal contraception alters a woman's biochemistry, preventing ovulation (release of the egg) from taking place and producing changes that make it more difficult for the sperm to reach the egg if ovulation does occur. Some hormonal contraceptives contain both estrogen and progestin (synthetic progesterone), and several products contain just progestin. Synthetic estrogen works to prevent the ovaries from releasing an egg. If no egg is released, there is nothing to be fertilized by the sperm and pregnancy cannot occur. Progestin thickens the cervical mucus, which hinders the movement of the sperm, inhibits the egg's ability to travel through the fallopian tubes, and suppresses the sperm's ability to unite with the egg. Progestin also thins the uterine lining, making it unlikely that an egg will be able to implant in the uterine wall.

Oral Contraceptives

Oral contraceptives pills were first marketed in the United States in 1960. Their convenience quickly made them the most widely used reversible method of fertility control. Most modern pills are more than 99 percent effective at preventing pregnancy with perfect use. Today, oral contraceptives are the most commonly used birth control method among college women.[3]

Most oral contraceptives work through the combined effects of synthetic estrogen and progestin (*combination pills*). Combination pills are taken in a cycle. At the end of each 3-week cycle, the user discontinues the drug or takes placebo pills for 1 week. The resultant drop in hormones causes the uterine lining to shed, and the user will have a menstrual period, usually within 1 to 3 days. Menstrual flow is generally lighter than it is for women who don't use the pill, because the hormones in the pill prevent thick endometrial buildup.

Several newer brands of pills have extended cycles, such as the 91-day Seasonale and Seasonique. A woman using this regimen takes active pills for 12 weeks, followed by 1 week of placebos. Under this cycle, women can expect to have a menstrual period every 3 months. Data indicate that women do have an increased occurrence of spotting or bleeding in the first few cycles.[4] Lybrel, another extended-cycle pill, supplies an active dose of hormones every day for 365 days. This eliminates menstruation completely during the time a woman takes it.

Advantages Combination pills are highly effective at preventing pregnancy: 99.7 percent with perfect use and 92 percent with typical use. It is easier to achieve perfect use with pills than it is with barrier contraceptives, as user error is less likely. Aside from its effectiveness, much of the pill's popularity is due to its convenience and ability to be used discreetly. Users like the fact that it does not interrupt or interfere with lovemaking, which can lead to enhanced sexual enjoyment.

In addition to preventing pregnancy, the pill may lessen menstrual difficulties, such as cramps and premenstrual syndrome (PMS). Oral contraceptives also lower the risk of several health conditions, including endometrial and ovarian cancers, noncancerous breast disease, osteoporosis, ovarian cysts, pelvic inflammatory disease (PID), and iron-deficiency anemia.[5] There are many different brands of combination pills on the market; some contain progestin, which offers additional benefits, such as reducing acne or minimizing fluid retention. Less-expensive generic versions are also available for many brands. With extended-cycle pills, the major additional benefit is the reduction in or absence of menstruation and any associated cramps or PMS symptoms. Users of these pills also like that they don't need to remember when to stop or start a cycle of pills or when to use placebos.

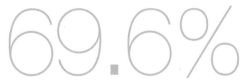

69.6%

of sexually active female college students use some form of hormonal contraception (pills, shot, patch, ring, or implant).

Disadvantages The estrogen in combination pills is associated with the risk of several serious health problems, including blood clots (which can lead to strokes or heart at-

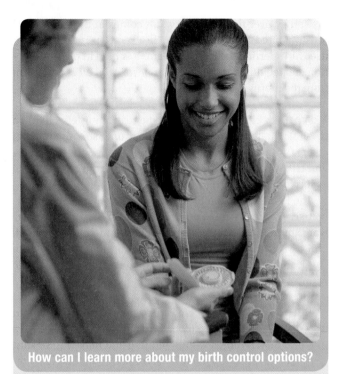

How can I learn more about my birth control options?

Studies show that college-age women are often familiar with only the birth control pill and the male condom. It's important to take the time to talk to your health care provider about all the options available to you and your partner so that you can make the decision that's best for you. Depending on your preferences, you might choose a hormonal, barrier, or other method of contraception.

tacks) and an increased risk of high blood pressure. The risk is low for most healthy women under the age of 35 who do not smoke; it increases with age and especially with cigarette smoking. Early warning signs of complications associated with oral contraceptives include severe abdominal, chest, or leg pain, severe headache, and/or eye problems.

Different brands of pills have varying minor side effects. Some of the most common are spotting between periods (particularly with extended-cycle regimens), breast tenderness, and nausea and vomiting. With most pills, these side effects clear up within a few months. Other, less common potential side effects include acne, weight gain, hair loss or growth, and a change in sexual desire. Because there are so many brands available, most women who wish to use the pill are able to find one that works for them without causing unpleasant side effects.

Apart from its risk factors and potential side effects, the pill's greatest disadvantage is that it must be taken every day (see the **Tech & Health** box on the next page). There is variation among brands, but in general, if a woman misses a pill, she should use an alternative form of contraception for the remainder of that cycle. A backup method of birth control is also necessary during the first week of use. After a woman discontinues the pill, return of fertility may be delayed, but the pill is not known to cause infertility. Another drawback is that the pill does not protect against STIs. Cost may also be a barrier for some women (see the **Money & Health** box on page

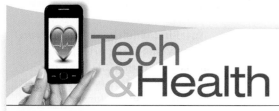

BIRTH CONTROL, PREGNANCY, AND NEWBORNS: APPS FOR ALL OPTIONS

The difference between the "perfect use" failure rates and "typical use" failure rates is most often human error. It is easy to leave your pills at home when you go out of town, to run out of condoms, or to forget to schedule an appointment to get your shot. In fact, the reason that implants and IUDs are so effective is that they remove human error from the equation.

Technology can help reduce this error. Reminder apps, such as Don't Forget The Pill and iPill (both for Android) send text messages or sound alarms to remind you to take your pill. Many ringtone options are discreet, but the "screaming baby" ringtone provides extra incentive to take your pill imme-

diately. Reminder apps can also help women remember to schedule their shot or visit the pharmacy to buy more pills.

For women trying to get pregnant, iChartMe and FemiCyle (both for the iPhone) help predict fertility cycles based on fertility awareness methods. While not perfect, because ovulation is not always predictable, they do simplify charting basal temperatures and predicting fertile periods. Once pregnant, there are many apps for women to choose from, such as I'm Expecting (Android and iPhone) and Baby Bump (iPhone). These apps provide many great tools, such as pregnancy countdowns, week-by-week information about fetal growth and development, and details on what a woman should

expect from each week of pregnancy. Some apps are more specific: Prenatal Smart (iPhone) lists which foods to avoid and which foods are safe to eat, and Baby Kicks, as the name implies, helps you track the number of times the baby kicks. Not to leave out dad, mPregnancy (iPhone) provides useful facts for men during pregnancy, not only about the baby, but also about what's going on with mom, too.

When the baby arrives, you can download all kinds of apps to chart growth, play white noise, and track nursing times and diaper changes, but don't forget to put down the phone and cuddle the baby!

---

173), and some young women report that the requirement to have a complete gynecological examination to obtain a pill prescription is an obstacle.

Progestin-Only Pills

Progestin-only pills (or minipills) contain small doses of progestin and no estrogen. These pills are available in 28-day packs of active pills (menstruation usually occurs during the fourth week even though the active dose continues through the entire month). Ovulation may occur, but the progestin prevents pregnancy by thickening cervical mucus and interfering with implantation of a fertilized egg.

Advantages Progestin-only pills are a good choice for women who are at high risk for estrogen-related side effects or who cannot take estrogen-containing pills because of diabetes, high blood pressure, or other cardiovascular conditions. They also can be used safely by women who are older than age 35 and by women who are currently breast-feeding. The effectiveness rate of these pills is 96 percent with perfect use, which is slightly lower than that of estrogen-containing pills. Progestin-only pills share some of the health benefits associated with combination pills, and they carry no estrogen-related cardiovascular risks. Also, some of the typical side effects of combination pills, including nausea and breast tenderness, usually do not occur with progestin-only pills, and menstrual periods generally become lighter or cease.

Disadvantages Because of the lower dose of hormones in progestin-only pills, it is especially important that they be taken at the same time each day. If a woman takes a pill 3 or more hours later than usual, she will need to use a backup method of contraception for the next 48 hours. The most common side effect of progestin-only pills is irregular menstrual bleeding or spotting. Less common side effects include headaches and changes in mood or sex drive. As with all oral contraceptives, progestin-only pills do not protect against STIs.

Contraceptive Skin Patch

Ortho Evra is a square transdermal (through the skin) adhesive patch, which is as thin as a plastic strip bandage. It is worn for 1 week and is replaced on the same day of the week for 3 consecutive weeks; during the fourth week, no patch is worn. Ortho Evra works by delivering continuous levels of estrogen and progestin through the skin and into the bloodstream. The patch can be worn on one of four areas of the body: buttocks, abdomen, upper torso (front or back, excluding the breasts), or upper outer arm. It should not be used by women over age 35 and is less effective in women who are obese.

Ortho Evra Patch that releases hormones similar to those in oral contraceptives; each patch is worn for 1 week.

Advantages Ortho Evra is 99.7 percent effective with perfect use. As with other hormonal methods, there is less room for user error than with barrier methods. Women who choose to use the patch often do so because they find it easier to remember to replace it than to take a daily pill, and they like the fact that they only need to change the patch once a week. Ortho Evra likely offers similar potential health benefits as combination pills (reduction in risk of certain cancers and diseases, lessening of PMS symptoms, etc.). Like other hormonal methods, the patch regulates a woman's menstrual cycle.

Disadvantages Using the patch requires an initial exam and prescription, weekly patch changes, and the ongoing expense of patch purchases. There is currently no generic version. A backup method is required during the first week of use. Similar to other hormonal birth control methods, the patch offers no protection against HIV or other STIs. Some women experience minor side effects such as those associated with combination pills. The estrogen in the patch is associated with cardiovascular risks, particularly in women who smoke and women over the age of 35. In 2005, amid evidence that the patch may increase the risk of life-threatening blood clots, the U.S. Food and Drug Administration (FDA) mandated an additional warning label explaining that patch use exposes women to about 60 percent more total estrogen than they would receive if they were taking a typical combination pill. The FDA released an updated warning, indicating more conclusive evidence of an increased risk of blood clots among regular users in 2010[6] and an even stronger warning in 2011.[7]

Vaginal Contraceptive Ring

NuvaRing is a soft, flexible plastic hormonal contraceptive ring about 2 inches in diameter. The user inserts the ring into the vagina, leaves it in place for 3 weeks, and removes it for 1 week, during which she will have a menstrual period. Once the ring is inserted, it releases a steady flow of estrogen and progestin.

NuvaRing Soft, flexible ring inserted into the vagina that releases hormones, preventing pregnancy.
Depo-Provera Injectable method of birth control that lasts for 3 months.

Advantages When used properly, the ring is 99.7 percent effective. Advantages of NuvaRing include less likelihood of user error, protection against pregnancy for 1 month, no pill to take daily or patch to change weekly, no need to be fitted by a clinician, no requirement to use spermicide, and rapid return of fertility when use is stopped. It also exposes the user to a lower dosage of estrogen than do the patch and some combination pills, so it may have fewer estrogen-related side effects. It likely offers some of the same potential health benefits as combination pills, and like other hormonal contraceptives, it regulates the menstrual cycle.

Ortho Evra is an adhesive patch that delivers estrogen and progestin through the skin for 1 week. Patches are changed weekly and worn for 3 out of 4 weeks.

Disadvantages NuvaRing requires an initial exam and prescription, monthly ring changes, and the ongoing expense of purchasing the ring (there is currently no generic version). A backup method must be used during the first week, and the ring provides no protection against STIs. Like combination pills, the ring poses possible minor side effects and potentially serious health risks for some women. Possible side effects unique to the ring include increased vaginal discharge and vaginal irritation or infection. Oil-based vaginal medicines to treat yeast infections cannot be used when the ring is in place, and a diaphragm or cervical cap cannot be used as a backup method for contraception.

Contraceptive Injections

Depo-Provera is a long-acting progestin that is injected intramuscularly every 3 months by a health care provider. It prevents ovulation, thickens cervical mucus, and thins the uterine lining, all of which prevent pregnancy.

Advantages Depo-Provera takes effect within 24 hours of the first shot so there is usually no need to use a backup method. There is little room for user error as the injection is administered by a clinician every 3 months. With perfect

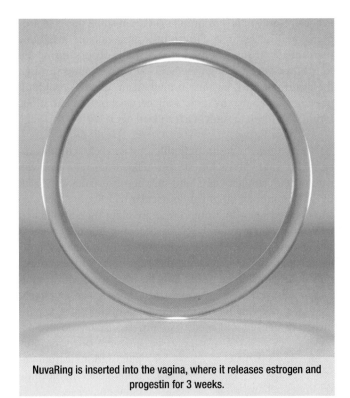

NuvaRing is inserted into the vagina, where it releases estrogen and progestin for 3 weeks.

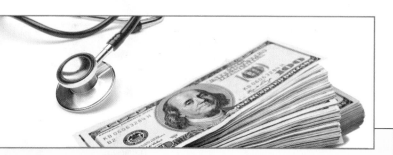

Money&Health

HEALTH CARE REFORM AND CONTRACEPTIVES

In March 2010, President Obama signed into law the Patient Protection and Affordable Care Act, which requires new private health insurance plans to cover "preventive services" with no co-payments or deductibles as of August 2012. Preventive services include: birth control, yearly "wellness visits" (physical exams), breast-feeding counseling and supplies, and screening for domestic violence and sexually transmitted infections. Abortions are not included, but emergency contraception is.

Family planning experts anticipate that the law will have impact in two ways. One, women who have been unable to afford birth control will now have access. Half of all young adult women report having been unable to afford birth control consistently at some point, and when women have to choose between paying the heat bill and paying for birth control, birth control usually loses. Two, this coverage will enable women to "upgrade" their birth control to a more reliable method. Women who would prefer to use an IUD or implant to reduce the risk of "user error" resulting in an unintended pregnancy but have been unable to because of the high upfront costs ($175–$1,000), will now be able to. Both of these changes should work to significantly reduce unintended pregnancy, a major win for reproductive health advocates!

The implementation of the new law has not been without debate. In February 2012, the Obama administration created a firestorm of controversy by limiting the religious institutions exempt from offering these "preventive services" to include only churches themselves, not religious-affiliated charities, hospitals, or universities. The debate boiled down to this question: Should institutions with religious ties (like Catholic hospitals) be required to offer insurance plans covering birth control despite their objection to its use? Those wanting to reduce unintended pregnancies and provide broad preventive health services to all women argued that it shouldn't matter where a woman works, she should have equal access to birth control. Religious lead-

ers argued that the requirement was an infringement on First Amendment rights and on religious liberty.

After days of political turmoil, President Obama announced a "compromise." Women who work directly for churches will continue to have no guarantee of any contraception coverage, and religiously affiliated institutions would not be required to offer contraception coverage to their employees; however, the insurance companies that cover those institutions would be required to offer contraceptive coverage free of charge to women working at such institutions. Unsatisfied with the "compromise," 43 Catholic institutions filed multiple federal lawsuits, arguing that the mandate's exception for religious groups was too narrow and charging that requiring most religious employers to provide health insurance that includes birth-control services violates their right to religious freedom. The lawsuits will likely remain unsettled for some time.

While birth control remains a highly contentious political topic, it is one that almost all Americans have stake in as 99 percent of American women use birth control at some point in their lives, including 98 percent of Catholic women. In the meantime, the benefits of birth control, including a reduction in unintended pregnancies, a reduction in abortions, and more opportunities for women are ones that most of us can agree upon.

Sources: WebMD, "No More Co-pay for Birth Control," August 2011, http://women.webmd.com/news/20110801/no-more-copay-for-womens-wellness-birth-control; Associated Press, "Free Birth Control: Insurance Now Covers It with No Copay," August 1, 2011, http://www.nola.com/health/index.ssf/2011/08/free_birth_control_insurance_c.html;Planned Parenthood, "Key Facts on Birth Control Coverage," Accessed February 15, 2012, http://www.plannedparenthood.org/files/PPFA/Myth_V_Fact_on_Birth_Control_coverage.pdf; A. Silverleib, "Obama Announces Contraception Compromise," February 10, 2012, http://articles.cnn.com/2012-02-10/politics/politics_contraception-controversy_1_contraception-religious-groups-religious-liberty?_s=PM:POLITICS; W. Richey, "Catholic Groups Take Fight against Obama Birth-Control Rules to Court," May 21, 2012, http://www.csmonitor.com/USA/2012/0521/Catholic-groups-take-fight-against-Obama-birth-control-rules-to-court.

use the shot is 99.7 percent effective, and with typical use it is 97 percent effective. Some women feel that Depo-Provera encourages sexual spontaneity because they do not have to remember to take a pill or insert a device. With continued use of this method, a woman's menstrual periods become lighter and may eventually cease. There are no estrogen-related health risks associated with Depo-Provera, and it offers the same potential health benefits as progestin-only pills. Unlike estrogen-containing hormonal methods, Depo-Provera can be used by women who are breast-feeding.

Disadvantages Using Depo-Provera requires an initial exam and prescription, then follow-up visits every 3 months to have the shot administered. It offers no protection against STIs. The main disadvantage of Depo-Provera use is irregular bleeding, which can be troublesome at first, but within a year, most women are amenorrheic (have no menstrual periods). Weight gain (an average of 5 pounds in the first year) is common. Prolonged use of Depo-Provera has been linked to loss of bone density. Other possible side effects include dizziness, nervousness, and headache. Unlike other methods of contraception, this method cannot be stopped immediately if problems arise, and the drug and its side effects may linger for up to 6 months after the last shot. A concern for women who want to get pregnant is that after the final injection it may take women up to a year to conceive.

Contraceptive Implants

A single-rod implantable contraceptive, Implanon is a small (about the size of a matchstick) soft plastic capsule that is inserted just beneath the skin on the inner side of a woman's upper underarm by a health care provider. Implanon continually releases a low, steady dose of progestin for up to 3 years, suppressing ovulation during that time.

Advantages After insertion, Implanon is generally not visible, making it a discreet method of birth control. The main advantages of Implanon are that it is highly effective (99.95%), it is not subject to user error, and it needs to be replaced only once every 3 years. It has benefits similar to other progestin-only forms of contraception, including the lightening or cessation of menstrual periods, the lack of estrogen-related side effects, and safety for use by breast-feeding women. Fertility usually returns immediately after removal of the implant.

intrauterine device (IUD) A device, often T-shaped, that is implanted in the uterus to prevent pregnancy.

Disadvantages Insertion and removal of Implanon must be performed by a clinician. There is a higher initial cost for this method, and it may not be covered by all health plans. Potential minor side effects include irritation, allergic reaction, swelling, or scarring around the area of insertion, and there is also a possibility of infection or complications with removal. As with other progestin-only contraceptives, users can experience irregular bleeding. Implanon offers no protection against STIs, and it may require a backup method during the first week of use.

Intrauterine Contraceptives

The **intrauterine device (IUD)** is a small plastic, flexible device, with a nylon string attached, that is placed in the

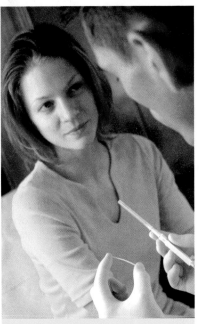
Implanon is inserted by a clinician beneath the skin of a woman's arm, where it releases progestin for up to 3 years.

uterus through the cervix and left there for 5 to 10 years. The exact mechanism by which it works is not clearly understood, but researchers believe that IUDs affect the way sperm and eggs move, thereby preventing fertilization and/or affecting the lining of the uterus to prevent a fertilized ovum from implanting. The IUD was once extremely popular in the United States; however, in the 1970s most brands were removed from the market because of serious complications, such as pelvic inflammatory disease and infertility. The IUD, redesigned for safe use, is very popular again worldwide, and it is experiencing a resurgence of popularity among U.S. women.

ParaGard and Mirena IUDs

Two IUDs are currently available in the United States. ParaGard is a T-shaped plastic device with copper around the shaft. It does not contain any hormones and can be left in place for 10 years. A newer IUD, Mirena, is effective for 5 years and releases small amounts of progestin. A physician must fit and insert an IUD. One or two strings extend into the vagina so the user can check to make sure that the device is in place. The IUD can be removed at any time by a practitioner. While IUDs were initially not recommended for women who had never had a baby, the American Congress of Obstetricians and Gynecologists now supports their use for all ages.[8]

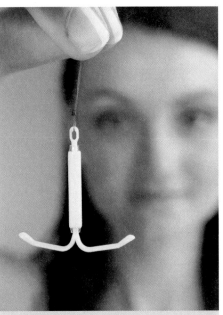
The Mirena IUD is a flexible plastic device inserted by a clinician into a woman's uterus, where it releases progestin for up to 5 years.

Advantages The IUD is a safe, discreet, and highly effective method (at least 99.4%) of birth control. It is effective immediately and needs to be replaced only every 5 years (Mirena) or every 10 years (ParaGard). ParaGard has the benefit of containing no hormones at all and so has none of the potential negative health impacts of hormonal contraceptives. Mirena, on the other hand, likely offers some of the same potential health benefits as other progestin-only methods. Both IUDs can be used by breast-feeding women. With Mirena, periods become lighter or stop completely. The IUDs are fully reversible; after removal, there is usually no delay in return of fertility. Both of these methods offer sexual spontaneity, as there is no need to keep supplies on hand or to interrupt lovemaking. The devices begin working immediately, and there is a low incidence of side effects.

Disadvantages Disadvantages of IUDs include possible discomfort, cost of insertion, and potential complications. Also, the IUD does not protect against STIs. In some women, the device can cause heavy menstrual flow and severe cramps for the first few months. With Mirena, menstrual periods tend to become shorter and lighter over time. Other side effects include acne, headaches, nausea, breast tenderness, mood changes, uterine cramps, and backache, which seem to occur most often in women who have never been pregnant. Women using IUDs have a higher risk of benign ovarian cysts.

Emergency Contraception

Emergency contraception is the use of a contraceptive to prevent pregnancy after unprotected intercourse, a sexual assault, or the failure of another birth control method. Combination estrogen-progestin pills and progestin-only pills are two common types of **emergency contraceptive pills (ECPs),** sometimes referred to as "morning-after pills." They are not the same as the "abortion pill," although the two are often confused. ECPs contain the same type of hormones as regular birth control pills and are used after unprotected intercourse but before a woman misses her period. A woman taking ECPs does so to prevent pregnancy; the method will not work if she is already pregnant, nor will it harm an existing pregnancy. In contrast, Mifeprex or mifepristone (formerly known as RU-486), the *early abortion pill,* is used to terminate a pregnancy that is already established—it is taken after a woman is sure she is pregnant (having taken a pregnancy test with a positive result). It and other abortion methods are discussed in detail later in the chapter.

ECPs prevent pregnancy the same way that other hormonal contraceptives do, by delaying or inhibiting ovulation, inhibiting fertilization, or blocking implantation of a fertilized egg, depending on the phase of the woman's menstrual cycle. Although ECPs use the same hormones as birth control pills, not all brands of birth control pills can be used for emergency contraception. When taken within 24 hours, ECPs reduce the risk of pregnancy by up to 95 percent; when taken 2 to 5 days later, ECPs reduce the risk of pregnancy by 75 to 89 percent.[9]

There are three brands of ECPs in the United States: Plan B One-Step, Next Choice, and ella. Plan B One-Step and Next Choice are available over the counter for those 17 and older. For anyone under 17, a prescription is still required to purchase them. Nine states have enacted laws that permit a pharmacist to provide emergency contraception to customers under 17 without a prescription under certain conditions. Seven states have laws allowing pharmacists to distribute it to minors if they are working in collaboration with a physician under state-approved protocols.[10] Plan B One-Step is a progestin-only pill that should be taken as soon as possible (but not later than 72 hours or 3 days) after unprotected intercourse. Next Choice is a generic equivalent of Plan B.

The newest ECP, ella, was approved by the FDA in August 2010. Unlike Plan B One-Step or Next Choice, ella is only available by prescription. A progesterone receptor modulator, ella works by inhibiting or preventing ovulation. It can prevent pregnancy when taken up to 120 hours (5 days) after unprotected intercourse.

emergency contraceptive pills (ECPs) Drugs taken within 3 to 5 days after unprotected intercourse to prevent fertilization or implantation.

withdrawal Contraceptive method that involves withdrawing the penis from the vagina before ejaculation; also called *coitus interruptus.*

Widespread availability of emergency contraception has the potential to significantly affect the rates of unintended pregnancies and abortions, particularly among young women. Although ECPs are no substitute for taking proper precautions before having sex (such as using a condom), their potential for reducing the rate of unintended pregnancy, and ultimately abortion, is very strong. According to a recent national survey, 16 percent of sexually active college students reported using emergency contraception within the past year (or reported their partner had used it).[11]

Behavioral Methods

Some methods of contraception rely on one or both partners altering their sexual behavior. In general, these methods require more self-control, diligence, and commitment, making them more prone to user error than hormonal and barrier methods.

Withdrawal

Withdrawal, also called *coitus interruptus,* involves removing the penis from the vagina just before ejaculation. In the 2011 American College Health Association's National College Health Assessment (ACHA-NCHA), 26.6 percent of respondents reported that withdrawal was their method of birth control the last time they had sexual intercourse.[12] This statistic is startlingly high, considering the very high risk of

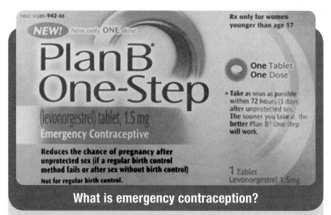

What is emergency contraception?

Emergency contraception involves the use of hormone-containing pills or an IUD after an act of unprotected intercourse. Plan B One-Step and Next Choice are the two brands of emergency contraceptive pills currently available without a prescription to American consumers age 17 or older. When taken within 120 hours of unprotected intercourse, they reduce the risk of pregnancy by 89%.

fertility awareness methods (FAMs) Several types of birth control that require alteration of sexual behavior rather than chemical or physical intervention in the reproductive process.

basal body temperature The lowest temperature the body reaches, usually during sleep.

pregnancy and contracting an STI associated with this method of birth control.

Advantages and Disadvantages Although withdrawal can be practiced when there is absolutely no other contraceptive available, it is highly unreliable, even with "perfect" use, because there are a half million sperm in just the drop of preejaculate fluid released *before* ejaculation. Timing withdrawal is also difficult, and males concentrating on accurate timing may not be able to relax and enjoy intercourse. Withdrawal offers no protection against STIs and requires a high degree of self-control, experience, and trust.

Abstinence and "Outercourse"

Strictly defined, *abstinence* means "deliberately avoiding intercourse." This definition would allow one to engage in forms of sexual intimacy such as massage, kissing, and masturbation. Couples who go beyond fondling and kissing to activities such as oral sex and mutual masturbation, but not vaginal or anal sex, are sometimes said to be engaging in "outercourse."

Advantages and Disadvantages Abstinence is the only method of avoiding pregnancy that is 100 percent effective. It is also the only method that is 100 percent effective against transmitting disease. Like abstinence, outercourse can be 100 percent effective for birth control as long as the male does not ejaculate near the vaginal opening. Unlike abstinence, however, outercourse is not 100 percent effective against STIs. Oral–genital contact can transmit disease, although the practice can be made safer by using a condom on the penis or a latex barrier, such as a dental dam, on the vaginal opening. Both abstinence and outercourse may be difficult for couples to sustain over long periods of time.

Fertility Awareness Methods

Fertility awareness methods (FAMs) of birth control rely on altering sexual behavior during certain times of the month (Figure 6.4). These techniques require observing female fertile periods and abstaining from sexual intercourse (or any penis–vagina contact) during these times.

Fertility awareness methods rely on knowledge of basic physiology. A released ovum can survive for up to 48 hours after ovulation. Sperm can live for as long as 5 days in the vagina. Natural methods of birth control help women to recognize their fertile times. Some of the more common forms include the following:

- **Cervical mucus method.** This method requires women to examine the consistency and color of their normal vaginal secretions. Prior to ovulation, vaginal mucus becomes slippery, thin, and stretchy, and normal vaginal secretions may

increase. To prevent pregnancy, partners must avoid sexual activity involving penis–vagina contact while this mucus is present and for several days afterward.

- **Body temperature method.** This method relies on the fact that a woman's **basal body temperature** rises between 0.4 and 0.8 degree after ovulation has occurred. For this method to be effective, a woman must chart her temperature for several months to learn to recognize her body's temperature fluctuations. To prevent pregnancy, partners must abstain from penis–vagina contact before the temperature rise until several days after the temperature rise is observed.
- **Calendar method.** This method requires the woman to record the exact number of days in her menstrual cycle. Because few women menstruate with complete regularity, this method involves keeping a record of the menstrual cycle for 12 months, during which time some other method of birth control must be used. This method assumes that ovulation occurs during the midpoint of the cycle. To prevent pregnancy, the couple must abstain from penis–vagina contact during the fertile time.

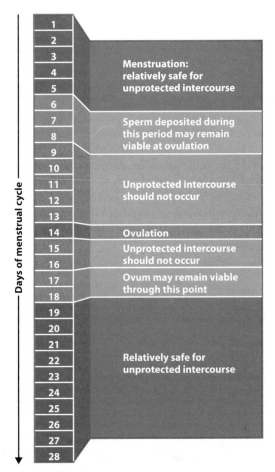

FIGURE 6.4 The Fertility Cycle
Fertility awareness methods (FAMs) can combine the use of a calendar, the cervical mucus method, and body temperature measurements to identify the fertile period. It is important to remember that most women do not have a consistent 28-day cycle.

Advantages and Disadvantages Fertility awareness methods are the only forms of birth control that comply with certain religious teachings, including those of the Roman Catholic Church. They don't require a medical visit or prescription, and there are no negative health effects. Women who are untrained in these techniques run a high risk of unintended pregnancy; anyone interested in using them is advised to take a class. Free classes are often offered by health centers and churches, and there is only minimal expense for supplies. The effectiveness of fertility awareness methods depends on diligence, commitment, and self-discipline; they are only 75 percent effective with typical use. These methods offer no STI protection, and they may not work for women with irregular menstrual cycles.

Surgical Methods

In the United States, **sterilization** has become the second leading method of contraception for women of all ages and the leading method of contraception among married women and women over age 35.[13] Because sterilization is permanent, anyone considering it should think through possibilities such as divorce and remarriage or a future improvement in financial status that might make pregnancy realistic or desirable.

Female Sterilization

One method of sterilization for women is **tubal ligation,** a surgical procedure in which the fallopian tubes are sealed shut to block the sperm's access to released eggs (see Figure 6.5). The operation is usually done laparoscopically on an outpatient basis. The procedure usually takes less than an hour, and the patient is usually allowed to return home within a short time.

A tubal ligation does not affect ovarian and uterine function. The woman's menstrual cycle continues, and released eggs simply disintegrate and are absorbed by the lymphatic system. As soon as her incision heals, the woman may resume sexual intercourse with no fear of pregnancy.

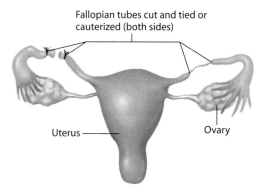

Fallopian tubes cut and tied or cauterized (both sides)

Uterus

Ovary

FIGURE 6.5 **Female Sterilization: Tubal Ligation**
In a tubal ligation, both fallopian tubes are cut and tied or sealed shut. This surgery is usually performed laparoscopically.

A newer sterilization procedure, Essure, involves the placement of small microcoils into the fallopian tubes via the vagina. The entire procedure takes about 35 minutes and can be performed in a physician's office. Once in place, the microcoils expand to the shape of the fallopian tubes. The coils promote the growth of scar tissue around the device and lead to a blockage in the fallopian tubes. Like traditional forms of tubal ligation, Essure is permanent. It is recommended for women who cannot have a tubal ligation because of chronic health conditions such as obesity or heart disease.

Adiana is another minimally invasive method of blocking a woman's fallopian tubes. A small flexible instrument is used to place a soft insert about the size of a grain of rice into each fallopian tube. The body's tissue begins to grow on and around the insert and eventually blocks the fallopian tubes. The insertion can be performed in a clinician's office in about 15 minutes.

A **hysterectomy,** or removal of the uterus, is a method of sterilization requiring major surgery. It is usually done only when a woman's uterus is diseased or damaged.

Advantages The main advantage to female sterilization is that it is highly effective and permanent. After the one-time expense of the procedure, there is no other cost or ongoing action required. Sterilization has no negative effect on a woman's sex drive. A potential advantage of the Essure and Adiana methods is that they do not require an incision.

Disadvantages As with any surgery, there are risks involved with a tubal ligation. Although rare, possible complications include infection, pulmonary embolism, hemorrhage, anesthesia complications, and ectopic pregnancy. Essure and Adiana do not require an incision, so the immediate risks are lower; however, because these are relatively new techniques, the long-term risks are unknown. Sterilization offers no protection against STIs, and it is initially expensive. The procedure is permanent and should be used only if both partners are certain they do not want more children.

Male Sterilization

Sterilization in men is less complicated than it is in women. A **vasectomy** is frequently done on an outpatient basis, using a local anesthetic (see Figure 6.6 on page 178). This procedure involves making a small incision in the side of the scrotum to expose a vas deferens, cutting the vas deferens and either tying off or cauterizing the ends, then repeating the procedure on the other side.

Many men are reluctant to consider sterilization because they fear the operation will affect their sexual performance. However, a vasectomy in no way affects sexual response. Because sperm constitute only a small part (about 2%) of the semen, the amount of ejaculate is not changed significantly.

sterilization Permanent fertility control achieved through surgical procedures.
tubal ligation Sterilization of a woman that involves cutting and tying off or cauterizing the fallopian tubes.
hysterectomy Surgical removal of the uterus.
vasectomy Male sterilization procedure that involves cutting and tying off of the vasa deferentia.

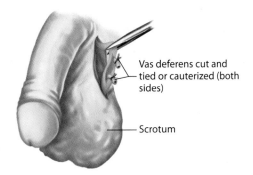

Vas deferens cut and
tied or cauterized (both
sides)

Scrotum

FIGURE 6.6 **Male Sterilization: Vasectomy**
In a vasectomy, the surgeon makes an incision in the
scrotum, then locates and cuts the vasa deferentia, either
sealing or tying both sides shut.

The testes continue to produce sperm, but the sperm can no longer enter the ejaculatory duct. Any sperm that are manufactured disintegrate and are absorbed into the lymphatic system.

Advantages A vasectomy is a highly effective and permanent means of preventing pregnancy. After 1 year, the pregnancy rate in women whose partners have had vasectomies is 0.15 percent.[14] A vasectomy is a fairly simple outpatient procedure requiring minimal recovery time, and after the one-time expense, there is no other cost or ongoing action required. A vasectomy has no negative effect on a man's sex drive or sexual performance.

Disadvantages In addition to its initial expense, male sterilization offers no protection against STI transmission. Also, a vasectomy is not immediately effective in preventing pregnancy. Because sperm are stored in other areas of the reproductive system besides the vasa deferentia, couples must use alternative birth control methods for at least 1 month after the vasectomy. The man must check with his physician (who will do a semen analysis) to determine when unprotected intercourse can take place. As with any surgery, there are some risks involved with a vasectomy. In a small percentage of cases, serious complications occur, such as formation of a blood clot in the scrotum, infection, or inflammatory reactions. Very infrequently the vas deferens may create a new path, negating the procedure.

Choosing a Method of Contraception

With all the options available, how does a person or a couple decide what method of contraception is best? Take some time to research the various methods, ask questions of your health care provider, and be honest with yourself about your own preferences. Questions to ask yourself are included below. Also, see the two **Student Health Today** boxes: one for tips on talking about contraception with your partner on page 179 and the other on men's involvement in making choices about contraception on page 180.

- **How comfortable would I be using a particular method?** If you aren't at ease with a method, you may not use it consistently, and it probably will not be a reliable choice for you. Think about whether the method may cause discomfort for you or your partner and consider your own comfort level with touching your body. For women, some methods, such as the diaphragm, sponge, or NuvaRing, require inserting a device into the vagina and taking it out. For men, using a condom requires rolling it onto the penis.
- **Will this method be convenient for me and my partner?** Some methods require more effort than others. Be honest with yourself about how likely you are to use the method consistently. Are you willing to interrupt lovemaking, to abstain from sex during certain times of the month, or to take a pill at the same time every day? You may feel condoms are easy and convenient to use, or you may prefer something that requires little ongoing thought, such as an IUD or an implant.
- **Am I at risk for the transmission of STIs?** If you have multiple sex partners or are uncertain about the sexual history or disease status of your current sex partner, then you are at risk of contracting HIV or other STIs. Condoms (male and female) are the *only* birth control method that protects against STIs and HIV (although some other barrier methods offer limited protection).
- **Do I want to have a biological child in the future?** If you are unsure about your plans for future childbearing, you should use a temporary birth control method rather than a permanent one such as sterilization. Keep in mind that you may regret choosing a permanent method if you are young, if you have few or no children, if you are choosing this method because you feel pressured by your partner, or if you believe this option will fix relationship problems. If you know you want to have children in the future, consider how soon that will be, as some methods, such as Depo-Provera, will cause a delay in return to fertility.
- **How would an unplanned pregnancy affect my life?** If an unplanned pregnancy would be a potentially devastating event for you or would have a serious impact on your plans for the future, then you should choose a highly effective birth control method, for example, the pill, patch, ring, implant, or IUD. If, however, you are in a stable relationship, have a reliable source of income, are planning to have children in the future, and would embrace a pregnancy should it occur now, then you may be comfortable with a less reliable method, such as the diaphragm, cervical cap, or spermicides.
- **What are my religious and moral values?** If your beliefs prevent you from considering other birth control methods, fertility awareness methods are a good option. When both partners are motivated to use these methods, they can be successful at preventing unintended pregnancy. If you are considering this option, sign up for a class to get specific training for using the method effectively.
- **How much will the birth control method cost?** Some contraceptive methods involve an initial outlay of money and few

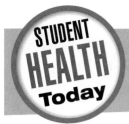

STUDENT HEALTH Today

LET'S TALK ABOUT (SAFER) SEX!

Communication is key to a healthy relationship, especially for those who are sexually intimate. It can be challenging to talk to your partner about using protection, but don't let embarrassment put your health at risk. The person that you're thinking about having sex with may or may not initially agree about using a condom or dental dam, so it's helpful to be prepared to discuss your concerns ahead of time. Research shows that individuals who set aside the time to have a conversation about safer sex are more likely to use condoms or dental dams. Remember: Communicating about sex is all about getting the most from your sex life and doing so safely.

WHY COMMUNICATING ABOUT SEX IS ESSENTIAL

Open communication about sexual health is a sign of care and respect for your own body and your partner's. It empowers both of you to be assertive about your needs, likes, limits, and desires in the sexual relationship. Open communication also creates a safe environment to ask about your partner's sexual history, STI testing, and expectations.

You may feel awkward or uncomfortable discussing sex, and you may believe that talking beforehand ruins spontaneity. Some people are concerned that their partner will misinterpret the conversation and feel accused of infidelity, promiscuity, or lack of love in the relationship. Try to address these concerns in an honest and open manner. And remember: Sexual communication is about protecting *both* of you and ensuring that you are clear about your needs and concerns.

If you are afraid that talking about sex beforehand is going to make your partner think you don't trust him or her, take some time to examine the strength of your relationship. Trust is about being open and honest. If you're afraid to talk with your partner, is it possible that you lack trust in him or her? If so, you might want to examine if this is a healthy relationship for you.

FINDING THE TIME AND PLACE FOR SEXUAL COMMUNICATION

Before you talk with your partner, it's a good idea to talk with your health care provider about your options for practicing safer sex. Remember, you need to think about preventing pregnancy *and* avoiding STIs.

Find a convenient time and a place where you are both comfortable and free of distractions. It's generally better to have this conversation outside of the bedroom, so that you're not pressured by the heat of the moment to do things you don't want to do.

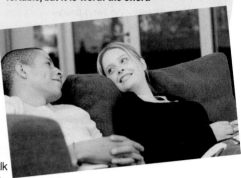

Don't let embarrassment put your health at risk! Talking about safer sex may be uncomfortable, but it is worth the effort.

FINDING THE WORDS FOR CONDOM/ DENTAL DAM NEGOTIATION

The table below lists some examples of how you can address potential excuses from your partner when you talk about using a condom or dental dam. While there is no perfect response for every situation, these may provide some helpful suggestions.

TIPS TO BOOST YOUR CONFIDENCE IN NEGOTIATING SAFER SEX

✳ Keep condoms and/or dental dams on hand, so when things start to heat up you will be ready.

✳ Practice makes perfect. The best way to learn how to use condoms correctly and guarantee their effectiveness is to practice putting them on yourself or your partner. A staggering 98 percent of all "condom malfunctions" (breaks, leaks, tears, slips) are due to user error. Consistency and correct use are the essential keys to successful condom usage.

✳ If you are concerned about the interruption factor, try to incorporate condoms or dental dams into foreplay; by doing this together, you both will stay aroused and in the moment.

Sources: M. K. Casey, L. Timmermann, M. Allen, S. Krahn, and K. L. Turkiewicz, "Response and Self-Efficacy in Condom Use: A Meta-Analysis of This Important Element of AIDS Education and Prevention," *Southern Communication Journal* 74, no. 1 (2009): 57–78; A. G. Lam, A. Mak, P. D. Lindsay, and S. T. Russell, "What Really Works? An Exploratory Study of Condom Negotiation Strategies," *AIDS Education and Prevention* 16, no. 2 (2004): 160–71.

Excuse	Response
Don't you trust me?	It's not an issue of trust; people can have sexually transmitted infections and not know it.
It doesn't feel as good with a condom/dental dam.	I'll feel more relaxed; if I'm more relaxed, I can make it feel better for you. We can also use lubricant to increase sensation for both of us.
I don't have a condom with me.	I do.
It's up to you.	It's your health. It should be your decision, too.
I'm on the pill; you don't need a condom.	I'd like to use one anyway. It will help to protect us from infections that we may not know we have.
Putting it on interrupts everything.	Not if I help put it on.
I guess you don't really love me.	I do, but I'm not willing to risk our futures to prove it.
I will pull out in time.	Preejaculate can still cause pregnancy and spread STIs.
I'm allergic to latex.	No problem, Student Health Services has a selection of nonlatex condoms and dental dams that we can get for free.
But I love you.	Then you'll help us protect ourselves.
Just this once.	Once is all it takes.

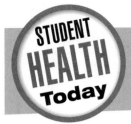
How Can Men Be More Involved in Birth Control?

The sexual health needs of young men have been largely overlooked in the field of reproductive health. Much of the focus on preventing teen pregnancy, sexually transmitted infections (STIs), and HIV/AIDS has been directed at young women.

On college campuses and in student health centers, the emphasis is also usually on women, leading to missed opportunities to emphasize the importance of *shared* responsibility for sexual health.

There are many reasons for the disparity: Men seek health care less often; it is sometimes incorrectly assumed that men are not interested in sexual health issues; and since women carry the baby, they are often seen as having a bigger stake in pregnancy prevention. However,

Some men are more comfortable discussing reproductive health issues with male clinicians.

healthy sexual relationships and ongoing reproductive health require that both partners be stakeholders. So, how can men be more involved in responsible sexual decision making?

✱ Initiate discussions with your partner about contraception and your sexual health histories.

✱ Take an active role in discussing and deciding what type of contraception is best for you and your partner.

✱ Buy and use condoms every time you have sex.

✱ Help pay for contraceptive costs.

✱ If an unintended pregnancy occurs, share in the responsibility and decision making about the best way to handle the situation.

---

continuing costs (e.g., sterilization, IUD), whereas others are fairly inexpensive but must be purchased repeatedly (e.g., condoms, spermicides, monthly pills). You should consider whether a method will be cost-effective for you in the long run. Remember that any prescription methods require routine checkups, which may involve some cost to you.

● **Do I have any health factors that could limit my choice?** Hormonal birth control methods can pose potential health risks to women with certain preexisting conditions, such as high blood pressure, a history of stroke or blood clots, liver disease, migraines, or diabetes. You should discuss this issue with your health care provider when considering birth control methods. In addition, women who smoke or are over age 35 are at risk from complications of combination hormonal contraceptives. Breast-feeding women can use progestin-only methods, but should avoid methods containing estrogen. Men and women with latex allergies can use barrier methods made of polyurethane or silicone.

● **Are there any additional benefits I'd like from my** contraceptive? Hormonal birth control methods may have desirable secondary effects, such as the reduction of acne or the lessening of premenstrual symptoms. Some hormonal birth control methods have been associated with reduced risks of certain cancers. Extended-cycle pills and some progestin-only methods cause menstrual periods to be less frequent or to stop altogether, which some women find desirable. Condoms carry the added health benefit of protecting against STIs.

Abortion

Women obtain abortions for a variety of reasons. The vast majority of abortions occur because of unintended pregnancies.[15] As we know, even the best birth control methods can fail. In addition, some pregnancies are terminated because they are a consequence of rape or incest. Other reasons commonly cited are not being ready financially or emotionally to care for a child.[16] When an unintended pregnancy does occur, a woman must decide whether to terminate the pregnancy, carry it to term and keep the baby, or carry it to term and give the baby up for adoption. This is a personal decision that each woman must make based on her personal beliefs, values, and resources and after carefully considering all alternatives.

In 1973, the landmark U.S. Supreme Court decision in *Roe v. Wade* stated that the "right to privacy . . . founded on the

---

what do you think?

Who do you think is responsible for deciding which method of contraception should be used in a sexual relationship?

● What are some examples of good opportunities for you and your partner to discuss contraceptives?

● What do you think are the biggest barriers in our society to the use of condoms?

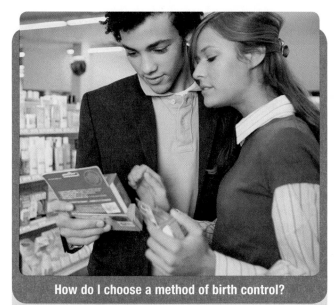

How do I choose a method of birth control?

There are many different methods of birth control on the market: barrier methods, hormonal methods, and other options (including surgery as a permanent option). When you choose a method, you'll need to consider several factors, including cost, comfort level, convenience, and health risks. All of these factors will influence your ability to consistently and correctly use the contraceptive and prevent unwanted pregnancy.

Fourteenth Amendment's concept of personal liberty . . . is broad enough to encompass a woman's decision whether or not to terminate her pregnancy."[17] The decision maintained that during the first trimester of pregnancy a woman and her health care provider have the right to terminate the pregnancy through **abortion** without legal restrictions. It allowed individual states to set conditions for second-trimester abortions. Third-trimester abortions were ruled illegal unless the mother's life or health was in danger. Prior to the legalization of first- and second-trimester abortions, women wishing to terminate a pregnancy had to travel to a country where the procedure was legal, consult an illegal abortionist, or perform their own abortions. These procedures sometimes led to death from hemorrhage or infection or infertility from internal scarring.

The Abortion Debate

Abortion is a highly charged and politically thorny issue in American society. In a recent poll, 26 percent of the population felt that abortion should be legal under any circumstances, 20 percent thought it should be illegal in all circumstances, and 51 percent thought it should be legal in some situations.[18] Pro-choice individuals feel that it is a woman's right to make decisions about her own body and health, including the decision to continue or terminate a pregnancy. On the other side of the issue, pro-life individuals believe that the embryo or fetus is a human being with rights that must be protected. The political debate contin-

ues as pro-life groups lobby for laws prohibiting the use of public funds for abortion and abortion counseling while pro-choice groups lobby for laws that make abortions more widely available. At times, violence has arisen as a result of this controversy in the form of attacks on clinics or on individual physicians who perform abortions.

In the past few years, new legislation has given states the right to impose certain restrictions on abortions. The procedure cannot be performed in publicly funded clinics in some states, and other states have laws requiring parental notification before a teenager can obtain an abortion. Ninety-two new abortion restrictions were passed 2011, shattering the previous record of 34 in 2005. Five states also recently passed restrictions banning abortion after the twentieth week, three states adopted waiting periods for women seeking abortions, five states adopted mandatory ultrasound provisions, and seven states limited the provision of medication abortions by prohibiting the use of telemedicine for patient counseling.[19]

At the federal level, the U.S. Congress has banned access to abortion for virtually all women who receive health care through the federal government. Since the Federal Abortion Ban was signed in 2003, it has been challenged by the American Civil Liberties Union (ACLU), the National Abortion Federation, Planned Parenthood, and the Center for Reproductive Rights in federal courts across the country on the grounds that it is unconstitutional. The two main reasons for these claims are that the broad language could ban abortion as early as the twelfth week in pregnancy and that it does not include exceptions to protect women's health.[20] The U.S. Supreme Court struck down an identical law as unconstitutional in 2000, and the ban was found unconstitutional by six federal courts before the Supreme Court ruled in 2007 that the ban was constitutional and could be enforced.[21] This decision represented a monumental departure from prior cases, and with it the Court effectively eliminated one of *Roe v. Wade*'s core protections: that a woman's health must always be paramount. For a discussion of how contraception and abortion are perceived in various countries, see the **Health in a Diverse World** box on the next page.

> **abortion** Termination of a pregnancy by expulsion or removal of an embryo or fetus from the uterus.

51%

of pregnancies that occur each year are unintended.

Emotional Aspects of Abortion

The best scientific evidence available indicates that among adult women who have an unplanned pregnancy, the risk of mental health problems is no greater if they have an abortion than if they deliver a baby. Although a variety of feelings such

CONTRACEPTIVE USE AND THE INCIDENCE OF ABORTION WORLDWIDE

Approximately 208 million pregnancies occur throughout the world every year, more than a third of which are unintended. Worldwide, about one-fifth of all pregnancies end in induced abortion, although reports have indicated a decline in the overall number of abortions in recent decades. This decline has been greater in developed nations than it has been in developing countries. In developed nations, where almost all abortions are safe and legal, the incidence of the procedure dropped from 39 per 1,000 women age 15 to 44 in 1995 to 24 per 1,000 women age 15 to 44 in 2008. In developing nations, the rate declined from 34 to 29 in the same period of time. The world's population is largely concentrated in developing nations, and, consequently, most abortions occur in those countries—38 million annually—often in places where abortion is illegal and access to contraception is limited.

The primary cause of abortion is unplanned pregnancy. Whether abortion is legal or not has little to do with its overall incidence. The abortion rate in Africa, where abortion is illegal in most countries, is higher than the rate in Europe, where abortion is generally legal. Illegal abortions are usually unsafe; nearly

50,000 women die of complications from unsafe abortions each year, nearly all in developing nations where abortion is illegal. Worldwide, 49 percent of all abortions are unsafe; however, only 8 percent of abortions in developed nations are unsafe, compared to 55 percent in developing nations.

When abortion is legalized, it also becomes safer. For example, after expanding the legalization of abortion in 1996, South Africa experienced a 52 percent reduction in the incidence of infections resulting from abortion. The general global trend is to remove legal restrictions on abortion: Since 1995, 17 countries have liberalized their abortion laws, compared to only 3 countries that have tightened them.

Access to voluntary family planning services, including contraception, is essential in helping to reduce the number of unintended pregnancies and the incidence of abortion. When modern contraceptives are unavailable, women often turn to abortion to end an unwanted pregnancy. Countries where contraceptive use is most prevalent usually have lower abortion rates.

The lowest abortion rates are in western Europe, where abortion is legal and contraceptives are widely accepted

and available at low cost. In eastern Europe and the former Soviet Union, abortion rates were high during the Cold War years, when the procedure was free and was the only reliable method of fertility control available to most women. Modern contraceptives manufactured in the West were not available until the fall of the Soviet Union. Since that time, contraceptives have become prevalent in eastern Europe and the former Soviet bloc countries, such that the abortion rate dropped 50 percent between 1995 and 2003. However, because of economic pressure to keep families small, the ratio of abortions to live births in eastern Europe is still the highest in the world: 105 abortions for every 100 live births.

Sources: Guttmacher Institute and WHO, "In Brief: Facts on Induced Abortion Worldwide," 2012, www.guttmacher.org/pubs/fb_IAW.html; S. Cohen, "Facts and Consequences: Legality, Incidence and Safety of Abortion Worldwide," *Guttmacher Policy Review* 12, no. 4 (2009); S. Cohen, "New Data on Abortion Incidence, Safety Illuminate Key Aspects of Worldwide Abortion Rate," *Guttmacher Policy Review* 10, no. 4 (2007); G. Sedgh et al., "Legal Abortions Worldwide: Incidence and Recent Trends," *International Family Planning Perspectives* 33, no. 3 (2007).

as regret, guilt, sadness, relief, and happiness are normal, no evidence has shown that an abortion causes long-term negative mental health outcomes.[22] Researchers found that the best predictor of a woman's emotional well-being following an abortion was her emotional well-being prior to the procedure.[23] The factors that place a woman at higher risk for negative psychological responses following an abortion include the following: perception of stigma, need for secrecy, low levels of social support for the abortion decision, prior history of mental health issues, low self-esteem, and avoidance and denial coping strategies.[24] The majority of women who have an abortion are able to view an abortion in context as one of life's events. Certainly the presence of a support network and the assistance of mental health professionals are

helpful to any woman who is struggling with the emotional aspects of her abortion decision.

Methods of Abortion

The choice of abortion procedure is determined by how many weeks the woman has been pregnant. Length of pregnancy is calculated from the first day of her last menstrual period.

Surgical Abortions The majority of abortions performed in the United States today are surgical. If performed during the first trimester, abortion presents a relatively low health risk to the mother. About 88 percent of abortions occur

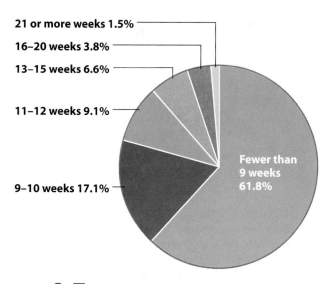

21 or more weeks 1.5%

16–20 weeks 3.8%

13–15 weeks 6.6%

11–12 weeks 9.1%

9–10 weeks 17.1%

Fewer than 9 weeks 61.8%

FIGURE 6.7 **When Women Have Abortions (in weeks from the last menstrual period)**

Source: Guttmacher Institute, *Facts on Induced Abortion in the United States*, New York: Guttmacher Institute, 2011, www.guttmacher.org/pubs/fb_induced_abortion.html, Accessed February 15, 2012.

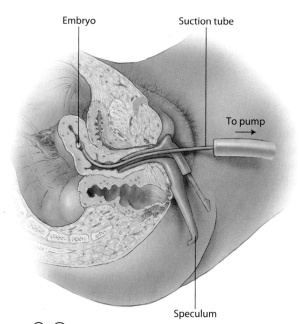

Embryo   Suction tube

To pump →

Speculum

FIGURE 6.8 **Suction Curettage Abortion**
This procedure, in which a long tube with gentle suction is used to remove fetal tissue from the uterine walls, can be performed until the twelfth week of pregnancy.

during the first 12 weeks of pregnancy (see Figure 6.7).[25] The most commonly used method of first-trimester abortion is **suction curettage** (also called vacuum aspiration) (Figure 6.8). The vast majority of abortions in the United States are done using this procedure, which is usually performed under local anesthesia. The cervix is dilated with instruments or by placing laminaria, a sterile seaweed product, in the cervical canal. The laminaria is left in place for a few hours or overnight and slowly dilates the cervix. After it is removed, a long tube is inserted through the cervix and into the uterus, and gentle suction removes fetal tissue from the uterine walls.

Pregnancies that progress into the second trimester (after week 12) can be terminated through **dilation and evacuation (D&E).** For this procedure, the cervix is dilated for 1 to 2 days, and a combination of instruments and vacuum aspiration is used to empty the uterus. Second-trimester abortions may be done under general anesthesia. The D&E can be performed on an outpatient basis (usually in a physician's office), with or without pain medication. Generally, however, the woman is given a mild tranquilizer to help her relax. This procedure may cause moderate to severe uterine cramping and blood loss. After a D&E, a return visit to the clinician is an important follow-up.

Two other methods used in second-trimester abortions, less common than D&E, are prostaglandin and saline **induction abortions**. Prostaglandin hormones or saline solution are injected into the uterus, which kills the fetus and initiates labor contractions. After 24 to 48 hours, the fetus and placenta are expelled from the uterus. A **hysterotomy,** or surgical removal of the fetus from the uterus, may be used during emergencies, when the mother's life is in danger, or when other types of abortions are deemed too dangerous.

One surgical method that abortion opponents specifically oppose is **intact dilation and extraction (D&X)**, sometimes referred to by the nonmedical term *partial-birth abortion*. The dilation and extraction procedure is used after 21 weeks of gestation. This procedure is rarely performed but is considered when other abortion methods could injure the mother and when there are severe fetal abnormalities. Two days before the procedure, laminaria is inserted vaginally to dilate the cervix. The woman's water should break on the third day, and she then returns to the clinic. The fetus is rotated to a breech (feet first) position, and forceps are used to pull the legs, shoulders, and arms through the birth canal. The head is collapsed to allow it to pass through the cervix. Then the fetus is completely removed.

The risks associated with surgical abortion include infection, incomplete abortion (when parts of the placenta remain in the uterus), excessive bleeding, and cervical and uterine trauma. Follow-up and attention to danger signs decrease the chances of long-term problems.

The mortality rate for women undergoing first-trimester abortions in the United States averages 1 death per every 1,000,000 procedures at 8 or fewer weeks. The risk of death increases with the length of pregnancy. At 16 to

suction curettage Abortion technique that uses gentle suction to remove fetal tissue from the uterus.

dilation and evacuation (D&E) Abortion technique that uses a combination of instruments and vacuum aspiration; fetal tissue is both sucked and scraped out of the uterus.

induction abortions Abortion technique in which chemicals are injected into the uterus through the uterine wall; labor begins, and the woman delivers a dead fetus.

hysterotomy Surgical removal of the fetus from the uterus.

intact dilation and extraction (D&X) Late-term abortion procedure in which the body of the fetus is extracted up to the head and then the contents of the cranium are aspirated.

20 weeks, the mortality rate is 1 per 29,000; at 21 weeks or more, it increases to 1 per 11,000.[26] This higher rate later in the pregnancy is due to the increased risk of uterine perforation, bleeding, infection, and incomplete abortion; these complications occur because the uterine wall becomes thinner as the pregnancy progresses.

Medical Abortions Unlike surgical abortions, a **medical abortion** (also called medication abortion) is performed without entering the uterus. Mifepristone, formerly known as RU-486 and currently sold in the United States under the brand name Mifeprex, is a steroid hormone that induces abortion by blocking the action of progesterone, the hormone produced by the ovaries and placenta that maintains the uterine lining. As a result, the lining and embryo are expelled from the uterus, terminating the pregnancy.

Mifepristone's nickname, "the abortion pill," may imply an easy process; however, this treatment actually involves more steps than a suction curettage abortion, which takes approximately 15 minutes followed by a physical recovery of about 1 day. With mifepristone, an initial visit to the clinic involves a physical exam and a dose of three tablets, which may cause minor side effects such as nausea, headaches, weakness, and fatigue. The patient returns 2 days later for a dose of prostaglandins (misoprostol; brand name Cytotec), which causes uterine contractions that expel the fertilized egg. The patient is required to stay under observation at the clinic for 4 hours and to make a follow-up visit 12 days later.[27]

Ninety-two percent of women who use mifepristone during the first 9 weeks of pregnancy will experience a complete abortion.[28] The side effects are similar to those reported during heavy menstruation and include cramping, minor pain, and nausea. Approximately 1 in 1,000 women requires a blood transfusion because of severe bleeding. The procedure does not require hospitalization; women may be treated on an outpatient basis.

medical abortion Termination of a pregnancy during the first 9 weeks using hormonal medications that cause the embryo to be expelled from the uterus.

preconception care Medical care received prior to becoming pregnant that helps a woman assess and address potential health issues.

Planning for Pregnancy as Well as for Parenthood

The many methods available to control fertility give you choices that did not exist when your parents—and even you—were born. If you are in the process of deciding whether or not to have children, take the time to evaluate your emotions, finances, and physical health.

Emotional Health

First and foremost, consider why you want to have a child. To fulfill an inner need to carry on the family? Because it's expected? Other reasons? Then, consider the responsibilities involved with becoming a parent. Are you ready to make all the sacrifices necessary to bear and raise a child? Can you care for this new human being in a loving and nurturing manner?

If you feel that you are ready to be a parent, the next step is preparation. You can prepare for this change in your life in several ways: Read about parenthood, take classes, talk to parents of children of all ages, spend time with friends' children, and join a support group. If you choose to adopt, you will find many support groups available to you as well.

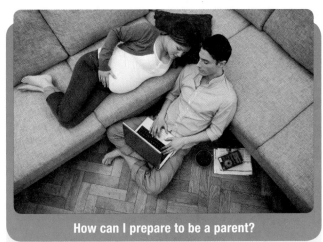

How can I prepare to be a parent?

Preparing to become a parent requires thoughtful evaluation of one's emotional, physical, social, and financial well-being. Both prospective mothers and prospective fathers should be willing to implement healthy change where needed to ready themselves for bringing a child into the world.

Maternal Health

Before becoming pregnant, a woman should have a thorough medical examination. **Preconception care** should include an assessment of potential complications that could occur during pregnancy. Medical problems such as diabetes and high blood pressure should be discussed, as well as any genetic disorders that run in the family. For suggestions on preparing for a healthy pregnancy, see the **Skills for Behavior Change** box on the following page.

Paternal Health

It is common knowledge that mothers-to-be should steer clear of toxic chemicals that can cause birth defects, should eat a healthy diet, and should stop smoking and drinking alcohol. Now, similar precautions are recommended for fathers-to-be. New research suggests that a man's exposure to chemicals influences not only his ability to father a child, but also the health of his future child as well.

Fathers-to-be have been overlooked in past preconception and prenatal studies for several reasons. Researchers assumed that the genetic damage leading to birth defects and other health problems occurred while a child was in the mother's womb or were caused by random errors of nature. However, it now appears that some disorders can be traced to sperm damaged by chemicals. Sperm are naturally vulnerable to toxic assault and genetic damage. Many drugs and ingested chemicals can readily invade the testes from the bloodstream; others ambush sperm after they leave the testes and pass through the epididymides, where they mature and are stored. By one route or another, half of 100 chemicals studied so far (including by-products of cigarette smoke) apparently harm sperm.[29] Chemical exposure can reduce the number of sperm, the sperms' ability to fertilize and egg, cause miscarriage, or cause health problems in the baby.

Financial Evaluation

Finances are another important consideration. Are you prepared to go out to dinner less often, forgo a new pair of shoes, or drive an older car? These are important questions to ask when considering the financial aspects of being a parent. Can you afford to give your child the life you would like him or her to enjoy?

First, check your medical insurance: Does it provide maternity benefits? If not, you can expect to pay, on average,

$14,000 for a normal delivery and up to $25,000 for a cesarean section. These costs don't include prenatal medical care, and complications can also increase the cost substantially. Both partners should investigate their employers' policies concerning parental leave, including length of leave available and conditions for returning to work.

The U.S. Department of Agriculture estimates that it will cost an average of $226,920 to raise a child born in 2010 to age 18 (housing costs and food are the two largest expenditures).[30] And these figures do not include college tuition, which currently averages about $8,000 per year for a state school and nearly $35,000 per year at a private institution, not including room and board.[31] When planning for children, potential parents must also consider the cost and availability of quality child care. How much family assistance can you realistically expect with a new baby, and is nonfamily child care available? Quality child care is expensive, although prices vary by region and type of care. According to the National Association of Child Care Resource and Referral Agencies (NAC-CRRA), full-time child care costs for an infant range from $4,650 in Mississippi to $18,200 a year in Washington, D.C.[32]

what do you think?

Have you thought about whether and when to have children?
● Is there a certain age at which you feel you will be ready to be a parent? ● What goals do you hope to achieve before undertaking parenthood? ● What are your biggest concerns about parenthood?

Contingency Planning

A final consideration is how to provide for your child should something happen to you and your partner. If both of you were to die, do you have relatives or close friends who could raise your child? If you have more than one child, would they have to be split up or could they be kept together? Although unpleasant to think about, this sort of contingency planning is crucial. Children who lose their parents are heartbroken and confused. A prearranged plan of action can smooth their transition into new families; without one, a judge will usually decide who will raise them.

Pregnancy

Pregnancy is an important event in a woman's life. The actions taken before as well as behaviors engaged in during pregnancy can significantly affect the health of both infant and mother.

Preconception Care

Every woman should be thinking about her health whether or not she is planning a pregnancy. The birth of a healthy baby depends in part on the mother's preconception health. Preconception health focuses on the conditions and risk factors that could affect a woman if she becomes pregnant.

Skills for Behavior Change

Preparing for Pregnancy

Before becoming pregnant, parents-to-be should assess and improve their own health to help ensure the health of their child. Among the most important factors to consider are the following:

FOR WOMEN:
❱ If you smoke, drink alcohol, or use drugs, stop.
❱ Reduce your caffeine intake or avoid it altogether.
❱ Maintain a healthy weight; lose or gain weight if necessary.
❱ Avoid X rays and environmental chemicals such as herbicides and pesticides.
❱ Get checked for sexually transmitted infections and seek treatment if you have one.
❱ Take prenatal vitamins, which are especially important for providing adequate folic acid.

FOR MEN:
❱ If you smoke, quit.
❱ Drink alcohol only in moderation, and avoid drug use.
❱ Get checked for sexually transmitted infections and seek treatment if you have one.
❱ Avoid exposure to toxic chemicals in your home, work, and school environment.
❱ Maintain a healthy weight; lose or gain weight if necessary.

These include factors such as taking prescription drugs or drinking alcohol. The key to promoting preconception health is to combine the best medical care, healthy behaviors, strong support, and safe environments at home and at work.[33] During a preconception care visit, a clinician talks with the woman about any conditions she might have, such as diabetes or high blood pressure, and finds out whether the woman has had any problems with prior pregnancies. The clinician will check to make sure the woman's immunizations are up to date and will encourage her to eliminate alcohol consumption and tobacco use, to follow a healthy diet, and to lead an active lifestyle.

human chorionic gonadotropin (HCG) Hormone detectable in blood or urine samples of a mother within the first few weeks of pregnancy.

Why is preconception care so important? Prenatal care, which usually begins at week 11 or 12 of a pregnancy, comes too late to prevent a number of serious maternal and child health problems. The fetus is most susceptible to developing certain problems in the first 4 to 10 weeks after conception, before prenatal care is normally initiated. Because many women are not aware that they are pregnant until after this critical period of time, they are unable to reduce the risks to their own and their baby's health unless intervention begins before conception.[34]

The Process of Pregnancy

The process of pregnancy begins the moment a sperm fertilizes an ovum in the fallopian tubes (Figure 6.9). From there, the single fertilized cell, now called a *zygote,* multiplies and becomes a sphere-shaped cluster of cells called a *blastocyst* that travels toward the uterus, a journey that may take 3 to 4 days. Upon arrival, the embryo burrows into the thick, spongy endometrium (implantation) and is nourished from this carefully prepared lining.

Pregnancy Testing A pregnancy test scheduled with your doctor or at a local family planning clinic will confirm a pregnancy. Women who wish to know immediately can purchase home pregnancy test kits, sold over the counter in drugstores. A positive test is based on the secretion of **human chorionic gonadotropin (HCG),** which is found in the woman's urine.

Home pregnancy tests can be used as early as 2 weeks after conception and are about 85 to 95 percent reliable. Instructions must be followed carefully. If the test is done too early in the pregnancy, it may show a false negative. Other causes of false negatives are unclean testing devices, ingestion of certain drugs, and vaginal or urinary tract infections.

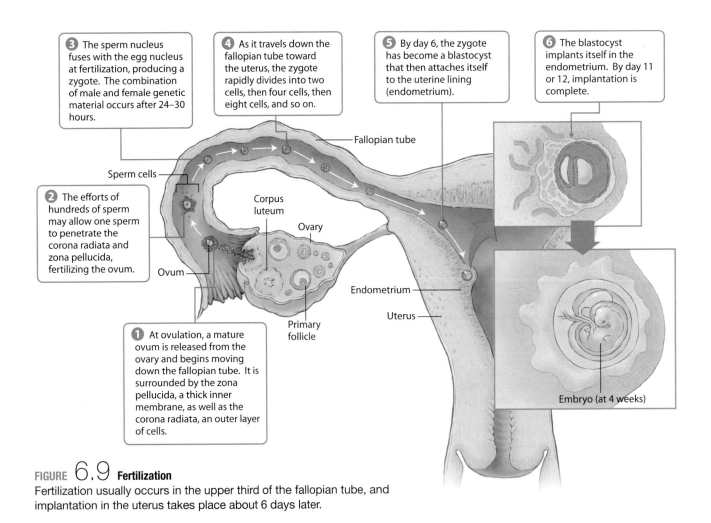

3 The sperm nucleus fuses with the egg nucleus at fertilization, producing a zygote. The combination of male and female genetic material occurs after 24–30 hours.

4 As it travels down the fallopian tube toward the uterus, the zygote rapidly divides into two cells, then four cells, then eight cells, and so on.

5 By day 6, the zygote has become a blastocyst that then attaches itself to the uterine lining (endometrium).

6 The blastocyst implants itself in the endometrium. By day 11 or 12, implantation is complete.

2 The efforts of hundreds of sperm may allow one sperm to penetrate the corona radiata and zona pellucida, fertilizing the ovum.

1 At ovulation, a mature ovum is released from the ovary and begins moving down the fallopian tube. It is surrounded by the zona pellucida, a thick inner membrane, as well as the corona radiata, an outer layer of cells.

Fallopian tube

Sperm cells

Corpus luteum

Ovary

Ovum

Primary follicle

Endometrium

Uterus

Embryo (at 4 weeks)

FIGURE 6.9 **Fertilization**
Fertilization usually occurs in the upper third of the fallopian tube, and implantation in the uterus takes place about 6 days later.

Accuracy also depends on the quality of the test itself and the user's ability to perform it and interpret the results. Blood tests administered and analyzed in a doctor's office are more accurate.

Early Signs of Pregnancy A woman's body undergoes substantial changes during a pregnancy (Figure 6.10). The first sign of pregnancy is usually a missed menstrual period (although some women "spot" in early pregnancy, which may be mistaken for a period). Other signs include breast tenderness, emotional upset, extreme fatigue, sleeplessness, and nausea and vomiting (especially in the morning).

Pregnancy typically lasts 40 weeks and is divided into three phases, or **trimesters,** of approximately 3 months each. The due date is calculated from the expectant mother's last menstrual period.

The First Trimester During the first trimester, few noticeable changes occur in the mother's body. She may urinate more frequently and experience morning sickness, swollen breasts, or undue fatigue. These symptoms may not be frequent or severe, so she may not even realize she is pregnant.

During the first 2 months after conception, the **embryo** differentiates and develops its various organ systems, beginning with the nervous and circulatory systems. At the start of the third month, the embryo is called a **fetus,** indicating that all organ systems are in place. For the rest of the pregnancy, growth and refinement occur in each body system so that at birth they can function independently, yet in coordination with all the

trimesters A 3-month segment of pregnancy.

embryo Fertilized egg from conception through the eighth week of development.

fetus Developing human from the ninth week until birth.

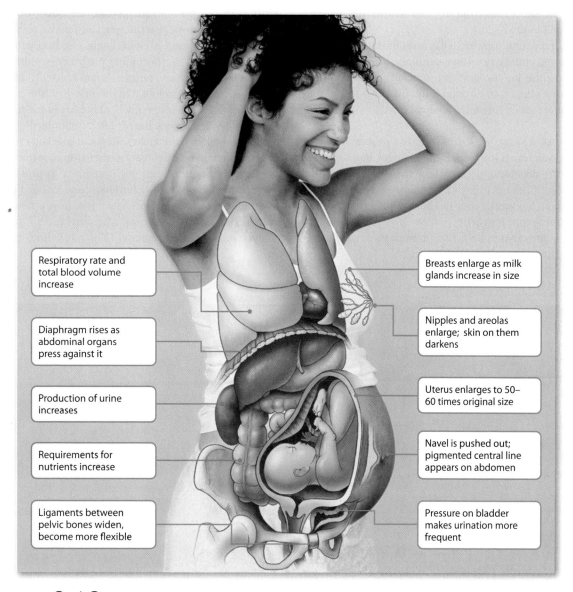

Respiratory rate and total blood volume increase

Diaphragm rises as abdominal organs press against it

Production of urine increases

Requirements for nutrients increase

Ligaments between pelvic bones widen, become more flexible

Breasts enlarge as milk glands increase in size

Nipples and areolas enlarge; skin on them darkens

Uterus enlarges to 50–60 times original size

Navel is pushed out; pigmented central line appears on abdomen

Pressure on bladder makes urination more frequent

FIGURE 6.10 **Changes in a Woman's Body during Pregnancy**

others. The photos in Figure 6.11 illustrate physical changes during fetal development.

The Second Trimester At the beginning of the second trimester, physical changes in the mother become more visible. Her breasts swell, and her waistline thickens. During this time, the fetus makes greater demands on the mother's body. In particular, the **placenta,** the network of blood vessels that carries nutrients and oxygen to the fetus and fetal waste products to the mother, becomes well established.

placenta Network of blood vessels connected to the umbilical cord that transports oxygen and nutrients to a developing fetus and carries away fetal wastes.

The Third Trimester From the end of the sixth month through the ninth is the third trimester. This is the period of greatest fetal growth, when the fetus gains most of its weight. During this time, the fetus must get large amounts of calcium, iron, and protein from food the mother eats. Approximately 85 percent of the calcium and iron the mother digests goes into the fetal bloodstream.

Although the fetus may live if it is born during the seventh month, it needs the layer of fat it acquires during the eighth month and time for the organs (especially the respiratory and digestive organs) to develop fully. Infants born prematurely usually require intensive medical care.

Emotional Changes Of course, the process of pregnancy involves much more than the changes in a woman's body and the developing fetus. Many important emotional changes occur from the time a woman learns she is pregnant through the first 6 weeks after her baby's birth (postpartum period). Throughout pregnancy, women may experience fear of complications, anxiety about becoming a parent, and wonder and excitement over the developing baby.

Prenatal Care

A successful pregnancy depends on a mother who takes good care of herself and her fetus. Good nutrition and exercise; avoiding drugs, alcohol, and other harmful substances; and regular medical checkups from the beginning of pregnancy are essential. Early detection of fetal abnormalities, identification of high-risk mothers and infants, and screening for possible complications are the major purposes of prenatal care.

A woman should carefully choose the health care provider who will attend her pregnancy and delivery. If possible, she should do this before she becomes pregnant. Recommendations from friends and from one's family physician are a good starting point. She should also consider a practitioner's philosophy about pain management during labor, experience in handling complications, and willingness to accommodate her personal beliefs on these issues. Several types of practitioners are qualified to care for a woman through pregnancy, birth, and the postpartum period, including obstetrician-gynecologists, family practitioners, and midwives (Table 6.3).

Ideally, a woman should begin medical checkups as soon as possible after becoming pregnant (within the first 3 months). This early care reduces infant mortality and the likelihood of low birth weight. On the first visit, the practitioner should obtain a complete medical history of the mother and her family and note any hereditary conditions that could put a woman or her fetus at risk. Regular checkups to measure weight gain and blood pressure and to monitor the fetus's size and position should continue throughout the pregnancy. The American Congress of Obstetricians and Gynecologists recommends seven or eight prenatal visits for women with low-risk pregnancies. Unfortunately, prenatal care is not available to everyone. American Indian, Hispanic/Latina, and African American women have the lowest rates of prenatal care in the

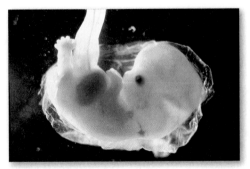

ⓐ A human embryo during the first trimester. The embryonic period lasts from the third to the eighth week of development. By the end of the embryonic period, all organs have formed.

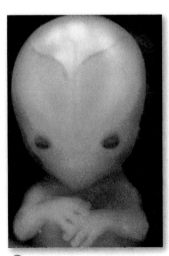

ⓑ A human fetus during the second trimester. Growth during the fetal period is very rapid.

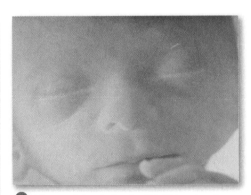

ⓒ A human fetus during the third trimester. By the end of the fetal period, the growth rate of the head has slowed relative to the growth rate of the rest of the body.

FIGURE 6.11 **Fetoscopic Photographs Showing Development in the First, Second, and Third Trimesters of Pregnancy**

Practitioner/Description	Advantages	Disadvantages
Obstetrician/Gynecologist: MD who specializes in obstetrics (care of a woman and child during pregnancy, birth, and the postpartum period) and gynecology (care of the reproductive system of women)	Trained to handle all types of pregnancy- and delivery-related emergencies.	Generally can perform deliveries only in a hospital setting. Cannot serve as the baby's physician after birth.
Family Practitioner: MD or nurse practitioner who provides comprehensive care for people of all ages	No need to change physicians; can refer to a specialist if necessary, can serve as the baby's physician after birth.	Some provide pregnancy care only to low-risk pregnancies; rarely perform home births.
Midwife: Experienced practitioner who can assist with pregnancies and deliveries. Midwives can oversee delivery of babies in non-hospital birthing sites, such as home deliveries or birthing centers. Most strive to help women have a natural childbirth experience.		
Certified Nurse Midwife: RN or NP with specialized training in pregnancy and delivery; most work in private practice or in conjunction with physicians.	Certified nurse midwives have formal training and accreditation. They may work with physicians and have access to traditional medical facilities, but are often able to offer more personal attention than a MD could.	RNs cannot provide medication without physician approval, but NPs can in many states; need to refer to clinician when the pregnancy is deemed high risk.
Lay Midwives: Uncertified or unlicensed midwife who was educated through informal routes such as self-study or apprenticeship rather than through a formal program.	Midwives tend to view pregnancy and childbirth as a family event. They usually offer low intervention, highly personalized birth plans. Home birth can lower costs.	Cannot administer any medication; would need to refer to a clinician. May not have extensive training in handling an emergency. Women should carefully evaluate the credentials of a prospective lay midwife and seriously consider the risks related to delivery outside a hospital.

United States with 14 percent, 12.9 percent, and 12.6 percent, respectively, receiving no prenatal care at all or none until the third trimester, compared to only 5.5 percent of non-Hispanic whites who receive no or late care.[35]

Nutrition and Exercise A pregnant woman needs additional protein, calories, vitamins, and minerals, so specific dietary needs and guidance should be discussed with her health care provider. Special attention should be paid to getting enough folic acid (found in dark leafy greens), iron (dried fruits, meats, legumes, liver, egg yolks), calcium (nonfat or low-fat dairy products and some canned fish), and fluids.

Vitamin supplements can correct some deficiencies, but there is no substitute for a well-balanced diet. Babies born to poorly nourished mothers run high risks of substandard mental and physical development. Folic acid, when consumed before and during early pregnancy, reduces the risk of spina bifida, a congenital birth defect resulting from failure of the spinal column to close. U.S. manufacturers of breads, pastas, rice, and other grain products are now required to add folic acid to their foods as a prevention measure to reduce neural tube defects in newborns.

Weight gain during pregnancy helps nourish a growing baby. For a woman of normal weight before pregnancy, the recommended gain during pregnancy is 25 to 35 pounds. Weight gain of 15 to 25 pounds is recommended for overweight women and a gain of 11 to 20 pounds for obese women. Underweight women should gain 28 to 40 pounds, and women carrying twins should gain about 35 to 45 pounds. Gaining too much or too little weight can lead to complications. With higher weight gains, women may develop gestational diabetes, hypertension, or increased risk of delivery complications. Gaining too little increases the chance of a low birth weight baby.

Of the total number of pounds gained during pregnancy, about 6 to 8 are the baby. The baby's birth weight is important, because low birth weight can mean health problems during labor and the baby's first few months and beyond. Pregnancy is not the time for a woman to think about losing weight—doing so may endanger the fetus.

As in all other stages of life, exercise is an important factor in overall health during pregnancy. Regular exercise is recommended for pregnant women; however, they should consult with their health care provider before starting any exercise program. Exercise can help control weight, make labor easier, and help with a faster recovery due to increased strength and endurance. Physical activity includes regular, moderate physical activity such as brisk walking and/or swimming. Women can usually maintain their customary level of activity during most of the pregnancy, although there are some cautions: pregnant women should avoid exercise that puts her at risk of falling or having an abdominal injury, such as horseback riding, soccer, or skiing, and in the third trimester, exercises that involve lying on the back should be avoided as blood flow to the uterus can be restricted.

Drugs and Alcohol

A woman should avoid all types of drugs during pregnancy. Even common over-the-counter medications such as aspirin can damage a developing fetus. During the first 3 months of pregnancy, the fetus is especially subject to the **teratogenic** (birth defect–causing) effects of drugs, environmental chemicals, X rays, or diseases. The fetus can also develop an addiction to or tolerance for drugs that the mother is using.

Maternal consumption of alcohol is detrimental to a growing fetus. Birth defects associated with **fetal alcohol syndrome (FAS)** include developmental disabilities, neural and cardiac impairments, and cranial and facial deformities. The exact amount of alcohol that causes FAS is not known; therefore, researchers recommend completely avoiding alcohol during pregnancy.

Smoking

Tobacco use, and smoking in particular, harms every phase of reproduction. Women who smoke have more difficulty becoming pregnant and have a higher risk of being infertile. Women who smoke during pregnancy have a greater chance of complications, premature births, low birth weight infants, stillbirth, and infant mortality.[36] Smoking restricts the blood supply to the developing fetus and thus limits oxygen and nutrition delivery and waste removal. Tobacco use also appears to be a significant factor in the development of cleft lip and palate.

Studies also show that secondhand smoke is detrimental. The exposed fetus is more likely to experience low birth weight, increased susceptibility to childhood diseases, and sudden infant death syndrome.[37]

teratogenic Causing birth defects; may refer to drugs, environmental chemicals, radiation, or diseases.

fetal alcohol syndrome (FAS) Pattern of birth defects, learning, and behavioral problems in a child caused by the mother's alcohol consumption during pregnancy.

toxoplasmosis Disease caused by an organism found in cat feces that, when contracted by a pregnant woman, may result in stillbirth or birth defects.

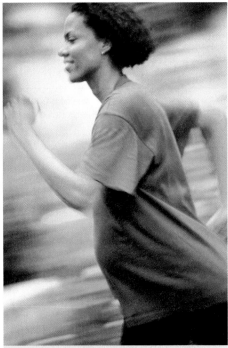

A doctor-approved exercise program during pregnancy can help control weight, make delivery easier, and have a healthy effect on the fetus.

Other Teratogens

A pregnant woman should avoid exposure to X rays, toxic chemicals, heavy metals, pesticides, gases, and other hazardous compounds. She should avoid cleaning litter boxes, if possible, because cat feces can contain organisms that cause **toxoplasmosis.** If a pregnant woman contracts this disease, the baby may be stillborn or suffer mental retardation or other birth defects. If a partner is not available to help, a friend, neighbor, or pet sitter could be asked for assistance, or the woman can clean the box by wearing rubber gloves and washing her hands thoroughly afterward.

If she has never had rubella (German measles), a woman should be immunized for it prior to becoming pregnant. A rubella infection can kill the fetus or cause blindness or hearing disorders in the infant. Sexually transmitted infections such as genital herpes or HIV are also risk factors. A woman should inform her physician of any infectious condition so proper precautions and treatment can be provided. For example, contact with an active herpes infection during birth can be fatal to the baby; thus, the physician may want to deliver the baby by cesarean section, especially if a woman has active lesions.

Several recent studies have shown that caffeine can increase the risk of miscarriage and stillbirth.[38] Based on these and other studies, women who are pregnant are advised to cut back on their caffeine consumption. The American Congress of Obstetricians and Gynecologists recommend pregnant women who drink caffeine-containing beverages limit intake to less than 200 mg a day, or about 12 ounces of coffee.[39]

Maternal Age

The average age at which a woman has her first child has been creeping up (from 21 in 1970 to 25 today), so a woman who becomes pregnant after age 35 has plenty of company. Although births to women in their twenties are declining, the rate of first births to women between the ages of 30 and 39 are the highest reported in four decades, and

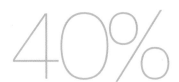

40%

of genetic abnormalities can be identified through amniocentesis, the most common being Down syndrome.

births to women over 39 have continued to increase slightly over previous years.[40] Many doctors note that older mothers tend to be more conscientious about following medical advice during pregnancy and are more psychologically mature and ready to include an infant in their family than are some younger women.

Statistically, the chances of having a baby with birth defects do rise after the age of 35. Researchers believe that there is a decline in both the quality and viability of eggs after this age. The incidence of **Down syndrome** increases with the mother's age.[41]Another concern is that a woman's fertility begins to decline as she ages. Fewer than 10 percent of women in their early twenties have issues with infertility, compared to nearly 30 percent of women in their early forties.

Prenatal Testing and Screening Modern technology enables medical practitioners to detect health defects in a fetus as early as the fourteenth to eighteenth weeks of pregnancy. One common test is **ultrasonography or ultrasound**, which uses high-frequency sound waves to create a *sonogram,* or visual image, of the fetus in the uterus. The sonogram is used to determine the fetus's size and position. Knowing the baby's position helps health care providers perform other tests and deliver the infant. Sonograms can also detect birth defects in the nervous and digestive systems.

Chorionic villus sampling (CVS) involves snipping tissue from the developing fetal sac. Chorionic villus sampling can be used at 10 to 12 weeks of pregnancy. This is an attractive option for couples who are at high risk for having a baby with Down syndrome or a debilitating hereditary disease.

The **triple marker screen** (often called the TMS or AFT [alpha-fetoprotein] test) is a commonly used maternal blood test that is optimally conducted between the sixteenth and eighteenth weeks of pregnancy. The TMS is a screening test, not a diagnostic tool; it can detect susceptibility for a birth defect or genetic abnormality, but it is not meant to confirm a diagnosis of any condition. A quad screen test (or AFP-plus test) is also available. By screening for an additional protein in maternal blood, a false-positive result is less likely than for the triple marker screen.

Amniocentesis is a common testing procedure that is strongly recommended for women over age 35. This test involves inserting a long needle through the mother's abdominal and uterine walls into the **amniotic sac**, the protective pouch surrounding the fetus. The needle draws out 3 to 4 teaspoons of fluid, which is analyzed for genetic information about the baby (Figure 6.12). Amnio-

centesis can be performed between weeks 14 and 18.

If any of these tests reveals a serious birth defect, parents are advised to undergo genetic counseling. In the case of a chromosomal abnormality such as Down syndrome, the parents are usually offered the option of a therapeutic abortion. Some parents choose this option; others research the condition and decide to continue the pregnancy.

Childbirth

Prospective parents need to make several key decisions long before the baby is born. These include where to have the baby, whether to use pain medication during labor and delivery, which childbirth

Down syndrome Syndrome caused by the presence of an extra chromosome that results in mental retardation and distinctive physical characteristics.

ultrasonography (ultrasound) Common prenatal test that uses sound waves to create a visual image of a developing fetus.

chorionic villus sampling (CVS) Prenatal test that involves snipping tissue from the fetal sac to be analyzed for genetic defects.

triple marker screen (TMS) Common maternal blood test that can be used to identify fetuses with certain birth defects and genetic abnormalities.

amniocentesis Medical test in which a small amount of fluid is drawn from the amniotic sac to test for Down syndrome and other genetic abnormalities.

amniotic sac Protective pouch surrounding the fetus.

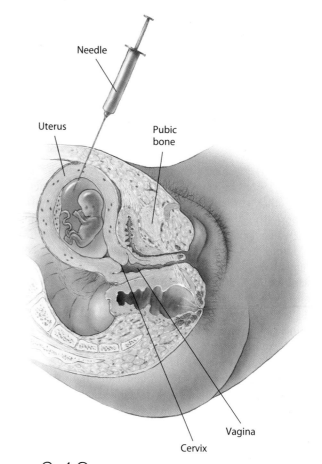

FIGURE 6.12 **Amniocentesis**
The process of amniocentesis, in which a long needle is used to withdraw a small amount of amniotic fluid for genetic analysis, can detect certain congenital problems as well as the fetus's sex.

what do you think?
Would you want to know if you or your partner were carrying a child with a genetic birth defect or other abnormality? ● Would you consider having your genes tested before starting a family? ● What would you do if both you and your partner were carriers of a genetic disorder that could be passed to your children?

method to choose, and whether to breast-feed or use formula. Answering these questions in advance will ensure a smoother passage into parenthood.

Labor and Delivery

During the few weeks preceding delivery, the baby normally shifts to a head-down position, and the cervix begins to dilate (widen). The junction of the pubic bones loosens to permit expansion of the pelvic girdle during birth. The exact mechanisms that initiate labor are unknown. A change in the hormones in the fetus and mother cause strong uterine contractions to occur, signaling the beginning of labor. Another common early signal is the breaking of the amniotic sac, which causes a rush of fluid from the vagina (commonly referred to as "water breaking").

The birth process has three stages, shown in Figure 6.13, which can last from several hours to more than a day. In some cases, toward the end of the second stage, the attending health care provider may perform an *episiotomy*, a straight incision in the mother's perineum (the area between the vulva and the anus) to prevent the baby's head from tearing vaginal tissues and to speed the baby's exit from the vagina. Upon exit, the baby takes its first breath, which is generally accompanied by a loud wail. After delivery, the attending practitioner assesses the baby's overall condition, cleans the baby's mucus-filled breathing passages, and ties and severs the umbilical cord. The mother's uterus continues to contract in the third stage of labor until the placenta is expelled.

Managing Labor Pain medication given to the mother during labor can cause sluggish responses in the newborn and other complications. For this reason, many women choose drug-free labor and delivery—but it is important to keep a flexible attitude about pain relief, because each labor is different. Use of pain medication during a delivery is not a sign of weakness. One person is not a "success" for delivering without medication or another a "failure" for using medical measures. Remember, pain is to be expected. In fact, many experts say that the pain of labor is the most intense in the human experience. There is no one right answer for managing that pain.

The Lamaze method is the most popular technique of childbirth preparation in the United States. It discourages the use of pain medication. Prelabor classes teach the mother to control her pain through special breathing patterns, focusing exercises, and relaxation. Lamaze births usually take place in a hospital or birthing center with a physician or midwife in attendance. The partner (or labor coach) assists by giving emotional support, physical comfort, and coaching for proper breath control during contractions.

Cesarean Section (C-Section) If labor lasts too long or if a baby is in physiological distress or is about to exit the uterus any way but headfirst, a **cesarean section (C-section)** may be necessary. This surgical procedure involves making an incision across the mother's abdomen and through the uterus to remove the baby. A C-section may also be performed if labor is extremely difficult, maternal blood pressure falls rapidly, the placenta separates from the uterus too soon, the mother has diabetes, or other problems occur. A C-section can be traumatic for the mother if she is not prepared for it. Risks are the same as for any major abdominal surgery, and recovery from birth takes considerably longer after a C-section.

The rate of delivery by C-section in the United States has increased from 5 percent in the mid-1960s to 32 percent in 2007.[42] Although this procedure is necessary in certain cases,

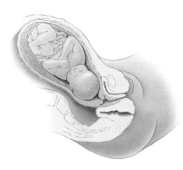

❶ Stage I: Dilation of the cervix Contractions in the abdomen and lower back push the baby downward, putting pressure on the cervix and dilating it. The first stage of labor may last from a couple of hours to more than a day for a first birth, but it is usually much shorter during subsequent births.

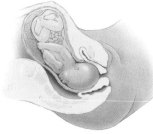

❷ End of Stage I: Transition The cervix becomes fully dilated, and the baby's head begins to move into the vagina (birth canal). Contractions usually come quickly during transition, which generally lasts 30 minutes or less.

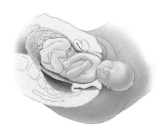

❸ Stage II: Expulsion Once the cervix has become fully dilated, contractions become rhythmic, strong, and more intense as the uterus pushes the baby headfirst through the birth canal. The expulsion stage lasts 1 to 4 hours and concludes when the infant is finally pushed out of the mother's body.

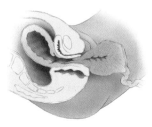

❹ Stage III: Delivery of the placenta In the third stage, the placenta detaches from the uterus and is expelled through the birth canal. This stage is usually completed within 30 minutes after delivery.

FIGURE 6.13 **The Birth Process**
The entire process of labor and delivery usually takes from 2 to 36 hours. Labor is generally longer for a woman's first delivery and shorter for subsequent births.

some physicians and critics, including the Centers for Disease Control and Prevention (CDC), feel that C-sections are performed too frequently in this country. Natural birth advocates suggest that hospitals, driven by profits and worried about malpractice, are too quick to intervene in the birth process. Some doctors say that the increase is due to maternal demand: busy mothers want to schedule their deliveries. Late preterm delivery (34 to 36 weeks) is also on the rise in the United States, with an increase from 7.3 to 12.3 percent between 1990 and 2008.[43] It is not clear how much of the increase is due to maternal or physician choice rather than medical necessity. Parents need to be aware that inducing labor early can have negative impacts on the baby's health and should be avoided unless essential.

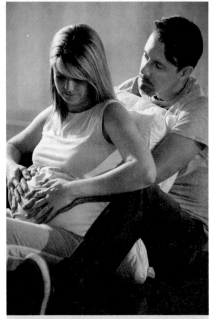
Expectant parents often take part in childbirth classes to learn what to expect during labor and delivery and to practice techniques for breathing and relaxation during labor.

Complications of Pregnancy and Childbirth

Pregnancy carries the risk for potential complications and problems that can interfere with the proper development of the fetus or threaten the health of the mother and child. Some complications may result from a preexisting health condition of the mother, such as diabetes or an STI, and others can develop during pregnancy and may result from physiological problems, genetic abnormalities, or exposure to teratogens.

Preeclampsia and Eclampsia
Preeclampsia is a condition characterized by high blood pressure, protein in the urine, and edema (fluid retention), which usually causes swelling of the hands and face. Symptoms may include sudden weight gain, headache, nausea or vomiting, changes in vision, racing pulse, mental confusion, and stomach or right shoulder pain. If preeclampsia is not treated, it can cause strokes and seizures, a condition called *eclampsia*. Potential problems can include liver and kidney damage, internal bleeding, stroke, poor fetal growth, and fetal and maternal death.

Preeclampsia tends to occur in the late second or third trimester. The cause is unknown; however, the incidence is higher in first-time mothers; women over 40 or under 18 years of age; women carrying multiple fetuses; and women with a history of chronic hypertension, diabetes, kidney disorder, or previous history of preeclampsia. Family history of preeclampsia is also a risk factor, whether the history is on the father's or mother's side. Treatment for preeclampsia ranges from bed rest and monitoring for mild cases to hospitalization and close monitoring for more severe cases.

Miscarriage Even when a woman does everything "right," not every pregnancy ends in delivery. In fact, in the United States, between 15 to 20 percent of known pregnancies end in **miscarriage** (also referred to as *spontaneous abortion*).[44] Most miscarriages occur during the first trimester.

Reasons for miscarriage vary. In some cases, the fertilized egg has failed to divide correctly. In others, genetic abnormalities, maternal illness, or infections are responsible. Maternal hormonal imbalance may also cause a miscarriage, as may a weak cervix, toxic chemicals in the environment, or physical trauma to the mother. In most cases, the cause is not known.

Rh Factor A rare blood incompatibility between mother and fetus can cause **Rh factor** problems, sometimes resulting in miscarriage. Rh is a blood protein, and problems occur when the mother is Rh-negative and the fetus is Rh-positive. During a first birth, some of the baby's blood passes into the mother's bloodstream. An Rh-negative mother may manufacture antibodies to destroy the Rh-positive blood introduced into her bloodstream at the time of birth. Her first baby will be unaffected, but subsequent babies with positive Rh factor will be at risk for a severe anemia called *hemolytic disease,* because the mother's Rh antibodies will attack the fetus's red blood cells. Prevention is preferable to treatment. Women with Rh-negative blood should be injected with a medication called RhoGAM within 72 hours after any birth, miscarriage, or abortion. The injection prevents the mother from developing Rh antibodies.

Ectopic Pregnancy The implantation of a fertilized egg outside the uterus, usually in the fallopian tube or occasionally in the pelvic cavity, is called an **ectopic pregnancy**. Because these structures are not capable of expanding and nourishing a developing fetus, the pregnancy must be terminated surgically or a miscarriage will occur. Ectopic pregnancy is generally accompanied by pain in the lower abdomen or aching in the shoulders as blood flows upward toward the diaphragm. If bleeding is significant, blood pressure drops, and the woman can go into shock. If an ectopic pregnancy progresses undiagnosed and untreated, the fallopian tube will rupture, which puts the woman at great risk of hemorrhage, peritonitis (infection

preeclampsia Pregnancy complication characterized by high blood pressure, protein in the urine, and edema.

miscarriage Loss of the fetus before it is viable; also called *spontaneous abortion.*

Rh factor Antigen present in the red blood cells of 85% of people; those with the Rh factor are known as Rh positive (Rh⁺); those without it are Rh negative (Rh⁻).

ectopic pregnancy Dangerous condition that results from the implantation of a fertilized egg outside the uterus, usually in a fallopian tube.

in the abdomen), and even death. Ectopic pregnancy occurs at a rate of 6.4 cases per 1,000 pregnancies in North America and is a leading cause of maternal mortality in the first trimester.[45] Ectopic pregnancy is a potential side effect of pelvic inflammatory disease, which has become increasingly common. The scarring or blockage of the fallopian tubes that occurs with this disease prevents a fertilized egg from passing to the uterus.

Stillbirth One of the most traumatic events a couple can face is a **stillbirth**. Stillbirth is the death of a fetus *after* the twentieth week of pregnancy but before delivery. A stillborn baby is born dead, often for no apparent reason. Each year in the United States, there is about 1 stillbirth in every 160 births.[46] Birth defects, placental problems, poor fetal growth, infections, and umbilical cord accidents are known contributing factors.

The Postpartum Period

The postpartum period typically lasts 4 to 6 weeks after delivery. During this period, many women experience fluctuating emotions. For many new mothers, the physical stress of labor, dehydration and blood loss, and other stresses challenge their stamina. Many new mothers experience what is called the "baby blues," characterized by periods of sadness, anxiety, headache, sleep disturbances, and irritability. For most women, these symptoms disappear after a short while. About 10 percent of new mothers experience **postpartum depression**, a more disabling syndrome characterized by mood swings, lack of energy, crying, guilt, and depression. It can happen any time within the first year after childbirth. Mothers who experience postpartum depression should seek professional treatment. Counseling is the most common type of treatment, but sometimes medication is recommended.[47]

Breast-Feeding Although the new mother's milk will not begin to flow for 2 or more days after delivery, her breasts secrete a yellow fluid called *colostrum* beginning immediately after birth. Because colostrum contains vital antibodies to help fight infection and boost the baby's immune system, the newborn should be allowed to suckle.

The American Academy of Pediatrics strongly recommends that infants be exclusively breast-fed for 6 months and breast-fed as a supplement for 12 months. Scientific findings indicate there are many advantages to breast-feeding. Breast-fed babies have fewer illnesses and a much lower hospitalization rate because breast milk contains maternal antibodies and immunological cells that stimulate the infant's immune system. When breast-fed babies do get sick, they recover more quickly. They are also less likely to be obese later in life than are babies fed formula, and they have fewer allergies. They may even be more intelligent: A recent study found that the longer a baby was breast-fed, the higher the IQ in adulthood. Researchers theorize that breast milk contains substances that enhance brain development.[48] Breast-feeding also has the added benefit of helping mothers lose weight after birth because the production of milk burns hundreds of calories a day. Breast-feeding also causes the hormone oxytocin to be released, which makes the uterus return to its normal size faster.

This does not mean that breast milk is the only way to nourish a baby. Some women are unable or unwilling to breast-feed; women with certain medical conditions or who are receiving certain medications are advised not to breast-feed. Prepared formulas can provide nourishment that allows a baby to grow and thrive. When deciding whether to breast-feed or formula-feed, mothers must consider their own desires and preferences, too. Both feeding methods can supply the physical and emotional closeness essential to the parent–child relationship.

Infant Mortality After birth, infant death can be caused by birth defects, low birth weight, injuries, or unknown causes. In the United States, the unexpected death of a child under 1 year of age, for no apparent reason, is called **sudden infant death syndrome (SIDS)**. SIDS is responsible for about 2,500 deaths a year. It is the leading cause of death for children age 1 month to 1 year and most commonly occurs in babies less than 6 months old.[49] It is not a specific disease; rather, it is ruled a cause of death after all other possibilities are ruled out. A SIDS death is sudden and silent; death occurs quickly, often during sleep, with no signs of suffering.

The exact cause of SIDS is unknown, but researchers have discovered trends in SIDS deaths that may help them understand these mysterious deaths. For instance, infants placed to sleep on their backs are less likely to die from SIDS than those placed on their stomachs. Babies are more likely to die from SIDS when they are placed on or covered by soft bedding. Troublingly, African American babies are twice as likely to die from SIDS than white babies, and the SIDS rate among American Indian babies is nearly three times that of white babies.[50]

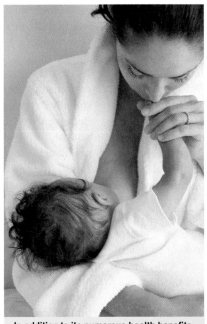

In addition to its numerous health benefits, breast-feeding enhances the development of intimate bonds between mother and child.

The American Academy of Pediatrics sponsors the Back to Sleep educational campaign that provides the following advice when putting a baby down to sleep: Lay infants down on their backs; place them on a firm sleep surface; keep soft objects, toys, and bedding out of the sleep area; don't allow smoking around the baby; don't use "wedges" to keep the baby from rolling over, and give the baby a clean, dry pacifier.

Infertility

For the couple desperately wishing to conceive, the road to parenthood may be frustrating. An estimated 1 in 6 American couples experiences **infertility**, usually defined as the inability to conceive after trying for a year or more. In the United States, it affects about 10 to 20 percent of the reproductive-age population. Although the focus is often on women, in about 20 percent of cases, infertility is due to a cause involving only the male partner, and in about 30 to 40 percent of cases, infertility is due to causes involving both partners.[51] Because of the likelihood of this, it is important for both partners to be evaluated.

Reasons for the high level of infertility in the United States include the trend toward delaying childbirth (as a woman gets older, she is less likely to conceive), endometriosis, the rising incidence of pelvic inflammatory disease, and low sperm count. Environmental contaminants known as *endocrine disrupters,* including some pesticides and emissions from burning plastics, appear to affect fertility in both men and women. Stress and anxiety (in general and about fertility) can also interfere with getting pregnant. The linked conditions of obesity and diabetes that affect such a high percentage of the U.S. population also have reproductive implications.

Causes in Women

Most cases of infertility in women result from problems with ovulation. The most common cause for female infertility is polycystic ovary syndrome (PCOS). A woman's ovaries have follicles, which are tiny, fluid-filled sacs that hold the eggs. When an egg is mature, the follicle breaks open to release the egg so it can travel to the uterus for fertilization. In women with PCOS, immature follicles bunch together to form large cysts or lumps. The eggs mature within the bunched follicles, but the follicles don't break open to

10%

of infertility cases have no known cause.

release them. As a result, women with PCOS often don't have menstrual periods, or they have periods infrequently. Because eggs are not released, most women with PCOS have trouble getting pregnant. Researchers estimate that 5 to 10 percent of women of child-bearing age—as many as 5 million women in the United States—have PCOS.[52]

In some women the ovaries stop functioning before natural menopause, a condition called *premature ovarian failure.* Other causes of infertility include **endometriosis**. With this very painful disorder, parts of the lining of the uterus implant outside the uterus, blocking the fallopian tubes. The disorder can be treated surgically or with hormonal therapy.

Pelvic inflammatory disease (PID) is a serious infection that scars the fallopian tubes and blocks sperm migration. (See **Chapter** 14 for more on PID.) Infection-causing bacteria (chlamydia or gonorrhea) can invade the fallopian tubes, causing normal tissue to turn into scar tissue. This scar tissue blocks or interrupts the normal movement of eggs into the uterus. If the fallopian tubes are totally blocked by scar tissue, a woman becomes infertile. Infertility also can occur if the fallopian tubes are partially blocked or even slightly damaged. About 1 in 10 women with PID becomes infertile, and if a woman has multiple episodes of PID, her chance of becoming infertile increases.[53]

Causes in Men

Among men, the single largest fertility problem is **low sperm count**.[54] Although only one viable sperm is needed for fertilization, research has shown that all the other sperm in the ejaculate aid in the fertilization process. There are normally 60 to 80 million sperm per milliliter of semen. When the count drops below 20 million, fertility declines.

Low sperm count may be attributable to environmental factors (such as exposure of the scrotum to intense heat or cold, radiation, certain chemicals, or altitude) or even to wearing excessively tight underwear or clothing. Other factors, such as the mumps virus, can damage the cells that make sperm. Varicose veins above one or both testicles can also render men infertile.

Infertility Treatments

Medical procedures can identify the cause of infertility in about 90 percent of cases. Once the cause has been determined, the chances of becoming pregnant range from 30

infertility Inability to conceive after a year or more of trying.

endometriosis Disorder in which endometrial tissue establishes itself outside the uterus.

pelvic inflammatory disease (PID) Inflammation of the female genital tract that may cause scarring or blockage of the fallopian tubes, resulting in infertility.

low sperm count Sperm count below 20 million sperm per milliliter of semen.

to 70 percent, depending on the reason for infertility.[55] The numerous tests and the invasion of privacy that are often involved in efforts to conceive can put stress on an otherwise strong, healthy relationship. A good physician or fertility team will take the time to ascertain a couple's level of motivation and coping skills.

Workups to determine the cause of infertility can be expensive, and the costs are not usually covered by health insurance. Fertility workups for men include a sperm count, a test for sperm motility, and an analysis of any disease processes present. Women are thoroughly examined by an obstetrician-gynecologist to determine the composition of cervical mucus and evidence of tubal scarring or endometriosis.

Fertility Drugs Fertility drugs stimulate ovulation in women who are not ovulating. Of women who use these drugs, 60 to 80 percent will begin to ovulate; of those who ovulate, about half will conceive.[56] Fertility drugs can have many side effects, including headaches, depression, fatigue, fluid retention, and abnormal uterine bleeding. Women using fertility drugs are also at increased risk of developing multiple ovarian cysts (fluid-filled growths) and liver damage. The drugs sometimes trigger the release of more than one egg, so a woman taking fertility drugs has a 1 in 10 chance of having multiple births. Most such births are twins, but triplets and even quadruplets are not uncommon.

Alternative Insemination Another treatment option is **alternative insemination** (also known as *artificial insemination*) of a woman with her partner's sperm. The couple may also choose insemination by an anonymous donor through a sperm bank. Donated sperm are medically screened, classified according to the donor's physical characteristics (such as hair and eye color), and then frozen for future use.

Assisted Reproductive Technology Assisted reproductive technology (ART) includes several different medical procedures that help a woman become pregnant. The most common is **in vitro fertilization (IVF)**. During IVF, eggs and sperm are mixed in a laboratory dish to fertilize, and some of the fertilized eggs (zygotes) are then transferred to the woman's uterus.

Other types of assisted reproductive technologies include:

- **Intracytoplasmic sperm injection (ICSI)**, which involves the injection of a single sperm into an egg. The fertilized egg is then placed in the woman's uterus or fallopian tube. Used with IVF, ICSI is often a successful treatment for men with impaired sperm.
- **Gamete intrafallopian transfer (GIFT)**, which involves collecting eggs from the ovaries, then placing them into a thin flexible tube with the sperm. This is then injected into the woman's fallopian tubes, where fertilization takes place.

alternative insemination
Fertilization procedure accomplished by depositing semen from a partner or donor into a woman's vagina via a thin tube.

in vitro fertilization (IVF)
Fertilization of an egg in a nutrient medium and subsequent transfer back to the mother's body.

- **Zygote intrafallopian transfer (ZIFT)**, which combines IVF and GIFT. Eggs and sperm are mixed outside the body. The fertilized eggs (zygotes) are then returned to the fallopian tubes, through which they travel to the uterus.

Other Infertility Treatments In *nonsurgical embryo transfer*, a donor egg is fertilized by the man's sperm and implanted in the woman's uterus. In *embryo transfer,* an ovum from a donor is artificially inseminated by the man's sperm, allowed to stay in the donor's body for a time, and then transplanted into the woman's body. Infertile couples have another alternative—embryo adoption programs. Fertility treatments such as IVF often produce excess fertilized eggs that couples may choose to donate for other infertile couples to adopt.

There are many ethical and moral questions surrounding infertility treatments. Before deciding on a treatment, couples must ask themselves important questions: Has infertility been confirmed? Are reputable fertility counseling services accessible? Have we explored all alternatives and considered potential risks? Have we examined our attitudes, values, and beliefs about conceiving a child in this manner? Finally, will we tell our child about the method of conception, and if so, how?

what do you think?

If you or your partner had infertility problems, how much time and money would you be willing to invest in treatment?
- Do you think that single women should have equal access to alternative methods of insemination?
- What about lesbian couples—should they have equal access to alternative methods of insemination? ● Do you think single men and women and gay couples should have equal opportunities to adopt?
- Do you think society views these adoptions differently?

Surrogate Motherhood

Many infertile couples are able to conceive after treatment. Those who cannot conceive may choose to live without children, or they may decide to adopt or to pursue surrogate motherhood. In the latter case, the couple hires a woman to be alternatively inseminated by the male partner. The surrogate then carries the baby to term and surrenders it to the couple at birth. Couples considering surrogate motherhood are advised to consult a lawyer before entering into this type of contract.

Adoption

Adoption serves several important purposes. It provides a way for individuals and couples who may not be able to have a biological child to form a legal parental relationship with a child who needs a home. As such, it benefits children whose birth parents are unable or unwilling to raise them and provides adults who are unable to conceive or carry a pregnancy to term a means to create a family. It is estimated that approximately 2 percent of the U.S. adult population has adopted children.[57]

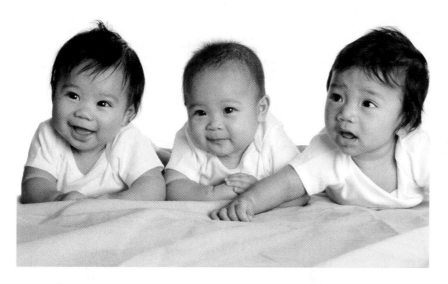

There are two types of adoption: *confidential* and *open*. In confidential adoption, the birth parents and the adoptive parents never know each other. Adoptive parents are given only basic information about the birth parents, such as medical background, that they need to care for the child. In open adoption, birth parents and adoptive parents know some information about each other. There are different levels of openness. Both parties must agree to this plan, and it is not available in every state.

Increasingly, couples are choosing to adopt children from other countries. In 2011, U.S. families adopted more than 9,000 foreign-born children.[58] The cost of overseas adoption varies widely, but can cost more than $30,000, including agency fees, dossier and immigration processing fees, travel, and court costs.[59] However, it may be a good alternative for many couples, especially those who want to adopt an infant rather than an older child. Some families find it beneficial to serve as foster parents prior to deciding to adopt, and others choose to adopt older children from the foster system in the United States rather than wait for an infant placed through international adoption.

Are You Comfortable with Your Contraception?

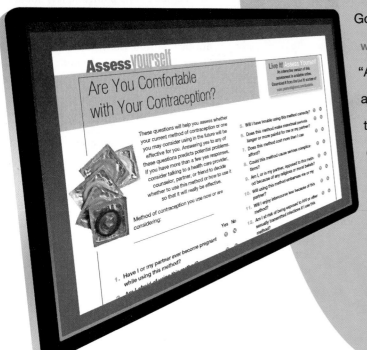

Go online to the **Live It!** section of www.pearsonhighered.com/donatelle to take the "Are You Comfortable with Your Contraception?" assessment.* This activity gives you the chance to assess your comfort and confidence with the contraceptive method you are using now or one you may use in the future. Depending on the results, you may consider changing your birth control method. If that's the case, then follow the steps outlined in the **YOUR PLAN FOR CHANGE** box.

*If your instructor so chooses, Assess Yourself Activities are available as a printed supplement or as assignable homework online at www.pearsonhighered.com/myhealthlab.

MyHealthLab®

YOUR PLAN FOR CHANGE

The **Assess yourself** activity gave you the chance to look at your contraception preferences and habits. If you'd like to explore new contraception options,

Today you can:

○ Visit your local drugstore and study the forms of contraception that are available without a prescription. Think about those you would consider using and why.

○ If you are not currently using any contraception or are not in a sexual relationship now, but might be in the future, purchase a package of condoms (or pick up free samples from your campus health center) to keep on hand just in case.

Within the next 2 weeks, you can:

○ Make an appointment for a checkup with your health care provider. Be sure to ask him or her any questions you have about contraception.

○ Sit down with your partner and discuss contraception. Talk about how your current method is working for both of you, if the effectiveness level of the method you are using is high enough, and if you aren't using birth control consistently, what you can do together to improve.

By the end of the semester, you can:

○ Periodically reevaluate whether your new or continued contraception is still effective for you. Review your experiences, and take note of any consistent problems you may have encountered.

○ Always keep a backup form of contraception on hand. Check this supply periodically and throw out and replace any supplies that have expired.

Summary

* Latex or polyurethane male and female condoms, when used correctly for oral sex or intercourse, provide the most effective protection in preventing sexually transmitted infections (STIs). Other contraceptive methods include spermicides, the diaphragm, the cervical cap, the contraceptive sponge, oral contraceptives, Ortho Evra, NuvaRing, Depo-Provera, Implanon, and intrauterine devices. Emergency contraception may be used within 72 hours of unprotected intercourse or the failure of another contraceptive method. Fertility awareness methods rely on altering sexual practices to avoid pregnancy, as do abstinence, outercourse, and withdrawal. While all these methods of contraception are reversible, sterilization is permanent.

* Abortion is legal in the United States, but strongly opposed by many Americans. Abortion methods include suction curettage, dilation and evacuation (D&E), intact dilation and extraction (D&X), hysterotomy, induction abortion, and medical abortions.

* Parenting is a demanding job that requires careful planning. Prospective parents must consider emotional health, maternal and paternal health, and financial resources.

* Full-term pregnancy has three trimesters. Prenatal care includes a complete physical exam within the first trimester, follow-up checkups throughout the pregnancy, healthy nutrition and exercise, and avoidance of all substances that could have teratogenic effects on the fetus, such as alcohol and drugs, tobacco smoke, X rays, and harmful chemicals. Prenatal tests, including ultrasonography, chorionic villus sampling, triple marker screen, quad screen, and amniocentesis, can be used to detect birth defects.

* Childbirth occurs in three stages. Partners should jointly choose a labor method early in the pregnancy to be better prepared when labor occurs. Possible complications of pregnancy and childbirth include preeclampsia and eclampsia, miscarriage, Rh factor problems, ectopic pregnancy, and stillbirth.

* Infertility in women may be caused by pelvic inflammatory disease (PID) or endometriosis. In men, it may be caused by low sperm count. Treatments may include fertility drugs, alternative insemination, in vitro fertilization (IVF), assisted reproductive technology (ART), embryo transfer, and embryo adoption programs. Surrogate motherhood and adoption are also options.

Pop Quiz

1. Which type of lubricant could you safely use with a latex condom?
   a. Mineral oil
   b. Water-based lubricant
   c. Body lotion
   d. Petroleum jelly

2. Which of the following is a barrier contraceptive?
   a. Seasonale
   b. FemCap
   c. Ortho Evra
   d. Contraceptive patch

3. What is the most commonly used method of first-trimester abortion?
   a. Suction curettage
   b. Dilation and evacuation (D&E)
   c. Medical abortion
   d. Induction abortion

4. What is meant by the *failure rate* of contraceptive use?
   a. The number of times a woman fails to get pregnant when she wanted to
   b. The number of times a woman gets pregnant when she did not want to
   c. The number of pregnancies that occurs in women using a particular method of birth control
   d. The number of times a couple fails to use birth control

5. Toxic chemicals, pesticides, X rays, and other hazardous compounds that cause birth defects are referred to as
   a. carcinogens.
   b. teratogens.
   c. mutants.
   d. environmental assaults.

6. In an ectopic pregnancy, the fertilized egg implants in the woman's
   a. fallopian tube.
   b. uterus.
   c. vagina.
   d. ovaries.

7. What is the recommended pregnancy weight gain for a woman who is at a healthy weight before pregnancy?
   a. 15 to 20 pounds
   b. 20 to 30 pounds
   c. 25 to 35 pounds
   d. 30 to 45 pounds

8. Which prenatal test involves snipping tissue from the developing fetal sac?
   a. Triple marker screen
   b. Ultrasound
   c. Amniocentesis
   d. Chorionic villus sampling

9. Why is it recommended not to use condoms made of lambskin?
   a. They are less elastic than latex condoms.
   b. They cannot be stored for as long as latex condoms.
   c. They do not protect against the transmission of STIs.
   d. They are likely to cause allergic reactions.

10. The number of American couples who experience infertility is
    a. 1 in 6.
    b. 1 in 24.
    c. 1 in 60.
    d. 1 in 100.

Answers to these questions can be found on page A-1.

Think about It!

1. List the most effective contraceptive methods. What are their drawbacks? What medical conditions would keep a person from using each one? Which methods do you think would be most effective for you? Why?
2. What are the various methods of abortion? What are the two opposing viewpoints concerning abortion? What is *Roe v. Wade,* and what impact has it had on the abortion debate in the United States?
3. What are the most important considerations in deciding whether the time is right to become a parent? If you choose to have children, what factors will you consider in regard to the right time to have them and the number to have?
4. Discuss the growth of the fetus through the three trimesters. What medical checkups or tests should be done during each trimester?
5. Discuss the emotional aspects of pregnancy. What types of emotional reactions are common during each trimester and the postpartum period?
6. If you and your partner are unable to have children, what alternative methods of conception would you consider? Would you consider adoption?

Accessing Your Health on the Internet

The following websites explore further topics and issues related to personal health. For links to the websites below, visit the Companion Website for *Access to Health,* 13th Edition, at www.pearsonhighered.com/donatelle.

1. *Guttmacher Institute.* This is a nonprofit organization focused on sexual and reproductive health research, policy analysis, and public education. www.guttmacher.org
2. *Association of Reproductive Health Professionals.* This organization was originally founded by Alan Guttmacher as the educational arm of Planned Parenthood. Now an independent organization, it provides education for health care professionals and the general public. The Patient Resources portion of the website includes information on various methods of birth control and an interactive tool to help you choose a method that will work for you. www.arhp.org
3. *Planned Parenthood.* This site offers a range of up-to-date information on sexual health issues, such as birth control, the decision of when and whether to have a child, sexually transmitted infections, abortion, and safer sex. www.plannedparenthood.org
4. *The American Pregnancy Association.* This is a national organization offering a wealth of resources to promote reproductive and pregnancy wellness. The website includes educational materials and information on the latest research. www.americanpregnancy.org
5. *Centers for Disease Control and Prevention.* The CDC provides up-to-date information on preconception care, pregnancy, breast-feeding, infant care, infertility, and contraception, all in one well-organized website. www.cdc.gov/ncbddd/pregnancy_gateway/index.html
6. *American College of Nurse-Midwives.* If the concept of midwifery is new to you, learn more about it at their website. www.mymidwife.org
7. *International Council on Infertility Information Dissemination.* This site includes current research and information on infertility. www.inciid.org

References

1. American College Health Association, *American College Health Association—National College Health Assessment III (ACHA-NCHA III): Reference Group Data Report Spring 2011* (Baltimore: American College Health Association, 2012), www.achancha.org/docs/ACHA-NCHA-II_ReferenceGroup_DataReport_Spring2011.pdf.
2. R. A. Hatcher et al., *Contraceptive Technology,* 19th rev. ed. (New York: Ardent Media, 2007).
3. ACHA-NCHA III, *Reference Group Data Report,* 2012.
4. Drug Information Online, Drugs.com, "Seasonale," February 2012, www.drugs.com/seasonale.html.
5. R. A. Hatcher et al., *Contraceptive Technology,* 2007.
6. U.S. Food and Drug Administration, "Safety Labeling Changes Approved By FDA Center for Drug Evaluation and Research (CDER)—April 2010: Ortho Evra (Norelgestromin/Ethinyl Estradiol) Transdermal System," May 2010, www.fda.gov/Safety/MedWatch/SafetyInformation/ucm211821.htm.
7. Janssen Pharmaceuticals, "Important Safety Update for U.S. Health Care Professionals ORTHO EVRA," March 2011, www.orthoevra.com/isi-hcp.html.
8. The American Congress of Obstetricians and Gynecologists, ACOG Committee Opinion-Intrauterine Device and Adolescents," December 2007, www.acog.org/Resources_And_Publications/Committee_Opinions/Committee_on_Adolescent_Health_Care/Intrauterine_Device_and_Adolescents.
9. Office of Population Research & Association of Reproductive Health Professionals, Emergency Contraception Website, "Answers to Frequently Asked Questions about Effectiveness," March 2010, http://ec.princeton.edu/questions/eceffect.html.
10. Guttmacher Institute, "State Policies in Brief—Emergency Contraception," February 2012, www.guttmacher.org/statecenter/spibs/spib_EC.pdf.
11. ACHA-NCHA III, *Reference Group Data Report,* 2012.
12. Ibid.
13. Guttmacher Institute, "Facts on Contraceptive Use in the United States," June 2010, www.guttmacher.org/pubs/fb_contr_use.html.
14. R. A. Hatcher et al., *Contraceptive Technology,* 2007.
15. Guttmacher Institute, "Facts on Induced Abortion in the United States," January 2011, www.guttmacher.org/pubs/fb_induced_abortion.html.
16. American Psychological Association (APA), Task Force on Mental Health and

Abortion, *Report of the Task Force on Mental Health and Abortion* (Washington, DC: American Psychological Association, 2008), www.apa.org/pi/wpo/mental-health-abortion-report.pdf.

17. Boston Women's Health Collective, *Our Bodies, Ourselves: 40th Anniversary Rev. Ed.* (New York: Simon & Schuster, 2011).

18. Gallup, "Abortion," May 2011, www.gallup.com/poll/1576/abortion.aspx

19. Guttmacher Institute, "States Enact Record Number of Abortion Restrictions in 2011," January 2012, www.guttmacher.org/media/inthenews/2012/01/05/endofyear.html.

20. NARAL Pro Choice America, "The Bush Administration's Federal Abortion Ban," January 2010, www.naral.org/media/publications.

21. Guttmacher Institute, "Supreme Court Upholds Federal Abortion Ban, Opens Door for Further Restrictions by States," *Guttmacher Policy Review* 10, no. 2 (2007): 19.

22. APA, *Report of the Task Force*, 2008.

23. Ibid.

24. Ibid.

25. Guttmacher Institute, "Facts on Induced Abortions," 2011.

26. Ibid.

27. Planned Parenthood. "The Abortion Pill (Medical Abortion)," 2011, www.plannedparenthood.org/health-topics/abortion/abortion-pill-medication-abortion-4354.asp.

28. Ibid.

29. D. Wigle et al., "Epidemiologic Evidence of Relationships between Reproductive and Child Health Outcomes and Environmental Chemical Contaminants," *Journal of Toxicology* 11, no. 5–6 (2008): 373–517.

30. M. Lino, *Expenditures on Children by Families, 2010* (Alexandria, VA: U.S. Department of Agriculture, Center for Nutrition Policy and Promotion, 2011), www.cnpp.usda.gov/ExpenditureonChildrenbyFamilies.htm.

31. College Board, "What It Costs to Go to College," 2011, www.collegeboard.com/student/pay/add-it-up/4494.html.

32. National Association of Child Care Resource and Referral Agencies, "Parents and the High Cost of Child Care, 2011 Report," August 2011, www.naccrra.org/sites/default/files/default_site_pages/2011/cost_report_2011_full_report_0.pdf.

33. Centers for Disease Control and Prevention, "Preconception Care Questions and Answers," January 2012, www.cdc.gov/ncbddd/preconception/QandA.htm.

34. Ibid.

35. National Center for Health Statistics, "Health, United States, 2010: With Special Feature on Death and Dying," 2011, www.cdc.gov/nchs/data/hus/hus10.pdf.

36. National Center for Chronic Disease Prevention and Health Promotion, "Tobacco Use and Pregnancy," May 2009, www.cdc.gov/reproductivehealth/TobaccoUsePregnancy/index.htm; U.S. Department of Health and Human Services, *How Tobacco Smoke Causes Disease: The Biology and Behavioral Basis for Smoking-Attributable Disease: A Report of the Surgeon General* (Atlanta: U.S. Department of Health and Human Services, Centers for Disease Control and Prevention, National Center for Chronic Disease Prevention and Health Promotion, Office on Smoking and Health, 2010).

37. M. Kharrazi et al., "Environmental Tobacco Smoke and Pregnancy Outcome," *Epidemiology* 15, no. 6 (November 2006): 660–70.

38. D. Greenwood et al., "Caffeine Intake during Pregnancy, Late Miscarriage, and Stillbirth," *European Journal of Epidemiology* 25, no. 4 (2010): 275–80; B. Zhang et al., "Risk Factors for Unexplained Recurrent Spontaneous Abortion in a Population from Southern China," *International Journal of Gynaecology and Obstetrics* 108, no. 2 (2010): 135–38; A. Pollack, L. Buck, R. Sundaram, and K. Lum, "Caffeine Consumption and Miscarriage: A Prospective Cohort Study," *Fertility and Sterility* 93, no. 1 (2010): 304–06.

39. The American Congress of Obstetricians and Gynecologists, "Committee Opinion: Moderate Caffeine Consumption During Pregnancy," August 2010, www.acog.org/Resources_And_Publications/Committee_Opinions/Committee_on_Obstetric_Practice/Moderate_Caffeine_Consumption_During_Pregnancy.

40. U.S. Department of Health and Human Services, Health Resources and Services Administration, Maternal and Child Health Bureau, *Child Health USA 2010* (Rockville, MD: U.S. Department of Health and Human Services, 2010), http://mchb.hrsa.gov/chusa10/popchar/pages/109ma.html.

41. National Institute of Child Health and Human Development, "Down Syndrome," March 2010, www.nichd.nih.gov/health/topics/down_syndrome.cfm.

42. F. Menacker and B. Hamilton, *Recent Trends in Cesarean Delivery in the United States*, NCHS Data Brief no. 35 (Hyattsville, MD: National Center for Health Statistics, 2010), DHHS Publication no. (PHS) 2010-1209, www.cdc.gov/nchs/data/databriefs/db35.htm.

43. J. A. Martin, M. J. K. Osterman, and P. D. Sutton, "Are Preterm Births on the Decline in the United States? Recent Data from the National Vital Statistics System," May 2010, www.cdc.gov/nchs/data/databriefs/db39.htm.

44. E. Puscheck, "Early Pregnancy Loss," eMedicine from WebMD, February 2010, http://emedicine.medscape.com/article/266317-overview.

45. K. W. Hoover, G. Tao, and C. K. Kent, "Trends in the Diagnosis and Treatment of Ectopic Pregnancy in the United States," *Obstetrics and Gynecology*, 115, no. 3, (2010) 495-502; V. P. Sepilian et al., "Ectopic Pregnancy," eMedicine from WebMD, March 2011, http://emedicine.medscape.com/article/258768-overview.

46. March of Dimes, "Loss and Grief: Stillbirth," February 2010, www.marchofdimes.com/Baby/loss_stillbirth.html.

47. U.S. Department of Health and Human Services, Office on Women's Health, "Frequently Asked Questions: Depression During and After Pregnancy," March 2009, www.womenshealth.gov/faq/depression-pregnancy.cfm.

48. American Academy of Pediatrics, "Benefits of Breastfeeding for Mom," April 2010, www.healthychildren.org/English/ages-stages/baby/breastfeeding/pages/Benefits-of-Breastfeeding-for-Mom.aspx.

49. National Institute on Child and Human Development, "Research on Sudden Infant Death Syndrome," October 2009, www.nichd.nih.gov/womenshealth/research/pregbirth/sids.cfm.

50. Ibid.

51. Mayo Clinic Staff, MayoClinic.com, "Infertility: Causes," June 2009, www.mayoclinic.com/health/infertility/DS00310/DSECTION=causes.

52. U.S. Department of Health and Human Services, Office on Women's Health, "Frequently Asked Questions: Polycystic Ovary Syndrome (PCOS)," March 2010, www.womenshealth.gov/faq/polycystic-ovary-syndrome.cfm.

53. Centers for Disease Control and Prevention (CDC), "Pelvic Inflammatory Disease CDC Fact Sheet," April 2008, www.cdc.gov/std/PID/STDFact-PID.htm.

54. Centers for Disease Control and Prevention (CDC), "Assisted Reproductive Technology," November 2009, www.cdc.gov/ART.

55. Ibid.

56. WebMD Medical Reference, "Fertility Drugs," February 2010, www.webmd.com/infertility-and-reproduction/guide/fertility-drugs.

57. J. Jones, *Who Adopts? Characteristics of Women and Men Who Have Adopted Children*, NCHS Data Brief no. 12 (Hyattsville, MD: National Center for Health Statistics, 2009) DHHS Publication No. (PHS) 2009-1209, www.cdc.gov/nchs/data/databriefs/db12.htm.

58. Intercountry Adoption, U.S. Department of State, "Statistics: Adoptions by Year," February 2012, http://adoption.state.gov/about_us/statistics.php.

59. Intercountry Adoption, U.S. Department of State, "How to Adopt" February 2012, http://adoption.state.gov/adoption_process/how.php.

7 Eating for a Healthier You

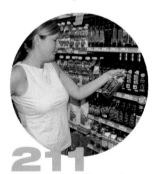

208
Why are whole grains better than refined grains?

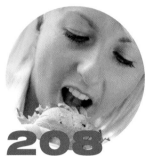

211
Are all fats bad for me?

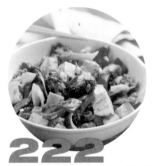

222
Are vegetarian diets healthy?

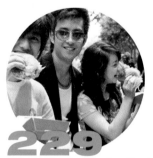

229
How can I eat well when I'm in a hurry?

OBJECTIVES

✳ Understand the factors that influence decisions about nutrition.

✳ List the six classes of nutrients, and explain the primary functions of each and their roles in maintaining long-term health.

✳ Discuss how to eat healthfully, including the characteristics of a healthful diet, how to use the MyPlate plan, the role of dietary supplements, and how to read food labels.

✳ Discuss the unique challenges that college students face when trying to eat healthy foods and the actions they can take to eat healthfully.

✳ Explain food safety concerns facing Americans and people in other regions of the world.

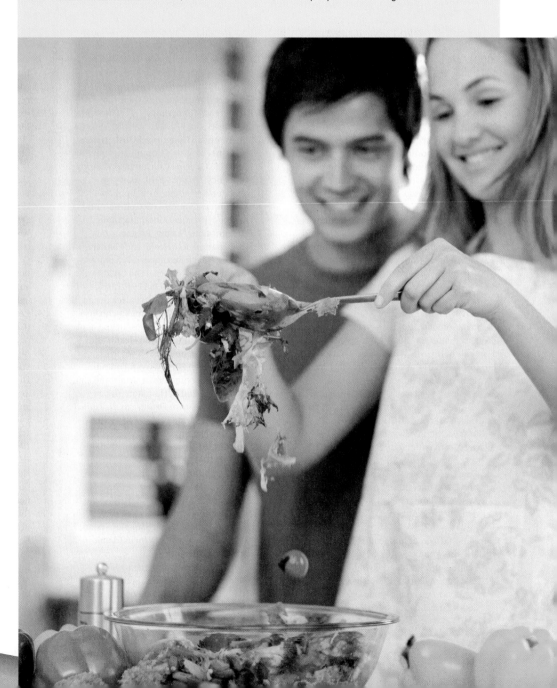

Advice about food comes at us from all directions: from the Internet, popular magazines, television, and friends and neighbors. Everyone is eager to offer "expert" advice, but this advice can be contradictory. For example, Dr. Atkins' recommendations for a diet high in protein and fat but low in carbohydrates contradict the advice of experts such as Dr. Dean Ornish and the American Heart Association, who advocate low-fat diets. Knowing what to eat, how much to eat, and how to choose from a media-driven array of food and advice can be mind-boggling. For some, this can cause a phenomenon known as *eating anxiety* and lead to a lifetime of cycling on and off diets.[1] Why does something that can be so good, ultimately end up being a problem for so many of us? What influences our eating habits and how can we learn to eat more healthfully?

The answers to these questions aren't as simple as they may seem. When was the last time you ate because you felt truly hungry? True **hunger** occurs when there is a lack of basic foods. When we are hungry, our brains initiate a physiological response that prompts us to seek food for the energy and **nutrients** that our bodies require to maintain proper functioning. Most people in the United States don't know true hunger—most of us eat because of **appetite,** a learned psychological desire to consume food. Hunger and appetite are not the only forces involved in our physiological drive to eat. Other factors include cultural and social meanings attached to food, convenience and advertising, habit or custom, emotional eating, perceived nutritional value, social interaction, and financial means.

Nutrition is the science that investigates the relationship between physiological function and the essential elements of the foods we eat. With an understanding of nutrition, you will be able to distinguish fact from fiction about trends in nutrition. Your health depends largely on what you eat, how much you eat, and the amount of exercise that you get throughout your life. The next few chapters focus on fundamental principles of nutrition, weight management, and exercise.

Before the body can use foods, the digestive system must break down the larger food particles into smaller, more usable forms. The **digestive process** is the sequence of functions by which the body breaks down foods into molecules small enough to be absorbed, and excretes the wastes. (See **Figure 7.1** on the next page.)

Essential Nutrients for Health

Food provides the chemicals we need for activity and body maintenance. Our bodies cannot synthesize certain *essential nutrients* (or cannot synthesize them in adequate amounts)—we must obtain them from the foods we eat. Of the six groups of essential nutrients, the four we need in the largest amounts—water, carbohydrates, fats, and proteins—are called *macronutrients*. The other two groups—vitamins and minerals—are needed in smaller amounts, so they are called *micronutrients*.

Recommended Intakes for Nutrients

Ahead, we discuss each of the six groups of nutrients and identify how much of each nutrient you need. These recommended amounts are known as the *Dietary Reference Intakes (DRIs)* and are published by the Food and Nutrition Board of the Institute of Medicine. The DRIs identify the intake of each essential nutrient that research suggests will prevent deficiency or reduce the risk for chronic disease. The DRIs are considered the umbrella guidelines under which the following categories fall:

- **Recommended Dietary Allowances (RDAs)** are daily nutrient intake levels meeting the nutritional needs of 97 to 98 percent of healthy individuals.
- **Adequate Intakes (AIs)** are daily intake levels assumed to be adequate for most healthy people. AIs are used when there isn't enough research to support establishing an RDA.
- **Tolerable Upper Intake Levels (ULs)** are the highest amounts of a nutrient that an individual can consume daily without risking adverse health effects.
- **Acceptable Macronutrient Distribution Ranges (AMDRs)** are the intakes of proteins, carbohydrates, and fats that provide adequate nutrition, and they are associated with a reduced risk for chronic disease.

Whereas the RDAs, AIs, and ULs are expressed as amounts—usually milligrams (mg) or micrograms (μg)—AMDRs are expressed as percentages. The AMDR for protein, for example, is 10 to 35 percent, meaning that no less than 10 percent and no more than 35 percent of the calories you consume should come from proteins. But that raises a new question: What are calories?

Calories

A *kilocalorie* is a unit of measure used to quantify the amount of energy in food. On nutrition labels and in consumer publications, the term is shortened to **calorie.** *Energy* is defined as the capacity to do work. We derive energy

hunger The physiological impulse to seek food, prompted by the lack or shortage of basic foods needed to provide the energy and nutrients that support health.

nutrients The constituents of food that sustain humans physiologically: water, proteins, carbohydrates, fats, vitamins, and minerals.

appetite The desire to eat; normally accompanies hunger but is more psychological than physiological.

nutrition The science that investigates the relationship between physiological function and the essential elements of foods eaten.

digestive process The process by which the body breaks down foods and either absorbs or excretes them.

calorie A unit of measure that indicates the amount of energy obtained from a particular food.

"Why Should I Care?"

The nutritional choices you make during college can have both immediate and lasting effects on your health. Thousands of studies associate what we eat with chronic diseases such as diabetes, heart disease, hypertension, stroke, and many types of cancer.

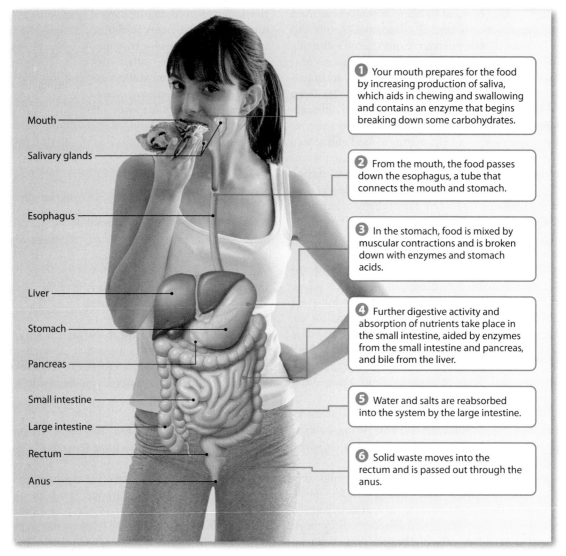

FIGURE 7.1 **The Digestive Process**
The entire digestive process takes approximately 24 hours.

① Your mouth prepares for the food by increasing production of saliva, which aids in chewing and swallowing and contains an enzyme that begins breaking down some carbohydrates.

② From the mouth, the food passes down the esophagus, a tube that connects the mouth and stomach.

③ In the stomach, food is mixed by muscular contractions and is broken down with enzymes and stomach acids.

④ Further digestive activity and absorption of nutrients take place in the small intestine, aided by enzymes from the small intestine and pancreas, and bile from the liver.

⑤ Water and salts are reabsorbed into the system by the large intestine.

⑥ Solid waste moves into the rectum and is passed out through the anus.

Mouth
Salivary glands
Esophagus
Liver
Stomach
Pancreas
Small intestine
Large intestine
Rectum
Anus

from the energy-containing nutrients in the foods we eat. These energy-containing nutrients—carbohydrates, fats, and proteins—provide calories. Vitamins, minerals, and water do not. Table 7.1 shows the caloric needs for various individuals.

Water: A Crucial Nutrient

Humans can survive for several weeks without food but only for about 1 week without water. **Dehydration,** a state of abnormal depletion of body fluids, can develop within a single day, especially in a hot climate. Too much water can also pose a serious risk to your health. This condition, *hyponatremia,* is characterized by low sodium levels.

dehydration Abnormal depletion of body fluids; a result of lack of water.

The human body consists of 50 to 70 percent water by weight. The water in our system bathes cells; aids in fluid, electrolyte, and acid-base balance; and helps regulate body temperature. Water is the major component of our blood, which carries oxygen, nutrients, and hormones and other substances to body cells and removes metabolic wastes.

Individual needs for water vary drastically according to dietary factors, age, size, overall health, environmental temperature and humidity levels, and exercise. For the most part, scientists now refute the conventional wisdom that everyone needs to drink eight glasses of water per day.[2] The latest DRIs suggest that most people can meet their hydration needs simply by eating a healthy diet and drinking in response to thirst. The general recommendations for women are approximately 11 cups of total water from all beverages and foods each day and for men an average of 16 cups.[3]

We usually get the fluids we need each day through the food, water, and other beverages we consume. About 20 percent of our daily water needs are met through the food we eat. In fact, fruits and vegetables

Hear It! Podcast

Want a study podcast for this chapter? Download the podcast **Nutrition: Eating for Optimum Health** at www.pearsonhighered.com/donatelle.

Estimated Daily Calorie Needs

	Calorie Range		
	Sedentary[a]		Active[b]
Children			
2–3 years old	1,000	→	1,400
Females			
4–8 years old	1,200	→	1,800
9–13	1,400	→	2,200
14–18	1,800	→	2,400
19–30	1,800	→	2,400
31–50	1,800	→	2,200
51+	1,600	→	2,200
Males			
4–8 years old	1,200	→	2,000
9–13	1,600	→	2,600
14–18	2,000	→	3,200
19–30	2,400	→	3,000
31–50	2,200	→	3,000
51+	2,000	→	2,800

[a] A lifestyle that includes only the light physical activity associated with typical day-to-day life.
[b] A lifestyle that includes physical activity equivalent to walking more than 3 miles per day at 3 to 4 miles per hour, in addition to the light physical activity associated with typical day-to-day life.

Source: U.S. Department of Agriculture and U.S. Department of Health and Human Services, *Dietary Guidelines for Americans, 2010*, 7th ed. (Washington, DC: U.S. Government Printing Office).

are 80 to 95 percent water, meats are more than 50 percent water, and even dry bread and cheese are about 35 percent water! Contrary to popular opinion, caffeinated drinks, including coffee, tea, and soda, also count toward total fluid intake. Caffeinated beverages have not been found to dehydrate people whose bodies are used to caffeine.

There are situations in which a person needs to take in additional fluids in order to stay properly hydrated. It is important to drink extra fluids when you have a fever or an illness in which there is vomiting or diarrhea. Anyone with kidney function problems or who tends to develop kidney stones may need more water, as may people with diabetes or cystic fibrosis. The elderly and very young also may have increased water needs. When the weather heats up, or when you exercise, work, or engage in other activities in which you sweat profusely, extra water is needed to keep your body's core temperature within a normal range. If you are an athlete and wonder about water consumption, visit the American College of Sports Medicine's website (www.acsm.org) to view its position on exercise and fluid replacement.[4]

Proteins

Next to water, **proteins** are the most abundant substances in the human body. Proteins are major components of living cells and are called the "body builders" because of their role in developing and repairing bone, muscle, skin, and blood cells. They are the key elements of antibodies that protect us from disease, enzymes that control chemical activities in the body, and many hormones that regulate body functions. Proteins also supply an alternative source of energy to cells when fats and carbohydrates are not available. Specifically, every gram of protein you eat provides 4 calories. (There are about 28 grams in an ounce.) Adequate protein in the diet is vital to many body functions and ultimately to survival.

Your body breaks down proteins into smaller nitrogen-containing molecules known as **amino acids,** the building blocks of protein. Nine of the 20 different amino acids needed by the body are termed **essential amino acids,** which means the body must obtain them from the diet; the other 11 can be produced by the body. Dietary protein that supplies all the essential amino acids is called **complete protein.** Typically, protein from animal products is complete.

Nearly all proteins from plant sources are **incomplete proteins** that lack one or more of the essential amino acids. However, it is easy to combine plant foods to produce a complete protein meal (Figure 7.2). Plant foods rich in incomplete proteins include *legumes* (beans, lentils, peas, peanuts, and soy products); *grains* (e.g., wheat, corn, rice, and oats); and *nuts and seeds.* Certain vegetables, such as leafy green vegetables and broccoli, also contribute valuable plant proteins. Mixing foods from these categories in the same meal will provide all the essential amino acids.

Although protein deficiency poses a threat to the global population (see the **Health in a Diverse World** box on page 207), few Americans suffer from protein deficiencies. In fact, the average American consumes more than 78 grams of protein daily, much of it from high-fat animal flesh and dairy products.[5] The AMDR for protein is 10 to 35 percent of calories. Adults should consume about 0.8 gram (g) per kilogram (kg) of body weight. To calculate your protein needs divide your body weight (in pounds) by 2.2 to get your weight in kilograms, then multiply by 0.8. The result is your recommended protein intake per day. For example, a woman who weighs 130 pounds should consume about 47 grams of protein each day. A 6-ounce steak provides 53 grams of protein—more than she needs!

People who need to eat extra protein include pregnant women and patients fighting a serious infection, recovering from surgery or blood loss, or recovering from burns. In these instances, proteins that are lost to cellular repair and development need to be replaced. There is considerable controversy over whether someone in high-level physical training needs additional protein to build and repair muscle fibers or whether normal daily requirements suffice. In

proteins Large molecules made up of chains of amino acids; essential constituents of all body cells.

amino acids The nitrogen-containing building blocks of protein.

essential amino acids Nine of the basic nitrogen-containing building blocks of human proteins, which must be obtained from foods

complete proteins Proteins that contain all nine of the essential amino acids.

incomplete proteins Proteins that lack one or more of the essential amino acids.

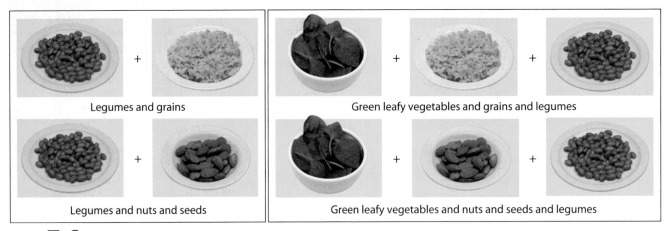

FIGURE 7.2 **Foods Providing Complementary Amino Acids**
Eaten in complementary combinations, plant-based foods can provide all essential amino acids. In some cases, you might need to combine three sources of protein to put together a complete meal. Two of the limited amino acids in leafy green vegetables are supplied by either grains or nuts and seeds, and the third is found in legumes.

Legumes and grains

Legumes and nuts and seeds

Green leafy vegetables and grains and legumes

Green leafy vegetables and nuts and seeds and legumes

addition, a sedentary person may find it easier to stay in energy balance when consuming a diet with a higher percentage of protein and a lower percentage of carbohydrate. Why? Because proteins make a person feel full for a longer period of time.

78.1 grams

of protein is what the average American consumes daily—much more than the recommended amount.

Carbohydrates

Carbohydrates supply us with the energy we need to sustain normal daily activity. The human body metabolizes carbohydrates more quickly and efficiently than it does proteins for a quick source of energy. Carbohydrates are easily converted to glucose, the primary fuel for many body cells. They are the best fuel for moderate to intense exercise because they can be broken down quickly, even when we're breathing hard and our muscle cells are getting less oxygen. Like proteins, carbohydrates provide 4 calories per gram. The RDA for adults is 130 grams of carbohydrate per day. There are two major types: simple and complex.

carbohydrates Basic nutrients that supply the body with glucose, the energy form most commonly used to sustain normal activity.

simple carbohydrates A carbohydrate made up of only one sugar molecule, or of two sugar molecules bonded together; also called simple sugars.

monosaccharides Simple sugars that contain only one molecule of sugar.

disaccharides Combinations of two monosaccharides.

complex carbohydrates A carbohydrate consisting of long chains of sugar molecules; also called a polysaccharide.

Simple Carbohydrates **Simple carbohydrates** or *simple sugars* are found naturally in fruits, many vegetables, and milk. The most common form is *glucose*. Eventually, the human body converts all types of simple sugars to glucose to provide energy to cells. Another simple sugar is *fructose* (commonly called *fruit sugar*), which is found in fruits and berries. Glucose and fructose are **monosaccharides.**

Disaccharides are combinations of two monosaccharides. Perhaps the best-known example is *sucrose* (granulated table sugar). *Lactose* (milk sugar), found in milk and milk products, and *maltose* (malt sugar) are other examples of common disaccharides. Disaccharides must be broken down into monosaccharides before the body can use them.

Sugar is found in high amounts in a wide range of processed food products. A classic example is the amount of sugar in one can of soda: more than 10 teaspoons per can! Moreover, such diverse items as ketchup, barbecue sauce, and flavored coffee creamers derive 30 to 65 percent of their calories from sugar. Read food labels carefully before purchasing. If *sugar* or one of its aliases (including *high fructose corn syrup* and *cornstarch*) appears near the top of the ingredients list, then that product contains a lot of sugar and is probably not your best nutritional bet. Also, most labels list the amount of sugar as a percentage of total calories.

1/3 of calories

Americans consume come from junk foods with no nutritional value, such as sweets, soft drinks, and alcoholic beverages.

Complex Carbohydrates: Starches and Glycogen **Complex carbohydrates** are found in grains, cereals, and vegetables. Also called *polysaccharides*, they are formed by long chains of monosaccha-

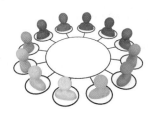

GLOBAL MALNUTRITION: ARE BUGS THE ANSWER?

Millions of people in the developed and developing world suffer from malnutrition. Consider the following:

✽ Poor nutrition contributes to 1 out of 2 deaths (53%) associated with infectious diseases among children under age 5 in developing countries.
✽ One out of 4 preschool children in the global population suffers from undernutrition.
✽ One in 3 people in developing countries is affected by vitamin and mineral deficiencies and therefore is at greater risk for infection, birth defects, and impaired physical and intellectual development.

But even as malnutrition plagues the world, there is an unlimited source of more than 1,400 species of edible insects, which could be propagated and harvested to fight global hunger. Health professionals point out that:

✽ Insects are high in protein, ranging from 45 to 80 percent of their body weight, depending on the species.
✽ Insects such as termites and silkworms are good sources of fats and amino acids.
✽ Insects such as grubs or palmworms are rich in riboflavin, thiamin, zinc, and iron.
✽ Unlike cattle and pigs, insects reproduce quickly and take little space to grow.
✽ Insects are more environmentally friendly than cattle and pigs because

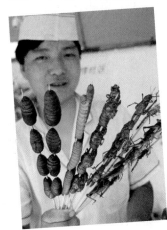

In many countries, insects are already a common food source. This vendor is selling insects in Rizhao, China.

they produce significantly less methane gas.
✽ Insects, including larvae of houseflies, silkworms, and mealworms, are an economical source of food for fish, poultry, and pigs.

The practice of consuming bugs, called *entomophagy,* is already common in areas of Africa, Asia, and Mexico. Mopani worms and termites are popular snacks in Africa. Japanese restaurants serve boiled wasp larvae called *hachi-no-ko* or fried cicada called *semi.* Dragonflies are cooked in coconut milk in Bali. Grasshoppers, known as *chapulines* in Mexico, are harvested,

cooked, sold, and consumed at local markets.

Entomophagy is still considered socially unacceptable in the United States and Europe, although most Westerners unknowingly consume about a pound of insects a year that are accidently mixed into processed foods. The acceptable limit of bugs in processed foods established by the FDA includes 30 insect parts per 100 grams in peanut butter or 60 insect parts per 100 grams of chocolate. The food industry also extracts food dyes from insects, including the red dye cochineal used to color imitation crab. Will Americans ever accept insects as part of a healthy diet? Perhaps if they could be processed into more conventional food forms. Bug Butter, anyone?

Sources: World Health Organization, "Nutrition: Challenges," Accessed April 2010, www.who .int/nutrition/challenges/en/index.html; M. Nord, M. Andrews, and S. Carlson, *Household Food Security in the United States, 2008,* Economic Research Report no. 83, U.S. Department of Agriculture, Economic Research Service, November 2009, www.ers.usda.gov/Publications/ ERR83; Department of Entomology, University of Kentucky College of Agriculture, 2010, www .ca.uky.edu/entomology/dept/bugfood2.asp; M. Dickie and A. Van Huis, "The Six Legged Meat of the Future," *Wall Street Journal,* 2011, http://online.wsj.com/article/SB100014240527 48703293204576106072340020728.html; UN News Centre, "Edible Insects Provide Food for Thought at a UN-organized Meeting," 2008, www.un.org/apps/news/story.asp?newsid=2566 2&cr=insects&cr1=food.

---

rides. Like disaccharides, they must be broken down into simple sugars before the body can use them. *Starches, glycogen,* and *fiber* are the main types of complex carbohydrates.

Starches make up the majority of the complex carbohydrate group and come from flours, breads, pasta, rice, corn, oats, barley, potatoes, and related foods. The body breaks down these complex carbohydrates into the monosaccharide glucose, which can be easily absorbed by cells and used as energy.

When not needed for energy, glucose can be stored in body muscles and the liver as a polysaccharide called **glycogen.**

When the body requires a sudden burst of energy, it breaks glycogen back down into glucose.

Complex Carbohydrates: Fiber Sometimes referred to as "bulk" or "roughage," **fiber** is the indigestible portion of plant foods that helps move foods through the digestive system, delays absorption of cholesterol and other nutrients, and softens stools

starch Polysaccharide that is the storage form of glucose in plants.

glycogen The polysaccharide form in which glucose is stored in the liver and, to a lesser extent, in muscles.

fiber The indigestible portion of plant foods that helps move food through the digestive system and softens stools by absorbing water.

by absorbing water. Dietary fiber is found only in plant foods, such as fruits, vegetables, nuts, and grains. The Food and Nutrition Board of the Institute of Medicine distinguishes three types of fiber: dietary, functional, and total.[6] *Dietary fiber* comprises the nondigestible parts of plants—the leaves, stems, and seeds. *Functional fiber* consists of nondigestible forms of carbohydrates that may come from plants or may be manufactured in the laboratory and have known health benefits. *Total fiber* is the sum of dietary fiber and functional fiber in a person's diet.

A more user-friendly classification of fiber types is either *soluble* or *insoluble.* Soluble fibers, such as pectins, gums, and mucilages, dissolve in water, form gel-like substances, and can be digested easily by bacteria in the colon. Major food sources of soluble fiber include citrus fruits, berries, oat bran, dried beans, and some vegetables. Insoluble fibers, such as lignins and cellulose, typically do not dissolve in water and cannot be fermented by bacteria in the colon. They are found in most fruits and vegetables, and in **whole grains,** such as brown rice, wheat, bran, and whole-grain breads and cereals (see Figure 7.3). The AMDR for carbohydrates is 45 to 60 percent of total calories, and heath experts recommend that the majority of this intake be fiber-rich carbohydrates. Find out more about the benefits of fiber in the **Student Health Today** box on the following page.

Despite growing evidence supporting the benefits of whole grains and high-fiber diets, intake among the general public remains low. Most experts believe that Americans should double their current consumption of dietary fiber. The AI for fiber is 25 grams per day for women and 38 grams per day for men. What's the best way to increase your intake of dietary fiber? Eat fewer refined carbohydrates in favor of more fiber-rich carbohydrates, including whole-grain breads and cereals, fresh fruits and vegetables, legumes, nuts, and seeds. As with most nutritional advice, however, too

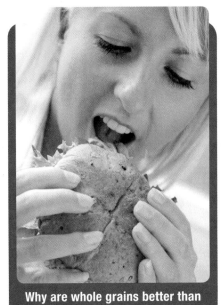

Why are whole grains better than refined grains?

Whole-grain foods contain fiber, a crucial form of carbohydrate that protects against some gastrointestinal disorders and may reduce your risk for certain cancers. Fiber is also associated with lowered blood cholesterol levels; studies have shown that eating 2.5 servings of whole grains per day can reduce cardiovascular disease risk by as much as 21%. But are people getting the message? One nutrition survey showed that only 8% of U.S. adults consume three or more servings of whole grains each day, and 42% ate no whole grains at all on a given day.

much of a good thing can pose problems. A sudden increase in dietary fiber may cause flatulence (intestinal gas), cramping, or bloating. Consume plenty of water or other (sugar-free!) liquids to reduce such side effects.

Fats

Fats, perhaps the most misunderstood nutrient, are the most energy dense, providing 9 calories per gram. Fats are a significant source of our body's fuel not only when we're at rest, but also during exercise. The body can store only a limited amount of carbohydrate, so the longer you exercise, the more fat your body burns. Fats also play a vital role in maintaining healthy skin and hair, insulating body organs against shock, maintaining body temperature, and promoting healthy cell function. Fats make foods taste better and carry the fat-soluble vitamins A, D, E, and K to the cells. They also make you feel full after eating. If fats perform all these functions, why are we constantly urged to cut back on them? Because some fats are less healthy than others and because excessive consumption of fats can lead to weight gain.

Triglycerides, which make up about 95 percent of total body fat, are also the most common form of

whole grains Grains that are milled in their complete form and thus include the bran, germ, and endosperm, with only the husk removed.

fats Essential nutrients needed for energy, cell function, insulation of body organs, maintenance of body temperature, and healthy skin and hair.

triglycerides The most common form of fat in foods and in the body; made up of a molecule called glycerol and three fatty acid chains.

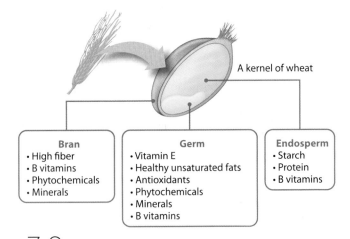

A kernel of wheat

Bran	**Germ**	**Endosperm**
• High fiber • B vitamins • Phytochemicals • Minerals	• Vitamin E • Healthy unsaturated fats • Antioxidants • Phytochemicals • Minerals • B vitamins	• Starch • Protein • B vitamins

FIGURE 7.3 **Anatomy of a Whole Grain**
Whole grains are more nutritious than refined grains because they contain the bran, germ, and endosperm of the seed—sources of fiber, vitamins, minerals, and beneficial phytochemicals (chemical compounds that occur naturally in plants).

Source: Adapted from Joan Salge Blake, Kathy D. Munoz, and Stella Volpe, *Nutrition: From Science to You,* 1st ed. © 2010, page 138. Printed and electronically reproduced by permission of Pearson Education, Inc., Upper Saddle River, New Jersey.

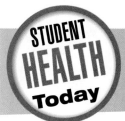

WHY FIBER IS YOUR FRIEND

Fiber may seem like something only your grandparents need to be concerned about. However, getting the recommended amount of fiber in your diet can help you feel your best right now and avoid problems in the future. Research supports many benefits of fiber:

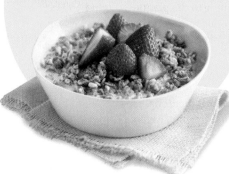

Cereal can be a good source of whole grains and fiber.

✳ **Protection against constipation.** When consumed with adequate fluids, fiber absorbs moisture and produces softer, bulkier stools that are more easily passed.

✳ **Protection against diverticulosis.** Diverticulosis is a condition in which pressure generated to pass compacted stools causes tiny bulges or pouches to form in the wall of the large intestine. These bulges can become irritated and infected and cause intense pain. Adequate fiber intake helps to prevent constipation and diverticulosis.

✳ **Protection against heart disease.** Many studies have indicated that soluble fiber helps delay or reduce the absorption of dietary cholesterol, a factor in heart disease.

✳ **Protection against type 2 diabetes.** Some studies suggest that soluble fiber slows the movement of food through the digestive tract and thereby slows the release of glucose into the bloodstream. This helps the body control blood glucose levels and may reduce the risk for type 2 diabetes.

✳ **Protection against obesity.** Because most high-fiber foods are low in fat, they help control caloric intake. Many take longer to chew, which slows you down at the table. Because fiber stays in the digestive tract longer than other nutrients, making you feel full longer, fiber can help you succeed in your weight-loss efforts.

✳ **May reduce the risk of colorectal cancer.** One of the leading causes of cancer deaths in the United States, colorectal cancer is much rarer in countries whose populations eat diets high in fiber and low in animal fat. Although some studies have suggested that fiber-rich diets, particularly those including insoluble fiber, may prevent the development of precancerous growths in the colon (the large intestine), other studies have not supported this claim.

Below are some ways for you to incorporate more fiber into your daily diet:

✳ Whenever possible, select whole-grain breads, especially those that are low in fat and sugars. Choose breads with 3 or more grams of fiber per serving. Read labels—just because bread is brown doesn't mean it is better for you.

✳ Eat whole, unpeeled fruits and vegetables rather than drinking their juices.

✳ Substitute whole-grain pastas, bagels, and pizza crust for the refined, white flour versions.

✳ Add wheat crumbs or grains to meat loaf and burgers to increase fiber intake.

✳ Toast grains to bring out their nutty flavor and make foods more appealing.

✳ Sprinkle ground flaxseed on cereals, yogurt, and salads, or add to casseroles, burgers, and baked goods. Flaxseed has a mild flavor and is also high in essential fatty acids.

Sources: K. Maki et al., "Whole-Grain Ready-to-Eat Oat Cereal, as Part of a Dietary Program for Weight Loss, Reduces Low-Density Lipoprotein Cholesterol in Adults with Overweight and Obesity More than a Dietary Program Including Low-Fiber Control Foods," *Journal of the American Dietetic Association* 110, no. 2 (2010): 205–14; E. J. Brunner et al., "Dietary Patterns and 15 Year Risks of Major Coronary Events, Diabetes and Mortality," *American Journal of Clinical Nutrition* 87, no. 5 (2008): 1414–21; A. E. Millen et al., "Fruit and Vegetable Intake and Prevalence of Colorectal Adenoma in Cancer Screening Trial," *American Journal of Clinical Nutrition* 86, no. 6 (2007): 1754–64; P. Newby et al., "Intake of Whole Grains, Refined Grains and Cereal Fiber Measured with 7-d Diet Records and Associations with Risk Factors for Chronic Disease," *American Journal of Clinical Nutrition* 86, no. 6 (2007): 1745–53.

fat in foods. When we consume too many calories from any source, the liver converts the excess into triglycerides, which are stored in fat cells throughout our bodies. Another oily substance in foods derived from animals is **cholesterol.** We don't need to consume any dietary cholesterol because our liver can make all that we need. Moreover, cholesterol contributes to a buildup of fatty plaque inside our blood vessels, the first stage of heart disease. Thus, the recommended intake for cholesterol is less than 300 milligram a day (one egg contains about 215 milligrams).

Because oil and water don't mix, neither triglycerides nor cholesterol can travel independently in the bloodstream. Instead, they are "packaged" inside protein coats to form compounds called lipoproteins (*lipo-* refers to lipids, a diverse group of oily substances). The levels of two types of lipoproteins in a blood sample help clinicians determine the patient's risk for heart disease:

High-density lipoproteins (HDLs) are relatively high in protein and low in cholesterol and triglycerides. A high level of HDLs in the blood is healthful because

cholesterol A lipid found in foods and synthesized by the body. Although essential to functioning, cholesterol circulating in the blood can accumulate on the inner walls of blood vessels.

high-density lipoproteins (HDLs) Compounds that facilitate the transport of cholesterol in the blood to the liver for metabolism and elimination from the body.

HDLs remove cholesterol from dying cells and from plaques within blood vessels. Their cholesterol load is eventually transported to the liver and eliminated from the body.

Low-density lipoproteins (LDLs) are much higher in both cholesterol and triglycerides than HDLs. They travel in the bloodstream delivering cholesterol to body cells; however, LDLs not taken up by cells degrade and release their cholesterol into the bloodstream. This cholesterol can then stick to the lining of blood vessels, contributing to the plaque that causes heart disease. (See **Chapter 15** for more on the role cholesterol plays in cardiovascular health.)

low-density lipoproteins (LDLs) Compounds that transport cholesterol in the blood to the body's cells.

saturated fats Fats that are unable to hold any more hydrogen in their chemical structure; derived mostly from animal sources; solid at room temperature.

unsaturated fats Fats with one or more chemical bonds that exclude hydrogen; derived mostly from plants; liquid at room temperature.

trans fats (trans fatty acids) Fatty acids that are produced when polyunsaturated oils are hydrogenated to make them more solid.

Types of Dietary Fats Triglycerides include *fatty acid* chains of oxygen, carbon, and hydrogen atoms. Fatty acid chains that cannot hold any more hydrogen in their chemical structure are called **saturated fats.** They generally come from animal sources, such as meat, dairy, and poultry products, and are solid at room temperature. **Unsaturated fats** have room for additional hydrogen atoms in their chemical structure, and are liquid at room temperature. They come from plants and include most vegetable oils.

The terms *monounsaturated fatty acids* (*MUFAs*) and *polyunsaturated fatty acids* (*PUFAs*) refer to the relative number of hydrogen atoms that are missing in a fatty acid chain. Peanut and olive oils are high in monounsaturated fats. Corn, sunflower, and safflower oils are high in polyunsaturated fats.

There is controversy about which type of unsaturated fat is most beneficial. Monounsaturated fatty acids, which are especially abundant in olive, canola, and peanut oils, seem to lower LDL levels and increase HDL levels and thus are considered more healthful. They also resist oxidation, a process that leads to cell and tissue damage. For a breakdown of the types of fats in common vegetable oils, see **Figure 7.4**.

Two types of polyunsaturated fatty acids essential to a healthful diet are *omega-3 fatty acids* (found in many types of fatty fish; dark green, leafy vegetables; walnuts; and flaxseeds) and *omega-6 fatty acids* (found in corn, soybean, peanut, sunflower, and cottonseed oils). Both are classified as *essential fatty acids*—that is, those we must receive from our diets—because the body cannot synthesize them yet requires them for functioning. The most important fats within these groups are *linoleic acid*, an omega-6 fatty acid, and *alpha-linolenic acid,* an omega-3 fatty acid. The body needs these to make hormone-like compounds that

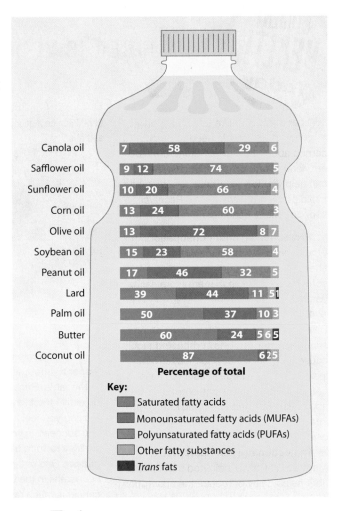

FIGURE 7.4 **Percentages of Saturated, Polyunsaturated, Monounsaturated, and Trans Fats in Common Vegetable Oils**

control immune function, pain perception, and inflammation, to name a few key benefits.[7] You may also have heard of EPA and DHA. These are derivatives of alpha-linolenic acid that are found abundantly in oily fish such as salmon and tuna and are associated with a reduced risk for heart disease.[8]

The AMDR for fats is 20 to 35 percent of calories, with 5 to 10 percent coming from the essential fatty acids. Within this range, we should minimize our intake of saturated fats.

Avoiding Trans Fatty Acids For decades, Americans shunned butter, red meat, and other foods because of the saturated fats found in them. What they didn't know is that some processed foods low in animal fats, such as margarine, could be just as harmful. These processed foods contain **trans fatty acids.** Research shows that just a 2 percent caloric intake of these fats is associated with a 23 percent increased risk for heart disease and a 47 percent increased chance of sudden cardiac death.[9]

"Why Should I Care?"

Cholesterol can accumulate on the inner walls of arteries and narrow the channels through which blood flows. This buildup, called plaque, is a major cause of *atherosclerosis*, a component of cardiovascular disease.

Do It! Nutritools

Go to the Do It! section of www.pearsonhighered.com/donatelle to complete the **Know Your Fat Sources** activity.

Although a small amount of *trans* fatty acids do occur in some animal products, the great majority are produced when food manufacturers add hydrogen to a plant oil such as corn oil. This solidifies the oil and helps it resist rancidity, giving the food in which it is used a longer shelf life. The hydrogenation process straightens out the fatty acid chain so that it is more like a saturated fatty acid, and it has similar harmful effects, lowering HDLs and raising LDLs. *Trans* fats have been used in margarines, many commercial baked goods, and restaurant deep-fried foods.

In 2006, the U.S. Food and Drug Administration (FDA) began to require *trans* fat labeling on all foods. California has become the first state to ban *trans* fats from restaurant food: all oils, margarines, and shortenings used for frying must contain less than 0.5 percent *trans* fat per serving.[10] Other bans have been implemented in New York City, Philadelphia, and parts of Maryland. Today, *trans* fats are being removed from most foods, and if they are present, they must be clearly indicated. If you see the words *partially hydrogenated oils, fractionated oils, shortening, lard,* or *hydrogenation* on a food label, then *trans* fats are present.

228,000 deaths from coronary heart disease could be averted each year by reducing Americans' consumption of *trans* fats, according to some estimates.

New Fat Advice: Is More Fat Ever Better? Some researchers worry that we have gone too far in our anti-fat frenzy. In fact, some studies have shown that when comparing low-fat diets to other diets, there are few improvements in weight loss and blood fat measures.[11]

Moderation is the key. No more than 7 to 10 percent of your total calories should come from saturated fat, and no more than 35 percent should come from all forms of fat. Follow these guidelines to add more healthy fats to your diet:

- Eat fatty fish (bluefish, herring, mackerel, salmon, sardines, or tuna) at least twice weekly. The **Be Healthy, Be Green** box on the next page provides tips for making sustainable seafood choices.
- Use olive, peanut, soy, and canola oils instead of butter or lard.
- Add healthy doses of green leafy vegetables, walnuts, walnut oil, and ground flaxseed to your diet.

Follow these guidelines to reduce your overall intake of less-healthy fats:

- Read the nutrition facts panel on food labels to find out how much fat is in your food.
- Chill meat-based soups and stews and scrape off any fat that hardens on top, and then reheat to serve.
- Fill up on fruits and vegetables.
- Hold the creams and sauces.
- Avoid margarine products with *trans* fatty acids. Whenever possible, opt for other condiments on your bread, such as fresh vegetable spreads, bean spreads, nut butters, sugar-free jams, fat-free cheese, and other healthy toppings.
- Choose lean meats, fish, or skinless poultry. Broil or bake whenever possible. Drain off fat after cooking.
- Choose fewer cold cuts, bacon, sausages, hot dogs, and organ meats.
- Select nonfat and low-fat dairy products.
- When cooking, use substitutes for butter, margarine, oils, sour cream, mayonnaise, and full-fat salad dressings. Chicken or beef broth, fresh herbs, wine, vinegar, and low-calorie dressings provide flavor with less fat.

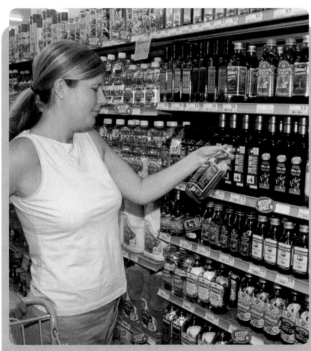

Are all fats bad for me?

All fats are not the same, and your body needs some fat to function. Try to reduce saturated fats, which are in meat, full-fat dairy, and poultry products, and avoid *trans* fats, which typically come in stick margarines, commercially baked goods, and deep-fried foods. Replace these with unsaturated fats, such as those in plant oils, fatty fish, and nuts and seeds.

Vitamins

Vitamins are potent and essential organic compounds that promote growth and help maintain life and health. Every minute of every day, vitamins help maintain nerves and skin, produce blood cells, build bones and teeth, heal wounds, and convert food energy to body energy— and they do all this without adding any calories to your diet.

vitamins Essential organic compounds that promote metabolism, growth, and reproduction and help maintain life and health.

BE HEALTHY, BE GREEN

TOWARD SUSTAINABLE SEAFOOD

The 2010 MyPlate food guidance system recommends consuming fish twice a week to reduce saturated fat and cholesterol levels and to increase omega-3 fatty acid levels. However, there are many environmental concerns surrounding the seafood industry today that call into question the sustainability and safety of such consumption. More than 70 percent of the world's natural fishing grounds have been overfished, and whole stretches of the oceans are, in fact, dead zones where fish and shellfish can no longer live. The FDA is also keeping a close eye on the safety of fish and shellfish affected by oil spills. Fish and shellfish from areas not affected by oil disasters are considered safe for consumers to eat.

To counteract the loss of wild fish populations, increasing numbers of fish are being farmed, which poses additional health risks and environmental concerns. Some farmed fish are laden with antibiotics. Other fish farms allow highly con-

centrated levels of parasites and bacteria from runoff to enter the ocean and rivers. Some farmed fish are fed wild fish, resulting in a net loss of fish from the sea.

At the same time that fish populations are threatened, high levels of toxins are being found in many of the fish available on the market. Mercury, a waste product of many industries, binds to proteins and stays in an animal's body, accumulating as it moves up the food chain; in humans, mercury can damage the nervous system and kidneys and cause birth defects and developmental problems in fetuses and children. Polychlorinated biphenyls (PCBs), chemicals that can build up in the fatty tissue of fish, are another cause of major concern.

So what is a savvy fish consumer to do? Know where your fish are caught and the methods by which they are caught. Several environmental groups have developed guides to inform consumers of safe and sustainable seafood choices. The Monterey Bay Aquarium in California pro-

vides a national guide for seafood available for purchase in the United States. You can find the guide online at www.montereybayaquarium.org/cr/cr_seafoodwatch/download.aspx. This guide is also available as a free iPhone or Android application, or it can be accessed on other mobile devices at http://mobile.seafoodwatch.org. Another great resource is the FishPhone service offered by the Blue Ocean Institute. Simply send a text message to 30644 with the word FISH and the type of fish you want to know about, and it will send you information about whether it is safe to eat.

Remember: Your consumer choices make a difference. Purchasing seafood from environmentally responsible sources will support fisheries and fish farms that are healthier for you and the environment.

Source: Food and Drug Administration, "Gulf of Mexico Oil Spill: Questions and Answers," 2011, www.fda.gov/Food/FoodSafety/Product-SpecificInformation/Seafood/ucm221563.htm.

Vitamins are classified as either *fat soluble,* which means they are absorbed through the intestinal tract with the help of fats, or *water soluble,* which means they are dissolved easily in water. Vitamins A, D, E, and K are fat soluble; B-complex vitamins and vitamin C are water soluble. Fat-soluble vitamins tend to be stored in the body, and toxic accumulations in the liver may cause cirrhosis-like symptoms. Water-soluble vitamins generally are excreted and cause fewer toxicity problems. See **Tables 7.2** and **7.3** on pages 213 and 214, respectively, for recommended intake amounts, food sources, functions, and potential dangers of specific vitamins.

Antioxidants Foods that may confer health benefits beyond the nutrients they contribute to the diet are called **functional foods** (see the **Health Headlines** box on page 215). Some of the most popular functional foods today are those containing **antioxidants.** Among the more commonly cited antioxidants are vitamin C, vitamin E, and beta-carotene, a precursor to vitamin A, as well as the minerals copper, iron, manganese, selenium, and zinc.

functional foods Foods believed to have specific health benefits and/or to prevent disease.

antioxidants Substances believed to protect against oxidative stress and resultant tissue damage.

These substances appear to protect people from the ravages of oxidative stress, a complex process in which *free radicals* (atoms with unpaired electrons that are produced during normal metabolism, as well as when the body is stressed) destabilize other atoms and molecules. This prompts a chain reaction that can damage cells, cell proteins, or genetic material in the cells. Free radical formation is a natural process that cannot be avoided, but antioxidants can combat it by donating their electrons to stabilize free radicals, activating enzymes that convert free radicals to less damaging substances, or by reducing or repairing the damage due to oxidative stress.

To date, many claims about the benefits of antioxidants in reducing the risk of heart disease and cancer, improving vision, and slowing the aging process have not been fully investigated, and conclusive statements about their true benefits are difficult to find. Large, longitudinal epidemiological studies support the hypothesis that antioxidants consumed in whole foods, mostly fruits and vegetables, may provide some protection against certain diseases, whereas antioxidant supplements do not confer such a benefit.[12]

Some studies indicate that when people's diets include foods rich in vitamin C, they seem to develop fewer cancers, but other

TABLE

7.2 A Guide to Water-Soluble Vitamins

Vitamin Name and Recommended Intake	Reliable Food Sources	Primary Functions	Toxicity/Deficiency Symptoms
Thiamin (vitamin B_1) RDA: Men = 1.2 mg/day Women = 1.1 mg/day	Pork, fortified cereals, enriched rice and pasta, peas, tuna, legumes	Required as enzyme cofactor for carbohydrate and amino acid metabolism	*Toxicity:* none known *Deficiency:* beriberi, fatigue, apathy, decreased memory, confusion, irritability, muscle weakness
Riboflavin (vitamin B_2) RDA: Men = 1.3 mg/day Women = 1.1 mg/day	Beef liver, shrimp, milk and dairy foods, fortified cereals, enriched breads and grains	Required as enzyme cofactor for carbohydrate and fat metabolism	*Toxicity:* none known *Deficiency:* ariboflavinosis, swollen mouth and throat, seborrheic dermatitis, anemia
Niacin, nicotinamide, nicotinic acid RDA: Men = 16 mg/day Women = 14 mg/day UL = 35 mg/day	Beef liver, most cuts of meat/fish/poultry, fortified cereals, enriched breads and grains, canned tomato products	Required for carbohydrate and fat metabolism; plays role in DNA replication and repair and cell differentiation	*Toxicity:* flushing, liver damage, glucose intolerance, blurred vision differentiation *Deficiency:* pellagra; vomiting, constipation, or diarrhea; apathy
Vitamin B_6 (pyridoxine, pyridoxal, pyridoxamine) RDA: Men and women 19–50 = 1.3 mg/day Men > 50 = 1.7 mg/day Women > 50 = 1.5 mg/day UL = 100 mg/day	Chickpeas (garbanzo beans), most cuts of meat/fish/ poultry, fortified cereals, white potatoes	Required as enzyme cofactor for carbohydrate and amino acid metabolism; assists synthesis of blood cells	*Toxicity:* nerve damage, skin lesions *Deficiency:* anemia; seborrheic dermatitis; depression, confusion, and convulsions
Folate (folic acid) RDA: Men = 400 µg/day Women = 400 µg/day UL = 1,000 µg/day	Fortified cereals, enriched breads and grains, spinach, legumes (lentils, chickpeas, pinto beans), greens (spinach, romaine lettuce), liver	Required as enzyme cofactor for amino acid metabolism; required for DNA synthesis; involved in metabolism of homocysteine	*Toxicity:* masks symptoms of vitamin B_{12} deficiency, specifically signs of nerve damage *Deficiency:* macrocytic anemia; neural tube defects in a developing fetus; elevated homocysteine levels
Vitamin B_{12} (cobalamin) RDA: Men = 2.4 µg/day Women = 2.4 µg/day	Shellfish, all cuts of meat/fish/poultry, milk and dairy foods, fortified cereals	Assists with formation of blood; required for healthy nervous system function; involved as enzyme cofactor in metabolism of homocysteine	*Toxicity:* none known *Deficiency:* pernicious anemia; tingling and numbness of extremities; nerve damage; memory loss, disorientation, and dementia
Pantothenic acid AI: Men = 5 mg/day Women = 5 mg/day	Meat/fish/poultry, shiitake mushrooms, fortified cereals, egg yolks	Assists with fat metabolism	*Toxicity:* none known Deficiency: rare
Biotin RDA: Men = 30 µg/day Women = 30 µg/day	Nuts, egg yolks	Involved as enzyme cofactor in carbohydrate, fat, and protein metabolism	*Toxicity:* none known *Deficiency:* rare
Vitamin C (ascorbic acid) RDA: Men = 90 mg/day Women = 75 mg/day Smokers = 35 mg more per day than RDA UL = 2,000 mg	Sweet peppers, citrus fruits and juices, broccoli, strawberries, kiwi	Antioxidant in extracellular fluid and lungs; regenerates oxidized vitamin E; assists with collagen synthesis; enhances immune function; assists in synthesis of hormones, neurotransmitters, and DNA; enhances iron absorption	*Toxicity:* nausea and diarrhea, nosebleeds, increased oxidative damage, increased formation of kidney stones in people with kidney disease *Deficiency:* scurvy, bone pain and fractures, depression, and anemia

Note: RDA = Recommended Daily Allowance; AI = Adequate Intakes; UL = Tolerable Upper Level Intakes. Values are for all adults aged 19 and older, except as noted. Values increase among women who are pregnant or lactating.

Source: Janice Thompson and Melinda Manore, *Nutrition for Life,* 3rd edition, © 2013. Printed and electronically reproduced by permission of Pearson Education, Inc., Upper Saddle River, New Jersey.

TABLE
7.3

A Guide to Fat-Soluble Vitamins

Vitamin Name and Recommended Intake	Reliable Food Sources	Primary Functions	Toxicity/Deficiency Symptoms
Vitamin A (retinol, retinal, retinoic acid) RDA: Men = 900 µg Women = 700 µg UL = 3,000 µg/day	Preformed retinol: beef and chicken liver, egg yolks, milk Carotenoid precursors: spinach, carrots, mango, apricots, cantaloupe, pumpkin, yams	Required for ability of eyes to adjust to changes in light; protects color vision; assists cell differentiation; required for sperm production in men and fertilization in women; contributes to healthy bone and healthy immune system	*Toxicity:* fatigue; bone and joint pain; spontaneous abortion and birth defects of fetuses in pregnant women; nausea and diarrhea; liver damage; nervous system damage; blurred vision; hair loss; skin disorders *Deficiency:* night blindness, xerophthalmia; impaired growth, immunity, and reproductive function
Vitamin D (cholecalciferol) RDA (assumes that person does not get adequate sun exposure): Adult 19–50 = 600 IU/day Adult 50–70 = 600 IU/day Adult > 70 = 800 IU/day UL = 4,000 IU/day	Canned salmon and mackerel, milk, fortified cereals	Regulates blood calcium levels; maintains bone health; assists cell differentiation	*Toxicity:* hypercalcemia *Deficiency:* rickets in children; osteomalacia and/or osteoporosis in adults
Vitamin E (tocopherol) RDA: Men = 15 mg/day Women = 15 mg/day UL = 1,000 mg/day	Sunflower seeds, almonds, vegetable oils, fortified cereals	As a powerful antioxidant, protects cell membranes, polyunsaturated fatty acids, and vitamin A from oxidation; protects white blood cells; enhances immune function; improves absorption of vitamin A	*Toxicity:* rare *Deficiency:* hemolytic anemia; impairment of nerve, muscle, and immune function
Vitamin K (phylloquinone, menaquinone, menadione) AI: Men = 120 µg/day Women = 90 µg/day	Kale, spinach, turnip greens, brussels sprouts	Serves as a coenzyme during production of specific proteins that assist in blood coagulation and bone metabolism	*Toxicity:* none known *Deficiency:* impaired blood clotting; possible effect on bone health

Note: RDA = Recommended Daily Allowance; AI = Adequate Intakes; UL = Tolerable Upper Level Intakes. Values are for all adults aged 19 and older, except as noted. Values increase among women who are pregnant or lactating.

Source: Janice Thompson and Melinda Manore, *Nutrition for Life*, 3rd edition, © 2013. Printed and electronically reproduced by permission of Pearson Education, Inc., Upper Saddle River, New Jersey.

studies detect no effect from dietary vitamin C.[13] Recent studies indicate that high-dose vitamin C given intravenously, rather than orally, may be effective in treating cancer and protecting from diseases affecting the central nervous system.[14]

Possible effects of vitamin E intake are even more controversial. Researchers have long theorized that because many cancers result from DNA damage, and because vitamin E appears to protect against such damage, vitamin E would also reduce cancer risk. Surprisingly, the great majority of studies have demonstrated no effect or, in some cases, a negative effect.[15] However, it can be difficult to compare studies on vitamin E because several different forms of vitamin E exist.

carotenoids Fat-soluble plant pigments with antioxidant properties.

Carotenoids are part of the red, orange, and yellow pigments found in fruits and vegetables. They are fat soluble, transported in the blood by lipoproteins, and stored in the fatty tissues of the body. Beta-carotene, the most researched carotenoid, is a precursor of vitamin A. This means that vitamin A can be produced in the body from beta-carotene; like vitamin A, beta-carotene has antioxidant properties.

Although there are over 600 carotenoids in nature, two that have received a great deal of attention are *lycopene* (found in tomatoes, tomato pastes, and tomato sauces; papaya; pink grapefruit; and guava) and *lutein* (found in green leafy vegetables such as spinach, broccoli, kale, and brussels sprouts). The National Cancer Institute and the American Cancer Society have endorsed lycopene as a possible factor in reducing the risk of cancer. A landmark study reported that men who ate ten or more servings of lycopene-rich foods per week had a 45 percent lower risk of prostate cancer.[16] However, subsequent studies have questioned the benefits of lycopene, and some professional groups are modifying their endorsements

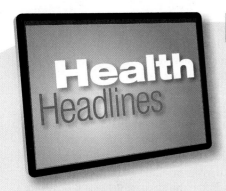
HEALTH CLAIMS OF FUNCTIONAL FOODS

Functional foods are those that may provide a health benefit beyond basic nutrition. They include a wide variety of foods that are believed to improve over-all health, reduce disease, or minimize health concerns. For example, probiotics are living, beneficial bacteria found in fermented milk products such as yogurt and kefir. You will see them labeled as *Lactobacillus* or *Bifidobacterium* in a product's list of ingredients. Probiotics colonize the large intestine, where they are thought to reduce the risk of diarrhea, irritable bowel syndrome, and inflammatory bowel disease.

Other examples of functional foods include the following: chocolate! Cocoa is particularly rich in a class of chemicals called flavanols that have been shown in many studies to reduce the risk for cardiovascular disease. Dark chocolate has a higher level of flavanols than milk chocolate. Whole-grain cereals, breads, and pastas may reduce the risk of cardiovascular disease and some types of cancer and may help maintain healthy blood glucose levels. Soy proteins, whether from soy milk, tofu, or other soy products, have also been associated with a reduced risk for cardiovascular disease. Note that functional foods don't have to come in fancy packages. For example, fruits, vegetables, and fish are all considered functional foods.

Want to incorporate more functional foods in your diet? Be aware that in the United States, the Food and Drug Administration (FDA) does not currently provide a specific definition or regulation for functional foods. However, the FDA does regulate health claims on the labels of food products sold in the U.S. See the Read Food Labels section on page 222

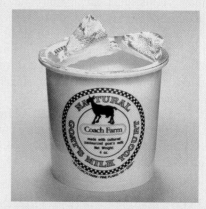

Yogurt and kefir (a fermented milk drink) are dairy products containing beneficial bacteria called *probiotics*.

for the types of health claims that the FDA allows food manufacturers to make.

Sources: E. M. Quigley, "Prebiotics and Probiotics: Modifying and Mining the Microbiota," *Pharmacological Research* 61, no. 3 (2010):213–18; J. W. Erdman et. al., "Health Benefits of Chocolate," *Asia Pacific Journal of Clinical Nutrition*, 17: Supplement no. 1 (2008):284–87; International Food Information Council, "Background on Functional Foods Backgrounder," September 2009, www.foodinsight.org/Resources/Detail.aspx?topic=Background_on_Functional_Foods.

---

of tomato-based products.[17] Lutein is most often touted as a means of protecting the eyes, particularly from age-related macular degeneration, a leading cause of blindness for people aged 65 and older.

Vitamin D Vitamin D, the sunshine vitamin, is formed from a compound in the skin when exposed to the sun's ultraviolet rays. In most people, an adequate amount of vitamin D can be synthesized with 10 to 30 minutes of sun on the face, neck, hands, arms, and legs twice a week. However, the sun is not high enough in the sky during late fall to early spring in northern climates to allow for vitamin D synthesis. Moreover, the skin must be bare, without clothing or sunscreen.[18] For people who cannot rely on the sun to meet their daily vitamin D needs, vitamin D–fortified milk, yogurt, soy milk, cereals, and fatty fish, such as salmon, can also supply this vitamin.

Vitamin D is essential for the body's regulation of calcium, the primary mineral component of bone. It also assists in the process of calcification by which bone minerals are crystallized. For these reasons, a deficiency of vitamin D can promote loss of bone density and strength, a condition

called *osteoporosis*. Two other bone disorders, *rickets* in children, and its adult version, *osteomalacia,* can also be prevented with adequate intake of vitamin D.[19] Vitamin D also helps fight infections, lowers blood pressure, reduces the risk of developing diabetes mellitus, and may reduce the growth of cancer cells. Breast and prostate cancer, heart disease, and stroke have also been connected to inadequate vitamin D.

More is not always better, however.[20] Too much vitamin D, generally from excessive intake of vitamin D supplements, can reduce appetite and cause nausea, vomiting, and constipation. Excess vitamin D can also affect the nervous system, cause depression, and deposit calcium in the soft tissues of the kidneys, lungs, blood vessels, and heart.

Blueberries are a great source of antioxidants.

Folate One of the B vitamins, folate is needed for the production of compounds necessary for DNA synthesis in body cells. It is particularly important for proper cell division during embryonic development; folate deficiencies during the first few weeks of pregnancy, typically before a woman even realizes she is pregnant, can prompt a neural tube defect (NTD), in which the primitive tube that eventually forms the brain and spinal cord fails to close properly. A common NTD is spina bifida, a birth defect in which a portion of the newborn's spinal cord protrudes through the vertebral column. In 1998, the FDA began requiring that all bread, cereal, rice, and pasta products sold in the United States be fortified with folic acid, the synthetic form of folate, to reduce the incidence of spina bifida and other neural tube defects.

Folate is also important for the synthesis of several amino acids and for the production of healthy red blood cells. The DRI for folate is 400 micrograms daily for both males and females throughout adulthood. During pregnancy, this increases to 600 micrograms per day.

Minerals

Minerals are the inorganic, indestructible elements that aid physiological processes within the body. Without minerals, vitamins could not be absorbed. Minerals are readily excreted and, with a few exceptions, are usually not toxic. *Major minerals* are the minerals that the body needs in fairly large amounts: sodium, calcium, phosphorus, magnesium, potassium, sulfur, and chloride. *Trace minerals* include iron, zinc, manganese, copper, fluoride, selenium, chromium, and iodine. Only very small amounts of trace minerals are needed, and serious problems may result if excesses or deficiencies occur (see Tables 7.4 and 7.5 on pages 217 and 218).

minerals Inorganic, indestructible elements that aid physiological processes.

Sodium Sodium is necessary for the regulation of blood volume and blood pressure, fluid balance, transmission of nerve impulses, heart activity, and certain metabolic functions. It enhances flavors, acts as a preservative, and tenderizes meats, so it's often present in high quantities in the foods we eat. A common misconception is that table salt and sodium are the same thing: Table salt is a compound containing both sodium and chloride. It accounts for only 15 percent of our sodium intake. The majority of sodium in our diet comes from processed foods that are infused with sodium to enhance flavor and preservation. Pickles, fast foods, salty snacks, processed cheeses, canned soups and frozen dinners, many breads and bakery products, and smoked meats and sausages often contain several hundred milligrams of sodium per serving.

Many health professionals believe that Americans need to reduce sodium.[21] The Institute of Medicine, the American Heart Association, and the U.S. Department of Agriculture (USDA) are among the professional and governmental organizations that recommend that healthy people consume fewer than 2,300 milligrams of sodium each day. What does that really mean? For most

Even if you never use table salt, you still may be getting excess sodium in your diet.

of us, less than 1 teaspoon of table salt per day is all we need! The latest National Health and Nutrition Examination Survey (NHANES) estimated that the average American over 2 years of age consumes 3,436 milligrams per day.[22]

Why is high sodium intake a concern? Salt-sensitive individuals respond to a high-sodium diet with an increase in blood pressure (hypertension). Although the cause of the majority of cases of hypertension is unknown, researchers recommend that hypertensive Americans cut back on sodium to reduce their risk for a heart attack, stroke, and other health problems.[23] See the Skills for Behavior Change box for tips on how to reduce your sodium intake.

Calcium Calcium is the primary mineral component of bones and teeth. It is also essential for muscle contraction, nerve impulse transmission, and regulation of the heartbeat. An alkaline mineral, calcium is an important buffer, reducing blood acidity and helping to maintain pH balance. It's also important for blood clotting and other functions. The issue of calcium consumption has gained national attention with the rising incidence of osteoporosis among older adults. Most Americans do not consume the recommended 1,000 to 1,200 milligrams of calcium per day.[24]

Dairy products, as well as calcium-fortified juices and milk alternatives are excellent sources of calcium. So are many leafy green vegetables, including broccoli, collard greens, and kale. Although the amount of calcium vegetables provide is lower, it is better absorbed than the calcium from dairy products. Spinach, chard, and beet greens are not particularly good sources of calcium because they contain oxalic acid, which interferes with calcium absorption. Many peas and beans also offer good supplies.

For optimal absorption, consume calcium throughout the day by eating foods and drinking beverages containing protein, vitamin D, and vitamin C. Many dairy products and milk alternatives are fortified with vitamin D, which is necessary for calcium regulation.

Do you consume carbonated soft drinks? Be aware that the added phosphoric acid (phosphate) in these drinks can cause you to excrete extra calcium, which may result in

Mineral Name and Recommended Intake	Reliable Food Sources	Primary Functions	Toxicity/Deficiency Symptoms
Sodium AI: Adults = 1.5 g/day (1,500 mg/day)	Table salt, pickles, most canned soups, snack foods, cured luncheon meats, canned tomato products	Fluid balance; acid–base balance; transmission of nerve impulses; muscle contraction	*Toxicity:* water retention, high blood pressure, loss of calcium *Deficiency:* muscle cramps, dizziness, fatigue, nausea, vomiting, mental confusion
Potassium AI: Adults = 4.7 g/day (4,700 mg/day)	Most fresh fruits and vegetables: potato, banana, tomato juice, orange juice, melon	Fluid balance; transmission of nerve impulses; muscle contraction	*Toxicity:* muscle weakness, vomiting, irregular heartbeat *Deficiency:* muscle weakness, paralysis, mental confusion, irregular heartbeat
Phosphorus RDA: Adults = 700 mg/day	Milk/cheese/yogurt, soy milk and tofu, legumes (lentils, black beans), nuts (almonds, peanuts), poultry	Fluid balance; bone formation; component of ATP, which provides energy for our bodies	*Toxicity:* muscle spasms, convulsions, low blood calcium *Deficiency:* muscle weakness, muscle damage, bone pain, dizziness
Chloride AI: Adults = 2.3 g/day (2,300 mg/day)	Table salt	Fluid balance; transmission of nerve impulses; component of stomach acid (HCL); antibacterial	*Toxicity:* none known *Deficiency:* dangerous blood acid–base imbalances, irregular heartbeat
Calcium AI: Adults 19–50 = 1,000 mg/day Adults > 50 = 1,200 mg/day UL = 2,500 mg	Milk/yogurt/cheese (best absorbed form of calcium), sardines, collard greens and spinach, calcium-fortified juices	Primary component of bone; acid–base balance; transmission of nerve impulses; muscle contraction	*Toxicity:* mineral imbalances, shock, kidney failure, fatigue, mental confusion *Deficiency:* osteoporosis, convulsions, heart failure
Magnesium RDA: Men 19–30 = 400 mg/day Men > 30 = 420 mg/day Women 19–30 = 310 mg/day Women > 30 = 320 mg/day UL = 350 mg/day	Greens (spinach, kale, collards), whole grains, seeds, nuts, legumes (navy and black beans)	Component of bone; muscle contraction; assists more than 300 enzyme systems	*Toxicity:* none known *Deficiency:* low blood calcium; muscle spasms or seizures; nausea; weakness; increased risk of chronic diseases such as heart disease, hypertension, osteoporosis, and type 2 diabetes
Sulfur No DRI	Protein-rich foods	Component of certain B vitamins and amino acids; acid–base balance; detoxification in liver	*Toxicity:* none known Deficiency: none known

Note: RDA = Recommended Daily Allowance; AI = Adequate Intakes; UL = Tolerable Upper Level Intake. Values are for all adults aged 19 and older, except as noted.

Source: Janice Thompson and Melinda Manore, *Nutrition for Life,* 3rd edition, © 2013. Printed and electronically reproduced by permission of Pearson Education, Inc., Upper Saddle River, New Jersey.

calcium loss from your bones. One study of 2,500 men and women found that in women who consumed at least three cans of cola per week, even diet cola, bone density of the hip was 4 to 5 percent lower than in women who drank fewer than one cola per month. Colas did not seem to have the same effect on men.[25] There may also be a "milk displace-ment effect," meaning that people who consume soda are not consuming milk, thereby decreasing their calcium intake.

Iron Worldwide, iron deficiency is the most common nu-trient deficiency, affecting nearly 30 percent of the world's population.[26] In the United States iron deficiency is less

A Guide to Trace Minerals

Mineral Name and Recommended Intake	Reliable Food Sources	Primary Functions	Toxicity/Deficiency Symptoms
Selenium RDA: Adults = 55 µg/day UL = 400 µg/day	Nuts, shellfish, meat/fish/poultry, whole grains	Required for carbohydrate and fat metabolism	*Toxicity:* brittle hair and nails, skin rashes, nausea and vomiting, weakness, liver disease *Deficiency:* specific forms of heart disease and arthritis, impaired immune function, muscle pain and wasting, depression, hostility
Fluoride AI: Men = 4 mg/day Women = 3 mg/day UL = 2.2 mg/day for children 4–8 years; children > 8 years = 10 mg/day	Fluoridated water and other beverages made with this water	Development and maintenance of healthy teeth and bones	*Toxicity:* fluorosis of teeth and bones *Deficiency:* dental caries, low bone density
Iodine RDA: Adults = 150 µg/day UL = 1,100 µg/day	Iodized salt and foods processed with iodized salt	Synthesis of thyroid hormones; temperature regulation; reproduction and growth	*Toxicity:* goiter *Deficiency:* goiter, hypothyroidism, cretinism in infant of mother who is iodine deficient
Chromium AI: Men 19–50 = 35 µg/day Men > 50 = 30 µg/day Women 19–50 = 25 µg/day Women > 50 = 20 µg/day	Grains, meat/fish/poultry, some fruits and vegetables	Glucose transport; metabolism of DNA and RNA; immune function and growth	*Toxicity:* none known *Deficiency:* elevated blood glucose and blood lipids, damage to brain and nervous system
Manganese AI: Men = 2.3 mg/day Women = 1.8 mg/day UL = 11 mg/day for adults	Whole grains, nuts, legumes, some fruits and vegetables	Assists many enzyme systems; synthesis of protein found in bone and cartilage	*Toxicity:* impairment of neuromuscular system *Deficiency:* impaired growth and reproductive function, reduced bone density, impaired glucose and lipid metabolism, skin rash
Iron RDA: Men = 8 mg/day Women 19–50 = 18 mg/day Women > 50 = 8 mg/day	Meat/fish/poultry (best absorbed form of iron), fortified cereals, legumes, spinach	Component of hemoglobin in blood cells; component of myoglobin in muscle cells; assists many enzyme systems	*Toxicity:* nausea, vomiting, and diarrhea; dizziness, confusion; rapid heartbeat; organ damage; death *Deficiency:* iron-deficiency microcytic anemia, hypochromic anemia
Zinc RDA: Men 11 mg/day Women = 8 mg/day UL = 40 mg/day	Meat/fish/poultry (best absorbed form of zinc), fortified cereals, legumes	Assists more than 100 enzyme systems; immune system function; growth and sexual maturation; gene regulation	*Toxicity:* nausea, vomiting, and diarrhea; headaches; depressed immune function; reduced absorption of copper *Deficiency:* growth retardation, delayed sexual maturation, eye and skin lesions, hair loss, increased incidence of illness and infection
Copper RDA: Adults = 900 µg/day UL = 10 mg/day	Shellfish, organ meats, nuts, legumes	Assists many enzyme systems; iron transport	*Toxicity:* nausea, vomiting, and diarrhea; liver damage *Deficiency:* anemia, reduced levels of white blood cells, osteoporosis in infants and growing children

Note: RDA = Recommended Daily Allowance; AI = Adequate Intakes; UL = Tolerable Upper Intake Level. Values are for all adults aged 19 and older, except as noted.

Source: Janice Thompson and Melinda Manore, *Nutrition for Life,* 3rd edition, © 2013. Printed and electronically reproduced by permission of Pearson Education, Inc., Upper Saddle River, New Jersey.

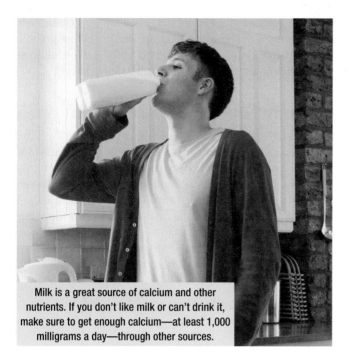

Milk is a great source of calcium and other nutrients. If you don't like milk or can't drink it, make sure to get enough calcium—at least 1,000 milligrams a day—through other sources.

prevalent, but it is still the most common micronutrient deficiency.[27] Women aged 19 to 50 need about 18 milligrams of iron per day, and men aged 19 to 50 need about 8 milligrams.

Iron deficiency can lead to *iron-deficiency anemia*. **Anemia** results from the body's inability to produce adequate amounts of hemoglobin (the oxygen-carrying component of the blood). When iron-deficiency anemia occurs, body cells receive less oxygen. As a result, the iron-deficient person feels tired. Iron is also important for energy metabolism, DNA synthesis, and other body functions. Iron deficiency in the diet is not the only cause of anemia; anemia can also result from blood loss, cancer, ulcers, and other conditions.

Iron overload or iron toxicity due to ingesting too many iron-containing supplements is the leading cause of accidental poisoning in small children in the United States. Symptoms of toxicity include nausea, vomiting, diarrhea, rapid heartbeat, weak pulse, dizziness, shock, and confusion. Excess iron intake, especially from supplements, is also associated with gastrointestinal distress, constipation, and other problems: A recent study of over 45,000 men indicated that those who consumed excess heme iron—the kind found in meat, seafood, and poultry—had a 20 percent higher risk of gallstones than those who consumed low-iron foods or got their iron from supplements.[28]

How Can I Eat More Healthfully?

Americans today overall eat more food than ever before. From 1970 to 2008, average calorie consumption increased from 2,157 to 2,673 calories per day (see Figure 7.5).[29] In general, it isn't the actual amount of food, but the number of calories in the foods we choose to eat that has increased. When these

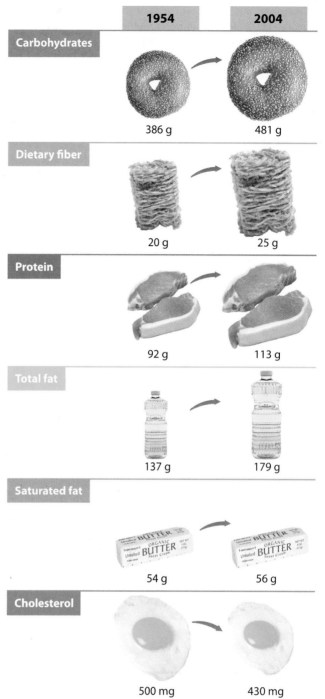

	1954	2004
Carbohydrates	386 g	481 g
Dietary fiber	20 g	25 g
Protein	92 g	113 g
Total fat	137 g	179 g
Saturated fat	54 g	56 g
Cholesterol	500 mg	430 mg

FIGURE 7.5 **Trends in Per Capita Nutrient Consumption**
Since 1954, Americans' daily caloric intake has increased by about 25%, as has daily consumption of carbohydrates, fiber, and protein. Daily total fat intake has increased by 30%.

Source: Data are from USDA Economic Research Service, Nutrient Availability, Updated February 2010, www.ers.usda.gov/Data/FoodConsumption/NutrientAvailIndex.htm.

trends are combined with our increasingly sedentary lifestyle, it is not surprising that we have seen a dramatic rise in obesity.[30]

anemia Condition that results from the body's inability to produce adequate hemoglobin.

Fortunately, the Center for Nutrition Policy and Promotion at the U.S. Department of Agriculture publishes two dietary tools created for consumers to make healthy eating easy: the Dietary Guidelines for Americans and the MyPlate food guidance system.

Dietary Guidelines for Americans, 2010

The Dietary Guidelines for Americans are a set of recommendations for healthy eating. They are revised every 5 years. The 2010 Dietary Guidelines for Americans are designed to help bridge the gap between the standard American diet and the key recommendations that aim to combat the growing obesity epidemic by balancing calories with adequate physical activity.[31] They provide advice about consuming fewer calories, making informed food choices, and being physically active to attain and maintain a healthy weight, reduce your risk for chronic disease, and improve your overall health. The 2010 Dietary Guidelines for Americans are presented as an easy-to-follow graphic and guidance system called MyPlate, which can be found at www.choosemyplate.gov and is illustrated in Figure 7.6.

MyPlate Food Guidance System

The MyPlate food guidance system takes into consideration the dietary and caloric needs for a wide variety of individuals, such as pregnant or breast-feeding women, those trying to lose weight, and adults with different activity levels. When you visit the interactive website, you can create personalized dietary and exercise recommendations based on the information you enter.

MyPlate also encourages consumers to eat for health through three general areas of recommendation:

1. Balance calories:
- Enjoy your food, but eat less.
- Avoid oversized portions.

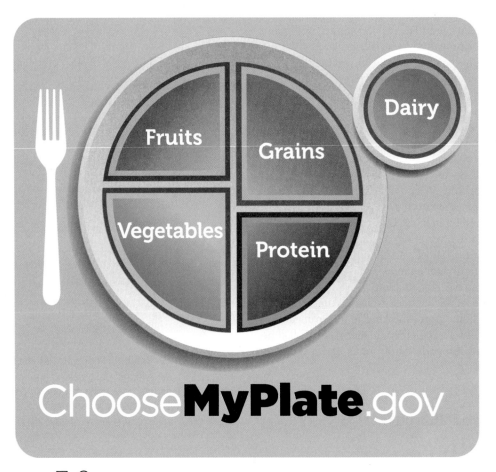

FIGURE 7.6 **MyPlate Plan**
The USDA MyPlate food guidance system takes a new approach to dietary and exercise recommendations. Each colored section of the plate represents a food group, and an interactive tool at www.choosemyplate.gov provides individualized recommendations.
Source: U.S. Department of Agriculture, 2010, www.choosemyplate.gov.

2. Increase foods:
- Fill half your plate with fruits and vegetables.
- Make at least half your grains whole.
- Switch to fat-free or 1 percent milk.

3. Reduce foods:

- Compare sodium in foods such as soup, bread, and frozen meals, and choose the foods with lower numbers.
- Drink water instead of sugary drinks.

Understand Serving Sizes MyPlate presents personalized dietary recommendations based on servings of particular nutrients. But how much is one serving? Is it different from a portion? Although these two terms are often used interchangeably, they actually mean very different things. A *serving* is the recommended amount you should consume, whereas a *portion* is the amount you choose to eat at any one time. Most of us select portions that are much bigger than recommended servings. In a survey conducted by the American Institute for Cancer Research, respondents were asked to estimate the standard servings for eight different foods. Only 1 percent of those surveyed correctly answered all serving size questions, and nearly 65 percent answered five or more of them incorrectly.[32] See **Figure 7.7** for a handy pocket guide with tips on recognizing serving sizes.

Unfortunately, we don't always get a clear picture from food producers and advertisers about what a serving really is. Consider a bottle of soda: The food label may list one serving size as 8 fluid ounces and 100 calories. However, note the size of the entire bottle. If the bottle holds 20 ounces, drinking the whole thing serves up 250 calories.

Eat Nutrient-Dense Foods Although eating the proper number of servings from MyPlate is important, it is also important to recognize that there are large caloric, fat, and energy differences among foods within a given food group. For example, salmon and hot dogs provide vastly different nutrient levels per calorie. Salmon is rich in essential fatty acids, and is considered nutrient dense. Hot dogs are loaded with saturated fats, cholesterol, and sodium—all substances we should limit. It is important to eat foods that have a high nutritional value for their caloric content.

Reduce Empty Calorie Foods Avoid *empty calories*, that is, high-calorie foods and beverages that have little nutritional value. MyPlate recommends we limit these sugar- and fat-laden items, including the following:[33]

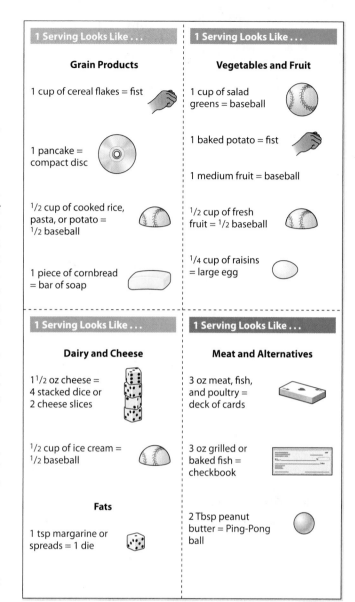

FIGURE 7.7 **Serving Size Card**
One of the challenges of following a healthy diet is judging how big a portion size should be and how many servings you are really eating. The comparisons on this card can help you recall what a standard food serving looks like. For easy reference, photocopy or cut out this card, fold on the dotted lines, and keep it in your wallet. You can even laminate it for long-term use.

Source: National Heart, Lung and Blood Institute, "Serving Size Card," Accessed April 2010, http://hp2010.nhlbihin.net/portion/servingcard7.pdf.

What's Working for You?

Maybe you already eat a healthful, balanced diet. Below are a few aspects of a healthful approach to eating. Which of these are you already incorporating into your life?

☐ I choose whole-grain breads and cereals.

☐ I try to avoid eating saturated fats.

☐ I limit my salt intake.

- **Cakes, cookies, pastries, and donuts:** Just one slice of chocolate cake contains 77 percent empty calories.
- **Sodas, energy drinks, sports drinks, and fruit drinks:** For soda, 12 fluid ounces contain 192 calories or 100 percent empty calories.
- **Cheese:** Switching from whole milk mozzarella cheese to nonfat mozzarella cheese saves you 76 empty calories per ounce.

● **Pizza:** One slice of pepperoni pizza adds 139 empty calories to your meal.

● **Ice cream:** For ice cream, 76 percent of the 275 calories are empty calories.

● **Sausages, hot dogs, bacon, and ribs:** Adding a sausage link to your breakfast adds 96 empty calories.

● **Wine, beer, and all alcoholic beverages:** A whopping 155 empty calories are consumed with each 12 fluid ounces of beer.

● **Refined grains, including crackers, cookies, white rice:** Switching from snack crackers to whole wheat can save you 25 fat-laden empty calories per serving.

Physical Activity Strive to be physically active for at least 30 minutes daily, preferably with moderate to vigorous activity levels on most days. Physical activity does not mean you have to go to the gym, jog 3 miles a day, or hire a personal trainer. Any activity that gets your heart pumping counts, including gardening, playing basketball, heavy yard work, and dancing. MyPlate personalized plans offer recommendations for weekly physical activity. (For more on physical fitness, see **Chapter 9**.)

Read Food Labels

How do you know what nutrients the packaged foods you eat are contributing to your diet? To help consumers evaluate the nutritional values of packaged foods, the FDA and the USDA developed the **percent daily values (%DVs)** list that you see on food and supplement labels. The %DV is calculated based on a 2,000 calorie per day diet, so your values may be different from those listed on a label (lower if you eat a higher calorie diet and higher if you eat a lower calorie diet). In addition to the percentage of nutrients found in a serving of food, labels also include information on the serving size and calories. **Figure 7.8** on page 223 walks you through a typical food label.

% Daily Values (%DVs) Percentages listed as "% DV" on food and supplement labels; identify how much of each listed nutrient a serving of food contributes to a 2,000 calorie/day diet.

vegetarian A person who follows a diet that excludes some or all animal products.

Food labels can contain other information as well, such as health claims. Health claims may assist you in selecting functional foods that meet your nutritional needs. The FDA allows five types of health-related claims on the packages of foods and dietary supplements:[34]

● **Nutrient content claims** that indicate a specific nutrient is present at a certain level. For example, a product label might say "High in fiber" or "Low in fat" or "This product contains 100 calories per serving." Nutrient content claims can use the following words: *more, less, fewer, good source of, free, light, lean, extra lean, high, low, reduced.*

● **Structure and function claims** that describe the effect that a dietary component has on the body. An example of a structure/function claim is "Calcium builds strong bones."

● **Dietary guidance claims** describe health benefits or health effects of a broad category of foods rather than a specific nutrient. An example is "Diets rich in fruits and vegetables may reduce the risks of some types of cancer."

● **Qualified health claims** convey a relationship between diet and the risk for disease. These must be approved by the FDA and supported by scientific research. You will find qualified health claims about cancer risk, cardiovascular disease, cognitive function, diabetes, and hypertension, for example, "Diets low in sodium may reduce the risk of high blood pressure, a disease associated with many factors."

● **Health claims** confirm a relationship between components in the diet and health promotion or disease prevention. These must be approved by the FDA and supported by evidence. For example, an approved health claim on a package of whole-grain bread may state, "In a low-fat diet, whole-grain foods like this bread may reduce the risk of heart disease."

Vegetarianism: A Healthy Diet?

More than 3 percent of U.S. adults, approximately 6 to 8 million people, are vegetarians.[35] In addition, nearly 23 million Americans are "vegetarian inclined," or "flexitarians," meaning that they are omnivores who are trying to eat more vegetarian meals and reducing meat consumption in favor of other "faceless" forms of protein.[36] The word **vegetarian** means different things to different people. See **Table 7.6** on page 223 for a complete listing of vegetarian types and the foods each type eats.

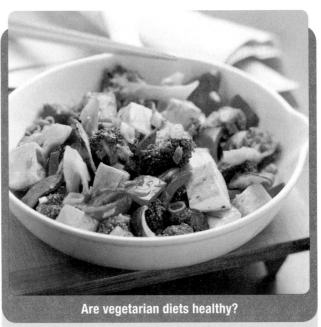

Are vegetarian diets healthy?

Adopting a vegan or vegetarian diet can be a very healthy way to eat. Take care to prepare your food healthfully by avoiding added sugars and excessive sodium. Make sure you get complementary essential amino acids by eating meals like this tofu and vegetable stir-fry. To further enhance it, add a whole grain, such as brown rice.

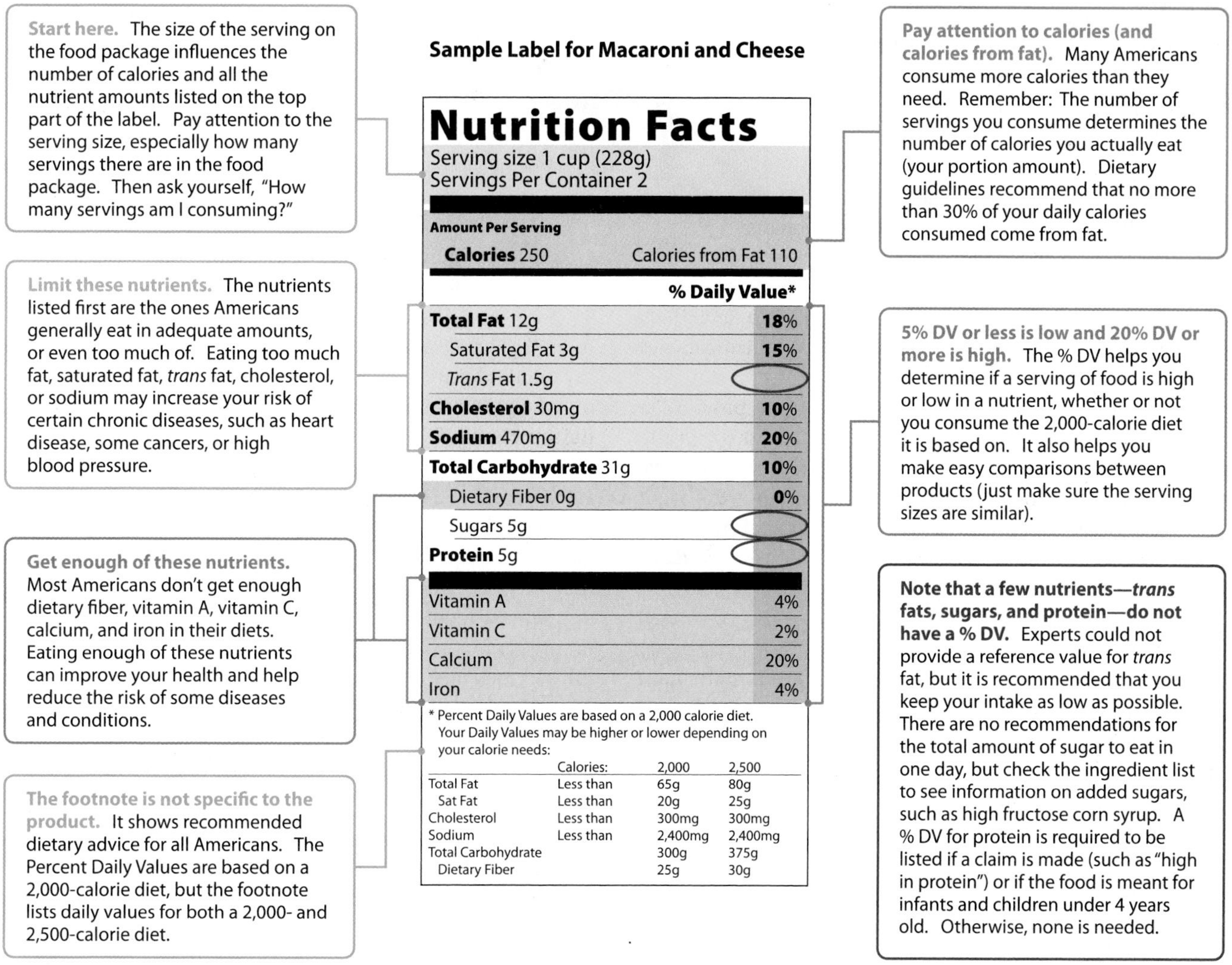

Start here. The size of the serving on the food package influences the number of calories and all the nutrient amounts listed on the top part of the label. Pay attention to the serving size, especially how many servings there are in the food package. Then ask yourself, "How many servings am I consuming?"

Limit these nutrients. The nutrients listed first are the ones Americans generally eat in adequate amounts, or even too much of. Eating too much fat, saturated fat, *trans* fat, cholesterol, or sodium may increase your risk of certain chronic diseases, such as heart disease, some cancers, or high blood pressure.

Get enough of these nutrients. Most Americans don't get enough dietary fiber, vitamin A, vitamin C, calcium, and iron in their diets. Eating enough of these nutrients can improve your health and help reduce the risk of some diseases and conditions.

The footnote is not specific to the product. It shows recommended dietary advice for all Americans. The Percent Daily Values are based on a 2,000-calorie diet, but the footnote lists daily values for both a 2,000- and 2,500-calorie diet.

Sample Label for Macaroni and Cheese

Nutrition Facts

Serving size 1 cup (228g)
Servings Per Container 2

Amount Per Serving

Calories 250   Calories from Fat 110

% Daily Value*

Total Fat 12g	**18%**
Saturated Fat 3g	**15%**
Trans Fat 1.5g	
Cholesterol 30mg	**10%**
Sodium 470mg	**20%**
Total Carbohydrate 31g	**10%**
Dietary Fiber 0g	**0%**
Sugars 5g	
Protein 5g	
Vitamin A	4%
Vitamin C	2%
Calcium	20%
Iron	4%

* Percent Daily Values are based on a 2,000 calorie diet. Your Daily Values may be higher or lower depending on your calorie needs:

		2,000	2,500
Total Fat	Less than	65g	80g
Sat Fat	Less than	20g	25g
Cholesterol	Less than	300mg	300mg
Sodium	Less than	2,400mg	2,400mg
Total Carbohydrate		300g	375g
Dietary Fiber		25g	30g

Pay attention to calories (and calories from fat). Many Americans consume more calories than they need. Remember: The number of servings you consume determines the number of calories you actually eat (your portion amount). Dietary guidelines recommend that no more than 30% of your daily calories consumed come from fat.

5% DV or less is low and 20% DV or more is high. The % DV helps you determine if a serving of food is high or low in a nutrient, whether or not you consume the 2,000-calorie diet it is based on. It also helps you make easy comparisons between products (just make sure the serving sizes are similar).

Note that a few nutrients—*trans* fats, sugars, and protein—do not have a % DV. Experts could not provide a reference value for *trans* fat, but it is recommended that you keep your intake as low as possible. There are no recommendations for the total amount of sugar to eat in one day, but check the ingredient list to see information on added sugars, such as high fructose corn syrup. A % DV for protein is required to be listed if a claim is made (such as "high in protein") or if the food is meant for infants and children under 4 years old. Otherwise, none is needed.

FIGURE 7.8 **Reading a Food Label**

Source: Center for Food Safety and Applied Nutrition, "A Key to Choosing Healthful Foods: Using the Nutrition Facts on the Food Label," Updated May 2009, www.fda.gov/Food/Resources-ForYou/Consumers/ucm079449.htm.

Video Tutor: Understanding Food Labels

TABLE 7.6 **Types of Vegetarians**

Type of Vegetarian	Does Eat	Doesn't Eat
Vegan	Vegetables, grains, fruits, nuts, seeds, and legumes	Meat, poultry, seafood, dairy products, eggs, any other animal-based products
Lacto-vegetarian	Vegetables, grains, fruits, nuts, seeds, legumes, and dairy products	Meat, poultry, seafood, and eggs
Ovo-vegetarian	Vegetables, grains, fruits, nuts, seeds, legumes, and eggs	Meat, poultry, seafood, and dairy products
Lacto-ovo-vegetarian	Vegetables, grains, fruits, nuts, seeds, legumes, dairy products, and eggs	Meat, poultry, and seafood
Pesco-vegetarian	Vegetables, grains, fruits, nuts, seeds, legumes, dairy products, eggs, and seafood	Meat and poultry
Semi-vegetarian (or "non–red meat eater")	Vegetables, grains, fruits, nuts, seeds, legumes, dairy products, eggs, seafood, and poultry (occasional)	Red meat

Source: Data are from Centers for Disease Control and Prevention, CDC Estimates of Foodborne Illness in the United States, CDC 2011 Estimates: Findings, Accessed February 7, 2012, from www.cdc.gov/foodborneburden/2011-foodborne-estimates.html.

Common reasons for pursuing a vegetarian lifestyle include concern for animal welfare, improving health, environmental concerns, natural approaches to wellness, food safety, weight loss, and weight maintenance. Generally, people who follow a balanced vegetarian diet weigh less and have better cholesterol levels, fewer problems with irregular bowel movements (constipation and diarrhea), and a lower risk of heart disease than do non-vegetarians. The benefits of vegetarianism also include a reduced risk of some cancers, particularly colon cancer, and a reduced risk of kidney disease.[37]

With proper meal planning, vegetarianism provides a healthful alternative to a meat-based diet. Although in the past some vegetarians suffered from nutrient deficiencies, most vegetarians today are adept at combining the right types of foods and eating a variety of different foods to ensure proper nutrient intake. Vegan diets are of greater concern than diets that include dairy products and eggs. Vegans may be deficient in vitamins B_2 (riboflavin), B_{12}, and D, as well as calcium, iron, zinc, and other minerals; however, many foods are fortified with these nutrients, or vegans can obtain them from supplements. Vegans also have to pay more attention to the amino acid content of their foods, but by eating complementary combinations of plant products, they can receive adequate amounts of protein. In fact, whereas vegans typically get 50 to 60 grams of protein per day, lacto-ovo-vegetarians normally consume 70 to 90 grams per day, well beyond the recommended amounts. Pregnant women, older adults, sick people, and families with young children who are vegans need to take special care to ensure that their diets are adequate. In all cases, seek advice from a health care professional if you have questions.

Supplements: Research on the Daily Dose

Dietary supplements are products containing one or more dietary ingredients taken by mouth and intended to supplement existing diets. Ingredients range from vitamins, minerals, and herbs to enzymes, amino acids, fatty acids, and organ tissues. They can come in tablet, capsule, liquid, powder, and other forms. Because of dietary supplements' potential for influencing health, their sales have skyrocketed.

It is important to note that dietary supplements are not regulated like foods or drugs. The FDA does not evaluate the

dietary supplements Products taken by mouth and containing dietary ingredients such as vitamins and minerals that are intended to supplement existing diets.

safety and efficacy of supplements prior to their marketing, and it can take action to remove a supplement from the market only after the product has been proved harmful. Currently, the United States has no formal guidelines for supplement marketing and safety, and supplement manufacturers are responsible for self-monitoring their activities.

Do you really need to take dietary supplements? The Office of Dietary Supplements, part of the National Institutes of Health, states that some supplements may help ensure that you get adequate amounts of essential nutrients if you don't consume a variety of foods, as recommended in the Dietary Guidelines for Americans. However, dietary supplements are not intended to prevent or treat disease, and they should be used under the guidance of your health care provider.[38] Populations who may benefit from using supplements include pregnant and breast-feeding women, older adults, vegans, people on a very low-calorie weight–loss diet, alcohol-dependent individuals, and patients with malabsorption problems or other significant health problems.

Recently, Canadian researchers raised a concern about toxicity from taking high-dose supplements of fat-soluble vitamins. They recommended that the fat-soluble vitamins A, D, and E, as well as the B vitamins folic acid and niacin, be categorized as over-the-counter medications and that vitamin A should be removed from multivitamins.[39] The Academy of Nutrition and Dietetics recommends that, whereas there are benefits for some people in taking supplements, a healthy diet is the best way to give your body what it needs.[40]

52% of adults

in the United States take multivitamins at an annual cost of over $23 billion.

Eating Well in College

Many college students find it hard to fit a well-balanced meal into the day, but eating breakfast and lunch are important if you are to keep energy levels up and get the most out of your classes. If your campus is like many others, you've probably noticed a distinct move toward fast-food restaurants in your student union. However, eating a complete breakfast that includes complex carbohydrates, protein, and healthy unsaturated fat (such as a banana, peanut butter, and whole-grain bread sandwich or a dry fruit and nut mix without added sugar or salt) is key. If you are short on time, you can bring these items to class to ensure your meals fit into your day. Generally speaking, you can eat more healthfully and for less money if you bring food from home or your campus dining hall. If you must eat fast food, follow the tips below to get more nutritional bang for your buck:

- Ask for nutritional analyses of items. Most fast-food chains now have them.
- Order salads, but be careful about what you add to them. Taco salads and Cobb salads are often high in fat, calories, and sodium. Ask for dressing on the side, and use it sparingly. Try vinaigrette or low-fat dressings. Stay away from high-fat add-ons, such as bacon bits, croutons, and crispy noodles.
- If you crave french fries, try baked "fries," which may be lower in fat.
- Avoid giant sizes, and refrain from ordering extra sauce, bacon, cheese, and other toppings that add calories, sodium, and fat.
- Limit sodas and other beverages that are high in added sugars.
- At least once per week, substitute a vegetable-based meat substitute into your fast-food choices. Most places now offer veggie burgers and similar products, which provide excellent sources of protein and often have considerably less fat and fewer calories.

In the dining hall, try these ideas:

- Choose lean meats, grilled chicken, fish, or vegetable dishes. Avoid fried chicken, fatty cuts of red meat, or meat dishes smothered in creamy or oily sauce.
- Hit the salad bar and load up on leafy greens, beans, tuna, or tofu. Choose items such as avocado or nuts for a little "good" fat, and go easy on the dressing.
- Get creative: Top your baked potato with salsa, or add grilled chicken to your salad. Top toast with a nut butter or hummus.
- When choosing items from a made-to-order food station, ask the preparer to hold the butter or oil, mayonnaise, sour cream, or cheese- or cream-based sauces.
- Avoid going back for seconds and consuming large portions.
- If there is something you'd like but don't see in your dining hall, speak to your food service manager and provide suggestions.
- Pass on high-calorie, low-nutrient foods such as sugary cereals, ice cream, and other sweet treats. Choose fruit or low-fat yogurt to satisfy your sweet tooth.

Maintaining a nutritious diet within the confines of student life can be challenging. However, if you take the time to plan healthy meals, you

Healthy Eating Simplified

Does all this information leave you scratching your head about how to eat healthfully? When it all starts to feel too complicated, here are some simple tips to follow:

❯ You don't need foods from fancy packages to improve your health. Fruits, vegetables, and whole grains should make up the bulk of your diet. Shop the perimeter of the store and the bulk foods aisle.

❯ Let the MyPlate method guide you. Your meal should be mostly vegetables and grains. Less than a quarter of your meal should be lean protein. Include a calcium-rich beverage. A serving of fruit should be dessert.

❯ Avoid or limit processed and packaged foods. This will help you limit added sodium, sugar, and fat. If you can't make sense of the ingredients, don't eat it.

❯ Eat natural snacks such as fresh or dried fruit, nuts, string cheese, yogurt without added sugar, hard-boiled eggs, and vegetables.

❯ Be mindful of your eating. Eat until you are satisfied but not overfull.

❯ Bring healthful foods with you when you head out the door. Whether to class, on a road trip, or going to work, you *can* control the foods that are available. Don't put yourself in a position to buy from a vending machine or convenience store.

Source: M. Pollan, *Food Rules: An Eater's Manual* (New York: Penguin Books, 2010).

will find that you are eating better, enjoying it more, and actually saving money. The **Skills for Behavior Change** box, above, boils down healthy eating into some simple tips to follow, and the **Student Health Today** box on page 226 suggests ways to continue your healthy eating when dining at a variety of ethnic restaurants. The **Money & Health** box on page 227 examines ways to include fruits and vegetables in your diet without breaking the bank.

Choosing Organic or Locally Grown Foods

Concerns about food safety, genetically modified foods, and the health impacts of chemicals used to grow and produce food have led many people to turn to foods that are **organic**—foods and beverages developed, grown, or raised without the use of toxic and persistent synthetic pesticides, chemicals, or hormones. Any food sold in the United States as organic has to meet criteria set by the USDA under the National Organic Rule and can carry a USDA seal verifying

organic Grown without use of toxic and persistent pesticides, chemicals, or hormones.

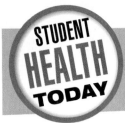
WHAT'S HEALTHY ON THE MENU?

No matter what type of cuisine you enjoy, there will always be healthier and less healthy options on the menu. To help you order wisely, here are lighter options and high-fat pitfalls. "Best" choices contain fewer than 30 grams of fat, a generous meal's worth for an active, medium-sized woman. "Worst" choices have up to 100 grams of fat.

Italian

Best Linguini with red or white clam sauce
        Spaghetti with marinara or tomato-and-meat sauce
Worst Eggplant parmigiana
        Fettuccine Alfredo
        Fried calamari
        Lasagna
Tips Stick with plain bread instead of garlic bread made with butter or oil. Ask for the waiter's help in avoiding cream- or egg-based sauces. Try vegetarian pizza, and don't ask for extra cheese.

Mexican

Best Bean burrito (no cheese)
        Chicken fajitas
Worst Beef chimichanga
        Quesadilla
        Chile relleno
        Refried beans
Tips Choose soft tortillas (not fried) with fresh salsa, not guacamole. Special-order grilled shrimp, fish, or chicken. Ask for beans made without lard or fat, and have cheeses and sour cream provided on the side or left out altogether.

Chinese

Best Hot-and-sour soup
        Stir-fried vegetables
        Shrimp with garlic sauce
        Szechuan shrimp
        Wonton soup
Worst Crispy chicken
        Kung pao chicken
        Moo shu pork
        Sweet-and-sour pork
Tips Share a stir-fry; help yourself to steamed rice. Ask for vegetables steamed or stir-fried with less oil. Order moo shu vegetables instead of pork. Avoid fried rice, breaded dishes, egg rolls and spring rolls, and items loaded with nuts. Avoid high-sodium sauces.

Japanese

Best Steamed rice and vegetables
        Tofu as a substitute for meat
        Broiled or steamed chicken and fish
Worst Fried rice dishes
        Miso (very high in sodium)
        Tempura
Tips Avoid soy sauces. Use caution in eating sashimi (raw fish) and sushi dishes to avoid possible bacteria or parasites.

Thai

Best Clear broth soups
        Stir-fried chicken and vegetables
        Grilled meats
Worst Coconut milk
        Peanut sauces
        Deep-fried dishes
Tips Avoid coconut-based curries. Ask for steamed, not fried, rice.

Korean

Best Soups, like hot fish soup (mehoon-tang) or stews (chigae) or chigae also known as soft tofu soup
        Kimchee-fermented cabbage
Worst Pork bulgogi
        Barbeque
Tips Avoid high sugar and sodium BBQ and opt for dishes with lots of vegetables.

Peruvian

Best Grilled fish
        Steamed fish
        Seafood
Worst Dishes with heavy milk
        Deep-fried items
Tips Select boiled or steamed dishes, limit cheese and milk.

Ethiopian

Best Vegetable stews
        Lentils
        Potatoes
Worst Ketfo (raw or rare beef)
        Deep-fried foods
Tips Choose vegetables and lentils, fish, and leaner meats such as chicken and goat.

Moroccan

Best Eggplant and tomato salads
        Couscous
        Fish and broth soups
Worst Pastilla or meat pie
        Beef dishes
        Pastry

Tips Look for tagines of slow-cooked lean meats and vegetables and avoid pastry and fried foods.

Indian

Best Baked fish
        Vegetable dishes
        Dal (lentils)
        Roti (flatbread)
Worst Samosas (stuffed and fried vegetable turnovers)
        Butter chicken
        Coconut oil
        Ghee (clarified butter)
Tips Limit foods cooked in coconut oil or ghee. Enjoy modest amounts of white rice. Avoid dishes that are deep fried.

American Breakfast

Best Hot or cold cereal with 2 percent milk
        Pancakes or French toast with syrup
        Scrambled eggs with hash browns and plain toast
Worst Belgian waffle with sausage
        Sausage and eggs with biscuits and gravy
        Ham-and-cheese omelet with hash browns and toast
Tips Ask for whole-grain cereal or shredded wheat with 2 percent milk or whole wheat toast without butter or margarine. Order omelets without cheese, and order fried eggs without bacon or sausage.

Sandwiches

Best Ham and Swiss cheese
        Roast beef
        Turkey
Worst Tuna salad
        Reuben
        Submarine
Tips Ask for mustard; hold the mayonnaise and high-fat cheese. See if turkey-ham is available.

Seafood

Best Broiled bass, halibut, or snapper-
        Grilled scallops
        Steamed crab or lobster
Worst Fried seafood platter
        Blackened catfish
Tips Order fish broiled, baked, grilled, or steamed—not pan fried or sautéed. Ask for lemon instead of tartar sauce. Avoid creamy and buttery sauces.

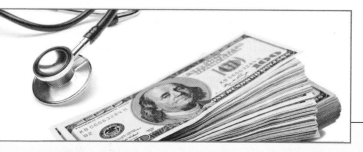

Money&Health

ARE FRUITS AND VEGGIES BEYOND YOUR BUDGET?

Many people on a tight budget, including college students, think that fruits and vegetables are beyond their budget. Maybe a carton of orange juice and a package of carrots are affordable, but five to nine servings a day? No way.

If that sounds like you, it's time for some facts. In 2011, the U.S. Department of Agriculture published data showing that the average American family spends more money on food than is necessary to consume a nutritious diet—one that includes the recommended servings of fruits and vegetables. The report concluded that, contrary to popular opinion, people on a tight budget can eat healthfully, including plenty of fruits and vegetables, and spend less on food.

So how do you do it? Here are some tips:

✻ Focus on five fresh favorites. Throughout the United States, five of the least expensive, perennially available fresh vegetables are carrots, eggplant, lettuce, potatoes, and summer squash. Five fresh fruit options are apples, bananas, pears, pineapple, and watermelon.

✻ Buy small amounts frequently. Most items of fresh produce keep only a few days, so buy amounts that you know you'll be able to eat or freeze.

✻ Celebrate the season. From apples to zucchini, when fruits and veggies are in season, they cost less. If you can freeze them, stock up. If not, enjoy them fresh while you can.

✻ Do it yourself. Avoid prewashed, precut fruits and vegetables, including salad greens. They cost more and often spoil faster. Also choose frozen 100% juice concentrate and add the water yourself.

✻ Buy canned or frozen on sale, in bulk. Canned and frozen produce, especially when it's on sale, may be much less expensive than fresh. Most frozen items are just as nutritious as fresh, and can be even more so, depending on how long ago the fresh food was harvested. For canned items, choose fruits without added sugars and vegetables without added salt or sauces. Bear in mind that beans are legumes and count as a vegetable choice. Low-sodium canned beans are one of the most affordable, convenient, and nutritious foods you can buy.

✻ Fix and freeze. Make large batches of homemade soup, vegetable stews, and pasta sauce and store them in single-serving containers in your freezer.

✻ Grow your own. All it takes is one sunny window, a pot, soil, and a packet of seeds. Lettuce, spinach, and fresh herbs are particularly easy to grow indoors in small spaces.

Sources: U.S. Department of Agriculture, *Eating Healthy on a Budget: The Consumer Economics Perspective*, September 2011, www.choosemyplate.gov/food-groups/downloads/ConsumerEconomicsPerspective.pdf; U.S. Department of Agriculture, *Smart Shopping for Veggies and Fruits,* Center for Nutrition Policy and Promotion, June 2011, www.choosemyplate.gov/food-groups/downloads/TenTips/DGTipsheet9SmartShopping.pdf; U.S. Centers for Disease Control and Prevention, *30 Ways in 30 Days to Stretch Your Fruit & Vegetable Budget,* Fruits & Veggies: More Matters, September 2011, www.fruitsandveggiesmatter.gov/downloads/Stretch_FV_Budget.pdf.

---

products as "certified organic." Under this rule, a product that is certified may carry one of the following terms: "100 percent Organic" (100% compliance with organic criteria), "Organic" (must contain at least 95% organic materials), "Made with Organic Ingredients" (must contain at least 70% organic ingredients), or "Some Organic Ingredients" (contains less than 70% organic ingredients—usually listed individually). To be labeled with any of the above terms, the foods also must be produced without hormones, antibiotics, or genetic modification. However, reliable monitoring systems to ensure credibility are still under development.

The market for organic foods has been increasing by more than 20 percent per year—five times faster than food sales in general. Where only a small subset of the population once bought organic, nearly all U.S. consumers now occasionally reach for something labeled organic. In 2010, annual organic food sales were estimated to be $25 billion.[41]

Is organic food really better? A review of the research published over the past 50 years found no evidence of a difference in nutrient quality of organic versus traditionally grown foods.[42] However, pesticide residues do remain on conventionally grown produce. In 2011, the USDA reported that 3 percent of food samples harvested in 2009 had pesticide residues that exceeded the established tolerance level or for which no tolerance level has been established. The USDA advises that consumers always rinse fruits and vegetables before cooking or consuming them.[43]

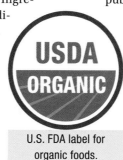

U.S. FDA label for organic foods.

EATING FOR A HEALTHY ENVIRONMENT

Food politics affect us all, even if we don't realize it. Much of the food politics debate focuses on controversies over which foods are best for you, for the environment, and for other living species.

For example, a commonly cited estimate is that it takes up to 16 pounds of grain and soybeans to produce 1 pound of beef and that far too much water, land, and food-based resources are used in doing so. It is argued that it would be better to eat the grains and soybeans, rather than eating the cow fed on them. Critics counter that these numbers are incorrect and that it's probably closer to 2.6 pounds of grain and soybeans to 1 pound of beef; they feel that, nutritionally, lean beef is an efficient, environmentally friendly resource. Proponents of grass-fed beef advocate raising cattle and producing beef in a more humane and ecologically sound manner. Others argue that all food production takes a toll on the environment and that even crops raised for vegan diets can have a significant effect on wild animals, water supplies, soil nutrients, insects, and other aspects of a locale's ecology.

One of the most significant forces shaping the nature of food production in the United States, and its environmental and human impacts, is the Farm Bill, properly known as the Food, Conservation, and Energy Act, which is renewed every 5 years by Congress (most recently in 2008). Essentially, the Farm Bill determines which crops the federal government will subsidize and at what levels. The 2008 bill includes subsidies for commodities such as wheat, feed grains, rice, and oilseeds, whereas fruits and vegetables are considered specialty crops and receive little financial support. Critics argue that the bill benefits corporate farms that have huge negative environmental impacts and that it puts small, local, and organic farms at a disadvantage. The Farm Bill can also have a major impact on food availability, pricing, and distribution in various geographical locations, including internationally.

How does agricultural legislation affect you personally? There is no easy answer, but here are a few actions to consider to enhance your health and that of other species and the environment:

✳ During your region's growing season, challenge yourself to a 100-mile diet. This means eating food that is shipped no farther than a 100-mile radius from where you live. If your food is transported to your local store, there is always an environmental cost involved, for example, the fuel that is needed to transport that food.

✳ Know where your meat comes from. Avoid large meat-producing superfarms where animals live in unhealthy conditions and the potential for water and air pollution is great. Buy from farmers who provide the best conditions for producing healthy animals and follow humane slaughtering practices.

✳ Remember that the Food, Conservation, and Energy Act is reexamined and renewed every 5 years by the federal government. Get involved in shaping our food landscape by becoming informed on the provisions of the bill, contacting your congressperson, and joining or organizing community education.

The word **locavore** has been coined to describe people who eat mostly food grown or produced locally, usually within close proximity to their homes. Farmers' markets or home-grown foods or those grown by independent farmers are thought to be fresher and to require far fewer resources to get them to market and keep them fresh for longer periods of time. Locavores believe that locally grown organic food is preferable to foods produced by large corporations or supermarket-based organic foods, as they make a smaller impact on the environment. Although there are many reasons organic farming is better for the environment, the fact that pesticides, herbicides, and other products are not used is perhaps the greatest benefit. The **Be Healthy, Be Green** box discusses some of the issues surrounding food politics and agriculture in the United States.

locavore A person who primarily eats food grown or produced locally.

Food Safety: A Growing Concern

Eating unhealthy food is one thing. Eating food that has been contaminated with a microorganism, toxin, or other harmful substance is quite another. As outbreaks of foodborne illness (commonly called food poisoning) make the news, the food industry has come under fire. The Food Safety Modernization Act, passed into law in 2011, included new requirements for food processors to take actions to prevent contamination of foods. The act gave the U.S. Food and Drug Administration greater authority to inspect food-manufacturing facilities and to recall contaminated foods.[44]

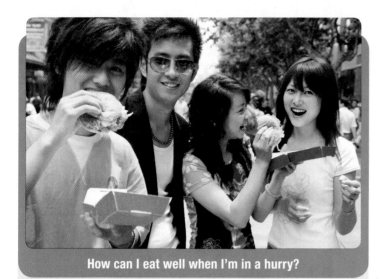

How can I eat well when I'm in a hurry?

Meals like this one may be convenient, but they are high in saturated fat, sodium, refined carbohydrates, and calories. Even when you are short on time and money, it is possible—and worthwhile—to make healthier choices. If you are ordering fast food, opt for foods prepared by baking, roasting, or steaming; ask for the leanest meat option; and request that sauces, dressings, and gravies be served on the side.

See It! Videos

Worried about mercury in your fish? Watch **Which Fish Is Safest to Eat?** at www.pearsonhighered.com/donatelle.

(over 48 million people) and cause some 128,000 hospitalizations and 3,000 deaths in the United States annually.[45] These numbers have remained fairly constant since 2004, despite increased attention to prevention in the United States.[46]

Table 7.7 lists some of the most common microbial culprits behind foodborne illness. Bear in mind that foodborne illness can be caused by multiplication of the microbe itself or by the presence in the food of a toxin that was originally produced by a microbe. These toxins can produce illness even if the microbes that produced them are no longer there. For example, botulism is caused by a deadly toxin produced by the bacterium *Clostridium botulinum*. This bacterium is widespread in soil, water, plants, and intestinal tracts, but it can grow only in environments with limited or no oxygen. Potential food sources include improperly canned food and vacuum-packed or tightly wrapped foods. Though rare, botulism is fatal if untreated.

Signs of foodborne illnesses vary tremendously but usually include diarrhea, nausea, abdominal cramping, and vomiting. Depending on the amount and virulence of the microbe, symptoms may appear as early as 30 minutes after eating contaminated food or as long as several days or weeks later. Most of the time, symptoms occur 5 to 8 hours after eating and last only a day or two. For certain populations,

Foodborne Illnesses

Are you concerned that the chicken you are buying doesn't look pleasingly pink or your "fresh" fish smells a little *too* fishy? You may have good reason to be worried. Scientists estimate that foodborne illnesses sicken 1 in 6 Americans

TABLE 7.7 Five Most Common Foodborne Illnesses

Microbe	Illnesses per Year	Description
Norovirus	5.4 million	Transmitted through contact with the vomit or stool of infected people, norovirus is the most common cause of foodborne illness in the United States annually. Symptoms include nausea, vomiting, and diarrhea. Most cases are self-limiting, but about 800 Americans die of infection each year. There is no treatment, but washing hands and all kitchen surfaces can help prevent transmission.
Salmonella	1 million	Commonly found in the intestines of birds, reptiles, and mammals, it can spread to humans through foods of animal origin. Infection by *Salmonella* usually consists of fever, diarrhea, and abdominal cramps. Salmonellosis can be life threatening if the bacteria invade the bloodstream, as is more likely in people with poor underlying health or weakened immune systems.
Clostridium perfringens	966,000	Bacterial species found in the intestinal tracts of humans and animals, as well as in the environment. Infection causes abdominal cramping and diarrhea.
Campylobacter	845,000	Most raw poultry has *Campylobacter* in it, and this bacterial infection most frequently results from eating undercooked chicken, raw eggs, or foods contaminated with juices from raw chicken. Shellfish and unpasteurized milk are also sources. Infection causes fever, diarrhea, and abdominal cramps.
Staphylococcus aureus	241,000	*Staph* lives on human skin, in infected cuts, and in the nose and throat. Infection causes severe nausea, vomiting, and diarrhea that lasts 1–3 days.

Source: Data are from Centers for Disease Control and Prevention, CDC Estimates of Foodborne Illness in the United States, CDC 2011 Estimates: Findings, Accessed February 7, 2012, from www.cdc.gov/foodborneburden/2011-foodborne-estimates.html.

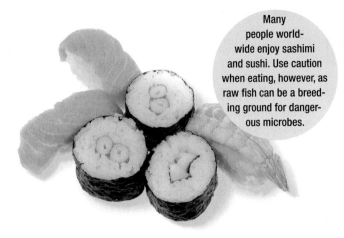

Many people worldwide enjoy sashimi and sushi. Use caution when eating, however, as raw fish can be a breeding ground for dangerous microbes.

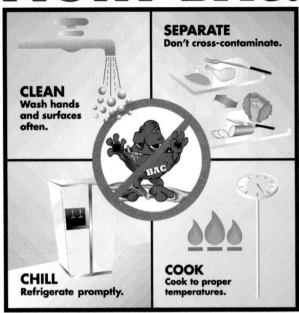

FIGHT BAC!

CLEAN Wash hands and surfaces often.

SEPARATE Don't cross-contaminate.

CHILL Refrigerate promptly.

COOK Cook to proper temperatures.

Keep Food Safe From Bacteria™

FIGURE 7.9 **The USDA's Fight BAC!** This logo reminds consumers how to prevent foodborne illness.

such as the very young; older adults; or people with severe illnesses such as cancer, diabetes, kidney disease, or AIDS, foodborne diseases can be fatal.

Several factors contribute to foodborne illnesses. Since fresh foods are not in season much of the year, we must import fresh fruits and vegetables from great distances. Depending on the season, up to 70 percent of the fruits and vegetables consumed in the United States come from Mexico. Although we are told when we travel to developing countries to "boil it, peel it, or don't eat it," we bring these foods into our kitchens at home and eat them, often without washing them. Food can become contaminated in the field by being watered with tainted water, fertilized with animal manure, or harvested by people who have not washed their hands properly after using the toilet. Food-processing equipment, facilities, or workers may contaminate food, or it can become contaminated if not kept clean and cool during transport or on store shelves. To give you an idea of the implications, studies have shown that the bacterium *Escherichia coli* can survive in cow manure for up to 70 days and can multiply in crops grown with manure unless heat or additives such as salt or preservatives are used to kill the microbes.[47] There are no regulations that prohibit farmers from using animal manure to fertilize crops. In addition, *E. coli* quickly reproduces in summer months as cows await slaughter in crowded, overheated pens. This increases the chances of meat coming to market already contaminated.

food irradiation Exposing foods to low doses of radiation to kill microorganisms or keep them from reproducing.

Avoiding Risks in the Home

Part of the responsibility for preventing foodborne illness lies with consumers—more than 30 percent of all such illnesses result from unsafe handling of food at home. Four basic steps reduce the likelihood of contaminating your food (see **Figure 7.9**). Among the most basic precautions are to wash your hands and to wash all produce before eating it. Also, avoid cross-contamination in the kitchen by using separate cutting boards and

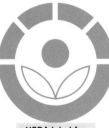

USDA label for irradiated foods.

utensils for meats and produce. Temperature control is also important—refrigerators must be set at 40°F or lower. Cook meats to the recommended temperature to kill contaminants before eating. Keep hot foods hot and cold foods cold to avoid unchecked bacterial growth. Eat leftovers within 3 days, and if you're unsure how long something has been sitting in the fridge, don't take chances. When in doubt, throw it out. See the **Skills for Behavior Change** box on page 231 for more tips about reducing risk of foodborne illness.

Food Irradiation

Food irradiation is a process that exposes foods to low doses of radiation, or ionizing energy, to break down the DNA of harmful bacteria, destroying them or keeping them from reproducing. Essentially, the rays pass through the food without leaving any radioactive residue.[48]

Irradiation lengthens food products' shelf life and prevents the spread of deadly microorganisms, particularly in high-risk foods such as ground beef and pork. Thus, the minimal costs of irradiation result in lower overall costs to consumers and reduce the need for toxic chemicals to preserve foods. Use of food irradiation is limited because of consumer concerns about safety and because irradiation facilities are expensive to build. Still, food irradiation is now common in over 40

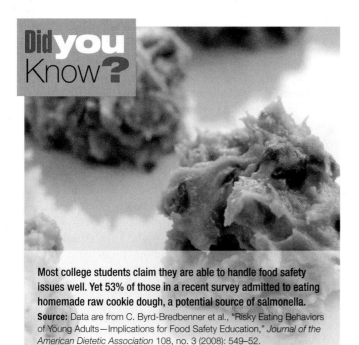

countries. Foods that have been irradiated are marked with the "radura" logo.

Food Sensitivities

About 33 percent of people today *think* they have a food allergy; however, only 4 to 8 percent of children and 2 percent of adults actually do. Still, there may be reason to be concerned. From 1997 through 2007 the prevalence of reported food allergies rose 18 percent.[49]

A **food allergy,** or hypersensitivity, is an abnormal response to a component—usually a protein—in food that is triggered by the immune system. Symptoms of an allergic reaction vary in severity and may include a tingling sensation in the mouth; swelling of the lips, tongue, and throat; difficulty breathing; skin hives; vomiting; abdominal cramps; and diarrhea. Approximately 200 deaths per year occur as a result of more severe reactions called *anaphylaxis* that cause widespread inflammation and cardiovascular problems such as a sudden drop in blood pressure. Anaphylaxis may occur within seconds to hours after eating the foods to which one is allergic.[50]

The Food Allergen Labeling and Consumer Protection Act (FALCPA) requires food manufacturers to label foods clearly to indicate the presence of (or possible contamination by) any of the eight major food allergens: milk, eggs, peanuts, wheat, soy, tree nuts (walnuts, pecans, cashews, pistachios, etc.), fish, and shellfish. Although over 160 foods have been identified as allergy triggers, these eight foods account for 90 percent of all food allergies in the United States.[51]

Celiac disease is an inherited autoimmune disorder that causes malabsorption of nutrients from the small intestine. Affecting over 3 million Americans, most of whom are undiagnosed, it is a growing problem, particularly for those under the age of 20.[52] When a person with celiac disease consumes gluten—a protein found in wheat, rye, and barley—the person's immune system responds with inflammation. This degrades the lining of the small intestine and reduces nutrient absorption. Pain, abdominal cramping, often diarrhea, and other symptoms follow in the short term. Untreated, celiac disease can lead to long-term health problems, such as osteoporosis, nutritional deficiencies, seizures, and cancer of the small intestine. Individuals diagnosed with celiac disease

food allergy Overreaction by the immune system to normally harmless proteins, which are perceived as allergens. In response, the body produces antibodies, triggering allergic symptoms.

celiac disease An inherited autoimmune disorder causing malabsorption of nutrients from the small intestine and triggered by the consumption of gluten.

Skills for Behavior Change

Reduce Your Risk for Foodborne Illness

❭ When shopping, put perishable foods in your cart last. Check for cleanliness throughout the store, especially at the salad bar and at the meat and fish counters. Never buy dented cans of food. Check the "sell by" or "use by" date on foods.

❭ Once you get home, put dairy products, eggs, meat, fish, and poultry in the refrigerator immediately. If you don't plan to eat meats within 2 days, freeze them. You can keep an unopened package of hot dogs or luncheon meats for about 2 weeks.

❭ When refrigerating or freezing raw meats, make sure their juices can't spill onto other foods.

❭ Never thaw frozen foods at room temperature. Put them in the refrigerator to thaw or thaw in the microwave, following manufacturer's instructions.

❭ Wash your hands with soap and warm water before preparing food. Wash fruits and vegetables before peeling, slicing, cooking, or eating them—but not meat, poultry, or eggs! Wash cutting boards, countertops, and other utensils and surfaces with detergent and hot water after food preparation.

❭ Use a meat thermometer to ensure that meats are completely cooked. To find out proper cooking temperatures for different types of meat, visit http://foodsafety.gov/keep/charts/mintemp.html.

❭ Refrigeration slows the secretion of bacterial toxins into foods. Never leave leftovers out for more than 2 hours. On hot days, don't leave foods out for longer than 1 hour.

See It! Videos

What's the big deal with farmers' markets? Watch **Going Green** at www.pearsonhighered.com/donatelle.

food intolerance Adverse effects that result when people who lack the digestive chemicals needed to break down certain substances eat those substances.

genetically modified (GM) foods Foods derived from organisms whose DNA has been altered using genetic engineering techniques.

are encouraged to consult a dietitian for help designing a gluten-free diet.

Food intolerance can cause you to have symptoms of digestive upset, but the upset is not the result of an immune system response. Probably the best example of a food intolerance is *lactose intolerance,* a problem that affects about 1 in every 10 American adults. Lactase is an enzyme in the lining of the small intestine that degrades lactose, a sugar in dairy products. If you don't have enough lactase, you cannot digest lactose, and it remains in the gut to be used by bacteria. Gas is formed, and you experience bloating, abdominal pain, and sometimes diarrhea. Populations in which fresh milk consumption continues into adulthood typically have rates of lactose intolerance as low as 2 to 3 percent, whereas 80 percent or more of non–milk-drinking populations are lactose intolerant.[53] Food intolerance also occurs in response to some food additives, such as the flavor enhancer monosodium glutamate (MSG), certain dyes, sulfites, gluten, and other substances. In some cases, the food intolerance may have psychological triggers.

If you suspect that you have a food allergy, celiac disease, or a food intolerance, see your doctor. Because there diseases can have some common symptoms, as well as share symptoms with other gastrointestinal disorders, clinical diagnosis is essential.

Peanuts are among the eight most common food allergens: 0.6% of the general population are allergic to them, with slightly higher rates in children.

Genetically Modified Food Crops

Genetic modification involves the insertion or deletion of genes into the DNA of an organism. In the case of **genetically modified (GM) foods,** usually this genetic cutting and pasting is done to enhance production, for example, by making disease- or insect-resistant plants, improving yield, or controlling weeds. In addition, GM foods are sometimes created to improve the color and appearance of foods or to enhance specific nutrients. For example, in regions where rice is a staple and vitamin A deficiency and iron-deficiency anemia are leading causes of morbidity and mortality, GM technology has been used to create varieties of rice high in vitamin A and iron. Another use under development is the production and delivery of vaccines through GM foods.

Farmers in the United States have widely accepted GM crops.[54] Soybeans and cotton are the most common GM crops, followed by corn. On supermarket shelves, about 75 percent of the soy and about 40 percent of the corn used in processed foods are genetically modified.

The long-term safety of GM foods is still a question. In a recent report, three strains of maize (corn) showed signs of causing liver and kidney toxicity.[55] These claims were refuted by producers. In addition, unintentional transfer of potentially allergy-provoking proteins has occurred, and rigorous, validated tests of crops are necessary to protect allergic consumers.[56] However, according to the World Health Organization, no adverse effects on human health have been shown from consumption of GM foods in countries that have approved their use.[57] The debate surrounding GM foods is not likely to end soon.

Assess yourself

How Healthy Are Your Eating Habits?

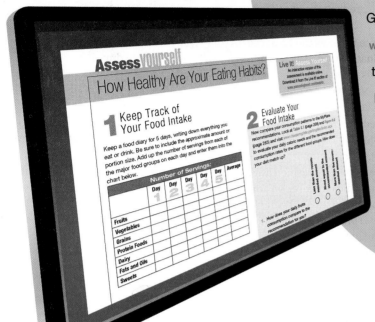

Go online to the **Live It!** section of

www.pearsonhighered.com/donatelle

to take the "How Healthy Are Your Eating Habits?" assessment.* If you feel you need to change your eating habits, use the tips outlined in the **YOUR PLAN FOR CHANGE** box to help you.

* If your instructor so chooses, Assess Yourself Activities are available as a printed supplement or as assignable homework online at www.pearsonhighered.com/myhealthlab.

MyHealthLab®

YOUR PLAN FOR CHANGE

The **Assess yourself** activity "How Healthy Are Your Eating Habits?" is available at www.pearsonhigher.com/myhealthlab. This activity gives you the chance to evaluate your current nutritional habits. Once you have considered these results, you can decide whether you need to make changes in your daily eating for long-term health.

Today, you can:

○ Start keeping a more detailed food log. Take note of the nutritional information of the various foods you eat and write down particulars about the number of calories, grams of saturated fat, grams of sugar, milligrams of sodium, and so on of each food. Try to find specific weak spots: Are you consuming too many calories or too much salt or sugar? Do you eat too little calcium or iron?

○ Take a field trip to the grocery store. Forgo your fast-food dinner and instead spend some time in the produce section of the supermarket. Purchase your favorite fruits and vegetables, and try something new to expand your tastes.

Within the next 2 weeks, you can:

○ Plan at least three meals that you can make at home or in your dorm room, and purchase the ingredients you'll need ahead of time. Something as simple as a chicken sandwich on whole-grain bread will be more nutritious, and probably cheaper, than heading out for a fast-food meal.

○ Start reading labels. Be aware of the amount of calories, sodium, sugars, and saturated fats in prepared foods; aim to buy and consume those that are lower in all of these and are higher in micronutrients and fiber.

By the end of the semester, you can:

○ Get in the habit of eating a healthy breakfast every morning. Combine whole grains, proteins, and fruit in your breakfast—for example, eat a bowl of cereal with soy milk and bananas or a cup of low-fat yogurt with granola and berries. Eating a healthy breakfast will jump-start your metabolism, prevent drops in blood glucose levels, and keep your brain and body performing at their best through those morning classes.

○ Commit to one or two healthful changes to your eating patterns for the rest of the semester. You might resolve to eat five servings of fruits and vegetables every day, to switch to low-fat or nonfat dairy products, to stop drinking soft drinks, or to use only olive oil in your cooking. Use your food diary to help you spot places where you can make healthier choices on a daily basis.

Summary

✳ Recognizing that we eat for more reasons than just survival is a step toward improving our eating habits.

✳ The Dietary Reference Intakes (DRIs) are recommended nutrient intakes for healthy people.

✳ The essential nutrients include water, proteins, carbohydrates, fats, vitamins, and minerals. Water makes up 50 to 60 percent of our body weight and is necessary for nearly all life processes. Proteins are major components of our cells and tissues and are key elements of antibodies, enzymes, and hormones. Carbohydrates are our primary sources of energy. Fats provide energy while we are at rest and for long-term activity. They also play important roles in maintaining body temperature and cushioning and protecting organs. Vitamins are organic compounds, and minerals are inorganic elements. We need both in relatively small amounts to maintain healthy body function.

✳ The Dietary Guidelines for Americans and the MyPlate food guidance system provide guidelines for healthy eating.

✳ Food labels provide information on the serving size, number of calories in a food, as well as the amounts of various nutrients and the percentage of recommended daily values those amounts represent.

✳ With a little menu planning, vegetarianism can be a healthful lifestyle choice, providing plenty of nutrients, plus fiber and phytochemicals, typically with less saturated fat and fewer calories.

✳ College students face unique challenges in eating healthfully. Learning to make better choices at fast-food restaurants, to eat healthfully on a budget, and to eat nutritionally in the dorm are all possible when you use the information in this chapter.

✳ Organic foods are grown and produced without the use of toxic and persistent synthetic pesticides, chemicals, or hormones. The USDA offers certification of organic farms and regulates claims regarding organic ingredients used on food labels.

✳ Foodborne illnesses can be traced to contamination of food at any point from fields to the consumer's kitchen. To keep food safe at home, follow four steps: Clean, separate, cook, and chill.

✳ Food irradiation, food allergies, celiac disease, food intolerances, GM foods, and other food safety and health concerns are becoming increasingly important to health-wise consumers. Recognizing potential risks and taking steps to prevent problems are part of a sound nutritional plan.

Pop Quiz

1. Triglycerides
   a. provide 4 calories per gram.
   b. are the primary component of the plaque that clogs blood vessels and leads to cardiovascular disease.
   c. are only found in meat, dairy, and poultry products.
   d. include saturated fats, unsaturated fats, and *trans* fats.

2. Which of the following foods would be considered a healthy, *nutrient-dense* food?
   a. Nonfat milk
   b. Cheddar cheese
   c. Soft drink
   d. Potato chips

3. What is the most crucial nutrient for life?
   a. Water
   b. Protein
   c. Minerals
   d. Starch

4. Which of the following substances helps move food through the digestive tract?
   a. Folate
   b. Fiber
   c. Minerals
   d. Starch

5. Which of the following nutrients is critical for the repair and growth of body tissue?
   a. Carbohydrates
   b. Proteins
   c. Vitamins
   d. Fats

6. What substance provides energy, promotes healthy skin and hair, insulates body organs, helps maintain body temperature, and contributes to healthy cell function?
   a. Fats
   b. Fibers
   c. Proteins
   d. Carbohydrates

7. Which vitamin helps maintain bone health?
   a. B_{12}
   b. D
   c. B_6
   d. Niacin

8. What is the most common nutrient deficiency worldwide?
   a. Fat deficiency
   b. Iron deficiency
   c. Fiber deficiency
   d. Calcium deficiency

9. Carrie eats dairy products and eggs, but she does not eat fish, poultry, or meat. Carrie is considered a(n)
   a. vegan.
   b. lacto-ovo-vegetarian.
   c. ovo-vegetarian.
   d. pesco-vegetarian.

10. Which of the following fats is a healthier fat to include in the diet?
    a. *Trans* fat
    b. Saturated fat
    c. Unsaturated fat
    d. Hydrogenated fat

Answers to these questions can be found on page A-1.

Think about It!

1. Which factors influence a person's dietary patterns and behaviors? What factors have been the greatest influences on your eating behaviors?
2. What are the major food groups in the MyPlate plan? From which groups do you eat too few servings? What can you do to increase or decrease your intake of selected food groups?
3. What are the major types of nutrients that you need to obtain from the foods you eat? What happens if you fail to get enough of some of them? Are there significant differences between men and women in particular areas of nutrition?
4. Distinguish between the different types of vegetarianism. Which types are most likely to lead to nutrient deficiencies? What can be done to ensure that even the most strict vegetarian receives enough of the major nutrients?
5. What are the major problems that many college students face when trying to eat the right foods? List five actions that you and your classmates could take immediately to improve your eating.
6. What are the major risks for foodborne illnesses, and what can you do to protect yourself?
7. How does a food intolerance differ from a food allergy?

Accessing Your Health on the Internet

The following websites explore further topics and issues. For live links, visit *Access to Health,* 13th Edition, at www.pearsonhighered.com/donatelle.

1. *Academy of Nutrition and Dietetics* (formerly the American Dietetic Association). The Academy provides information on a full range of dietary topics, including sports nutrition, healthful cooking, and nutritional eating; the site also links to scientific publications and information on scholarships and public meetings. www.eatright.org
2. *U.S. Food and Drug Administration (FDA).* The FDA provides information for consumers and professionals in the areas of food safety, supplements, and medical devices. There are links to other sources of information about nutrition and food. www.fda.gov
3. *Food and Nutrition Information Center.* This site offers a wide variety of information related to food and nutrition. http://fnic.nal.usda.gov
4. *National Institutes of Health: Office of Dietary Supplements.* This is the site of the International Bibliographic Database of Information on Dietary Supplements (IBDIDS), updated quarterly. http://dietary-supplements.info.nih.gov
5. *U.S. Department of Agriculture, USDA: Choose MyPlate.* The USDA offers a personalized nutrition and physical activity plan based on the MyPlate program, sample menus and recipes, and a full discussion of the Dietary Guidelines for Americans. http://www.choosemyplate.gov
6. *U.S. Department of Health and Human Services: Food Safety.* This is the offificial gateway site to food safety information provded by the federal government, including recalls and alerts, news, and tips for reporting problems. www.foodsafety.gov
7. *Linus Pauling Institute.* This is a key U.S. research center for studies on macro- and micronutrients, and it is a leader in antioxidant research. http://lpi.oregonstate.edu

References

1. F. Bruni, "Eating Anxiety: Is Anyone to Blame?" *The Atlantic,* September 8, 2009, Available at www.theatlantic.com/food/archive/2009/09/eating-anxiety-is-any-one-to-blame/24615.
2. D. Negoianu and S. Goldfarb, "Just Add Water," *Journal of the American Society of Nephrology* 19, no. 6 (2008): 1041–43; E. Jéquier and F. Constant, "Water as an Essential Nutrient: The Physiological Basis of Hydration," *European Journal of Clinical Nutrition* 64, no. 2 (2010): 115–23.
3. Institute of Medicine of the National Academies, Food and Nutrition Board, *Dietary Reference Intakes for Water, Potassium, Sodium, Chloride, and Sulfate* (Washington, DC: The National Academies Press, 2004), Available at http://iom.edu/Reports/2004/Dietary-Reference-Intakes-Water-Potassium-Sodium-Chloride-and-Sulfate.aspx.
4. American College of Sports Medicine (ACSM), "Exercise and Fluid Replacement," *Medicine and Science in Sports and Exercise* 39, no. 2 (2007): 377–90.
5. U.S. Department of Agriculture, Agricultural Research Service, Beltsville Human Nutrition Research Center, Food Surveys Research Group (Beltsville, MD) and U.S. Department of Health and Human Services, Centers for Disease Control and Prevention, National Center for Health Statistics (Hyattsville, MD), *What We Eat in America, NHANES 2007–2008 Data: Table 1. Nutrient Intakes from Food: Mean Amounts Consumed per Individual by Gender and Age, in the United States, 2007–2008,* Revised August 2010, Available at www.ars.usda.gov/Services/docs.htm?docid=18349.
6. Institute of Medicine of the National Academies, "Dietary, Functional, and Total Fiber," in *Dietary Reference Intakes for Energy, Carbohydrate, Fiber, Fat, Fatty Acids, Cholesterol, Protein, and Amino Acids* (Washington, DC: The National Academies Press, 2005), 339–421, Available at www.nap.edu/openbook.php?isbn=0309085373.
7. N. D. Riediger, R. A. Othman, M. Suh, and M. H. Moghadasian, "A Systemic Review of the Roles of n-3 Fatty Acids in Health and Disease," *Journal of the American Dietetic Association* 109 (2009): 668–79; B. McKevith, "Review: Nutritional Aspects of Oilseeds," *Nutrition Bulletin* 30, no. 1 (2005): 13–14.
8. A. H. Stark, M. A. Crawford, and R. Reifen, "Update on Alpha-Linolenic Acid," *Nutrition Reviews* 66, no. 6 (2008): 326–32.
9. W. Willet, "Dietary Fats and Coronary Heart Disease," *Journal of Internal Medicine,* 2012 (1): 13–24; N. Bendson, R. Christensen, E. Bartels, A. Astup, "Consumption of Industrial and Ruminant Trans Fatty Acids and Risk of CHD: A Systemic Review and Meta-Analysis of Cohort Studies," *European Journal of Clinical Nutrition,* 2011, 65: 773–783.
10. C. Scott-Thomas, "Californian *Trans* Fat Ban Takes Effect," FoodNavigator-USA.com, January 4, 2010, www.foodnavigator-usa.com/Legislation/Californian-trans-fat-ban-takes-effect.
11. F. Sacks et al., "Comparison of Weight-Loss Diets with Different Compositions of Fat, Protein, and Carbohydrates," *New England*

Journal of Medicine 360, no. 9 (2009): 859–73; M. Hession et al., "Systematic Review of Randomized Controlled Trials of Low-carbohydrate vs. Low-fat/Low-calorie Diets in the Management of Obesity and its Comorbidities," *Obesity Reviews* 10, no. 1 (2008): 36–50.

12. H. D. Sesso et al., "Vitamins E and C in the Prevention of Cardiovascular Disease in Men: The Physicians' Health Study II Randomized Controlled Trial," *Journal of the American Medical Association,* 300, no. 18: 2123–33.

13. D. Albanes, "Vitamin Supplements and Cancer Prevention: Where Do Randomized Controlled Trials Stand?" *Journal of the National Cancer Institute* 101, no. 1 (2009): 2–4; J. Lin et al., "Vitamins C and E and Beta Carotene Supplementation and Cancer Risk: A Randomized Controlled Trial," *Journal of the National Cancer Institute* 101, no. 1 (2009): 14–23.

14. Ibid.

15. C. G. Slatore, A. J. Littman, D. H. Au, J. A. Satia, and E. White, "Long-Term Use of Supplemental Multivitamins, Vitamin C, Vitamin E, and Folate Does Not Reduce the Risk of Lung Cancer," *American Journal of Respiratory and Critical Care Medicine* 177 (2008): 524–30; Linus Pauling Institute, Oregon State University, "Micronutrient Information Center: Vitamin E," Updated January 2009, http://lpi.oregon state.edu/infocenter/vitamins/vitaminE.

16. J. Chan and E. Giovannucci, "Vegetables, Fruits, Associated Micronutrients and Risk of Prostate Cancer," *Epidemiology Review* 23, no. 1 (2001): 82–86.

17. F. M. Haseen, M. Cantwell, J. M. O'Sullivan, and L. J. Murray, "Is There A Benefit From Lycopene Supplementation in Men With Prostate Cancer? A Systematic Review," *Prostate Cancer and Prostatic Diseases* 12, no. 4 (2009): 325–32.

18. National Institutes of Health Office of Dietary Supplements, "Dietary Supplement Fact Sheet: Vitamin D." Updated May 2008.

19. C. L. Wagner and F. R. Greer, American Academy of Pediatrics Section on Breastfeeding, American Academy of Pediatrics Committee on Nutrition, "Prevention of Rickets and Vitamin D Deficiency in Infants, Children, and Adolescents," *Pediatrics* 122 (2008): 1142–52.

20. Institute of Medicine, "Dietary Reference Intakes for Calcium and Vitamin D," 2010, www.iom.edu/Reports/2010/Dietary-Reference-Intakes-for-Calcium-and-Vitamin-D.aspx.

21. L. J. Appel and C. A. Anderson, "Compelling Evidence for Public Health Action to Reduce Salt Intake," *New England Journal of Medicine* 362, no. 7 (2010): 650–52.

22. U.S. Department of Agriculture, *What We Eat in America*, NHANES 2007-2008 Data: Table 1, 2010; C. Ayala et al., "Application of Lower Sodium Intake Recommendations to Adults—United States, 1999–2006," *Morbidity and Mortality Weekly* (*MMWR*) 58, no. 11 (2009): 281–83.

23. J. Hu et al., "Effects of Salt Substitute on Pulse Wave Analysis among Individuals at High Cardiovascular Risk in Rural China: A Randomized Controlled Study," *Hypertension Research* 32, no. 4 (2009): 282–88; J. Feng et al., "Salt Intake and Cardiovascular Mortality," *American Journal of Medicine* 120, no. 1 (2007): e5–e7.

24. J. Ma, R. Johns, and R. Stafford, "Americans Are Not Meeting Current Calcium Recommendations," *American Journal of Clinical Nutrition* 85 (2007): 1361–66.

25. K. Tucker et al., "Colas, but Not Other Carbonated Beverages, Are Associated with Low Bone Mineral Density in Older Women: The Framingham Osteoporosis Study," *American Journal of Clinical Nutrition* 84 (2006): 936–42.

26. World Health Organization, "Micronutrient Deficiencies: Iron Deficiency Anemia," Accessed February 2012, www.who.int/nutrition/topics/ida/en/index.html.

27. U.S. Centers for Disease Control and Prevention (CDC), "Iron and Iron Deficiency," Accessed February 23, 2011, from http://www.cdc.gov/nutrition/everyone/basics/vitamins/iron.html.

28. C. Tsai et al., "Heme and Non-Heme Iron Consumption and Risk of Gallstone Disease in Men," *American Journal of Clinical Nutrition* 85 (2007): 518–22.

29. U.S. Department of Agriculture, Economic Research Service, "U.S. Per Capita Loss-Adjusted Food Availability: Total Calories," Updated April 2010, www.ers.usda.gov/Data/FoodConsumption/app/reports/displayCommodities.aspx?reportName=Total+Calories&id=36#startForm.

30. D. Grotto and E. Zied, "The Standard American Diet and Its Relationship to the Health Status of Americans," *Nutrition in Clinical Practice* 25, (2010): 603–12.

31. U.S. Department of Agriculture, "Dietary Guidelines for Americans 2010," www.cnpp.usda.gov/dietaryguidelines.htm.

32. B. Black, "Health Library: Just How Much Food Is on That Plate? Understanding Portion Control," Last reviewed February 2009, EBSCO Publishing, www.ebscohost.com/healthLibrary.

33. U.S. Department of Agriculture, "Empty Calories: How Do I Count the Empty Calories I Eat?," Updated June 4, 2011, http://www.choosemyplate.gov/foodgroups/emptycalories_count_table.html.

34. U.S. Food and Drug Administration, "Food Labeling Guide," Updated May 2009, www.fda.gov/Food/GuidanceComplianceRegulatoryInformation/GuidanceDocuments/FoodLabelingNutrition/FoodLabelingGuide.

35. "How Many Vegetarians Are There?" Vegetarian Resource Group, Press Release, May, 15, 2009, www.vrg.org/press/2009poll.htm.

36. "Vegetarian Times Study Shows 7.3 Million Americans Are Vegetarians," *Vegetarian Times,* Press Release, April 15, 2008, www.vegetariantimes.com/features/667.

37. American Dietetic Association, "Position of the American Dietetic Association: Vegetarian Diets," *Journal of the American Dietetic Association* 109, no. 7 (2009): 1266–82.

38. Office of Dietary Supplements, "Frequently Asked Questions," Accessed June 6, 2011, from http://ods.od.nih.gov/Health_Information/ODS_Frequently_Asked_Questions.aspx#Need

39. A. L. Rogovik, S. Vohra, and R. D. Goldman, "Safety Considerations and Potential Interactions of Vitamins: Should Vitamins Be Considered Drugs?" *Annals of Pharmacotherapy* 44, no. 2 (2010): 311–24.

40. Academy of Nutrition and Dietetics, "Dietary Supplements," 2012, Retrieved from http://www.eatright.org/public/content.aspx?id=7918.

41. U.S. Department of Agriculture, Economic Research Services, "Organic Agriculture: Organic Market Overview," 2009, www.ers.usda.gov/briefing/organic/demand.htm.

42. A. D. Dangour, S. K. Dodhia, A. Hayter, E. Allen, K. Lock, and R. Uauy, "Nutrition-related Health Effects of Organic Foods: A Systematic Review," *American Journal of Clinical Nutrition,* 92, no. 1 (2010): 203–10.

43. U.S. Department of Agriculture, Pesticide Data Program: 19th Annual Summary, Calendar Year 2009, Agricultural Marketing Service, Accessed May 2011, from http://www.ams.usda.gov/AMSv1.0/getfile?dDocName=STELPRDC5091055.

44. U.S. Department of Health and Human Services, "Food Safety Modernization Act (FSMA)," 2011, www.fda.gov/Food/FoodSafety/fsma/default.htm.

45. CDC, "Estimates of Food-Borne Illnesses in the United States," 2010, www.cdc.gov/foodborneburden/index.html.

46. CDC, "Preliminary FoodNet Data on the Incidence of Infection with Pathogens Transmitted Commonly through Food—10 States, 2008," *Morbidity and Mortality Weekly Report* 58, no. 13 (2009): 333–37.

47. National Center for Infectious Diseases, Division of Bacterial and Mycotic Diseases, "*E. coli,*" Modified March 2010, www.cdc.gov/ecoli; CDC, "Preliminary FoodNet," 2009.

48. U.S. Food and Drug Administration, "Food Irradiation: What You Need to Know," Accessed October 25, 2011, from http://www.fda.gov/Food/ResourcesForYou/Consumers/ucm261680.htm.

49. A. M. Branum and S. L. Lukacs, "Food Allergy among U.S. Children: Trends in Prevalence and Hospitalizations," *National Center for Health Statistics Data Brief,* no. 10 (Hyattsville, MD: 2008).

50. Food Allergy and Anaphylaxis Network, "Food Allergy Facts and Statistics," 2008, Available at www.foodallergy.org/section/helpful-information.

51. Food Allergy and Anaphylaxis Network, "Advocacy: FALCPA FAQ," 2010, Available at www.foodallergy.org/page/falcpa-faq.

52. University of Chicago Celiac Disease Center, *Celiac Disease Facts and Figures* (Chicago, University of Chicago Celiac Disease Center, 2010), Available at www.celiacdisease.net/factsheets.

53. A. Ranciaro and S. A. Tishkoff, "Population Genetics: Evolutionary History of Lactose Intolerance in Africa," NIH Consensus Development Conference: Lactose Intolerance and Health, February 2010, http://consensus.nih.gov/2010/lactoseabstracts.htm#q1

54. U.S. Department of Agriculture, Economic Research Service, "Adoption of Genetically Engineered Crops in the U.S.," Updated July 2009, www.ers.usda.gov/Data/BiotechCrops.

55. A. Coghlan, "Engineered Maize Toxicity Claims Roundly Rebuffed," *New Scientist* 2744 (January 22, 2010).

56. R. E. Goodman, et al., "Allergenicity Assessment of Genetically Modified Crops—What Makes Sense?," *Nature Biotechnology* 26, no. 1 (2008): 73–81.

57. World Health Organization, "20 Questions on Genetically Modified Foods," Accessed April 2010, www.who.int/foodsafety/publications/biotech/20questions/en.

8 Reaching and Maintaining a Healthy Weight

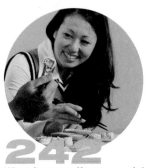

242
What factors affect my weight?

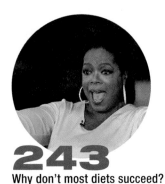

243
Why don't most diets succeed?

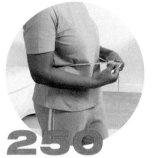

250
How can I tell if I am overweight or overfat?

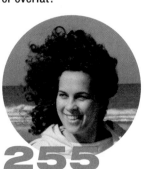

255
How important is exercise to weight management?

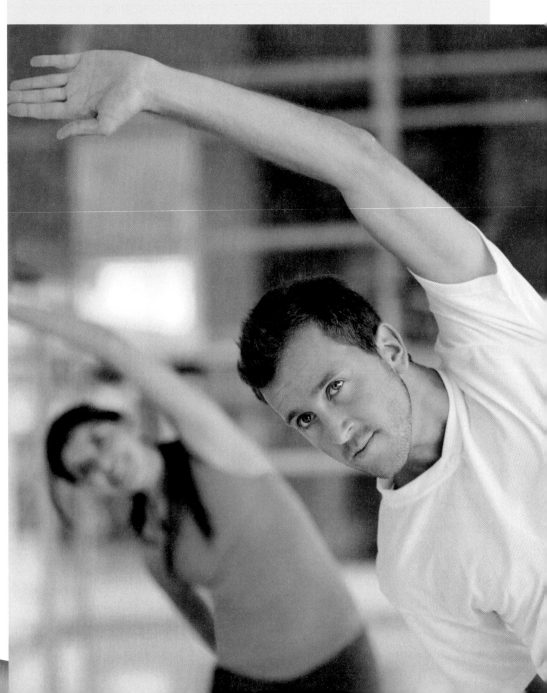

OBJECTIVES

✳ Define *overweight* and *obesity*, describe the current epidemic of overweight/obesity in the United States and globally, and understand risk factors associated with weight problems.

✳ Describe factors that place people at risk for problems with obesity. Distinguish between controllable and uncontrollable factors.

✳ Learn reliable options for determining your percentage of body fat and a healthy weight.

✳ Discuss the roles of exercise, diet, lifestyle modification, fad diets, and which weight-control strategies are most effective.

"The surge in obesity in this country is nothing short of a public health crisis that is threatening our children, our families, and our futures. In fact, the health consequences are so severe that medical experts have warned that our children could be on track to live shorter lives than their parents."

—*First Lady Michelle Obama, Introduction of New Plan to Combat Overweight and Obesity, Press Conference, Alexandria, Virginia, January 28, 2010*

The United States currently has the dubious distinction of being among the fattest nations on Earth. Young and old, rich and poor, rural and urban, educated and uneducated Americans share one thing in common—they are fatter than virtually all previous generations.[1] The word **obesogenic,** meaning "characterized by environments that promote increased food intake, nonhealthful foods, and physical inactivity," has become an apt descriptor of our society. Obesogenic comes from the word *obesity*, meaning body weight that is more than 20 percent above recommended levels for health. Less extreme but still damaging is *overweight*, which is body weight more than 10 percent above healthy levels. The U.S. maps in Figure 8.1 illustrate the increasing levels of obesity that have occurred in the past two decades. Indeed, the prevalence of obesity has tripled among children and doubled among adults in recent decades.[2] Research indicates that the rate of increase in obesity began to slow between 1999 and 2008 for many populations.[3] However, although the rate of increase has slowed, current rates are still extremely high, with more than 68 percent of U.S. adults overall (72.3% of men and 64.1% of women) considered to be overweight or obese.[4]

This translates into over 72 million adults—32 percent of men and 35.5 percent of women—who are classified as obese. This has staggering implications for increased risks from heart disease, diabetes, and other health complications associated with obesity.[5] The prospect is even more bleak for certain populations within the United States. Research points to higher obesity risks among adults of different ethnicities, most notably African American women, who have been found to have rates of overweight/obesity as high as 80 percent.[6] Similar racial disparities exist for both children and adolescents, particularly among Native American/Alaskan Natives and Hispanic populations.[7] However, it is important to note that obesity rates have increased and remain high for both sexes, all ages, all racial/ethnic groups, all educational levels, and all smoking levels, since 1960 when the details of these rates began to be widely recorded.[8]

While smoking is the leading cause of preventable death in America, obesity is second and gaining ground. Obesity and inactivity increase the risks from three of our leading killers: heart disease, cancer, strokes, and disability from arthritis and other ailments. Diabetes, another major obesity-associated problem, is a major concern. In 2010,

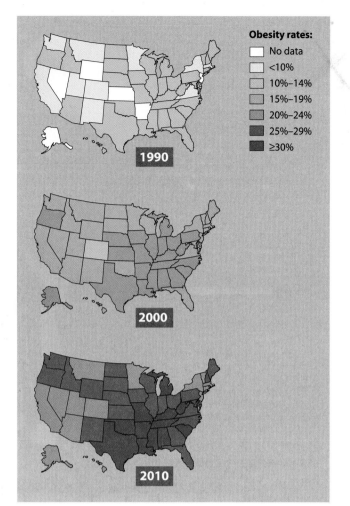

FIGURE 8.1 **Obesity Trends among U.S. Adults, 1990, 2000, and 2010**

These maps indicate the percentage of population in each state that is considered obese, based on a body mass index of 30 or higher, or about 30 pounds overweight for a person 5 feet 4 inches tall.

Source: Centers for Disease Control and Prevention, "U.S. Obesity Trends: 1999-2010," 2012, www.cdc.gov/obesity/data/trends.html

nearly 26 million Americans had diabetes and another 57 million adults had prediabetes.[9] Other health risks associated with obesity include gallstones, sleep apnea, osteoarthritis, and several cancers.

Health consequences of obesity are not our only concern: The estimated annual cost of obesity in the United States exceeds $147 billion in medical expenses and lost productivity. Overall, obese individuals average $1,500 more per year in medical costs, about 42 percent more than an average weight individual.[10] Of course, it is impossible to place a dollar value on a life lost prematurely due to diabetes, stroke, or heart attack or to assess the cost of the social isolation, diminished quality of life, and discrimination against overweight individuals. Of

obesogenic Characterized by environments that promote increased food intake, nonhealthful foods, and physical inactivity; refers to conditions that lead people to become excessively fat.

Hear It! Podcasts

Want a study podcast for this chapter? Download **Managing Your Weight: Finding a Health Balance** at www.pearsonhighered.com/donatelle.

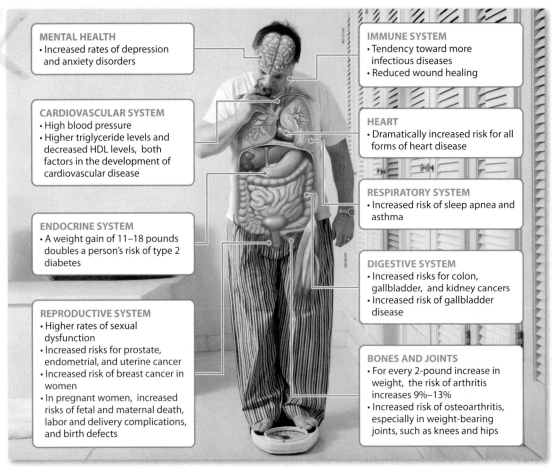

MENTAL HEALTH
- Increased rates of depression and anxiety disorders

CARDIOVASCULAR SYSTEM
- High blood pressure
- Higher triglyceride levels and decreased HDL levels, both factors in the development of cardiovascular disease

ENDOCRINE SYSTEM
- A weight gain of 11–18 pounds doubles a person's risk of type 2 diabetes

REPRODUCTIVE SYSTEM
- Higher rates of sexual dysfunction
- Increased risks for prostate, endometrial, and uterine cancer
- Increased risk of breast cancer in women
- In pregnant women, increased risks of fetal and maternal death, labor and delivery complications, and birth defects

IMMUNE SYSTEM
- Tendency toward more infectious diseases
- Reduced wound healing

HEART
- Dramatically increased risk for all forms of heart disease

RESPIRATORY SYSTEM
- Increased risk of sleep apnea and asthma

DIGESTIVE SYSTEM
- Increased risks for colon, gallbladder, and kidney cancers
- Increased risk of gallbladder disease

BONES AND JOINTS
- For every 2-pound increase in weight, the risk of arthritis increases 9%–13%
- Increased risk of osteoarthritis, especially in weight-bearing joints, such as knees and hips

FIGURE 8.2 **Potential Negative Health Effects of Overweight and Obesity**

Video Tutor: Obesity Health Effects

growing importance is the recognition that obese individuals suffer significant disability during their lives, in terms of both mobility and activities of daily living.[11] (Figure 8.2 summarizes these and other potential health consequences of obesity.)

The United States is not alone. During the past 20 years, the world's population has grown progressively heavier. Globally, there are more than 1.5 billion overweight adults; of these, at least 200 million men and nearly 300 million women are obese. Of increasing concern is that over 43 million of the world's children under the age of 5 were overweight in 2010.[12] Childhood obesity is associated with a higher chance of obesity, disability, and premature death in adulthood. In addition to increased future risks, obese children have more breathing difficulties, increased risk of fractures, hypertension, early markers of cardiovascular disease, more diabetes, and are more likely to suffer stigma and bullying in schools.[13] Since 1980, rates have risen three-fold or more in some areas of North America, the United Kingdom, eastern Europe, the Middle East, the Pacific Islands, Australasia, and China. Many developing regions of the world are demonstrating even faster rising rates of obesity.[14] The **Health in a Diverse World** box on page 241 looks at strategies to combat obesity around the globe, a problem sometimes referred to as *globesity*.

Factors Contributing to Overweight and Obesity

What factors predispose us to excess weight? Although diet and exercise are clearly two of the major contributors, other factors, including genetics and physiology, are also important. In addition, the environment you live in, eat in, exercise in, and play and work in has a significant influence on what you eat, how much you eat, and when you eat.[15]

Genetic and Physiological Factors

Are some people born to be fat? Genes, hormones, and other aspects of a person's physiology seem to influence whether you become fat or thin.

Genes: A Variety of Theories In spite of decades of research, the exact role of genes in one's predisposition toward obesity remains in question. Children whose parents are obese also tend to be overweight. In fact, countless observational studies back up the idea that a family history of obesity increases one's chances of being becoming obese. But, is that due to their learned eating and exercise behaviors,

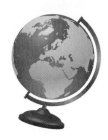

COMBATING GLOBESITY

The United States is not alone in being a "fat" country. During the past decade, epidemic rates of obesity and diabetes have emerged as global health problems. Today, more than 1.5 billion adults worldwide are overweight, and 500 million of them are obese. Add to that the 155 million children worldwide—43 million under age 5—who are overweight or obese and the vastness of the problem is clear. The World Health Organization (WHO) projects that by 2015 approximately 2.3 billion adults will be overweight and more than 700 million will be obese. The figure shows some of the world's most and least overweight countries. What factors do you think influence average weights in these nations? If we continue at our current rate, what do you think this graph will look like in another decade?

Sources: P. Hossain, K. Bisher, and M. El Nahas, "Obesity and Diabetes in the Developing World—A Growing Challenge," *New England Journal of Medicine* 356, no. 3 (2007): 312–15; World Health Organization, "Obesity and Overweight," Fact sheet no. 311, Updated March 2011, www.who .int/mediacentre/factsheets/fs311/en/index .html.

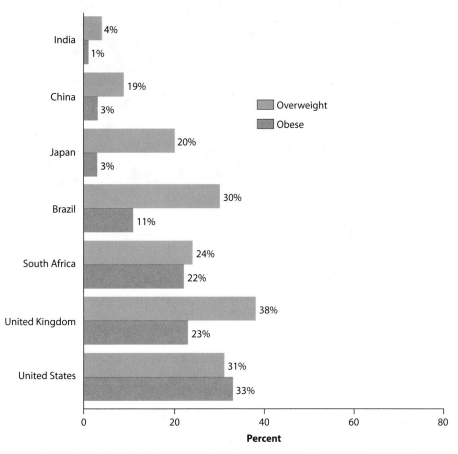

Source: Adapted from World Health Organization, "Global Database on Body Mass Index (BMI)," 2012, http://apps.who.int/bmi/index.jsp.

environmental cues, genes, or a combination of these factors? Supporting the genetic basis for obesity, researchers found that adopted individuals tend to be similar in weight to their biological parents and that identical twins are twice as likely to weigh the same as are fraternal twins, even if they are raised separately.[16] Newer meta-analyses of twin studies indicate that although genetics seems to play a role in body composition, the environment plays a substantial role in one's obesity-prone future.[17]

Although the exact mechanism remains unknown, researchers continue to explore whether genes are important in setting metabolic rates, influencing how the body balances calories and energy, or causing us to crave certain foods.[18] A growing number of experts believe that genes probably do play a role. Rather than acting individually, their effect may be in clusters, influencing the regulation of food intake through action in the central nervous system, as well as influencing fat cell synthesis and functioning.

If genetic factors are found to play a role in a tendency to obesity, are you doomed to a lifelong battle with your weight? Probably not, based on exciting new research that points to the fact that even if obesity does run in your family, a healthy lifestyle can override "obesity" genes. Results of a major European study found that the effects of the *FTO* gene on obesity is over 30 percent less among physically active adults. Those who seemed to be beating their obesity tendencies exercised at least 90 minutes a day compared to those who exercised 30 minutes.[19]

One potential genetic basis for obesity has been identified by observational studies of certain Indian and African tribes. Labeled the thrifty gene theory, researchers noted higher

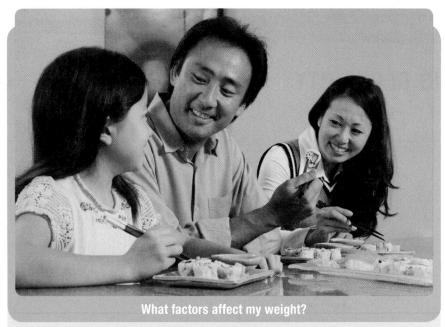

What factors affect my weight?

Many factors help determine weight and body type, including heredity and genetic makeup, environment, and learned eating patterns, which are often connected to family habits.

body fat and obesity levels in some of these tribes than in the general population.[20] Because their ancestors struggled through centuries of famine, members of the tribes appear to have survived by adapting metabolically to periods of famine with slowed metabolism, storing fat for the proverbial "rainy day." Over time, ancestors may have passed on a genetic, hormonal, or metabolic predisposition toward fat storage that makes losing fat more difficult. In short, it was thought that people may have been genetically programmed to burn fewer calories. Today, critics of this theory believe that there are many other factors that influence obesity development, most of which have not yet been discovered. There is growing consensus that only 2 to 5 percent of childhood obesity cases are caused by a defect that impairs function in a gene and that the common forms of childhood obesity seem to result from a predisposition that primarily favors obesogenic behaviors in an obesogenic environment.[21]

basal metabolic rate (BMR) The rate of energy expenditure by a body at complete rest in a neutral environment.

resting metabolic rate (RMR) The energy expenditure of the body under BMR conditions plus other daily sedentary activities.

exercise metabolic rate (EMR) The energy expenditure that occurs during exercise.

adaptive thermogenesis Theoretical mechanism by which the brain regulates metabolic activity according to caloric intake.

Metabolic Rates Several aspects of your metabolism also help determine whether you gain, maintain, or lose weight. Each of us has an innate energy-burning capacity that hums along even when we are in the deepest levels of sleep. This **basal metabolic rate (BMR)** is the minimum rate at which the body uses energy when at complete rest in a neutrally temperate environment, activities such as digestion are not occurring, and the body is simply working to maintain basic vital functions. Technically, to measure BMR, a person would

be awake, but all major stimuli, including stressors to the sympathetic nervous system, would be at rest. Usually, the best time to measure BMR is after 8 hours of sleep and after a 12-hour fast. A BMR for the average, healthy adult is usually between 1,200 and 1,800 calories per day.

A more practical way of assessing your energy expenditure levels is the **resting metabolic rate (RMR).** Slightly higher than the BMR, the RMR includes the BMR plus any additional energy expended through daily sedentary activities such as food digestion, sitting, studying, or standing. The **exercise metabolic rate (EMR)** accounts for the remaining percentage of all daily calorie expenditures. It refers to the energy expenditure that occurs during physical activity. For most of us, these calories come from light daily activities, such as walking, climbing stairs, and mowing the lawn.

Your BMR (and RMR) can fluctuate considerably. In general, the younger you are, the higher your BMR will be, partly because cells undergo rapid subdivision during periods of growth, an activity that consumes a good deal of energy. The BMR is highest during infancy, puberty, and pregnancy, when bodily changes are most rapid. After age 30, a person's BMR slows down by about 1 to 2 percent a year. Therefore, people over age 30 commonly find that they must work harder to burn off an extra helping of ice cream than they did in their teens. A slower BMR, coupled with less activity, shifting priorities (family and career become more important than fitness), and loss in muscle mass, contribute to the weight-gain of many middle-aged people.

75%

of dieters regain lost weight within 2 years.

Theories abound concerning the mechanisms that regulate metabolism and food intake. Some sources indicate that the hypothalamus (the part of the brain that regulates appetite) closely monitors levels of certain nutrients in the blood. When these levels fall, the brain signals us to eat. According to one theory, the monitoring system in obese people does not work properly, and the cues to eat are more frequent and intense than they are in people of normal weight. Another theory is that thin people send more effective messages to the hypothalamus. This concept, called **adaptive thermogenesis,** states that thin people can consume large amounts of food without gaining weight because the appetite center of their brains speeds up metabolic activity to compensate for the increased consumption.

On the other side of the BMR equation is the **set point theory,** which suggests that our bodies fight to maintain our weight around a narrow range or at a set point. If we go on a drastic starvation diet or fast, our bodies slow down our BMR to conserve energy. Set point theory suggests that our own bodies may sabotage our weight loss efforts by holding on to calories as a form of protection. The good news is that set points can be changed; however, these changes may take time to be permanent. Healthy diet, steady weight loss, and exercise appear to be the best methods of sustaining weight loss.

Yo-yo diets, in which people repeatedly gain weight and then starve themselves to lose it all quickly, are doomed to fail. When dieters resume eating after their weight loss, their BMR is set lower, making it almost certain that they will regain the pounds they just lost. After repeated cycles of dieting and regaining weight, these people find it increasingly hard to lose weight and increasingly easy to regain it, so they become heavier and heavier.

Hormonal Influences: Ghrelin and Leptin

Obese people may be more likely than thin people to satisfy their appetite and eat for reasons other than nutrition.[22] Over the years, many people have attributed obesity to problems with their thyroid gland and resultant hormone imbalances that made it hard for them to burn calories. Today, most authorities agree that less than 2 percent of the obese population have a thyroid problem and can trace their weight problems to a metabolic or hormone imbalance.[23] Should physicians test obese patients for low thyroid hormones and put those with low thyroid levels on medications to improve these levels as an edge against obesity? An increasing number of researchers believe that there is more to the thyroid-obesity interaction than we currently know and that more research is necessary to determine best practice in this area.[24] While hormones may have an impact on a person's ability to lose weight, control appetite, and sense fullness, the problem with overconsumption may be related more to **satiety** and to environmental cues than it is to appetite or hunger. People generally feel satiated, or full, when they have satisfied their nutritional needs and their stomach signals "no more."

One hormone that researchers suspect may influence satiety and play a role in our ability to keep weight off is *ghrelin,* sometimes referred to as "the hunger hormone," which is produced in the stomach. Initial interest in ghrelin was the result of an early study that focused on a small group of obese people who had lost weight over a 6-month period.[25] They noted that ghrelin levels rose before every meal and fell drastically shortly afterward, suggesting that the hormone plays a role in appetite stimulation. Since that early research, ghrelin has been shown to be an important growth hormone that plays a key role in the regulation of appetite and food intake control, gastrointestinal motility, gastric acid secretion, endocrine and exocrine pancreatic secretions, glucose and lipid metabolism, and cardiovascular and immunological processes.[26]

Another hormone gaining increased attention and research is *leptin,* which has long been recognized as an appetite regulator in mammals. Leptin is produced by fat cells; its levels in the blood increase as fat tissue increases. Scientists believe leptin serves as a form of satiety signal, telling the brain when you are full.[27] When levels of leptin in the blood rise, appetite levels drop. Although obese people have adequate amounts of leptin and leptin receptors, the receptors do not seem to work properly. The exact reasons leptin levels seem to be high in obese individuals but appetite level is not suppressed remains a mystery. It may be simply that environmental cues are stronger than our hunger pangs.

Fat Cells and Predisposition to Fatness

Some obese people may have excessive numbers of fat cells. An average-weight adult has approximately 25 to 35 billion fat cells, a moderately obese adult 60 to 100 billion, and an extremely obese adult as many as 200 billion.[28] This type of obesity, **hyperplasia,** usually appears in early childhood and perhaps, due to the mother's dietary habits, even prior to birth. The most critical periods for the development of hyperplasia seem to be the last 2 to 3 months of fetal development,

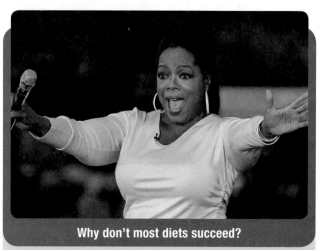

Why don't most diets succeed?

Just about any calorie-cutting diet can produce weight loss in the short term, often through water-weight loss. However, without improved nutrition and sustained exercise and activity, lost weight will return and the overall dieting process will have failed. Oprah Winfrey has been candid about her struggles with this pattern of weight cycling, or yo-yo dieting. Such a pattern disrupts the body's metabolism and makes future weight loss more difficult and permanent changes even harder to maintain.

set point theory Theory that a form of internal thermostat controls our weight and fights to maintain this weight around a narrowly set range.

yo-yo diets Cycles in which people diet and regain weight.

satiety The feeling of fullness or satisfaction at the end of a meal.

hyperplasia A condition characterized by an excessive number of fat cells.

See It! Videos

Frozen meals may not be the key to dieting success. Watch **Miscounting Calories** at www.pearsonhighered.com/donatelle.

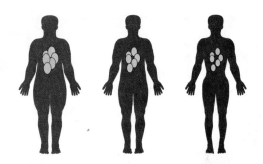

	Before body weight reduction	Initial weight reduction	Second weight reduction
Body weight	328 lb	227 lb	165 lb
Fat cell size	0.9 µg/cell	0.6 µg/cell	0.2 µg/cell
Fat cell number	75 billion	75 billion	75 billion

FIGURE 8.3 One Person at Various Stages of Weight Loss
Note that, according to the hyperplasia theory, the number of fat cells remains constant, but their size decreases when weight is lost.

the first year of life, and between the ages of 9 and 13. Central to this theory is the belief that the number of fat cells in a body does not increase appreciably during adulthood. However, the ability of each of these cells to swell (**hypertrophy**) and shrink does carry over into adulthood. People who add large numbers of fat cells to their bodies in childhood may be able to lose weight by decreasing the size of each cell in adulthood, but the total number of cells will remain the same. With the next calorie binge, the cells swell and sabotage weight-loss efforts. Weight gain may be tied to both the number of fat cells in the body and the capacity of individual cells to enlarge. See Figure 8.3.

hypertrophy The act of swelling or increasing in size, as with cells.

Environmental Factors

With all our twenty-first-century conveniences, environmental factors have come to play a large role in weight maintenance. Automobiles, remote controls, desk jobs, and long sessions on the Internet all cause us to sit more and move less, and this lack of physical activity causes a decrease in energy expenditure. Time our grandparents spent going for a walk after dinner we now spend watching TV shows or on Facebook. Coupled with our culture of eating, it's a recipe for weight gain.

Greater Access to High-Calorie Foods There are more high-calorie, low-nutrient-density foods on the market than ever

before. Even though most Americans report that they are trying to cut back on portion sizes and high fat, high-sugar foods, by most indications they find these behavioral changes difficult to sustain. A long list of environmental factors prompt us to eat what we shouldn't and eat too much:

● Advertising is designed to increase energy intake—ads promote high-calorie foods at a low price and market super-sized portions. See the **Student Health Today** box on page 245.
● Prepackaged, high-fat meals; fast food; and sugar-laden soft drinks are widespread. High-calorie coffee lattes and energy drinks add to daily caloric intake.
● The number of working women has grown, leading to less home cooking and greater consumption of restaurant meals, fast foods, and convenience foods. As society eats out more, higher-calorie, high-fat foods become the norm, and increased weight is the result.
● Bottle-feeding infants may increase energy intake relative to breast-feeding.
● Misleading food labels confuse consumers about portion and serving sizes.
● Fast-food restaurants, cafes, vending machines, and quick-stop markets are everywhere, offering easy access to high-calorie foods and beverages.
● Larger dishes, cups, and serving utensils inflate serving sizes and lead to increased calorie and fat intake.

Early Sabotage: A Youthful Start on Obesity

Children have always loved junk food. However, today's youth tend to eat larger portions and, from their earliest years, exercise less than any previous generation.[29] Video games, television, cell phones, and the Internet often keep them exercising their fingers more than any other part of their bodies, and children are subject to the same environmental, social, and cultural factors that influence obesity in their elders.

In addition, youth are at risk because of factors that are only beginning to be understood. Epidemiological studies suggest that maternal undernutrition, obesity, and diabetes during gestation and lactation are strong predictors of obesity in children.[30] Research also shows that race and ethnicity

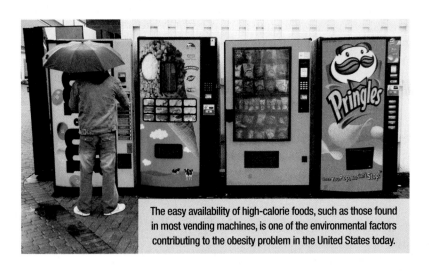

The easy availability of high-calorie foods, such as those found in most vending machines, is one of the environmental factors contributing to the obesity problem in the United States today.

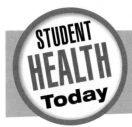

Portion Inflation

Would you be surprised to learn that today's serving portions are significantly larger than those of past decades? From burgers and fries to meat-and-potato or pasta meals, today's popular restaurant foods dwarf their earlier counterparts. For example, a 25-ounce prime-rib dinner served at one local steak chain contains nearly 3,000 calories and 150 grams of fat! That's half again the calories and more than three times the fat that most adults need in a whole day, and it's just the meat part of the meal.

Many researchers believe that the main reason Americans are gaining weight is that people no longer recognize a normal serving size. The National Heart, Lung, and Blood Institute has developed a pair of "Portion Distortion" quizzes that show how today's portions compare with those of 20 years ago. Test yourself online at http://hp2010.nhlbihin.net/portion to see whether you can guess the differences between today's meals and those previously considered normal.

To make sure you're not over-eating when you dine out, follow these strategies:

✳ Order the smallest size available. Focus on taste, not quantity. Get used to eating less and enjoy what you eat.
✳ Take your time, and let your fullness indicator have a chance to kick in while there is still time to quit.
✳ Dip your food in dressings, gravies, and sauces on the side rather than pouring these extra calories over the top.
✳ Order an appetizer as your main meal.
✳ Split your main entrée with a friend, and order a side salad for each of you. Alternatively, eat only half your dinner and take the rest home for another day.
✳ Avoid buffets and all-you-can-eat establishments.

Today's bloated portions.

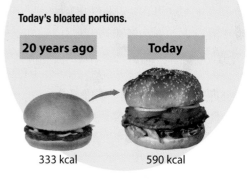

20 years ago	Today
333 kcal	590 kcal

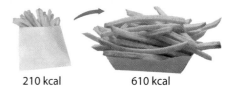

210 kcal   610 kcal

Source: Data are from National Heart, Lung, and Blood Institute, "Portion Distortion," last accessed May 8, 2012, http://hp2010.nhlbihin.net/portion.

---

seem to be intricately interwoven with environmental factors in increasing risks to young people.[31]

Obese kids not only suffer from the potential physical problems of obesity, they also often face weight-related stigma and hateful comments about their size from their peers (see the **Health Headlines** box on page 246). As a result, overweight and obese children may suffer lasting blows to their self-esteem, feelings of social acceptance, and emotional health, affecting personal identity and fostering mistrust and fear of others. New research indicates that obese youth who feel that they are picked on and discriminated against experience more stress and more negative health outcomes long term than their normal weight friends.[32]

Psychosocial and Economic Factors

The relationship of weight problems to deeply rooted emotional insecurities, needs, and wants remains uncertain. What is certain is that eating tends to be a focal point of people's lives; it has become a social ritual associated with companionship, celebration, and enjoy-

ment. It can also be used to help you feel good when other things in life are not going well, hence the term *comfort food*. Our friends and loved ones are often key influences in our eating behaviors. In fact, according to recent research, young adults who are overweight and obese tend to befriend and date people who are also overweight and obese and who like to socialize around food in much the same way that smokers or exercisers tend to hang out with smokers or exercisers.[33] Having "foodies" in your main social group may be a major obstacle in the psychological battle to control food intake.

Socioeconomic factors can provide obstacles or aids to weight control, as well. When economic times are tough, people tend to eat more inexpensive, high-calorie processed foods.[34] Unsafe neighborhoods and poor infrastructure (lack of recreational areas, for example) make it difficult for less-affluent people to exercise.[35] New research suggests that the more educated you are, the lower your body mass index and overall obesity profile are likely to be. In a study of comparative international data, highly educated men and, in particular, highly educated women in the United States have a lower average BMI than their less-educated counterparts.

See It! Videos
One town combats obesity beginning in elementary school. Watch **Obesity in America** at www.pearsonhighered.com/donatelle.

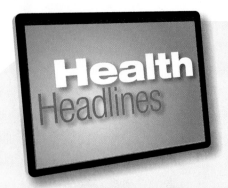

Health Headlines

OBESITY STIGMA: HAVE WE GONE TOO FAR?

Obesity stigma (or *weight bias*) refers to negative weight-related attitudes toward an overweight or obese individual. It can be subtle or overt, with examples ranging from negative stereotyping, social rejection, and prejudice to bullying and physical aggression. According to the experts, weight bias exists because of pervasive societal beliefs that shame will motivate people to diet and lose weight. Our culture values thinness and perpetuates the message that obesity is the mark of a weak-willed person, blaming the victim rather than addressing environmental and social conditions that increase our risks of obesity.

An extension of weight bias in our society is *weight discrimination,* or the unequal, unfair treatment of people because of weight. Weight discrimination might mean being qualified for a job but not being hired because of your weight, receiving unequal treatment in health care, being denied scholarships or awards due to appearance, or not being allowed to rent a particular home.

One example of the debate over obesity stigma was the reaction to an advertising campaign entitled Strong4Life, which urged

viewers in Georgia to acknowledge the issues that obese children face related to their weight. Heavy kids talked about the impact of their obesity in a series of stark, somber, black-and-white interviews, describing being victimized by others or asking their parents how they gotten so fat. Some think that the ads are a valuable first step, with the conversations that have been generated being worthwhile if not enough. Others look at the ads and suggest that parents with obese children should lose custody of them, have their children put in foster care, or face criminal charges. Still others think that the advertisements offer no positive benefits and may contribute to "shaming" kids for actions that are largely outside of their control.

Currently, the United States has no federal laws that protect overweight or obese individuals from discrimination and, as of this writing, only one state, Michigan, has state laws that ban discrimination in employment based weight The cities of Santa Cruz and San Francisco in California and the District of Columbia have ordinances that ban weight-based discrimination. There are many people who argue that making weight discrimination illegal would lead to countless irresolvable court cases. Others argue that weight discrimination laws are just as necessary as disability protection and anti-hate laws and would have an equally positive impact on society.

What do you think? Should there be laws against obesity stigma and discrimination? Do you think treating obese people differently—by requiring them to pay higher health care premiums or purchase a second airline seat, or excluding them

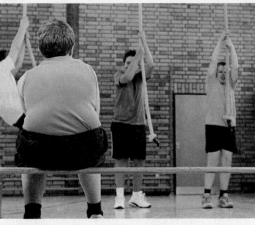

Stigmatization of people who are obese can contribute to depression and low self-esteem.

from certain jobs and social settings—is ever justified? Do the ads shown in Georgia sound like a useful step in opening up a conversation or an excuse to stigmatize obese children? Besides enacting laws, what do you think can be done to address weight stigma and discrimination in our society?

Sources: B. Rochman, "Ads Featuring Overweight Children Make Some Uncomfortable," *Time: Healthland,* January 4, 2012, http://healthland.time.com/2012/01/04/ads-featuring-overweight-children-make-some-uncomfortable; R. Puhl and C. Heuer, "Public Opinion About Laws to Prohibit Weight Discrimination in the United States," *Obesity* 19, no.1 (2011):74–82; The Council on Weight and Size Discrimination, "Weight Discrimination Laws," Accessed February 14, 2012, www.cswd.org/docs/legalaction; R. Puhl, Obesity Action Coalition, "Weight Discrimination: A Socially Acceptable Injustice," 2010, www.obesityaction.org/magazine/oac-news12/obesityanddiscrimination.php; R. Puhl and C. Heuer, "The Stigma of Obesity: A Review and Update," *Obesity* 17, no. 5 (2009): 941–64; Rudd Center for Food Policy and Obesity, Yale University, *Rudd Report: Weight Bias: A Social Justice Issue: Policy Brief* (New Haven, CT: Rudd Center for Food Policy and Obesity, 2009), Available at www.yaleruddcenter.org/briefs.aspx.

Lifestyle Factors

Although heredity, metabolism, and environment all have an impact on weight management, the increasingly high rate of overweight and obesity in the past decades is largely due to the way we live our lives. In general, Americans are eating more and moving less than ever before, and becoming overfat as a result. Weight management can be much harder when it feels like a chore.

Of all the factors affecting obesity, perhaps the most critical is the relationship between activity level and calorie intake. Obesity rates are rising, but aren't more people exercising than ever before? One big problem in determining activity levels is that data are largely based on self-report, and people overestimate their daily exercise level and intensity. Although 31 percent of U.S. adults report that they engage in 30 minutes or more of moderate physical activity on 5 or more days per week, when physical activity is measured by a device that detects movement (accelerometer), only 3 to 5 percent of adults are actually obtaining this amount of exercise.[36]

Data from the National Health Interview Survey show that over one third of U.S. adults aged 18 and over *never* engage in any leisure time activity (no sessions of light/moderate physical activity for at least 10 minutes). Inactivity was higher among women than men (35.2 percent versus 29.7 percent) and highest among non-Hispanic blacks (43.2 percent) and Hispanic adults (44.7 percent). Perhaps even more alarming is the fact that only 21.3 percent of non-Hispanic whites, 17.2 percent of non-Hispanic Blacks, and only 14.4 percent of Hispanics or Latinos met the most recent federal physical activity guidelines.[37] The **Skills for Behavior Change** box offers some ideas for making exercising and healthy eating more fun.

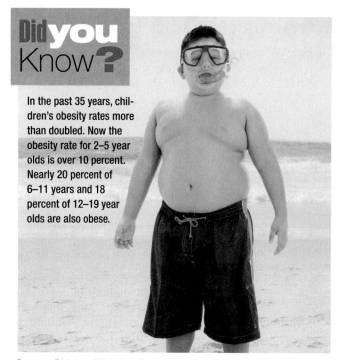

Source: Division of Nutrition, Physical Activity and Obesity, National Center for Chronic Disease Prevention and Health Promotion, "Overweight and Obesity: NHANES Surveys (1976–1980 and 2003–2008)," Updated September 2010, www.cdc.gov/obesity/childhood/prevalence.html.

Assessing Body Weight and Body Composition

Everyone has his or her own ideal weight, based on individual variables such as body structure, height, and fat distribution. Traditionally, experts used measurement techniques such as height–weight charts to determine whether an individual fell into the ideal weight, overweight, or obese category. However, these charts can be misleading because they don't take body composition—that is, a person's ratio of fat to lean muscle—or fat distribution into account. In fact, weight can be a deceptive indicator. Many a muscular athlete or middle-aged woman who brags that she weighs the same as she did in high school is shocked to find out that he or she has relatively high fat levels based on BMI. More accurate measures of evaluating healthy weight and disease risk focus on a person's percentage of body fat and how that fat is distributed in his or her body.

It's important to remember that fat isn't all bad. In fact, some fat is essential for healthy body functioning. Fat regulates body temperature, cushions and insulates organs and tissues, and is the body's main source of stored energy. Body fat is composed of two types: essential fat and storage fat. *Essential fat* is that fat necessary for maintenance of life and reproductive functions. *Storage fat,* the nonessential fat that many of us try to shed, makes up the remainder of our fat reserves.

Overweight and Obesity

In general, **overweight** is increased body weight due to excess fat that exceeds healthy recommendations, whereas **obesity** refers to body weight that greatly exceeds health recommendations. Traditionally, *overweight* was defined as being 1 to 19 percent above one's ideal weight, based on a standard height–weight chart, and *obesity* was defined as being 20 percent or more above one's ideal weight. Morbidly obese people are 100 percent or more above their ideal weight. Experts now usually define *overweight* and *obesity* in terms of BMI, a measure discussed below, or percentage of body fat, as determined by some of the methods we'll discuss shortly. Although opinion varies somewhat, most experts agree that men's bodies should contain between 8 and 20 percent total body fat, and women should be within the range of 20 to 30 percent. At various ages and stages of life, these ranges also vary, but generally, men who exceed 22 percent body fat and women who exceed 35 percent are considered overweight (see Table 8.1).

overweight Having a body weight more than 10 percent above healthy recommended levels; in an adult, having a BMI of 25 to 29.

obesity A body weight more than 20 percent above healthy recommended levels; in an adult, a BMI of 30 or more.

underweight Having a body weight more than 10 percent below healthy recommended levels; in an adult, having a BMI below 18.5.

body mass index (BMI) A number calculated from a person's weight and height that is used to assess risk for possible present or future health problems.

Underweight

There are percentages of body fat below which a person is considered **underweight,** and health is compromised. In men, this lower limit is approximately 3 to 7 percent of total body weight, and in women it is approximately 8 to 15 percent. Extremely low body fat can cause a host of problems, including hair loss, visual disturbances, skin problems, a tendency to fracture bones easily, digestive system disturbances, heart irregularities, gastrointestinal problems, difficulties in maintaining body temperature, and amenorrhea (in women). Problems with being underweight and having a percentage of body fat that is too low are on the increase today, particularly as our culture's obsession with appearance continues. (See Focus On: Enhancing Your Body Image beginning on page 266 for an in-depth discussion of eating disorders and body image issues.)

Body Mass Index (BMI)

Although people have a general sense that BMI is an indicator of how "fat" a person is, most do not really know what it is assessing. **Body mass index (BMI)** is a description of body weight relative to height, numbers that are highly correlated with your total body fat. Body mass index is not sex specific, and it does not directly measure percentage of body fat, but it provides a more accurate measure of overweight and obesity

TABLE 8.1 | Body Fat Percentage Norms for Men and Women*

MEN

Age	Very Lean	Excellent	Good	Fair	Poor	Very Poor
20–29	<7%	7%–10%	11%–15%	16%–19%	20%–23%	>23%
30–39	<11%	11%–14%	15%–18%	19%–21%	22%–25%	>25%
40–49	<14%	14%–17%	18%–20%	21%–23%	24%–27%	>27%
50–59	<15%	15%–19%	20%–22%	23%–24%	25%–28%	>28%
60–69	<16%	16%–20%	21%–22%	23%–25%	26%–28%	>28%
70–79	<16%	16%–20%	21%–23%	24%–25%	26%–28%	>28%

WOMEN

Age	Very Lean	Excellent	Good	Fair	Poor	Very Poor
20–29	<14%	14%–16%	17%–19%	20%–23%	24%–27%	>27%
30–39	<15%	15%–17%	18%–21%	22%–25%	26%–29%	>29%
40–49	<17%	17%–20%	21%–24%	25%–28%	29%–32%	>32%
50–59	<18%	18%–22%	23%–27%	28%–30%	31%–34%	>34%
60–69	<18%	18%–23%	24%–28%	29%–31%	32%–35%	>35%
70–79	<18%	18%–24%	25%–29%	30%–32%	33%–36%	>36%

*Assumes nonathletes. For athletes, recommended body fat is 5 to 15 percent for men and 12 to 22 percent for women. Please note that there are no agreed-upon national standards for recommended body fat percentage.

Source: Based on data from The Cooper Institute, Dallas TX, www.cooperinstitute.org.

than weight alone.[38] Find your BMI in inches and pounds in Figure 8.4, or calculate your BMI now by dividing your weight in kilograms by height in meters squared. The mathematical formula is

$$BMI = weight\ (kg)/height\ squared\ (m^2)$$

A BMI calculator is also available from the National Heart, Lung, and Blood Institute at http://nhlbisupport.com/bmi/bmicalc.htm.

Desirable BMI levels may vary with age and by sex; however, most BMI tables for adults do not account for such variables. *Healthy weights* are defined as those with BMIs of 18.5 to 25, the range of lowest statistical health risk.[39] A BMI of 25 to 29.9 indicates overweight and potentially significant health risks. A BMI of 30 to 39.9 is classified as *obese,* a BMI of 40 to 49.9 is **morbidly obese,** and a new category of BMI of 50 or higher has been labeled as *super obese.*[40] Nearly 3 percent

BMI	19	20	21	22	23	24	25	26	27	28	29	30	31	32	33	34	35	36	37	38	39	40	41	42
Height							Weight in pounds																	
4'10"	91	96	100	105	110	115	119	124	129	134	138	143	148	153	158	162	167	172	177	181	186	191	196	201
4'11"	94	99	104	109	114	119	124	128	133	138	143	148	153	158	163	168	173	178	183	188	193	198	203	208
5'	97	102	107	112	118	123	128	133	138	143	148	153	158	163	168	174	179	184	189	194	199	204	209	215
5'1"	100	106	111	116	122	127	132	137	143	148	153	158	164	169	174	180	185	190	195	201	206	211	217	222
5'2"	104	109	115	120	126	131	136	142	147	153	158	164	169	175	180	186	191	196	202	207	213	218	224	229
5'3"	107	113	118	124	130	135	141	146	152	158	163	169	175	180	186	191	197	203	208	214	220	225	231	237
5'4"	110	116	122	128	134	140	145	151	157	163	169	175	180	186	192	197	204	209	215	221	227	232	238	244
5'5"	114	120	126	132	138	144	150	156	162	168	174	180	186	192	198	204	210	216	222	228	234	240	246	252
5'6"	118	124	130	136	142	148	155	161	167	173	179	186	192	198	204	210	216	223	229	235	241	247	253	260
5'7"	121	127	134	140	146	153	159	166	172	178	185	191	198	204	211	217	223	230	236	242	249	255	261	268
5'8"	125	131	138	144	151	158	164	171	177	184	190	197	204	210	216	223	230	236	243	249	256	262	269	276
5'9"	128	135	142	149	155	162	169	176	182	189	196	203	210	216	223	230	236	243	250	257	263	270	277	284
5'10"	132	139	146	153	160	167	174	181	188	195	202	209	216	222	229	236	243	250	257	264	271	278	285	292
5'11"	136	143	150	157	165	172	179	186	193	200	208	215	222	229	236	243	250	257	265	272	279	286	293	301
6'	140	147	154	162	169	177	184	191	199	206	213	221	228	235	242	250	258	265	272	279	287	294	302	309
6'1"	144	151	159	166	174	182	189	197	204	212	219	227	235	242	250	257	265	275	280	288	295	302	310	318
6'2"	148	155	163	171	179	186	194	202	210	218	225	233	241	249	256	264	272	280	287	295	303	311	319	326
6'3"	152	160	168	176	184	193	200	208	216	224	232	240	248	256	264	272	279	287	295	303	311	319	327	335
6'4"	156	164	172	180	189	197	205	213	221	230	238	246	254	263	271	279	287	295	304	312	320	328	336	344
	Healthy weight BMI 18.5–24.9						Overweight BMI 25–29.9					Obese BMI 30–39.9										Morbidly obese BMI ≥40		

FIGURE 8.4 **Body Mass Index (BMI)**
Locate your height, read across to find your weight, then read up to determine your BMI. Any weight less than those listed for a given height would yield a BMI of less than 18.5, classified as underweight.

Source: National Institutes of Health/National Heart, Lung, and Blood Institute (NHLBI), *Evidence Report of Clinical Guidelines on the Identification, Evaluation, and Treatment of Overweight and Obesity in Adults,* 1998, www.nhlbi.nih.gov/guidelines/obesity/ob_gdlns.htm.

of obese men and almost 7 percent of obese women are morbidly obese.[41]

Limitations of BMI Although a useful indicator, the BMI does have limitations. Base metabolism index levels don't account for the fact that muscle weighs more than fat and thus a well-muscled person could weigh enough to be classified as obese according to his or her BMI, nor are bone mass and water weight considered in BMI calculations. For people who are under 5 feet tall, are highly muscled, or who are older and have little muscle mass, BMI levels can be inaccurate. More precise methods of determining body fat, described below, should be used for these individuals.

Youth and BMI Today, over 30 percent of youth in America are obese, three times higher than rates in the 1980s.[42] Although the labels *obese* and *morbidly obese* have been used for years for adults, there is growing concern that such labels increase bias and stigma against youth.[43] BMI ranges above a normal weight for children and teens are often labeled differently, as "at risk of overweight" and "overweight," to avoid the sense of shame such words may cause. In addition, BMI ranges for children and teens are defined so that they take into account normal differences in body fat between boys and girls and the differences in body fat that occur at various ages. Specific guidelines for calculating youth BMI are available at the Centers for Disease Control and Prevention website, www.cdc.gov.

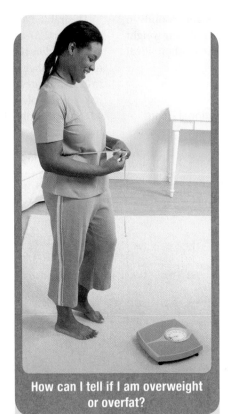

How can I tell if I am overweight or overfat?

Observing the way you look and how your clothes fit can give you a general idea of whether you weigh more or less than in the past. But for evaluating your weight and body fat levels in terms of potential health risks, it's best to use more scientific measures, such as BMI, waist circumference, waist-to-hip ratio, or a technician-administered body composition test.

Waist Circumference and Ratio Measurements

Knowing where your fat is carried may be more important than knowing how much you carry. Men and postmenopausal women tend to store fat in the upper regions of the body, particularly in the abdominal area. Premenopausal women usually store fat in the lower regions of their bodies, particularly the hips, buttocks, and thighs. Waist circumference measurement is increasingly recognized as a useful tool in assessing abdominal fat, which is considered more threatening to health overall than fat in other regions of the body. In particular, as waist circumference increases, there is a greater risk for diabetes, cardiovascular disease, and stroke.[44]

morbidly obese Having a body weight 100 percent or more above healthy recommended levels; in an adult, having a BMI of 40 or more.

waist-to-hip ratio Waist circumference divided by hip circumference; a high ratio indicates increased health risks due to unhealthy fat distribution.

A waistline greater than 40 inches (102 centimeters) in men and 35 inches (88 centimeters) in women may be particularly indicative of greater health risk.[45] If a person is less than 5 feet tall or has a BMI of 35 or above, waist circumference standards used for the general population might not apply.

The **waist-to-hip ratio** measures regional fat distribution. A waist-to-hip ratio greater than 1 in men and 0.8 in women indicates increased health risks.[46] Waist-to-hip ratios have been used extensively in the past, and the popularity of the technique is again increasing. It's relatively inexpensive and accurate; however, it is less practical to use in clinical settings and many believe that for most people, waist circumference and BMI are sufficient.[47]

Measures of Body Fat

There are numerous ways besides BMI calculations and waist measurements to assess whether your body fat levels are too high. One low-tech way is simply to look in the mirror or consider how your clothes fit now compared with how they fit the last season you wore them. For those who wish to take a more precise measurement of their percentage of body fat, more accurate techniques are available, several of which are described and depicted in Figure 8.5 on page 251. These methods usually involve the help of a skilled professional and typically must be done in a lab or clinical setting. Before undergoing any procedure, make sure you understand the expense, potential for accuracy, risks, and training of the tester. Also, consider why you are seeking this assessment and what you plan to do with the results.

Managing Your Weight

At some point in our lives, almost all of us will decide to lose weight or modify our diet. Many will have mixed success. Failure is often related to thinking about losing weight in terms of short-term "dieting" rather than carefully analyzing individual risks for obesity and adjusting long-term eating behaviors (such as developing the habit of healthy snacking). Low-calorie diets produce only temporary losses and may actually lead to disordered binge eating or related problems.[48] Repeated bouts of restrictive dieting may be physiologically harmful; moreover, the sense of failure we experience each time we don't meet our goal can exact far-reaching psychological costs. Drugs and intensive counseling can contribute to positive weight loss, but even then, many people regain weight after treatment. Maintaining a healthful body takes constant attention and nurturing over the course of your lifetime.

Improving Your Eating Habits

Before you can change a behavior, such as unhealthy eating habits, you must first determine what causes or triggers it. Many people find it helpful to keep a chart of their eating patterns: when they feel like eating, where they are when they decide to eat, the amount of time they spend eating, other activities they engage in during the meal (watching television or reading), whether they eat alone or with others, what and how much they consume, and how they felt before they took their first bite. If you keep a detailed daily log of eating triggers for at least a week, you will discover useful clues about what in your environment or your emotional makeup causes you to want food. Typically, these dietary triggers center on patterns and problems in everyday living rather than on real hunger pangs. Many people eat compulsively when stressed; however, for other people, the same circumstances diminish their appetite, causing them to lose weight. See the Skills for Behavior Change box for tips on healthy snacking.

Once you have evaluated your behaviors and determined your triggers, you can begin to devise a plan for improved eating. If you are unsure of where to start, seek assistance from reputable sources in selecting a dietary plan that is nutritious and easy to follow, such as the MyPlate plan at www.choosemyplate.gov. Registered dietitians (RDs), some physicians (not all doctors have a strong background in nutrition), health educators, exercise physiologists with nutritional training, and other health professionals can provide reliable

Underwater (hydrostatic) weighing:
Measures the amount of water a person displaces when completely submerged. Fat tissue is less dense than muscle or bone, so body fat can be computed within a 2%–3% margin of error by comparing weight underwater and out of water.

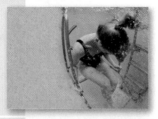

Skinfolds:
Involves "pinching" a person's fold of skin (with its underlying layer of fat) at various locations of the body. The fold is measured using a specially designed caliper. When performed by a skilled technician, it can estimate body fat with an error of 3%–4%.

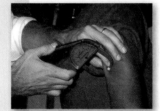

Bioelectrical impedance analysis (BIA):
Involves sending a very low level of electrical current through a person's body. As lean body mass is made up of mostly water, the rate at which the electricity is conducted gives an indication of a person's lean body mass and body fat. Under the best circumstances, BIA can estimate body fat with an error of 3%–4%.

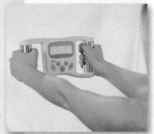

Dual-energy X-ray absorptiometry (DXA):
The technology is based on using very-low-level X ray to differentiate between bone tissue, soft (or lean) tissue, and fat (or adipose) tissue. The margin of error for predicting body fat is 2%–4%.

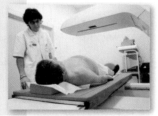

Bod Pod:
Uses air displacement to measure body composition. This machine is a large, egg-shaped chamber made from fiberglass. The person being measured sits in the machine wearing a swimsuit. The door is closed and the machine measures how much air is displaced. That value is used to calculate body fat, with a 2%–3% margin of error.

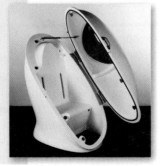

FIGURE 8.5 **Overview of Various Body Composition Assessment Methods**
Source: Adapted from J. Thompson and M. Manore, *Nutrition: An Applied Approach My Plate Edition*, 3rd edition, © 2012. Printed and electronically reproduced by permission of Pearson Education, Inc., Upper Saddle River, New Jersey.

Tips for Sensible Snacking

❭ **Keep healthy munchies around.** Buy 100 percent whole wheat breads, and if you need something to spice that up, use low-fat or soy cheese, low-fat cream cheese, peanut butter, hummus, or other high-protein healthy favorites. Some baked crackers or chips are low in fat and calories and high in fiber.

❭ **Keep "crunchies" on hand.** Apples, pears, green or red pepper sticks, popcorn, snap peas, and celery all are good choices. Wash the fruits and vegetables and cut them up to carry with you; eat them when a snack attack comes on.

❭ **Choose natural beverages.** Drink plain water, 100 percent juice in small quantities, or other low-sugar choices to satisfy your thirst. Hot tea, coffee (black), or soup broths are also good choices. Avoid juices, energy drinks, and soft drinks that have added sugars, low fiber, and no protein.

❭ **Eat nuts instead of candy.** Although relatively high in calories, nuts are also loaded with healthy fats and are healthy when consumed in moderation.

❭ **If you must have a piece of chocolate, keep it small and dark.** Dark chocolate has more antioxidants.

❭ **Avoid high-calorie energy bars.** Eat these only if you are exercising hard and don't have an opportunity to eat a regular meal. Select ones with a good mixture of fiber and protein and that are low in fat, sugar, and calories.

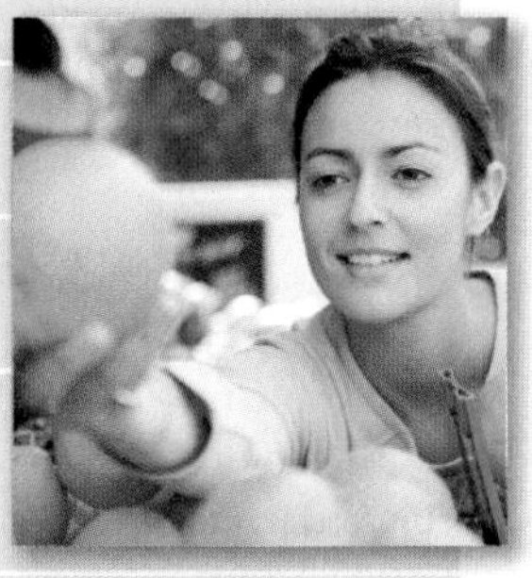

If your trigger is . . .	then try this strategy . . .
A stressful situation	Acknowledge and address feelings of anxiety or stress, and develop stress management techniques to practice daily.
Feeling angry or upset	Analyze your emotions and look for a noneating activity to deal with them, such as taking a quick walk or calling a friend.
A certain time of day	Change your eating schedule to avoid skipping or delaying meals and overeating later; make a plan of what you'll eat ahead of time to avoid impulse or emotional eating.
Pressure from friends and family	Have a response ready to help you refuse food you do not want, or look for healthy alternatives you can eat instead when in social settings.
Being in an environment where food is available	Avoid the environment that causes you to want to eat: Sit far away from the food at meetings, take a different route to class to avoid passing the vending machines, shop from a list and only when you aren't hungry, arrange nonfood outings with your friends.
Feeling bored and tired	Identify the times when you feel low energy and fill them with activities other than eating, such as exercise breaks; cultivate a new interest or hobby that keeps your mind and hands busy.
The sight and smell of food	Stop buying high-calorie foods that tempt you to snack, or store them in an inconvenient place, out of sight; avoid walking past or sitting or standing near the table of tempting treats at a meeting, party, or other gathering.
Eating mindlessly or inattentively	Turn off all distractions, including phones, computers, television, and radio, and eat more slowly, savoring your food and putting your fork down between bites so you can become aware of when your hunger is satisfied.
Spending time alone in the car	Get a book on tape to listen to, or tape your class notes and use the time for studying. Keep your mind off food. Don't bring money into the gas station where snacks are tempting.
Alcohol use	Drink plenty of water and stay hydrated. Seek out healthy snack choices. After a night out, brush your teeth immediately upon getting home and stay out of the kitchen.
Feeling deprived	Allow yourself to eat "indulgences" in moderation, so you won't crave them; focus on balancing your calorie input to calorie output.
Eating out of habit	Establish a new routine to circumvent the old, such as taking a new route to class so you don't feel compelled to stop at your favorite fast-food restaurant on the way.
Watching television	Look for something else to occupy your hands and body while your mind is engaged with the screen: Ride an exercise bike, do stretching exercises, doodle on a pad of paper, or learn to knit.

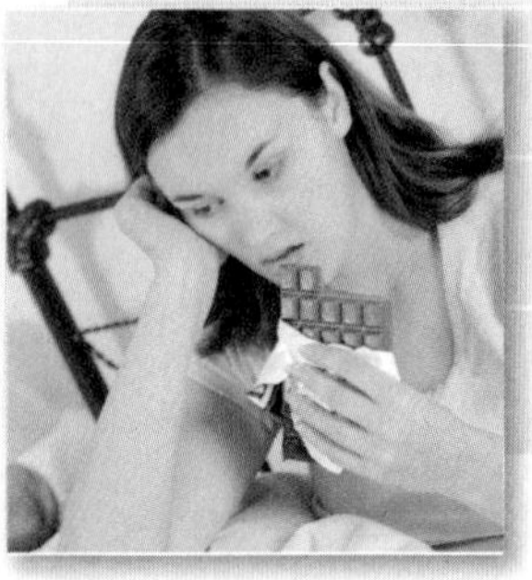

FIGURE 8.6 **Avoid Trigger-Happy Eating**
Learn what triggers your "eat" response—and what stops it—by keeping a daily log.

information. Beware of people who call themselves nutritionists or nutritional life coaches. There is no formal credential for those titles. Check the formal nutritional training of people who give advice. Avoid weight-loss programs that promise quick, "miracle" results or that are run by "trainees," often people with short courses on nutrition and exercise that are designed to sell products or services. See Figure 8.6 for ways you can adjust your eating triggers and snack more healthfully in order to manage your weight.

Assess the nutrient value of any prescribed diet; verify that dietary guidelines are consistent with reliable nutrition research; and analyze the suitability of the diet to your tastes,

budget, and lifestyle. Any diet that requires radical behavior changes or sets up artificial dietary programs through prepackaged products that don't teach you how to eat healthfully is likely to fail. Supplements and fad diets that claim fast weight loss will invariably mean fast weight regain. The most successful plans allow you to make food choices in real-world settings and do not ask you to sacrifice everything you enjoy. See Table 8.2 for an analysis of some of the popular diet books being marketed today. For information on other books, check out the regularly

See It! Videos
A new trick for weight loss? Watch **Food Diary Diet Writing** at www.pearsonhighered.com/donatelle.

Diet Book	Author Credentials	Claims	What You Eat	Science Validity	Cautions
The Best Life Diet, revised and updated	Bob Greene (Oprah Winfrey's personal fitness trainer)	• Prepares "festive foods" • Watch weight go away • Emphasis on lifestyle change	• Three phases 1. Adopt healthy habits and increase activity; regular meals; no food before bed; ditch problem foods 2. Weekly weigh-ins; get rid of emotional eating 3. Rest of life	• Sensible multi-pronged approach • Sticks to good science • No quick weight loss	• None evident
The Complete Beck Diet for Life: The Five-Stage Program for Permanent Weight Loss	Judith S. Beck, PhD	• Teaches self-motivation • Teaches how to handle hunger and cravings • Teaches how to create time for dieting	• Five-stage program • Meal plans • 1,600–2,400 daily calories • Recipes	• Sensible approach • Well-balanced meals • Flexible "bonus" calories • Behavior based	• None evident
The Flexitarian Diet: The Mostly Vegetarian Way to Lose Weight, Be Healthier, Prevent Disease, and Add Years to Your Life	Dawn Jackson Blatner, RD, LDN	• Be healthier • Prevent disease; add years to your life	• 5 × 5 Flex Plan • Vegetarian • Occasional meat, poultry, fish	• In the beginning, small amounts of meat allowed	• No direction on how to wean self off meat • No step-by-step instruction on how to include meat in a mostly vegetarian diet
You: On a Diet: The Owner's Manual for Waist Management	Michael F. Roizen, MD and Mehmet C. Oz, MD	• Shaves inches off waistline: 2 inches in 2 weeks	• 14-Day Rebooting Plan • Whole grains • Nuts • Lean meat • Fish	• Simplified science • Daily exercise • Strength training • Describes how emotions, hormones, and other variables affect eating behaviors	• 2 inches in 2 weeks are mostly water • Inch mentality not as relevant as BMI and health
The DUKAN Diet by Dr. Pierre Dukan	Jenna Bergen	• Focus on fast weight loss • Consists of phases: Attack, Cruise, Consolidation, and Permanent Stabilization. Includes exercise,	• Emphasis on lean animal protein and supplements of oat bran, also allows eggs, tofu, seitan, and nonfat dairy. • Salt reduction key.	• Not the most versatile • High protein can result in water loss • Restricted carbs • Body burns fat for fuel • Could result in ketosis, kidney damage, or gout	• Highly restricted nature of diet, • Emphasis on high protein only could be an issue in early phases. • Diabetics, those with kidney problems and others need to monitor closely.
The All-New Atkins Advantage: The 12-Week Low-Carb Program to Lose Weight, Achieve Peak Fitness and Health, and Maximize Your Willpower to Reach Life Goals	Stuart L. Trager, MD, with Colette Heimowitz, MSc	• Achieve peak fitness and health • Maximize will power	• 12-week meal plan • 20–80 grams of net carbohydrates • Multivitamin supplement recommended	• Vague approach	• Unproven claims to control cravings • Misleading regarding intake of saturated fats • Eating fewer whole grains, fruits, and vegetables reduces natural vitamins and minerals • Emphasis on carbohydrate cuts is questionable

(continued)

TABLE
8.2

Analyzing Popular Diet Books (*continued*)

The Biggest Loser: The Weight Loss Program to Transform Your Body, Health, and Life—Adapted from NBC's Hit Show!	Maggie Greenwood-Robinson, PhD, et al.	• Lower cholesterol • Strengthen body	4-3-2-1 Daily Pyramid: • 4 servings of fruits and vegetables • 3 servings of proteins • 2 servings of whole grains • 1,200 calories from "extra" category	• Sensible approach • Gaining health through diet and exercise • Explains how to choose healthy, low-fat foods	• Does not explain how to choose daily calorie intake range • Fewer than 1,200 calories puts body in semistarvation mode • Makes it difficult to obtain necessary vitamins and nutrients
The New Sonoma Diet: Trimmer Waist, More Energy in Just 10 Days	Connie Guttersen, PhD., RD.	• Simplicity, flavors of food and health lifestyle	• Divided into WAVES, avoiding refined sugars and processed foods • Focus on healthy Grains, fruits, veggies and lean proteins • Includes menus and detailed plans	• Consistent with scientific evidence, • Balanced • Includes healthy choices • Easy to use	• Book doesn't address specific goals but recommended by nutritional experts overall
The Mayo Clinic Diet: Eat Well, Enjoy Life, Lose Weight	Mayo Foundation for Medical Education and Research	• Lifestyle approach • Long-term success	• Reduce calories and fats • Increase fruits and vegetables • Lean protein	• Sound and sensible, based on ADA recommendations • Lifestyle emphasis • Creative strategies to remove barriers and ensure success	• Short on detail • Large print

Source: Adapted from the Academy of Nutrition and Dietetics Diet and Lifestyle Book Reviews, 2012, www.eatright.org/dietreviews.

updated list of the diet book reviews on the website of the Academy of Nutrition and Dietetics (formerly the American Dietetic Association) at www.eatright.org.

Understanding Calories and Energy Balance

A *calorie* is a unit of measure that indicates the amount of energy gained from food or expended through activity. Each time you consume 3,500 calories more than your body needs to maintain weight, you gain a pound of storage fat. Conversely, each time your body expends an extra 3,500 calories, you lose a pound of fat. If you consume 140 calories (the amount in one can of regular soda) more than you need every single day and make no other changes in diet or activity, you would gain 1 pound in 25 days (3,500 calories ÷ 140 calories ÷ day = 25 days). Even when you think you are watching fat intake by ordering your Starbucks vanilla latte with skim milk, you are still consuming a whopping 230 calories with every 16 ounces. Assuming you start hav-

"Why Should I Care?"

It may be easy to grab a fast-food meal, but unless you are very physically active, your body will likely store that "super-sized" meal as fat, which is anything but easy to lose. Remember—it takes only 3,500 unused calories to create a pound of body fat, so eating 500 extra calories a day—less than the average hamburger—can lead to a pound of weight gain in just a week's time.

ing the same drink every day and do nothing else differently, you'll gain 1 pound every 15 days! Conversely, if you walk for 30 minutes each day at a pace of 15 minutes per mile (172 calories burned) in addition to your regular activities, you would lose 1 pound in 20 days (3,500 calories ÷ 172 calories ÷ day = 20.3 days). This is an example of the concept of energy balance described in Figure 8.7; see page 255. Of course, these are generic formulas. If you weigh more, you will burn more calories moving your body through the same exercise routine than someone who is thinner.

Including Exercise

Increasing metabolic rate will help burn calories. Any increase in the intensity, frequency, and duration of daily exercise levels can have a significant impact on total calorie expenditure because lean (muscle) tissue is more metabolically active than fat tissue. Exact estimates vary, but experts currently feel that 2–50 more calories per day are burned per pound of muscle compared to every pound of fat tissue. Thus, the base level of calories needed to maintain a healthy weight varies greatly from person to person, depending on activity levels.

Physical activity makes a greater contribution to metabolic rate when large muscle groups are used. The energy spent on physical activity is the energy used to move the body's muscles and the extra energy used to speed up heartbeat and respiration rate. The number of calories spent depends on three factors:

1. The number and proportion of muscles used
2. The amount of weight moved
3. The length of time the activity takes

An activity involving both the arms and legs burns more calories than one involving only the legs. An activity performed by a heavy person burns more calories than the same activity performed by a lighter person. And, an activity performed for 40 minutes requires twice as much energy as the same activity performed for only 20 minutes. Thus, an obese person walking for 1 mile burns more calories than does a slim person walking the same distance. It also may take overweight people longer to walk the mile, which means that they are burning energy for a longer time and therefore expending more overall calories than the thin walkers.

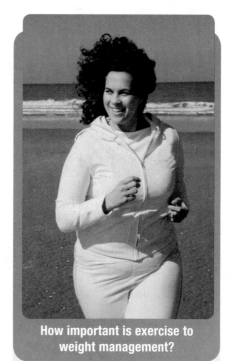

How important is exercise to weight management?

Participating in daily physical activity is key to managing your weight. Go for a jog on your own for some quiet time, or join a soccer game for social, fast-moving fun, but get out there and move!

Keeping Weight Control in Perspective

Weight loss is difficult for many people and may require supportive friends, relatives, and community resources, plus extraordinary efforts to prime the body for burning extra calories. People of the same age, sex, height, and weight can have resting metabolic rates that differ by as much as 1,000 calories a day. This may explain why one person's gluttony is another's starvation. Other factors such as depression, stress, culture, and available foods can also affect a person's ability to lose weight. In other words, being overweight does not mean people are weak willed or lazy.

To reach and maintain the weight at which you will be healthy and feel your best, you must develop a program of exercise and healthy eating behaviors that will work for you now and over the long term. Remember that you didn't gain your weight in 1 week, so you're not likely to lose it all in the week or two before spring break. It is unrealistic and potentially dangerous to punish your body by trying to lose weight in a short period of time. Instead, try to lose a healthy 1 to 2 pounds during the first week, and stay with this slow and easy regimen. Making permanent changes to your lifestyle by adding exercise and cutting back on calories to expend about 500 calories more than you consume each day will help you lose weight at a rate of 1 pound per week. You may find tracking your intake and activity easier with one of the apps described in the **Tech & Health** box on page 256.

Considering Drastic Weight-Loss Measures

When nothing seems to work, people often become frustrated and may take significant risks to lose weight. Dramatic weight loss may be recommended in cases of extreme health risk. However, even in such situations, drastic dietary, pharmacological, or surgical measures should be considered carefully and discussed with several knowledgeable health professionals.

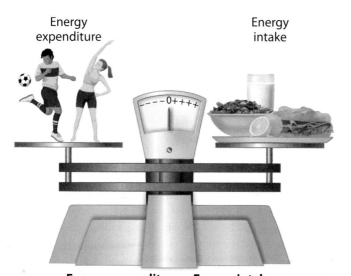

Energy expenditure

Energy intake

Energy expenditure = Energy intake

FIGURE 8.7 **The Concept of Energy Balance**
If you consume more calories than you burn, you gain weight. If you burn more than you consume, you lose weight. If both are equal, your weight will not change.

3,500

calories equal approximately 1 pound of body fat.

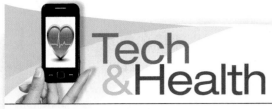

Tech & Health

TRACKING YOUR DIET OR WEIGHT LOSS? THERE'S AN APP FOR THAT

Until recently, those seeking feedback on their diet would have to keep an accurate food journal for a week or two and then consult a professional at a diet program or health-related institution. Getting personal analysis and advice could be expensive and took lots of effort. But today, anyone with a computer, tablet, or smart phone can easily keep tabs on what he or she eats and set weight loss or weight maintenance goals.

Many free and low-cost programs include large databases of foods and related nutritional information you can use to accurately log meals. Most programs also include calculators and other tools to help determine healthy weight goals and how daily activities and exercise affect how much you can eat.

The number of apps and available platforms continues to grow. Here are just a few of the options out there:

✳ **Lose It!** (Free: Android, iPhone, Nook tablet, PCs), www.loseit.com
Simple to use, comprehensive database of foods and activities designed to help you log meals and track exercise.

✳ **Restaurant Weight Watcher.** (Modest cost; Android only), https://play.google.com/store/apps/details?id=com.ellisapps.wwrestaurant&hl=en
Lists nutrition information for the menus of over 200 restaurants and continues to add new ones.

✳ **Weight Watchers Mobile.** (Free trial, but full version only available to Weight Watchers members: Android, iPhone, iPod), www.weightwatchers.com/help/index.aspx?pageid=1107041
Notable for its ability to scan food purchases with its barcode app.

✳ **Calorie Counter & Diet Tracker by MyFitnessPal.** (Free: iPhone, Android, Blackberry, PCs) www.myfitnesspal.com
A combination of diet and fitness goals as well as a nutritional analysis of what you are eating

✳ **MyPlate Calorie Tracker by LIVESTRONG.** (Modest cost: Android, iPhone, Blackberry) www.livestrong.com/thedailyplate
Comprehensive information for tracking diet and exercise, analyzing nutrients, setting goals and finding resources.

Very-Low-Calorie Diets

In severe cases of obesity that are not responsive to traditional dietary strategies, medically supervised, powdered formulas with daily values of 400 to 700 calories plus vitamin and mineral supplements may be given to patients. Such **very-low-calorie diets (VLCDs)** should never be undertaken without strict medical supervision. These severe diets do not teach healthy eating, and persons who manage to lose weight on them may experience significant weight regain. More important, fasting, starvation diets, and other forms of VLCDs have been shown to cause significant health risks and can, in fact, be deadly. Problems associated with any form of severe caloric restriction include blood sugar imbalance, cold intolerance, constipation, decreased BMR, dehydration, diarrhea, emotional problems, fatigue, headaches, heart irregularities, kidney infections and failure, loss of lean body tissue, weakness, and the potential for coma and death.

very-low-calorie diets (VLCDs) Diets with a daily caloric value of 400 to 700 calories.

One particularly dangerous potential complication of VLCDs or starvation diets is *ketoacidosis.* After a prolonged period of inadequate carbohydrate or food intake, the body will have depleted its immediate energy stores and will begin metabolizing fat stores through *ketogenesis* in order to supply the brain and nervous system with an alternative fuel known as *ketones.* Ketogenesis is one of the body's normal processes for metabolizing fat and may help provide energy to the brain during times of fasting, low carbohydrate intake, or vigorous exercise. However, ketones may also suppress appetite and cause dehydration at a time when a person should feel hungry and seek out food. The condition of having increased levels of ketones in the body is *ketosis*; if enough ketones accumulate in the blood, it may lead to *ketoacdiosis,* in which the blood becomes more acidic.[49] People with untreated type 1 diabetes and individuals with anorexia nervosa or bulimia nervosa are at risk of developing ketoacidotic symptoms as damage to body tissues begins.

If fasting continues, the body will turn to its last resort—protein—for energy, breaking down muscle and organ tissue to stay alive. As this occurs, the body loses weight rapidly. At the same time, it also loses significant water stores. Eventually, the body begins to run out of liver tissue, heart muscle, and so on. Within about 10 days after the typical adult begins a complete fast, the body will have depleted its energy stores, and death may occur.

Drug Treatment Individuals looking for help in losing weight often turn to thousands of commercially marketed weight-loss supplements, which are available on the Internet and at drug and health-food stores. U.S. Food and Drug Administration (FDA) approval is not required for over-the-counter "diet aids" or supplements, and many manufacturers simply feed off people's desperation. Most of these supplements contain stimulants, such as caffeine, or diuretics, and their effectiveness in promoting weight loss has been largely untested and unproved by any scientific studies. In many cases, the only thing that users lose is money they might have put to better use.

Virtually all persons who used diet pills in review studies regained their weight once they stopped taking them.[50]

In contrast, FDA-approved diet pills have historically been available only by prescription. These lines were blurred in 2007 when the FDA approved the first over-the-counter weight loss pill—a half-strength version of the prescription drug orlistat (brand name Xenical), marketed as Alli. This drug inhibits the action of lipase, an enzyme that helps the body to digest fats, causing about 30 percent of fats consumed to pass through the digestive system undigested, leading to reduced overall caloric intake. Known side effects of orlistat include gas with watery fecal discharge; oily stools and spotting; frequent, often unexpected, bowel movements; and possible deficiencies of fat-soluble vitamins. There have also been several FDA warnings issued about fake Alli products being sold at reduced prices online. In 2012 the FDA approved the weight loss drugs Belviq and Qsymia. You should discuss risks, benefits, and options with your doctor.

In general, diet pills have been shown to be most effective when used as part of comprehensive lifestyle change, including diet and exercise The challenge is to develop an effective drug that can be used over time without adverse effects or abuse, and no such drug currently exists. A classic example of supposedly safe drugs that were later found to have dangerous side effects is *fen phen* (a combined drug made up of fenfluramine and phentermine, two drugs that had individual FDA approval, but were not approved in combination). Despite being widely prescribed, the drugs were recalled when they were found to cause severe pulmonary hypertension and lasting heart valve damage.[51] Metabolife, a drug that increased metabolism and energy using the herbal supplement *Ephedra*, had warnings issued against it when it was suspected of causing over 100 deaths and 800 heart attacks. A similar over-the-counter natural product, *Hydroxycut,* was pulled in 2009 when there were over 23 reported cases of serious liver damage and one reported death.

See the **Skills for Behavior Change** box for strategies to make your weight management program succeed.

Another diet drug that has recently gained a great deal of attention is hCG (see the **Health Headlines** box on page 258). Other currently available diet drugs and supplements that you should view with caution include:

Sibutramine (Meridia). This prescription-only medication suppresses appetite by inhibiting the uptake of serotonin in the brain. It works best with a reduced-calorie diet and exercise, but side effects include dry mouth, headache, constipation, insomnia, and high blood pressure. Although research has shown positive effects on blood glucose control, the FDA has issued warnings about use of Meridia for people who have hypertension or heart disease.[52]

Hoodia gordonii. This African cactus-like plant is a purported appetite suppressant. No convincing evidence has been shown for or against it; to date, it is not FDA approved and has not been tested in clinical trials.[53] Supplements containing *Hoodia gordonii* have become popular in recent years, and there are many off-market brands produced,

Keys to Successful Weight Management

The key to successful weight management is finding a sustainable way to control what you eat and to make exercise a priority. First:

❱ Write down the positive things about your diet and exercise behaviors. Then write down the things that need changing. For each big change you need to make, list three or four small things you could change right now.
❱ Ask yourself why you want to make this change right now. What are your ultimate goals? Plan non-food rewards for meeting your goals each week.
❱ What campus or community resources are available where you could go for help? Could any friends or family members help you?
❱ Keep a food and exercise log for 2 or 3 days. Note the good things you are doing, the things that need improvement, and the triggers you need to address.
❱ Talk.

MAKE A PLAN

❱ Set realistic short- and long-term goals.
❱ Establish a plan. What are the diet and exercise changes you can make this week? Once you do 1 week, plot a course for 2 weeks, and so on.
❱ Look for balance. Remember it's calories taken in and burned over time that make the difference.

CHANGE YOUR HABITS

❱ Be adventurous. Expand your usual meals and snacks to enjoy a wider variety of options.
❱ Do not constantly deprive yourself or set unrealistic guidelines. If you blow it and overconsume, get right back on track. Cut yourself some slack and remember that you are in this for the long run.
❱ Notice whether you are hungry before starting a meal. Eat slowly, noting when you start to feel full, and STOP before you are full.
❱ Eat breakfast, especially low-fat foods with whole grains and protein. This will prevent you from being too hungry and overeating at lunch.
❱ Keep healthful snacks on hand for when you get hungry.

INCORPORATE EXERCISE

❱ Be active and slowly increase your time, speed, distance, or resistance levels.
❱ Vary your physical activity. Find activities that you really love and try things you haven't tried before.
❱ Find an exercise partner to help you stay motivated.
❱ Make it a fun break. Go for a walk in a place that interests you. Tune in to your surroundings to take your mind off of your sweating and heavy breathing!

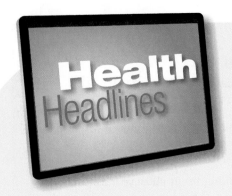
HCG-BASED DIETS: BUYER BEWARE

Human chorionic gonadotropin (hCG) is a hormone produced by the placenta during pregnancy that, in prescription form, is also a federally approved treatment for some female fertility problems. Recently, hCG has become known as a crash-diet miracle drug. Some individuals, notably a few celebrities, tout using it while undertaking extremely low-calorie diets. They claim to benefit from fat-burning and hunger-suppressant qualities. Is there any merit to the hype?

Human chorionic gonadotropin has not been approved by the Federal Drug Administration (FDA) for weight loss. In fact, after more than 50 years of extensive, double-blind research, results consistently show that hCG is no more effective for weight loss than cutting calories. Today, all hCG prescription labels and advertising must clearly state it does not reset metabolism, decrease hunger, or reduce the discomfort associated with a low-calorie diet. According to experts such Elizabeth Miller, acting director of FDA's Division of Non-Prescription Drugs and Health Fraud, "the data do not support that it is hCG causing the weight loss; any weight loss is due to the extremely low-calorie, potentially dangerous diet that goes along with the typical hCG regimen." Severe caloric restrictions in any starvation diet such as this one can cause electrolyte imbalances, muscle wasting, digestive irregularities, gallstone formation, cardiac irregularities, liver and kidney failure, skin problems, lowered immunity, and a host of other problems. Each of these risks could lead to serious problems for the user. Long-term risks are not known, and death is a possibility.

As of December 2011, hCG products have been the focus of increased FDA and Federal Trade Commission warnings for some companies and outright hCG homeopathic product bans for others. These actions are the first steps in warning companies that they are violating federal law by selling drugs that have not been approved by the FDA and making unsupported claims for the substances in the media. Don't fall for fraudulent claims. So far there is no miracle pill to replace good diet and lots of exercise when it comes to losing weight.

Sources: Federal Drug Administration, " Consumer Updates: Beware of Fraudulent Weight-Loss Dietary Supplements," Accessed February 10, 2012, from www.fda.gov/ForConsumerUpdates/ucm246742.htm; Federal Drug Administration, "FDA Consumer Updates: HCG Diet Products are Illegal," Accessed February 10, 2012 from www.fda.gov/ForCOnsumers/ConsumerUpdates/ucm281333.htm.

---

including some that contain more unproven ingredients such as bitter orange and other stimulants.

- **Herbal weight-loss aids.** Products containing *Ephedra* can cause rapid heart rate, tremors, seizures, insomnia, headaches, and raised blood pressure, all without significant effects on long-term weight control. *St. John's wort* and other alternative medicines reported to enhance serotonin, suppress appetite, and reduce the side effects of depression have not been shown to be effective in weight loss, either.

Surgery When all else fails, particularly for people who are severely overweight and have weight-related diseases such as diabetes or hypertension, a person may be a candidate for weight-loss surgery. Generally, these surgeries fall into one of two major categories: *restrictive surgeries,* such as gastric banding or lap banding, that limit food intake, and *malabsorption surgeries,* such as gastric bypass, which decrease the absorption of food into the body (**Figure 8.8**, on page 259).

To select the best option, a physician will consider that operation's benefits and risks, the patient's BMI, eating behaviors, obesity-related health conditions, and previous operations. Some health advocates have proposed that obesity be classified as a disability (see the **Points of View** box on page 260), which could potentially affect a physician's decision on recommending surgery.

In gastric banding and other restrictive surgeries, the surgeon uses an inflatable band to partition off part of the stomach. The band is wrapped around that part of the stomach and is pulled tight, like a belt, leaving only a small opening between the two parts of the stomach. The upper part of the stomach is smaller, so the person feels full more quickly, and food digestion slows so that the person also feels full longer. Although the bands are designed to stay in place, they can be removed surgically. They can also be inflated to different levels to adjust the amount of restriction.

In contrast to the restrictive surgeries, gastric bypass is designed to drastically decrease the amount of food a person can eat and absorb. Results are fast and dramatic, but there are many risks, including blood clots in the legs, a leak in a staple line in the stomach, pneumonia, infection, and death. According to the Agency for Healthcare Research and Quality, 19 percent of patients experience dumping syndrome, which is involuntary vomiting or defecation.[54] Because the stomach pouch that remains after surgery is only the size of a lime, the person can drink only a few tablespoons of liquid and consume only a very small amount of food at a time. For this reason, other possible side effects include nausea, vitamin and mineral deficiencies, and dehydration. Additional risks include

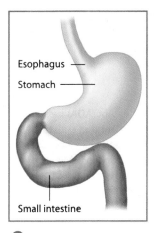

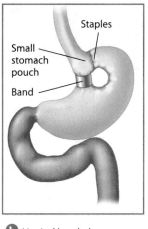

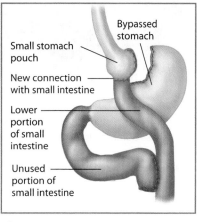

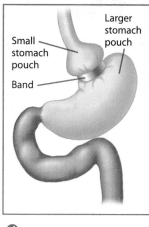

ⓐ Normal anatomy

ⓑ Vertical banded gastroplasty

ⓒ Gastric bypass

ⓓ Gastric banding

FIGURE 8.8 **Weight-Loss Surgery Alters the Normal Anatomy of the Stomach**

Source: Adapted from J. Thompson and M. Manore, *Nutrition: An Applied Approach My Plate Edition*, 3rd edition, © 2012. Printed and electronically reproduced by permission of Pearson Education, Inc., Upper Saddle River, New Jersey.

the potential for excess bleeding, ulcers, hernia, and the typical risks from anesthesia. These risks must be considered against the risks of obesity. Because the surgery and follow-up is very expensive and insurance may or may not cover it, many people do not have the resources to have this procedure.

A technique gaining in popularity is the *duodenal switch procedure,* which combines elements of restrictive and malabsorption surgeries. The patient receives a partial gastrectomy to reduce the size of the stomach while maintaining normal stomach function. The pyloric valve remains intact, which helps prevent dumping syndrome, ulcers, blockages, and other problems that can occur with other techniques.

Aftercare for gastric surgery patients often includes counseling to help them cope with the urge to eat after the ability to eat normal portions has been removed, as well as other adjustment problems. Keep in mind that it is always best to lose weight by eating a healthy diet and getting regular physical activity. Ironically, even after undergoing surgery, people must learn to eat healthy foods and exercise. Otherwise, they can continue to gain weight, even returning to their original weight.

Recent research has demonstrated exciting, unexpected results from gastric surgeries: Even prior to weight loss, patients have shown complete remission of type 2 diabetes in the majority of cases, with drastic reductions in blood glucose levels in others.[55] In one study, nearly 99 percent of the morbidly obese who had gastric bypass and had a previous history of type 2 diabetes were free of the disease after surgery, even before they began to lose weight. This finding has caused much excitement in the scientific community as researchers explore surgical options for prevention of diabetes in other populations.[56] For those at high risk from these diseases, the choice of undergoing a high-risk surgery may ultimately be similar to the risk of maintaining their current weight.

Unlike restrictive and malabsorption surgeries, which facilitate overall weight loss, *liposuction* is a surgical procedure in which fat cells are removed from specific areas of the body. Generally, liposuction is considered cosmetic surgery rather than weight-loss surgery and is used for spot reducing and body contouring. Although this technique has garnered much attention, it too is not without risk: Infections, severe scarring, and even death have resulted. In many cases, people who have liposuction regain fat in those areas or require multiple surgeries to repair lumpy, irregular surfaces from which the fat was removed.

Trying to Gain Weight

For some people, trying to gain weight is a challenge for a variety of metabolic, hereditary, psychological, and other reasons. If you are one of these individuals, the first priority is to determine why you cannot gain weight. Perhaps you're an athlete and you burn more calories than you manage to eat. Perhaps you're stressed out and skip meals to increase study time. Among older adults, the senses of taste and smell may decline, which makes food taste different and therefore less pleasurable to eat. Visual problems and other disabilities may make meals more difficult to prepare, and dental problems may make eating more difficult. People who engage in extreme energy-burning sports and exercise routines may be at risk for caloric and nutritional deficiencies, which can lead not only to weight loss, but also to immune system problems and organ dysfunction; weakness, which leads to falls and fractures; slower recovery from diseases; and a host of other problems as well. People who are too thin need to take the same steps as those who are overweight or obese to find out what their healthy weight is and attain that weight.

Obesity:
IS IT A DISABILITY?

A person who is 150 to 200 pounds overweight can have difficulty walking, running, standing, and doing other simple daily tasks. Some people believe obesity should be considered a disability that legally entitles individuals to certain health benefits and other accommodations. Other people believe that labeling obesity as a disability would add to its stigma and create more problems than it would solve.

The federal Americans with Disabilities Act (ADA) defines *disability* as "a physical or mental impairment that substantially limits one or more of the major life activities of [an] individual." Currently, people must have body mass indexes (BMIs) over 40 or be at least 100 pounds overweight, and also have an underlying disorder that caused the obesity, before the ADA classifies them as disabled. These strict criteria means that the ADA currently receives few valid complaints relating to obesity.

Arguments Favoring Disability Status for Obese People

◯ Labeling obesity as a disability would provide obese individuals with better insurance coverage.

◯ A disability label would protect individuals against discrimination based on their weight.

◯ An obese person can have many related medical conditions including arthritis, high blood pressure, diabetes, diabetic-related vascular diseases, and a weakened cardiovascular system. All of these conditions can lead to the need for walkers, wheelchairs, and other mobility devices, as well as special health accommodations at home or in the workplace.

Arguments Opposing Disability Status for Obese People

◯ Some doctors worry that defining obesity as a disability would make them vulnerable to lawsuits from obese patients who don't want doctors to discuss their weight. The threat of such lawsuits would prevent doctors from discussing obesity with their overweight patients and recommending specific actions.

◯ Issues of unfair insurance or job practices could be handled with antidiscrimination laws, not disability status.

◯ Not all obese people are disabled by their weight, so labeling them all as such would be discriminatory.

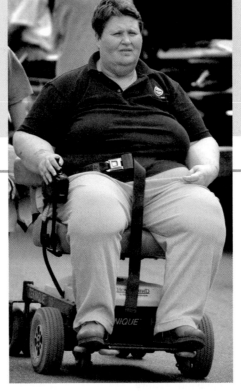

Where Do You Stand?

◯ In your opinion, what positive results could come from classifying overweight or obese individuals as disabled?

◯ What negative consequences do you foresee from classifying overweight or obese people as disabled?

◯ How would you determine whether an individual is disabled because of his or her weight?

◯ Are there legitimate situations where a person who is overweight or obese should be labeled as disabled?

◯ Do you think labeling obesity as a disability would alter the way our society perceives and behaves toward overweight and obese individuals? If so, in what way?

Assess Yourself

Are You Ready to Start a Weight-Loss Program?

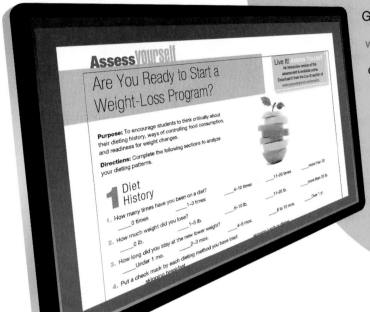

Go online to the **Live It!**
www.peasonhighered.com/donatelle to fill out the "Are You Ready to Start a Weight-Loss Program?" assessment.* Use the steps outlined in the **YOUR PLAN FOR CHANGE** box to help you take action.

*If your instructor so chooses, Assess Yourself Activities are available as a printed supplement or as assignable homework online at www.pearsonhighered.com/myhealthlab.

MyHealthLab®

YOUR PLAN FOR CHANGE

The **Assess Yourself** activity found at www.pearsonhighered.com/donatelle allows you to gauge if you are prepared to lose weight. The worksheet identifies six areas of importance in determining your readiness for weight loss. If you wish to lose weight to improve your health, understanding your attitudes about food and exercise will help you succeed in your plan.

Today, you can:

○ Set "SMART" goals for weight loss and give them a reality check: Are they **s**pecific, **m**easurable, **a**chievable, **r**elevant, and **t**ime oriented? For example, rather than aiming to lose 15 pounds this month (which probably wouldn't be healthy or achievable), set a comfortable goal to lose 5 pounds. Realistic goals will encourage weight-loss success by boosting your confidence in your ability to make lifelong healthy changes.

○ Begin keeping a food log and identifying the triggers that influence your eating habits. Think about what you can do to eliminate or reduce the influence of your two most common food triggers.

Within the next 2 weeks, you can:

○ Get in the habit of incorporating more fruits, vegetables, and whole grains in your diet and eating less fat. The next time you make dinner, look at the proportions on your plate. If vegetables and whole grains do not take up most of the space, substitute 1 cup of the meat, pasta, or cheese in your meal with 1 cup of legumes, salad greens, or a favorite vegetable. You'll reduce the number of calories while eating the same amount of food!

○ Aim to incorporate more exercise into your daily routine. Visit your campus rec center or a local gym, and familiarize yourself with the equipment and facilities that are available. Try a new machine or

sports activity, and experiment until you find a form of exercise you really enjoy.

By the end of the semester, you can:

○ Get in the habit of grocery shopping every week and buying healthy, nutritious foods while avoiding high-fat, high-sugar, or overly processed foods. As you make healthy foods more available and unhealthy foods less available, you'll find it easier to eat better.

○ Chart your progress and reward yourself as you meet your goals. If your goal is to lose weight and you successfully take off 10 pounds, reward yourself with a new pair of jeans or other article of clothing (which will likely fit better than before!).

Summary

* Overweight, obesity, and weight-related health problems have reached epidemic levels in the United States. *Globesity,* or global rates of obesity, is also on an epidemic rise, particularly among the developing regions of the world. Obesogenic behaviors in an obesogenic environment are key reasons for our weight-related problems.

* Societal costs from obesity include increased health care costs, lowered worker productivity, low self-esteem, increased depression, discrimination, and stigma. Individual health risks from overweight and obesity include increased chance of developing diabetes and other chronic or infectious diseases. Overweight individuals are also at risk of struggling with depression, low self-esteem, and high levels of stress.

* Factors contributing to one's risk for obesity include the physical and social environment, poverty, education level, genetics, developmental factors, endocrine influences, psychosocial factors, eating cues, metabolic changes, and lifestyle.

* Percentage of body fat is a fairly reliable indicator for levels of overweight and obesity. There are many different methods of assessing body fat. Body mass index (BMI) is one of the most commonly accepted measures of weight based on height. *Overweight* is most commonly defined as a BMI of 25 to 29 and *obesity* as a BMI of 30 or greater. Waist circumference, or the amount of fat in the belly region, is believed to be related to the risk for several chronic diseases, particularly type 2 diabetes.

* Exercise, dieting, diet pills, surgery, and other strategies are used to maintain or lose weight. However, sensible eating behavior and aerobic exercise and exercise that builds muscle mass offer the best options for weight loss and maintenance.

Pop Quiz

1. The proportion of your total weight that is made up of fat is called
   a. body composition.
   b. lean mass.
   c. percentage of body fat.
   d. BMI.

2. All of the following statements are true *except* which?
   a. A slowing basal metabolic rate may contribute to weight gain after age 30.
   b. Hormones are increasingly implicated in hunger impulses and eating behavior.
   c. The more muscles you have, the fewer calories you will burn.
   d. Overweight and obesity among young adults can have serious health consequences even before they reach middle age.

3. All of the following statements about BMI are true *except* which?
   a. BMI is based on height and weight measurements.
   b. BMI is accurate for everyone, including athletes with high amounts of muscle mass.
   c. Very low and very high BMI scores are associated with greater risk of mortality.
   d. BMI stands for "body mass index."

4. Which of the following BMI ratings is considered overweight?
   a. 20
   b. 25
   c. 30
   d. 35

5. Which of the following body circumferences is most strongly associated with risk of heart disease and diabetes?
   a. Hip circumference
   b. Chest circumference
   c. Waist circumference
   d. Thigh circumference

6. One pound of additional body fat is created through consuming how many extra calories?
   a. 1,500 calories
   b. 3,500 calories
   c. 5,000 calories
   d. 7,000 calories

7. To lose weight, you must establish a(n)
   a. negative caloric balance.
   b. isocaloric balance.
   c. positive caloric balance.
   d. set point.

8. The rate at which your body consumes food energy to sustain basic functions is your
   a. basal metabolic rate.
   b. resting metabolic rate.
   c. body mass index.
   d. set point.

9. Successful weight maintainers are most likely to do which of the following?
   a. Eat two large meals a day before 1 P.M.
   b. Skip meals
   c. Drink diet sodas
   d. Eat high-volume but low-calorie density foods

10. Successful, healthy weight loss is characterized by
    a. a lifelong pattern of healthful eating and exercise.
    b. cutting out all fats and carbohydrates and eating a lean, mean, high-protein diet.
    c. never eating foods that are considered bad for you and rigidly adhering to a plan.
    d. a pattern of repeatedly losing and regaining weight.

Answers to these questions can be found on page A-1.

Think about It!

1. Discuss the pressures, if any, you feel to change your body's shape.

Do these pressures come from media, family, friends, and other external sources, or from concern for your personal health?

2. Are you satisfied with your body weight right now? Why or why not? Are other members of your family suffering from weight-related health problems? How much do you worry that you will have a similar problem in the next 10 years? 20 years?

3. Which measurement would you choose to assess your fat levels? Why?

4. List the risk factors for your being overweight or obese right now. Which seem most likely to determine whether you will be obese in middle age?

5. Why do you think that obesity rates are rising in both developed and less-developed regions of the world? What strategies can we take collectively and individually to reduce risks of obesity?

Accessing Your Health on the Internet

The following websites explore further topics and issues related to personal health. For links to these websites, visit the Companion Website for *Access to Health*, 13th Edition, at www.pearsonhighered.com /donatelle.

1. *Academy of Nutrition and Dietetics.* This site includes recommended dietary guidelines and other current information about weight control. www.eatright.org

2. *Duke University Diet and Fitness Center.* This site includes information about one of the best programs in the country focused on helping people live healthier, fuller lives through weight control and lifestyle change. www.dukedietcenter.org

3. *F as in Fat: How Obesity Policies Are Failing in America.* This report provides an excellent summary of the current status of obesity, obesity policies, and programs in the United States, as well as suggestions for new strategies and policies to reduce risks. http://healthyamericans.org/ reports/obesity2009

4. *Weight Control Information Network.* This is an excellent resource for diet and weight-control information. http://win.niddk.nih.gov/index.htm

5. *The Rudd Center for Foods Policy and Obesity.* This website provides excellent information on the latest in obesity research, public policy, and ways we can stop the obesity epidemic at the community level. www.yaleruddcenter.org

References

1. C. L. Ogden, M. M. Lamb, M. D. Carroll, and K. M. Flegal, "Obesity and Socioeconomic Status in Adults: United States, 2005–2008," *NCHS Data Brief*, 50 (2010): 1–8; C.L. Ogden, M.M. Lamb, M. D. Carroll, and K. M. Flegal, "Obesity and Socioeconomic Status in Children and Adolescents: United States, 2005–2008," *NCHS Data Brief*, 51 (2010): 1–8.

2. U.S. Department of Health and Human Services, *The Surgeon General's Vision for a Healthy and Fit Nation* (Rockville, MD: U.S. Department of Health and Human Services, Office of the Surgeon General, 2010), Available at www.surgeongeneral .gov/library/obesityvision.

3. C. Ogden, M. Carrol, B. Kit and K. Flegal. "Prevalence of Obesity in the United States, 2009–2010," *NCHS Data Brief*, 82 (2012).

4. NIDDK, Weight Loss Information Network. Overweight and Obesity Statistics, 2011, www.win.niddk.nih.gov/statistics/ index.

5. S. Steward et al., "Forecasting the Effects of Obesity and Smoking on U.S. Life Expectancy," *New England Journal of Medicine* 361, no. 23 (2009): 2252–60; NIDDK, Weight Loss Information Network. Overweight and Obesity Statistics, 2011, www .win.niddk.nih.gov/statistics/index.

6. C. Ogden, "Disparities in Obesity Prevalence in the United States: Black Women at Risk," *American Journal of Clinical Nutrition* 89, no. 4 (2009): 10001–02.

7. C. Ogden et al., "Prevalence of High Body Mass Index in U.S. Children and Adolescents, 2007–2008," *JAMA: The Journal of the American Medical Association* 303, no. 3 (2010):242–49.

8. Ibid.

9. Centers for Disease Control and Prevention, "National Diabetes Fact Sheet: National Estimates and General Information on Diabetes and Prediabetes in the United States, 2011," (Atlanta, GA: U.S. Department of Health and Human Services, Centers for Disease Control and Prevention, 2011).

10. NIDDK, Weight Loss Information Network. Overweight and Obesity Statistics, 2011, www.win.niddk.nih.gov/statistics/ index.

11. K. Froehlich-Grobe and D. Lollar, "Obesity and Disability: Time to Act," *American Journal of Preventive Medicine* 41, no. 5 (2011): 541–45; C. Murtaugh, B. Spillman, and X. Wang, "Lifetime Risk and Duration of Chronic Disease and Disability," *Journal of Aging and Health* 23, no. 3 (2011): 554–77; E. Stallard, "The Impact of Obesity and Diabetes on LTC Disability and Mortality: Population Estimates from the National Long Term Care Survey," 2011, Paper presented at the Living to 110 Symposium, Society of Actuaries (Orlando, Florida).

12. World Health Organization, "Obesity and Overweight Fact Sheet," 2011, www.who .int/mediacentre/factsheets/fs311/en/ index.html

13. Ibid.

14. World Health Organization, "Global Strategy on Diet, Physical Activity, and Health: Obesity and Overweight," 2009, www.who.int/dietphysicalactivity/ publications/facts/obesity/en.

15. J. Spence et al., "Relation between Local Food Environments and Obesity among Adults," *BMC Public Health* 9, no. 1 (2009): 192; D. Spruijt-Metz, "Etiology, Treatment, and Prevention of Obesity in Childhood and Adolescence: A Decade in Review," *Journal of Research on Adolescence* 21 (2011): 129–52, DOI: 10.1111/j.1532-7795.2010.00719.x.

16. D. Cummings and M. Schwartz, "Genetics and Pathophysiology of Human Obesity," *Annual Review of Medicine* 54 (2003): 453–71.

17. K. Silventoinen et al., "The Genetic and Environmental Influences on Childhood Obesity: A Systematic Review of Twin and Adoption Studies," *International Journal of Obesity* 34, no. 1 (2010): 29–40.

18. S. Li et al., "Cumulative and Predictive Value of Common Obesity—Susceptibility Variants Identified by Genome-wide Association Studies," *American Journal of Clinical Nutrition* 91, no. 1 (2010): 184–90.

19. C. Bouchard, "Defining the Genetic Architecture of the Predisposition to Obesity: A Challenging but Not Insurmountable Task," *American Journal of Clinical Nutrition* 91, no. 1 (2010): 5–6; T. O. Kilpelainen et al., "Physical Activity Attenuates the Influence of *FTO* Variants on Obesity Risk: A

Meta-Analysis of 218,166 Adults and 19,268 Children," 2012, *PLoS Medicine* 8, no.11 (2012), e1001116. doi:10.1371/journal. pmed.1001116; S. Li et al. "Cumulative Effects and Predictive Value of Common Obesity-Susceptibility Variants Identified by Genome-wide Association Studies," *American Journal of Clinical Nutrition* 91 (2010): 184–190; B. Herera and C. Lindgren, "The Genetics of Obesity," *Current Diabetes Report* 10, no. 6 (2010): 498–505; S. Li. et al., "Genetic Predisposition to Obesity Leads to Increased Risk of Type 2 Diabetes," *Diabetologia* 54, no. 4 (2011): 776–82.

20. C. Bouchard, "Thrifty Gene Hypothesis: Maybe Everyone Is Right?" *International Journal of Obesity* 32, no. 4 (2008): 25–27; R. Stoger, "The Thrifty Epigenotype: An Acquired and Heritable Predisposition for Obesity and Diabetes?" *Bioessays* 30, no. 2 (2008): 156–66.

21. U. Baig, P. Belsare, M. Watve, and M. Jog, "Can Thrifty Gene(s) or Predictive Fetal Programming for Thrtifiness Lead to Obesity?" *Journal of Obesity* (2011), DOI: 10.1155/2011/861049; S. Li. et al., "Physical Activity Attenuates the Genetic Predisposition to Obesity in 20,000 Men and Women from the EPIC-Norfolk Prospective Population Study," *PLoS Medicine* 7, no. 8 (2010): e1000322, DOI:10.1371/journal.pmed.1000332; J. Wells, "The Thrifty Phenotype: An Adaptation in Growth or Metabolism?" *American Journal of Human Biology* 23, no. 1 (2011): 65–75; C. Bouchard, "Defining the Genetic Architecture of the Predisposition to Obesity," 2010; S. Li et al., "Cumulative and Predictive Value of Common Obesity," 2010.

22. B. Biondi, "Thyroid and Obesity: An Intriguing Relationship," *Journal of Clinical Endocrinology and Metabolism* 95, no. 8 (2010): 3614–17; T. Reinehr, "Obesity and Thyroid Function," *Molecular and Cellular Endocrinology* 316, no. 2 (2010): 165–71; E. Kaptein, E. Beale, and L. Chan, "Thyroid Hormone Therapy for Obesity and Nonthyroidal Illnesses: A Systematic Review," *The Journal of Clinical Endocrinology and Metabolism* 94, no. 10 (2009): 3663–75; E. Schuer et al., "Activation in Brain Energy Regulation and Reward Centers by Food Cues Varies with Choice of Visual Stimulation," *International Journal of Obesity* 33, no. 6 (2009): 653–61.

23. M. Rotondi, F. Magri, and L. Chiovato, "Thyroid and Obesity: Not a One Way Interaction," *The Journal of Clinical Endocrinology and Metabolism* 96, no. 2 (2011): 344–56.

24. Ibid.

25. D. E. Cummings et al., "Plasma Ghrelin Levels after Diet-Induced Weight Loss or Gastric Bypass Surgery," *New England Journal of Medicine* 346, no. 21 (2002): 1623–30.

26. C. DeVriese et al., "Focus on the Short- and Long-Term Effects of Ghrelin on Energy Homeostasis," *Nutrition* 26, no. 6 (2010): 579–84; T. Castaneda et al., "Ghrelin in the Regulation of Body Weight and Metabolism," *Frontiers in Neuroendocrinology* 31, no. 1 (2010): 44–60.

27. P. Marzullo et al. "Investigations of Thyroid Hormones and Antibodies in Obesity: Leptin Levels are Associated with Thyroid Autoimmunity Independent of Bioanthropometric, Hormonal and Weight-related Determinants," *The Journal of Clinical Endocrinology and Metabolism* 95, no. 8 (2010): 3965–72; Y. Friedlander et al., "Leptin, Insulin, and Obesity-Related Phenotypes: Genetic Influences on Levels and Longitudinal Changes," *Obesity* 17, no. 7 (2009): 1458–60.

28. L. K. Mahan and S. Escott-Stump, *Krause's Food, Nutrition, and Diet Therapy*, 13th ed. (New York: W. B. Saunders, 2012).

29. M. Treuth et al., "A Longitudinal Study of Sedentary Behavior and Overweight in Adolescent Girls," *Obesity* 17, no. 5 (2009): 1003–08.

30. B. Levin, "Synergy of Nurture and Nature in the Development of Childhood Obesity," *International Journal of Obesity* 33, Supplement 1 (2009): S53–S56.

31. S. Anderson and R. Whitaker, "Prevalence of Obesity among U.S. Preschool Children in Different Racial and Ethnic Groups," *Archives of Pediatrics and Adolescent Medicine* 163, no. 4 (2009): 344–48.

32. M. H. Schafer and K.F. Ferraro, "The Stigma of Obesity: Does Perceived Weight Discrimination Affect Identity and Physical Health?" *Social Psychology Quarterly* 74, no. 1 (2011): 76–97.

33. T. Lehey, J. LaRose, J. Fave, and R. Wing. "Social Influences are Associated with BMI and Weight Loss Intentions in Young Adults," *Obesity* 19, no. 6 (2011): 1157–62.

34. M. Beydoun et al., "The Association of Fast Food, Fruit, and Vegetable Prices with Dietary Intakes among U.S. Adults: Is There Modification by Family Income?" *Social Science and Medicine* 66, no. 11 (2008): 2218–29; J. Tillotson, "Americans' Food Shopping in Today's Lousy Economy," *Nutrition Today* 44, no. 5 (2009): 218–21.

35. F. Li et al., "Built Environment, Adiposity, and Physical Activity in Adults Aged 50–75," *American Journal of Preventive Medicine* 35, no. 1 (2008): 38–46.

36. R. P. Troiano et al., "Physical Activity in the United States Measured by Acceler-ometer," *Medicine and Science in Sports and Exercise* 40, no. 1 (2008): 181–88.

37. V. Roger et al., on behalf of the American Heart Association, "Heart Disease and Stroke Statistics, 2012 Update: A Report from the American Heart Association," *Circulation* (2012), published online before print, December 15, 2011, 10.1161/CIR.Ob013e31823ac046.

38. American Heart Association, "Body Composition Tests," 2010, www .americanheart.org/presenter .jhtml?identifier=4489.

39. Obesity Society, "What Is Obesity?" Accessed November 2009, www.obesity .org/information/what_is_obesity.asp.

40. Centers for Disease Control and Prevention, "Defining Overweight and Obesity," Updated June 2010, www.cdc.gov/ obesity/defining.html.

41. K. Flegal et al., "Prevalence and Trends in Obesity among U.S. Adults, 1999–2008," 2010.

42. Centers for Disease Control and Prevention, "Childhood Obesity Facts," 2011, www.cdc.gov/healthyyouth/obesity/facts. htm; C. Ogden et al., "Prevalence of High Body Mass Index in US Children," 2010.

43. R. Puhl and J. Latner, "Weight Bias: New Science on a Significant Social Problem" *Obesity* 16 (2008): S1–S2, DOI: 10.1038/ oby.2008.460; R. Puhl, "Weight Stigmatization toward Youth: A Significant Problem in Need of Societal Solutions," *Childhood Obesity* 7, no.5 (2011): 359–63; R. Puhl and C. Heuer, "Obesity Stigma: Important Considerations for Public Health," *American Journal of Public Health* 100, no.6 (2010): 1019–1028.

44. J. Kizer et al., "Measures of Adiposity and Future Risk of Ischemic Stroke and Coronary Heart Disease in Older Men and Women," *American Journal of Epidemiology* 173, no. 1 (2010): 10–25; A. Taylor, S. Ebrahim, and Y. Ben-Shlomo, "Comparisons of the Associations of Body Mass Index and Measures of Central Adiposity and Fat Mass with Coronary Heart Disease, Diabetes, and All-cause Mortality: A Study Using Data from 4 UK Cohorts," *American Journal of Clinical Nutrition*, 91, no. 3 (2010): 547–56, First published online January 20, 2010, DOI:10.3945/ajcn.2009.28757

45. National Heart, Lung, and Blood Institute, "Classification of Overweight and Obesity by BMI, Waist Circumference and Associated Disease Risks," 2012, www.nhlbi.nih.gov/health/public/heart/ obesity/lose_wt/bmi_dis.htm.

46. Rush University, "Waist-to-Hip Ratio Calculator," Accessed May 2010, www .rush.edu/itools/hip/hipcalc.html.

47. World Health Organization, "Waist Circumference and Waist-Hip Ratio:

Report of WHO Expert Counsultation," 2011, http://whqlibdoc.who.int/publications/2011/9789241501491_eng.pdf.

48. F. Fernandez-Aranda et al., "Individual and Family Eating Patterns during Childhood and Early Adolescence: An Analysis of Associated Eating Disorder Factors," *Appetite* 49, no. 2 (2007): 476–85.

49. J. Thompson and M. Manore, *Nutrition: An Applied Approach,* 2d ed. (San Francisco: Benjamin Cummings, 2009), 126.

50. L. Gray, N. Cooper, A. Dunkley et al., "A Systematic Review and Mixed Treatment Comparison of Pharmacological Interventions for the Treatment of Obesity," *Obesity Reviews* 13, no. 6 (2012): 483–498.

51. U.S. Food and Drug Administration, "Fen-Phen Safety Update Information," Updated September 2009, www.fda.gov/Drugs/DrugSafety/PostmarketDrugSafetyInformationforPatientsandProviders/ucm072820.htm; FDA Recall Statement for Fen Phen, Uploaded February 20, 2012, www.ronw.org/fda-fen-phen.htm.

52. U.S. Food and Drug Administration, "Follow-Up to the November 2009 Early Communication about an Ongoing Safety Review of Sibutramine, Marketed as Meridia," January 2010, www.fda.gov/Drugs/DrugSafety/PostmarketDrugSafetyInformationforPatientsandProviders/DrugSafetyInformationforHeathcareProfessionals/ucm198206.htm.

53. ConsumerSearch, "Diet Pills: Reviews," 2012, www.consumersearch.com/diet-pills.

54. Mayo Clinic, "Gastric ByPass Surgery," www.mayoclinic.com/health/gastric-bypass/MY00825/.

55. F. Rubino et al., "Metabolic Surgery to Treat Type 2 Diabetes: Clinical Outcomes and Mechanisms of Action," *Annual Review of Medicine* 61 (2010): 393–411; E. Karra et al., "Mechanisms Facilitating Weight Loss and Resolution of Type 2 Diabetes Following Bariatric Surgery," *Trends in Endocrinology and Metabolism* 21, no. 6 (2010): 227–344.

56. C. Mottin et al., "Behavior of Type 2 Diabetes Mellitus in Morbid Obese Patients Submitted to Gastric Bypass," *Obesity Surgery* 18, no. 2 (2008): 179–82.

Enhancing Your Body Image

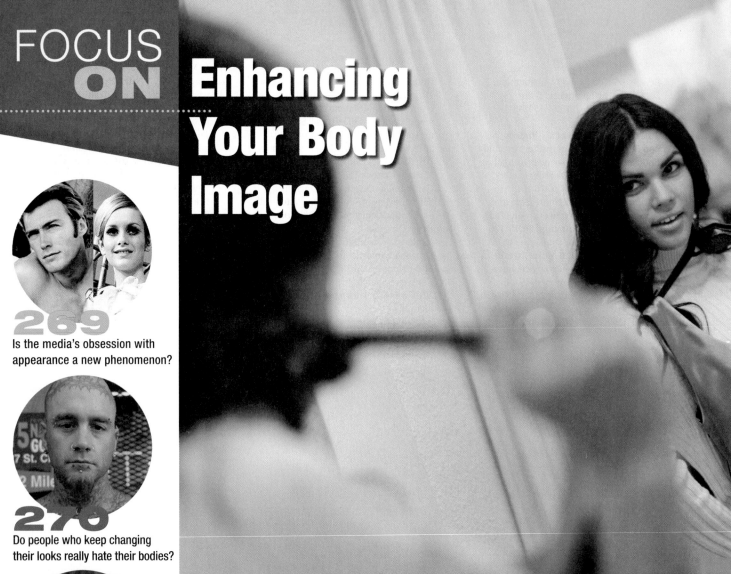

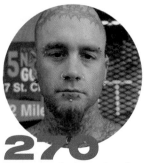

269

Is the media's obsession with appearance a new phenomenon?

270

Do people who keep changing their looks really hate their bodies?

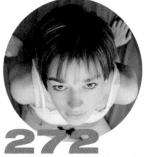

272

Can eating disorders be fatal?

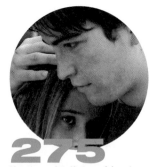

275

How can I talk to a friend about an eating disorder?

As he began his arm curls, Ali checked his form in the full-length mirror on the weight-room wall. His biceps were bulking up, but after 6 months of regular weight training, he expected more. His pecs, too, still lacked definition, and his abdomen wasn't the washboard he envisioned. So after a 45-minute upper-body work-out, he added 200 sit-ups. Then he left the gym to shower back at his apart-ment: No way was he going to risk any of the gym regulars seeing his flabby torso unclothed. But by the time Ali got home and looked in the mirror, frustration had turned to anger. He was just too fat! To punish himself for his slow progress, instead of taking a shower, he went for a 4-mile run.

When you look in the mirror, do you like what you see? If you feel dis-appointed, frustrated, or even angry like Ali, you're not alone. A major-ity of adults are dissatisfied with their bodies. A UK study found that 93 per-cent of the women reported having negative thoughts about their appear-ance during the past week.[1] Approxi-mately 79 percent of them also said they would like to lose weight—even though the majority of the women sampled (78.37%) were actually within

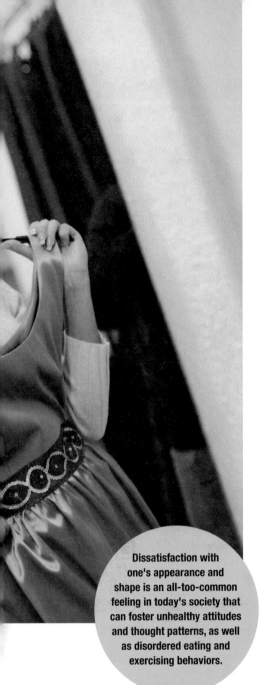

Dissatisfaction with one's appearance and shape is an all-too-common feeling in today's society that can foster unhealthy attitudes and thought patterns, as well as disordered eating and exercising behaviors.

the underweight or "normal" weight ranges. Over half of American females aged 12–23 years are unhappy with their bodies. One third of high-school students think they are overweight even when they are not.[2] Tragically, negative feelings about one's body can contribute to behaviors that can threaten your health—and your life. A healthy body image is a key indicator of self-esteem, and can contribute to reduced stress, an increased sense of personal empowerment, and joyful living.

80%
of adult American women report dissatisfaction with their appearance.

What Is Body Image?

This chapter text focuses on body image because it's so fundamental to our sense of who we are. The term **body image** refers to more than what you see when you look in a mirror, such as the following:[3]

- How you see yourself in your mind
- What you believe about your own appearance (including your memories, assumptions, and generalizations)
- How you feel about your body, including your height, shape, and weight
- How you sense and control your body as you move

A *negative body image* is defined as either a distorted perception of your shape, or feelings of discomfort, shame, or anxiety about your body. You may be convinced that only other people are attractive, whereas your own body is a sign of personal failure. Does this attitude remind you of Ali? It should, because he clearly exhibits signs of a negative body image.

In contrast, a *positive body image* is a true perception of your appearance: You see yourself as you really are. You understand that everyone is different, and you celebrate your uniqueness—including your "flaws," which you know have nothing to do with your value as a person.

Is your body image negative or positive—or somewhere in between? Researchers have developed a body image continuum that may help you decide (see Figure 1 on page 268). Like a spectrum of light, a continuum represents a series

body image Most fundamentally, what you believe about your overall body and how you feel subjectively about your body, including shape, weight, and how you picture yourself in your mind.

of stages that aren't entirely distinct. Notice that the continuum identifies behaviors associated with particular states, from total dissociation with one's body to body acceptance and ownership.

Many Factors Influence Body Image

You're not born with a body image, but you do begin to develop one at an early age as you compare yourself against images you see in the world around you and interpret the responses of family members and peers to your appearance. Let's look more closely at the factors that probably played a role in the development of your body image.

The Media and Popular Culture Images and celebrities in the media set the standard for what we find attractive, leading some people to go to dangerous extremes to have the biggest biceps or fit into size 2 jeans. Most of us think of this obsession with appearance as a recent phenomenon. The truth is, it has long been part of American culture. During the early twentieth century, while men idolized the hearty outdoorsman President Teddy Roosevelt, women pulled their corsets ever tighter to achieve unrealistically tiny waists. In the 1920s and 1930s, men emulated the burly cops and robbers in gangster films, while women dieted and bound their breasts to achieve the boyish "flapper" look. By the 1960s, tough guys like Clint Eastwood and Marlon Brando were the male ideal, whereas rail-thin supermodel Twiggy embodied the nation's standard of female beauty.

Today, more than 68 percent of American adults are overweight or obese; thus, a significant disconnect exists between the media's idealized images of male and female bodies and

Body hate/ dissociation	Distorted body image	Body preoccupied/ obsessed	Body acceptance	Body ownership
I often feel separated and distant from my body—as if it belongs to someone else. I don't see anything positive or even neutral about my body shape and size. I don't believe others when they tell me I look OK. I hate the way I look in the mirror and often isolate myself from others.	I spend a significant amount of time exercising and dieting to change my body. My body shape and size keep me from dating or finding someone who will treat me the way I want to be treated. I have considered changing or have changed my body shape and size through surgical means so I can accept myself.	I spend a significant amount of time viewing my body in the mirror. I spend a significant amount of time comparing my body to others. I have days when I feel fat. I am preoccupied with my body. I accept society's ideal body shape and size as the best body shape and size.	I base my body image equally on social norms and my own self-concept. I pay attention to my body and my appearance because it is important to me, but it only occupies a small part of my day. I nourish my body so it has the strength and energy to achieve my physical goals.	My body is beautiful to me. My feelings about my body are not influenced by society's concept of an ideal body shape. I know that the significant others in my life will always find me attractive.

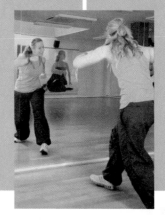

FIGURE 1 | **Body Image Continuum**

This is part of a two-part continuum, the second part of which is shown in Figure 2. Individuals whose responses fall to the far left side of the continuum have a highly negative body image, whereas responses to the right indicate a positive body image.

Source: Adapted from Smiley/King/Avery, Campus Health Service. Original continuum, C. Schislak, *Preventive Medicine and Public Health.* Copyright © 1997 Arizona Board of Regents. Used with permission of Dr. Lynne Smiley, Ph.D.

Video Tutor: Body Image Continuum

the typical American body.[4] At the same time, the media—in the form of television, the Internet, movies, and print publications—is more pervasive than ever before, bombarding us with messages telling us that we just don't measure up. In fact, one study of 26 countries with more than 7,400 participants concluded that exposure to Western media was significantly associated with body weight ideals and body dissatisfaction.[5]

Family, Community, and Cultural Groups The members of society with whom we most often interact—family, friends, and others—strongly influence the way we see ourselves. Parents are especially influential in body image development.

For instance, it's common and natural for fathers of adolescent girls to experience feelings of discomfort related to their daughters' changing bodies. If they are able to navigate these feelings successfully and validate the acceptability of their daughters' appearance throughout puberty, it's likely that they'll help their daughters maintain a positive body image. In contrast, if they verbalize or indicate even subtle judgments about their daughters' changing bodies, girls may begin to question how members of the opposite sex view their bodies in general. In addition, mothers who model body acceptance or body ownership may be more likely to foster a similar positive body image in their daughters, whereas mothers who are frustrated with or ashamed of

their own bodies may foster these negative attitudes.

Interactions with siblings and other relatives, peers, teachers, coworkers, and

What's Working for You?

Maybe you're already focusing on building a positive body image. Below is a list of some behaviors that can contribute to your positive body image. Which of these is true for you?

☐ I surround myself with people who are supportive of me and help to build me up, rather than being critical of me or others.

☐ I ignore media messages that emphasize physical appearance.

☐ I remind myself that beauty is not just outer appearance.

other community members can also influence body image development. For instance, peer harassment (teasing and bullying) is widely acknowledged to contribute to a negative body image. Associations within one's cultural group are also a factor. For example, studies have found that European American females experience the highest rates of body dissatisfaction, and as a minority group becomes more acculturated into the mainstream, the body dissatisfaction levels of women in that group increase.[6]

Body image also reflects the larger culture in which you live. In parts of Africa, for example, obesity has been associated with abundance, erotic desirability, and fertility. Girls in Mauritania traditionally were force-fed to increase their body size in order to signal a family's wealth, although the practice has become much less common in recent years.[7]

Physiological and Psychological Factors Recent neurological research suggests that people who have been diagnosed with a body image disorder show differences in the brain's ability to regulate chemicals called *neurotransmitters,* which are linked to mood.[8] Poor regulation of neurotransmitters is also involved in depression and in anxiety disorders, including obsessive-compulsive disorder. One study linked distortions in body image, particularly the face, to a malfunction in the brain's visual processing region that was revealed by MRI scanning.[9]

How Can I Build a More Positive Body Image?

If you want to develop a more positive body image, your first step might be to challenge some commonly held attitudes in contemporary society. Have you been accepting these four myths?[10]

Myth 1: **How you look is more important than who you are.** Do you think your weight is important in defining who you are? How much does it matter to you to have friends who are

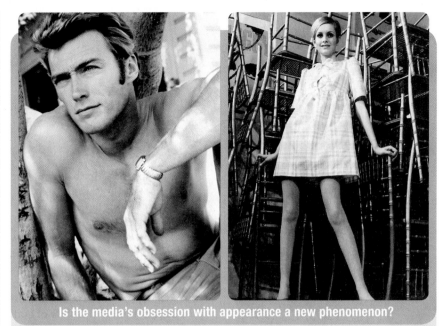

Is the media's obsession with appearance a new phenomenon?

Although the exact nature of the "in" look may change from generation to generation, unrealistic images of both male and female celebrities are nothing new. For example, in the 1960s, images of brawny film stars such as Clint Eastwood and ultrathin models such as Twiggy dominated the media.

thin and attractive? How important do you think being thin is in trying to attract your ideal partner?

Myth 2: **Anyone can be slender and attractive if they work at it.** When you see someone who is extremely thin, what assumptions do you make about that person? When you see someone who is overweight or obese, what assumptions do you make? Have you ever berated yourself for not having the "willpower" to change some aspect of your body?

Myth 3: **Extreme dieting is an effective weight-loss strategy.** Do you believe in trying fad diets or "quick-weight-loss" products? How far would you be willing to go to attain the "perfect" body?

Myth 4: **Appearance is more important than health.** How do you evaluate whether a person is healthy? Do you believe it's possible for overweight people to be healthy? Is your desire to change some aspect of your body motivated by health reasons or by concerns about appearance?

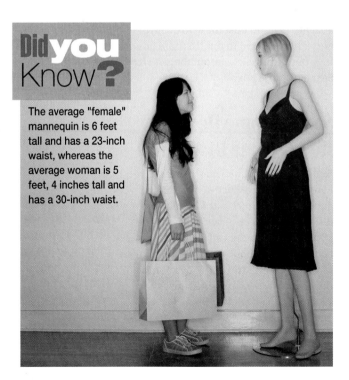

Did you Know?

The average "female" mannequin is 6 feet tall and has a 23-inch waist, whereas the average woman is 5 feet, 4 inches tall and has a 30-inch waist.

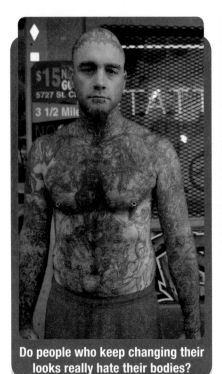

Do people who keep changing their looks really hate their bodies?

It's not always easy to spot people who are highly dissatisfied with their bodies, as they don't necessarily stick out in a crowd. For instance, people who cover their bodies with tattoos may have a strong sense of self-esteem. On the other hand, extreme tattooing can be an outward sign of a severe body image disturbance known as *body dysmorphic disorder.*

To learn ways to bust these toxic myths and attitudes, and to build a more positive body image, check out the **Skills for Behavior Change** box.

Some People Develop Body Image Disorders

Although most Americans are dissatisfied with some aspect of their appearance, very few have a true body image disorder. However, several diagnosable body image disorders affect a small percentage of the population. Two of the most common are body dysmorphic disorder and social physique anxiety.

body dysmorphic disorder (BDD) Psychological disorder characterized by an obsession with a minor or imagined flaw in appearance.

Ten Steps to a Positive Body Image

One list cannot automatically tell you how to turn negative thoughts into positive, but it can help you think about new ways to look more healthfully and happily at yourself and your body. The more you do that, the better you will feel about who you are and the body you naturally have.

❭ **Step 1.** Appreciate all that your body can do. Every day your body carries you closer to your dreams. Celebrate all of the amazing things your body does for you—running, dancing, breathing, laughing, dreaming.

❭ **Step 2.** Make a list of things you like about yourself—things that aren't related to how much you weigh or how you look. Read your list often. Add to it as you become aware of more things to like about yourself.

❭ **Step 3.** Remind yourself that true beauty is not simply skin deep. When you feel good about yourself and who you are, you carry yourself with a sense of confidence, self-acceptance, and openness that makes you beautiful. Beauty is a state of mind, not a state of body.

❭ **Step 4.** Look at yourself as a whole person. When you see yourself in a mirror or in your mind, choose not to focus on specific body parts. See yourself as you want others to see you—as a whole person.

❭ **Step 5.** Surround yourself with positive people. It is easier to feel good about yourself when you are around others who are supportive and who recognize the importance of liking yourself just as you naturally are.

❭ **Step 6.** Shut down those voices in your head that tell you your body is not "right" or that you are a "bad" person. You can overpower those negative thoughts with positive ones.

❭ **Step 7.** Wear comfortable clothes that make you feel good about your body. Work with your body, not against it.

❭ **Step 8.** Become a critical viewer of social and media messages. Pay attention to images, slogans, and attitudes that make you feel bad about your appearance. Protest these messages: Write a letter to the advertiser. Talk back to the image or message.

❭ **Step 9.** Do something nice for yourself—something that lets your body know you appreciate it. Take a bubble bath, make time for a nap, or find a peaceful place outside to relax.

❭ **Step 10.** Use the time and energy that you might have spent worrying about food, calories, and your weight to do something to help others. Reaching out to other people can help you feel better about yourself and make a positive change in our world.

Source: Reprinted with permission from the National Eating Disorders Association, www.NationalEatingDisorders.org.

Body Dysmorphic Disorder (BDD) Approximately 1 percent of people in the United States suffer from **body dysmorphic disorder (BDD).**[11] Persons with BDD are obsessively concerned with their appearance, and they have a distorted view of their own body shape, size, weight, perceived lack of muscles, facial blemishes, size of body parts, and so on. Although the cause of the disorder isn't known, an anxiety disorder such as obsessive-compulsive disorder is often present as well. (Anxiety disorders are discussed in Chapter 2.) Contributing factors may include genetic susceptibility, childhood teasing, physical or sexual abuse, low self-esteem, and rigid sociocultural expectations of beauty.[12]

People with BDD may try to fix their perceived flaws through abuse of steroids, excessive bodybuilding, repeated cosmetic surgeries, extreme tattooing, or other appearance-altering behaviors. It is estimated that 10 percent of people seeking dermatology or cosmetic treatments have BDD.[13] Not only do such actions fail to address the underlying problem, but they are also actually considered diagnostic signs of BDD. Psychiatric treatment, including psychotherapy and/or antidepressant medications, is often successful.

Social Physique Anxiety An emerging problem, seen in both young men and women, is **social physique anxiety (SPA).** The desire to "look good" becomes so strong that it has a destructive and sometimes disabling effect on the person's ability to function effectively in relationships and interactions with others. People suffering from SPA spend a disproportionate amount of time fixating on their bodies, working out, and performing tasks that are ego centered and self-directed, rather than focusing on interpersonal relationships and general tasks.[14] Experts speculate that this anxiety may contribute to disordered eating (discussed next).

What Is Disordered Eating?

As we've seen, people with a negative body image can fixate on a wide range of self-perceived "flaws." The "flaw"

social physique anxiety (SPA) A desire to look good that has a destructive effect on a person's ability to function well in social interactions and relationships.

disordered eating A pattern of atypical eating behaviors that is used to achieve or maintain a lower body weight.

that distresses the majority of people with negative body image is feeling overweight.

Some people channel their anxiety about their weight into self-defeating thoughts and harmful behaviors. Check out the eating issues continuum in **Figure 2**: The far left identifies a pattern of thoughts and behaviors associated with **disordered eating.** These behaviors can include chronic dieting, abusing diet pills and laxatives, self-induced vomiting, and many others.

Eating disordered	Disruptive eating patterns	Food preoccupied/obsessed	Concerned well	Food is not an issue
I regularly stuff myself and then exercise, vomit, or use diet pills or laxatives to get rid of the food or calories.	I have tried diet pills, laxatives, vomiting, or extra time exercising in order to lose or maintain my weight.	I think about food a lot.	I pay attention to what I eat in order to maintain a healthy body.	I am not concerned about what others think regarding what and how much I eat.
My friends and family tell me I am too thin.	I have fasted or avoided eating for long periods of time in order to lose or maintain my weight.	I feel I don't eat well most of the time.	I may weigh more than what I like, but I enjoy eating and balance my pleasure with eating with my concern for a healthy body.	When I am upset or depressed, I eat whatever I am hungry for without any guilt or shame.
I am terrified of eating fatty foods.	I feel strong when I can restrict how much I eat.	It's hard for me to enjoy eating with others.	I am moderate and flexible in goals for eating well.	Food is an important part of my life but only occupies a small part of my time.
When I let myself eat, I have a hard time controlling the amount of food I eat.	Eating more than I wanted to makes me feel out of control.	I feel ashamed when I eat more than others or more than what I feel I should be eating.	I try to follow the USDA's Dietary Guidelines for healthy eating.	
I am afraid to eat in front of others.		I am afraid of getting fat.		
		I wish I could change how much I want to eat and what I am hungry for.		

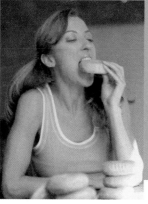

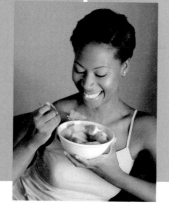

FIGURE 2 Eating Issues Continuum
This second part of the continuum shown in Figure 1 suggests that the progression from normal eating to eating disorders also occurs on a continuum.

Source: Adapted from Smiley/King/Avery, Campus Health Service. Original continuum, C. Schislak, *Preventive Medicine and Public Health*. Copyright © 1997 Arizona Board of Regents. Used with permission of Dr. Lynne Smiley, Ph.D.

Some People Develop Eating Disorders

Only some people who exhibit disordered eating patterns progress to a clinical **eating disorder.** The diagnosis of an eating disorder can be applied only by a physician to a patient who exhibits severe disturbances in thoughts, behavior, and body functioning—disturbances that can prove fatal. The American Psychiatric Association (APA) classifies eating disorders as *anorexia nervosa, bulimia nervosa, binge-eating disorder,* and a cluster of less distinct conditions collectively referred to as *eating disorders not otherwise specified* (*EDNOS*).

In the United States, as many as 25 million people of all ages meet the criteria for an eating disorder.[15] Although anorexia nervosa and bulimia nervosa used to affect people primarily in their teens and twenties, children as young as 6 and women as old as 76 have been diagnosed. In 2011, 2.3 percent of college students reported that they were dealing with either anorexia or bulimia.[16] Disordered eating and eating disorders are also common among ballet dancers and athletes, particularly athletes in sports with an aesthetic component (e.g., figure skating or gymnastics) or are tied to a weight class (e.g., tae kwon do, judo, or wrestling).[17]

Eating disorders are on the rise among men, who currently represent up to 25 percent of anorexia and bulimia patients.[18] Many men suffering from eating disorders fail to seek treatment.

What factors put individuals at risk? Many people with eating disorders feel disenfranchised in other aspects of their lives and try to gain a sense of control through food. Many are clinically depressed, suffer from obsessive-compulsive disorder, or have other psychiatric problems. In addition, individuals with low self-esteem, negative body image, and a high tendency for perfectionism are at risk.[19] Figure 3 shows how individual and social factors can interact to increase the risk of an eating disorder.

Anorexia Nervosa

Anorexia nervosa is a persistent, chronic eating disorder characterized by deliberate food restriction and severe, life-threatening weight loss. It involves self-starvation motivated by an intense fear of gaining weight and an extremely distorted body image. Initially, most people with anorexia nervosa lose weight by reducing total food intake, particularly of high-calorie foods. Eventually, they progress to restricting their intake of almost all foods. The little they do eat, they may purge through vomiting or using laxatives. Although they lose weight, people with anorexia nervosa never feel thin enough.

An estimated 0.3 percent of females suffer from anorexia nervosa in their lifetime.[20] The APA criteria for anorexia nervosa are as follows:[21]

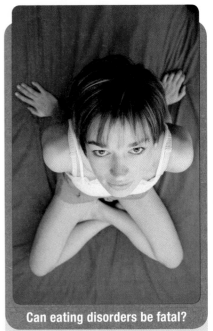

Can eating disorders be fatal?

People with anorexia nervosa put themselves at risk for starving to death. In addition, people with anorexia nervosa or bulimia nervosa may die from sudden cardiac arrest caused by electrolyte imbalances. About 20 percent of people with a serious eating disorder die from it.

- Refusal to maintain body weight at or above a minimally normal weight for age and height
- Intense fear of gaining weight or becoming fat, even though considered underweight by all medical criteria
- Disturbance in the way in which one's body weight or shape is experienced, undue influence of body weight or shape on self-evaluation, or denial of the seriousness of the current low body weight

Figure 4 on page 273 illustrates physical symptoms and negative health consequences associated with anorexia nervosa. Because it involves starvation and can lead to heart attacks and seizures, anorexia nervosa has the highest death rate (20%) of any psychological illness.

The causes of anorexia nervosa are complex and variable. Many people

Sociocultural factors
- Family and personal relationships
- History of being teased
- History of abuse
- Cultural norms
- Media influences
- Economic status

Psychological factors
- Low self-esteem
- Feelings of inadequacy or lack of control
- Unhealthy body image
- Perfectionism
- Lack of coping skills

Biological factors
- Inherited personality traits
- Genes that affect hunger, satiety, and body weight
- Depression or anxiety
- Brain chemistry

FIGURE 3 **Factors That Contribute to Eating Disorders**

with anorexia have other coexisting psychiatric problems, including low self-esteem, depression, an anxiety disorder such as obsessive-compulsive disorder, and substance abuse. Some people have a history of being physically or sexually abused, and others have troubled interpersonal relationships with family members. Cultural norms that value appearance and glorify thinness are, of course, a factor, as are weight-based teasing and weight bias.[22] Physical factors are thought to include an imbalance of neurotransmitters and genetic susceptibility.[23]

Bulimia Nervosa Individuals with **bulimia nervosa** often binge on huge amounts of food and then engage in some kind of purging, or "compensatory behavior," such as vomiting, taking laxatives, or exercising excessively, to lose the calories they have just consumed. People with bulimia are obsessed with their bodies, weight gain, and appearance, but unlike those with anorexia, their problem is often "hidden" because their weight may fall within a normal range or they may be overweight.

Up to 3 percent of adolescents and young women are bulimic; rates among men are about 10 percent of the rate among women.[24] The APA diagnostic criteria for bulimia nervosa are as follows:[25]

● Recurrent episodes of binge eating (defined as eating, in a discrete period of time, an amount of food that is larger than most people would eat during a similar period of time and under similar circumstances, and experiencing a sense of lack of control over eating during the episode)
● Recurrent inappropriate compensatory behavior to prevent weight gain, such as self-induced vomiting; misus-

bulimia nervosa Eating disorder characterized by binge eating followed by inappropriate measures, such as vomiting, to prevent weight gain.
binge-eating disorder A type of eating disorder characterized by binge eating once a week or more, but not typically followed by a purge.

ing laxatives, diuretics, or other medications; fasting; or excessive exercise
● Binge eating and inappropriate compensatory behavior occurs on average at least once a week for 3 months
● Body shape and weight unduly influence self-evaluation
● The disturbance does not occur exclusively during episodes of anorexia nervosa

Figure 5 on page 274 illustrates the physical symptoms and negative health consequences associated with bulimia nervosa. One of the more common symptoms is tooth erosion, which results from excessive vomiting. Bulimics who vomit are also at risk for electrolyte imbalances and dehydration, both of which can contribute to a heart attack and sudden death.

A combination of genetic and environmental factors is thought to cause bulimia nervosa.[26] A family history of obesity, an underlying anxiety disorder, and an imbalance in neurotransmitters are all possible contributing factors. In support of the role of neurotransmitters, a recent study showed that brain circuitry involved in regulating impulsive behavior seems to be less active in women with bulimia than in healthy women.[27] However, it is unknown whether such differences exist before bulimia develops or arise as a consequence of the disorder.

Binge-Eating Disorder Individuals with **binge-eating disorder** gorge like their bulimic counterparts but do not take excessive measures to lose the weight that they gain. Thus, they are often clinically obese. As in bulimia, binge-eating episodes are typically characterized by eating large amounts of food rapidly, even when not feeling hungry, and feeling guilty or depressed after overeating.[28]

A national survey reported a lifetime prevalence of binge-eating disorder in

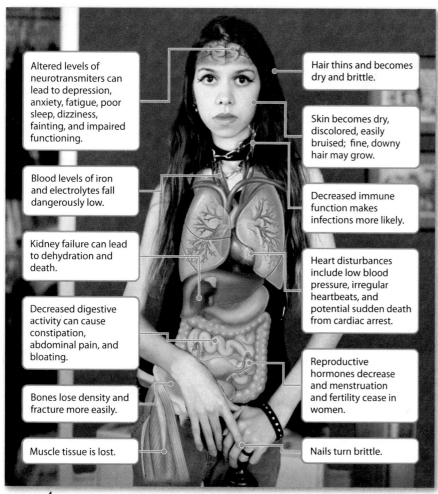

Altered levels of neurotransmitters can lead to depression, anxiety, fatigue, poor sleep, dizziness, fainting, and impaired functioning.

Blood levels of iron and electrolytes fall dangerously low.

Kidney failure can lead to dehydration and death.

Decreased digestive activity can cause constipation, abdominal pain, and bloating.

Bones lose density and fracture more easily.

Muscle tissue is lost.

Hair thins and becomes dry and brittle.

Skin becomes dry, discolored, easily bruised; fine, downy hair may grow.

Decreased immune function makes infections more likely.

Heart disturbances include low blood pressure, irregular heartbeats, and potential sudden death from cardiac arrest.

Reproductive hormones decrease and menstruation and fertility cease in women.

Nails turn brittle.

FIGURE 4 **What Anorexia Nervosa Can Do to the Body**

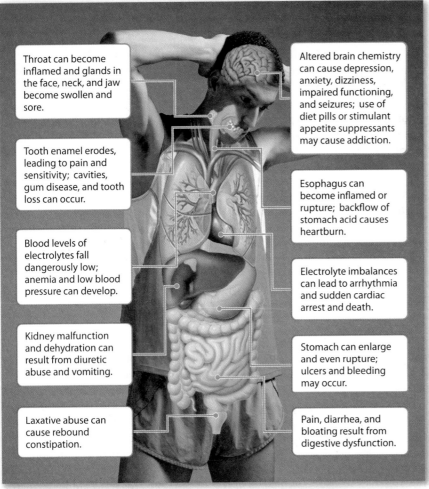

Throat can become inflamed and glands in the face, neck, and jaw become swollen and sore.

Tooth enamel erodes, leading to pain and sensitivity; cavities, gum disease, and tooth loss can occur.

Blood levels of electrolytes fall dangerously low; anemia and low blood pressure can develop.

Kidney malfunction and dehydration can result from diuretic abuse and vomiting.

Laxative abuse can cause rebound constipation.

Altered brain chemistry can cause depression, anxiety, dizziness, impaired functioning, and seizures; use of diet pills or stimulant appetite suppressants may cause addiction.

Esophagus can become inflamed or rupture; backflow of stomach acid causes heartburn.

Electrolyte imbalances can lead to arrhythmia and sudden cardiac arrest and death.

Stomach can enlarge and even rupture; ulcers and bleeding may occur.

Pain, diarrhea, and bloating result from digestive dysfunction.

FIGURE 5 **What Bulimia Nervosa Can Do to the Body**

the study participants of 1.6%.[29] APA criteria for binge-eating disorder are as follows:[30]

● Recurrent episodes of binge eating (defined as eating, in a discrete period of time, an amount of food that is larger than most people would eat during a similar period of time and under similar circumstances, and experiencing a sense of lack of control over eating during the episode)
● Binge-eating episodes are associated with three (or more) of the following: (1) eating much more rapidly than normal; (2) eating until feeling uncomfortably full; (3) eating large amounts of food when not feeling physically hungry; (4) eating alone because of embarrassment over how much one is eating; (5) feeling disgusted with oneself, depressed, or guilty after overeating
● Experiencing marked distress regarding binge eating
● The binge eating occurs, on average, at least once a week for 3 months
● The binge eating is not associated with the recurrent use of inappropriate compensatory behavior (i.e., purging) and does not occur exclusively during the course of bulimia nervosa or anorexia nervosa

Eating Disorders Not Otherwise Specified The APA recognizes that some patterns of disordered eating qualify as a legitimate psychiatric illness but don't fit into the strict diagnostic criteria for anorexia, bulimia, or binge-eating disorder. These are the

eating disorders not otherwise specified (EDNOS). This group of disorders can include night eating syndrome and recurrent purging in the absence of binge eating.

Treatment for Eating Disorders Because eating disorders are caused by a combination of many factors, there are no simple solutions. The bad news is that without treatment, approximately 20 percent of people with a serious eating disorder will die from it; with treatment, long-term full recovery rates range from 44 to 76 percent for anorexia nervosa and from 50 to 70 percent for bulimia nervosa.[31]

Treatment often focuses first on reducing the threat to life; once the patient is stabilized, long-term therapy focuses on the psychological, social, environmental, and physiological factors that have led to the problem. Therapy allows the patient to work on adopting new eating behaviors, building self-confidence, and finding other ways to deal with life's problems. Support groups can help the family and the individual learn positive actions and interactions. Treatment of an underlying anxiety disorder or depression may also be a focus.

How Can You Help Someone with Disordered Eating?

Although every situation is different, there are several things you can do if you suspect someone you know is struggling with disordered eating:[32]

What Do You Think?

Is the national attention to the obesity epidemic likely to worsen the problems with eating disorders? Why or why not?
● What do you think can be done to increase awareness of eating disorders in the United States?
● Can you think of ways to prevent eating disorders?

eating disorders not otherwise specified (EDNOS) Eating disorders that are a true psychiatric illness but that do not fit the strict diagnostic criteria for anorexia nervosa, bulimia nervosa, or binge-eating disorder.

- **Learn** as much as you can about disordered eating through books, articles, brochures, and trustworthy websites.
- **Know the facts** about weight, nutrition, and exercise. Being armed with accurate information can help you reason against any inaccurate ideas that your friend may be using as excuses to maintain a disordered eating pattern.
- **Be honest.** Talk openly and honestly about your concerns with your friend who is struggling with eating problems.
- **Be caring, but be firm.** Caring about your friend does not mean allowing him or her to manipulate you. Your friend must be responsible for his or her actions and the consequences of those actions. Avoid making statements that you cannot or will not uphold, such as, "I promise not to tell anyone," or, "If you do this one more time, I'll never talk to you again."
- **Compliment** your friend's personality, successes, and accomplishments.
- **Be a good role model** in regard to healthy eating, exercise, and self-acceptance.
- **Tell someone.** It may seem difficult to know when, or if, to tell someone else about your concerns. Your friend needs as much support as

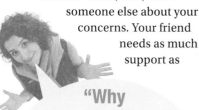

"Why Should I Care?"

Although exercising is generally beneficial to your health, doing it compulsively can lead to broken bones, joint injuries, and even depression—all of which can put you out of commission for the other things you enjoy. Remember that moderation is essential and taking rest days is important to your health.

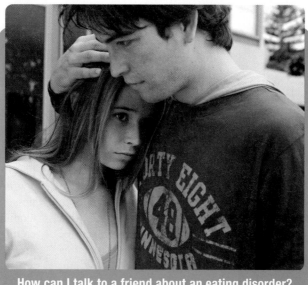

How can I talk to a friend about an eating disorder?

When talking to a friend about an eating disorder or disordered eating patterns, avoid casting blame, preaching, or offering unsolicited advice. Instead, be a good listener, let the person know that you care, and offer your support.

possible, the sooner the better. Don't wait until the situation is so severe that your friend's life is in danger. Addressing disordered eating patterns in their beginning stages offers your friend the best chance for working through these issues and becoming healthy again.

Can Exercise Be Unhealthy?

Although exercise is generally beneficial, in excess it can be a problem. In addition to being a common compensatory behavior used by people with anorexia or bulimia, exercise can become a compulsion or contribute to more complex disorders such as muscle dysmorphia or the female athlete triad.

Some People Develop Exercise Disorders

A study of almost 600 college students revealed that 18 percent met the criteria for **compulsive exercise.**[33] Also called *anorexia athletica,* compulsive exercise is characterized not by a *desire* to exercise but a *compulsion* to do so. That is, the person struggles with guilt and anxiety if he or she doesn't work out. Compulsive exercisers, like people with eating disorders, often define their self-worth externally. They overexercise in order to feel more in control of their lives. Disordered eating or a true eating disorder is often part of the picture.

Compulsive exercise can contribute to a variety of other injuries. It can also put significant stress on the heart, especially if combined with disordered eating. Psychologically, people who engage in compulsive exercise are often plagued by anxiety and/or depression. Their social life and academic success can suffer as they fixate more and more on exercise.

Muscle Dysmorphia **Muscle dysmorphia** appears to be a relatively new form of body image disturbance and exercise disorder among men in which a man believes that his body is insufficiently lean or muscular.[34] Men with muscle dysmorphia believe that they look "puny," when in reality they look normal or even unusually muscular. As a result of their adherence to a meticulous diet and time-consuming workout schedule, and their shame over their perceived appearance flaws, they may neglect important social or occupational activities.

Other behaviors characteristic of muscle dysmorphia include comparing oneself unfavorably to others, checking one's appearance in the mirror, and camouflaging one's appearance. Men with muscle dysmorphia

---

compulsive exercise Disorder characterized by a compulsion to engage in excessive amounts of exercise and feelings of guilt and anxiety if the level of exercise is perceived as inadequate.

muscle dysmorphia Body image disorder in which men believe that their body is insufficiently lean or muscular.

FOCUS ON! | ENHANCING YOUR BODY IMAGE | 275

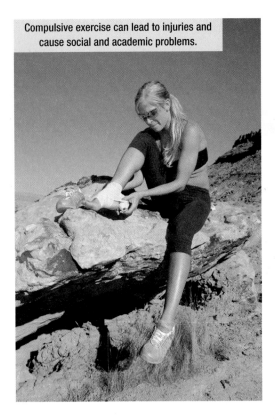

Compulsive exercise can lead to injuries and cause social and academic problems.

See It! Videos

Can you go too far with healthy eating? Watch **Extreme Healthy Eating: What Is Orthorexia?** at www.pearsonhighered.com/donatelle.

alters normal body functions. For example, when an athlete restricts her eating, she can deplete her body stores of nutrients essential to health. At the same time, her body begins to burn its stores of fat tissue for energy. Adequate body fat is essential to maintaining healthy levels of the female reproductive hormone *estrogen*; when an athlete isn't getting enough food, estrogen levels decline. This can manifest as amenorrhea: The body is using all calories to keep the athlete alive, and

The female athlete triad is particularly prevalent in women who participate in highly competitive individual sports or activities that emphasize leanness and require body-contouring clothing. Gymnasts, figure skaters, cross-country runners, and ballet dancers are among those at highest risk for the female athlete triad.

1 million

American males are estimated to struggle with some form of eating disorder.

also are likely to abuse anabolic steroids and dietary supplements.[35]

The Female Athlete Triad Female athletes in competitive sports often strive for perfection. In an effort to be the best, they may do more damage than good and put themselves at risk for a syndrome called the **female athlete triad.** *Triad* means "three," and the three interrelated problems are as follows (Figure 6):[36]

- Low energy intake, typically prompted by disordered eating behaviors
- Menstrual dysfunction, such as amenorrhea
- Poor bone density

How does the female athlete triad develop, and what makes it so dangerous? First, a chronic pattern of low energy intake and intensive exercise

nonessential body functions such as menstruation cease.

In addition, fat-soluble vitamins, calcium, and estrogen are all essential for dense, healthy bones, so their depletion weakens the athlete's bones, leaving her at high risk for fracture.

Warning signs of the female athlete triad include dry skin; light-headedness/fainting; lanugo (fine, downy hair covering the body); multiple injuries; and changes in endurance, strength, or speed.

In addition, behaviors associated with the disorder include preoccupation with

female athlete triad A syndrome of three interrelated health problems seen in some female athletes: disordered eating, amenorrhea, and poor bone density.

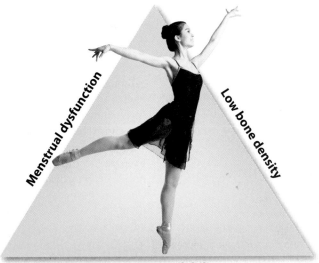

FIGURE 6 **The Female Athlete Triad**
The female athlete triad is a cluster of three interrelated health problems.

food and weight, compulsive exercise, use of weight-loss products or laxatives, trips to the bathroom during or immediately after eating, decreased ability to concentrate, self-criticism, anxiety, and depression. Treatment can be challenging, and it requires a multidisciplinary approach involving the athlete's coach and trainer, a sports medicine team, psychologist, and other professionals, as well as family members and friends.

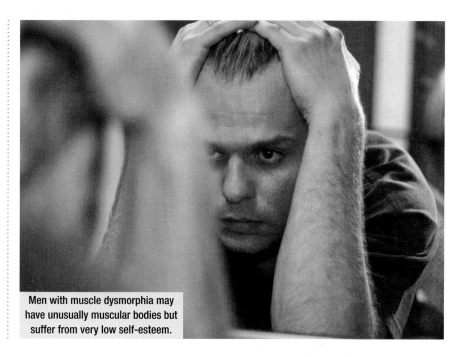

Men with muscle dysmorphia may have unusually muscular bodies but suffer from very low self-esteem.

Assess yourself

Are Your Efforts to Be Thin Sensible— Or Spinning Out of Control?

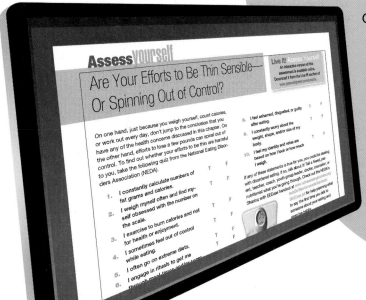

Go online to the **Live It!** section of www.pearsonhighered.com/donatelle to take the "Are Your Efforts to Be Thin Sensible?" assessment.* Afterward, you can follow the steps outlined in the **YOUR PLAN FOR CHANGE** box to work on building a more positive body image.

*If your instructor so chooses, Assess Yourself Activities are available as a printed supplement or as assignable homework online at www.pearsonhighered.com/myhealthlab.

MyHealthLab®

YOUR PLAN FOR CHANGE

The **Assessyourself** activity gives you a chance to evaluate your feelings about your body and determine whether you might be engaging in eating or exercise behaviors that could undermine your health and happiness. Below are some steps you can take to improve your body image, starting today.

Today, you can:

○ Talk back to the media. Write letters to advertisers and magazines that depict unhealthy and unrealistic body types. Boycott their products or start a blog commenting on harmful body image messages in the media.

○ Visit www.mypyramid.gov and print out your personalized food plan. Just for today, eat the recommended number of servings from every food group at every meal, and don't count calories!

Within the next 2 weeks, you can:

○ Find a photograph of a person you admire for his or her contributions to humanity, *not* for his or her appearance. Paste it up next to your mirror to remind yourself that true beauty comes from within and benefits others.

○ Start a diary. Each day, record one thing you are grateful for that has nothing to do with your appearance. At the end of each day, record one small thing you did to make someone's world a little brighter.

By the end of the semester, you can:

○ Establish a group of friends who support you for who you are, not what you look like, and who get the same support from you. Form a group on a favorite social-networking site, and keep in touch, especially when you start to feel troubled by self-defeating thoughts or have the urge to engage in unhealthy eating or exercise behaviors.

○ Borrow from the library or purchase one of the many books on body image now available, and read it!

References

1. University of the West of England, "30% of Women Would Trade at Least One Year of Their Life to Achieve Their Ideal Body Weight and Shape," March 31, 2011, http://info.uwe.ac.uk/news/UWENews/news.aspx?id=1949.
2. American College of Obstetricians and Gynecologists Committee on Adolescent Health Care, "Media and Body Image: A Fact Sheet for Parents," FS 032, 2009, www.acog.org/departments/adolescentHealthCare/TeenCareToolKit/mediabody_4_parents.pdf. doi:10.1177/0146167209359702
3. Mayo Clinic, "Healthy Body Image," 2010, www.mayoclinic.com/health/healthy-body-image/MY01225; National Women's Information Network, "Body Image," 2009, www.womenshealth.gov/bodyimage/.
4. K. M. Flegal et al., "Prevalence and Trends in Obesity among U.S. Adults, 1999–2008," *Journal of the American Medical Association* 303, no. 3 (2010): 235–41.
5. V. Swami et al., "The Attractive Female Body Weight and Female Body Dissatisfaction in 26 Countries across 10 World Regions: Results of the International Body Project I," *Personality and Social Psychology Bulletin* 36, no. 3 (2010): 309–25.
6. Ibid.
7. Consultancy Africa Intelligence, 2010, "Force-feeding in Mauritania: Beauty in the Eye of the Male Beholders," Accessed April 21, 2012, from www.consultancyafrica.com/index.php?option=com_content&view=article&id=330&Itemid=222.
8. Mayo Clinic Staff, "Body Dysmorphic Disorder," November 2010, www.mayoclinic.com/health/body-dysmorphic-disorder/DS00559.
9. J. D. Feusner, J. Townsend, A. Bystritsky, M. McKinley, H. Moller, and S. Bookheimer, "Regional Brain Volumes and Symptom Severity in Body Dysmorphic Disorder," *Psychiatry Research* 172, no. 2 (2009): 161–67, www.psyn-journal.com/article/S0925-4927(08)00203-5/abstract.
10. University of Kansas Student Health, "Body Image Myths and Misconceptions," Accessed February 1, 2012, http://hawkhealth.ku.edu/?q=node/20; Women's Health Information Network, "Body Image," www.womenshealth.gov/bodyimage/.
11. I. Ahmed, L. Genen, and T. Cook, "Psychiatric Manifestations of Body Dysmorphic Disorder," Medscape Reference, Updated February 11, 2011, http://emedicine.medscape.com/article/291182-overview.
12. Mayo Clinic Staff, "Body Dysmorphic Disorder," 2010; KidsHealth, "Body Dysmorphic Disorder," October 2010, http://kidshealth.org/parent/emotions/feelings/bdd.html.
13. I. Ahmed, L. Genen, and T. Cook, "Psychiatric Manifestations of Body Dysmorphic Disorder," 2011.
14. O. Mülazimoğlu-Balli, C. Koka, and F. H. Asci, "An Examination of Social Physique Anxiety with Regard to Sex and Level of Sport Involvement," *Journal of Human Kinetics* 26, (2010): 115–22, www.johk.awf.katowice.pl/pdfy/nr26/014_Ozgor%20et%20al.pdf; S. R. Bratrud, M. M. Parmer, J. R. Whitehead, and R. C. Eklund, "Social Physique Anxiety, Physical Self-Perceptions and Eating Disorder Risk: A Two-sample Study," *Pamukkale Journal of Sport Sciences* 1, no. 3 (2010): 01–10, http://psbd.pau.edu.tr/index.php/pjss/article/viewFile/33/pdf_9.
15. Alliance for Eating Disorders, 2012, What are Eating Disorders?, Accessed April 21, 2012, from www.allianceforeatingdisorders.com/what-are-eating-disorders
16. American College Health Association, *National College Health Assessment II: Reference Group Executive Summary Spring 2011* (Linthicum, MD: American College Health Association, 2011), www.acha-ncha.org/reports_ACHA-NCHAII.html.
17. L. M. Gottschlich, "Female Athlete Triad," Medscape Reference, Drugs, Diseases & Procedures, January 25, 2012, http://emedicine.medscape.com/article/89260-overview#a0156.
18. Alliance for Eating Disorders, What Are Eating Disorders?, 2012.

19. Ibid.

20. S. A. Swanson, S. J. Crow, D. Le Grange, J. Swendsen, and K. R. Merikangas, "Prevalence and Correlates of Eating Disorders in Adolescents: Results from the National Comorbidity Survey Replication Adolescent Supplement," *Archives of General Psychiatry* 68, no. 7 (2011): 714–23, DOI: 10.1001/archgenpsychiatry.2011.22.

21. American Psychiatric Association, "DSM-5 Development: Proposed Revision: 307.1 Anorexia Nervosa," Updated October 2010, www.dsm5.org/ProposedRevisions/Pages/proposedrevision.aspx?rid=24.

22. A. L. Ahern et al., "Internalization of the Ultra-Thin Ideal: Positive Implicit Associations with Underweight Fashion Models Are Associated with Drive for Thinness in Young Women," *Eating Disorders* 16, no. 4 (2008): 294–307; M. Eisenberg and D. Neumark-Sztainer, "Peer Harassment and Disordered Eating," *International Journal of Adolescent Medicine and Health* 20, no. 2 (2008): 155–64.

23. National Association of Anorexia Nervosa and Associated Disorders, "Eating Disorders: General Information," Accessed February 1, 2012, from www.anad.org/get-information/about-eating-disorders/general-information/; Eating Disorder Institute, "What Are Neurotransmitters and How Do They Influence the Development of Eating Disorders?", 2009, www.eatingdisorder-institute.com/?tag=neurotransmitters.

24. National Alliance on Mental Illness, "Bulimia Nervosa," 2011, www.nami.org/template.cfm?Section=by_illness&template=/ContentManagement/ContentDisplay.cfm&ContentID=65839.

25. American Psychiatric Association, "DSM-5 Development: Bulimia Nervosa," 2010.

26. National Alliance on Mental Illness, "Bulimia Nervosa," 2010.

27. R. Marsh et al., "Deficient Activity in the Neural Systems That Mediate Self-Regulatory Control in Bulimia Nervosa," *Archives of General Psychiatry* 66, no. 1 (2009): 51–63.

28. National Association of Anorexia Nervosa and Associated Disorders, "Binge Eating Disorder," Accessed February 1, 2012, from www.anad.org/get-information/about-eating-disorders/binge-eating-disorder/.

29. S. A. Swanson et al. "Prevalence and Correlates of Eating Disorders in Adolescents," 2011.

30. American Psychiatric Association, "DSM-5 Development: Proposed Revision: Binge Eating Disorder," Updated October 2010, www.dsm5.org/ProposedRevisions/Pages/proposedrevision.aspx?rid=372.

31. K. N. Franco, Cleveland Clinic Center for Continuing Education, "Eating Disorders," Accessed February 1, 2012, from www.clevelandclinicmeded.com/medicalpubs/diseasemanagement/psychiatry-psychology/eating-disorders; Mirasol Eating Disorder Recovery Centers, "Eating Disorder Statistics," Accessed February 1, 2012, from www.mirasol.net/eating-disorders/information/eating-disorder-statistics.php.

32. College of Scholastica, "Helping a Friend," Accessed February 1, 2012, from www.css.edu/Administration/Health-and-Well-Being/Eating-Issues/Helping-a-Friend.html; California Institute of Technology, "Helping a Friend with an Eating Disorder," Accessed February 1, 2012, from www.counseling.caltech.edu/InfoandResources/Eating_Disorder.

33. J. Guidi et al., "The Prevalence of Compulsive Eating and Exercise among College Students: An Exploratory Study," *Psychiatry Research* 165, no. 1–2 (2009): 154–62.

34. J. J. Waldron, "When Building Muscle Turns into Muscle Dysmorphia," Association for Applied Psychology, 2011, http://appliedsportpsych.org/Resource-Center/health-and-fitness/articles/muscledysmorphia.

35. M. Silverman, "What is Muscle Dysmorphia?" Massachusetts General Hospital, February 18, 2011, https://mghocd.org/what-is-muscle-dysmorphia/; J. J. Waldron, "When Building Muscle Turns into Muscle Dysmorphia," 2011.

36. L. M. Gottschlich, "Female Athlete Triad," 2012.

Improving Your Physical Fitness

OBJECTIVES

* Describe the benefits of physical activity for health, fitness, and performance.

* Commit to getting physically fit by overcoming obstacles and participating in lifestyle fitness activities.

* Use the FITT guidelines (frequency, intensity, time, and type) to design a fitness program that meets your personal goals.

* Implement your safe and effective fitness program.

* Consume optimal foods and fluids for exercise and recovery.

* Prevent and treat common exercise injuries.

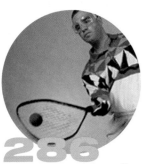

286

Can physical activity really reduce stress?

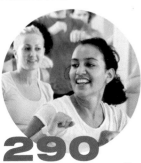

290

How can I motivate myself to get moving?

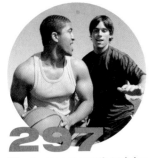

297

Why is core strength training important?

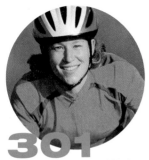

301

What can I do to avoid injury when I exercise?

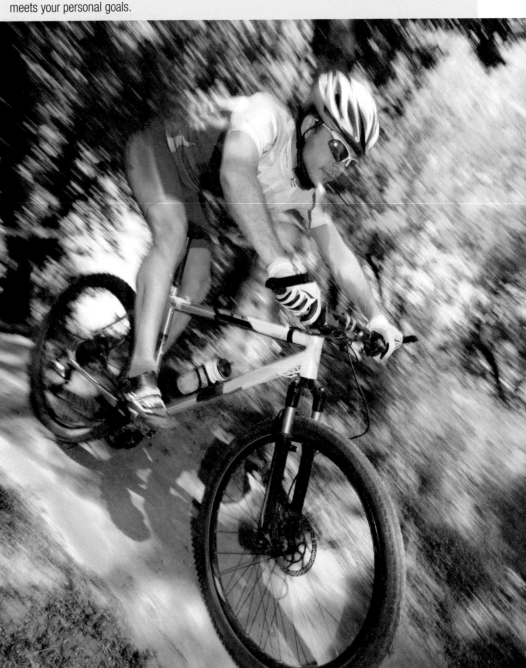

Most Americans are aware of the wide range of physical, social, and mental health benefits of physical activity and that they should be more physically active. The physiological body changes that result from regular physical activity reduce the likelihood of coronary artery disease, high blood pressure, type 2 diabetes, obesity, and other chronic diseases. Furthermore, engaging in regular physical activity helps control stress, increase self-esteem, and contribute to that "feel-good" feeling.

Despite knowing about the importance of physical activity for health and wellness, most people are not sufficiently active for optimal health benefits. Recent statistics indicate that 25.4 percent of American adults do not engage in any leisure-time physical activity or activity done during one's "down" time.[1] The growing percentage of Americans who live physically inactive lives has been linked to the current high incidences of obesity, type 2 diabetes, and other chronic and mental health diseases.[2]

In general, college students are more physically active than are older adults, but a recent survey indicated that 54 percent of college women and 48 percent of college men do not meet recommended guidelines for engaging in moderate or vigorous physical activities.[3]

College is a great time to develop positive attitudes and behaviors that can increase the quality and quantity of your life. Now is the time to get moving. It may not be easy to change a sedentary lifestyle, but it is definitely worth every effort made. This text will help you develop strategies to get moving.

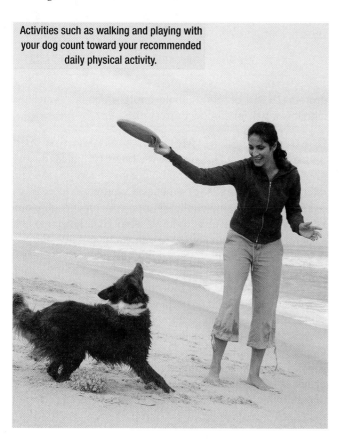

Activities such as walking and playing with your dog count toward your recommended daily physical activity.

Using Physical Activity for Health, Fitness, and Performance

Physical activity is any body movement that works your muscles, uses more energy than when resting, and enhances health.[4] Walking, swimming, strength training, dancing, and doing yoga are examples of physical activity. Physical activities can vary by intensity and thus are categorized as light, moderate, and vigorous. For example, walking to class typically requires little effort (light), while walking to class uphill is more intense and harder to do (moderate or vigorous). There are three general categories of physical activity defined by the purpose for which they are done: physical activity for health, physical activity for physical fitness, and physical activity for performance.

Exercise refers to a particular kind of physical activity. Although all exercise is physical activity, not all physical activity would be considered exercise. For example, walking from your car to class is physical activity, whereas going for a brisk 30-minute walk is considered exercise. *Exercise* is defined as planned, structured, and repetitive bodily movement done to improve or maintain one or more components of physical fitness, such as cardiorespiratory endurance, muscular strength or endurance, or flexibility.

physical activity Refers to all body movements produced by skeletal muscles resulting in substantial increases in energy expenditure.

exercise Planned, structured, and repetitive bodily movement done to improve or maintain one or more components of physical fitness.

Physical Activity for Health: What Are the Health Benefits of Regular Physical Activity?

From a major review of research on physical activity and health, researchers concluded that "there is irrefutable evidence of the effectiveness of regular physical activity in the primary and secondary prevention of several chronic diseases (e.g., cardiovascular disease, diabetes, cancer, hypertension, obesity, depression, and osteoporosis)."[5] Adding more physical activity to your day, like walking or cycling to school, can benefit your health.

In fact, if all Americans followed the 2008 Physical Activity Guidelines (see Table 9.1 on page 283) it is estimated that about one third of deaths related to coronary heart disease; one quarter of deaths related to stroke and osteoporosis; one fifth of deaths related to colon cancer, high blood pressure, and type 2 diabetes; and one seventh of deaths related to breast cancer could be prevented.[6]

Regular participation in physical activity improves more than 50 different physiological, metabolic, and psychological

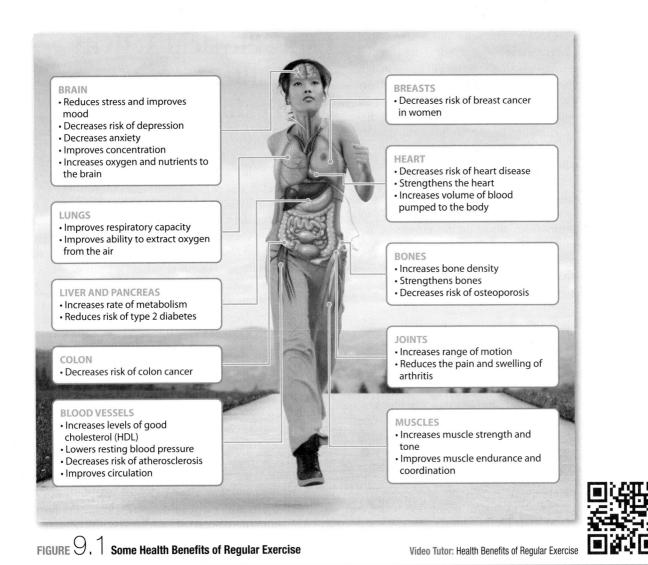

BRAIN
- Reduces stress and improves mood
- Decreases risk of depression
- Decreases anxiety
- Improves concentration
- Increases oxygen and nutrients to the brain

LUNGS
- Improves respiratory capacity
- Improves ability to extract oxygen from the air

LIVER AND PANCREAS
- Increases rate of metabolism
- Reduces risk of type 2 diabetes

COLON
- Decreases risk of colon cancer

BLOOD VESSELS
- Increases levels of good cholesterol (HDL)
- Lowers resting blood pressure
- Decreases risk of atherosclerosis
- Improves circulation

BREASTS
- Decreases risk of breast cancer in women

HEART
- Decreases risk of heart disease
- Strengthens the heart
- Increases volume of blood pumped to the body

BONES
- Increases bone density
- Strengthens bones
- Decreases risk of osteoporosis

JOINTS
- Increases range of motion
- Reduces the pain and swelling of arthritis

MUSCLES
- Increases muscle strength and tone
- Improves muscle endurance and coordination

FIGURE 9.1 **Some Health Benefits of Regular Exercise**

Video Tutor: Health Benefits of Regular Exercise

aspects of human life. **Figure 9.1** summarizes some of these major health-related benefits.

Reduced Risk of Cardiovascular Diseases Aerobic exercise is good for the heart and lungs and reduces the risk for heart-related diseases. It improves blood flow and eases the performance of everyday tasks. Regular exercise makes the cardiovascular and respiratory systems more efficient by strengthening the heart muscle, thus enabling more blood to be pumped with each stroke. The number of *capillaries* (small blood vessels that allow gas exchange between blood and surrounding tissues) in trained skeletal muscles is greater than in untrained, which allows for enhanced blood flow to working muscles. Exercise also improves the respiratory system by increasing the amount of oxygen that is inhaled and distributed to body tissues.[7]

Regular physical activity can reduce hypertension, or chronic high blood pressure, a form of cardiovascular disease and a significant risk factor for coronary heart disease and stroke.[8] Regular aerobic exercise also reduces low-density lipoproteins (LDLs, or "bad" cholesterol), total cholesterol, and triglycerides (a blood fat), thus reducing plaque buildup in the arteries, while increasing high-density lipo-

proteins (HDLs, or "good" cholesterol), which are associated with lower risk for coronary artery disease.[9]

Reduced Risk of Metabolic Syndrome and Type 2 Diabetes Regular physical activity reduces the risk of metabolic syndrome, a combination of heart disease and diabetes risk factors that produces a synergistic increase in risk.[10] Specifically, metabolic syndrome includes high blood pressure, abdominal obesity, low levels of HDLs, high levels of triglycerides, and impaired glucose tolerance.[11] Regular participation in moderate-intensity physical activities increases fitness, reduces obesity, and thus reduces the risk for each metabolic syndrome factor individually and collectively.[12]

Research indicates that a healthy dietary intake combined with sufficient physical activity could prevent many of the current cases of type 2 diabetes.[13] In a major national clinical trial, researchers found that exercising 150 minutes per week while eating fewer calories and less fat could prevent or delay the onset of type 2 diabetes.[14] (For more on diabetes prevention and management, see **Focus On: Minimizing Your Risk for Diabetes**).

Hear It! Podcasts

Want a study podcast for this chapter? Download the podcast **Personal Fitness: Improving Health through Exercise** at www.pearsonhighered.com/donatelle.

	Key Guidelines for Health*	For Additional Fitness or Weight Loss Benefits*	PLUS
Adults	150 min/week moderate-intensity physical activity OR 75 min/week of vigorous-intensity physical activity OR Equivalent combination of moderate- and vigorous-intensity (i.e., 100 min moderate-intensity + 25 min vigorous-intensity) physical activity	300 min/week moderate-intensity physical activity OR 150 min/week of vigorous-intensity physical activity OR Equivalent combination of moderate- and vigorous-intensity (i.e., 200 min moderate-intensity + 50 min vigorous-intensity) physical activity OR More than the previously described amounts	Muscle strengthening activities for ALL the major muscle groups at least 2 days/week
Older Adults	If unable to follow above guidelines, then as much physical activity as your condition allows	If unable to follow above guidelines, then as much physical activity as your condition allows	In addition to muscle strengthening activities, those with limited mobility should add exercises to improve balance and reduce risk of falling
Children and Youth	60 min or more of moderate- or vigorous-intensity physical activity daily	Add vigorous-intensity physical activities within the 60 daily minutes at least 3 days/week	Include muscle and bone strengthening activities within the 60 daily minutes at least 3 days/week Activities should be age-appropriate, enjoyable, and varied

*Avoid inactivity; some activity is better than none; accumulate physical activity in sessions of 10 minutes or more at one time; and spread activity throughout the week.

Source: Office of Disease Prevention and Health Promotion, U.S. Department of Health and Human Services, *2008 Physical Activity Guidelines for Americans: Be Active, Healthy, and Happy!* ODPHP Publication no. U0036 (Washington, DC: U.S. Department of Health and Human Services, 2008), Available at www.health.gov/paguidelines.

Reduced Cancer Risk After decades of research, most cancer epidemiologists believe that the majority of cancers are preventable and can be avoided by healthier lifestyle and environmental choices.[15] In fact, a report released by the World Cancer Research Fund, in conjunction with the American Institute for Cancer Research, stated that two thirds of all cancers could be prevented based on lifestyle changes.[16] More specifically, one third of cancers could be prevented by being physically active and eating well.

Regular physical activity appears to lower the risk for some specific cancers, particularly breast cancer. Research on exercise and breast cancer risk has found that the earlier in life a woman starts to exercise, the lower her breast cancer risk.[17] Regular exercise is also associated with lower risk for colon and rectal cancers.[18]

Improved Bone Mass *Osteoporosis,* a disease characterized by low bone mass, deterioration of bone tissue, and increased fracture risk, is becoming more prevalent among older populations. Regular weight-bearing and strength-building physical activities are recommended to maintain bone health and prevent osteoporotic fractures. Although men and women are both negatively affected by osteoporosis, it is more common in women. Both men and women have much to gain by being physically active and remaining physically active as they age—bone mass levels are significantly higher among active individuals than among sedentary persons.[19] However, it appears that the full bone-related benefits of physical activity can only be achieved with sufficient hormone levels (estrogen in women; testosterone in men) and adequate calcium, vitamin D, and total caloric intakes.[20]

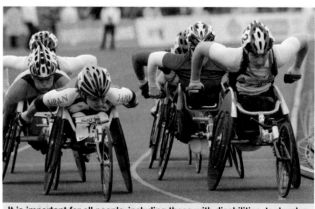

It is important for all people, including those with disabilities, to develop optimal levels of physical fitness to participate in physical activities they enjoy—including competitive sports.

Improved Weight Control For many people, the desire to lose weight is the main reason for their physical activity. On the most basic level, physical activity requires your body to generate energy through calorie expenditure; if calories expended exceed calories consumed over a span of time, the net result will be weight loss. Some activities are more intense or vigorous than others and result in more calories used. Figure 9.2 shows the caloric cost of various activities when done for 30 minutes.

In addition to the calories expended during activity, physical activity has a direct positive effect on metabolic rate, keeping it elevated for several hours following vigorous physical activities. This increase in metabolic rate can reduce body fat and lead to body composition changes that favor weight management. In addition to helping you lose weight, increased physical activity also improves your chances of maintaining the weight loss.[21]

Improved Immunity Research shows that regular moderate-intensity physical activity reduces individual susceptibility to disease.[22] Just how physical activity alters immunity is not well understood. We know that moderate-intensity physical activity temporarily increases the number of white blood cells (WBCs), which are responsible for fighting infection.[23] Often the relationship of physical activity to immunity, or more specifically to disease susceptibility, is described as a J-shaped curve. In other words, susceptibility to disease decreases with moderate activity, but then increases as you move to extreme levels of physical activity or exercise or if you continue to exercise without adequate recovery time and/or dietary intake.[24] Athletes engaging in marathon-type events or very intense physical training programs have been shown to be at greater risk for upper respiratory tract infections (cold and flu), particularly in the 8 hours immediately after an intense exercise session.[25]

Improved Mental Health and Stress Management Most people who engage in regular physical activity are likely to notice psychological benefits, such as feeling better about themselves and an overall sense of well-being. Although these mental health benefits are difficult to quantify, they are frequently mentioned as reasons for continuing to be physically active.

Physical activity contributes to mental health in more than one way. Learning new skills, developing increased ability and capacity in recreational activities, and sticking with a physical activity plan all improve an individual's self-esteem. In addition, regular physical activity can improve a person's physical appearance, thus increase self-esteem as a result.

Regular vigorous exercise has been shown to "burn off" the chemical by-products of the stress response and increase endorphins, giving your mood a natural boost. Elimination of these stress hormones reduces the stress response by accelerating the neurological system's return to a balanced state.[26] For these reasons, regular physical activity of moderate to vigorous intensity should be an integral component of your mental health and stress management plan.

Longer Life Span Experts have long debated the relationship between physical activity and longevity. Several studies indicate significant decreases in long-term health risk and increases in years lived, particularly among those who have several risk factors and who use physical activity as a means of risk reduction. Results from a study of nearly a million subjects showed that the greatest benefits from physical activity occurred in sedentary individuals who added a little physical activity to their lives, with additional benefits added as physical activity levels were increased.[27]

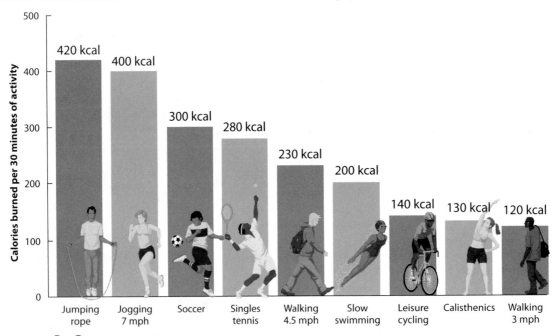

FIGURE 9.2 **Calories Burned by Different Activities**
The harder you exercise, the more energy you expend. Estimated calories burned for various moderate and vigorous activities are listed for a 30-minute bout of activity.

Physical Activity for Fitness: Health-Related Components of Physical Fitness

Physical fitness refers to a balance of physical attributes that are either health or performance related. The health-related attributes—cardiorespiratory fitness, muscular strength and endurance, flexibility, and body composition—allow you to perform moderate- to vigorous-intensity physical activities on a regular basis without getting too tired and with energy left over to handle physical or mental emergencies. **Figure 9.3** identifies the major health-related components of physical fitness.

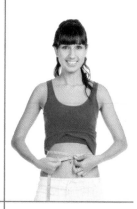

"Why Should I Care?"

You know being fit reduces your risk for many chronic diseases, right? Not an immediate concern? Remember, there are immediate benefits to staying active—improved physical appearance and self-esteem, protection from infectious diseases, a reduction in stress, and even an improvement in your sleep and ability to concentrate! All that, and it's fun, too—so drop the excuses—get out and play!

Cardiorespiratory Fitness

Cardiorespiratory fitness is the ability of the heart, lungs, and blood vessels to supply the body with oxygen efficiently. The primary category of physical activity known to improve cardiorespiratory fitness is **aerobic exercise.** The word *aerobic* means "with oxygen" and describes any type of exercise that increases your heart rate. Aerobic activities such as swimming, cycling, and jogging are among the best exercises for improving or maintaining cardiorespiratory fitness.

Cardiorespiratory fitness is measured by determining **aerobic capacity** (or **power**), the volume of oxygen the muscles consume during exercise. Maximal aerobic power (commonly written as VO_{2max}) is defined as the volume of oxygen that the muscles consume per minute during maximal exercise. The most common measure of maximal aerobic capacity is a walk or run test on a treadmill. For greatest accuracy, this is done in a lab with specialized equipment and technicians to measure the precise amount of oxygen entering and exiting the body during the exercise session. Submaximal tests can be used in the classroom or field to get a more general sense of cardiorespiratory fitness.

Muscular Strength

Muscular strength refers to the amount of force a muscle or group of muscles is capable of exerting in one contraction. The most common way to assess the strength of a particular muscle group is to measure the maximum amount of weight you can move one time (and no more), or your one repetition maximum (1 RM).

physical fitness A balance of health-related attributes that allow you to perform moderate to vigorous physical activities on a regular basis and complete daily physical tasks without undue fatigue.

cardiorespiratory fitness The ability of the heart, lungs, and blood vessels to supply oxygen to skeletal muscles during sustained physical activity.

aerobic exercise Any type of exercise that increases heart rate.

aerobic capacity (or power) The functional status of the cardiorespiratory system; refers specifically to the volume of oxygen the muscles consume during exercise.

muscular strength The amount of force that a muscle is capable of exerting in one contraction.

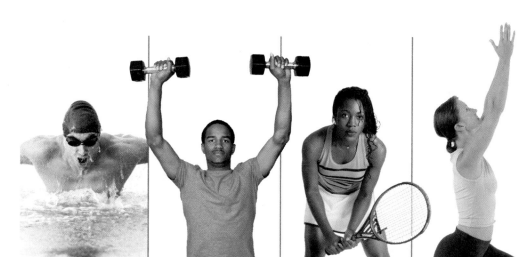

Cardiorespiratory fitness	Muscular strength	Muscular endurance	Flexibility	Body composition
Ability to sustain aerobic whole-body activity for a prolonged period of time	Maximum force able to be exerted by single contraction of a muscle or muscle group	Ability to perform muscle contractions repeatedly without fatiguing	Ability to move joints freely through their full range of motion	The relative proportions of fat mass and fat-free mass in the body

FIGURE 9.3 **Health-Related Components of Physical Fitness**

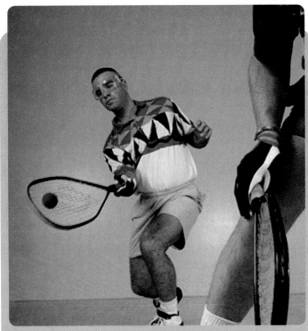

Can physical activity really reduce stress?

You bet it can! Physical activity actually stimulates the stress response, but a physically fit body adapts efficiently to the *eustress* of exercise and as a result is better able to tolerate and effectively manage *distress* of all kinds. In fact, a more physically fit body has a lower stress response and more effectively clears the chemical by-products associated with the stress response.

Muscular Endurance **Muscular endurance** is the ability of a muscle or group of muscles to exert force repeatedly without fatigue or the ability to sustain a muscular contraction. The more repetitions you can perform successfully (e.g., push-ups) or the longer you can hold a certain position (e.g., wall sit), the greater your muscular endurance. General muscular endurance is most often measured from the number of curl-ups or push-ups an individual can do. The **Assess Yourself** questionnaire found online at the text website (see the box at the end of this chapter for details) describes these tests.

Flexibility **Flexibility** refers to the range of motion, or the amount of movement possible, at a particular joint or series of joints. A larger range of motion in a joint means a greater level of flexibility in that particular body area. Various tests measure the flexibility of the body's joints, including range-of-motion tests for specific joints. One of the most common measures of general flexibility is the sit-and-reach test, described in the online Assess Yourself questionnaire.

Body Composition **Body composition** is the fifth and final component of a comprehensive fitness program. Body composition describes the relative proportions and distribution of fat and lean (muscle, bone, water, organs) tissues in the body.

muscular endurance A muscle's ability to exert force repeatedly without fatiguing or the ability to sustain a muscular contraction for a length of time.

flexibility The range of motion, or the amount of movement possible, at a particular joint or series of joints.

body composition Describes the relative proportions of fat and lean (muscle, bone, water, organs) tissues in the body.

47%

of American adults met cardiorespiratory physical activity guidelines in 2009, and 22% met muscle-strengthening physical activity guidelines; but only 19% met the guidelines for both cardiorespiratory and muscular fitness.

Physical Activity for Performance: Skill-Related Components of Physical Fitness

In addition to the five health-related components of physical fitness, physical fitness for athletes also involves attributes that improve their ability to perform athletic tasks. These attributes, called the *skill-related components* of physical fitness, can also help recreational athletes and general exercisers increase fitness levels and their ability to perform daily tasks. The skill-related components of physical fitness (also called sport skills) are *agility, balance, coordination, power, speed,* and *reaction time.*

Athletes will undertake specific exercises to increase their sport skills, and regular training results in significant improvements. Improving your sport skills can be as easy as participating regularly in any sport or activity. Playing football will increase reaction time and power, while dancing will increase balance, agility, and coordination. Another way to increase sport skills is to perform drills that mimic a sport-specific skill or work specifically on any of the skill-related components of fitness. You can practice

If you want to lose weight, you need to move more and move often!

drills in group exercise classes that incorporate sport skills, or you can work with a personal trainer.

Committing to Physical Fitness

What If I Have Been Inactive for a While?

If you have been physically inactive for the past few months or longer, first make sure that your physician clears you for exercise. Consider consulting a personal trainer or fitness instructor to help you get started. In this phase of your fitness program, known as *preconditioning,* you may begin at levels lower than those recommended for physical fitness. Starting slowly will ease you into a workout regime with a minimum of soreness. For example, you might start your cardiorespiratory program by simply getting moving each day. Take the stairs instead of the elevator, walk farther from your car to the store, and plan for organized movement each day, such as a 10- to 15-minute walk. In addition, you can start your muscle fitness program with simple body weight exercises, emphasizing proper technique and body alignment before adding any resistance.

Overcome Common Obstacles to Physical Activity

People give many excuses to explain why they do not exercise, ranging from personal ("I do not have time") to environmental ("I do not have a safe place to be active"). Some people may be reluctant to exercise if they are overweight, are embarrassed to work out with their more "fit" friends, or feel they lack the knowledge and skills required.

What keeps you from being more physically active? Think about your obstacles and write them down. Once you honestly evaluate why you are not as physically active as you want to be, review Table 9.2 for suggestions on overcoming your hurdles.

what do you think?
● Why is it hard to overcome your obstacles and get more physically active?
● What would be the immediate "pay-off" to getting active this week?

TABLE 9.2 | Overcoming Obstacles to Physical Activity

Obstacle	Possible Solution
Lack of time	• Look at your schedule. Where can you find 30-minute time slots? Perhaps you need to focus on shorter times (10 minutes or more) throughout the day. • Multitask. Read while riding an exercise bike or listen to lectures or podcasts while walking. • Be physically active during your lunch and study breaks as well as between classes. Skip rope or throw a Frisbee with a friend. • Select activities that require less time, such as brisk walking or jogging. • Ride your bike to class, or park (or get off the bus) farther from your destination.
Social influence	• Invite family and friends to be active with you. • Join a class to meet new people. • Explain the importance of exercise and your commitment to physical activity to people who may not support your efforts. • Find a role model to support your efforts. • Plan for physically active dates—go dancing or bowling.
Lack of motivation, willpower, or energy	• Schedule your workout time just as you would any other important commitment. • Enlist the help of an exercise partner to make you accountable for working out. • Give yourself an incentive. • Schedule your workouts when you feel most energetic. • Remind yourself that exercise gives you more energy. • Get things ready for your workout; for example, if you walk in the morning, set out your walking clothes the night before. Or pack your gym bag before going to bed.
Lack of resources	• Select an activity that requires minimal equipment, such as walking, jogging, jumping rope, or calisthenics. • Identify inexpensive resources on campus or in the community. • Use active forms of transportation. • Take advantage of no-cost opportunities, such as playing catch in the park/green space on campus.

Source: Adapted from National Center for Chronic Disease Prevention and Health Promotion, "How Can I Overcome Barriers to Physical Activity?" Updated February 2011, www.cdc.gov/physicalactivity/everyone/getactive/barriers.html.

BE HEALTHY, BE GREEN

TRANSPORT YOURSELF!

Before we became a car culture, much of our transportation was human powered. Historically, bicycling and walking were important means of transportation and recreation in the United States. These modes not only helped keep people in good physical shape, but they also had little impact on the environment. Since World War II, however, the development of automobile-oriented communities has led to a steady decline of bicycling and walking. Currently, only about 10 percent of trips are made by foot or bike.

The more we use our cars to get around, the more congested our roads, the more polluted our air, and the more sedentary we become. That is why many people are embracing a movement toward more active transportation. *Active transportation* means getting out of your car and using your own power to get from place to place—whether walking, riding a bike, skateboarding, or roller skating. Here are just a few of the many reasons to make active transportation a bigger part of your life:

✳ **You will be adding more exercise into your daily routine.** People who use active forms of transportation to complete errands are more likely to meet physical activity guidelines.

✳ **Walking or biking can save you money.** With rising gas prices, parking rates, car maintenance costs, and insurance payments, fewer automobile trips could add up to considerable savings. During the course of a year, bicycle commuters who ride 5 miles to work can save about $500 on fuel and more than $1,000 on other expenses related to driving.

✳ **Walking or biking may save you time!** Cycling is usually the fastest mode of travel door to door for distances up to 6 miles in city centers. Walking is simpler and faster for distances of about a mile.

✳ **You will enjoy being outdoors.** Research is emerging on the physical and mental health benefits of nature and being outdoors. So much of what we do is inside, with recirculated air and artificial lighting, that our bodies are deficient in fresh air and sunlight.

✳ **You will make a significant contribution to reducing air pollution.** Leaving your car at home just 2 days a week will reduce greenhouse gas emissions by an average of 1,600 pounds per year.

✳ **You will help reduce traffic.** The average traveler now wastes the equivalent of a full work week stuck in traffic every year. More active commuters means fewer cars on the roads and less traffic congestion.

✳ **You will contribute to global health.** Annually, personal transportation consumes approximately 136 billion gallons of gasoline, or the production of 1.2 billion tons of carbon dioxide. Reducing vehicle trips will help reduce overall greenhouse gas emissions and the need to source more fossil fuel.

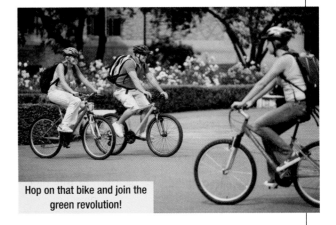

Hop on that bike and join the green revolution!

Source: T. Gotschi and K. Mills, *Active Transportation for America: The Case for Increased Federal Investment in Bicycling and Walking* (Washington, DC: Rails to Trails Conservancy, 2008), Available at www.railstotrails.org/ourwork/advocacy/active-transportation/makingthecase; D. Shinkle and A. Teigens, *Encouraging Bicycling and Walking: The State Legislative Role* (Washington, DC: National Conference of State Legislatures, 2008), Available at www.americantrails.org/resources/trans/Encourage-Bicycling-Walking-State-Legislative-Role.html; U.S. Environmental Protection Agency, "Climate Change: What You Can Do—On the Road," Updated May 2010, www.epa.gov/climatechange/wycd/road.html.

Incorporate Fitness into Your Life

When designing your fitness program, there are several factors to consider in order to boost your chances of achieving your goals. First, choose activities that are appropriate for you, that you genuinely like doing, and that are convenient. For example, choose jogging because you like to run and there are beautiful trails nearby versus swimming when you do not really like the water and the pool is difficult to get to. Likewise, choose activities that are suitable for your current fitness level. If you are overweight and have not exercised in months, do not sign up for advanced aerobics classes. Start slow, plan fun activities, and progress to more challenging physical activities as your physical fitness improves. You may choose to simply walk more in an attempt to achieve the recommended goal of 10,000 steps per day; keep track with a pedometer. (See Table 9.3 on page 289 for more on pedometers and other fitness equipment.) Try to make exercise a part of your routine by incorporating it into something you already have to do—such as getting to class or work. See the **Be Healthy, Be Green** box for more on using your transportation for fitness.

TABLE 9.3 | Popular Fitness Equipment

Heart Rate Monitor

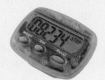

Pedometer

Stability Ball

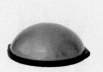

Balance Board

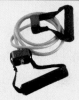

Resistance Band

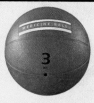

Medicine Ball

Heart Rate Monitor	Pedometer	Stability Ball	Balance Board	Resistance Band	Medicine Ball
A chest strap with a watch device that measures heart rate during training. • Provides instant and continuous feedback about the intensity of your workout. • Strap must fit well; can be uncomfortable (most women tuck the strap under the bottom strap of their sport bra). Cost: $50–$200	A battery-operated device, usually worn on your belt, that measures the number of steps taken. Some models also monitor calories, distance, and speed. • Great motivation and feedback regarding the recommended 10,000 steps per day. • Must be calibrated for your height, weight, and stride length. Cost: $25–$50	Ball made of burst-resistant vinyl that can be used for strengthening core muscles or to improve flexibility. • Balls must be inflated correctly to be most effective. Cost: $25–$50	A board with a rounded bottom that can be used to improve balance, core muscle strength, and flexibility. • Great for improving agility, coordination, reaction skills, and ankle strength. • Can be difficult initially for new users. Caution new users with weak ankles, as there is risk of straining ligaments and tendons. Cost: $40–$80	Rubber or elastic material, sometimes with handles that can be used to build muscular strength and endurance. Also can be used in yoga or Pilates to provide assistance in flexibility training. • Improves muscular strength and endurance, balance, coordination, and flexibility. • Lightweight, durable, and portable. • Breaks down over time; need to inspect regularly to avoid injury if it breaks during use. Cost: $5–$15	A heavy ball, about 14 inches in diameter, used in rehabilitation and strength training. Weight varies from 2 to 25 lb. Some made with handles. • Can be used effectively to increase explosive power. • Also used to develop core body strength. • If used incorrectly, there is potential for lower back injuries. Cost: $10–$150

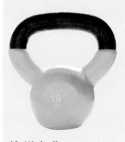

Kettlebell

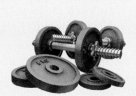

Free Weights

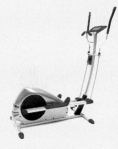

Elliptical Trainer

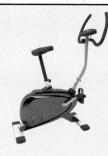

Stationary Bike

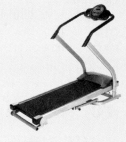

Treadmill

Kettlebell	Free Weights	Elliptical Trainer	Stationary Bike	Treadmill
A heavy ball with a handle used for full-body muscular strength and endurance exercises. Weight varies from 5 to 100 lb • Can be used effectively to increase muscular fitness, core strength, and explosive power. • Movements can be complex, and if used incorrectly, there is potential for lower back and/or wrist injuries. Cost: $10–$150	Rubber, plastic, or metal dumbbells or barbells, often with adjustable weight; can be used with a weight bench. • Traditional method for building muscular strength and endurance. • A full set allows you to increase resistance as you train, allowing for greater improvements in muscular strength. • Potential for injury if form is incorrect; must concentrate on body alignment and ensuring sufficient core body strength. Cost: $10–$300	A stationary exercise machine that simulates walking or running without impact on the bones and joints. Some machines include arm movements. • Nonimpact; less wear and tear on the joints and risk of shin splints. • Readout and programs vary. Cost: $300–$4,000	A lower-body exercise machine designed to simulate bike riding. • Generally easy to use; does not require balance. • Comes with varied resistance programs. • Recumbent styles offer less strain on back and knees and are useful for individuals struggling with back pain. Cost: $200–$2,000	Exercise machine for walking or running on a moving platform while remaining in one place. • Generally easy to use; comes with an emergency shutoff. • Different models have varied readouts and programmability. • Less impact on joints than running on most pavements. Cost: $500–$4,000

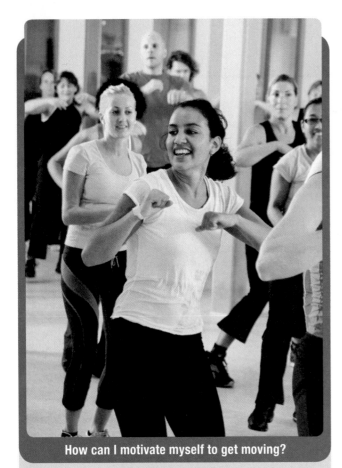

How can I motivate myself to get moving?

One great way to motivate yourself to get moving is to sign up for an exercise class. Find something that interests you—dance, yoga, aerobics, martial arts, acrobatics—and get involved. The structure, schedule, social interaction, and challenge of learning a new skill can be terrific motivators that make exercising and being physically active exciting and fun.

Create Your Own Fitness Program

FITT Acronym for **F**requency, **I**ntensity, **T**ime, and **T**ype; the terms that describe the recommended levels of exercise to improve a health-related component of physical fitness.

frequency As part of the FITT prescription, refers to how many days per week a person should exercise.

intensity As part of the FITT prescription, refers to how hard or how much effort is needed when a person exercises.

time As part of the FITT prescription, refers to how long a person needs to exercise each time.

type As part of the FITT prescription, refers to what kind of exercises a person should do.

The first step in creating a personal physical fitness program is identifying your goals. Take some time to reflect on your personal circumstances and desires regarding physical fitness. Do you want to be better at sports or feel better about your body? Is your goal to manage stress, improve health, and reduce your risk of chronic diseases? Perhaps your most vital goal will be to commit to physical fitness for the long haul—to establish a realistic schedule of diverse physical activities that you can maintain and enjoy throughout

your life. Your physical fitness goals and objectives should be both achievable for you and in line with what you truly want. Achievable, truly desired goals increase motivation, and this, in turn, leads to a better chance of success.

To set successful goals, try using the *SMART* system. SMART goals are **s**pecific, **m**easurable, **a**ction-oriented, **r**ealistic, and **t**ime-oriented.

A vague goal would be "Get into better shape by exercising more." A SMART goal would be as follows:

- *Specific*—"Start weight training."
- *Measurable*—"Increase the amount of weight I can safely lift."
- *Action-oriented*—"I'll go to the gym three times per week."
- *Realistic*—"I'll increase the weight I can lift by 20 percent (not 200 percent)."
- *Time-oriented*—"I'll try my new weight program for 8 weeks, then reassess."

Use the FITT Principle

Now that you've set realistic goals and are motivated to improve your physical fitness, the next step is to learn about the fitness recommendations and principles involved so that you can devise your own workout plan. What is the best approach to take? Where should you start? Assuming your intention is to improve your health-related physical fitness (although the principles can also be applied to performance-related physical fitness), the **FITT (frequency, intensity, time, and type)** principle should be used to define your exercise program (**Figure 9.4** on page 291):

- Exercise **frequency** refers to the number of times per week you need to engage in particular exercises to achieve the desired level of physical fitness in a particular component.
- **Intensity** refers to how hard your workout must be to achieve the desired level of physical fitness.
- How much **time**, or the *duration,* refers to how many minutes or repetitions of an exercise are required at a specified intensity during any one session.
- **Type** refers to what kind of exercises should be performed to improve the various components of physical fitness.

The FITT Principle for Cardiorespiratory Fitness

The most effective aerobic exercises for building cardiorespiratory fitness are total body activities involving the large muscle groups of your body. The FITT prescription for cardiorespiratory fitness includes 3 to 5 days per week of vigorous, rhythmic, continuous activity, at 64 to 95 percent of your estimated maximal heart rate, for 20 to 60 minutes.[28]

Frequency To improve your cardiorespiratory fitness, exercise at least three times a week at a moderate to vigorous level. If you are a newcomer to exercise, you can still improve by doing less intense exercise (light to moderate level) but doing it more

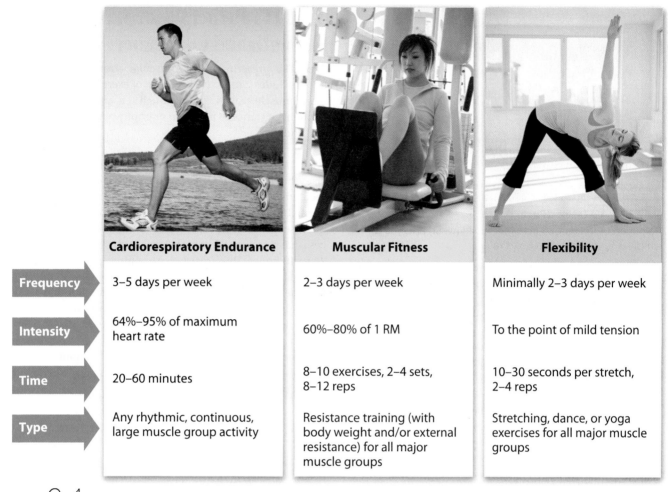

	Cardiorespiratory Endurance	**Muscular Fitness**	**Flexibility**
Frequency	3–5 days per week	2–3 days per week	Minimally 2–3 days per week
Intensity	64%–95% of maximum heart rate	60%–80% of 1 RM	To the point of mild tension
Time	20–60 minutes	8–10 exercises, 2–4 sets, 8–12 reps	10–30 seconds per stretch, 2–4 reps
Type	Any rhythmic, continuous, large muscle group activity	Resistance training (with body weight and/or external resistance) for all major muscle groups	Stretching, dance, or yoga exercises for all major muscle groups

FIGURE 9.4   **The FITT Principle Applied to Cardiorespiratory Fitness, Muscular Strength and Endurance, and Flexibility**

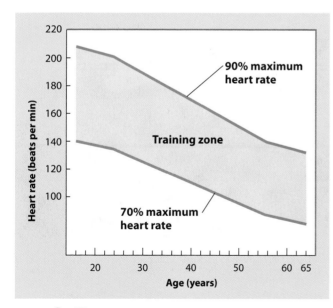

FIGURE 9.5 **Target Heart Rate Ranges**
These ranges are based on calculating the maximum heart rate as 220 – age and the training zone as 64% to 95% of maximum heart rate. Individuals with low fitness levels should start below or at the low end of these ranges.

days during a week. In this case, follow the recommendations from the Centers for Disease Control and Prevention (CDC) for moderate physical activity (refer to Table 9.1 on page 283).

Intensity The most common methods used to determine the intensity of cardiorespiratory endurance exercises are target heart rate, rating of perceived exertion, and the talk test. The exercise intensity required to improve cardiorespiratory endurance is a heart rate between 64 and 95 percent of your maximum heart rate. To calculate your **target heart rate**, start by subtracting your age from 220 to get your predicted maximum heart rate. Your target heart rate would be 64 to 96 percent of that predicted maximum heart rate. For example, if you are a 20-year-old male, your estimated maximum heart rate is 200 (220 − 20 = 200). Your target heart rate would be somewhere between 140 (200 × 0.64 = 128) and 180 (200 × 0.95 = 190) beats per minute. Figure 9.5 shows a range of target heart rates for various ages.

target heart rate The heart rate range of aerobic exercise that leads to improved cardiorespiratory fitness (i.e., 64% to 95% of maximal heart rate).

Take your pulse during your workout to determine how close you are to your target heart rate. Lightly place your index and middle fingers (not your thumb) over one of the

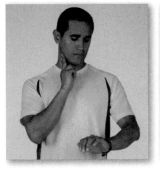

ⓐ Carotid pulse

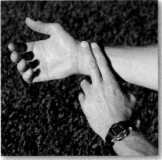

ⓑ Radial pulse

FIGURE 9.6 **Taking a Pulse**
Palpation of the carotid (neck) or radial (wrist) artery is a simple way to determine heart rate.

major arteries in your neck or on the artery on the inside of your wrist (Figure 9.6). Count your pulse while exercising, if possible, or start counting your pulse immediately after you stop exercising, as your heart rate decreases rapidly when you stop. Using a watch or a clock, take your pulse for 10 seconds (the first pulse is "0") and multiply this number by 6 to get the number of beats per minute.

Another way to determine the intensity of cardiorespiratory exercise intensity is to use Borg's rating of perceived exertion (RPE) scale. Perceived exertion refers to how hard you feel you are working, which you might base on your heart rate, breathing rate, sweating, and level of fatigue. This scale uses a rating from 6 (no exertion at all) to 20 (maximal exertion). An RPE of 12 to 16 is generally recommended for training the cardiorespiratory system.

The easiest, but least scientific, method of measuring cardiorespiratory exercise intensity is the "talk test." A "moderate" level of exercise (heart rate at 64 to 76 percent of maximum) is a conversational level of exercise. At this level you are able to talk with a partner while exercising. If you can talk but prefer brief statements, you may be at a "vigorous" level of exercise (heart rate at 77 to 95 percent of maximum). If you are breathing so hard that speaking at all is difficult, the intensity of your exercise may be too high. Conversely, if you are able to sing or laugh heartily while exercising, the intensity of your exercise is light and may be insufficient for maintaining or improving cardiorespiratory fitness.

Time For cardiorespiratory fitness benefits, the American College of Sports Medicine (ACSM) recommends that vigorous activities be performed for at least 20 minutes at a time, and moderate activities for at least 30 minutes.[29] See also the **Health in a Diverse World** box for recommendations for individuals with chronic diseases or conditions that require alterations to the FITT prescription.

Type Any sort of rhythmic, continuous, and vigorous physical activity that can be done for 20 or more minutes will improve cardiorespiratory fitness. Examples include walking briskly, cycling, jogging, fitness classes, and swimming.

The FITT Principle for Muscular Strength and Endurance

The FITT prescription for muscular strength and endurance includes 2 to 3 days per week of exercises that train the major muscle groups, using enough sets and repetitions and enough resistance to maintain or improve muscular strength and endurance.[30]

Frequency For frequency, performing eight to ten exercises that train the major muscle groups 2 to 3 days a week is recommended. It is believed that overloading the muscles, a normal part of resistance training described below, causes microscopic tears in muscle fibers, and the rebuilding process that increases the muscle's size and capacity takes about 24 to 48 hours. Thus, resistance-training exercise programs should include at least one day of rest between workouts before the same muscles are overloaded again. But don't wait too long between workouts: One of the important principles of strength training is the idea of *reversibility*. Reversibility means that if you stop exercising, the body responds by deconditioning. Even after as little as 4 days without training, muscles begin to revert to their untrained state.[31] The saying "use it or lose it" applies!

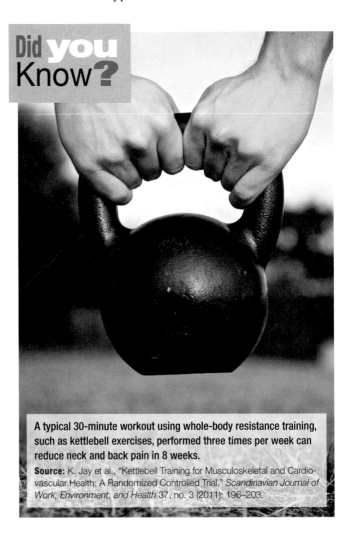

Did you Know?

A typical 30-minute workout using whole-body resistance training, such as kettlebell exercises, performed three times per week can reduce neck and back pain in 8 weeks.

Source: K. Jay et al., "Kettlebell Training for Musculoskeletal and Cardiovascular Health: A Randomized Controlled Trial," *Scandinavian Journal of Work, Environment, and Health* 37, no. 3 (2011): 196–203.

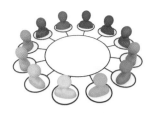
PHYSICAL ACTIVITY AND EXERCISE FOR SPECIAL POPULATIONS

In some cases, modifications to the FITT prescription may be suggested. For people with the special considerations mentioned below, as for all individuals, it is recommended that you consult with your physician before beginning any exercise program.

ASTHMA

Regular physical activity provides benefits for individuals with asthma. It strengthens the respiratory muscles, making it easier to breathe; improves immune system functioning; and helps maintain weight.

Before engaging in exercise, ensure that your asthma is under control. Ask about adjusting your medications (your doctor may recommend you use your inhaler 15 minutes prior to exercise, for example). Keep your inhaler nearby. Warm up and cool down properly; it is particularly important that you allow your lungs and breathing rate to adjust slowly. Protect yourself from your asthma triggers when exercising. If you have symptoms while exercising, stop and use your inhaler; if an asthma attack persists, call 9-1-1.

OBESITY

Obese individuals may have limitations such as heat intolerance, shortness of breath during physical activity, lack of flexibility, frequent musculoskeletal injuries, and difficulty with balance. Programs should emphasize physical activities that can be sustained for longer periods of time such as walking, swimming, or bicycling, with caution recommended for performing these activities in hot or humid environments. Although it is recommended to start slow (5 to 10 minutes of activity) and at a lower intensity (55% to 65% of maximal heart rate), the ultimate goal is to obtain at least 30 minutes per exercise session resulting in over 250 minutes per week to enhance weight loss and prevent

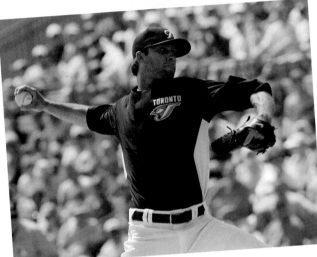

Athletes like Brandon Morrow, a Major League Baseball pitcher and a type 1 diabetic, are living proof that chronic conditions needn't prevent you from achieving your physical activity goals.

weight re-gain. Regardless of weight loss, evidence suggests that individuals who are obese improve their health with cardiorespiratory and resistance training activities.

CORONARY HEART DISEASE

Although regular physical activity reduces risk of coronary heart disease, vigorous-intensity activity acutely increases risk of sudden cardiac death and myocardial infarction (heart attack). Individuals with coronary heart disease must consult their physicians.

HYPERTENSION

Using the FITT prescription, individuals who are hypertensive should engage in physical activity on most, if not all, days of the week, at a moderate intensity (12 to 13 on the Borg RPE scale), for 30 minutes or more.

DIABETES

Physical activity benefits individuals with diabetes in many ways. It controls blood glucose (for individuals with type 2) by improving transport into the cells, controls body weight, and reduces risk for heart disease.

Before people with type 1 diabetes engage in physical activity, they must learn how to manage their resting blood glucose levels. Individuals should have an exercise partner; eat 1 to 3 hours prior to the activity; eat complex carbohydrates after the activity; avoid late-evening exercise; and monitor their blood glucose before, during, and after activity.

One of the most important factors for individuals with type 2 diabetes is the time or length of their physical activity. Because a critical objective of the management of type 2 diabetes is to reduce body fat (obesity), the recommendations for time are longer—reaching 60 minutes per session. For sessions of this length, it is prudent to reduce the intensity of the activity to a target heart rate range of 40 to 60 percent of maximal heart rate.

Sources: J. E. Donnelly et al., "American College of Sports Medicine Position Stand: Appropriate Physical Activity Intervention Strategies for Weight Loss, and Prevention of Weight Regain for Adults," *Medicine and Science in Sports and Exercise* 41, no. 2 (2009): 459–71; L. S. Pescatello et al., "American College of Sports Medicine Position Stand: Exercise and Hypertension," *Medicine and Science in Sports and Exercise* 36, no. 3 (2004): 533–53; B. A. Franklin et al., "American College of Sports Medicine and American Heart Association Joint Position Stand: Exercise and Acute Cardiovascular Events: Placing the Risks into Perspective," *Medicine and Science in Sports and Exercise* 39, no. 5 (2007): 886–97; W. J. Chodzko-Zajko et al., "American College of Sports Medicine Position Stand: Exercise and Physical Activity for Older Adults," *Medicine and Science in Sports and Exercise* 41, no. 7 (2009): 1510–30; The Canadian Lung Association, "Asthma: Exercise and Asthma," Updated April 2010, www.lung.ca/diseases-maladies/asthma-asthme/exercise-exercice/index_e.php; Office of Disease Prevention and Health Promotion, U.S. Department of Health and Human Services, *2008 Physical Activity Guidelines for Americans*, 2008.

TABLE
9.4 **Methods of Providing Muscular Resistance**

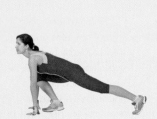

Calisthenics (Body Weight Resistance)

- Uses your own body weight to develop muscular strength and endurance.
- Improves overall muscular fitness, in particular core body strength and overall muscle tone.

Examples: Push-ups, pull-ups, curl-ups, dips, leg raises, chair sits, etc. For an extra challenge, you can do these exercises on a stability ball or balance board.

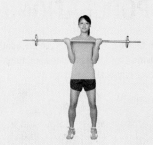

Free Weights (Fixed Resistance)

- Provides a constant resistance throughout the full range of movement.
- Requires balance and coordination; promotes development of core body strength.

Examples: Barbells, dumbbells, medicine balls, and kettlebells. Resistance bands can be used for resistance instead of weights.

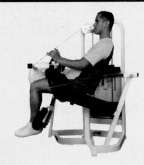

Weight Machines (Variable Resistance)

- Resistance altered so that the muscle's effort is consistent throughout the full range of motion.
- Provides more controlled motion and isolates certain muscle groups.

Examples: Weight machines in gyms, homes (Nautilus or Bowflex), and rehabilitation centers.

Intensity To determine the intensity of exercise needed to improve muscular strength and endurance, you need to know the maximum amount of weight you can lift (or move) in one contraction. This value is called your **one repetition maximum (1 RM)** and can be individually determined or predicted from a 10 RM test. Once your 1 RM is determined, it is used as the basis for intensity recommendations for improving muscular strength and endurance. Muscular strength is improved when resistance loads are greater than 60 percent of your 1 RM, whereas muscular endurance is improved using loads less than 50 percent of your 1 RM.

---
one repetition maximum (1 RM) The amount of weight or resistance that can be lifted or moved only once.

Everyone begins a resistance-training program at an initial level of strength. To become stronger, you must *overload* your muscles, that is, regularly create a degree of tension in your muscles that is greater than what they are accustomed to. Overloading them forces your muscles to adapt by getting larger, stronger, and capable of producing more tension. If you "underload" your muscles, you will not increase strength. If you create too great an overload, you may experience muscle injury, muscle fatigue, and potentially a loss in strength. Once your strength goal is reached, no further overload is necessary; your challenge at that point is to maintain your level of strength by engaging in a regular (once or twice per week) total-body resistance exercise program.

Time The time recommended for muscular strength and endurance exercises is measured not in minutes of exercise, but rather in repetitions and sets.

- **Repetitions and sets.** To increase muscular strength, you need higher intensity and fewer repetitions and sets: Use a resistance of at least 60 percent of your 1 RM (or at least 40 percent if you are new to resistance training), performing 8 to 12 repetitions per set, with two to four sets performed overall. If improving muscular endurance is your goal, use less resistance and more repetitions. The recommendations for improving muscular endurance are to perform one to two sets of 15 to 25 repetitions using a resistance that is less than 50 percent of your 1 RM.

- **Rest periods.** Varying the amount of rest between exercises is another way to adjust the intensity of your resistance training workout. Resting between exercises is crucial to reduce fatigue and help with performance and safety in subsequent sets. A rest period of 2 to 3 minutes is recommended. Note that this "rest period" refers specifically to the muscle group being exercised and it is possible to alternate muscle groups, thus taking advantage of your time available to train. For example, you can alternate a set of push-ups with curl-ups, as the muscle groups worked in one set can rest while you are working the other muscle groups.

Type To improve muscular strength or endurance, it is most often recommended that resistance training use either the body's weight or devices that provide a fixed or variable resistance (see Table 9.4). When selecting the type of strength-training exercises to do, there are three important principles to bear in mind: specificity, exercise selection, and exercise order. According to the *specificity principle,* the effects of resistance-exercise training are specific to the muscles exercised; thus to improve total body strength, include exercises for all the major muscle groups.

The second important concept is *exercise selection.* Exercises that work a single joint (e.g., bicep curls) are effective for building muscle-specific strength, while multiple-joint exercises (e.g., a squat coupled with an overhead press) are effective for increasing overall muscle strength. The ACSM recommends that while both exercise types can be included in a resistance training program, an emphasis should be placed upon multiple-joint exercises for opposing muscle groups in the lower and upper body and the trunk.[32]

Finally, for optimal training effects, pay attention to *exercise order*. When training all major muscle groups in a single workout, complete large muscle group exercises before small muscle group exercises, multiple-joint exercises before single-joint exercises, and high-intensity exercises before lower-intensity exercises.

The FITT Principle for Flexibility

Although often overshadowed by cardiorespiratory and muscular fitness training, flexibility is important. Improving your flexibility not only enhances the efficiency of your movements, it can enhance your sense of well-being, help you manage your stress effectively, and prevent or reduce pain in your joints as well. Furthermore, inflexible muscles are susceptible to injury, and flexibility training reduces the incidence and severity of lower back problems and muscle or tendon injuries that can occur during sports and everyday physical activities.[33] Improved flexibility also means less tension and pressure on joints, resulting in less joint pain

and joint deterioration.[34] This means that remaining flexible can help prevent the decreased physical function that often occurs with aging.[35] Figure 9.7 illustrates some basic stretching exercises to increase flexibility.

30 minutes of physical activity a day provide major health benefits.

Frequency The FITT principle calls for a minimum of 2 to 3 days per week for flexibility training.

Intensity Flexibility has the least formal method for identifying the intensity required for improvement. Specifically, the recommendations are that you perform or hold stretching positions at the "point of mild tension." This "point of mild tension" is individually determined. You should be able to feel tension or mild discomfort in the muscle(s) you are stretching, but the stretch should not hurt.[36]

Time The time recommended to improve flexibility is based upon time per stretch. Once you are in a stretching position, you should hold at the "point of tension" for 10 to 30 seconds for each stretch and repeat two or four times in close succession.[37]

Type The most effective exercises for increasing flexibility involve stretching the major muscle groups of your body when the body is already warm, such as after your cardiorespiratory workout. The safest exercises for improving flexibility involve **static stretching.** Static stretching techniques slowly and

static stretching Stretching techniques that slowly and gradually lengthen a muscle or group of muscles and their tendons.

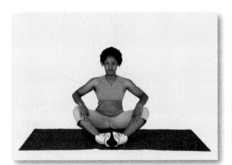

ⓐ Stretching the inside of the thighs

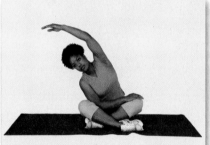

ⓑ Stretching the upper arm and the side of the trunk

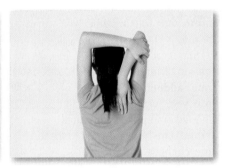

ⓒ Stretching the triceps

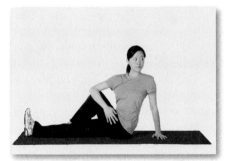

ⓓ Stretching the trunk and the hip

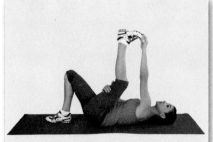

ⓔ Stretching the hip, back of the thigh, and the calf

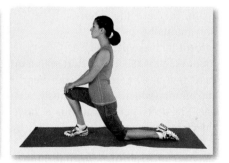

ⓕ Stretching the front of the thigh and the hip flexor

FIGURE 9.7 **Stretching Exercises to Improve Flexibility**
Use these stretches as part of your cool-down. Hold each stretch for 10 to 30 seconds and repeat two to four times.

gradually lengthen a muscle or group of muscles and their tendons. The primary strategy is to decrease the resistance to stretch (tension) within a tight muscle targeted for increased range of motion.[38] To do this, you repeatedly stretch the muscle and its two tendons of attachment to elongate them. With each repetition of a static stretch, your range of motion improves temporarily due to the slightly lessened sensitivity of tension receptors in the stretched muscles, and when done regularly, range of motion increases.[39]

Implementing Your Fitness Program

Develop a Progressive Plan

As your physical fitness improves, you will need to adjust the frequency, intensity, time, and type of your exercise to maintain or continue to improve your level of physical fitness. It is recommended that you begin an exercise regimen by picking an exercise and gradually increasing the frequency of your workouts. For week 1, you may exercise on 3 days, moving to 4 days in week 3 or 4, and so on. Once you are working out 5 or more days per week and that seems comfortable, then you increase the length of each workout. For safety and proper progression, increase your exercise time by no more than 10 percent each week. For example, if you are accustomed to walking for 20 minutes, then you would add 2 minutes to your walking time ($20 \text{ min} \times 0.10 = 2 \text{ min}$) so that you walk for a total of 22 minutes. Continue adding 10 percent until you reach the recommended amount of 30 minutes.

Once you have adjusted to these time changes and are working out 5 days per week, then you can increase the intensity of your workout. Again, increase the intensity gradually, using a 10 percent increase per week as your guideline. So, if you start with a target heart rate of 64 percent of your heart rate maximum (which, as previously shown, was 128 beats per minute for a 20-year-old male), you would increase that by 1 to 2 beats per minute each week until you reach your desired exercise intensity level.

For type of exercise, focus on variety, a fundamental principle in strength training that is also relevant to cardiorespiratory fitness and flexibility training. This principle

Resistance training to improve muscular strength and endurance can be done with free weights, machines, or even your own body weight.

identifies the need for changes in one or more parts of your workout on a regular basis, not only to produce a higher level of physical fitness (because different muscle groups are used), but also to keep you motivated and interested enough to continue training regularly.

Reevaluate your physical fitness goals and action plan monthly to ensure that the plan is still working for you. A mistake many people make when they decide to become more physically active (or to make any other behavior change) is putting so much effort into getting started that they allow their efforts to dwindle once in the action phase. Evaluate your progress, make changes if necessary, and continue to reevaluate regularly. The **Skills for Behavior Change** box on page 297 offers more tips on starting and sticking with an exercise plan.

Design Your Exercise Session

A well-designed exercise program should improve or maintain cardiorespiratory fitness, muscular strength and endurance, flexibility, and body composition. But what should you do when you begin your exercise routine? A comprehensive workout would include a warm-up, cardiorespiratory and/or resistance training, and then a cool-down to finish the session.

Warm-Up The warm-up prepares the body physically and mentally for the cardiorespiratory and/or resistance training that is to follow. A warm-up should involve large body movements, generally using light cardiorespiratory activities, followed by range-of-motion exercises of the muscle groups to be used during the exercise session. A warm-up usually lasts 5 to 15 minutes, but it is shorter when you are geared up and ready to go and longer when you are struggling with your motivation to get moving or your muscles are feeling

What's Working for You?

Maybe you're already improving your physical fitness. Which of the following are you already incorporating into your life?

- [ ] I go for a run several times a week.
- [ ] I bike to my classes.
- [ ] I participate in an intercollegiate or intramural sport.
- [ ] I go for hikes on the weekends.
- [ ] I lift weights at the gym several times a week.

what do you think?

What does "realistic goal" mean to you?

● How soon do you expect to see results from your increased activity levels?

● How can you change your food or fluid intake to enhance your fitness?

"cold" or tight. The important thing is to listen to your body and take the time needed to prepare for more intense activity. The warm-up provides a transition from rest to physical activity by slowly increasing heart rate, blood pressure, breathing rate, and body temperature. These gradual changes improve joint lubrication, increase muscle and tendon elasticity, and enhance blood flow throughout the body, facilitating performance during the next stage of the workout.

Cardiorespiratory and/or Resistance Training Immediately following your warm-up, move into the next stage of your workout. This stage may involve cardiorespiratory training, resistance training, or a little of both. If you are in a fitness center, you may choose to use one or more of the aerobic training devices for the recommended time frame. Before or after cardiorespiratory training, you may choose to follow your prescribed program for muscular strength and endurance

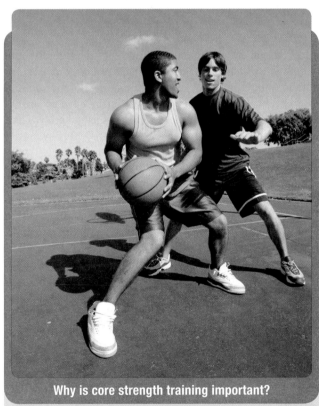

Why is core strength training important?

Your core muscles are essential for supporting your spine in everything you do—from standing to sitting, from dancing to playing basketball. Core muscles work together to effectively transmit forces between your upper and lower body, allowing you to twist, jump, lift, bend, and change directions. While weak core muscles can lead to back pain, strong core muscles can prevent back pain and improve physical performance in all of your activities.

Plan It, Start It, Stick with It!

The most successful physical activity program is one that is realistic and appropriate for your skill level and needs.

❭ **Make it enjoyable.** Pick something you like to do so you will make the effort and find the time to do it.

❭ **Start slowly.** If you have been physically inactive for a while or are a first-time exerciser, any type and amount of physical activity is a step in the right direction. Keep in mind that it is an achievement to get to the fitness center or to put your sneakers on for a walk! Make sure you start slowly—in fact, 5 minutes of walking or exercise may be plenty—letting your body adapt so that your new physical activity or exercise does not cause excess pain the next day (a real reaction to using muscles you have not used much or as intensely before). Do not be discouraged; you will be able to increase your activity each week and soon you will be on your way to meeting the physical activity recommendations and your personal physical fitness goals!

❭ **Make only one lifestyle change at a time.** It is not realistic to change everything at once. Furthermore, success with one behavioral change will increase your confidence and encourage you to make other positive changes.

❭ **Set reasonable expectations for yourself and your physical fitness program.** You will not become "fit" overnight. It takes several months to really feel the benefits of new physical activity. Be patient.

❭ **Choose a time to exercise and stick with it.** Set priorities and keep to a schedule. Try exercising at different times of the day to learn what works best for you. Yet, be flexible, so if something comes up that you cannot work around, you will find time later that day or evening to do some physical activity. Be careful of an all-or-none attitude.

❭ **Keep a record of your progress.** Include the intensity, time, and type of physical activity, your emotions, and your personal achievements.

❭ **Take lapses in stride.** Sometimes life gets in the way. Start again and do not despair; your commitment to physical fitness has ebbs and flows like everything else in life.

training. Regardless of what you choose, the bulk of the workout occurs in this section and can last 20 to 30 minutes or more.

Cool-Down and Stretching Just as you ease into a workout with a warm-up, you should slowly transition from activity to rest. A cool-down is an essential component of a fitness program involving another 10 to 15 minutes of activity time. Start your cool-down with 5 to 10 minutes of moderate- to low-intensity activity, and follow it with approximately 10 minutes of stretching. Because of the body's increased temperature, the cool-down is an excellent time to stretch to improve flexibility. The purpose of the cool-down is to gradually reduce your heart rate, blood pressure, and body temperature to pre-exercise levels. In addition, the cool-down reduces the risk of blood pooling in the extremities and facilitates quicker recovery between exercise sessions.

Explore Fitness Activities

Some forms of activity have the potential to improve several components of physical fitness and thus improve your everyday functioning ("functional" exercises). For example, yoga, tai chi, and Pilates improve flexibility, muscular strength and endurance, balance, coordination, and agility. They also focus on the mind–body connection through concentration on breathing and body position. Some people see these activities as strongly connected to the development of their spiritual health as well, particularly when time is spent relaxing, breathing deeply, and trying to clear the mind.

Core Strength Training Before we explore yoga, tai chi, and Pilates, let's consider core strength for a moment. The body's core muscles are the foundation for all movement.[40] These muscles include the deep back, abdominal, and hip muscles that attach to the spine and pelvis. The contraction of these muscles provides the basis of support for movements of the upper and lower body and powerful movements of the extremities. A weak core generally results in poor posture, low back pain, and muscle injuries. A strong core provides a more stable center of gravity and as a result more stable platform for movements, thus reducing the chance of injury.

You can develop core strength by doing various exercises, including calisthenics, yoga, or Pilates. Holding yourself in a front or reverse plank ("up" and reverse of a push-up position) and holding or doing abdominal curl-ups are examples of exercises that increase core strength. Increasing core strength does not happen from one single exercise, but rather from a structured regime of postures and exercises.[41] The use of instability devices (stability ball, wobble boards, etc.) and exercises to train the core have become popular.[42] Although research suggests instability training is effective for improving core strength and reducing back pain, it should not replace traditional programs completely; it should rather be used in conjunction with and become part of the FITT prescription.[43]

Yoga Yoga originated in India about 5,000 years ago. It blends the mental and physical aspects of exercise, a union of mind and body that participants often find relaxing and satisfying. If done regularly, yoga improves flexibility, vitality, posture, agility, balance, coordination, and muscular strength and endurance. Many people also report an improved sense of general well-being.

The practice of yoga focuses attention on controlled breathing

and physical exercise, and it incorporates a complex array of static stretching and balance exercises expressed as postures (*asanas*). During a session, participants move to different asanas and hold them for 30 seconds or longer. Asanas, singly or in combination, can be changed and adapted for young and old or to accommodate physical limitations or disabilities. Asanas can also be combined to provide well-conditioned athletes with a challenging workout!

Some forms of yoga are more meditative in their practice, whereas other forms, such as Ashtanga and Bikram, are more athletic. *Ashtanga yoga,* also called "power yoga," is an energetic form of yoga that focuses on a series of poses done in a continuous, repeated flow, with controlled breathing. *Bikram yoga,* also known as *hot yoga,* is unique in that classes are held in rooms heated to 105°F. The theory behind this practice is that performing yoga in a "hot" environment allows the muscles to easily stretch to their point of tension with a greater potential for increasing flexibility.

Tai Chi Tai chi is an ancient Chinese form of exercise that combines stretching, balance, muscular endurance, coordination, and meditation. It increases range of motion and flexibility while reducing muscular tension. Based on Qigong, a Taoist philosophy dedicated to spiritual growth and good health, tai chi was developed about AD 1000 by monks who wanted to defend themselves against bandits and warlords. It involves a series of positions called *forms* that are performed continuously. Tai chi is often described as "meditation in motion" because it promotes serenity through gentle movements, connecting the mind and body.

Pilates Developed by Joseph Pilates in 1926, Pilates is an exercise style that combines stretching with movement against resistance, frequently aided by devices such as tension springs or heavy rubber bands. It teaches body awareness, good posture,

Tai chi and other styles of exercise that strengthen core body muscles can also enhance flexibility and help lower stress levels.

and easy and graceful body movements while improving flexibility, coordination, core strength, muscle tone, and economy of motion.

Pilates differs from yoga and tai chi in that it includes a component specifically designed to increase strength. The method consists of a sequence of carefully performed movements. Some are carried out on specially designed equipment, whereas others can be performed on mats. Each exercise stretches and strengthens the muscles involved and has a specific breathing pattern associated with it.

Taking in Proper Nutrition for Exercise

Foods for Exercise and Recovery

To make the most of your workouts, follow the recommendations from the MyPlate plan, and make sure that you eat sufficient carbohydrates, the body's main source of fuel. Your body stores carbohydrates as glycogen primarily in the muscles and liver and then uses this stored glycogen for energy when you are physically active. Fats are also an important source of energy, packing more than double the energy per gram compared to carbohydrates. Protein plays a role in muscle repair and growth, but is not normally a source of energy.

When you eat is almost as important as what you eat. Eating a large meal before exercising can cause upset stomach, cramping, and diarrhea, because your muscles have to compete with your digestive system for energy. After a large meal, wait 3 to 4 hours before you begin exercising. Smaller meals (snacks) can be eaten about an hour before activity. Not eating at all before a workout can cause low blood sugar levels that in turn cause weakness and slower reaction times.

It is also important to refuel after your workout. Help your muscles recover and prepare for the next bout of activity by eating a snack or meal that contains plenty of carbohydrates and a little protein, too. Today there is a burgeoning market for dietary supplements that claim to deliver the nutrients needed for muscle recovery, as well as additional "performance-enhancing" ingredients; see Table 9.5 on page 300 for some of the most popular performance-enhancing drugs and supplements, their purported benefits, and associated risks.

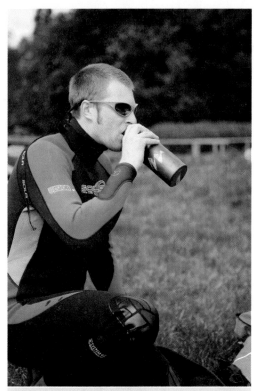

The American College of Sports Medicine and the National Athletic Trainers' Association recommend consuming 14 to 22 ounces of fluid several hours prior to exercise and about 6 to 12 ounces per 15 to 20 minutes during—assuming you are sweating.

Fluids for Exercise and Recovery

In addition to eating well, staying hydrated is also crucial. How much fluid do you need? Keep in mind that the goal of fluid replacement is to prevent excessive dehydration (greater than 2% loss of body weight). The ACSM and the National Athletic Trainers Association recommend consuming 5 to 7 milliliters per kilogram of body weight (approximately 0.7 to 1.07 oz per 10 lb body weight) 4 hours prior to exercise.[44] Drinking fluids during exercise is also important, but it is difficult to provide guidelines for how much or when because intake should be based on time, intensity, and type of activity performed. A good way to monitor how much fluid you need to replace is to weigh yourself before and after your workout. The difference in weight is how much you should drink. So, for example, if you lost 2 pounds during a training session, you should drink 32 ounces of fluid.[45]

What are the best fluids to drink? For exercise sessions lasting less than 1 hour, plain water is sufficient for rehydration. If your exercise session exceeds 1 hour—and you sweat profusely—consider a sports drink containing electrolytes. The electrolytes in these products are minerals and ions such as sodium and potassium that are needed for proper functioning of your nervous and muscular systems. Replacing electrolytes is particularly important for endurance athletes engaging in long bouts of exercise or competition. In endurance events lasting more than 4 hours, an athlete's overconsumption of plain water can dilute the sodium concentration in the blood with potentially fatal results, an effect called **hyponatremia** or **water intoxication**.

hyponatremia or water intoxication Overconsumption of water, which leads to a dilution of sodium concentration in the blood with potentially fatal results.

What is the best choice to replenish fluids after a workout? Although water is the best choice in most cases, there are situations in which you might need to choose something different. Some people are likely to consume more when their drink is flavored, a point that may be significant in ensuring proper hydration. Recently, research has considered chocolate milk as a recovery drink. Chocolate milk is a liquid that not only hydrates, but also is a source of sodium, potassium, carbohydrates, and protein. Consuming carbohydrates and protein immediately after exercise will help replenish muscle and liver glycogen stores and stimulate muscle protein synthesis for better recovery from

Performance-Enhancing Dietary Supplements and Drugs—Their Uses and Effects

	Primary Uses	Side Effects
Creatine Naturally occurring compound that helps supply energy to muscle	• Improve postworkout recovery • Increase muscle mass • Increase strength • Increase power	• Weight gain, nausea, muscle cramps • Large doses can impair kidney function
Ephedra and ephedrine Stimulant that constricts blood vessels and increases blood pressure and heart rate *Illegal; banned by FDA in 2006; banned by sports organizations	• Lose weight • Increase performance	• Nausea, vomiting • Anxiety and mood changes • Hyperactivity • Rarely seizures, heart attack, stroke, psychotic episodes
Anabolic steroids Synthetic versions of the hormone testosterone *Nonmedical use is illegal; banned by major sports organizations	• Improve strength, power, and speed • Increase muscle mass	• In adolescents, stops bone growth; therefore reduced adult height • Masculinization of females; feminization of males • Mood swings • Severe acne, particularly on the back • Sexual dysfunction • Aggressive behavior • Potential heart and liver damage
Steroid precursors Substances that the body converts into anabolic steroids, e.g., androstenedione (andro), dehydroepiandrosterone (DHEA) *Nonmedical use is illegal; banned by major sports organizations	• Converted in the body to anabolic steroids to increase muscle mass	• In addition to side effects noted with anabolic steroids: • Body hair growth, increased risk of pancreatic cancer
Human growth hormone Naturally occurring hormone secreted by the pituitary gland that is essential for body growth *Nonmedical use is illegal; banned by major sports organizations	• Antiaging agent • Improve performance • Increase muscle mass	• Structural changes to the face • Increased risk of high blood pressure • Potential for congestive heart failure

Sources: Mayo Clinic Staff, "Performance-Enhancing Drugs and Your Teen Athlete," MayoClinic.com, January 2009, www.mayoclinic.com/health/performance-enhancing-drugs/SM00045; Office of Diversion Control, Drug and Chemical Evaluation Section, "Drugs and Chemicals of Concern: Human Growth Hormone," August 2009, www.deadiversion.usdoj.gov/drugs_concern/hgh.htm; Office of Dietary Supplements, National Institutes of Health, "Ephedra and Ephedrine Alkaloids for Weight Loss and Athletic Performance," Updated July 2010, http://ods.od.nih.gov/factsheets/EphedraandEphedrine.

traumatic injuries Injuries that are accidental and occur suddenly and violently.

overuse injuries Injuries that result from the cumulative effects of day-after-day stresses placed on tendons, muscles, and joints.

exercise. The protein in milk, whey protein, is ideal because it contains all of the essential amino acids and is rapidly absorbed by the body. Low-fat chocolate milk provides a low-cost way to hydrate and recover after exercise.

Preventing and Treating Common Exercise Injuries

There are two basic types of exercise injuries: traumatic and overuse injuries. **Traumatic injuries** occur suddenly

and violently, typically by accident. Typical traumatic injuries are broken bones, torn ligaments and muscles, contusions, and lacerations. Many traumatic injuries are unavoidable—for example, spraining your ankle by landing on another person's foot after jumping up for a rebound in basketball. Others are preventable through proper training, appropriate equipment and clothing, and common sense. If your traumatic injury causes a noticeable loss of function and immediate pain or pain that does not go away after 30 minutes, consult a physician.

Overtraining is the most frequent cause of injuries related to physical fitness training. Doing too much intense exercise, too much exercise without variation, or not allowing for sufficient rest and recovery time increase the likelihood of **overuse injuries.** Overuse injuries occur because of cumulative, day-after-day stresses placed on tendons, muscles, and joints.

Common Overuse Injuries

Three of the most common overuse injuries are plantar fasciitis, shin splints, and runner's knee.

Plantar Fasciitis *Plantar fasciitis* is an inflammation of the plantar fascia, a broad band of dense, inelastic tissue (fascia) that runs from the heel to the toe on the bottom of your foot. The main function of the plantar fascia is to protect the nerves, blood vessels, and muscles of the foot from injury. In repetitive weight-bearing physical activities such as walking and running, the plantar fascia may become inflamed. Common symptoms are pain and tenderness under the ball of the foot, at the heel, or at both locations.[46] The pain of plantar fasciitis is particularly noticeable during your first steps in the morning. If not treated properly, this injury may progress until weight-bearing activities are too painful to endure.

Shin Splints *Shin splints,* a general term for any pain that occurs on the front part of the lower legs, describes more than 20 different medical conditions. The most common type of shin splints occurs along the inner side of the tibia and is usually a combination of muscle irritation and irritation of the tissues that attach the muscles to the bone. Specific pain on the tibia or on the fibula (the adjacent smaller bone) should be examined for a possible stress fracture.

Sedentary people who start a new weight-bearing physical activity program are at the greatest risk for shin splints, although even well-conditioned aerobic exercisers who rapidly increase their distance or pace may also be at risk.[47] Running and exercise classes are the most frequent cause of shin splints, but those who do a great deal of walking (such as postal carriers and restaurant workers) may also develop them.

Runner's Knee *Runner's knee* describes a series of problems involving the muscles, tendons, and ligaments of the knee. The most common cause is abnormal movements of the patella (or kneecap), and women are more commonly affected due to greater dynamic flexibility in their hips and knees. In women (and some men), the abnormal patella

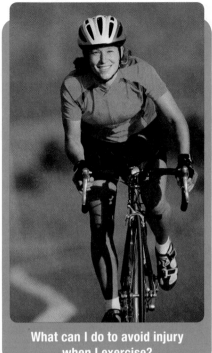

What can I do to avoid injury when I exercise?

Reducing risk for exercise injuries requires common sense and some preventative measures. Wear protective gear (helmets, knee pads, elbow pads, eyewear) and footwear that is appropriate for your activity. Vary your activities to avoid overuse injuries. Dress for the weather, try to avoid exercising in extreme conditions, and always stay properly hydrated. Finally, respect your personal physical limitations, listen to your body, and if needed, reevaluate and change your exercise program.

movements irritate the cartilage on the back of the patella and nearby tendons and ligaments. The main symptom is the pain experienced when downward pressure is applied to the kneecap after the knee is straightened fully. Additional symptoms include pain, swelling, redness, and tenderness around the patella, and a dull aching pain in the center of the knee.[48]

Prevent Exercise Injuries

There are steps you can take to reduce your risk of overuse or traumatic injuries. Use common sense and the proper gear and equipment. Vary your physical activities throughout the week, setting appropriate and realistic short- and long-term goals. Listen to your body when working out. Warning signs include muscle stiffness and soreness, bone and joint pains, and whole-body fatigue that simply does not go away.

Appropriate Footwear Proper footwear can decrease the likelihood of foot, knee, or back injuries. Biomechanics research has revealed that running is a collision sport—with each stride, the runner's foot collides with the ground with a force three to five times the runner's body weight.[49] The force not absorbed by the running shoe is transmitted upward into the foot, leg, thigh, and back. Our bodies can absorb forces such as these but may be injured by the cumulative effect of repetitive impacts (such as running 40 miles per week). Thus, the shoes' ability to absorb shock is critical—not just for runners, but for anyone engaged in weight-bearing activities.

In addition to absorbing shock, an athletic shoe should provide a good fit for maximal comfort and performance. To get the best fit, shop at a sports or fitness specialty store where there is a large selection and the salespeople are trained in properly fitting athletic shoes. Try on shoes later in the day when your feet are largest, and check to make sure there is a little extra room in the toe and that the width is appropriate. Because different

what do you think?

In what ways do your physical activities put you at risk of injury?

● What changes can you make in terms of your training program, equipment, or footwear to reduce these risks?

activities place different stresses on your feet and joints, you should choose shoes specifically designed for your sport or activity. Shoes of any type should be replaced once they lose their cushioning. Continuing to use a shoe that is worn out will increase your risk of injury. Replace athletic shoes after 6 to 9 months of moderate use or after 3 to 6 months of heavy use.

Appropriate Protective Equipment It is essential to use well-fitted, appropriate protective equipment for your physical activities. For example, using the correct racquet with the proper tension helps prevent the general inflammatory condition known as "tennis elbow." As another example, eye injuries can occur in virtually all physical activities, although some are more risky than others. As many as 90 percent of the eye injuries resulting from racquetball and squash could be prevented by wearing appropriate eye protection, such as goggles with polycarbonate lenses.[50]

> **heat cramps** Involuntary and forcible muscle contractions that occur during or following exercise in hot and/or humid weather.
>
> **heat exhaustion** A heat stress illness caused by significant dehydration resulting from exercise in hot and/or humid conditions.
>
> **heatstroke** A deadly heat stress illness resulting from dehydration and overexertion in hot and/or humid conditions.

Wearing a helmet while bicycle riding is an important safety precaution. An estimated 45 to 88 percent of head injuries among cyclists can be prevented by wearing a helmet. Of the college students who rode a bike in the past 12 months, 43 percent reported never wearing a helmet, and 22.8% said they wore one only sometimes or rarely.[51] The direct medical costs from cyclists' failure to wear helmets is an estimated $81 million a year.[52] Cyclists aren't the only ones who should be wearing helmets. People who skateboard, ski, in-line skate, snowboard, play contact sports, or use kick-scooters should also wear helmets. Look for helmets that meet the standards established by the American National Standards Institute or the Snell Memorial Foundation. The **Money & Health** box on page 303 offers suggestions for evaluating and choosing a fitness center, equipment, and fitness clothing.

Exercising in the Heat Exercising in hot or humid weather increases your risk of a heat-related injury. In these conditions, your body's rate of heat production can exceed its ability to cool itself. The three different heat stress illnesses, progressive in their level of severity, are heat cramps, heat exhaustion, and heatstroke.

Heat cramps (heat-related involuntary and forcible muscle contractions that cannot be relaxed), the least serious problem, can usually be prevented by adequate fluid replacement and a dietary intake that includes the electrolytes lost through sweating. **Heat exhaustion** is actually a mild form of shock, in which the blood pools in the arms and legs away from the brain and major organs of the body. It is caused by excessive water loss because of intense or prolonged exercise or work in a hot and/or humid environment. Symptoms of heat exhaustion include nausea, headache, fatigue, dizziness and faintness, and, paradoxically, "goosebumps" and chills. When suffering from heat exhaustion, your skin will be cool and moist. **Heatstroke**, often called *sunstroke,* is a life-threatening emergency condition with a high morbidity and mortality rate.[53] Heatstroke occurs during vigorous exercise when the body's heat production significantly exceeds its cooling capacities. Core body temperature can rise from normal (98.6°F) to 105°F to 110°F within minutes after the body's cooling mechanism shuts down. A rapid increase in core body temperature can cause brain damage, permanent disability, and death. Common signs of heatstroke are dry, hot, and usually red skin; very high body temperature; and rapid heart rate. If you experience any of the symptoms mentioned here, stop exercising immediately. Move to the shade or a cool spot to rest and drink plenty of cool fluids for heat cramps and exhaustion. If heatstroke is suspected, seek medical attention immediately.

Heat stress illnesses may also occur in situations in which the danger is not so obvious. Serious or fatal heat stroke may result from prolonged immersion in a sauna, hot tub, or steam bath or from exercising in a plastic or rubber head-to-toe "sauna suit." Similarly, exercising or training in the heat with lots of heavy clothing and equipment, such as a football uniform, including the helmet, puts an individual at risk.[54]

You can prevent heat stress by following certain precautions. First, acclimatize yourself to hot or humid conditions. The process of heat acclimatization, which increases your body's cooling efficiency, requires about 10 to 14 days of gradually increased physical activity in the hot environment. Second, reduce your risk of dehydration by replacing fluids before, during, and after exercise. Third, wear clothing appropriate for the activity and the environment—for example, light-colored nylon shorts and a mesh tank top. Finally, use common sense—for example, on a day when the temperature

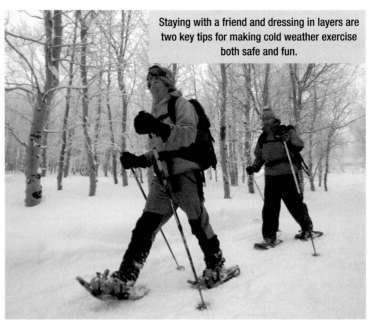

Staying with a friend and dressing in layers are two key tips for making cold weather exercise both safe and fun.

Money&Health

INVESTING IN YOUR PHYSICAL HEALTH! HOW TO SHOP FOR FITNESS FACILITIES, EQUIPMENT, AND CLOTHING

Do you really need to belong to the best gym or have the latest equipment and fashionable clothing to meet your physical fitness goals? The short answer is no. You can achieve your personal goals without joining a fitness center, without buying equipment, and without spending lots of money on the latest fitness fashions. All you need is a good pair of shoes, comfortable clothing to suit the environment you will be physically active in, your own body to use as resistance, and a safe place for activity. However, you may enjoy the experience of going to a wellness center or prefer to buy exercise equipment for your home, and you may need new exercise clothing. Use the following tips to help guide you through this process.

CHOOSING A FACILITY

✳ Visit several facilities before making a decision, if possible during the time when you intend to use them (so you can see how busy or crowded they are at that time).
✳ Determine the location and hours of operation; are these convenient for you?
✳ Consider the exercise classes offered. What is the schedule? Can you try one for free?
✳ Evaluate their equipment. Is it sufficient to cover your training needs (i.e., aerobic exercise machines, resistance-training equipment, including both free weights and machines, mats, and other items to assist with stretching)?

Before you sign on the dotted line, check out the classes, equipment, and personnel a fitness center offers.

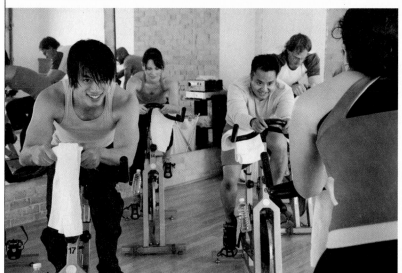

✳ Consider the personnel (including training in first aid and CPR), options for working with a personal trainer, and how friendly and approachable they are.
✳ Consider the financial implications. What membership benefits, student rates, or other discounts are available? Steer clear of clubs that pressure you for a long-term commitment and do not offer trial memberships or grace periods that allow you to get a refund.

BUYING EQUIPMENT

✳ Ignore claims that an exercise device provides lasting "no sweat" results in a short time.
✳ Question claims that an exercise device can target or burn fat.
✳ Read the fine print. Advertised results may be based on more than just using this machine; they may also involve caloric restriction.
✳ Be skeptical of testimonials and before-and-after pictures of satisfied customers.
✳ Calculate the total cost by including shipping and handling fees, sales tax, delivery and setup charges, or long-term commitments.
✳ Ask about warranties, guarantees, and return policies.
✳ Try the equipment at a gym, if you can, or borrow it from someone.
✳ Consider how this piece of equipment will fit in your home. Where will you store it? Will you be able to get to it easily?
✳ Check out consumer reviews or online resources for the best product ratings.

BUYING EXERCISE CLOTHING

✳ Choose your exercise clothing based on comfort, not looks. It should be neither too loose nor too tight.
✳ Consider the environment (temperature, humidity, ventilation) when making your selection.
✳ Dress in layers, ensuring that your skin can breathe in the cold (see also the section Exercising in the Cold).
✳ Dress to allow for optimal heat dissipation in hot and humid environments (see also the section Exercising in the Heat).
✳ Choose clothing that helps you to feel good about yourself and the activity you are undertaking.

is 85°F and the humidity is 80 percent, postpone your lunchtime run until the evening when it is cooler.

Exercising in the Cold

When you exercise in cool weather, especially in windy conditions, your body's rate of heat loss is frequently greater than its rate of heat production. These conditions may lead to **hypothermia**—a situation where the body's core temperature drops below 95°F.[55] Temperatures need not be frigid for hypothermia to occur; it can also result from prolonged, vigorous exercise in 40°F to 50°F temperatures, particularly if there is rain, snow, or a strong wind.

As body core temperature drops from its normal 98.6°F to about 93.2°F, shivering begins. Shivering—the involuntary contraction of nearly every muscle in the body—increases body temperature by using the heat given off by muscle activity. You may also experience cold hands and feet, poor judgment, apathy, and amnesia. Shivering ceases in most hypothermia victims as body core temperatures drop to between 87°F and 90°F, a sign that the body has lost its ability to generate heat. Death usually occurs at body core temperatures between 75°F and 80°F.[56]

To prevent hypothermia, analyze weather conditions before engaging in outdoor physical activity. Remember that wind and humidity are as significant as temperature. Have a friend join you for your cold-weather outdoor activities and wear layers of appropriate clothing to prevent excessive heat loss (polypropylene or woolen undergarments, a windproof outer garment, and a wool hat and gloves). Keep your head, hands, and feet warm. Finally, do not allow yourself to become dehydrated.[57]

Treat Exercise Injuries

First-aid treatment for virtually all fitness-training related injuries involves **RICE: r**est, **i**ce, **c**ompression, and **e**levation.

- **Rest**—is required to avoid further irritation of the injured body part.
- **Ice**—is applied to relieve pain and constrict the blood vessels to reduce internal or external bleeding. To prevent frostbite, wrap the ice or cold pack in a layer of wet toweling or elastic bandage before applying to your skin. A new injury should be iced for approximately 20 minutes every hour for the first 24 to 72 hours.
- **Compression**—of the injured body part can be accomplished with a 4- or 6-inch-wide elastic bandage; this applies indirect pressure to damaged blood vessels to help stop bleeding. Be careful, though, that the compression wrap does not interfere with normal blood flow. Throbbing or pain indicates that the compression wrap should be loosened.
- **Elevation**—of an injured extremity above the level of your heart also helps control internal or external bleeding by making the blood flow upward to reach the injured area.

Applying ice to an injury such as a sprain can help relieve pain and reduce swelling, but never apply the ice directly to the skin, as that could lead to frostbite.

How Physically Fit Are You?

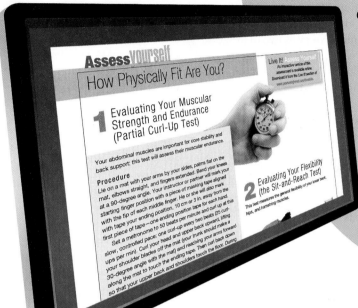

Assess yourself

How Physically Fit Are You?

1 Evaluating Your Muscular Strength and Endurance (Partial Curl-Up Test)

Your abdominal muscles are important for core stability and back support; this test will assess their muscular endurance.

Procedure
Lie on a mat with your arms by your sides, palms flat on the mat, elbows straight, and fingers extended. Bend your knees at a 90-degree angle. Your instructor or partner will mark your starting finger position with a piece of masking tape aligned with the tip of each middle finger. He or she will also mark with tape your ending position, 10 cm or 3 in. away from the first piece of tape—one ending position tape for each hand.

Set a metronome to 50 beats per minute and curl up at this slow, controlled pace: one curl-up every two beats (25 curl-ups per min). Curl your head and upper back upward, lifting your shoulder blades off the mat (your trunk should make a 30-degree angle with the mat) and reaching your arms forward along the mat to touch the ending tape. Then curl back down so that your upper back and shoulders touch the floor. During

2 Evaluating Your Flexibility (the Sit-and-Reach Test)

This test measures the general flexibility of your lower back, hips, and hamstring muscles.

Live It! Assess Yourself
An interactive version of this assessment is available online. Download it from the Live It! section of www.pearsonhighered.com/donatelle.

Go online to the **Live It!** section of www.pearsonhighered.com/donatelle for an assessment that will help you evaluate your fitness level.* To make improvements, follow the plan outlined in the **YOUR PLAN FOR CHANGE** box.

*If your instructor so chooses, Assess Yourself Activities are available as a printed supplement or as assignable homework online at www.pearsonhighered.com/myhealthlab.

MyHealthLab®

YOUR PLAN FOR CHANGE

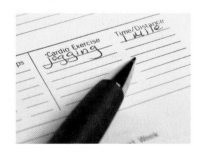

The **Assess yourself** activity mentioned above should help you determine your current level of physical fitness. Based on your results, you may decide that you should take steps to improve one or more components of your physical fitness.

Today, you can:

○ Visit your campus fitness facility (or its website) and familiarize yourself with the equipment and resources. Find out what classes they offer, and take home a copy of the schedule. Alternately, visit the website of your campus facility (if available) to find out what facilities and classes are offered.

○ Walk between your classes; make an extra effort to take the long way to get from building to building. Use the stairs instead of the elevator or escalator.

○ Take a stretch break. Spend 5 to 10 minutes between homework projects or just before bed doing some whole-body stretches to release tension.

Within the next 2 weeks, you can:

○ Shop for comfortable workout clothes and appropriate athletic footwear.

○ Look into group activities on your campus or in your community that you might enjoy.

○ Ask a friend to join you in your workout once a week. Agree on a date and time in advance so you'll both be committed to following through.

○ Plan for a physically active outing with a friend or date; perhaps you can go dancing or bowling, or shoot hoops. Use active transportation (i.e., walk or cycle) to get to a movie or go out for dinner.

By the end of the semester, you can:

○ Establish a regular routine of engaging in physical activity or exercise at least three times a week. Mark your exercise times on your calendar and keep a log to track your progress.

○ Take your workouts to the next level. If you have been working out at home, try going to a gym or participating in an exercise class. If you are walking, try walking up hills, intermittent jogging, or sign up for a fitness event such as a charity 5K.

Summary

* Health benefits of regular physical activity include reduced risk of heart attack, some cancers, hypertension, and type 2 diabetes and improved blood profile, bone mass, weight control, immunity to disease, mental health, and stress management. Regular physical activity also enhances physical fitness and may in turn increase life span.

* Physical fitness involves achieving minimal levels in the health-related components of fitness: cardiorespiratory, muscular strength, muscular endurance, flexibility, and body composition. Skill-related components of fitness, such as agility, balance, reaction time, speed, coordination, and power, are essential for elite and recreational athletes to increase performance and enjoyment in sport.

* Commit to your new lifestyle of physical activity and increased fitness levels by incorporating fitness activities into your life. If you are new to exercise, start slowly, keep your fitness program simple, and consider consulting your physician and/or a fitness instructor for recommendations. Overcome your barriers or obstacles to exercise by identifying them and then planning specific strategies to address them. Choose activities that are fun and convenient to increase your likelihood of sticking with them.

* The FITT principle can be used to develop a progressive program of physical fitness. For general health benefits, every adult should participate in moderate-intensity activities for 30 minutes at least 5 days a week. To improve cardiorespiratory fitness, you should engage in vigorous, continuous, and rhythmic activities 3 to 5 days per week at an exercise intensity of 64 to 95 percent of your maximum heart rate for 20 to 30 minutes.

* Three key principles for developing muscular strength and endurance are overload, specificity of training, and variation. Muscular strength is improved by engaging in resistance training exercises two to three times per week, using an intensity of greater than 60 percent of 1 RM and completing two to four sets of 8 to 12 repetitions. Muscular endurance is improved by engaging in resistance training exercises two to three times per week, using an intensity of less than 50 percent of 1 RM and completing one to two sets of 15 to 25 repetitions.

* Flexibility is improved by engaging in two to four repetitions of static stretching exercises at least 2 to 3 days a week, where each stretch is held for 10 to 30 seconds.

* Planning to improve your physical fitness involves setting goals and designing a program to achieve these goals. A comprehensive workout repeated regularly will increase physical fitness and should include a warm-up with some light stretching, strength-development exercises, aerobic activities, and a cool-down period with a heavier emphasis on stretching exercises. Core strength training is important for mobility, stability, and preventing back injury. The popular exercise forms of yoga, tai chi, and Pilates all develop core strength as well as flexibility, strength, and endurance.

* Fueling properly for exercise involves eating a balance of healthy foods 3 to 4 hours before exercise. In exercise sessions lasting an hour or more, performance can benefit from some additional calories ingested during the exercise session. Hydrating properly for exercise is important for performance and injury prevention. Chocolate milk is a good source of carbohydrates and protein for postexercise recovery.

* Exercise injuries are generally caused by overuse or trauma; the most common are plantar fasciitis, shin splints, and runner's knee. Proper footwear and equipment can help prevent injuries. Exercising in the heat or cold requires taking special precautions. Minor exercise injuries should be treated with RICE (rest, ice, compression, and elevation).

Pop Quiz

1. The volume of oxygen consumed by the muscles during maximal exercise defines
   a. target heart rate.
   b. muscular strength.
   c. aerobic capacity.
   d. muscular endurance.

2. What is physical fitness?
   a. The ability to respond to routine physical demands
   b. Having enough physical reserves to cope with a sudden challenge
   c. A balance of cardiorespiratory, muscle, and flexibility fitness
   d. All of the above

3. Type 2 diabetes risk can be reduced by
   a. reading about it.
   b. getting your blood sugar level tested.
   c. engaging in daily physical activity.
   d. It cannot be reduced.

4. Muscular endurance is defined by your ability to
   a. contract muscles repeatedly over time.
   b. lift a heavy weight one time.
   c. hike for 8 hours.
   d. reach your toes during a muscle-stretching test.

5. The "talk test" measures
   a. exercise intensity.
   b. exercise time.
   c. exercise frequency.
   d. exercise type.

6. At the start of an exercise session you should always
    a. stretch.
    b. do 50 crunches to activate your core muscles.
    c. warm-up with light cardiorespiratory activities.
    d. eat a meal to ensure that you are fueled for the activity.

7. Theresa wants to lower her ratio of fat to her total body weight. She wants to work on her
    a. flexibility.
    b. muscular endurance.
    c. muscular strength.
    d. body composition.

8. Miguel is a cross-country runner and is therefore able to sustain moderate-intensity, whole-body activity for continuous, extended periods of time. This ability relates to what component of physical fitness?
    a. Flexibility
    b. Body composition
    c. Cardiorespiratory fitness
    d. Muscular strength and endurance

9. Janice has been lifting 95 pounds while doing three sets of ten leg curls. To become stronger, she began lifting 105 pounds while doing leg curls. What principle of strength development does this represent?
    a. Reversibility
    b. Overload
    c. Flexibility
    d. Specificity of training

10. Overuse injuries can best be prevented by
    a. monitoring the quantity and quality of your workouts.
    b. engaging in only one type of aerobic training.
    c. working out daily.
    d. working out with a friend.

Answers to these questions can be found on page A-1.

Think about It!

1. How do you define *physical fitness*? What are the key components of a physical fitness program? What should you consider when planning and starting a physical fitness program?
2. What do you do to motivate yourself to engage in physical activity on a regular basis? What and who helps you to be physically active?
3. Describe the FITT prescription for cardiorespiratory fitness, muscular strength and endurance, and flexibility training.
4. Why is flexibility important in everyday activities? What is the best time to stretch for increased flexibility?
5. Your roommate has decided to start running to improve cardiorespiratory fitness. What advice would you give to make sure your roommate gets off to a good start, does not get injured, and continues the program throughout the year?
6. Identify at least four physiological and psychological benefits of physical activity. How would you promote these benefits to nonexercisers?

Accessing Your Health on the Internet

The following websites explore further topics and issues related to personal health. For links to the websites below, visit the Companion Website for *Access to Health*, 13th Edition, at www.pearsonhighered.com/donatelle.

1. *ACSM Online.* This site is the link to the American College of Sports Medicine and all its resources. www.acsm.org
2. *American Council on Exercise.* Information is found here on exercise and disease prevention. www.acefitness.org
3. *Centers for Disease Control and Prevention, National Center for Chronic Disease Prevention and Health Promotion, Division of Nutrition, Physical Activity, and Obesity.* This site is a great resource for current information on exercise and health. www.cdc.gov/nccdphp/dnpao/index.html
4. *National Strength and Conditioning Association.* This site is a resource for personal trainers and others interested in conditioning and fitness. www.nsca.com
5. *The President's Council on Physical Fitness and Sports.* Look here for information on fitness programs. www.fitness.gov

References

1. Centers for Disease Control and Prevention, "Physical Activity Statistics," Updated February 2010, http://apps.nccd.cdc.gov/PASurveillance/StateSumResultV.asp; Centers for Disease Control and Prevention, "QuickStats: Percentage of Adults Aged ≥ 18 Years Who Engaged in Leisure Time Strengthening Activities, by Age Group and Sex—National Health Interview Survey, United States, 2008," *Morbidity and Mortality Weekly Report* 58, no. 34 (2009): 955.
2. Office of Disease Prevention and Health Promotion, U.S. Department of Health and Human Services, *2008 Physical Activity Guidelines for Americans: Be Active, Healthy, and Happy!* ODPHP Publication no. U0036 (Washington, DC: U.S. Department of Health and Human Services, 2008), www.health.gov.paguidelines; F. B. Hu, "Globalization of Diabetes: The Role of Diet, Lifestyle, and Genes," *Diabetes Care* 34, no. 6 (2011): 1249–57.
3. American College Health Association, *American College Health Association-National College Health Assessment II (ACHA-NCHA II) Reference Group Executive Summary Spring 2011* (Linthicum, MD: American College Health Association, 2012), http://www.acha-ncha.org/docs/ACHA-NCHA-II_ReferenceGroup_ExecutiveSummary_Spring2011.pdf.
4. National Heart, Lung, and Blood Institute, U.S. Department of Health and Human Services, National Institutes of Health, "What Is Physical Activity," Updated September 2011, www.nhlbi.nih.gov/health/health-topics/topics/phys/; Office of Disease Prevention and Health Promotion, *2008 Physical Activity Guidelines for Americans, 2008.*

5. P. Kokkinos, H. Sheriff, and R. Kheirbek, "Physical Inactivity and Mortality Risk," *Cardiology Research and Practice,* published online January 20, Volume 11 (2011): 924–49. Article ID 924945 http://www.hindawi.com/journals/crp/2011/924945/.

6. D. E. R. Warburton et al., "Evidence-Informed Physical Activity Guidelines for Canadian Adults," *Canadian Journal of Public Health* 98, Supplement 2 (2007): S16–S68.

7. S. Plowman and D. Smith, *Exercise Physiology for Health, Fitness, and Performance,* 3rd ed. (Philadelphia: Lippincott Williams & Wilkins, 2011).

8. S. Grover et al., "Estimating the Benefits of Patient and Physician Adherence to Cardiovascular Prevention Guidelines: The MyHealthCheckup Survey," *Canadian Journal of Cardiology* 27, no. 2 (2011): 159–66.

9. American Heart Association, "About Cholesterol," Updated November 2011, www.heart.org/HEARTORG/Conditions/Cholesterol/AboutCholesterol/About Cholesterol_UCM_001220_Article.jsp.

10. A. Mehta, "Management of Cardiovascular Risk Associated with Insulin Resistance, Diabetes, and the Metabolic Syndrome," *Postgraduate Medicine* 122, no. 3 (2010): 61–70.

11. Ibid.

12. D. C. Lee, X. Sui, T. S. Church, C. J. Lavie, A. S. Jackson, and S. N. Blair.. "Changes in Fitness and Fatness on the Development of Cardiovascular Disease Risk Factors Hypertension, Metabolic Syndrome, and Hypercholesterolemia," *Journal of the American College of Cardiology* 59, no. 7 (2012): 665–72.

13. M. Uusitupa, J. Tuomilehto, and P. Puska, "Are We Really Active in the Prevention of Obesity and Type 2 Diabetes at the Community Level?" *Nutrition and Metabolism in Cardiovascular Diseases,* published online April 4 (2011), DOI: 21470836.

14. National Diabetes Information Clearinghouse, U.S. Department of Health and Human Services, *Diabetes Prevention Program (DPP),* NIH Publication no. 09–5099 (Bethesda, MD: National Diabetes Information Clearinghouse, 2008), Available at http://diabetes.niddk.nih.gov/dm/pubs/preventionprogram.

15. N. Magné et al., "Recommendations for a Lifestyle Which Could Prevent Breast Cancer and Its Relapse: Physical Activity and Dietetic Aspects," *Critical Review of Oncology and Hematology,* published online February 18 (2011): DOI: 21334920.

16. World Cancer Research Fund/American Institute for Cancer Research, *Policy and Action for Cancer Prevention. Food, Nutrition, and Physical Activity: A Global Perspective* (Washington, DC: American Institute for Cancer Research, 2009), www.wcrf.org/cancer_research/policy_report/preventability_estimates_food.php.

17. C. M. Friedenreich and A. E. Cust, "Physical Activity and Breast Cancer Risk: Impact of Timing, Type, and Dose of Activity and Population Subgroup Effects," *British Journal of Sports Medicine* 42, no. 8 (2008): 636–47.

18. World Cancer Research Fund/American Institute for Cancer Research, *Policy and Action for Cancer Prevention, 2009;* A. Shibata, K. Ishii, and K. Oka, "Psychological, Social, and Environmental Factors of Meeting Recommended Physical Activity Levels for Colon Cancer Prevention among Japanese Adults," *Journal of Science and Medicine in Sport* 12, no. 2 (2010): e155–e156; K. Y. Wolin, Y. Yan, G. A. Colditz, and I. M. Lee, "Physical Activity and Colon Cancer Prevention: A Meta-Analysis," *British Journal of Cancer* 100, no. 4 (2009): 611–16.

19. M. Nilsson, C. Ohlsson, A. Odén, D. Mellström, and M. Lorentzon, "Increased Physical Activity Is Associated with Enhanced Development of Peak Bone Mass in Men: A Five Year Longitudinal Study," *Journal of Bone and Mineral Research,* electronically published ahead of print January 13 (2012): DOI: 10.1002/jbmr.1549; M. Callréus, F. McGuigan, K. Ringsberg, and K. Akesson, "Self-Reported Recreational Exercise Combining Regularity and Impact Is Necessary to Maximize Bone Mineral Density in Young Adult Women: A Population-Based Study of 1,061 Women 25 Years of Age," *Osteoporosis International* electronically published ahead of print January 13 (2012) www.springerlink.com/content/173253mk02vq3221/; S. Tolomio et al., "Short-Term Adapted Physical Activity Program Improves Bone Quality in Osteopenic/Osteoporotic Postmenopausal Women," *Journal of Physical Activity and Health* 5, no. 6 (2008): 844–53.

20. T. Post et al., "Bone Physiology, Disease and Treatment: Towards Disease System Analysis in Osteoporosis," *Clinical Pharmacokinetics,* 49, no. 2 (2010): 89–118.

21. J. G. Thomas and R. R. Wing, "Maintenance of Long-Term Weight Loss," *Medicine & Health Rhode Island* 92, no. 2 (2009): 56–57.

22. A. Koch, "Immune Response to Resistance Exercise," *American Journal of Lifestyle Medicine* 4, no. 3 (2010): 244–52.

23. MedLine Plus, National Institutes of Health, "Exercise and Immunity," Updated May 2010, www.nlm.nih.gov/medlineplus/ency/article/007165.htm.

24. N. P. Walsh et al., "Position Statement. Part Two: Maintaining Immune Health," *Exercise and Immunology Review* 17 (2011): 64–103.

25. M. W. Kakanis et al., "The Open Window of Susceptibility to Infection After Acute Exercise in Healthy Young Male Elite Athletes," *Exercise Immunology Review* 16 (2010): 119–37.

26. M. Cardinale et al., "Hormonal Responses to a Single Session of Whole-body Vibration Exercise in Older Individuals," *British Journal of Sports Medicine* 44, no. 4 (2010): 284–88.

27. J. Berry et al., "Lifetime Risks for Cardiovascular Disease Mortality by Cardiorespiratory Fitness Levels Measured at Ages 45, 55, and 65 Years in Men: The Cooper Center Longitudinal Study," *Journal of the American College of Cardiology* 57, no. 15 (2011): 1604–10; J. Woodcock, O. Franco, N. Orsini, and I. Roberts, "Non-Vigorous Physical Activity and All-Cause Mortality: Systematic Review and Meta-Analysis of Cohort Studies," *International Journal of Epidemiology* 40, no. 1 (2011): 121–38.

28. C. E. Garner et al., "American College of Sports Medicine Position Stand: Quantity and Quality of Exercise for Developing and Maintaining Cardiorespiratory, Musculoskeletal and Neuromotor Fitness in Apparently Healthy Adults: Guidance for Prescribing Exercise," *Medicine and Science in Sports and Exercise* 33, 7 (2011): 1334–59.

29. Ibid.

30. Ibid.

31. W. D. McArdle et al., *Exercise Physiology: Energy, Nutrition, and Human Performance,* 7th ed. (Baltimore, MD: Lippincott Williams & Wilkins, 2010); K. Kubo et al., "Time Course of Changes in Muscle and Tendon Properties During Strength Training and Detraining," *Journal of Strength and Conditioning Research* 24, no. 2 (2010): 322–31.

32. C. E. Garner et al., "American College of Sports Medicine Position Stand, 2011."

33. L. Y. Lee, D. T. Lee, and J. Woo, "Tai Chi and Health-Related Quality of Life in Nursing Home Residents," *Journal of Nursing Scholarship* 41, no. 1 (2009): 35–43.

34. Arthritis Foundation, "Exercise and Arthritis: Introduction to Exercise," 2010, www.arthritis.org/conditions/exercise.

35. M. J. Spink et al., "Foot and Ankle Strength, Range of Motion, Posture, and Deformity are Associated with Balance and Functional Ability in Older Adults," *Archives of Physical Medicine and Rehabilitation* 92, no. 1 (2011): 68–75.

36. C. E. Garner et al., "American College of Sports Medicine Position Stand," 2011.

37. Ibid.

38. D. G. Behm and A. Chaouachi, "A Review of the Acute Effects of Static and Dynamic Stretching on Performance," *European Journal of Applied Physiology* 111, no. 11 (2011): 2633–51.

39. K. Small, L. McNaughton, and M. Matthews, "A Systematic Review into the Efficacy of Static Stretching as Part of a Warm-Up for the Prevention of Exercise-Related Injury," *Research in Sports Medicine* 16, no. 3 (2008): 213–31.

40. V. Baltzpoulos, "Isokinetic Dynamometry," in *Biomechanical Evaluation of Movement in Sport and Exercise: The British Association of Sport and Exercise Sciences Guidelines,* eds. C. Payton and R. Bartlett (New York: Routledge, 2008), 105.

41. J. R. Fowles, "What I Always Wanted to Know about Instability Training," *Applied Physiology, Nutrition, and Metabolism* 35, no. 1 (2010): 89–90: D. G. Behm et al., "The Use of Instability to Train the Core Musculature," *Applied Physiology, Nutrition, and Metabolism* 35, no. 1 (2010): 91–108.

42. J. R. Fowles, "What I Always Wanted to Know about Instability Training," 2010.

43. D. G. Behm et al., "Canadian Society for Exercise Physiology Position Stand: The Use of Instability to Train the Core in Athletic and Nonathletic Conditioning," *Applied Physiology, Nutrition, and Metabolism* 35, no. 1 (2010): 109–12.

44. M. N. Sawka et al., "American College of Sports Medicine Position Stand: Exercise and Fluid Replacement," *Medicine and Science in Sports and Exercise* 39, no. 2 (2007): 377–90.

45. bid.

46. D. Ritchie, "Plantar Fasciitis: Treatment Pearls," American Academy of Podiatric Sports Medicine, Accessed July 2010 from, www.aapsm.org/plantar_fasciitis .html.

47. M. H. Moen et al., "Medial Tibial Stress Syndrome: A Critical Review," *Sports Medicine* 39, no. 7 (2009) 523–46.

48. M. A. Schiff, D. J. Caine, and R. O'Halloran, "Injury Prevention in Sport," *American Journal of Lifestyle Medicine* 4, no. 1 (2010): 42–64.

49. K. B. Fields, J. C. Sykes, K. M. Walker, and J. C. Jackson, "Prevention of Running Injuries," *Current Sports Medicine Reports* 9, no. 3 (2010): 176–82.

50. American Academy of Ophthalmology, "Protective Eyewear," Updated February 2009, www.aao.org/eyesmart/injuries/ eyewear.cfm.

51. American College Health Association, *American College Health Association-National College Health Assessment II: Reference Group Data Report Spring 2011* (Baltimore: American College Health Association, 2012).

52. Bicycle Helmet Safety Institute, "Helmet-Related Statistics from Many Sources," Revised July 2010, www.helmets.org/ stats.htm.

53. N. G. Nelson, C. L. Collins, R. D. Comstock, and L. B. McKenzie, "Exertional Heat-Related Injuries Treated in Emergency Departments in the U.S., 1997–2006," *American Journal of Preventive Medicine* 40, no. 1 (2011): 54–60.

54. L. E. Armstrong et al., "The American Football Uniform: Uncompensable Heat Stress and Hyperthermic Exhaustion," *Journal of Athletic Training* 45, no. 2 (2010): 117–27.

55. E. E. Turk, "Hypothermia," *Forensic Science Medical Pathology* 6, no. 2 (2010): 106–15.

56. Ibid.

57. American Council on Exercise, "Exercising in the Cold," 2010, www .acefitness.org/fitfacts/fitfacts_display .aspx?itemid=24.

10 Recognizing and Avoiding Addiction

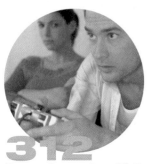

312

How can I recognize addiction in a loved one or even myself?

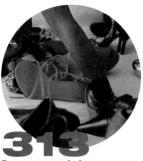

313

Do some people have a more addictive personality than others?

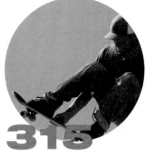

315

Is my roommate's constant exercising an addiction?

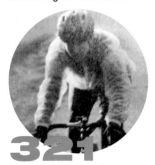

321

How can I approach someone who needs help?

OBJECTIVES

* Define and discuss *addiction*.

* Distinguish addictions from habits, and identify the signs of addiction.

* Discuss the addictive process, the physiology of addiction, the biopsychosocial model of addiction, as well as codependence.

* Describe types of addictions, including disordered gambling, compulsive buying, compulsive Internet or technology use, work addiction, compulsive exercise, and sexual addiction.

* Evaluate treatment and recovery options for addicts, including intervention, individual therapy, group therapy, family therapy, and 12-step programs.

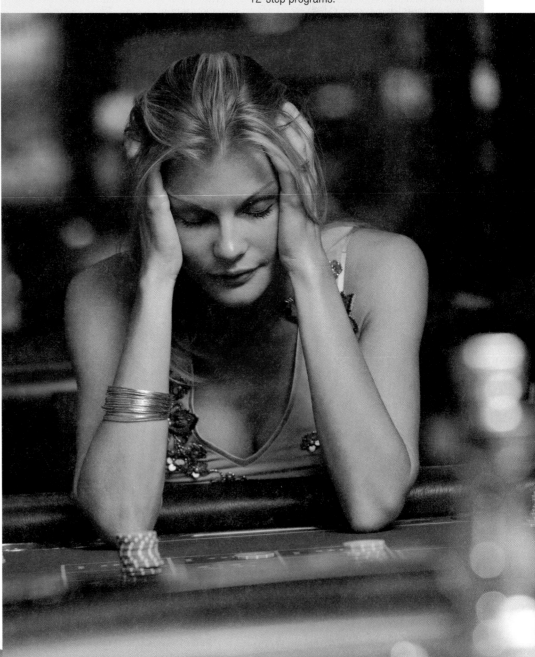

These days, it's easy to find high-profile cases of compulsive and destructive behavior. Stories of celebrities and politicians struggling with addictions to alcohol, drugs, and sex are splashed in the headlines and profiled on TV news programs. But millions of "everyday" people throughout the world are waging their own battles with addiction as well. People with addictions can sometimes be unaware that they have a problem, because many potentially addictive activities may actually enhance the lives of those who engage in them moderately. In addition to alcohol and drugs, the most commonly recognized addictions include food, sex, relationships, shopping, work, exercise, gambling, and using the Internet.

What Is Addiction?

Addiction is a persistent, compulsive dependence on a behavior or substance, including mood-altering behaviors or activities, despite ongoing negative consequences. Some researchers speak of two types of addictions: *substance addictions* (e.g., alcoholism, drug abuse, and smoking) and *process addictions* (e.g., gambling, spending, shopping, eating, and sexual activity). There is a growing recognition that many addicts, such as polydrug abusers, are addicted to more than one substance or process. Addictive behaviors initially provide a sense of pleasure or stability that is beyond the addict's power to achieve in other ways. Eventually, the addicted person needs to do the behavior in order to feel normal.

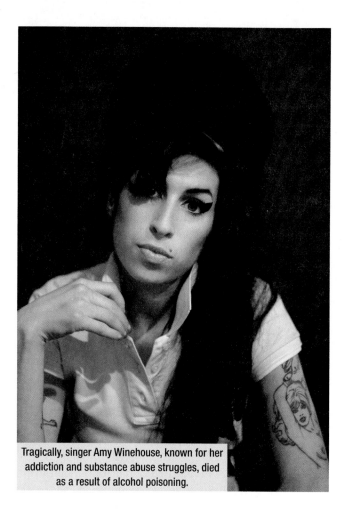

Tragically, singer Amy Winehouse, known for her addiction and substance abuse struggles, died as a result of alcohol poisoning.

47%

of college students admitted for substance abuse treatment list alcohol as their primary problem.

In this text, *addiction* is used interchangeably with *physiological addiction*. However, **physiological dependence,** the adaptive state that occurs with regular addictive behavior and results in withdrawal syndrome, is only one indicator of addiction. Psychological dynamics play an important role, which explains why behaviors not related to chemicals may also be additive. To be addictive, a behavior must have the potential to produce a positive mood change. Chemicals are responsible for the most profound addictions because they produce dramatic mood changes and cause cellular changes to which the body adapts so well that it eventually requires the chemical in order to function normally. Yet other behaviors, such as gambling, spending money, working, and sex, also create changes at the cellular level along with positive mood changes. A person with an intense, uncontrollable urge to continue engaging in a particular activity is said to have developed a psychological dependence. In fact, psychological and physiological dependence are so intertwined

that it is not really possible to separate the two. Although the mechanism is not well understood, all forms of addiction probably reflect dysfunction of certain biochemical systems in the brain.[1]

Studies show that most animals share the same basic pleasure and reward circuits in the brain that turn on when they encounter addictive substances or engage in something pleasurable, such as eating or orgasm. We all engage in potentially addictive behaviors to some extent, because some are essential to our survival and are highly reinforcing, such as eating, drinking, and sex. At some point along the continuum, however, some individuals are not able to engage in these or other behaviors moderately—they become addicted.

Addiction has four common symptoms: (1) **compulsion,** which is characterized by **obsession,** or excessive preoccupation, with the behavior and an overwhelming need to perform it; (2) **loss of control,** the inability to reliably

addiction Persistent, compulsive dependence on a behavior or substance, including mood-altering behaviors or activities, despite ongoing negative consequences.

physiological dependence The adaptive state that occurs with regular addictive behavior and results in withdrawal syndrome.

compulsion Preoccupation with a behavior and an overwhelming need to perform it.

obsession Excessive preoccupation with an addictive object or behavior.

loss of control Inability to reliably predict whether a particular instance of involvement with the addictive substance or behavior will be healthy or damaging.

predict whether any isolated occurrence of the behavior will be healthy or damaging; (3) **negative consequences,** such as physical damage, legal trouble, financial problems, academic failure, and family dissolution, which do not occur with healthy involvement in any behavior; and (4) **denial,** the inability to perceive that the behavior is self-destructive. These four components are present in all addictions, whether chemical or behavioral.

Habit versus Addiction

How do we distinguish between a harmless habit and an addiction? Addiction certainly involves elements of **habit,** a repeated behavior in which the repetition may be unconscious. A habit can be annoying, but it can be broken without too much discomfort by simply becoming aware of its presence and choosing not to do it. Addiction also involves repetition of a behavior, but the repetition occurs by compulsion, and considerable discomfort is experienced if the behavior is not performed. Habits are behaviors that occur through choice and typically do not cause negative health consequences. In contrast, no one decides to become addicted, even though people make choices that contribute to the development of an addiction.

negative consequences Severe problems associated with addiction, such as physical damage, legal trouble, financial problems, academic failure, or family dissolution.

denial Inability to perceive or accurately interpret the self-destructive effects of the addictive behavior.

habit A repeated behavior in which the repetition may be unconscious.

codependence A self-defeating relationship pattern in which a person is controlled by an addict's addictive behavior.

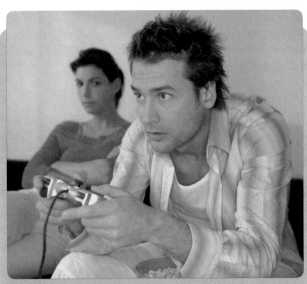

How can I recognize addiction in a loved one or even myself?

Addiction can be difficult to recognize or acknowledge. Symptoms to look for are an obsession or compulsion with a behavior or activity, a loss of control, and negative consequences as a result of the behavior. Another symptom, denial of a problem, may be easy to see in another person but difficult to recognize in yourself.

To understand addiction, we must look beyond the amount and frequency of the behavior because what happens when a person is involved in the behavior is far more meaningful. For example, someone who drinks only rarely and then engages in a night of heavy drinking may experience personality changes, blackouts (drug-induced amnesia), and other negative consequences (e.g., failing a test, missing an important appointment, getting into a fight) that would never have occurred otherwise. On the other hand, someone who has a few martinis every evening may never do anything out of character while under the influence of alcohol but may become irritable, manipulative, and aggressive without those regular drinks. For both of these people, alcohol performs a function (mood control) that they should be able to achieve without the aid of chemicals, which is a possible sign of addiction.

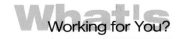
Addiction Affects Family and Friends

The family and friends of an addicted person can suffer many negative consequences. Often they struggle with **codependence,** a self-defeating relationship pattern in which a person is controlled by an addict's addictive behavior.

Codependence is often the result of growing up in an environment of addiction. Codependents find it hard to set healthy boundaries and often live in the chaotic, crisis-oriented mode that occurs around addicts. They assume responsibility for meeting others' needs to the point that they subordinate or even cease being aware of their own needs. They may be unable to perceive their needs because they have been taught that their needs are inappropriate or less important than someone else's. Although the word *codependent* is used less frequently today, treatment professionals still recognize the importance of helping addicts see how

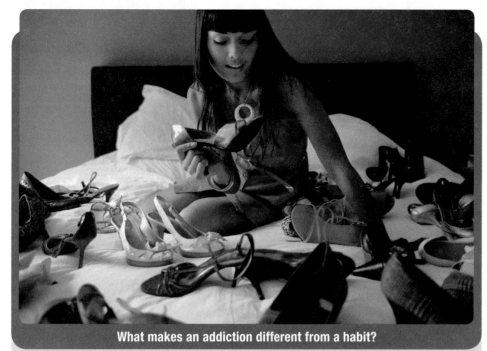

What makes an addiction different from a habit?

Once a person recognizes a habit and decides to change it, the habit can usually be broken. With an addiction, however, there is a sense of compulsion so strong that the addict is no longer in control of his or her behavior. For example, you may like to hit the stores when the latest fashions arrive or spend time online hunting for bargains, but your shopping isn't considered an addiction unless you have lost control over where and when you shop—and how much—and you are experiencing negative impacts on the rest of your life as a result.

their behavior affects those around them and of working with family and friends to establish healthier relationships.

Family and friends can play an important role in getting an addict to seek treatment. They are most helpful when they refuse to be enablers. **Enablers** are people who knowingly or unknowingly protect addicts from the natural consequences of their behavior. If they don't have to deal with the consequences, addicts cannot see the self-destructive nature of their behavior and will therefore continue it. Codependents are the primary enablers of their addicted loved ones, although anyone who has contact with an addict can be an enabler and thus contribute to continuation of the addictive behavior. Enablers are generally unaware that their behavior has this effect. In fact, enabling is rarely conscious and certainly not intentional.

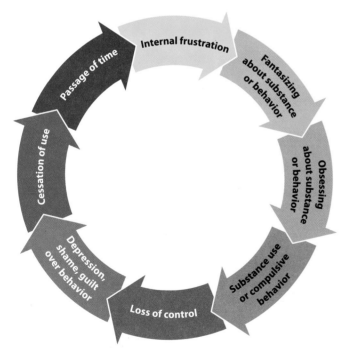

FIGURE 10.1 **Cycle of Psychological Addiction**

Source: Adapted from Recovery Connection, Cycle of Addiction, 2012, www.recoveryconnection.org/cycle-of-addiction/.

Video Tutor: Addiction Cycle

How Addiction Develops

Addiction is a process that evolves over time. It begins when a person repeatedly seeks the illusion of relief to avoid unpleasant feelings or situations. This pattern is known as *nurturing through avoidance* and is a maladaptive way of taking care of emotional needs. As a person becomes increasingly dependent on the addictive behavior, there is a corresponding deterioration in relationships with family, friends, and coworkers; in performance at work or school; and in personal life. Eventually, addicts do not find the addictive behavior pleasurable but consider it preferable to the unhappy realities they are seeking to escape. Figure 10.1 illustrates the cycle of psychological addiction.

The Physiology of Addiction

Virtually all intellectual, emotional, and behavioral functions occur as a result of biochemical interactions between nerve cells in the body. Biochemical messengers, called **neurotransmitters,** exert their influence at specific receptor sites on nerve cells. Drug use and chronic stress can alter these receptor sites and cause the production and breakdown of neurotransmitters. Some people's bodies naturally produce insufficient quantities of these neurotransmitters, which predisposes

enablers People who knowingly or unknowingly protect addicts from the natural consequences of their behavior.

neurotransmitters Biochemical messengers that bind to specific receptor sites on nerve cells.

them to seek out chemicals, such as alcohol, as substitutes or pursue behaviors, such as exercise, that increase natural production. Thus, some may be "wired" to look for substances or experiences that increase pleasure or reduce discomfort, making them more susceptible to addiction.

Mood-altering substances and experiences produce **tolerance,** a phenomenon in which progressively larger doses of a drug or more intense involvement in an experience are needed to obtain the desired effects. All of us develop some degree of tolerance to any mood-altering experience. But because addicts tend to seek intense mood-altering experiences, they eventually increase their amount and intensity to the point of causing negative side effects.

An addictive substance or activity replaces or causes an effect that the body should normally provide on its own. If the experience is repeated often enough, the body adjusts: It starts requiring the experience to obtain that effect. Stopping the behavior will cause **withdrawal,** because the body can no longer create the same effect naturally. Mood-altering chemicals, for example, fill up the receptor sites for the body's natural "feel-good" neurotransmitters (endorphins), and nerve cells shut down production of these substances temporarily. When the drug use stops, those receptor sites sit empty, resulting in uncomfortable feelings that remain until the body resumes normal neurotransmitter production or the person consumes more of the drug.

Withdrawal symptoms of chemical dependencies are generally the opposite of the effects of the drugs. For example, a cocaine addict who feels a high while using the drug will experience a characteristic "crash" (depression and lethargy) when he or she stops taking it. Conversely, a heroin addict experiences drowsiness, slowed speech and reactions, and uninhibited behavior while using the drug. When withdrawing from heroin, the addict experiences anxiety, elevated heart rate, trembling, irritability, insomnia, and convulsions. Withdrawal symptoms for addictive behaviors are usually less dramatic. They typically involve psychological discomfort such as anxiety, depression, irritability, guilt, anger, and frustration, with an underlying preoccupation with or craving for the behavior. Withdrawal syndromes range from mild to severe. The most severe form is delirium tremens (DTs), which occurs in approximately 5 to 10 percent of dependent individuals withdrawing from alcohol.[2]

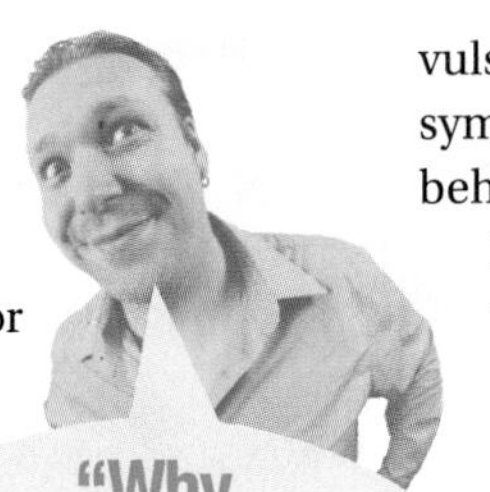

"Why Should I Care?"

Addictions of any kind limit your ability to make good decisions and maintain your focus, making it hard for you to meet your full potential as a student and a member of the community. A seemingly harmless habit may actually be progressing into an addiction that prevents you from attending classes, meeting new people, or participating in other activities that you might find enjoyable.

tolerance Phenomenon in which progressively larger doses of a drug or more intense involvement in a behavior is needed to produce the desired effects.

withdrawal A series of temporary physical and biopsychosocial symptoms that occurs when an addict abruptly abstains from an addictive chemical or behavior.

biopsychosocial model of addiction Theory of the relationship between an addict's biological (genetic) nature and psychological and environmental influences.

See It!

What behavior are you addicted to, and how can you stop it? Go to the See It! section of www.pearsonhighered.com/donatelle to view the **Kick Your Habit** videos.

The Biopsychosocial Model of Addiction

The most effective treatment today is based on the **biopsychosocial model of addiction,** which proposes that addiction is caused by a variety of factors operating together. The biopsychosocial model was developed to explain the complex interaction between the biological, psychological, and social aspects of addiction. Biological, psychological, and environmental factors all contribute to its development. Although one factor may play a larger role than another in a specific individual, it is rarely sufficient to explain an addiction. Figure 10.2 lists risk factors for addiction.

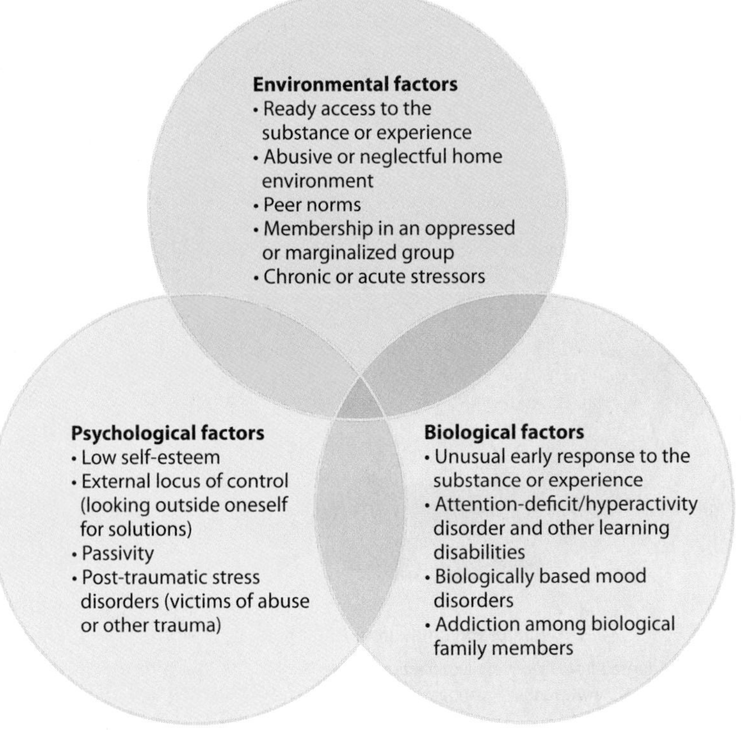
Environmental factors
• Ready access to the substance or experience
• Abusive or neglectful home environment
• Peer norms
• Membership in an oppressed or marginalized group
• Chronic or acute stressors
Psychological factors
• Low self-esteem
• External locus of control (looking outside oneself for solutions)
• Passivity
• Post-traumatic stress disorders (victims of abuse or other trauma)
Biological factors
• Unusual early response to the substance or experience
• Attention-deficit/hyperactivity disorder and other learning disabilities
• Biologically based mood disorders
• Addiction among biological family members

FIGURE 10.2 **Risk Factors for Addiction**

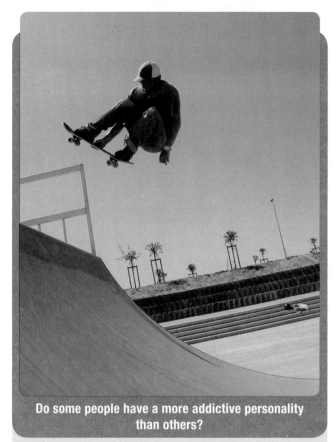

Do some people have a more addictive personality than others?

Psychological factors may make some people more prone to addiction than others. Low self-esteem, poor coping skills, or a tendency toward risk-taking behavior may put you at higher risk of developing an addiction than someone without these traits.

Biological or Disease Influences For many people, addiction is thought to be based in the brain and involves memory, motivation, and emotional state. The processes that control these aspects of brain function are thus logical subjects for genetic research into a biologically based risk for addiction, particularly to mood-altering substances. Studies show that drug addicts metabolize these substances differently than do nonaddicted people. Genes affecting the activity of the neurotransmitters serotonin and GABA (gamma-aminobutyric acid) are likely involved in the risk for alcoholism.[3]

Addiction may also develop outside the typical, expected models. For example, see the Health Headlines box on page 316 for the story of some Parkinson's disease sufferers who had no history of addictive behaviors until they began taking medication to treat body tremors, then developed behaviors such as compulsive buying or pathological gambling.

Research also supports a genetic influence on addiction. It has been known for centuries that alcoholism runs in families. Recent studies have confirmed that identical twins, who share the same genes, are about twice as likely as fraternal twins, who share an average of 50 percent of their genes, to resemble each other in terms of the presence of alcoholism. Studies also show that 50 to 60 percent of the risk for alcoholism is genetically determined for both men and women.[4]

Psychological Factors A person's psychological make-up also factors into the potential for addiction. People with low self-esteem, a tendency toward risk-taking behavior, or poor coping skills are more likely to develop addictive patterns. Individuals who consistently look outside themselves for solutions and explanations for life events (who have an external locus of control) are more likely to experience addiction.

Environmental Influences Social expectations and mores help determine whether people engage in certain behaviors. For example, although many Italians use alcohol abundantly, there is a low incidence of alcoholism in this culture. Low rates of alcoholism typically exist in countries and cultures where children are gradually introduced to alcohol in diluted amounts, on special occasions, and within a strong family group. There is deep disapproval of intoxication, which is not viewed as socially acceptable, stylish, or funny.[5] Such cultural traditions and values are less widespread in the United States, where the incidence of alcohol addiction and alcohol-related problems is very high.

Societal attitudes and messages also influence addictive behavior. The media's emphasis on appearance and the ideal body plays a significant role in exercise addiction. Societal glorification of money and material achievement can lead to work addiction, which is often admired. Societal changes, in turn, influence individual norms. People living in cities characterized by rapid social change or social disorganization often feel less connected to civic and religious institutions. The resulting disenfranchisement leads to increased destructive behaviors, including addiction.[6]

Social learning theory proposes that people learn behaviors by watching role models—parents, caregivers, and significant others. The effects of modeling, imitation, and identification with behavior from early childhood on are well documented. Modeling is especially influential when it involves behavior that is mood altering. Many studies show that modeling

social learning theory Theory that people learn behaviors by watching role models—parents, caregivers, and significant others.

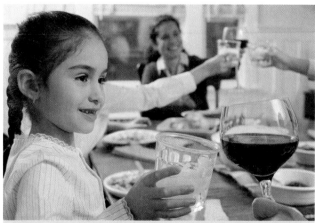

One predisposing factor for whether a person develops an addiction might be environmental influences such as the norms and cultural values he or she was taught during childhood.

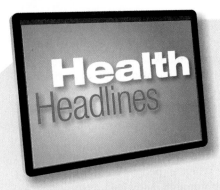

Health Headlines

CAN MEDICATION FOR PARKINSON'S DISEASE CAUSE SEX OR GAMBLING ADDICTION?

Parkinson's disease (PD) is a degenerative brain disorder with symptoms that include body tremors, rigid muscles, and impaired balance. Generally speaking, PD patients have a very low incidence of drug abuse and display a personality type that is the opposite of the typical addictive personality. Yet since a certain treatment was introduced, the incidence of pathological gambling has been estimated to be as high as 8 percent in PD patients who use it versus 1 percent of the general population. It has also been documented that some PD patients develop impulse control disorders such as disordered gambling,

compulsive shopping, or compulsive sexual behaviors. Others report becoming addicted to their own medication.

How could a medication used to improve shaking and movement control cause gambling, sex, or shopping addictions? The answer has to do with the neurotransmitter dopamine. Parkinson's disease patients lack dopamine and are often treated with dopamine agonists, medication that mimics dopamine action. Dopamine is involved in brain processes controlling movement, but it also plays a part in emotional response, the experience of pleasure and pain, and reward-based learning. Studies show that that dopamine acts in an area of the brain known as the ventral striatum, which receives input from other areas such as the hippocampus and amygdala. It may be through this region that dopamine promotes addictive behaviors. Also, researchers have found that the decision-making process is dysregulated by dopamine agonists, increasing the likelihood of vulnerability to compulsive behaviors; this finding provides clues to the mechanisms that underlie the escalation of addictive behaviors.

In PD patients who develop addictive disorders, the problems usually start soon after beginning dopamine agonist therapy and stop when treatment is discontinued. It was found that adjusting the dosage

and combination of medication resolved the addictive symptoms while maintaining the same motor benefit. Understanding the brain function that leads to drug addiction may help in the development of drugs to block drug-craving and drug-seeking behaviors in the general population as well as refine disease treatment for PD patients.

The phenomenon of addiction induced by dopamine medications can also tell us something about vulnerability to addiction in the general population. Not everyone is equally vulnerable, and it now appears that the propensity to become addicted is in part hereditary. Many of the genes implicated in addiction appear to affect brain levels of dopamine.

Sources: McGill University, "Addiction: Insights From Parkinson's Disease," *ScienceDaily*, February 25, 2009, Retrieved February 15, 2012, from http://www.sciencedaily.com/releases/2009/02/090225132341.htm; National Institute of Neurological Disorders and Stroke, 2012, NINDS Parkinson's Disease Information Page, 2012, Accessed February 17, 2012, from http://www.ninds.nih.gov/disorders/parkinsons_disease/parkinsons_disease.htm; D. Weintraub et. al., "Impulse Control Disorders in Parkinson Disease: A Cross-Sectional Study of 3,090 Patients, *Archives of Neurology* 67 (2010): 589–95; A. Dagher and T. Robbins, "Personality, Addiction, Dopamine: Insights from Parkinson's Disease.," *Neuron Review* 61 (2009): 502–10.

---

process addictions Behaviors such as disordered gambling, compulsive buying, compulsive Internet or technology use, work addiction, compulsive exercise, and sexual addiction that are known to be addictive because they are mood altering.

by parents and by idolized celebrities exerts a profound influence on young people.[7]

On an individual level, major stressful life events—uch as marriage, divorce, change in work status, or death of a loved one—may trigger addictive behaviors. Traumatic events in general often instigate addictive behaviors, as traumatized people seek to medicate their pain—pain they may not even be aware of because they've repressed it. One thing that makes addictive behaviors so powerfully attractive is that they reliably alleviate personal pain for a short time. However, over the long term, addictive behaviors actually cause more pain than they relieve.

Family members whose needs for love, security, and affirmation are not consistently met; who are refused permission to express their feelings; and who frequently submerge their personalities to "keep the peace" are prone to addiction.

Children whose parents are not consistently available to them (physically or emotionally); who are subjected to sexual abuse, physical abuse, neglect, or abandonment; or who receive inconsistent or disparaging messages about their self-worth may experience psychosocial or physical illness and addiction in adulthood.

Addictive Behaviors

Thus far in this chapter, we have examined the fundamental concepts and processes of addiction and its associated problems. Clearly, tobacco, alcohol, and other drugs are addictive, and addictions to them create multiple problems for addicted individuals and for their families and society. Later chapters will discuss these substance-related addictions.

Here we will look at **process addictions**—behaviors known to be addictive because they are mood altering. Traditionally, the word *addiction* has been used mainly with alcohol and other psychoactive substances. However, this is changing. New knowledge about the brain's reward system suggests that, as far as the brain is concerned, a reward is a reward, whether it is brought on by a chemical or a behavior.[8] Examples of process addictions include disordered gambling, compulsive buying, compulsive Internet or technology use, work addiction, compulsive exercise, and sexual addiction.

Disordered or Pathological Gambling

Gambling is a form of recreation and entertainment for millions of Americans. Most people who gamble do so casually and moderately to experience the excitement of anticipating a win. However, more than 2 million Americans suffer from pathological or **disordered gambling,** and 6 million more are considered to be at risk for developing a gambling addiction.[9] The American Psychiatric Association (APA), which previously used the term *pathological gambling,* has proposed the term *disordered gambling* for this addiction and recognizes it as a mental disorder. As proposed for the APA's *Diagnostic and Statistical Manual of Mental Disorders,* 5th edition (*DSM-V,* to be published in May 2013), the revised APA definition lists nine characteristic behaviors, including preoccupation with gambling, unsuccessful efforts to cut back or quit, using gambling to escape problems, and lying to family members to conceal the extent of gambling.

Gamblers and drug addicts describe many similar cravings and highs. A recent study supports what many experts believe to be true: Disordered gambling is like drug addiction.[10]

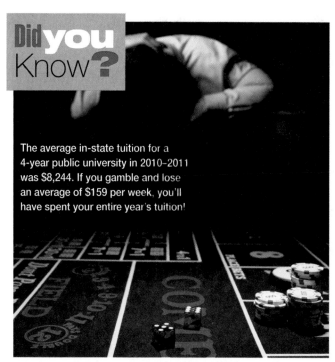

Did you Know?

The average in-state tuition for a 4-year public university in 2010–2011 was $8,244. If you gamble and lose an average of $159 per week, you'll have spent your entire year's tuition!

Source: The College Board, *Trends in College Pricing, 2010–2011* (New York: The College Board, 2011), available at www.trends-collegeboard.com/college_pricing.

26%

of college men report gambling at least once a week, compared to 5.5% of college women.

Disordered gamblers in this study were found to have decreased blood flow to a key section of the brain's reward system. It is thought that disordered gamblers, like people who abuse drugs, compensate for this deficiency in their brain's reward system by overdoing it and getting hooked.[11] Most disordered gamblers state that they seek excitement even more than money. They place increasingly larger bets to obtain the desired level of excitement. Like drug addicts, they live from fix to fix. Their subjective cravings can be as intense as those of drug abusers; they show tolerance in their need to increase the amount of their bets; and they experience highs rivaling that of a drug high. Up to half of disordered gamblers show withdrawal symptoms similar to a mild form of drug withdrawal, including sleep disturbance, sweating, irritability, and craving.

Who is at risk for getting hooked on the rush of gambling? Men are more likely to have gambling problems than are women. Women, however, tend to begin gambling later than do men, but they develop gambling problems more rapidly. Gambling prevalence is also higher among lower-income individuals; those who are widowed, separated, or divorced; African Americans; individuals who begin gambling at a younger age; and older adults. Gambling disorders tend to run in families. If they are regularly exposed to gambling, family members of disordered gamblers are more susceptible to disordered gambling than are individuals without disordered gambling family members.

Disordered gamblers are much more likely to have mental disorders and/or substance use disorders than are those without gambling disorders. It is not uncommon for gamblers to suffer from mood disorders such as depression, anxiety, or post-traumatic stress disorder. A significant number of disordered gamblers are more likely to be alcoholics, drug use abusers, and/or smokers.[12]

Although gambling is illegal for anyone under the age of 21, college students have easier access to gambling opportunities than ever before. Approximately 75 percent of college students reported gambling in the past year (whether legally or illegally), with about 18 percent gambling weekly or more frequently.[13] With the advent of online gambling, televised poker tournaments, and a growing number of casinos, scratch tickets, lotteries, and sports-betting networks, there are many opportunities for college students to gamble. However, a recent study found that non-college students gambled more frequently than did college students.[14] However, students at most risk for problem gambling were males, African American, with lower socioeconomic status. It is estimated that 6 percent of college students in the United States have a serious

disordered gambling Compulsive gambling that cannot be controlled.

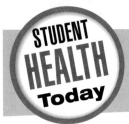
Although many people gamble occasionally without it ever becoming a problem, even model students can find themselves caught up in it. Consider John,* an ex–Lehigh University sophomore and class president, the son of a Baptist minister, a former fraternity member, and cellist in the university orchestra—the epitome of a responsible student. When John was arrested for robbing a bank in Pennsylvania, making off with $2,781, many wondered why he would be driven to such an act. His lawyer stated that John had run up about $5,000 in debt playing online poker. In a desperate move to feed his gambling addiction, John turned to bank robbery. He has been sentenced to 22 months to 10 years in prison.

Disordered gambling on college campuses has become a big concern. It is estimated that each year during March Madness (the men's college basketball tournament), there is an estimated $12 billion that is wagered over 3 weeks on The National Collegiate Athletic Association (NCAA) basketball tournament. Over $3 billion is from office pools. More and more of these dollars come from the pockets of college students. There is growing evidence, in fact, that betting is interfering with students' financial and academic futures. In a recent survey, approximately 75 percent of students reported they had gambled during the past year, whether legally or illegally. Consider the following:

*Not his real name.

✳ Almost 53 percent of college students have participated in most forms of gambling, including casino gambling, lottery tickets, racing, and sports betting in the past month.
✳ At least 78 percent of youths have placed a bet by the age of 18.
✳ An estimated 6 percent of college students could be classified as problem gamblers.
✳ The three most common reasons college students give for gambling are risk, excitement, and the chance to make money.

Although most college students who gamble are able to do so without developing a problem, warning signs of disordered gambling include the following:

✳ Frequent talk about gambling; encouraging or challenging others to gamble
✳ Spending more time or money on gambling than he or she can afford
✳ Borrowing money, using financial aid money or other money, or committing crimes to finance gambling
✳ "Chasing" losses with more gambling
✳ Secretive about his or her gambling habits, and defensive when confronted.
✳ Possessing gambling paraphernalia such as lottery tickets or poker items
✳ Missing or being late for school, work, or family activities due to gambling
✳ Feeling sad, anxious, fearful, or angry about gambling losses

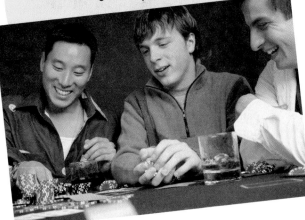

Call, fold, or raise? For increasing numbers of college students, gambling and the debts it can incur are becoming serious problems.

Sources: Task Force on College Gambling Policies, Division on Addictions at the Cambridge Health Alliance and the National Center for Responsible Gambling, *A Call to Action: Addressing College Gambling: Recommendations for Science-Based Policies and Programs* (Cambridge, MA: Cambridge Health Alliance and the National Center for Responsible Gambling, 2009), Available at www.ncrg.org/public_education/task-force-college-gambling-policies.cfm; R. Schachter, "Targeting Student Gambling," *University Business* (January 2008): 35–38; J. Welte et al., "The Prevalence of Problem Gambling among U.S. Adolescents and Young Adults: Results from a National Survey," *Journal of Gambling Studies* 24, no. 2 (2008): 119–33; National Council on Problem Gambling, "March Madness Gambling Brings Out Warnings from NCAA to Tournament Players," 2011, Available at www.ncpgambling.org/i4a/headlines/headlinedetails.cfm?id=791&archive=1; Prevention Lane, Problem Gambling Prevention: College Problem Gambling, 2011, Available at http://prevention-lane.org/gambling/college-signs-pg.htm.

---

compulsive shoppers People who are preoccupied with shopping and spending.

gambling problem that can result in psychological difficulties, debt, and failing grades.[15]

The most popular forms of gambling reported for college males are the lottery, card games, pools and raffles, sports betting, and games of skill. The most popular forms of gambling for women are lottery, card games, pools and raffles, and bingo. What is interesting is that Internet gambling is not as common among college students as once thought.

Whereas casual gamblers can stop anytime they wish and are capable of seeing the necessity to do so, disordered gamblers are unable to control the urge to gamble even in the face of devastating consequences: high debt; legal problems; and the loss of everything meaningful, including homes, families, jobs, health, and even their lives. The **Student Health Today** box discusses student gambling in more detail.

Compulsive Buying Disorder

In our society, people often use shopping as a way to make themselves feel better. However, **compulsive shoppers** are preoccupied with shopping and spending and exercise little control over their impulses to buy. Shopping actually makes them feel worse, not better. Compulsive buying is

See It!

How do you battle compulsive shopping? Go to the See It! section of www.pearsonhighered.com/donatelle to view the **Money Rehab** video.

estimated to afflict up to 5 percent of adults. The vast majority of compulsive buyers are women.[16]

Compulsive buying has many of the same characteristics as alcoholism, gambling, and other addictions. Symptoms that signal that a person has crossed the line into compulsive buying include preoccupation with shopping and spending, buying more than one of the same item, shopping for longer periods than intended, repeatedly buying much more than he or she needs or can afford, and buying to the point that it interferes with social activities or work and creates financial problems (e.g. indebtedness or bankruptcy). Compulsive buying frequently results in psychological distress such as depression and feelings of guilt, conflict with friends and between couples.[17]

Compulsive buying disorders are reported to begin in a person's late teens and early twenties, coinciding with the age that people first establish credit and independence from their parents. Thanks to easy buying capabilities via the Internet, compulsive buyers can begin their adult life in substantial debt.

Compulsive buying can be seasonal, such as shopping during the winter months, to alleviate feelings of anxiety and depression. It can also occur when people feel depressed, lonely, or angry. Shopping and spending will not assure more love, increase self-esteem, or heal the problems of daily living. It generally makes people feel worse because of increased debt. Like disordered gambling, compulsive buying can lead to compulsive borrowing to support the addiction. People may borrow money repeatedly from family, friends, or institutions in spite of the problems this causes.

Technology Addictions

As technology becomes more integrated into our daily lives, the risk of overexposure grows for people of all ages. Some people, in fact, become addicted to new technologies, such as smartphones, video games, networking sites, and the Internet in general. Have you ever opened your Web browser to check something quickly, and an hour later found yourself still blogging or checking your Facebook

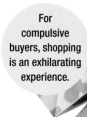

For compulsive buyers, shopping is an exhilarating experience.

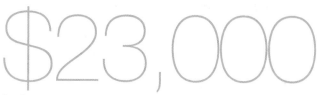

is the average amount of debt that a compulsive shopper owes.

page? Do you have friends who seem more concerned with texting or surfing the Internet than with eating, going out, studying, or having a face-to-face conversation? These behaviors are not unusual; many experts suggest that technology addiction is real and can present serious problems. An estimated 1 in 8 Internet users will likely experience **Internet addiction**.[18] Younger people are more likely to be addicted to the Internet than middle-aged users.[19] Approximately 12 percent of college students report that Internet use and computer games have interfered with their academic performance.[20] To read about the experiences of students taking part in an "unplug from technology day," see the **Tech & Health** box on the following page.

> **Internet addiction** Compulsive use of the computer, PDA, cell phone, or other forms of technology to access the Internet for activities such as e-mail, games, shopping, social networking, or blogging.

So how important is technology to college students? To provide some insight into this question, it is reported that 98 percent of college students own at least one digital device. In a recent survey, 38 percent of students said they couldn't even go 10 minutes without switching on some sort of electronic device. Three out of 4 college students say they wouldn't be able to study without technology. The average minutes a day a college student spends texting on a cell phone is 181.5 minutes, followed by 131 minutes searching the Web, 101 minutes on Facebook, and just under 60 minutes on e-mail.[21] Remember, what you do when using technology may be as important as how long you spend using it. Some people find themselves texting constantly, while others update their status repeatedly on Facebook and other social networking sites. You may follow numerous Twitter feeds or engage in extended gaming sessions. Some online activities, such as gaming and cybersex, seem to be more potentially addictive than others.

Technology addicts typically exhibit symptoms such as general disregard for their health, sleep deprivation, depression, neglecting family and friends, lack of physical activity, euphoria when online, lower grades in school, and poor job performance. Internet addicts may feel moody or uncomfortable when they are not online. They may be using their behavior to compensate for loneliness, marital or work problems, a poor social life, or financial problems.

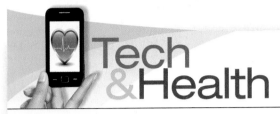

Tech & Health

MOBILE DEVICES, MEDIA, AND THE INTERNET: COULD YOU UNPLUG?

Today college students typically have many interactions with traditional media (such as radio, television, or print sources) as well as the Internet and social media throughout their day. Usually this happens via phones or tablet computers, which allow us to check the weather, take photos, submit homework assignments, communicate with friends and family, and kill time by watching a favorite show or playing a game. If someone asked you to give up your mobile devices, media, and the Internet for 24 hours, how hard would it be?

Based on the results of a study by the International Center for Media & the Public Agenda (ICMPA) at the University of Maryland, it's very difficult to unplug, even for just a day. Students from Maryland and 11 other university partners of the Salzburg Academy on Media & Global Change participated in the study. Altogether there were nearly 1,000 study participants hailing from 37 different countries on six continents. All students followed the same assignment: give up Internet, newspapers, magazines, TV, radio, phones, iPods/MP3 players, movies, Facebook, chat, Twitter, video games, and any other form of electronic or social media for 24 hours.

Students' "addiction" to media may not be clinically diagnosed, but the cravings seem real—as does the anxiety and the depression.

✳ Students around the world repeatedly used the term *addiction* to speak about their dependence on media. "Media is my drug; without it I was lost," said one student from the UK. Sharing analogies and metaphors made explicit the depths of their distress and likened their reactions to feelings of a drug withdrawal. As a student from the United States noted: "I was itching, like a crackhead, because I could not use my phone." A student from Argentina observed: *"Sometimes I*

felt 'dead,'" and a student from Slovakia simply noted:

"I felt sad, lonely and depressed."

✳ Students reported that media—especially their mobile phones—have virtually become an extension of themselves. Going without media, therefore, made it seem like they had lost part of themselves. "It was an unpleasant surprise to realize that I am in a state of constant distraction, as if my real life and my virtual life were coexisting in different planes, but in equal time," said a student from Mexico.

Despite the withdrawal symptoms, many students found there were definite benefits to being unplugged. Some students said they were able to simplify their

lives, "revert to simple pleasures" when they gave up media for 24 hours. Others found they had time to talk, to fully hear what was being said. They experienced more time to share themselves with others. Students also reported feeling liberated. They took time to do things they normally would not do, such as visiting relatives, playing board games, or having face-to-face conversations.

Have you thought at all about what going "unplugged" might mean for you? What are the opportunities that you would have if you did not use media for 24 hours?

Source: The World Unplugged, *Going 24 Hours Without Media,* 2011, Available at http://theworldunplugged.wordpress.com/.

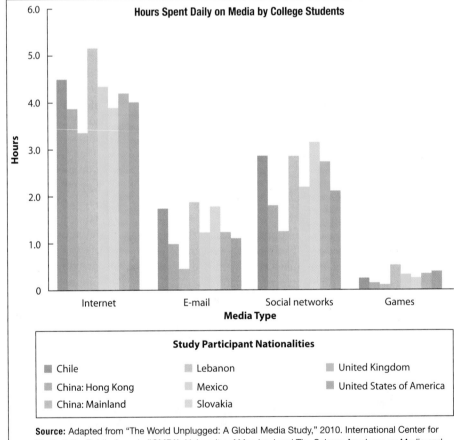

Hours Spent Daily on Media by College Students

Study Participant Nationalities
- Chile
- China: Hong Kong
- China: Mainland
- Lebanon
- Mexico
- Slovakia
- United Kingdom
- United States of America

Source: Adapted from "The World Unplugged: A Global Media Study," 2010. International Center for Media & the Public Agenda (ICMPA), University of Maryland and The Salzurg Academy on Media and Global Change. http://theworldunplugged.wordpress.com.

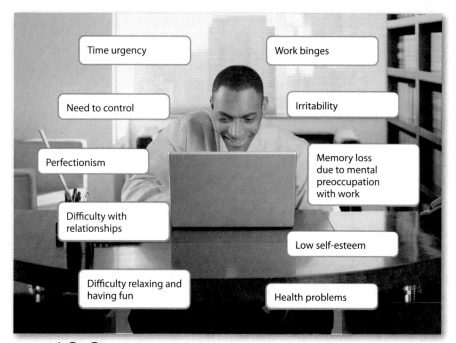

- Time urgency
- Work binges
- Need to control
- Irritability
- Perfectionism
- Memory loss due to mental preoccupation with work
- Difficulty with relationships
- Low self-esteem
- Difficulty relaxing and having fun
- Health problems

FIGURE 10.3 **Signs of Work Addiction**

and chest pain or more chronic health conditions such as heart disease and asthmatic attacks. Figure 10.3 identifies other signs of work addiction.

Work addiction is found among all age, racial, and socioeconomic groups, but it typically develops in people in their forties and fifties. Male work addicts outnumber female work addicts, but this is changing as women gain more equality in the workforce. Most work addicts come from homes that were alcoholic, rigid, violent, or otherwise dysfunctional.

Work addiction can bring admiration from society at large, as addicts often excel in their professions. However, the negative effects on individuals and those around them are far-reaching. Work addiction is a major source of marital discord and family breakup in addition to the cause of relationship problems with friends.[24]

Work Addiction

To understand work addiction, we must first understand the concept of healthy work. Healthy work provides a sense of identity; helps develop our strengths; and is a means of satisfaction, accomplishment, and mastery of problems. Healthy workers may work passionately for long hours. Although they have occasional projects that keep them away from family, friends, and personal interests for short periods of time, they generally maintain balance in their lives and full control of their schedules. Healthy work does not "consume" the worker.

Conversely, **work addiction** is the compulsive use of work and the work persona to fulfill needs of intimacy, power, and success. Work addicts usually set an intense work schedule, are unable to set boundaries regarding work, and feel driven to work even when they are away from work. Work addiction is more than being unable to relax when not doing something considered "productive."[22] The disorder is characterized by obsession, perfectionism, overachievement, anxiety, stress, anger, and burnout.[23] Work addicts may feel too busy to take care of their health, and there is some evidence work addiction may cause physical symptoms such as ulcers

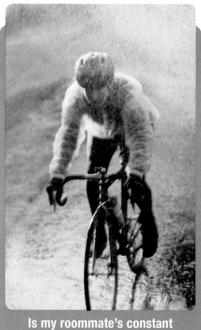

Is my roommate's constant exercising an addiction?

Obsession with a substance or behavior, even a generally positive activity such as exercise, can eventually develop into an addiction. If there are negative consequences from exercising, such as overuse injuries or withdrawal from friends and other activities, then addiction is a possibility.

Exercise Addiction

It may seem odd that a personal health text that advocates exercise would also identify it as a potential addiction. Yet, as a powerful mood enhancer, exercise can be addictive. Firm statistics on the incidence of exercise addiction are not available, but one indication of its prevalence is that a large percentage of Americans with the eating disorders anorexia nervosa and bulimia nervosa use exercise to purge instead of, or in addition to, self-induced vomiting.[25] **Exercise addicts** use exercise compulsively to try to meet needs—for nurturance, intimacy, self-esteem, and self-competency—that an object or activity cannot truly meet. Consequently, addictive or compulsive exercise results in negative consequences similar to those found in other addictions: alienation of family and friends, injuries from overdoing it, and a craving for more. Warning signs of exercise addiction include increasing the desired amount of exercise to feel the desired effect, be it a buzz or sense of accomplishment; feeling anxious, irritable, and restless,

work addiction The compulsive use of work and the work persona to fulfill needs for intimacy, power, and success.

exercise addicts People who exercise compulsively to try to meet needs of nurturance, intimacy, self-esteem, and self-competency.

50%

of Americans or more would give up chocolate, alcohol, and caffeine for a week before parting temporarily with their phones.

or having sleep problems in the absence of exercise; being unable to reduce the level of exercise or not exercise for a certain period of time; being unable to stick to the intended exercise routine by exceeding the amount of time spent exercising; spending a great deal of time preparing for, engaging in, and recovering from exercise; exercising to the point that it interferes with classes, social plans, work, and other activities; and continuing to exercise despite knowing that this activity is creating or increasing physical, psychological, and/or interpersonal problems.[26]

Traditionally, women have been perceived as being more at risk for exercise addiction. However, more men are overexercising and abusing steroids to attain an ideal frame. *Muscle dysmorphia*, sometimes referred to as *bigarexia*, is a pathological preoccupation with being larger and more muscular.[27] Sufferers view themselves as small and weak, even though they may be quite the opposite. Consequences of muscle dysmorphia include excessive weight lifting and exercising as well as steroid or supplement abuse. (See Focus On: Enhancing Your Body Image beginning on page 266 for further discussion of these disorders and the body image issues associated with them.)

Compulsive Sexual Behavior

Everyone needs love and intimacy, but the sexual practices of people addicted to sex involve neither. **Sexual addiction** is compulsive involvement in sexual activity.

Compulsive sexual behavior may involve a normally enjoyable sexual experience that becomes an obsession, or it may involve fantasies or activities outside the bounds of culturally, legally, or morally acceptable sexual behavior.[28] In fact, people with compulsive sexual behavior do not necessarily seek partners to obtain sexual arousal; they may be satisfied by masturbation, whether alone, during phone sex, or while reading or watching erotica. They may participate in a wide range of sexual activities, including affairs, sex with strangers, prostitution, voyeurism, exhibitionism, rape, incest, or pedophilia. People with compulsive sexual behavior frequently experience crushing episodes of depression and anxiety, fueled by the fear of discovery. The toll that compulsive sexual behavior exacts is most clearly seen in loss of intimacy with loved ones, which frequently leads to family disintegration.

sexual addiction Compulsive involvement in sexual activity.

intervention A planned process of confronting an addict; carried out by close family, friends, and significant others.

Compulsive sexual behaviors affect men and women of all ages, although it is more common in men, whether married or single, and it can affect anyone, regardless of sexual preference. Compulsive sexual behavior often occurs in people who experience other psychological conditions such as a mood disorder, impulse control disorders, or have alcohol or drug abuse problems. Many may have been physically and emotionally abused. People with compulsive sexual behaviors often have a history of sexual abuse.[29]

Multiple Addictions

Addicts often depend on more than one chemical or behavior. Although they tend to have a favorite drug or behavior—one that is most effective at meeting their needs—60 to 75 percent of people in treatment have problems with more than one addiction. For example, alcohol addiction and eating disorders are commonly paired in women. Individuals trying to break a chemical dependency frequently resort to compulsive eating to keep themselves from taking drugs. Although multiple addictions complicate recovery, they do not make it impossible. As with single addictions, recovery begins with recognizing that there is a problem.

> ### what do you think?
> Do you think any behavior can be addictive?
> ● Can one be a chocolate addict, a study addict, or a shoe addict?
> ● Why or why not?
> ● What dangers lie in using the word *addiction* too loosely?

Recovering from Addiction

Recovery from addiction is a lifelong process. Before treatment can begin, the individual must recognize the addiction. This can be difficult because denial—the inability to see the truth—is the hallmark of addiction. Denial can be so powerful that intervention is sometimes necessary to break down the addict's defenses.

Intervention

Intervention is a planned process of confrontation by people who are important to the addict, including spouses, parents, children, bosses, and friends. Its purpose is to break down the denial compassionately so that the person can see the addiction's destructive nature. Getting addicts to admit they have a problem is not enough. They must perceive that the behavior is destructive and requires treatment.

Individual confrontation is difficult and often futile. However, an addict's defenses generally crumble when significant others collectively share their observations and concerns. Effective intervention includes (1) emphasizing care and concern for the addicted person; (2) describing the behavior that is the cause for concern; (3) expressing how the behavior affects the addict, each person taking part in the intervention, and others; and (4) outlining specifically what those participating in the intervention would like to see happen.

It is critical that those involved in the intervention clarify how they plan to end their enabling. For example, there have been instances in which a wife has stated in public, or put notices in the local paper, that she will no longer cover bounced checks or be responsible for her gambling-addicted husband's antisocial behavior. Some spouses have even closed their joint bank accounts and opened personal accounts so they are not legally responsible for irresponsible acts. Whether these actions hold up under legal scrutiny may depend on state laws. Regardless of the type of intervention, all parties involved in the intervention should obtain advice about the legality of specific actions before jumping into a complicated situation. In addition, persons contemplating interventions must choose consequences they are ready to stick to if the addict refuses treatment. Significant others must also be ready to give support if the addict is willing to begin a recovery program.

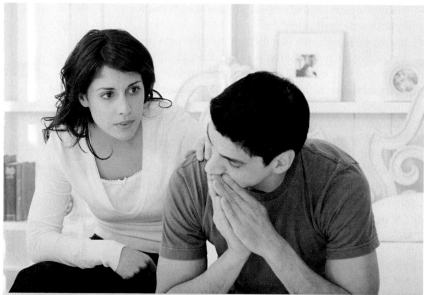

Confronting a person about addiction is a difficult task, and one that usually requires intervention by a group of family members and friends. It is more effective for an addict to be faced with the facts from a group of the people most important to him or her than by one person. In a planned intervention, the goal is to break down the addict's denial compassionately and to get him or her to recognize the addiction's destructive nature. Most addiction treatment centers have specialists who can help plan an intervention.

Intervention is a serious step that should be well planned and rehearsed. Most addiction treatment centers have specialists on staff who can help plan an intervention. In addition, books and Internet resources are available. Once the problem has been recognized, recovery can begin.

Treatment for Addiction

Treatment and recovery for any addiction generally begin with **abstinence**—refraining from the addictive behavior. Whereas complete abstinence is possible for people addicted to chemicals, it obviously is not feasible for people addicted to behaviors such as work and sex. For these addicts, abstinence means restoring balance to their lives through noncompulsive engagement in the behaviors.

Detoxification refers to an early abstinence period during which an addict adjusts physically and cognitively to being free from the addiction's influence. It occurs in virtually every recovering addict, and, while it is uncomfortable for all addicts, it can be dangerous for some. This is primarily true for those addicted to chemicals, especially alcohol, heroin, and painkillers such as OxyContin. For these people, early abstinence may involve profound withdrawal symptoms that require medical supervision. Therefore, most inpatient treatment programs provide a pretreatment component of supervised detoxification to achieve abstinence safely before treatment begins.

Abstinence alone does little to change the psychological, biological, and environmental dynamics that underlie the addictive behavior. Without treatment, an addict is apt to relapse repeatedly or simply change addictions. Treatment involves learning new ways of looking at oneself, others, and the world. It may require exploring a traumatic past so that psychological wounds can be healed. It also involves developing communication skills and new ways of having fun.

Finding a Quality Treatment Program For a large number of addicts, recovery begins with a period of formal treatment. The best programs provide a combination of therapies (behavioral therapy, medications, or both) and other services to meet an addict's needs. A good treatment program includes the following:

- Professional staff familiar with the specific addictive disorder for which help is being sought
- A flexible schedule of inpatient and outpatient services
- Access to medical personnel who can assess the addict's health and treat all medical concerns as needed

40%

of college students report feeling lonely without the Internet.

abstinence Refraining from a behavior.

detoxification The early abstinence period during which an addict adjusts physically and cognitively to being free from the influences of the addiction.

- Medical supervision of addicts who are at high risk for a complicated detoxification
- Involvement of family members in the treatment process
- A coordinated team approach to treating addictive disorders (for example, medical staff, counselors, psychotherapists, social workers, clergy, educators, dietitians, and fitness counselors)
- Both group and individual therapy options
- Peer-led support groups that encourage the addict to continue involvement after treatment ends
- Structured aftercare and relapse-prevention programs
- Accreditation by the Joint Commission (a national organization that accredits and certifies health care organizations and programs) and a license from the state in which the program operates. Matching treatment settings, programs, and services to a person's unique problems and level of need is a key to their success.

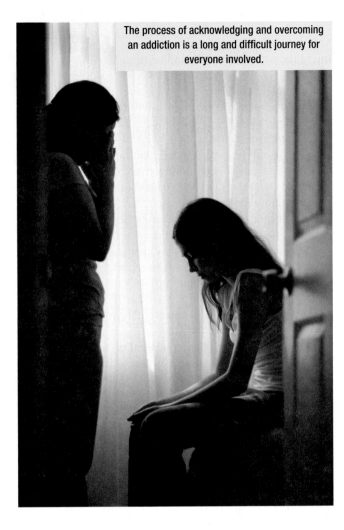

The process of acknowledging and overcoming an addiction is a long and difficult journey for everyone involved.

what do you think?

Why might addicts resist seeking treatment, even when they may admit they have a problem?

● What factors need to be considered in helping prevent relapse?

Most programs apply a combination of family, individual, and group counseling, supplemented with attendance at a 12-step support group. Individuals may also wish to explore alternatives to 12-step groups. Organizations such as Rational Recovery and the Secular Organization for Sobriety provide support without the spiritual emphasis of 12-step groups such as Alcoholics Anonymous.

Relapse

Relapse is an isolated occurrence of or full return to addictive behavior. It is one of the defining characteristics of addiction. A person who does not relapse or have powerful urges to do so was probably not addicted in the first place. Addicts are set up to relapse long before they actually do so because of their tendency to meet change and stress with the same kind of denial they once used to justify their addictive behavior (for example, thinking, "I don't have a problem; I can handle this"). This sets off a series of events involving immediate or gradual abandonment of structured recovery plans. For example, the addict may quit attending support group meetings and slip into situations that previously triggered the addictive behavior.

relapse The tendency to return to the addictive behavior after a period of abstinence.

Because those who facilitate treatment programs recognize this strong tendency to relapse, they routinely teach clients and significant others to recognize the signs of imminent relapse and develop a plan for responding to these signs. Without such a plan, recovering addicts are likely to relapse more frequently, more completely, and perhaps permanently.

Relapse should not be interpreted as failure to change or lack of desire to stay well. The appropriate response to relapse is to remind addicts that they are addicted and to redirect them to the strategies that have previously worked for them. In addition to teaching skills, relapse prevention may involve aftercare planning such as connecting the recovering person with support groups, career counselors, or community services.

Are You Addicted?

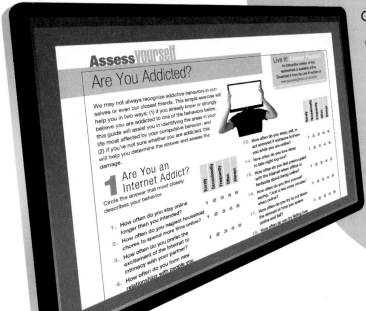

Go online to the **Live It!** section of www.pearsonhighered.com/donatelle to take the "Are You Addicted?" assessment.*

Follow the strategies in the **YOUR PLAN FOR CHANGE** box to help change any problems you uncover.

*If your instructor so chooses, the Assess Yourself Activities are available as a printed supplement or as assignable homework online at www.pearsonhighered.com/myhealthlab.

MyHealthLab®

YOUR PLAN FOR CHANGE

The online **Assess yourself** activity gave you a chance to evaluate signs of Internet, gambling, and shopping addictions. Depending on your results, you may need to take steps toward changing certain behaviors that could be detrimental to your health.

Today, you can:

○ Identify any problem areas in which you may have an addiction. Be honest with yourself about your behaviors and commit to addressing the issue. The first step in beating an addiction is admitting you have a problem.

○ Write a list of the things that contribute to the behavior you feel may be addictive. Include your reasons for engaging in the behavior and the things about it that are reinforcing. Why do you want to change it? Try to identify barriers that would make it hard to break away from the behavior or bring it under control. What would help you address these barriers?

Within the next 2 weeks, you can:

○ Look into support groups in your area that could possibly help you, such as Gamblers Anonymous or Debtors Anonymous. Visit your student health center to find out about programs that may be available on campus.

○ Begin tracking your addictive behavior. Keep a log of dates, time spent engaging in the behavior, the way you are feeling, the amount of money spent (if pertinent), other people involved, and anything else you think is relevant. Look for patterns, such as particular times of day when you are most vulnerable to the addiction, a specific mood related to it, or certain people or places that trigger your compulsion.

By the end of the semester, you can:

○ Take positive steps to address some of the patterns you noted in your log. Come up with a distraction to turn to when you begin feeling the addictive urge, and try to avoid settings or situations that trigger your addictive behavior.

○ Establish new limits for your addictive behavior and strive to enforce them for several days at a time. For example, this could mean setting a time limit on Internet use. Enlist a trusted friend to help you enforce these limits—for example, by making plans to play Frisbee after your allotted half hour of Internet surfing.

Summary

✱ Addiction is the continued use of a substance or activity despite ongoing negative consequences. Addiction develops over time through a pattern known as *nurturing through avoidance*. Mood-altering substances and experiences produce biochemical reactions that make the body feel good; when they are absent, the person feels the effects of withdrawal. All addictions share four common symptoms: compulsion, loss of control, negative consequences, and denial.

✱ Habits are repeated behaviors, whereas addiction is behavior resulting from compulsion; without the behavior, the addict experiences withdrawal.

✱ Codependents are friends or family members who are controlled by an addict's addictive behavior. Enablers are people who knowingly or unknowingly protect addicts from the consequences of their behavior.

✱ The biopsychosocial model of addiction takes into account biological (genetic) factors as well as psychological and environmental influences in understanding the addiction process.

✱ Addictive behaviors include disordered gambling, compulsive buying, compulsive technology use, work addiction, compulsive exercise, and sexual addiction.

✱ Treatment begins with abstinence from the addictive behavior or substance, usually instituted through intervention by close family, friends, or other loved ones. Treatment programs may include individual, group, or family therapy, as well as 12-step programs.

Pop Quiz

1. Which of the following is not a characteristic of addiction?
   a. Compulsion
   b. Loss of control
   c. Habit
   d. Withdrawal

2. Gina is addicted to the Internet. She is so preoccupied with surfing websites that she skips classes and misses important exams. What symptom of addiction does her preoccupation characterize?
   a. Denial
   b. Compulsion
   c. Loss of control
   d. Negative consequences

3. Which of the following is the definition of *denial*?
   a. The body's rejection of a drug or chemical
   b. The inability to perceive that a behavior is self-destructive
   c. The need to consume more drugs to get the same high
   d. A person's ability to handle a toxic amount of drugs in the body

4. Chemical dependency *relapse* refers to
   a. a person who is experiencing a blackout.
   b. a gap in one's drinking or drug-taking patterns.
   c. a full return to addictive behavior.
   d. the failure to change one's behavior.

5. People who excessively and compulsively exercise to meet needs of nurturance, intimacy, and self-esteem have a(n)
   a. money addiction.
   b. work addiction.
   c. buying addiction.
   d. exercise addiction.

6. When a person repeatedly seeks the illusion of relief to avoid unpleasant feelings, this pattern is known as
   a. neurotransmitter deficiency.
   b. nurturing through avoidance.
   c. a bad habit.
   d. compulsive behavior.

7. The current theory of addiction relies on the biopsychosocial model of addiction. This model proposes that most addictive conditions are influenced by
   a. biological or disease influences.
   b. psychological influences.
   c. environmental influences.
   d. All of the above

8. Chris is obsessed with his weight-lifting program and constantly checks to see if his six-pack abs and lean muscles are nicely sculpted. He suffers from
   a. anorexia.
   b. muscle dysmorphia.
   c. muscle atrophy.
   d. tolerance.

9. The first step in treating an addiction is to
   a. organize an intervention.
   b. recognize the addiction.
   c. enter a rehabilitation facility.
   d. find a psychotherapist.

10. An individual who knowingly tries to protect an addict from natural consequences of his or her destructive behaviors is
    a. enabling.
    b. coddling.
    c. practicing intervention.
    d. controlling.

Answers to these questions can be found on page A-1.

Think about It!

1. What factors distinguish a habit from an addiction? Is it possible for you to tell whether someone else is truly addicted?
2. Explain why the biopsychosocial model is an effective treatment mode for addiction.
3. Explain the potential genetic, environmental, and psychological risk factors for addiction.
4. Discuss how addiction affects family and friends. What role do family and friends play in helping the addict get help and maintain recovery?
5. What are some key components of an effective treatment program? Do you think the components might vary for men and women? Why or why not?

Accessing Your Health on the Internet

The following websites explore further topics and issues related to personal health. For links to the websites below, visit the Companion Website for *Access to Health,* 13th Edition, at www.pearsonhighered.com/donatelle.

1. *Center for Online and Internet Addiction.* This site provides information and assistance for those dealing with Internet addiction. www.netaddiction.com
2. *National Center for Responsible Gambling, College Gambling.org.* A resource for gambling information pertinent to college campuses. www.collegegambling.org
3. *National Council on Problem Gambling.* This site provides information and help for people with gambling problems and their families, including a searchable directory for counselors. www.ncpgambling.org

4. *Society for the Advancement of Sexual Health.* This site provides information, resources, and a self-quiz relating to sexual addiction. www.sash.net

References

1. R. Goldberg, *Drugs across the Spectrum,* 6th ed. (Belmont, CA: Brooks/Cole, 2009).
2. J. Kinney, *Loosening the Grip: A Handbook of Alcohol Information,* 9th ed. (Boston: McGraw-Hill, 2009), 175.
3. A. Agrawal et al., "Linkage Scan for Quantitative Traits Identifies New Regions of Interest for Substance Dependence in the Collaborative Study on the Genetics of Alcoholism (COGA) Sample," *Drug and Alcohol Dependence* 93, no. 1-2 (2008): 12-20.
4. A. Agrawal et al., "Linkage Scan for Quantitative Traits Identifies New Regions of Interest" 2008.
5. J. Kinney, *Loosening the Grip,* 2009, 106.
6. G. Hansen and P. Venturelli, *Drugs and Society,* 10th ed. (Sudbury, MA: Jones and Bartlett, 2009), 49.
7. Ibid, 4.
8. J. Grant et al., "Introduction to Behavioral Addictions," *American Journal of Behavioral Addictions* 36, no. 5 (2010): 233-41; National Institute on Drug Abuse, National Institutes of Health, U.S. Department of Health and Human Services, *Drugs, Brains, and Behavior: The Science of Addiction,* NIH Publication no. 07-5605 (Bethesda, MD: National Institute on Drug Abuse, 2007), Available at www.nida.nih.gov/scienceofaddiction.
9. National Council on Problem Gambling, "FAQs—Problem Gamblers," Accessed September 28, 2011 www.ncpgambling.org/i4a/pages/index.cfm?pageid=3390.
10. C. Holden, "Behavioral Addictions Debut in Proposed DSM-V," *Science 347,* no. 5968 (2010): 935.
11. Ibid.
12. H. Shaffer and R. Martin, "Disordered Gambling: Etiology, Trajectory and Clinical Considerations," *Annual Review Clinical Psychology* 7, (2011): 483-510.
13. National Center for Responsible Gambling, College Students: Facts and Stats, Accessed February 5, 2012, from http://www.collegegambling.org/just-facts/gambling-college-campuses.
14. G. M. Barnes et al., "Comparisons of Gambling and Alcohol Use Among College Students and Noncollege Young People in the United States," *American Journal of College Health* 58, no. 5 (2010): 443-52.
15. National Center for Responsible Gambling, "Fact Sheet: Gambling Disorders among College Students," Accessed February 5, 2012, from http://www.collegegambling.org/just-facts/gambling-disorders-among-college-students.
16. M. Lejoyeux and A. Weinstein, "Compulsive Buying," *The American Journal of Drug and Alcohol Issues* 36, no.5 (2010): 248-53.
17. Ibid.
18. The Center for Internet Addiction, "The Growing Epidemic," 2010, www.netaddiction.com.
19. C. Morrison and H. Gore, "The Relationship between Excessive Internet Use and Depression: A Questionnaire-Based Study of 1,319 Young People and Adults," *Psychopathology* 43, no. 2 (2010): 121-26.
20. American College Health Association, *American College Health Association—National College Health Assessment II: Reference Group Data Report Spring 2011* (Baltimore: American College Health Association, 2012).
21. J. Dunn, "Students Addicted to Technology: The Good and Bad News," *Edudemic* (2011), Accessed February 5, 2012, from http://edudemic.com/2011/08/students-technology-stats/.
22. C. Chamberlin and N. Zhang, "Workaholism, Health and Self-Acceptance," *Journal of Counseling and Development* 87, no. 2 (2009): 159-69.
23. Ibid.
24. Ibid.
25. B. Cook and H. A. Hausenblas, "The Role of Exercise Dependence for the Relationship between Exercise Behavior and Eating Pathology: Mediator or Moderator?," *Journal of Health Psychology* 13, no. 4 (2008): 495-502.
26. J. Dunn, "Students Addicted to Technology," 2011.
27. J. F. Morgan, *The Invisible Man: A Self-Help Guide for Men with Eating Disorders, Compulsive Exercise and Bigorexia* (New York: Routledge, 2008), 36.
28. Mayo Clinic, "Compulsive Sexual Behavior," September 15, 2011, Accessed February 5, 2012, from http://www.mayoclinic.com/health/compulsive-sexual-behavior/DS00144.
29. Ibid.

11

Drinking Alcohol Responsibly

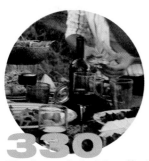
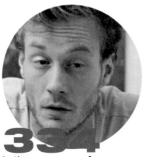
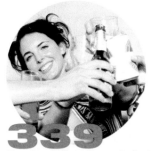
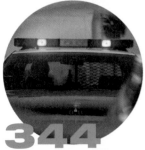
OBJECTIVES

✳ Describe the alcohol use patterns of college students and overall trends in consumption.

✳ Explain the physiological and behavioral effects of alcohol, including blood alcohol concentration, absorption, metabolism, and immediate and long-term effects of alcohol consumption.

✳ Describe practical strategies for drinking responsibly and coping with campus and societal pressures to drink.

✳ Explain the causes of alcoholism, its symptoms, and the cost to society.

✳ Explain how alcoholism affects family members and how families sometimes play a role in getting an alcoholic into treatment.

✳ Describe the various types of treatment programs for alcoholism.

✳ Explain the concepts of relapse and recovery.

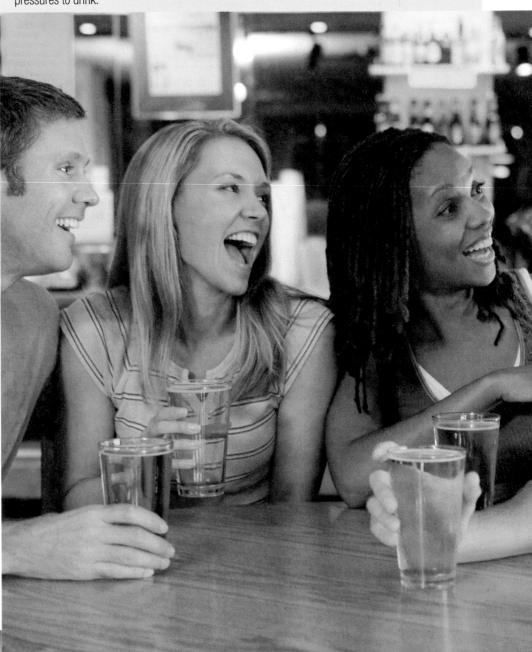

Throughout history, humans have used alcohol for everything from social gatherings to religious ceremonies. The consumption of alcoholic beverages is part of many traditions, and moderate use of alcohol can enhance celebrations or special times. Research even shows that very low levels of alcohol consumption, particularly red wine, may actually lower some health risks in older adults. Potential benefits include reduced risks of cardiovascular diseases and osteoporosis, though some critics of these studies argue that confounding factors, such as socioeconomic status, may account for the apparent benefits.[1] However, while alcohol can sometimes play a positive role in some people's lives, it is first and foremost a chemical substance that affects both physical and mental functions. Alcohol is a drug, and if it is not used responsibly, it can become dangerous.

An estimated half of Americans consume alcoholic beverages regularly, and about 21 percent abstain from drinking alcohol altogether.[2] Among those who drink, consumption patterns vary. More men are regular drinkers, and men typically drink more than women. White drinkers are more likely to drink daily or nearly daily than are nonwhites. As age increases, the number of people who consume alcohol regularly decreases.[3]

However, new estimates show that binge drinking is a bigger problem now than previously thought. More than 38 billion U.S. adults binge drink (or approximately 1 in 6), about four times a month, and the largest number of drinks per binge is on average eight. Binge drinking prevalence (28%) and intensity of drinking (9.3 drinks) were highest among persons ages 18 to 24. Interestingly, those households with incomes over $75,000 had the highest drinking prevalence (20%), but those with household incomes below $25,000 had the highest frequency (5.0 episodes per month) and intensity (8.5 drinks on occasion).[4]

90%

of people who drink alcohol are classified as moderate, light, or infrequent drinkers.

Alcohol consumption among Americans has declined steadily since the late 1970s. This downward trend has been tied to a stronger focus on personal health, weight management, and physical activity. The alcohol industry has responded by introducing beers and wines with fewer calories and carbohydrates and, in some cases, reduced alcohol content.

Alcohol in the Body

Learning about the metabolism and absorption of alcohol can help you understand how it affects each person differently and how it is possible to drink safely. It is also key to understanding how to avoid life-threatening alcohol-related circumstances such as alcohol poisoning.

The Chemistry and Potency of Alcohol

The intoxicating substance found in beer, wine, liquor, and liqueurs is **ethyl alcohol,** or **ethanol.** It is produced during a process called **fermentation,** in which yeast organisms break down plant sugars, yielding ethanol and carbon dioxide. For beers, ales, and wines, the process ends with fermentation. Manufacturers then add other ingredients that dilute the alcohol content of the beverage. Hard liquor is produced through further processing called **distillation,** during which alcohol vapors are condensed and mixed with water to make the final product.

The **proof** of an alcoholic drink is a measure of the percentage of alcohol in the beverage and therefore the strength of the drink. Alcohol percentage is half of the given proof. For example, 80 proof whiskey or scotch is 40 percent alcohol by volume, and 100 proof vodka is 50 percent alcohol by volume. Lower-proof drinks will produce fewer alcohol effects than the same amount of higher-proof drinks. Most wines are between 12 and 15 percent alcohol, and most beers are between 2 and 8 percent, depending on state laws and the type of beer.

When discussing alcohol consumption, researchers usually talk in terms of "standard drinks." As defined by the National Institute on Alcohol Abuse and Alcoholism (NIAAA), a **standard drink** is any drink that contains about 14 grams of pure alcohol (about 0.6 fluid ounce or 1.2 tablespoons; see Figure 11.1 on page 330). The actual size of a standard drink depends on the proof: a 12-ounce can of beer and a 1.5-ounce shot of vodka are both considered one standard drink because they contain the same amount of alcohol—about 0.6 fluid ounce. If you are estimating your blood alcohol concentration using standard drinks as a measure (see the following sections), you need to keep in mind the size of your drinks as well as their proof. For example, you may have bought only one beer while you were at the ballpark last weekend, but if that beer came in a 22-ounce cup, then you actually consumed two standard drinks.

ethyl alcohol (ethanol) Addictive drug produced by fermentation that is the intoxicating substance in alcoholic beverages.

fermentation Process in which yeast organisms break down plant sugars to yield ethanol.

distillation Process in which alcohol vapors are condensed and mixed with water to make hard liquor.

proof Measure of the percentage of alcohol in a beverage; the proof is double the percentage of alcohol in the drink.

standard drink Amount of any beverage that contains about 14 grams of pure alcohol.

Absorption and Metabolism

Unlike the molecules found in most foods and drugs, alcohol molecules are sufficiently small and fat soluble to be absorbed throughout the entire gastrointestinal system. A

Standard drink equivalent (and % alcohol)		Approximate number of standard drinks in:
	Beer = 12 oz (~5% alcohol)	12 oz = 1 16 oz = 1.3 22 oz = 2 40 oz = 3.3
	Malt liquor = 8.5 oz (~7% alcohol)	12 oz = 1.5 16 oz = 2 22 oz = 2.5 40 oz = 4.5
	Table wine = 5 oz (~12% alcohol)	750-mL (25-oz) bottle = 5
	80 proof spirits (gin, vodka, etc.) = 1.5 oz (~40% alcohol)	mixed drink = 1 or more* pint (16 oz) = 11 fifth (25 oz) = 17 1.75 L (59 oz) = 39

FIGURE 11.1 **What Is a Standard Drink?**

*Note: It can be difficult to estimate the number of standard drinks in a single mixed drink made with hard liquor. Depending on factors such as the type of spirits and the recipe, a mixed drink can contain from one to three or more standard drinks.

Source: Adapted from National Institute on Alcohol Abuse and Alcoholism, *Tips for Cutting Down on Drinking*, NIH Publication no. 07–3769 (Bethesda, MD: National Institutes of Health, 2008), http://pubs.niaaa.nih.gov/publications/Tips/tips.htm.

negligible amount of alcohol is absorbed through the lining of the mouth. Approximately 20 percent of ingested alcohol diffuses through the stomach lining into the bloodstream, and nearly 80 percent passes through the lining of the upper third of the small intestine.

Several factors influence how quickly your body will absorb alcohol: the alcohol concentration in your drink; the amount of alcohol you consume; the amount of food in your stomach; pylorospasm (spasm of the pyloric valve in the digestive system); your metabolism, weight, and body mass index; and your mood.

The higher the concentration of alcohol in your drink, the more rapidly it will be absorbed. As a rule, wine and beer are absorbed more slowly than distilled beverages. "Fizzy" alcoholic beverages—such as champagne and carbonated wines—are absorbed more rapidly than those containing no sparkling additives. Carbonated beverages and drinks served with mixers cause the pyloric valve to relax, thereby emptying the stomach's contents more rapidly into the small intestine. Because the small intestine is the site of the greatest absorption of alcohol, carbonated beverages increase the rate of absorption. The Health Headlines box on the following page discusses the effects of mixing energy drinks with alcohol.

The more alcohol you consume, the longer absorption takes. Alcohol can irritate the digestive system, which causes pylorospasm. When the pyloric valve is closed, nothing can move from the stomach to the upper third of the small intestine, which slows absorption. If the irritation continues, it can cause vomiting. Alcohol also takes longer to absorb if there is food in your stomach, because the surface area exposed to alcohol is smaller, and because a full stomach retards the emptying of alcoholic beverages into the small intestine.

Mood is another factor, because emotions affect how long it takes for the stomach's contents to empty into the intestine. Powerful moods, such as stress and tension, are likely to cause the stomach to dump its contents into the small intestine more rapidly. This is why alcohol is absorbed much faster when people are tense than it is when they are relaxed.

Once it has been absorbed into the bloodstream, alcohol circulates throughout the body and is metabolized in the liver, where it is converted to *acetaldehyde* by the enzyme *alcohol dehydrogenase*. It is then rapidly oxidized to *acetate*, converted to carbon dioxide and water, and eventually excreted from the body. Acetaldehyde is a toxic chemical that can cause immediate symptoms, such as nausea and vomiting, as well as long-term effects, such as liver damage. A very small portion of alcohol is excreted unchanged by the kidneys, lungs, and skin.

Alcohol contains 7 calories (kcal) per gram. This means that the average regular beer contains about 150 calories. Mixed drinks may contain more if they are combined with sugary soda or fruit juice. The body uses the calories in alco-

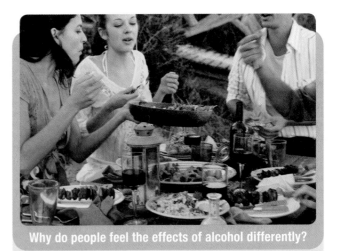

Why do people feel the effects of alcohol differently?

Many factors influence how rapidly a person's body absorbs alcohol and thus how quickly that person feels the effects of the alcohol. For example, eating while drinking slows the absorption of alcohol into your bloodstream. Other relevant factors include gender, body weight, body composition, and mood.

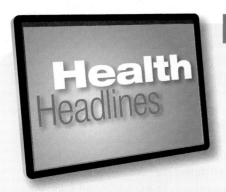
ALCOHOL AND ENERGY DRINKS: A DANGEROUS MIX

Energy drinks are aggressively marketed on college campuses, with manufacturers often giving away samples to promote their drinks. The success of these products is based on claims that they provide a burst of energy from caffeine and other plant-based stimulants and vitamins. Thirty-four percent of 18- to 24-year-olds are regular energy drink consumers.

The alcohol industry has used the popularity of energy drinks to promote its own products, introducing premixed alcohol and energy drink products such as Sparks, Rockstar 21, and Tilt. In addition, on their websites energy drink companies promote mixing energy drinks with alcohol products. Red Bull for example, promotes a top drinks list suggesting "Jaegerbombs" and "Tucker Death mix".

Because students often mix energy drinks with alcohol for the sake of masking the taste or effects of alcohol, these drinks can be particularly dangerous. One study found that students drinking alcohol with energy drinks consumed more than those who drank other types of alcoholic beverages (8.3 drinks vs. 6.1 drinks, respectively).

Students also report not noticing the signs of intoxication (dizziness, fatigue, headache, or lack of coordination) when they had consumed alcohol-mixed energy drinks. There are several reasons for this. Caffeine may delay the onset of normal sleepiness, increasing the amount of time a person would normally stay awake and drink. The caffeine in energy drinks also reduces the subjective feeling of drunkenness without actually reducing alcohol-related impairment

Students who reported drinking alcohol-mixed energy drinks were more likely to be taken advantage of sexually; they were twice as likely to take advantage of someone sexually, ride with a drunk driver, be hurt or injured, or require medical treatment. They were more than twice as likely than non-energy drink drinkers to

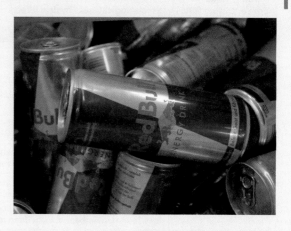

meet the criteria for alcohol dependency. Weekly or daily energy drink consumption is also strongly associated with alcohol dependency.

Sources: D. L. Thombs et al., "Event-level Analyses of Energy Drink Consumption and Alcohol Intoxication in Bar Patrons," *Addictive Behaviors* 35, no. 4 (2010): 325–30; M. C. O'Brien et al., "Caffeinated Cocktails: Energy Drink Consumption, High-Risk Drinking, and Alcohol-Related Consequences among College Students," *Society for Academic Emergency Medicine* 15 (2008): 1–8; Center for Science in the Public Interest, *Alcohol Policies Project Fact Sheet: Alcoholic Energy Drinks*, Updated September 2008, www.cspinet.org/booze/fctindex.htm; A.M. Arria et al., "Energy Drink Consumption and Increased Risk for Alcohol Dependence," *Alcoholism: Clinical and Experimental Research* 35, no. 2 (2011): 365–75; William W.I et al., "Energy Drinks: Psychological Effects and Impact on Well-being and Quality of Life: A Literature Review," *Innovations in Clinical Neuroscience*, 9, no. 1 (2012): 25–34.

---

hol in the same manner it uses those found in carbohydrates: for immediate energy or for storage as fat if not immediately needed.

The breakdown of alcohol occurs at a fairly constant rate of 0.5 ounce per hour (approximately equivalent to one standard drink). This amount of alcohol is equivalent to 12 ounces of 5 percent beer, 5 ounces of 12 percent wine, or 1.5 ounces of 40 percent (80 proof) liquor. Unmetabolized alcohol circulates in the bloodstream until enough time passes for the body to break it down.

Blood Alcohol Concentration

Blood alcohol concentration (BAC) is the ratio of alcohol to total blood volume. It is the factor used to measure the physiological and behavioral effects of alcohol. Despite individual differences, alcohol produces some general behavioral effects, depending on BAC (**Figure 11.2**, on page 332).

At a BAC of 0.02 percent, a person feels slightly relaxed and in a good mood. At 0.05 percent, relaxation increases, there is some motor impairment, and a willingness to talk becomes apparent. At 0.08 percent, a person feels euphoric, and there is further motor impairment. The legal limit for driving a motor vehicle is a 0.08 percent BAC in all states and the District of Columbia. At 0.10 percent, the depressant effects of alcohol become apparent, drowsiness sets in, and motor skills are further impaired, followed by a loss of judgment. Thus, a driver may not be able to estimate distance or speed, and some drinkers may do things they would not do when sober. As BAC increases, the drinker suffers increasingly negative physiological and psychological effects.

A drinker's BAC depends on weight and percentage of body fat, the water content in body tissues, the concentration of alcohol in the beverage consumed, the

blood alcohol concentration (BAC) The ratio of alcohol to total blood volume; the factor used to measure the physiological and behavioral effects of alcohol.

Blood Alcohol Concentration (BAC)	Psychological and Physical Effects
Not Impaired	
<0.01%	Negligible
Sometimes Impaired	
0.01–0.04%	Slight muscle relaxation, mild euphoria, slight body warmth, increased sociability and talkativeness
Usually Impaired	
0.05–0.07%	Lowered alertness, impaired judgment, lowered inhibitions, exaggerated behavior, loss of small muscle control
Always Impaired	
0.08–0.14%	Slowed reaction time, poor muscle coordination, short-term memory loss, judgment impaired, inability to focus
0.15–0.24%	Blurred vision, lack of motor skills, sedation, slowed reactions, difficulty standing and walking, passing out
0.25–0.34%	Impaired consciousness, disorientation, loss of motor function, severely impaired or no reflexes, impaired circulation and respiration, uncontrolled urination, slurred speech, possible death
0.35% and up	Unconsciousness, coma, extremely slow heartbeat and respiration, unresponsiveness, probable death

FIGURE 11.2 **The Psychological and Physical Effects of Alcohol**

rate of consumption, and the volume of alcohol consumed. Heavier people have larger body surfaces through which to diffuse alcohol; therefore, they have lower concentrations of alcohol in their blood than do thin people after drinking the same amount.

Blood Alcohol Concentration and Gender

Because alcohol does not diffuse as rapidly into body fat as it does into water, alcohol concentration is higher in a person with more body fat. Because women tend to have more body fat and less water in their tissues than men of the same weight, they will become more intoxicated after drinking the same amount of alcohol. Body fat is not the only contributor to the

differences in alcohol's effects on men and women. Women have half as much *alcohol dehydrogenase,* the enzyme that breaks down alcohol in the stomach before it reaches the bloodstream and the brain. So if a man and a woman drink the same amount of alcohol, the woman's BAC will be approximately 30 percent higher than the man's. Hormonal differences can also play a role: certain points in the menstrual cycle and the use of oral contraceptives are likely to contribute to longer periods of intoxication. This prolonged peak appears to be related to a woman's estrogen levels. Figure 11.3 compares blood alcohol levels in men and women by weight and number of drinks consumed.

Both breath analysis (breathalyzer test) and urinalysis are used to determine whether an individual is legally intoxicated, but blood tests are more accurate measures of BAC. An increasing number of states require blood tests for people suspected of driving under the influence of alcohol. In some states, refusal to take the breath or urine test results in immediate revocation of the person's driver's license.

People can develop physical and psychological tolerance of the effects of alcohol through regular use. The nervous system adapts over time, so greater amounts of alcohol are required to produce the same physiological and psychological effects.

what do you think?

What do you think the legal BAC for drivers should be?
● What should the penalty be for people arrested for driving under the influence of alcohol (DUI) for the first offense?
● For subsequent offenses?

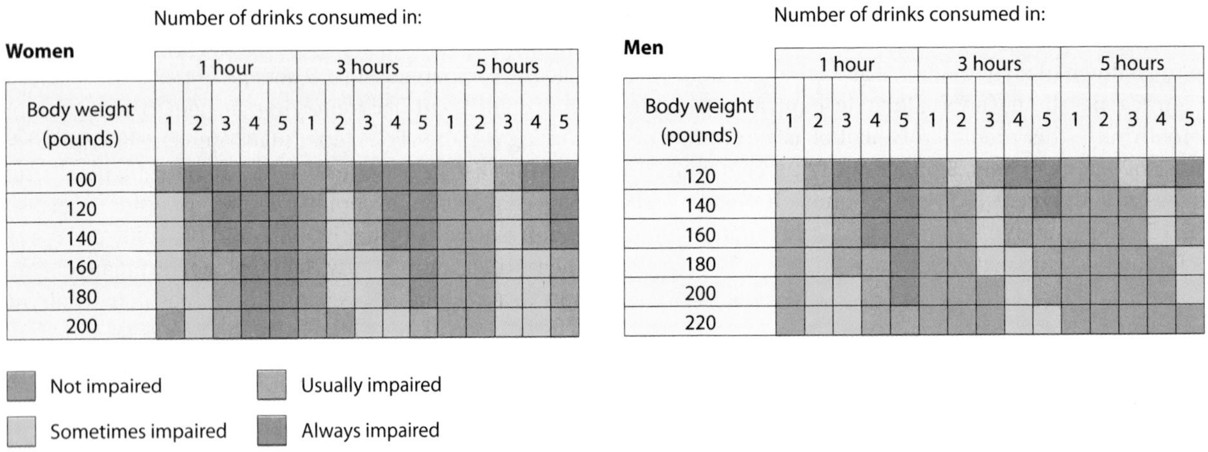

FIGURE 11.3 **Approximate Blood Alcohol Concentration (BAC) and the Physiological and Behavioral Effects**
Remember that there are many variables that can affect BAC, so this is only an estimate of what your BAC would be.

Though BAC may be quite high, the individual has learned to modify his or her behavior to appear sober. This ability is called **learned behavioral tolerance.**

Alcohol and Your Health

The immediate and long-term effects of alcohol consumption can vary greatly (Figure 11.4). Whether you experience any immediate or long-term consequences as a result of your alcohol use depends on you as an individual, the amount of alcohol you consume, and your circumstances.

Short-Term Effects of Alcohol

The most dramatic effects produced by ethanol occur within the central nervous system (CNS). Alcohol depresses CNS functions, which decreases respiratory rate, pulse rate, and blood pressure. As CNS depression deepens, vital functions become noticeably affected. In extreme cases, coma and death can result.

Alcohol is a diuretic that causes increased urinary output. Although this effect might be expected to lead to automatic **dehydration,** the body actually retains water, most of it in the muscles or in cerebral tissues. Because water is usually pulled out of the *cerebrospinal fluid* (fluid within the brain and spinal cord), drinkers may suffer symptoms that include the "morning-after" effects.

Alcohol irritates the gastrointestinal system and may cause indigestion and heartburn if consumed on an empty stomach. In addition, people who engage in brief drinking sprees during which they consume unusually high amounts of alcohol put themselves at risk for irregular heartbeat or

learned behavioral tolerance The ability of heavy drinkers to modify behavior so they appear to be sober even when they have high BAC levels.
dehydration Loss of water from body tissues.

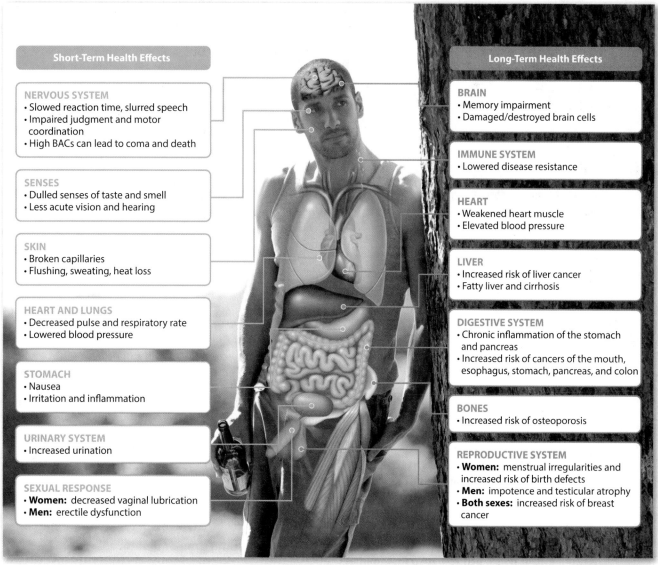

Short-Term Health Effects

NERVOUS SYSTEM
• Slowed reaction time, slurred speech
• Impaired judgment and motor coordination
• High BACs can lead to coma and death

SENSES
• Dulled senses of taste and smell
• Less acute vision and hearing

SKIN
• Broken capillaries
• Flushing, sweating, heat loss

HEART AND LUNGS
• Decreased pulse and respiratory rate
• Lowered blood pressure

STOMACH
• Nausea
• Irritation and inflammation

URINARY SYSTEM
• Increased urination

SEXUAL RESPONSE
• **Women:** decreased vaginal lubrication
• **Men:** erectile dysfunction

Long-Term Health Effects

BRAIN
• Memory impairment
• Damaged/destroyed brain cells

IMMUNE SYSTEM
• Lowered disease resistance

HEART
• Weakened heart muscle
• Elevated blood pressure

LIVER
• Increased risk of liver cancer
• Fatty liver and cirrhosis

DIGESTIVE SYSTEM
• Chronic inflammation of the stomach and pancreas
• Increased risk of cancers of the mouth, esophagus, stomach, pancreas, and colon

BONES
• Increased risk of osteoporosis

REPRODUCTIVE SYSTEM
• **Women:** menstrual irregularities and increased risk of birth defects
• **Men:** impotence and testicular atrophy
• **Both sexes:** increased risk of breast cancer

FIGURE 11.4 **Effects of Alcohol on the Body and Health**

Video Tutor: Long- and Short-Term Effects of Alcohol

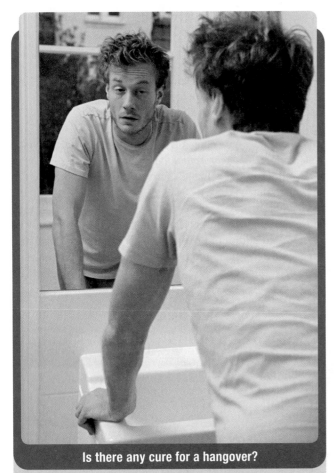

Is there any cure for a hangover?

The only cure for a hangover is abstaining from excessive alcohol use in the first place.

Alcohol and Injuries Alcohol use plays a significant role in the types of injuries people experience. Approximately 40,000 youths ages 15 to 20 are hospitalized annually after drinking alcohol, and 13 percent of emergency room visits by undergraduate college students are related to alcohol. When it comes to hospitalizations, 34 percent are the result of acute intoxication.[5] One study found that injured patients with a BAC over 0.08 percent who were treated in emergency rooms were 3.2 times more likely to have a violent intentional injury than an unintentional injury.[6] Most people admitted to emergency rooms are men 21 years or older, mostly as the result of accidents or fights in which alcohol was involved.[7] Alcohol use is involved in up to half of fatal injuries during activities such as swimming and boating and in 40 percent of fatal injuries due to house fires.[8] Alcohol use is also a key factor in many suicides and rapes. About two thirds of all completed suicides involve alcohol, and more than 30 percent of rape victims reported that their assailant was under the influence of alcohol.[9]

Alcohol and Sexual Decision Making Because it lowers inhibitions, alcohol has a clear influence on one's ability to make good decisions about sex, and you may do things you might not do when sober. People who are intoxicated are less likely to use safer sex practices and are more likely to engage in high-risk sexual activity. About 1 in 5 college students report engaging in sexual activity, including having sex with someone they just met and having unprotected sex, after drinking.[10] The chance of acquiring a sexually transmitted infection or experiencing an unplanned pregnancy also increases among students who drink more heavily compared with those who drink moderately or not at all. In one study, heavy drinking was associated with dating violence by men in their first year in college. Among women, heavy drinking in their sophomore year predicted dating violence in their junior year.[11]

Alcohol Poisoning **Alcohol poisoning** (also known as *acute alcohol intoxication*) occurs much more frequently than people realize, and all too often it can be fatal. Drinking large amounts of alcohol in a short period of time can cause the blood alcohol level to quickly reach the lethal range. Alcohol, used either alone or in combination with other drugs, is responsible for more toxic overdose deaths than any other substance.

3 in 10

Americans will be involved in an alcohol-related accident at some time in their lives.

The amount of alcohol that causes a person to lose consciousness is dangerously close to the lethal dose. Death from alcohol poisoning can be caused by CNS and respiratory depression or by the inhalation of vomit or fluid into the

even total loss of heart rhythm, which can disrupt blood flow and damage the heart muscle.

Hangover A **hangover** is often experienced the morning after a drinking spree. Its symptoms are familiar to most people who drink: headache, muscle aches, upset stomach, anxiety, depression, diarrhea, and thirst. **Congeners,** forms of alcohol that are metabolized more slowly than ethanol and are more toxic, are thought to play a role in the development of a hangover. The body metabolizes the congeners after the ethanol is gone from the system, and their toxic by-products may contribute to the hangover. Alcohol also upsets the water balance in the body, which results in excess urination, dehydration, and thirst the next day. Increased production of hydrochloric acid can irritate the stomach lining and cause nausea. Recovery from a hangover usually takes 12 hours. Bed rest, solid food, and aspirin may help relieve a hangover's discomforts, but the only sure way to avoid one is to abstain from excessive alcohol use in the first place.

hangover Physiological reaction to excessive drinking, including headache, upset stomach, anxiety, depression, diarrhea, and thirst.

congeners Forms of alcohol that are metabolized more slowly than ethanol and produce toxic by-products.

alcohol poisoning Potentially lethal blood alcohol concentration that inhibits the brain's ability to control consciousness, respiration, and heart rate; usually occurs as a result of drinking a large amount of alcohol in a short period of time. Also known as *acute alcohol intoxication.*

lungs. Alcohol depresses the nerves that control involuntary actions such as breathing and the gag reflex (which prevents choking). As BAC levels reach higher concentrations, eventually these functions can be completely suppressed. If a drinker becomes unconscious and vomits, there is a danger of asphyxiation through choking to death on the vomit. Blood alcohol concentration can continue rising even after a drinker becomes unconscious because alcohol in the stomach and intestine continues to empty into the bloodstream.

The **Skills for Behavior Change** box describes the signs of alcohol poisoning. If you are with someone who has been drinking heavily and who exhibits these symptoms, or if you are unsure about the person's condition, call your local emergency number (9-1-1 in most areas) for immediate assistance.

Long-Term Effects

Alcohol is distributed throughout most of the body and may affect many organs and tissues. Problems associated with long-term, habitual alcohol abuse include diseases of the nervous system, cardiovascular system, and liver, as well as some cancers.

Effects on the Nervous System The nervous system is especially sensitive to alcohol. Even people who drink moderately experience shrinkage in brain size and weight and a loss of some degree of intellectual ability.

Research suggests that developing brains in adolescents are much more prone to damage than was previously thought. Alcohol appears to damage the frontal areas of the adolescent brain, which are crucial for controlling impulses and thinking through consequences of intended actions.[12] In addition, researchers suggest that people who begin drinking at an early age are at much higher risk of experiencing alcohol abuse or dependence, drinking five or more drinks per drinking occasion, and driving under the influence of alcohol at least weekly.[13]

Cardiovascular Effects Alcohol affects the cardiovascular system in a number of ways. Numerous studies have associated light to moderate alcohol consumption (no more than two drinks a day) with a reduced risk of coronary artery disease.[14] Several mechanisms have been proposed to explain how this might happen. The strongest evidence points to an increase in high-density lipoprotein (HDL) cholesterol, which is known as "good" cholesterol. Studies have shown that moderate drinkers have higher levels of HDL.[15] Alcohol's effects on blood clotting, insulin sensitivity, and inflammation are also thought to play a role in protecting against heart disease. However, alcohol consumption is not a preventive measure against heart disease: It causes many more cardiovascular health hazards than benefits. Drinking too much alcohol contributes to high blood pressure and higher calorie intake, both of which are risk factors for cardiovascular disease.[16]

Liver Disease One of the most common diseases related to alcohol abuse is **cirrhosis** of the liver (see **Figure 11.5** on page 336). It is among the top ten causes of death in the United States. One result of heavy drinking is that the liver begins to store fat—a condition known as *fatty liver*. If there is insufficient time between drinking episodes, this fat cannot be transported to storage sites, and the fat-filled liver cells stop functioning. Continued drinking can cause a further stage of liver deterioration called *fibrosis*, in which the damaged area of the liver develops fibrous scar tissue. Cell function can be partially restored at this stage with proper nutrition and abstinence from alcohol. However, if the person continues to drink, cirrhosis results. At this point, liver cells die and the damage becomes permanent. **Alcoholic hepatitis** is another serious condition resulting from prolonged alcohol use. A chronic inflammation of the liver develops, which may be fatal in itself or progress to cirrhosis.

cirrhosis The last stage of liver disease associated with chronic heavy alcohol use, during which liver cells die and damage becomes permanent.

alcoholic hepatitis Condition resulting from prolonged use of alcohol in which the liver is inflamed; can be fatal.

Cancer Alcohol is considered a carcinogen. The repeated irritation caused by long-term alcohol use has been linked to cancers of the esophagus, stomach, mouth, tongue, and liver. In one study,

"Why Should I Care?"

Going out drinking may be fun at the time, but excessive alcohol consumption can result in a hangover that ruins the day after you overindulge. Feeling sick with a hangover can lead you to skip class and to miss out on other activities you had planned for the day.

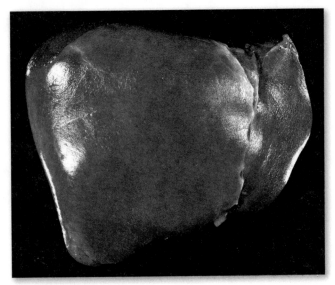

(a) A normal liver

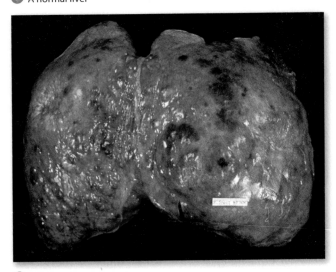

(b) A liver with cirrhosis

FIGURE 11.5 **Comparison of a Healthy Liver with a Cirrhotic Liver**
In cirrhosis, healthy liver cells are replaced with scar tissue that interferes with the liver's ability to perform its many vital functions.

NIAAA scientists discovered a possible link between acetaldehyde and DNA damage that could help explain the connection between drinking and certain types of cancer.[17]

There is substantial evidence that women who consume even low levels of alcohol (three to six drinks per week) have a higher risk of breast cancer compared with those who abstain. The risk for breast cancer is higher for women who consume more than 2 drinks per day. It also made no difference the type of alcohol consumed (beer, wine, or liquor).[18] Girls and young women who drink alcohol increase their risk of benign (noncancerous) breast disease. Benign breast disease increases the risk for developing breast cancer. In a recent study, girls and young women who drank 6 or 7 days a week were 5.5 times more likely to have benign breast disease than those who didn't drink or who had less than one drink per week. Those diagnosed with benign breast disease on average drank more often, drank more on each occasion, and had an average daily consumption that was two times that of those who did not have benign breast disease.[19]

fetal alcohol syndrome (FAS) Birth defect involving physical and mental impairment that results from the mother's alcohol consumption during pregnancy.

Other Effects Alcohol abuse is a major cause of chronic inflammation of the pancreas, the organ that produces digestive enzymes and insulin. Chronic alcohol abuse inhibits enzyme production, which further inhibits the absorption of nutrients. Drinking alcohol can block the absorption of calcium, a nutrient that strengthens bones. This should be of particular concern to women because of their risk for osteoporosis. Heavy consumption of alcohol worsens this condition. Evidence also suggests that alcohol impairs the body's ability to recognize and fight foreign bodies, such as bacteria and viruses.

Alcohol and Pregnancy

Teratogenic substances cause birth defects. Of the 30 known teratogens in the environment, alcohol is one of the most dangerous. If a woman ingests alcohol while pregnant, it will pass through the placenta and enter the growing fetus's bloodstream. A recent study found that more than 12 percent of children have been exposed to alcohol *in utero* and 2 percent of pregnant women reported binge drinking.[20] Consuming four or more drinks a day during pregnancy may significantly increase the risk of childhood mental health and learning problems. However, any use can result in varying degrees of effects, ranging from mild learning disabilities to major physical, mental, and intellectual impairment. Alcohol consumed during the first trimester poses the greatest threat to organ development; exposure during the last trimester, when the brain is developing rapidly, is most likely to affect CNS development.

A disorder called **fetal alcohol syndrome (FAS)** is associated with alcohol consumption during pregnancy. FAS is the third most common birth defect and the second leading cause of mental retardation in the United States, with an estimated incidence of 1 to 2 in every 1,000 live births.[21] It is the most common preventable cause of mental impairment in the Western world. Among the symptoms of FAS are mental retardation; small head size;

tremors; and abnormalities of the face, limbs, heart, and brain. Children with FAS may experience problems such as poor memory and impaired learning, reduced attention span, impulsive behavior, and poor problem-solving abilities, among others.

Some children may have fewer than the full physical or behavioral symptoms of FAS and may be diagnosed with disorders such as partial fetal alcohol syndrome (PFAS) or alcohol-related neurodevelopmental disorder (ARND); all of these disorders (including FAS) fall under the umbrella term *fetal alcohol spectrum disorder* (FASD). An estimated 40,000 infants in the United States are affected by FASD each year—more than those affected by spina bifida, Down syndrome, and muscular dystrophy combined.[22] Infants whose mothers habitually consumed more than 3 ounces of alcohol (approximately six drinks) in a short time period when pregnant are at high risk for FASD. Risk levels for babies whose mothers consume smaller amounts are uncertain. To avoid any chance of harming her fetus, any woman of childbearing age who is or may become pregnant is advised to refrain from consuming any amount of alcohol.

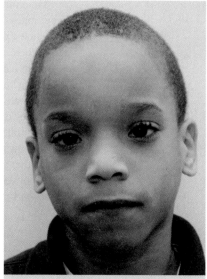

Characteristic facial features of FAS include a small, upturned nose with a low bridge and a thin upper lip.

Alcohol Use in College

Alcohol is the most popular drug on college campuses: Large numbers of students report having consumed alcoholic beverages in the past 30 days (Figure 11.6).[23] In a new trend

on college campuses, women's consumption of alcohol has come close to equaling men's.

Approximately 44 percent of all college students engage in **binge drinking.**[24] According to the NIAA, a binge is a pattern of drinking alcohol that brings blood alcohol concentration (BAC) to 0.08 gram-percent or above. For a typical adult, this pattern corresponds to consuming five or more drinks (men), or four or more drinks (women), in about 2 hours.[25] Therefore, students who might go out and drink only once a week are considered binge drinkers if they consume these amounts within 2 hours. Binge drinking is especially dangerous because it can lead to extreme intoxication, unconsciousness, alcohol poisoning, and even death. Drinking competitions, celebrations, or games and hazing rituals encourage this type of drinking.

College is a critical time to become aware of and responsible for drinking. Many students are away from home, often for the first time, and are excited by their newfound independence. For some students, this independence and the rite of passage into the college culture are symbolized by alcohol use. Many students say they drink to have fun. "Having fun," which often means drinking simply to get drunk, may really be a way of coping with stress, boredom, anxiety, or pressures created by academic and social demands.

binge drinking A pattern of drinking alcohol that brings blood alcohol concentration (BAC) to 0.08 grampercent or above; corresponds to consuming five or more drinks (adult male) or four or more drinks (adult female) in 2 hours.

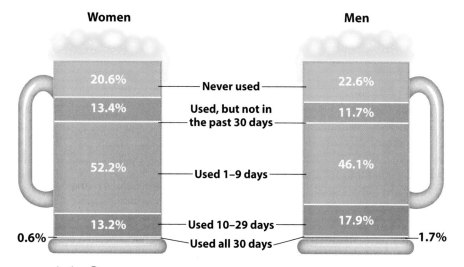

Women   **Men**

	Women		Men
Never used	20.6%		22.6%
Used, but not in the past 30 days	13.4%		11.7%
Used 1–9 days	52.2%		46.1%
Used 10–29 days	13.2%		17.9%
Used all 30 days	0.6%		1.7%

FIGURE 11.6 **College Students' Patterns of Alcohol Use in the Past 30 Days**
Source: Data from American College Health Association, *American College Health Association—National College Health Assessment II (ACHA-NCHA II) Reference Group Data Report Spring 2011* (Baltimore: American College Health Association, 2012).

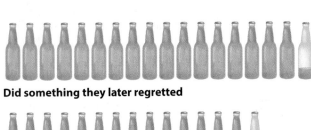

Did something they later regretted   34.6%

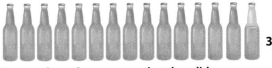

Forgot where they were or what they did   30.4%

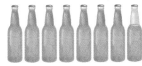

Had unprotected sex   16.5%

Physically injured self   14.9%

3.6%

Got in trouble with the police

2.3%

Physically injured another person

FIGURE 11.7 **Prevalence of Negative Consequences of Drinking among College Students, Past Year**
Source: Data from American College Health Association, *American College Health Association—National College Health Assessment II (ACHA-NCHA II) Reference Group Data Report Spring 2011* (Baltimore: American College Health Association, 2012).

A significant number of students experience negative consequences as a result of their alcohol consumption. Figure 11.7 shows some examples of alcohol-related problems. According to the American College Health Association (ACHA), in the past 12 months, about 35 percent of college students who drank reported doing something they later regretted; one third forgot where they were or what they did due to intoxication; almost 15 percent accidentally injured themselves; and 16.5 percent had unprotected sex.[26]

Alcohol use among college students also has consequences related to academic performance. Alcohol consumption tends to disrupt sleep, particularly the second half of the night's sleep, and these disruptive effects increase daytime sleepiness and decrease alertness. Research shows that daytime sleepiness as a result of alcohol use and disruptive sleep negatively impacts students' academic performance.[27]

On a more positive note, according to the ACHA survey, many college students reported always or usually practicing protective behaviors when consuming alcohol to reduce the risk of negative consequences as a result of their alcohol use. Seventy-two percent of students reported eating before or during drinking, about 65 percent said they usually or always stayed with the same group of friends the entire time they drank, 66 percent reported using a designated driver most or all of the time, and 63 percent always or usually kept track of how many drinks they consumed.[28] It is important to recognize that choices such as these can help reduce the risk of negative consequences as a result of drinking. The Skills for Behavior Change box provides additional strategies for drinking responsibly.

High-Risk Drinking and College Students

According to one study, 1,825 college students die each year because of alcohol-related unintentional injuries, including car accidents.[29] Consumption of alcohol is the number one cause of preventable death among undergraduate college students in the United States today.

Who Drinks? It's likely that students who enter college will drink at some point, but there are groups of students who are more likely to drink more and more often. For example, students who believe that their parents approve of their drinking are more likely to drink and to report a drinking-related problem.[30] Students who drank heavily in high school are also at risk for heavy drinking in college.[31] Most students have tried alcohol in high school. By their senior year, 23 percent of high school students report engaging in binge drinking, and 27 percent report having been drunk, while another 12 percent report having had at least one full drink during a month.[32]

Why Do College Students Drink So Much? Although everyone is at some risk for alcohol-related problems, college students are particularly vulnerable for the following reasons:

- Alcohol exacerbates their already high risk for suicide, automobile crashes, and falls.
- Some university celebrations encourage certain dangerous practices and patterns of alcohol use.
- The alcoholic beverage industry heavily targets university campuses with promotions and ads.
- College students have a strong need to be accepted by their peers and believe that alcohol will make them feel better and be less stressed, more sociable, and less self-conscious.
- College administrators often deny that alcohol problems exist on their campuses.

College Student Drinking Behavior College students are more likely than their noncollegiate peers to drink recklessly and to engage in drinking games and other dangerous practices. One such practice is **pre-gaming** (also called pre-loading or front-loading). Pre-gaming has become increasingly common and involves planned heavy drinking, usually in someone's home, apartment, or residence hall, prior to going out to a bar, nightclub, or sporting event. Sometimes it occurs prior to attending an event where alcohol is not available. In a recent study of pre-gaming, 55 percent of college men and 60 percent of college women drank before going to a bar or nightclub.[33] The goal of many pre-gamers is to get drunk. Some of the motivations for pre-gaming are to avoid paying for high-cost drinks, to socialize with friends, to reduce social anxiety, and to enhance male bonding. Pre-gamers have higher alcohol consumption during the evening and more negative consequences such as blackouts, hangovers, passing out, and alcohol poisoning.

More than 80 percent of college students drink alcohol to celebrate their twenty-first birthday, and they consume an average of nearly 13 drinks, with estimated BACs of 19 percent and higher. See the **Points of View** box on the following page on the issue of legal drinking age.

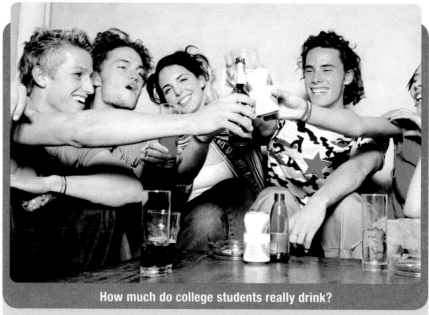

How much do college students really drink?

It may sometimes seem like your campus is crowded with heavy drinkers, but in fact, most college students—about 65%—drink only occasionally, and 21.3% don't drink at all. However, college students have high rates of binge drinking; when they do drink, they tend to drink a lot. Irresponsible consumption of alcohol can easily result in disaster, so it is important for you to take control of when you drink and how much.

Source: American College Health Association, *American College Health Association—National College Health Assessment II (ACHA-NCHA II) Reference Group Data Report Spring 2011* (Baltimore: American College Health Association, 2012).

Binge drinking is especially dangerous because it often involves drinking a lot of alcohol in a very short period of time. Two thirds of college students engage in drinking games that involve binge drinking.[34] Those who participate in drinking games are much less likely to monitor or regulate how much they are drinking and are at extreme risk for intoxication. Men more often than women participate in drinking games to consume larger amounts of alcohol.[35] Drinking games have been associated with alcohol-related injuries and deaths from alcohol poisoning. Easy access to alcohol also contributes to higher rates of binge drinking. Campus communities with a large number of bars and alcohol outlets have a higher rate of binge drinking than those with few bars and alcohol outlets located close to campus.[36]

pre-gaming Drinking heavily at home before going out to an event or other location.

To see whether your alcohol consumption is a problem, complete the **Assess Yourself** online activity; see more details on this in the related box at the end of the chapter.

What Is the Impact of Student Drinking? Unfortunately, recent studies confirm what students have been experiencing for a long time—drinking and binge drinkers cause problems not only for themselves, but also for those around them. One study indicated that more than 696,000 students between the ages of 18 and 24 were assaulted by another student who had been drinking.[37] There is significant

The Drinking Age:
IS THERE A RIGHT ONE?

The legal drinking age used to be different from state to state, with some areas setting it at 18 or 19 and others at 21 years old. But in 1984 Congress passed the National Minimum Drinking Age Act, setting the legal age at 21 for the entire country. In 2008 the Amethyst Initiative was founded by university and college presidents to call for the discussion of current drinking age laws and whether the appropriate minimum legal drinking age should be younger than 21. Below are the major points from both sides of the issue.

Arguments for Reducing the Legal Drinking Age

○ Many studies show educational programs advocating abstinence for those under age 21 have not resulted in significant behavioral change among underage students.

○ Adults under 21 can legally vote, marry, sign contracts, serve on juries, and enlist in the military, but they are deemed too immature to have a beer.

○ Widespread use of fake IDs for drinking means that students make ethical compromises that erode respect for the law.

○ Binge drinking often occurs off campus to avoid detection of underage drinkers, which makes it more difficult when a drinker needs medical attention.

Arguments for Keeping the Drinking Age 21

○ Higher drinking ages were associated with reduced consumption in 11 of 33 studies.

○ In evaluating the relationship between legal drinking ages and motor vehicle accidents, a majority of recent studies found a higher drinking age was associated with a decreased incidence of accidents.

○ Students are influenced to drink responsibly by their campus environment, so improving that environment will be more effective than changing the drinking age.

○ The public school system will be faced with an increased burden in dealing with those who are legal to drink and those who are not within the high school setting.

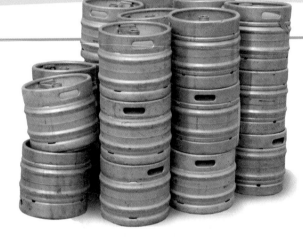

Where Do You Stand?

○ What do you think the legal drinking age should be? What potential problems would be created by changing it? What issues might be resolved by changing it?

○ Do you think that drinking ages should vary by state? Why or why not?

○ Do you think the laws should be changed in regard to underage drinking? Why or why not? Are laws effective deterrents?

Sources: Amethyst Initiative, "Statement," 2008, www.amethystinitiative.org/statement; Washington State University, College Coalition for Substance Abuse Prevention, "Response to Amethyst Initiative," August 2008, http://ccsap.wsu.edu/default.asp?PageID=2718; K. Kiewra, "Binge Drinking: Harvard College Alcohol Study Calls for Changes at U.S. Colleges," Harvard School of Public Health, Accessed June 2010, www.hsph.harvard.edu/news/hphr/winter-2009/winter09binge.html.

evidence that campus rape is linked to binge drinking. Women from colleges with medium to high binge drinking rates are 1.5 times more at risk of being raped than those from schools with a low binge drinking rate. Although exact numbers are hard to find, estimates are that more than 97,000 U.S. students between the ages of 18 and 24 experience alcohol-related sexual assault or date rape each year.[38]

The laws regarding sexual consent are clear: A person who is drunk or passed out cannot consent to sex. Anyone who has sex with a person who is drunk or unconscious is committing rape. Claiming you were also drunk when you had sex with someone who was intoxicated or unconscious does not absolve you of your legal and moral responsibility for this crime.

Some students report sleep disruptions and academic problems related to alcohol. The more students drink, the more likely they are to miss class, do poorly on tests and papers, have lower grade point averages, and fall behind on assigned work. Some students even drop out of school as a result of their drinking.

Efforts to Reduce Student Drinking

Some colleges are taking action to curb binge drinking and alcohol abuse by instituting strong policies against drinking. University policies include banning alcohol on campus, no alcohol at university events, and no advertising of alcohol in campus newspapers. Many fraternities have elected to have "dry" houses. At the same time, schools are making more help available to students with drinking problems. Today, most campuses offer both individual and group counseling and are directing more attention toward preventing alcohol abuse. Student organizations such as BACCHUS (Boost Alcohol Consciousness Concerning the Health of University Students) promote responsible drinking and party hosting.

The National Institute on Alcohol Abuse and Alcoholism (NIAAA) has studied interventions that effectively deal with the problem. Programs that have proven particularly effective include cognitive-behavioral skills training with *motivational interviewing,* a nonjudgmental approach to working with students to change behavior, and e-Interventions, which are electronically based alcohol education interventions using text messages.[39] Preventive podcasts and e-mails have become more common on campus.[40] Sending electronic twenty-first birthday cards about the negative consequences of excess drinking on that milestone birthday has actually shown to reduce the number of drinks taken and consequently resulted in lower BACs in women celebrating that day.[41]

Web-based education for first-year students, particularly those who are incoming, has become an increasingly important intervention used by universities to reduce both hazardous drinking and alcohol-related problems. Because first-year students are at increased risk for alcohol-related problems, schools ensure that students are made aware of risks and effects of alcohol. Colleges and universities are also trying a *social norms* approach to reducing alcohol consumption, sending a consistent message to students about actual drinking behavior on campus. Many students perceive that their peers drink more than they actually do, which may cause students to feel pressured to drink more themselves. This misperception includes inaccurately estimating the frequency and amount that students drink and the actual consequences of students' drinking. As a result of these social norms campaigns, heavy episodic alcohol consumption—binge drinking—has declined at campuses across the country. For example, Michigan State University, Florida State University, and the University of Arizona all reported 20 to 30 percent reductions in heavy episodic alcohol consumption within 3 years of implementing social norms campaigns, while Hobart and William Smith Colleges saw a 40 percent reduction in 5 years and Northern Illinois University saw a 44 percent reduction in 10 years.[42]

Drinking and Driving

Traffic accidents are the leading cause of accidental death for all age groups from 5 to 65 years old.[43] In the United States, adults drank too much and got behind the wheel approximately 112 million times in 2010.[44] Although the number of episodes of driving after drinking have gone down by 30 percent during the past 5 years, it remains a serious problem in the United States. Alcohol-impaired drivers are involved in about 1 in 3 crash deaths, resulting in nearly 11,000 deaths a year.[45] This number represents roughly one traffic fatality every 48 minutes.[46] Some groups are more likely to drink and drive than others. Most recently, men were responsible for 81 percent of the drinking and driving episodes. Also, it has been reported that of those drinking and driving episodes, 85 percent of people were reported to have been binge drinking.[47] Unfortunately, college students are overrepresented

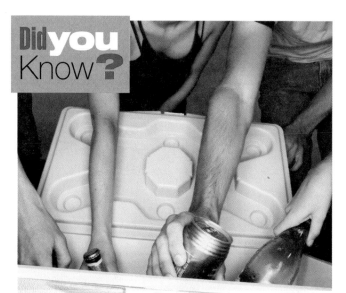

Did you Know?

The average college student spends about $900 per year on alcohol—compared to spending an average of about $450 a year on books.

Source: Data from Facts on Tap, "School Daze?" Accessed May 2011, www.factsontap.org.

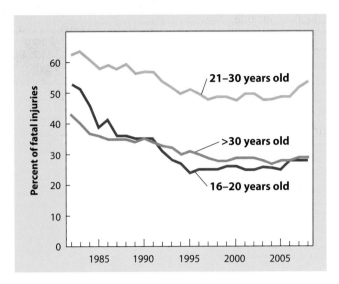

FIGURE 11.8 **Percentage of Fatally Injured Drivers with BACs Greater Than 0.08 Percent, by Driver Age, 1982–2009**
Source: Insurance Institute for Highway Safety, "Fatality Facts 2009: Alcohol," Copyright 2011. Reprinted with permission.

in alcohol-related crashes. A recent survey reported that 14 percent of college students have driven after drinking alcohol, and about 3 percent said that in the past 30 days they had driven after drinking five or more drinks.[48]

Over the past 20 years, the percentage of intoxicated drivers involved in fatal crashes decreased for all age groups (Figure 11.8). Several factors probably contributed to these reductions in fatalities: laws that raised the drinking age to 21, stricter law enforcement, laws prohibiting anyone under 21 from driving with any detectable BAC, increased automobile safety, and educational programs designed to discourage drinking and driving. Furthermore, all states have zero-tolerance laws for driving while intoxicated, and the penalty is usually suspension of the driver's license.[49]

Despite all these measures, the risk of being involved in an alcohol-related automobile crash remains substantial. Laboratory and test track research shows that the vast majority of drivers are impaired even at 0.08 BAC with regard to critical driving tasks. The likelihood of a driver being involved in a fatal crash rises significantly with a BAC of 0.05 percent and even more rapidly after 0.08 percent.[50]

Alcohol-related fatal car crashes occur more often at night than during the day; the hours between 9:00 PM and 6:00 AM are the most dangerous. Seventy-five percent of fatally injured drivers involved in nighttime single-vehicle crashes had detectable levels of alcohol in their blood.[51] The risk of being involved in an alcohol-related crash increases not only with the time of day, but also with the day of the week; 26 percent of all fatal crashes during the week were alcohol related, compared with 48 percent on weekends.[52] For information on phone apps that claim to help you estimate your blood alcohol level, presumably so you can judge whether it is safe to drive after drinking, see the **Tech & Health** box on the next page.

Ethnic Differences

Different ethnic and racial minority groups have their own patterns of alcohol consumption and abuse. Social or cultural factors, such as drinking norms and attitudes and, in some cases, genetic factors, may account for those differences. Better understanding of ethnic and racial differences in alcohol use patterns (Table 11.1) and factors that influence alcohol use can help guide the development of culturally appropriate prevention and treatment programs.

Among Native American populations, alcohol is the most widely used drug; the rate of alcoholism in this population is two to three times higher than the national average, and the death rate from alcohol-related causes is eight times higher than the national average.[53] When comparing other racial or ethnic groups, Native Americans have the highest alcohol-related motor vehicle crash and pedestrian fatalities, suicide, and falls.[54] Poor economic conditions and the cultural belief that alcoholism is a spiritual problem, not a physical disease, may partially account for high rates of alcoholism in this group.

African American and Latino populations also exhibit distinct patterns of abuse. On average, African Americans drink less than white Americans; however, those who do drink tend to be heavy drinkers.[55] Twice as many African Americans die of cirrhosis of the liver. Alcohol also contributes to high rates of hypertension, esophageal cancer, and homicide. Among Latino populations, men have a higher than average rate of alcohol abuse and alcohol-related health problems. In contrast, many the Latino cultures tend to discourage any drinking by women, therefore many Latinas abstain. Many researchers agree that a major factor for alcohol problems in this ethnic group is the key role that drinking plays in Latino culture.[56]

TABLE 11.1 **Prevalence of Heavy Alcohol Use* by Ethnicity**

Ethnic Group	Percent of Total Population
Whites	7.9
African Americans	4.5
Latino	5.2
Native Americans/Alaska Natives	8.3
Asian Americans	1.5
Persons reporting two or more races	6.4

*"Heavy alcohol use" is defined by the Substance Abuse and Mental Health Services Administration as five or more drinks on at least 5 days within the past month.

Source: Substance Abuse and Mental Health Services Administration, "Results from the 2009 National Survey on Drug Use and Health: National Findings," NSDUH Series H-38A, DHHS Publication no. SMA 10-4856 Findings (Rockville, MD: Office of Applied Studies, U.S. Department of Health and Human Services, 2010).

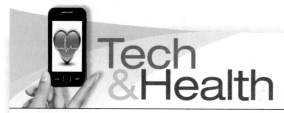

Tech & Health

SMART PHONE BAC APPLICATIONS AND DRIVING DON'T NECESSARILY MIX

Perhaps you have heard about smartphone applications that can estimate a person's blood alcohol concentration (BAC). You enter how many drinks you've consumed along with weight, gender, and total number of hours spent drinking. The apps estimate your BAC based on this information. They are designed to help people decide if they should avoid driving after drinking. Some even provide the phone number of a local taxi if a person has exceeded the legal BAC limit.

However, it is important to realize that these apps give general estimates, not your actual BAC. Many of these programs don't take into consideration elements such as food consumption, medication, general health, and

psychological conditions. It can also be hard to accurately input how many drink servings you consume when one mixed drink, such as a margarita, might contain two or three standard servings of alcohol, depending on its size and how it was mixed. Some programs also do not take into consideration that it can take time for the body to fully absorb and eliminate a drink and that blood alcohol levels can continue to rise for some time even after someone has stopped drinking. Additionally, keeping track of drinks is only as accurate as your memory. Given all these issues, there is a real chance your individual BAC could be higher than the legal driving limit, even if the app says otherwise.

These applications are great for giving you general information to use when thinking about your drinking habits, patterns, and decisions, but it isn't safe to rely on an app alone to decide if it's okay to drive after a night out. It's much better to arrange for a designated driver ahead of time or plan to take the bus or a taxi whenever you are mixing alcohol and going out.

Sources: Join Together, "New Smartphone App Estimates Blood Alcohol Concentration," Accessed August 22, 2011, www.drugfree.org/join-together/alcohol/new-smartphone-app-estimates-blood-alcohol-concentration; Blood Alcohol Content Gauging Apps, Available from http://appadvice.com/appguides/show/best-blood-alcohol-content-gauging-apps-for-the-iPhone.

Asian Americans have a very low rate of alcoholism.[57] When compared to other racial or ethnic groups, Asians have the lowest rates of alcohol-related injuries. Social and cultural influences, such as strong kinship ties, are thought to discourage heavy drinking in Asian American groups. Asians also have a genetic predisposition that might influence their low risk for alcohol abuse: Many possess a variant of the gene that codes for the enzyme aldehyde dehydrogenase, which plays a key role in the metabolism of alcohol.[58] People with this variant gene experience unpleasant side effects from consuming alcohol, making drinking a less pleasurable experience. Because of the presence of this gene, Asian populations tend to consume less alcohol and have lower rates of alcoholism than do other ethnic groups.

Abuse and Dependence

Alcohol use becomes **alcohol abuse** when it interferes with work, school, or social and family relationships or when it entails any violation of the law, including driving under the influence (DUI). **Alcoholism,** or **alcohol dependence,** results when personal and health problems related to alcohol use are severe and stopping alcohol use results in withdrawal symptoms.

Identifying an Alcoholic

As with other drug addictions, craving, loss of control, tolerance, psychological dependence, and withdrawal symptoms must be present to qualify a drinker as an addict (see **Chapter 10**). Irresponsible and problem drinkers, such as people who get into fights or embarrass themselves or others when they drink, are not necessarily alcoholics. Alcoholics can be found at all socioeconomic levels and in all professions, ethnic groups, geographical locations, religions, and races. Data indicate that about 15 percent of people in the United States are problem drinkers, and about 5 to 10 percent of male drinkers and 3 to 5 percent of females would be diagnosed as alcohol dependent.[59]

Recognizing and admitting the existence of an alcohol problem is often extremely difficult. Alcoholics deny their problem, often making statements such as, "I can stop any time I want to. I just don't want to right now." The fear of being labeled a "problem drinker" often prevents people from seeking help. People who recognize alcoholic behaviors in themselves may wish to seek professional help to determine whether alcohol has become a controlling factor in their lives.

Even though there is a high prevalence of alcohol disorders on

alcohol abuse Use of alcohol in a way that interferes with work, school, or personal relationships or that entails violations of the law.

alcoholism (alcohol dependence) Condition in which personal and health problems related to alcohol use are severe, and stopping alcohol use results in withdrawal symptoms.

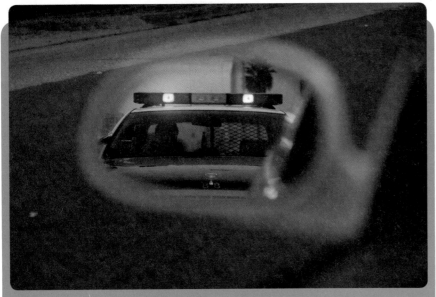

What are the legal consequences if you are caught drinking and driving?

Getting behind the wheel after drinking alcohol is a dangerous choice, with serious legal consequences. Underage drinkers with any detectable alcohol in their bloodstream can have licenses revoked. Other penalties for driving under the influence (DUI) include driving restrictions, fines, mandatory counseling, and jail time. In many states three DUI convictions make you a felon, meaning that you lose your right to vote and own a weapon, among other rights, and may also be permanently banned from driving. If you are involved in an accident in which someone is injured, the consequences are even more serious. If a person dies as a result of the accident, the drunk driver may be charged with manslaughter or second-degree murder.

campus, only 5 percent of affected students sought treatment in the prior year, and 3 percent thought they should seek help, but did not. The heaviest drinkers are the least likely to seek treatment, yet they experience and are responsible for the most alcohol-related problems on campus.[60]

Alcohol and Prescription Drug Abuse

When alcohol and prescription drugs are taken together, severe medical problems can result, including alcohol poisoning, unconsciousness, respiratory depression, and death. Recent studies have shown that people with alcohol use disorders are 18 times more likely to report nonmedical use of prescription drugs than those who do not drink at all.[61] Young adults aged 18 to 24 are at the highest risk for concurrent or simultaneous abuse of alcohol and drugs. In a study of college students, it was revealed that in the past year 12 percent had used both alcohol and prescription drugs nonmedically but at different times, and

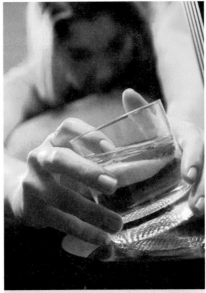

Drinking alone or in secret and using alcohol to cope with stress and emotional problems are all potential signs of alcohol dependency.

7 percent had taken them simultaneously.[62] Students who took prescription drugs while drinking were more likely to black out, vomit, and engage in other risky behaviors such as drunk driving and unplanned sex. The prescription drugs that are most commonly combined with alcohol include opioids (e.g., Vicodin, OxyContin, Percocet); stimulants (e.g., Ritalin, Adderall, Concerta); sedative/anxiety medications (e.g., Ativan, Xanax); and sleeping medications (e.g., Ambien, Halcion).

The Causes of Alcohol Abuse and Alcoholism

We know that alcoholism is a disease with biological and social/environmental components, but we do not yet know what role each component plays in the disease.

Biological and Family Factors
Research into the hereditary and environmental causes of alcoholism has found higher rates of alcoholism among children of alcoholics than in the general population. The development of alcoholism among individuals with a family history of alcoholism is about four to eight times more common than it is among individuals with no such family history.[63]

Despite evidence of heredity's role in alcoholism, scientists do not yet understand the precise role of genes and increased risk for alcoholism, nor have they identified a specific "alcoholism" gene. Adoption studies demonstrate a strong link between biological parents' substance use and their children's risk for addiction.[64] However, there is nothing deterministic about the genetic basis for addiction. Researchers have not yet identified a specific gene that puts people at risk for developing an addiction.

Social and Cultural Factors
Social and cultural factors may trigger the affliction for many people who are not genetically predisposed to alcoholism. Some people begin drinking as a way to dull the pain of an acute loss or an emotional or social problem. Unfortunately, they become even sadder as the depressant effect of alcohol begins to take its toll, even antagonizing friends and other social supports. Eventually, the drinker becomes physically dependent on the drug.

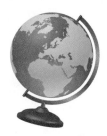

GLOBAL HEALTH AND ALCOHOL USE

Alcohol consumption comes with many serious social and developmental issues, including violence, child neglect and abuse, and absenteeism in the workplace. Throughout the world, alcohol is a factor in 60 types of diseases and injuries and a component cause in 200 others. Almost 4 percent of all deaths worldwide are attributed to alcohol, greater than deaths caused by HIV/AIDS, violence, or tuberculosis. Worldwide, the impact of alcohol use is as follows:

✳ The use of alcohol results in 2.5 million deaths each year.

✳ 320,000 people ages 15 to 29 die from alcohol-related causes annually—9 percent of all deaths for that age group.
✳ Alcohol is the world's third largest risk factor for disease burden.
✳ It is the leading risk factor for disease burden in the Western Pacific and the Americas and the second leading risk factor in Europe.

A large variation exists in adult per capita consumption. The highest consumption levels can be found in the developed world, mostly the Northern Hemisphere, but also in Argentina, Australia, and New Zealand. Medium consumption levels can be found in southern Africa, with Namibia and South Africa having the highest levels, and in North and South America. Low consumption levels can be found in the countries of North Africa and sub-Saharan Africa, the Eastern Mediterranean region, and southern Asia and the Indian Ocean. These regions represent large populations Muslims, who have high rates of abstention.

Sources: World Health Organization, "Global Status Report on Alcohol and Health," 2011, Available from www.who.int/substance_abuse/publications/global_alcohol_report/msbgsruprofiles.pdf.

Family attitudes toward alcohol also seem to influence whether a person will develop a drinking problem. It has been clearly demonstrated that people who are raised in cultures in which drinking is a part of religious or ceremonial activities or in which alcohol is a traditional part of the family meal are less prone to alcohol dependence. In contrast, in societies in which alcohol purchase is carefully controlled and drinking is regarded as a rite of passage to adulthood, the tendency for abuse appears to be greater.

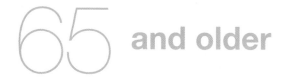

65 and older

Is the age group that most often binge drinks.

Apparently, then, some combination of heredity and environment plays a decisive role in the development of alcoholism. The **Health in a Diverse World** box discusses some of the patterns of alcohol use and abuse among different racial and ethnic groups.

The amount of alcohol a person consumes seems to be directly related to the drinking habits of that individual's social group. A recent study found that those whose friends and relatives drank heavily were 50 percent more likely to drink heavily themselves.[65] Even having friends of friends who drank heavily appeared to influence individual alcohol consumption. The opposite is also true, that people who were friends with abstinent individuals or had family members who were abstinent were less likely to drink themselves. This finding has increased importance for individuals who are in treatment or have been in treatment and their need to sever ties with heavy drinkers to successfully maintain their abstinence.

what do you think?

Why do you think women are drinking more heavily today than they did in the past?
● Does society look at men's and women's drinking habits in the same way?
● Can you think of ways to increase support for women in their recovery process?

Women and Alcoholism

Women are the fastest growing population of alcohol abusers. They tend to become alcoholics at later ages and after fewer years of heavy drinking than do male alcoholics. Women get addicted faster with less alcohol use and then suffer the consequences more profoundly. Women alcoholics have greater risks for cirrhosis; excessive memory loss and shrinkage of the brain; heart disease; and cancers of the mouth, throat, esophagus, liver, and colon than do male alcoholics.[66]

See It! Videos

Should high schools test students for alcohol to curb underage drinking? Watch **Teen Drinking Test** at www.pearsonhighered.com/donatelle.

Women at highest risk are those who are unmarried but living with a partner, are in their twenties or early thirties, or have a husband or partner who drinks heavily. Other risk factors for drinking problems among *all women* include a family history of drinking problems, pressure to drink from a peer or spouse, depression, and stress.

Effects on Family and Friends

In addition to harming themselves, people who abuse alcohol cause tremendous harm to their family and friends. Everyone close to an addicted person suffers and becomes a part of the dynamics of addiction. Alcoholism is a family disease, and friends, roommates, and fellow fraternity or sorority members can also be considered a family.

An estimated 7.5 million children in the United States live with a parent who has experienced an alcohol use disorder in the past year. Approximately 6 million of these children live with two parents, one or both of whom have experienced an alcohol use disorder. The other 1.4 million live in a single-parent household, with a parent who has had an alcohol use disorder. These children are at increased risk for a range of problems, including physical illness, emotional disturbances, behavioral problems, lower educational performance, and susceptibility to alcoholism or other addictions later in life.[67] In particular, children of alcoholic parents are four times more likely to develop alcohol problems themselves.[68]

In dysfunctional families, children learn certain rules from an early age: Don't talk, don't trust, and don't feel. These unspoken rules allow the family to avoid dealing with real problems and issues as family members adapt to the alcoholic's behavior by adjusting their own behavior. Unfortunately, these behaviors enable the alcoholic to keep drinking. Children in such dysfunctional families generally assume at least one of the following roles:

- **Family hero.** Tries to divert attention from the problem by being too good to be true
- **Scapegoat.** Draws attention away from the family's primary problem through misbehavior
- **Lost child.** Becomes passive and quietly withdraws from upsetting situations
- **Mascot.** Disrupts tense situations by providing comic relief

For children in alcoholic homes, life is a struggle. They have to deal with constant stress, anxiety, and embarrassment. Because the alcoholic is the center of attention, the child's needs are often ignored. It is not uncommon for these children to be victims of violence, abuse, neglect, or incest.

Living with a family member (or friend or roommate) who is an alcoholic can be extremely stressful. People in close proximity to alcoholics can find themselves in codependent relationships that are often emotionally destructive or abusive and that enable the alcoholic's addiction. Codependents try to cover up for the addicted person: They may phone a

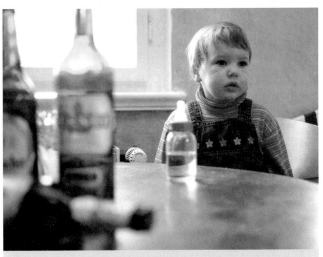

Adult children of alcoholics can have trouble developing social attachments and suffer low self-esteem and other problems from lack of parental nurturing. Fortunately, as they mature, many children of alcoholics can also develop resiliency in response to their families' problems.

professor to say that the alcoholic is sick and can't take an exam, make excuses for the drinker's behavior, or lie to cover for him or her. (For more information on how addiction can affect families and friends, see **Chapter 10**.)

Costs to Society

Alcohol-related costs to society are estimated to be well over $223.5 billion, $746 per person, or about $1.90 per drink, when health insurance, criminal justice costs, treatment costs, and lost productivity are factored in.[69] Alcoholism is directly or indirectly responsible for more than 25 percent of the nation's medical expenses and lost earnings.[70]

Workplace Prevalence of Alcohol Dependence and Abuse Most people with alcohol problems are employed. In fact, employed adults have a 27 percent greater risk of having an alcohol problem compared to adults not in the workforce. Among alcoholics, 75 percent work full-time, and 16 percent work part-time.[71] Rates of alcohol problems vary greatly from industry to industry, but it is estimated that alcohol problems contribute to 500 million lost workdays in the United States annually.[72]

The Cost of Underage Drinking A recent study estimated that underage drinking costs society $62 billion annually.[73] The largest costs were related to violence ($35 billion) and drunk-driving accidents ($9.955 billion), followed by high-risk sex ($5 billion), property crime ($3 billion), and addiction treatment programs (nearly $2.5 billion). By dividing the cost of underage drinking by the estimated number of underage drinkers, the study estimated that every underage drinker costs society an average of $2,070 a year.[74]

Treatment and Recovery

Despite growing recognition of our national alcohol problem, only 8 percent of alcoholics in the United States receive care in a special facility.[75] Factors contributing to this low figure include an inability or unwillingness to admit to an alcohol problem, the social stigma attached to alcoholism, potential loss of income, inability to pay for treatment, breakdowns in referral and delivery systems, and failure of the medical establishment to recognize and diagnose alcoholic symptoms among patients. Most problem drinkers who seek help have experienced a turning point such as a spouse walking out or a boss issuing an ultimatum to dry out or lose the job. The point at which an alcoholic seeks help occurs when the person recognizes that alcohol controls his or her life.

Alcoholics who quit drinking will experience *detoxification,* the process by which addicts end their dependence on a drug. Withdrawal symptoms include hyperexcitability, confusion, agitation, sleep disorders, convulsions, tremors, depression, headaches, and seizures. For a small percentage of people, alcohol withdrawal results in a severe syndrome known as **delirium tremens (DTs),** which is characterized by confusion, delusions, agitated behavior, and hallucinations.

The Family's Role in Recovery

Members of an alcoholic's family sometimes take action before the alcoholic does. An effective method of helping an alcoholic confront the disease is a process called **intervention.** Essentially, this is a planned confrontation with the alcoholic that involves family members and friends assisted by professional substance abuse counselors. (See **Chapter 10** for more on intervention.) See the **Skills for Behavior Change** box on the following page for additional guidelines.

Treatment Programs

The alcoholic who is ready for help has several avenues of treatment: psychologists and psychiatrists specializing in the treatment of alcoholism, private treatment centers, hospitals specifically designed to treat alcoholics, community mental health facilities, and support groups.

Private Treatment Facilities Upon admission to a private treatment facility, the patient receives a complete physical exam to determine whether underlying medical problems will interfere with treatment. Shortly after detoxification, alcoholics begin their treatment for psychological addiction. Most treatment facilities keep their patients from 3 to 6 weeks. Treatment at private facilities costs several thousand dollars, but some insurance programs or employers will assume most of this expense.

Therapy Several types of therapy, including family therapy, individual therapy, and group therapy, are commonly used in alcoholism recovery programs. In family therapy, the recovering alcoholic and family members examine the psychological reasons underlying the addiction. In individual and group therapy, alcoholics learn positive coping skills for situations that have regularly caused them to turn to alcohol.

On some college campuses, the problems associated with alcohol abuse are so great that student health centers are opening their own treatment programs. For example, the University of Texas offers a support service called Complete Recovery 101, and at other schools, students in recovery live together in special housing. Programs such as these aim to provide the support and comfortable environment recovering students need.

Pharmacological Treatment Disulfiram (trade name Antabuse) is a drug commonly used for treating alcoholism. It is given to deter drinking, as it causes an individual to become acutely ill when he or she consumes alcohol. Disulfiram inhibits the breakdown of acetaldehyde from the liver. If individuals taking this drug drink alcohol or consume any foods with alcohol content, acetaldehyde will build up in the liver and cause nausea and vomiting. Other unpleasant effects, such as headache, bad breath, drowsiness, and temporary impotence discourage drinking. Because disulfiram does not reduce the

delirium tremens (DTs) State of confusion, delusions, and agitation brought on by withdrawal from alcohol.

intervention A planned confrontation with an alcoholic led by a professional counselor in which family members and/or friends try to get the alcoholic to face the reality of his or her problem and to seek help.

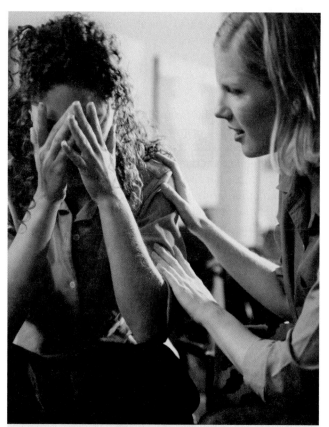

Most alcohol-dependent people need the help of others during their recovery, whether through support groups or individual, family, or group therapy.

Thinking and Talking about Alcohol Use

The following questions can help gauge whether you or a friend or relative could have an alcohol problem. The more questions you answer with a "yes," the more likely it is that there is a problem.

Does the person you are concerned about

❭ Lose time from classes, studying, or work because of drinking?

❭ Feel embarrassed about their behavior after sobering up?

❭ Drink to get drunk?

❭ Do dangerous things or get injured while drunk?

❭ Drink to cope with problems or stress?

HOW TO TALK TO SOMEONE ABOUT ALCOHOL ABUSE

❭ Talk when he or she is sober. Avoid lecturing.

❭ Restrict comments to what you have experienced of the person's behavior.

❭ Use concrete examples: "You started a fight," or "You were hung over and failed an exam."

❭ Contrast sober and drunk behavior: "You have the most wonderful sense of humor, but when you drink it turns into cruel sarcasm."

❭ Distinguish between the person you like and the behavior you don't.

❭ Encourage him or her to consult a professional. Offer to go along for support.

---

cravings for alcohol, this treatment works best in conjunction with ongoing psychotherapy and support groups.

Naltrexone is used to reduce the craving for alcohol and decrease the pleasant reinforcing effects of alcohol without making the user ill. It also works most effectively with counseling and other forms of psychotherapy. A recent pharmaceutical treatment for alcoholism approved by the U.S. Food and Drug Administration (FDA) is called acamprosate (Campral). Acamprosate helps people who have consumed large amounts of alcohol avoid drinking. Drinking large amounts of alcohol over a long period of time changes the way the brain works. Acamprosate helps stabilize the resulting chemical imbalance in the brain. It also helps to reduce the physical and emotional distress associated with the attempt to stay alcohol free. As with other pharmacological treatments, acamprosate should be used in conjunction with psychotherapy and support groups.

Alcoholics Anonymous (AA)
Organization whose goal is to help alcoholics stop drinking; includes auxiliary branches such as Al-Anon and Alateen.

Support Groups The support gained from talking with others who have similar problems is one of the greatest benefits derived from self-help/support groups. **Alcoholics Anonymous (AA)** is a private, nonprofit, self-help organization founded in 1935. The organization, which relies on group support to help people stop drinking, currently has branches all over the world and more than 1 million members. At meetings, participants do not give their last names, and no one is forced to speak. Members are taught that alcoholism is a lifetime problem and that they can never drink alcohol again. They share their struggles and talk about the devastating effects alcoholism has had on their personal and professional lives. AA established the concept of the 12-step program for recovery from addiction, and its guiding principles are now used by other recovery organizations. The 12 steps ask members to address recovery one step at a time and to place their faith and control of their habit into the hands of a "Higher Power."

Alcoholics Anonymous also has auxiliary groups to help spouses or partners, friends, and children of alcoholics. *Al-Anon* is the group dedicated to helping adult relatives and friends of alcoholics understand the disease and how they can contribute to the recovery process. *Alateen* helps adolescents living with alcoholic parents. They are taught that they are not at fault for their parents' problems. They develop their self-esteem to overcome their guilt and function better socially.

Other self-help groups include Women for Sobriety and Secular Organizations for Sobriety (SOS). Women for Sobriety addresses the specific needs of female alcoholics, who often have more severe problems than do males. Unlike AA meetings, where attendance can be quite large, each group has no more than ten members. These meetings focus on behavioral changes through positive reinforcement, cognitive strategies, relaxation techniques, meditation, diet, exercise, and dynamic group involvement. SOS was founded to help people who are uncomfortable with AA's spiritual emphasis. It is a self-empowerment approach to recovery and maintains that sobriety is a separate issue from all else. Like AA, SOS holds confidential meetings, celebrates sobriety anniversaries, and views recovery as a one-day-at-a-time process.

Relapse

Success in recovery varies with the individual. Over half of alcoholics relapse (resume drinking) within the first 3 months of treatment. Treating an addiction requires more than getting the addict to stop using a substance; it also requires getting the person to break a pattern of behavior that has dominated his or her life. Many alcoholics refer to themselves as "recovering" throughout their lifetime rather than "cured."

People seeking to regain a healthy lifestyle must not only confront their addiction, but also guard against the tendency to relapse. For alcoholics, it is important to identify situations that could trigger a relapse, such as becoming angry or frustrated and being around others who drink. During the initial recovery period, it can help to join a support group, maintain stability (resisting the urge to relocate, travel, take a new job, or make other drastic life changes), set aside time each day for reflection, and maintain a pattern of assuming responsibility for one's own actions. To be effective, recovery programs must offer alcoholics ways to increase self-esteem and resume personal growth.

Assess yourself

What's Your Risk of Alcohol Abuse?

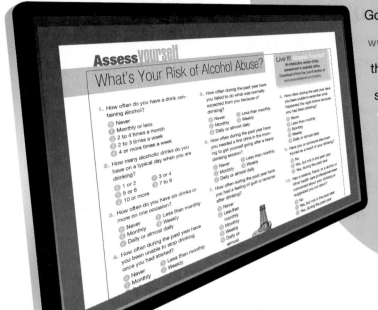

Go online to the **Live It!** section of www.pearsonhighered.com/donatelle to complete the "What's Your Risk for Alcohol Abuse?" assessment.* Follow the strategies outlined in the **YOUR PLAN FOR CHANGE** box to modify your drinking habits.

*If your instructor so chooses, Assess Yourself Activities are available as a printed supplement or as assignable homework online at www.pearsonhighered.com/myhealthlab.

MyHealthLab®

YOUR PLAN FOR CHANGE

If the results of your **Assess yourself** exercise concern you, consider taking these steps to change your behavior.

Today, you can:

◯ Start a diary of your drinking habits to track how much alcohol you consume and what you spend on it.

◯ If you have a family history of alcohol abuse or addiction, consider whether your current use is healthy or is likely to create problems for you in the future.

Within the next 2 weeks, you can:

◯ Make your first drink at a party something nonalcoholic.

◯ Intersperse alcoholic drinks with nonalcoholic beverages to help you pace yourself.

By the end of the semester, you can:

◯ Commit yourself to determining and limiting alcohol intake at every social function.

◯ Cultivate friendships and explore activities that do not center on alcohol. If your friends drink heavily you may need to step back from the group for a while or make an effort to meet new people who do not make drinking a major focus of their social activity.

Summary

* Alcohol is a central nervous system (CNS) depressant used by about half of all Americans. About 60 percent of all college students report drinking in the past 30 days. Although consumption trends are slowly creeping downward, college students are under extreme pressure to consume alcohol.
* Negative consequences associated with alcohol use among college students include academic problems, traffic accidents, unplanned sex, hangovers, alcohol poisoning, injury to self or others, and dropping out of school.
* Alcohol's effect on the body is measured by the blood alcohol concentration (BAC), the ratio of alcohol to total blood volume: The higher the BAC, the greater the drowsiness and impaired judgment and motor function.
* Excessive alcohol consumption can cause long-term damage to the nervous system and cardiovascular system, liver disease, and increased risk for cancer. Drinking during pregnancy can cause fetal alcohol spectrum disorders (FASD).
* Alcohol use becomes alcoholism when it interferes with school, work, or social and family relationships or entails violations of the law. Causes of alcoholism include biological, family, social, and cultural factors. Alcoholism has far-reaching effects on families, especially on children, who have problematic childhoods and may take those problems into adulthood.
* Most alcoholics do not admit to having a problem until reaching a major life crisis or until their families intervene. Treatment options include detoxification at private medical facilities, therapy (family, individual, or group), and self-help programs such as Alcoholics Anonymous. Most recovering alcoholics relapse (over half within 3 months) because alcoholism is a behavioral addiction as well as a chemical addiction.

Pop Quiz

1. If a man and a woman drink the same amount of alcohol, the woman's BAC will be approximately
   a. the same as the man's BAC.
   b. 60 percent higher than the man's BAC.
   c. 30 percent higher than the man's BAC.
   d. 30 percent lower than the man's BAC.

2. Which of the following is a *true* statement regarding how one can metabolize alcohol faster to lower one's blood alcohol level?
   a. Drink black coffee.
   b. Take a cold shower.
   c. Engage in vigorous exercise.
   d. Only time can metabolize and rid the body of high alcohol content.

3. BAC is the
   a. concentration of plant sugars in the bloodstream.
   b. percentage of alcohol in a beverage.
   c. level of alcohol content in the blood.
   d. ratio of alcohol to the total blood volume.

4. Which is a strategy you could take to avoid drinking too much alcohol?
   a. Alternate alcoholic beverages with nonalcoholic drinks.
   b. Eat before and during drinking.
   c. Pace your drinks to one or fewer per hour.
   d. All of the above

5. Which of the following statements is *false*?
   a. College students under 21 drink less often than older students but drink more heavily.
   b. College students tend to underestimate the amount that their peers drink.
   c. In the past 10 years, the number of female college students who report being drunk ten or more times has increased.
   d. Alcohol is involved in at least two thirds of suicides on campus.

6. Which of the following is *not* typical of a child born with fetal alcohol syndrome?
   a. A small head
   b. Deafness
   c. Impaired learning
   d. Abnormal facial features

7. The fastest-growing population of alcohol abusers is
   a. older adults.
   b. adolescents.
   c. women.
   d. immigrants.

8. When Amanda goes out with her friends on the weekends, she usually has four or five beers in a row. This type of high-risk drinking is called
   a. tolerance.
   b. alcoholic addiction.
   c. alcohol overconsumption.
   d. binge drinking.

9. Drinking large amounts of alcohol in a short period of time that leads to passing out is known as
   a. learned behavioral tolerance.
   b. alcoholic unconsciousness.
   c. alcohol poisoning.
   d. acute metabolism syndrome.

10. Jake was raised in an alcoholic family. To adapt to his father's alcoholic behavior, he played the good, obedient son. Which role did Jake assume?
    a. Family hero
    b. Mascot
    c. Scapegoat
    d. Lost child

Answers to these questions can be found on page A-1.

Think about It!

1 When it comes to drinking alcohol, how much is too much? How can you avoid drinking amounts that will affect your judgment? If you see a friend having too many drinks at a party, what actions could you take?

2 What are some of the most common negative consequences college students experience as a result of drinking? What are secondhand effects of binge drinking? Why do students tolerate the negative behaviors of students who have been drinking?

3 Would a person be more intoxicated after having four gin and tonics instead of four beers? Why or why not? At what point in your life should you start worrying about the long-term effects of alcohol abuse?

4 Describe the difference between a problem drinker and an alcoholic. What factors can cause someone to become an alcoholic? What effect does alcoholism have on an alcoholic's family?

5 Does anyone ever permanently recover from alcoholism? Why or why not? Do you think society's views on drinking have changed over the years? Explain your answer.

Accessing Your Health on the Internet

The following websites explore further topics and issues related to personal health. For links to the websites below, visit the Companion Website for *Access to Health,* 13th Edition, at www.pearsonhighered.com/donatelle.

1. *Alcoholics Anonymous (AA).* This website provides general information about AA and the 12-step program. www.aa.org

2. *College Drinking: Changing the Culture.* This online resource center targets three audiences: the student population as a whole, the college and its surrounding environment, and the individual at risk or alcohol-dependent drinker. www.collegedrinkingprevention.gov

3. *The Alcohol Calculators.* This link allows you to do the following calculations related to alcohol use: the cost of your drinking on a monthly and annual basis, the amount of calories you are regularly consuming from alcohol, and your BAC. www.collegedrinkingprevention.gov/CollegeStudents/calculator/default.aspx

4. *Had Enough.* This site is designed for college students who have suffered the secondhand effects of other students' drinking. http://gbgm-umc.org/mission_programs/cim/hadenough/home

5. *Higher Education Center for Alcohol, Drug Abuse, and Violence Prevention.* This website is funded through the U.S. Department of Education and provides information relevant to colleges and universities. A specific site exists for students who are seeking information regarding alcohol. www.higheredcenter.org

References

1. A. Klatsky, "Alcohol and Cardiovascular Health," *Physiology and Behavior* 100, no. 1 (2010): 76–81; K. Tucker et al., "Effects of Beer, Wine and Liquor Intakes on Bone Mineral Density in Older Men and Women," *American Journal of Clinical Nutrition* 89, no. 4 (2009): 1188–96; H. Macdonald, "Alcohol and Recommendations for Bone Health: Should We Still Exercise Caution?" *American Journal of Clinical Nutrition* 89, no. 4 (2009): 999–1000; W. Snow et al., "Alcohol Use and Cardiovascular Health Outcomes: A Comparison across Age and Gender in the Winnipeg Health and Drinking Survey Cohort," *Age and Ageing* 38, no. 2 (2009): 206–12.

2. National Center for Health Statistics, "Summary Health Statistics for U.S. Adults: National Health Interview Survey, 2010," *Vital and Health Statistics* 10, no. 252 (2012): 94.

3. Ibid.

4. Centers for Disease Control and Prevention, "Vital Signs: Binge Drinking Prevalence, Frequency and Intensity Among Adults," *Morbidity and Mortality Weekly Report* 61 (2012): 1–7.

5. J. Turner et al., "Serious Health Consequences Associated with Alcohol Use among College Students: Demographic and Clinical Characteristics of Patients Seen in the Emergency Department," *Journal of Studies on Alcohol* 65, no. 2 (2004): 179.

6. S. MacDonald, "The Criteria for Causation of Alcohol in Violent Injuries in Six Countries," *Addictive Behaviors* 30, no. 1 (2005): 103–13.

7. J. Turner et al., "Serious Health Consequences," 2004.

8. Centers for Disease Control and Prevention, "Injury Prevention and Control: Home and Recreational Safety: Unintentional Drowning: Fact Sheet," Updated June 2010, www.cdc.gov/HomeandRecreationalSafety/Water-Safety/waterinjuries-factsheet.html; Centers for Disease Control and Prevention, "Injury Prevention and Control: Home and Recreational Safety: Fire Deaths and Injuries: Fact Sheet," Updated October 2009, www.cdc.gov/HomeandRecreationalSafety/Fire-Prevention/fires-factsheet.html.

9. L. Sher, "Alcohol Consumption and Suicide," *QJM: An International Journal of Medicine* 99, no. 1 (2006): 57–61; Bureau of Justice Statistics, "Criminal Victimization in the United States, Table 32, Percent Distribution of Victimizations by Perceived Drug or Alcohol Use by Offender, 2007," Accessed June 2010, http://bjs.ojp.usdoj.gov/content/pub/html/cvus/alcohol.cfm.

10. K. Davis, "College Women's Sexual Decision Making: Cognitive Mediation of Alcohol Expectancy Results," *American Journal of College Health* 58, no. 5 (2010): 481–90.

11. C. Stappenbeck, "A Longitudinal Investigation of Heavy Drinking and Physical Dating Violence in Men and Women." *Addictive Behaviors* 35, no. 5 (2010): 479–85.

12. K. Butler, "The Grim Neurology of Teenage Drinking," *New York Times* (July 4, 2006).

13. R. W. Hingson et al., "Age at Drinking Onset and Alcohol Dependence," *Archives of Pediatric and Adolescent Medicine* 160 (2006): 739–46.

14. L. Arriola et al., "Alcohol Intake and the Risk of Coronary Heart Disease in Spanish EPIC Cohort Study," *Heart* 96, no. 10 (2010): 124–30; T. Wilson et al., eds., "Should Moderate Alcohol Consumption be Promoted?" *Nutrition and Health: Nutrition Guide for Physicians* (New York: Humana Press, 2010); The American Heart Association, "Alcohol and Cardiovascular Disease," 2011, www.heart.org/HEARTORG/Conditions/

Alcohol-and-Cardiovascular-Disease_
UCM_305173_Article.jsp.

15. Ibid.

16. The American Heart Association, "Alcohol and Cardiovascular Disease," 2011, www.heart.org/HEARTORG/Conditions/Alcohol-and-Cardiovascular-Disease_UCM_305173_Article.jsp.

17. H. K. Seitz and P. Becker, "Alcohol Metabolism and Cancer Risk," *NIAAA Publications*, http://pubs.niaaa.nih.gov/publications/arh301/38-47.htm.

18. W.Y. Chen et al., "Moderate Alcohol Consumption during Adult Life, Drinking Patterns, and Breast Cancer Risk," *Journal of the American Medical Association* 306 (2011): 1884; American Association for Cancer Research, "Excessive Alcohol Drinking Can Lead to Increased Risk of Breast Cancer, Study Suggests," *Science Daily*, April 14, 2008, www.sciencedaily.com/releases/2008/04/080413173510.htm; National Institute on Alcohol Abuse and Alcoholism, *Alcohol: A Women's Health Issue,* NIH Publication no. 03-4956 (Bethesda, MD: National Institutes of Health, revised 2008), Available at www.niaaa.nih.gov/Publications/Pamphlets BrochuresPosters/English/Pages/default.aspx.

19. C. S. Berkey et al., "Prospective Study of Adolescent Alcohol Consumption and Risk of Benign Breast Disease in Young Women," *Pediatrics* 125, no. 5 (2010): e1081-87.

20. Centers for Disease Control and Prevention, "Alcohol Use among Pregnant and Nonpregnant Women of Childbearing Age—United States, 1991-2005," *Morbidity and Mortality Weekly* 58, no. 19 (2009): 529-32.

21. Centers for Disease Control and Prevention, "Fetal Alcohol Spectrum Disorders (FASDs) Data and Statistics," Updated May 2010, www.cdc.gov/ncbddd/fasd/data.html.

22. Substance Abuse and Mental Health Services Administration, Fetal Alcohol Spectrum Disorders (FASD) Center for Excellence, "What Is FASD?" Accessed May 23, 2011, www.Fasdcenter.samhsa.gov.

23. American College Health Association, *American College Health Association—National College Health Assessment II: Reference Group Executive Summary Spring 2011* (Linthicum, MD: American College Health Association, 2012), Available at www.acha-ncha.org/reports_ACHA-NCHAII.html.

24. Substance Abuse and Mental Health Services Administration, *Results from the 2009 National Survey on Drug Use and Health: Volume I. Summary of National Findings,* NSDUH Series H-38A, DHHS Publication no. SMA 10-4856 Findings (Rockville, MD: Office of Applied Studies, U.S. Department of Health and Human Services, 2010).

25. U.S. Department of Health and Human Services, National Institute on Alcohol Abuse and Alcoholism, "What Colleges Need to Know: An Update on College Drinking Research," NIH Publication no. 07-5010, November 2007, Available at www.collegedrinkingprevention.gov.

26. American College Health Association, *American College Health Association—National College Health Assessment II,*2012.

27. R. Singleton, "Alcohol Consumption, Sleep, and Academic Performance among College Students," *Journal of Alcohol and Drugs* 70, no. 3 (2009): 355-63.

28. American College Health Association, *American College Health Association—National College Health Assessment II,* 2012

29. R. Hingson et al., "Magnitude of Alcohol-Related Mortality and Morbidity among U.S. College Students Ages 18–24: Changes from 1998 to 2005," *Journal of Studies on Alcohol and Drugs* (2009): 12–20.

30. R. R. Wetherill et al., "Perceived Awareness and Caring Influences Alcohol Use by High School and College Students," *Psychology of Addictive Behaviors* 21, no. 2 (2007): 147–54.

31. L. D. Johnston, *Monitoring the Future National Survey Results on Drug Use, 1975–2010: Volume II, College Students and Adults Ages 19–50* (Ann Arbor, MI: Institute for Social Research, The University of Michigan, 2011), Available at http://monitoringthefuture.org/pubs/monographs/mtf-vol2_2010.pdf.

32. L. D. Johnston, *Monitoring the Future National Survey Results on Drug Use, 1975–2010: Volume I, Secondary School Students* (Ann Arbor, MI: Institute for Social Research, The University of Michigan, 2011), Available at http://monitoringthefuture.org/pubs/monographs/mtf-vol1_2010.pdf.

33. "Policy Implications of the Widespread Practice of 'Pre-drinking' or 'Pre-gaming' before Going to Public Drinking Establishments—Are Current Prevention Strategies Backfiring?" *Addiction* 104 (2008): 4–9; L. D. Johnston, *Monitoring the Future National Survey Results on Drug Use, 1975–2008* (Ann Arbor, MI: Institute for Social Research, The University of Michigan, 2009).

34. N. R. Ahern et al., "Youth in Mind: Drinking Games and College Students," *Journal of Psychosocial Nursing and Mental Health Services* 48, no. 2 (2010): 17–20.

35. J. M. Cameron et al., "Drinking Game Participation among Undergraduate Students Attending National Alcohol Screening Day," *Journal of American College Health* 58, no. 5 (2010): 499–506.

36. National Center on Addiction and Substance Abuse at Columbia University, *Wasting the Best and the Brightest: Substance Abuse at America's Colleges and Universities,* March 2007, Available at www.casacolumbia.org/templates/publications_reports.aspx.

37. R. Hingson et al., "Magnitude of Alcohol-Related Mortality and Morbidity," 2009.

38. The Higher Education Center for Alcohol, Drug Abuse, and Violence Prevention, *Sexual Violence and Alcohol and Other Drug Use on Campus* (Newton, MA: The Higher Education Center for Alcohol, Drug Abuse, and Violence Prevention, 2008), Available at www.higheredcenter.org/services/publications/sexual-violence-and-alcohol-and-other-drug-use-campus.

39. Rollnick et al., *Motivational Interviewing in Health Care: Helping Patients Change Behavior.* (New York: Guilford Press, 2008); U.S. Department of Health and Human Services, National Institute on Alcohol Abuse and Alcoholism, "What Colleges Need to Know," 2007.

40. C. Elliott et al., "Computer-based Interventions for College Drinking: A Qualitative Review," *Addictive Behaviors*, 33, no. 8 (2008): 994–1005.

41. J. Labrie et al., "A Night to Remember: A Harm-Reduction Birthday Card Intervention Reduces High Risk Drinking During 21st Birthday Celebrations," *Journal of American College Health* 57, no. 6 (2009): 659–63.

42. National Social Norms Institute, "Case Studies: Alcohol," Accessed 2009, www.socialnorms.org/CaseStudies/alcohol.php.

43. Centers for Disease Control and Prevention, "Injury Mortality: Unintentional Injury: U.S. 2001–2006," 2009, http://205.207.175.93/HDI/TableViewer/tableView.aspx?ReportId=71.

44. National Highway Traffic Safety Administration, "Traffic Safety Facts Research Note: 2008 Traffic Safety Annual Assessment—Highlights," DOT HS 811 172, 2009, www-nrd.nhtsa.dot.gov/pubs/811016.pdf.

45. Centers for Disease Control and Prevention (CDC), "Drinking and Driving: A Threat to Everyone," *Vital Signs,* October 2011, www.cdc.gov/vitalsigns/drinkinganddriving.

46. Insurance Institute for Highway Safety, "Fatality Facts 2009: Alcohol," 2010, www

.iihs.org/research/fatality_facts_2009/
alcohol.html.

47. CDC, "Drinking and Driving: A Threat to Everyone," 2011.

48. American College Health Association, *American College Health Association—National College Health Assessment II*, 2012.

49. Ibid.

50. Insurance Institute for Highway Safety, "Fatality Facts 2009: Alcohol," 2010, www.iihs.org/research/fatality_facts_2009/alcohol.html.

51. Ibid.

52. Ibid.

53. Substance Abuse and Mental Health Services Administration, *Results from the 2009 National Survey on Drug Use and Health: National Findings*, 2010.

54. K. Keyes et al., "The Role of Race/Ethnicity in Alcohol-Attributable Injury in the United States," *Epidemiologic Reviews* (2011): 1–14

55. K. Chartier and R. Caetano, "Ethnicity and Health Disparities in Alcohol Research," *Alcohol Research and Health* 33, no. 1 and 2 (2010): 152–160.

56. Substance Abuse and Mental Health Services Administration, *Results from the 2009 National Survey on Drug Use and Health: National Findings*, 2010.

57. Ibid.

58. K. Chartier and R. Caetano, "Ethnicity and Health Disparities in Alcohol Research," 2010.

59. National Institutes of Health, Medline Plus, "Alcoholism and Alcohol Abuse," Updated May 2010, www.nlm.nih.gov/medlineplus/ency/article/000944.htm.

60. C. A. Presley et al., "The Introduction of the Heavy and Frequent Drinker: A Proposed Classification to Increase Accuracy of Alcohol Assessments in Postsecondary Education Settings," *Journal of Alcohol Studies on Alcohol* 67 (2006): 324–31.

61. National Institute on Drug Abuse, "Alcohol Abuse Makes Prescription Drug Abuse More Likely," *NIDA Notes* 21, no. 5 (2008), Available at www.drugabuse.gov/NIDA_notes/NNvol21N5/alcohol.html.

62. Ibid.

63. National Institute on Alcohol Abuse and Alcoholism, U.S. Department of Health and Human Services, *A Family History of Alcoholism: Are You at Risk?* NIH Publication no. 03–5340 (Bethesda, MD: National Institute on Alcohol Abuse and Alcoholism, 2007), Available at www.niaaa.nih.gov/Publications/PamphletsBrochuresPosters/English/Pages/default.aspx.

64. A. Agrawal and M. T. Lynskey, "Are There Genetic Influences on Addiction? Evidence from Family, Adoption and Twin Studies," *Addiction* 103 (2008): 1069–81.

65. J. Niels Rosenquist et al., "The Spread of Alcohol Consumption Behavior in a Large Social Network," *Annals of Internal Medicine* 152, no. 7 (2010): 426–33.

66. Centers for Disease Control and Prevention, Fact Sheet, "Excessive Alcohol Use and Risks to Women's Health: 2010," www.cdc.gov/alcohol/fact-sheets/womens-health.htm.

67. Join Together Staff, "7.5 Million Children in the U.S. Live With Alcoholic Parent," February 16, 2012, www.drugfree.org/join-together/alcohol/7-5-million-children-in-u-s-live-with-alcoholic-parent; Claudia Black, "Children of Addiction," The Many Faces of Addiction Blog, *Psychology Today*, February 8, 2010, www.psychologytoday.com/blog/the-many-faces-addiction/201002/children-addiction.

68. Ibid.

69. Centers for Disease Control and Prevention, "Excessive Drinking Costs U.S. $233.5 Billion," October 17, 2011, Available at www.cdc.gov/Features/AlcoholConsumption/.

70. Ensuring Solutions to Alcohol Problems, *Workplace Screening and Brief Intervention: What Employers Can and Should Do about Excessive Alcohol Use* (Washington, DC: The George Washington University Medical Center, 2008), Available at www.jointogether.org/resources/2008/workplace-sbi.html.

71. Ibid.

72. Ibid.

73. Underage Drinking Enforcement Training Center, Underage Drinking Costs, "Underage Drinking," September 2011, www.udetc.org/UnderageDrinkingCosts.asp.

74. Ibid.

75. Substance Abuse and Mental Health Services Administration, Office of Applied Studies, *The NSDUH Report—Alcohol Treatment: Need, Utilization, and Barriers*, (Rockville, MD: Substance Abuse and Mental Health Services Administration, 2009); E. Cohen et al., "Alcohol Treatment Utilization: Findings from the National Epidemiologic Survey on Alcohol and Related Conditions," *Drug and Alcohol Dependence* 86, nos. 2–3 (2007): 214–21.

12

Ending Tobacco Use

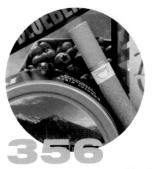

356
Why do people start smoking?

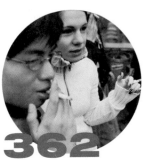

362
Is social smoking really that bad for me?

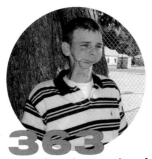

363
Is chewing tobacco as harmful as smoking?

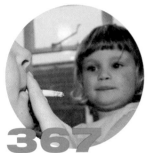

367
What are the health risks of secondhand smoke?

OBJECTIVES

✱ Describe the rate of tobacco use in the United States and on college campuses.

✱ Explain the social and political issues involved in tobacco use.

✱ Describe how the chemicals in tobacco products affect the body.

✱ Explain the health risks of smoking and using smokeless tobacco and the dangers created by environmental tobacco smoke.

✱ Describe various quitting strategies, including those aimed at ending the body's addiction to nicotine.

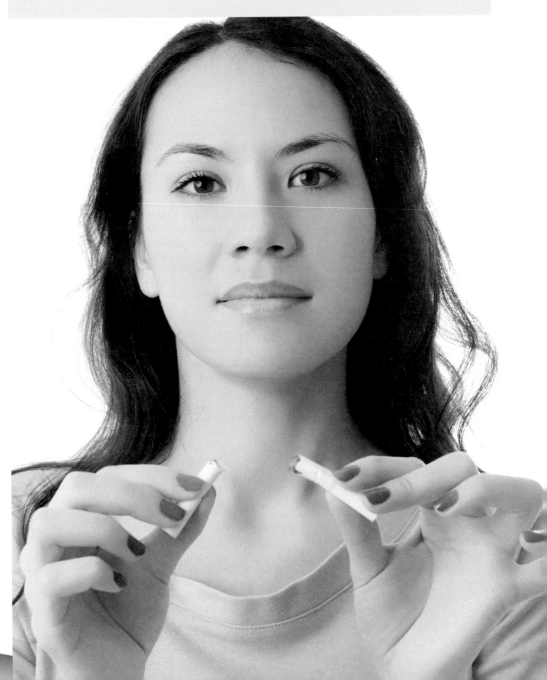

The prevalence of cigarette smoking among adults has declined significantly over the last 40 years.[1] However, tobacco use is still the single most preventable cause of death in the United States: Nearly 443,000 Americans die each year from tobacco-related diseases. Moreover, another 10 million people will suffer from health disorders caused by tobacco. To date, tobacco is known to cause more than 20 diseases, and about half of all regular smokers die of smoking-related causes. Smoking kills more Americans than alcohol, car accidents, suicide, AIDS, homicide, and illegal drugs combined.[2] Any contention by the tobacco industry that tobacco use is not dangerous is irresponsible and ignores the scientific evidence.

United States Tobacco Use

Approximately 70 million Americans age 12 and older report using tobacco products (cigarettes, cigars, smokeless tobacco, and pipe tobacco) at least once in the past month.[3] Declines in cigarette smoking over the past two decades have slowed compared with earlier periods. In 2010, 21.5 percent of men and 17.3 percent of women were current cigarette smokers. Adults 25 to 44 years old had the highest percentage of current cigarette smoking (22 percent), and the percentage continues to decrease with age, with 21.1 percent of adults 45 to 64 years old and 9.5 percent of adults aged 65 years and older reported to be current smokers.[4]

The rate of past-month cigarette use among those 12 to 17 years old declined from 13 percent in 2002 to 8.3 percent in 2010. The rate of past-month smokeless tobacco use among those 12 to 17 years old increased from 2 percent in 2002 to 2.3 percent in 2010. In addition, every day another 3,800 teens under the age of 18 smoke their first cigarette, and approximately 1,000 of them become daily smokers[5].

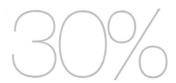

30%

of all cancer deaths have smoking

as a primary causal factor.

Education is closely linked to cigarette use: Adults with a bachelor's degree or higher education are two times *less* likely to smoke than are those with less than a high school education. Cigarette smoking also varies by ethnicity, with the highest rates of smoking found among and American Indian and Alaska Natives, with a prevalence of 31.4 percent.[6] Table 12.1 shows the percentage of Americans who smoke by demographic group.

More than 20 percent of Americans are former smokers, and about 60 percent have never smoked. The most commonly

TABLE 12.1	Percentage of Population That Smokes (Age 18 and Older) among Select Groups in the United States
	Percentage
United States overall	19.3
Race	
Asian	9.2
Black, non-Hispanic	20.6
Hispanic	12.5
Native American	31.4
White, non-Hispanic	21.1
Age	
18–24	20.1
25–44	22
45–64	21.1
65+	9.5
Gender	
Male	21.5
Female	17.3
Education	
Undergraduate	9.9
High school	23.8
GED diploma	45.2
9–11 years	33.8
Postgraduate	6.3
Income Level	
Below poverty level	28.9
At or above poverty level	18.3

Source: Centers for Disease Control and Prevention, "Adult Cigarette Smoking in the United States: Current Estimate," January 2012, www.cdc.gov/tobacco/data_statistics/fact_sheets/adult_data/cig_smoking/index.htm.

used tobacco product is cigarettes, followed by cigars and smokeless tobacco. Approximately 6 percent of Americans smoke cigars, and 7 percent of men and less than 1 percent of women use smokeless tobacco.[7]

Tobacco and Social Issues

The production and distribution of tobacco products involve many political and economic issues. Tobacco-growing states derive substantial income from tobacco production, and federal, state, and local governments benefit enormously from cigarette taxes.

Advertising The tobacco industry spends an estimated $36 million per day on advertising and promotional material.[8] With the number of smokers declining by about 1 million each year, the industry must actively recruit new smokers. Tobacco advertising also plays an important role in encouraging young people to begin a lifelong addiction to smoking before they are old enough to fully understand its long-term health risk.[9] Ninety percent of adults who smoke started by the age of 21, and half of them became regular smokers by their eighteenth birthday. Tobacco companies also target children and teens with tobacco products that have candy, fruit, or alcohol flavorings that mask the harshness of the tobacco, thus making these items more appealing and palatable to young people.[10]

Advertisements in women's magazines imply that smoking is the key to financial success, thinness, independence, and social acceptance. These ads have apparently been working. From the mid-1970s through the early 2000s, cigarette sales to women increased dramatically. Not coincidentally, by 1987 cigarette-induced lung cancer had surpassed breast cancer as the leading cancer killer among women and has remained the leading cancer killer in every year since.[11]

Women are not the only targets of gender-based cigarette advertisements. Men are depicted in locker rooms, charging over rugged terrain in off-road vehicles, or riding stallions into the sunset in blatant appeals to a need to feel and appear masculine. Minorities are also often targeted. Recent studies have shown a higher concentration of tobacco advertising in magazines aimed at African Americans, such as *Jet* and *Ebony*, than in similar magazines aimed at broader audiences, such as *Time* and *People*. Billboards and posters aiming the cigarette message at Hispanics have spotted the landscape in Hispanic communities for many years, especially in low-income areas. Recent innovations by tobacco companies have included sponsorship of community-based events such as festivals and annual fairs.

Financial Costs to Society

Estimates show that tobacco use causes over $193 billion in annual health-related economic losses. The economic burden of tobacco use totals more than $96 billion in medical expenditures and $97 billion in indirect costs (absenteeism, added cost of fire insurance, training costs to replace employees who die prematurely, disability payments, etc.).[12] The economic costs of smoking are estimated to be about $3,100 per smoker per year.[13] These costs far exceed the tax revenues on the sale of tobacco products, even though the average cigarette tax in 2011 was $1.46 per pack and is rising in some states.[14]

nicotine poisoning Symptoms often experienced by beginning smokers, including dizziness, diarrhea, lightheadedness, rapid and erratic pulse, clammy skin, nausea, and vomiting.

Tobacco Addiction

A recent study found that about half of high school students had experimented with smoking.[15] They might try a cigarette out of curiosity, because their parents smoke, or as a result of peer pressure. Why do some people walk away from cigarettes while others get hooked? This is a complicated question, but there are several possible reasons: Nicotine is a very addictive drug, people can become hooked on the behavior itself, weight control can be a motivating factor, and U.S. residents are bombarded with cigarette advertising messages every day.

Nicotine Addiction Beginning smokers usually feel the effects of nicotine with their first puff. These symptoms, called **nicotine poisoning,** can include dizziness, lightheadedness, rapid and erratic pulse, clammy skin, nausea, vomiting, and diarrhea. These symptoms cease as tolerance develops, which happens almost immediately in new users, perhaps after the second or third cigarette. In contrast, tolerance to most other drugs, such as alcohol, develops over a period of months or years. Regular smokers generally do not experience a "buzz"

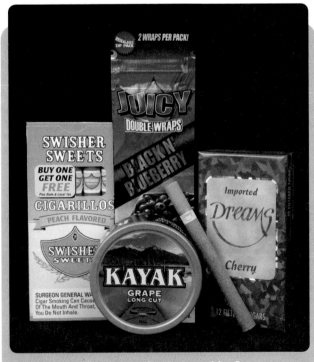

Why do people start smoking?

Peer pressure plays a large role, as do advertising and the portrayal of smoking in various media. Tobacco companies know that once a person starts smoking, chances are good that he or she will get hooked, so they make a concerted effort to attract children and teens by using colorful images and flavored products that mask the harshness of tobacco.

from smoking. They continue to smoke simply because quitting is so difficult.

Studies have found genetic factors to be significantly influential in smoking initiation and nicotine dependence. Specifically, one study found that teenagers carrying variants in two genes were three times more likely to become regular smokers in adolescence and twice as likely to be persistent smokers in adulthood, compared to noncarriers.[16] These two specific genes may influence smoking behavior by affecting the action of the brain chemical dopamine.[17] Understanding the influence of genetics on nicotine addiction could be crucial to developing more effective smoking-cessation treatments.[18]

Behavioral Dependence People who smoke are not just physically dependent on nicotine, they are also psychologically dependent. Nicotine "tricks" the brain into creating pleasurable memory associations between sensory stimuli or environmental cues that may trigger the urge for a cigarette.[19] Even those who smoke only occasionally might find it hard to quit because of associations between smoking and a behavior such as having a drink or a morning cup of coffee.

Many smokers have a difficult time imagining not smoking. They often describe their cigarette as their friend. For some smokers, simply holding a cigarette provides comfort and can have a calming effect. Some former smokers remain vulnerable to sensory and environmental cues, such as the smell of tobacco or driving a car, for years after they quit. For information on the growing number of women smokers, see the **Health in a Diverse World** box on the following page.

Weight Control Nicotine is an appetite suppressant and slightly increases the smoker's basal metabolic rate. People who start smoking often lose weight. After smoking, a smoker's metabolism increases right away and then returns to a normal level. Heavy smokers have surges in metabolism throughout the day. As a result, they experience less appetite than do those who smoke less

or not at all. When a smoker quits, the metabolic rate slows down and appetite returns. People tend to eat more (sweets in particular) when they stop smoking, with an average weight gain between 5 to 8 pounds. Fear of gaining weight is one of the biggest reasons smokers are reluctant to quit. Ways to avoid weight gain after quitting include avoiding crash diets, keeping low-calorie treats handy, and drinking plenty of water.

College Students and Tobacco Use

College students are the targets of heavy tobacco marketing and advertising campaigns. The tobacco industry has set up aggressive marketing promotions at bars, music festivals, and other events specifically targeted at the 18- to 24-year-old age group. Being placed in a new, often stressful social and academic environment makes college students especially vulnerable to outside influences. Peer influence can prompt students to start or continue smoking, and many colleges and universities still sell tobacco products in campus stores. However, cigarette smoking among U.S. college students has decreased in recent years (see **Figure 12.1**). In a 2011 study, about 15.2 percent of college students reported having smoked cigarettes in the past 30 days.[20] Among young adults 18 to 22 years old,

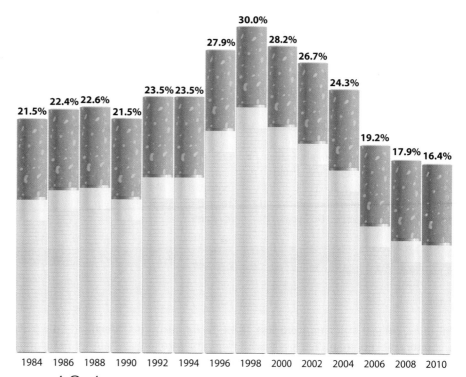

FIGURE 12.1 **Trends in Prevalence of Cigarette Smoking in the Past Month among College Students**
Source: Data from L. D. Johnston, P. M. O'Malley, J. G. Bachman, and J. E. Schulenberg, *Monitoring the Future National Survey Results on Drug Use, 1975–2009, Volume II: College Students and Adults Ages 19–50*, NIH Publication no. 10-7585 (Bethesda, MD: National Institute on Drug Abuse, 2010).

Have you noticed a change in the number of your friends who smoke?
● How many smoked prior to college compared to now?
● What are their reasons for smoking?
● What keeps your friends from quitting?

what do you think?

WOMEN AND SMOKING: CATCHING UP WITH MEN

Beginning during World War II and continuing to this day, tobacco marketers have used themes of social desirability, independence, and weight control to attract women smokers. Today, slightly more than 1 in 6 women in the United States smoke, and men's and women's smoking rates are nearly equal. Accordingly, women have assumed a much larger burden of smoking-related diseases than they did in the past. However, not all women are equally likely to smoke.

✳ Smoking among women differs by race and ethnicity: Rates for non-Latina white women are 19.6 percent; African American women, 17.1 percent; Latina women, 9 percent; Asian American women, 4.3 percent; and Native American/Alaskan Native women, 36 percent.
✳ Affluent women are less likely to smoke than are women who are poor. Thirty-two percent of women with incomes below the poverty line smoke.

Despite recent declines in smoking overall, the prevalence of tobacco-related disease continues to increase, especially among women. Consider the following:

✳ Every year, tobacco-related disease kills an estimated 174,000 women, making it the largest preventable cause of death among women in the United States.
✳ Women who die of a smoking-related disease lose, on average, 14.5 years of

Cigarette companies have become adept at marketing to women using "glamorous" packaging and ad campaigns borrowed from cosmetics, perfume (such as the famous Chanel scents evoked by this Camel No. 9 brand), and the fashion industry.

College students and young adults are the targets of heavy tobacco marketing and advertising campaigns. The tobacco industry has set up aggressive marketing promotions at bars and has sponsored concerts, music festivals, and other events targeted at the 18- to 24-year-old age group.

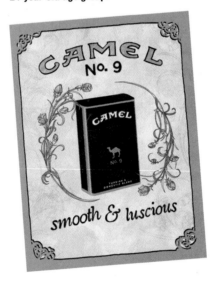

potential life. Men who die of a smoking-related disease lose 13 years of life, on average.

✳ Women who begin smoking at an early age (within 5 years of their first menstrual period) are at higher risk of developing breast cancer.
✳ Evidence suggests that breast cancer is more likely to spread to the lungs in women who smoke than it is in women who do not smoke.
✳ Recent data from the Centers for Disease Control and Prevention indicate that smoking-related cancer deaths are decreasing among men but are increasing among women.
✳ Postmenopausal women who smoke have lower bone density than do women who never smoked, putting these women at increased risk for osteoporosis.

Sources: American Cancer Society, "Women and Smoking: An Epidemic of Smoking-Related Cancer and Disease in Women," Revised November 2011, www.cancer.org/Cancer/CancerCauses/TobaccoCancer/WomenandSmoking/women-and-smoking-intro; American Heart Association, "Women, Heart Disease," 2012, www.heart.org/HEARTORG/Advocate/IssuesandCampaigns/QualityCare/Women-and-Heart-Disease_UCM_430484_Article.jsp; Office on Smoking and Health, Centers for Disease Control and Prevention, "Cigarette Smoking among Adults—United States, 2007," *Morbidity and Mortality Weekly Report* 57, no. 45 (2008): 1221–26; Centers for Disease Control and Prevention, "Smoking-Attributable Mortality, Years of Potential Life Lost, and Productivity Losses—United States, 2000–2004," *Morbidity and Mortality Weekly Report* 57, no. 45 (2008): 1226–28; Centers for Disease Control and Prevention, "Cigarette Smoking among Adults and Trends in Smoking Cessation—United States 2009," *Morbidity and Mortality Weekly Report* 59, no. 35 (2010): 1135–40.

full-time college students were less likely to be current cigarette smokers than their peers who were not enrolled full time in college. In 2010, cigarette use in the past month was reported by 24.8 percent of full-time college students, less than the rate of 39.9 percent for those not enrolled full time.[21] The same pattern was found among both males and females in this age range. Among males age 18 to 22 who were full-time college students in 2010, cigarette use

declined from 31.7 percent in 2009 to 27.1 percent in 2010. Rates of past-month use of smokeless tobacco did not differ significantly between males age 18 to 22 who were full-time college students and males of the same age group who were not enrolled full time in college, 12.0 and 12.7 percent, respectively. College men and women have nearly identical rates of cigarette smoking, but men use more cigars and smokeless tobacco.[22]

Why Do College Students Smoke?

In one survey (see **Figure 12.2**) the main reason students gave for smoking was to relax or to reduce stress (38%).[23] According to this study, smokers are more likely to have higher levels of perceived stress than do nonsmokers. Other key reasons provided by students were that they smoked to fit in or due to social pressure (16%) and because they cannot stop or are addicted (12%).

For some students weight control is an important motivator, and fear of weight gain is a common reason for smoking relapse. Students diagnosed or treated for depression are 7.5 times more likely to use tobacco compared to students who were never diagnosed or treated for depression.[24]

Social Smoking

Many college-age smokers identify themselves as "social smokers"—those who smoke when they are with people, rather than alone. Half of college smokers deny being smokers, even though they reported smoking in the past 30 days. Those students who deny being smokers are often younger males who are low-level smokers. Many of these students smoke in social situations where they also drink alcohol.[25] However, even occasional smoking is not without risks of damaging health effects. Social smoking in college can lead to a complete dependence on nicotine and thus to all the same health risks as smoking regularly.

Smoking less than a pack of cigarettes a week has been shown to damage blood vessels and to increase the risk of heart disease and cancer.[26] Occasional or social smokers also experience an increased occurrence of colds, sore throats, shortness of breath, and fatigue.[27] In women taking birth control pills, even a few cigarettes a week can increase the likelihood of heart disease, blood clots, stroke, liver cancer, and gallbladder disease.[28] Pregnant women who smoke only occasionally still run a risk of giving birth to unhealthy babies.

what do you think?

Should nicotine be regulated as a controlled substance?
● Should more resources be used for research into nicotine addiction?
● Why or why not?

Most Student Smokers Want to Quit

Unlike social smokers, most students who smoke regularly and are nicotine dependent do want to stop smoking. Unfortunately, in spite of their efforts or desire to quit, almost all daily smokers continue to smoke throughout college.[29] To reduce the incidence of smoking among students, colleges and universities need to engage in antismoking efforts, control tobacco advertising, provide smoke-free residence halls, and offer greater access to smoking-cessation programs. See the **Points of View** box on page 360 for a discussion of banning smoking on campuses.

nicotine Primary stimulant chemical in tobacco products that is highly addictive.

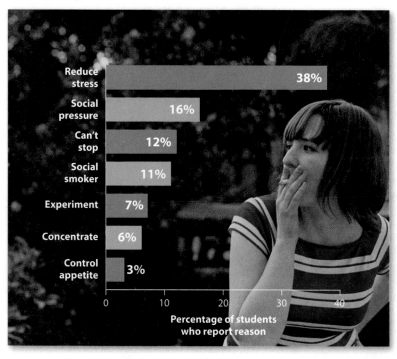

FIGURE 12.2 **Reasons Why College Students Smoke**
Source: National Center on Addiction and Substance Abuse at Columbia University, *Wasting the Best and the Brightest: Substance Abuse at America's Colleges and Universities* (New York: National Center on Addiction and Substance Abuse at Columbia University, March 2007), 48. Copyright © 2007. Used with permission.

Effects of Tobacco

Smoking, the most common form of tobacco use, delivers a strong dose of nicotine directly to the lungs, along with 7,000 other chemical substances, including arsenic, formaldehyde, and ammonia. Among these chemicals are at least 69 known or suspected carcinogens.[30] Some of the chemicals contained in tobacco smoke can also be found in chemical weapons, household cleaners, car exhaust, and embalming fluid (see **Table 12.2** on page 361). Inhaling toxic gases exposes sensitive mucous membranes to irritating chemicals that weaken the tissues and contribute to cancers of the mouth, larynx, and throat. The heat from tobacco smoke is also harmful to tissues.

Nicotine

The highly addictive chemical stimulant **nicotine** is the major psychoactive substance in all tobacco products. In its natural form, nicotine is a colorless liquid that turns brown upon exposure to air. When tobacco leaves are

Smoking on College & University Campuses:
SHOULD IT BE BANNED?

Approximately 20 percent of students begin smoking in college, and another 50 percent intensify their smoking behavior. In a recent study, 83 percent of students reported having been exposed to environmental tobacco smoke (ETS) at least once in the 7 days preceding the survey. Most of those exposures (65%) happened at a restaurant or bar, followed by exposure at home or in the same room as a smoker (55%) and in a car (38%).

Daily and occasional smokers were more likely than nonsmokers to report exposure, perhaps not surprising given that they are more likely to have friends who smoke and to frequent or live in locations where smoking occurs, according to the study. Similarly, students who binge drink were more likely than other students to report exposure to ETS. This is not surprising given there is a well-established link between smoking and drinking behaviors. Other factors that appeared to be associated with increased exposure to ETS included living in residence locations where smoking is allowed or locations associated with smoking, such as Greek houses and off-campus housing; being female; being white; having parents with higher education levels; and attending a public versus private school. Nearly all nonsmokers (93.9%) and the majority of smokers (57.8%) reported that ETS was somewhat or very annoying.

As a result, at least 381 campuses have all-out prohibitions or significant restrictions on tobacco use, with many more campuses pursuing becoming smoke free. The debate regarding tobacco-free campuses is contentious at many schools. Below are some of the major points for both sides of the question.

Arguments for Banning Tobacco on Campuses

- The majority of college students—4 out of 5—do not smoke.
- Two thirds of students prefer to attend classes held on a smoke-free campus.
- Most college employees prefer a smoke-free campus.
- Three quarters of students (both smokers and nonsmokers) say it is okay for colleges to prohibit smoking on campus to keep secondhand smoke away from students and staff.
- One in five students say they have experienced some immediate health impact from exposure to ETS.
- Nonsmokers are 40 percent less likely to become smokers if they live in smoke-free dorms.

Arguments against Banning Tobacco on Campuses

- There are so many other causes of potentially harmful fumes on campus—from diesel trucks, for example—that banning smoking wouldn't really affect the overall health and air quality on campus.
- Smoking is not illegal, so students should be able to do it somewhere on campus; it would be a violation of individual rights to not let adults do something that is legally allowed.
- The policy would be difficult if not impossible to enforce. For example, when visitors come to campus for athletic or community events, it would be unenforceable.
- Where can students go to smoke that is safe if they live in residence halls?
- Smoking bans in public and private places violate the rights of smokers and encourage discriminatory treatment of people addicted to nicotine.
- Colleges should focus more money and effort on smoking-cessation programs, not on implementing and enforcing smoking bans.

Where Do You Stand?

- Is smoking on a college campus a threat to public health?
- Do you think that smokers have the right to smoke in dorms, in campus buildings, in adjacent parks, or in other public places on campus? Why or why not?
- How do you feel when you are walking across campus and someone is smoking close to you? Do you feel as though you could or should ask smokers to put out their cigarettes?

City Campus

This is a smoke free area. Smoking is prohibited on University land. Thank you for not smoking on the University Campus.

- Would banning smoking be discriminatory? A violation of individual rights? Should student smokers be singled out for exclusion on college campuses?

Sources: American Cancer Society, "Smoke-Free College Campus Initiative," 2010, ww2.cancer.org/docroot/com/content/div_northwest/com_5_1x_smoke-free_college_campus_initiative.asp; Tobacco-Free Oregon, *Making Your College Campus Tobacco-Free*, 2010, http://smokefreeoregon.com/college/resources; M. Wolfson, T. McCoy, and E. Sutfin, "College Students' Exposure to Secondhand Smoke," *Nicotine and Tobacco Research* 11, no. 8 (2009): 977–84.

TABLE
12.2 What Exactly Are You Inhaling?

Chemical in Tobacco Smoke	Where Else Can You Find It?
Acetic acid	Vinegar
Acetone	Nail polish remover
Ammonia	Floor/toilet cleaner
Arsenic	Rat poison
Butane	Lighter fluid
Cadmium	Rechargeable batteries
Carbon monoxide	Car exhaust
DDT/dieldrin	Insecticides
Ethanol	Alcohol
Hexamine	Barbecue lighter
Hydrogen cyanide	Gas chamber poison, chemical weapons
Methane	Swamp gas, cow flatulence
Methanol	Rocket fuel
Naphthalene	Mothballs
Nicotine	Insecticide/addictive drug
Stearic acid	Candle wax
Toluene	Industrial solvent, paint thinner

Source: Utah Department of Health, TobaccoFreeUtah.org, "Chemicals Found in Tobacco Smoke," 2012, www.tobaccofreeutah.org/chemicals.html.

burned in a cigarette, pipe, or cigar, nicotine is released and inhaled into the lungs. Sucking or chewing tobacco releases nicotine into the saliva, and the nicotine is then absorbed through the mucous membranes in the mouth.

Nicotine is a powerful central nervous system stimulant that produces a variety of physiological effects. In the cerebral cortex, it produces an aroused, alert mental state. Nicotine stimulates the adrenal glands, which increases the production of adrenaline. It also increases heart and respiratory rates, constricts blood vessels, and, in turn, increases blood pressure because the heart must work harder to pump blood through the narrowed vessels.

tar Thick, brownish sludge condensed from particulate matter in smoked tobacco.

carbon monoxide Gas found in cigarette smoke that reduces the ability of blood to carry oxygen.

Tar and Carbon Monoxide

Cigarette smoke is a complex mixture of chemicals and gases produced by the burning of tobacco and its additives. Particulate matter condenses in the lungs to form a thick, brownish sludge called **tar,** which contains various carcinogenic agents, such as benzopyrene, and chemical irritants, such as phenol. Phenol has the potential to combine with other chemicals that contribute to developing lung cancer.

In healthy lungs, millions of tiny hairlike projections (*cilia*) on the surfaces lining the upper respiratory passages sweep away foreign matter, which is expelled from the lungs by coughing. However, the cilia's cleansing function is impaired in smokers' lungs by nicotine, which paralyzes the cilia for up to 1 hour following a single cigarette. This allows tars and other solids in tobacco smoke to accumulate and irritate sensitive lung tissue. **Figure 12.3** illustrates how tobacco smoke damages the lungs.

Cigarette smoke also contains poisonous gases, the most dangerous of which is **carbon monoxide,** the deadly gas emitted in car exhaust. Carbon monoxide reduces the oxygen-carrying capacity of the red blood cells by binding with the receptor sites for oxygen; this causes oxygen deprivation in many body tissues. It is at least partly

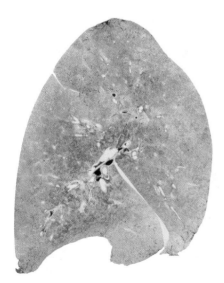

ⓐ A healthy lung

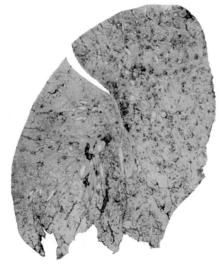

ⓑ A smoker's lung permeated with deposits of tar

FIGURE 12.3 **Lung Damage from Chemicals in Tobacco Smoke**
Smoke particles irritate lung pathways, causing extra mucus production, and nicotine paralyzes the cilia that normally function to keep the lungs clear of excess mucus. The result is difficulty breathing, "smoker's cough," and chronic bronchitis. At the same time, tar collects within the alveoli (air sacs), ultimately causing their walls to break, leading to emphysema. Tar and other carcinogens in tobacco smoke also cause cellular mutations that lead to cancer.

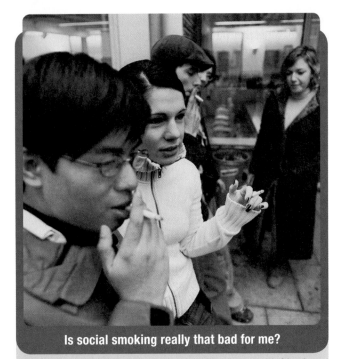

Is social smoking really that bad for me?

An occasional puff once in a while when you are out with friends can't hurt, right? Wrong! There is no "safe" amount of tobacco use—any smoking or exposure to smoke increases your risks for negative health effects such as heart disease and lung cancer. And even if you smoke only once or twice a week and consider yourself a social smoker, chances are you're on the road to dependence and a more frequent smoking habit.

responsible for the increased risk of heart attacks and strokes in smokers.

Tobacco Products

Tobacco comes in several forms. Cigarettes, cigars, pipes, and bidis are used for burning and inhaling tobacco. Smokeless tobacco is sniffed or placed in the mouth.

Cigarettes *Filtered cigarettes* are the most common form of tobacco available today. Almost all manufactured cigarettes have filters designed to reduce levels of gases such as hydrogen cyanide and carbon monoxide, but these products may actually deliver more hazardous gases to the user than nonfiltered brands. Some smokers use low-tar and low-nicotine products as an excuse to smoke more cigarettes. This practice is self-defeating because they wind up exposing themselves to more harmful substances than they would with a smaller number of regular-strength cigarettes.

Clove cigarettes contain about 40 percent ground cloves (a spice) and about 60 percent tobacco. Many users mistakenly believe that these products are made entirely of ground cloves and

that smoking them eliminates the risks associated with tobacco. In fact, clove cigarettes contain higher levels of tar, nicotine, and carbon monoxide than do regular cigarettes—and the numbing effect of eugenol, an ingredient in cloves, allows smokers to inhale more deeply. The same effect is true of *menthol cigarettes:* The throat-numbing effect of the menthol allows for deeper inhalation. Menthol cigarettes also have higher carbon monoxide concentrations than regular cigarettes.

Cigars Since 1997, cigar sales in the United States have increased dramatically, up nearly 240 percent between 1997 and 2007.[31] Many people believe that cigars are safer than cigarettes, when in fact the opposite is true. Cigar smoke contains 23 poisons and 43 carcinogens. Most cigars contain as much nicotine as several cigarettes, and when cigar smokers inhale, nicotine is absorbed as rapidly as it is with cigarettes. For those who don't inhale, nicotine is still absorbed through the mucous membranes in the mouth.

Pipes and Hookahs Pipes have had a long history of use throughout the world, including ritualistic and ceremonial use in many cultures. Often thought to be safer than cigarettes or cigars, pipes are not risk-free options. According to the National Cancer Institute and the American Cancer Society, pipe smoking carries risks similar to cigar smoking. Of concern in recent years is the increasing prevalence, particularly among college students, of the use of hookahs, or water pipes. Hookah smoking originated in the Middle East and involves burning flavored tobacco in a water pipe and inhaling the smoke through a long hose. Hookahs are marketed as a safe alternative to cigarettes because they reduce the risks from hazardous chemicals by filtering the smoke through water before it is inhaled. While water pipes may cool the smoke, they do not eliminate or filter out harmful substances.[32] In addition to the health risks associated with all tobacco products, risks associated

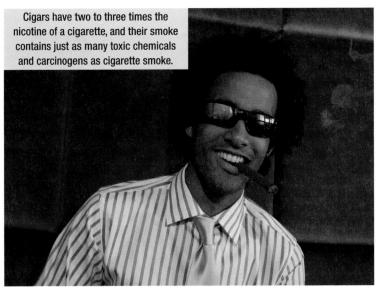

Cigars have two to three times the nicotine of a cigarette, and their smoke contains just as many toxic chemicals and carcinogens as cigarette smoke.

with hookah use include the possibility of infectious disease transmission by sharing a pipe.

Bidis Generally ma de in India or Southeast Asia, **bidis** are small, hand-rolled cigarettes that come in a variety of flavors, such as vanilla, chocolate, and cherry, and resemble a marijuana joint or a clove cigarette. They have become increasingly popular with college students because they are viewed as safer and cheaper than cigarettes. However, they are far more toxic than cigarettes. Smoke from a bidi contains three times more carbon monoxide and nicotine and five times more tar than cigarettes.[33] The leaf wrappers are nonporous, which means that smokers must suck harder to inhale and must inhale more to keep the bidi lit. During testing, it took an average of 28 puffs to smoke a bidi, compared to only 9 puffs for a regular cigarette. This results in increased exposure to higher amounts of tar, nicotine, and carbon monoxide, and bidis lack any sort of filter to reduce these levels. Bidi smoking increases the risk for oral cancer, lung cancer, stomach cancer, and esophageal cancer and is also associated with emphysema and chronic bronchitis.[34]

Smokeless Tobacco There are two types of smokeless tobacco: chewing tobacco and snuff.

Chewing tobacco comes in three forms—loose leaf, plug, or in a pouch—and contains tobacco leaves treated with molasses and other flavorings. The user dips the tobacco by placing a small amount between the lower lip and teeth to stimulate the flow of saliva and release the nicotine. **Dipping** rapidly releases nicotine into the bloodstream. Use of chewing tobacco by teenage boys, especially in rural areas, has increased by 30 percent in the past 10 years.[35]

Snuff is a finely ground form of tobacco that can be inhaled, chewed, or placed against the gums. It comes in dry or moist powdered form or sachets (tea bag–like pouches). In 2009, "snus" became the latest form of smokeless tobacco to hit the market in the United States. Popular for more than 100 years in Sweden, these small sachets of tobacco are placed inside the cheek and sucked. Some people prefer snus to chewing tobacco because it doesn't require the user to spit frequently.

Smokeless tobacco is just as addictive as cigarettes and actually contains more nicotine—holding an average-sized dip or chew in the mouth for 30 minutes delivers as much nicotine as smoking four cigarettes. A two-can-a-week snuff user gets as much nicotine as a 10-pack-a-week smoker.

Dental problems are common among users of smokeless tobacco. Contact with tobacco juice causes receding gums, tooth decay, bad breath, and discolored teeth. Damage to both the teeth and jawbone can contribute to loss of teeth.

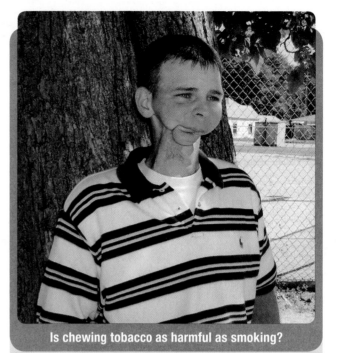

Is chewing tobacco as harmful as smoking?

No matter in what form you use it, tobacco is hazardous to your health. Chewing tobacco and snuff actually contain more nicotine than cigarettes and just as many toxic and carcinogenic chemicals. This young cancer survivor began using smokeless tobacco at age 13; by age 17, he was diagnosed with squamous cell carcinoma. He has undergone surgery to remove neck muscles, lymph nodes, and his tongue, and he now educates others about the dangers of chewing tobacco.

Health Hazards of Tobacco Products

Each day, cigarettes contribute to more than 1,200 deaths from cancer, cardiovascular disease, and respiratory disorders.[36] In addition, tobacco use can negatively affect the health of almost every system in your body. Figure 12.4 on page 364 summarizes some of the physiological and health effects of smoking.

Cancer

Lung cancer is the leading cause of cancer deaths in the United States. The American Cancer Society estimates that tobacco smoking causes 85 to 90 percent of all cases of lung cancer; fewer than 10 percent of cases occur among nonsmokers. There were an estimated 226,160 *new* cases of lung cancer in the United States in 2010 alone, and an estimated 160,340

what do you think?

Should smokeless tobacco be banned wherever smoking is forbidden?

● Why do you think smokeless tobacco is popular with many athletes and young men?

bidis Hand-rolled flavored cigarettes.

chewing tobacco Stringy form of tobacco that is placed in the mouth and then sucked or chewed.

dipping Placing a small amount of chewing tobacco between the lower lip and teeth for rapid nicotine absorption.

snuff Powdered form of tobacco that is sniffed or absorbed through the mucous membranes in the nose or placed inside the cheek and sucked.

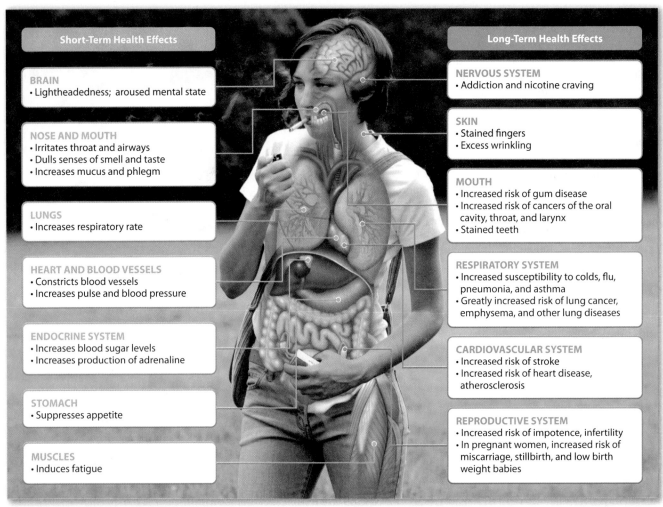

Short-Term Health Effects	Long-Term Health Effects

BRAIN
• Lightheadedness; aroused mental state

NOSE AND MOUTH
• Irritates throat and airways
• Dulls senses of smell and taste
• Increases mucus and phlegm

LUNGS
• Increases respiratory rate

HEART AND BLOOD VESSELS
• Constricts blood vessels
• Increases pulse and blood pressure

ENDOCRINE SYSTEM
• Increases blood sugar levels
• Increases production of adrenaline

STOMACH
• Suppresses appetite

MUSCLES
• Induces fatigue

NERVOUS SYSTEM
• Addiction and nicotine craving

SKIN
• Stained fingers
• Excess wrinkling

MOUTH
• Increased risk of gum disease
• Increased risk of cancers of the oral cavity, throat, and larynx
• Stained teeth

RESPIRATORY SYSTEM
• Increased susceptibility to colds, flu, pneumonia, and asthma
• Greatly increased risk of lung cancer, emphysema, and other lung diseases

CARDIOVASCULAR SYSTEM
• Increased risk of stroke
• Increased risk of heart disease, atherosclerosis

REPRODUCTIVE SYSTEM
• Increased risk of impotence, infertility
• In pregnant women, increased risk of miscarriage, stillbirth, and low birth weight babies

FIGURE 12.4 **Effects of Smoking on the Body and Health**

Video Tutor: Long- and Short-Term Effects of Tobacco

---

leukoplakia Condition characterized by leathery white patches inside the mouth, which is produced by contact with irritants in tobacco juice.

Americans died from the disease in 2012.[37]

Lung cancer can take 10 to 30 years to develop, and the outlook for its victims is poor. Most lung cancer is not diagnosed until it is fairly widespread in the body; at that point, the 5-year survival rate is only 16 percent. When a malignancy is diagnosed and recognized while still localized, the 5-year survival rate rises to 52 percent.[38]

If you are a smoker, your risk of developing lung cancer depends on several factors. First, the amount you smoke per day is important. Someone who smokes two packs a day is 15 to 25 times more likely to develop lung cancer than a nonsmoker. As little as one cigar per day can double the risk of several can-

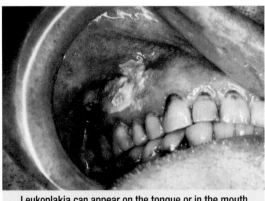

Leukoplakia can appear on the tongue or in the mouth, as shown here.

cers, including cancer of the oral cavity (lip, tongue, mouth, and throat); esophagus; larynx; and lungs. A second factor is the age at which you started smoking; if you started in your teens, you have a greater chance of developing lung cancer than do people who start later. And a third risk factor is whether you inhale deeply when you smoke. Smokers are also more susceptible to the cancer-causing effects of exposure to other irritants, such as asbestos and radon, than are nonsmokers.

A major risk of chewing tobacco is **leukoplakia,** a condition characterized by leathery white patches inside the mouth that are produced by contact with irritants in tobacco juice. Three to 17 percent of diagnosed leukoplakia cases develop into oral cancer.[39]

It is estimated that there were over 40,000 oral cancer cases in

2012.[40] Heavy alcohol and smokeless tobacco users are 30 times more likely to develop oral cancers than are nonusers. Warning signs include lumps in the jaw or neck; color changes or lumps inside the lips; white, smooth, or scaly patches in the mouth or on the neck, lips, or tongue; a red spot or sore on the lips or gums or inside the mouth that does not heal in 2 weeks; repeated bleeding in the mouth; and difficulty or abnormality in speaking or swallowing.

The lag time between first use and contracting cancer is shorter for smokeless tobacco users than for smokers because absorption through the gums is the most efficient route of nicotine administration. Many smokeless tobacco users eventually "graduate" to cigarettes and increase their risk for developing additional problems.

Tobacco is linked to other cancers as well. The rate of pancreatic cancer is more than twice as high for smokers as for nonsmokers. Typically, people diagnosed with pancreatic cancer live only about 3 months after their diagnosis. Smokers are at increased risk to develop cancers of the lip, tongue, salivary glands, and esophagus. A growing body of evidence suggests that long-term use of smokeless tobacco increases the risk of cancers of the larynx, esophagus, nasal cavity, pancreas, kidney, and bladder. Figure 12.5 shows the association between tobacco consumption rates and lung cancer deaths.

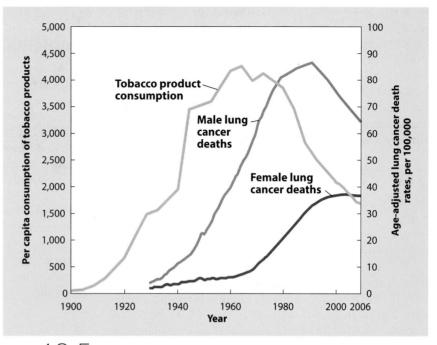

FIGURE 12.5 Correlation between Tobacco Consumption and Lung Cancer Deaths in the United States

A dramatic rise in lung cancer death rates echoed the rise in popularity of cigarettes and other tobacco products in the last century. After tobacco use and smoking rates began to decline in the 1980s, the lung cancer death rates began to decline as well.

Sources: Death rates data from U.S. Mortality Files, National Center for Health Statistics, Centers for Disease Control and Prevention, 2010; Cigarette consumption data from U.S. Department of Agriculture, 1900–2006.

Cardiovascular Disease

Over a third of all tobacco-related deaths occur from heart disease.[41] Smoking poses as great a risk for developing heart disease as high blood pressure and high cholesterol do. Daily cigar smoking, especially for people who inhale, also increases the risk of heart disease (cigar smokers double their risk of heart attack and stroke compared to nonsmokers).[42]

Smoking contributes to heart disease by aging the arteries.[43] This occurs because smoking and exposure to environmental tobacco smoke (ETS; see definition on page 366), encourage and accelerate the buildup of fatty deposits (plaque) in the heart and major blood vessels (*atherosclerosis*). Smokers can experience a 50 percent increase in plaque accumulation in the arteries as compared with exsmokers. People regularly exposed to ETS can have a 20 to 25 percent increase in plaque buildup.[44] For unknown reasons, smoking decreases blood levels of high-density lipoproteins (HDLs), the "good" cholesterol that helps protect against heart attacks.

Smoking also contributes to **platelet adhesiveness,** the sticking together of red blood cells that is associated with blood clots. The oxygen deprivation associated with smoking decreases the oxygen supplied to the heart and can weaken tissues. Smoking also contributes to irregular heart rhythms, which can trigger a heart attack. Both carbon monoxide and nicotine can precipitate angina attacks (chest pain due to the heart muscle not getting the blood supply it needs).

Smokers are two to four times as likely to suffer strokes as nonsmokers.[45]

A stroke occurs when a small blood vessel in the brain bursts or is blocked by a blood clot, denying oxygen and nourishment to vital portions of the brain. Depending on the area of the brain affected, stroke can result

platelet adhesiveness Stickiness of red blood cells associated with blood clots.

"Why Should I Care?"

If the life-threatening health consequences aren't enough to make you give up smoking, consider the negative impact smoking can have on your social (and romantic!) life. Popular media may make smoking seem glamorous and sexy, but in reality, smoking makes your breath, hair, and clothing smell bad; it causes your skin to age prematurely; it yellows your teeth; and it can interfere with a man's ability to achieve and maintain an erection.

in paralysis, loss of mental functioning, or death. Smoking contributes to strokes by raising blood pressure, which increases the stress on vessel walls. Platelet adhesiveness contributes to blood clot formation.

If a person quits smoking, the risk of dying from a heart attack falls by half after only 1 year without smoking and declines steadily thereafter. After about 15 years without smoking, an ex-smoker's risk of coronary heart disease is similar to that of people who have never smoked.[46]

Respiratory Disorders

Smoking quickly impairs the respiratory system. Smokers can feel its impact in a relatively short period of time—they are more prone to breathlessness, chronic cough, and excess phlegm production than are nonsmokers of the same age. Smokers tend to miss work one third more often than nonsmokers, primarily because of respiratory conditions. Over time, cumulative lung damage can lead to chronic obstructive pulmonary disease (COPD), including chronic bronchitis and emphysema. Ultimately, smokers are up to 18 times more likely to die of lung disease than are nonsmokers.[47]

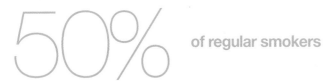

50% of regular smokers

eventually die of smoking-related diseases.

Chronic bronchitis may develop in smokers because their inflamed lungs produce more mucus, which they constantly try to expel along with foreign particles. This results in the persistent cough known as "smoker's hack." Smokers are also more prone to respiratory ailments such as influenza, pneumonia, and colds.

Emphysema is a chronic disease in which the alveoli (the tiny air sacs in the lungs) are destroyed, impairing the lungs' ability to obtain oxygen and remove carbon dioxide. As a result, breathing becomes difficult. While healthy people expend only about 5 percent of their energy in breathing, people with advanced emphysema expend nearly 80 percent. Because the heart has to work harder to do even the simplest tasks, it may become enlarged and death from heart damage may result. There is no known cure for emphysema, and the damage is irreversible. Approximately 80 percent of all cases of emphysema are related to cigarette smoking.[48]

emphysema Chronic lung disease in which the tiny air sacs in the lungs are destroyed, making breathing difficult.

environmental tobacco smoke (ETS) Smoke from tobacco products, including secondhand and mainstream smoke.

mainstream smoke Smoke that is drawn through tobacco while inhaling.

sidestream smoke Cigarette, pipe, or cigar smoke breathed by nonsmokers, commonly called *secondhand smoke.*

Sexual Dysfunction and Fertility Problems

Despite attempts by tobacco advertisers to make smoking appear sexy, research shows just the opposite: It can cause impotence in men. Several studies have found that male smokers are twice as likely as nonsmokers to suffer from some form of impotence.[49] Toxins in cigarette smoke damage blood vessels, reducing blood flow to the penis and leading to an inadequate erection. Impotence may indicate oncoming cardiovascular disease.

In women, smoking can lead to infertility and problems with pregnancy. Women who smoke increase their risk for infertility, ectopic pregnancy, miscarriage, and stillbirth. Smoking also increases the risk of sudden infant death syndrome and the chances of a baby being born with a cleft lip or cleft palate.[50] Smoking during pregnancy accounts for approximately 30 percent of premature births and increases the risk of low birth weight (less than 5.5 pounds), which in turn increases the likelihood of illness or death of an infant.[51]

Other Health Effects

Gum disease is three times more common among smokers than among nonsmokers, and smokers lose significantly more teeth.[52] In addition, smoking increases the risk of macular degeneration, one of the most common causes of blindness in older adults. It also causes premature skin wrinkling, staining of the teeth, yellowing of the fingernails, and bad breath. Nicotine speeds up the process by which the body uses and eliminates drugs, making medications less effective. In addition, recent research suggests that smoking significantly increases the risk of Alzheimer's disease.[53]

what do you think?
Why do most smokers continue despite knowing long-term hazards?
● What strategies might be effective in reducing the number of people who begin smoking?

Environmental Tobacco Smoke

Although fewer Americans smoke than in the past, air pollution from smoking in public places continues to be a problem. **Environmental tobacco smoke (ETS)** is divided into two categories: mainstream and sidestream smoke. **Mainstream smoke** refers to smoke drawn through tobacco while inhaling; **sidestream smoke** (commonly called *secondhand smoke*) refers to smoke from the burning end of a cigarette or smoke exhaled by a smoker. People who breathe smoke from someone else's smoking product are said to be *involuntary* or *passive* smokers.

Between 1988 and 2008, detectable levels of nicotine exposure in nonsmoking Americans has decreased from 87.9 percent

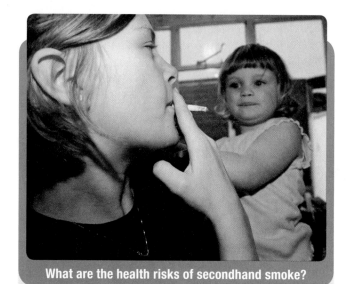

What are the health risks of secondhand smoke?

Every year, ETS is responsible for thousands of deaths from lung cancer and heart disease in nonsmoking adults, as well as hundreds of infant deaths from SIDS among babies who live with smokers. Because their bodies and brains are still developing, infants and children are particularly vulnerable to the toxins in secondhand smoke: It can cause respiratory problems, including lower respiratory infections and increased frequency and severity of asthma attacks, and other health concerns, such as greater risk of ear infections.

to 40.1 percent.[54] The decrease in exposure to secondhand smoke is due to the growing number of laws that ban smoking in workplaces and other public areas. As of 2010, 19 states, Puerto Rico, and the District of Columbia had laws in effect requiring workplaces, restaurants, and bars to be 100 percent smoke free. These laws, along with local laws, protect 41 percent of the U.S. population. Another 19 states ban smoking in some of these locations. Groups such as Action on Smoking and Health and Americans for Nonsmokers' Rights continue to push for policies and laws in support of smoke-free public places.[55]

Children are more heavily exposed to ETS than adults. More than 53 percent of U.S. children age 3 to 11 years—or 22 million children—are exposed to ETS.[56] Disparities in ETS also occur along ethnic and racial lines and by income level. African Americans have been found to have higher levels of exposure to ETS than whites and Latinos. ETS exposure is also higher among low-income persons.[57]

Risks from Environmental Tobacco Smoke

Although involuntary smokers breathe less tobacco than active smokers do, they still face risks from exposure. Secondhand smoke actually contains more carcinogenic substances than that which a smoker inhales, and it is the primary cause of indoor air pollution. According to the American Lung Association, secondhand smoke has about 2 times more tar and nicotine, 5 times more carbon monoxide, and 50 times more ammonia than mainstream smoke. Every year, ETS is estimated to be responsible for approximately 3,400 lung cancer deaths in nonsmoking adults, 46,000 coronary and heart disease deaths in nonsmoking adults who live with smokers, and higher risk of death in newborns from sudden infant death syndrome.[58]

The Environmental Protection Agency has designated secondhand smoke as a known carcinogen. There are more than 50 cancer-causing agents found in secondhand smoke.[59] There is also strong evidence that secondhand smoke interferes with normal functioning of the heart, blood, and vascular systems, significantly increasing the risk for heart disease. Studies indicate that nonsmokers exposed to secondhand smoke were 20 to 30 percent more likely to have coronary heart disease than nonsmokers not exposed to smoke.[60]

Children and ETS Exposure to ETS increases children's risk of lower respiratory tract infections. Consequently, there are an estimated 150,000 to 300,000 lower respiratory tract infections in children under 18 months of age and lung infections resulting in 7,500 to 15,000 hospitalizations each year.[61] In addition, children exposed to secondhand smoke have a greater chance of developing other respiratory problems such as coughing, wheezing, asthma, and chest colds, along with a decrease in lung function. The most significant effects of secondhand smoke are seen in children under the age of 5. Children exposed to secondhand smoke daily in the home miss 33 percent more school days and have 10 percent more colds and acute respiratory infections than do those not exposed.[62]

Secondhand smoke affects not only children's physical health, but also their cognitive abilities and academic success. One study found that children exposed to high levels of secondhand smoke were are twice as likely to develop learning disabilities, conduct disorders, and other behavioral disorders.[63] In addition, boys were more likely to be at risk of developing learning disabilities than girls.[64]

ETS and Additional Health Problems ETS in enclosed areas presents other hazards; it can cause allergic reactions such as itchy eyes, difficulty in breathing, headaches, nausea, and dizziness. Environmental tobacco smoke may also increase the risk of breast cancer in women; cancer of the nasal sinus cavity and of the pharynx in adults; and leukemia, lymphoma, and brain tumors in children.[65] The level of carbon monoxide in cigarette smoke in enclosed spaces is 4,000 times higher than that allowed in the clean-air standard recommended by the EPA.

what do you think?

What rights should smokers have to smoke in public?

● Does your campus allow smoking in residence halls?

● Does your community have nonsmoking restaurants or only designated nonsmoking sections?

● Are you more or less likely to frequent public places that allow smoking?

Tobacco Use and Prevention Policies

It has been more than 40 years since the U.S. government began warning that tobacco use was hazardous to health. Despite all the education on the health hazards of tobacco use, health care spending and lost productivity associated with smoking still exceeds $193 billion each year.[66]

In 1998, the tobacco industry reached the Master Settlement Agreement with 46 states. The agreement requires tobacco companies to pay more than $206 billion over 25 years. The agreement includes a variety of measures to support antismoking education and advertising and to fund research to determine effective smoking-cessation strategies. The agreement also curbs certain advertising and promotions directed at youth.

Unfortunately, most of the money designated for tobacco control and prevention at the state level has not been used for this purpose. Facing budget woes, many states have drastically cut spending on antismoking programs. In the few states that have spent the settlement money on smoking-cessation programs, there has been some success in decreasing cigarette use.[67] The Family Smoking Prevention and Tobacco Control Act of 2009 allows the U.S. Food and Drug Administration (FDA) to forbid advertising geared toward children, to lower the amount of nicotine in tobacco prod-

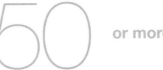

ucts, to ban sweetened cigarettes that appeal to young people, and to prohibit labels such as "light" and "low tar."[68] One of the most significant impacts of the law is that it requires more prominent health warnings on advertising of tobacco products. Smokeless tobacco ads must contain a warning that fills 20 percent of the advertising space. As of June 2012, cigarette packages and advertising are required to have larger, stronger warnings that must cover the top half of both the front and back of each package and include "color graphics depicting the negative health consequences of smoking." The graphics are to be modeled on ads already used in Canada, Australia, and New Zealand that depict the damaging effects of using tobacco products.

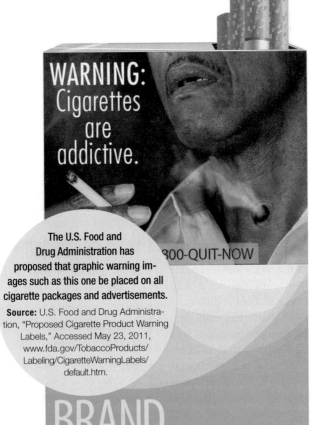

WARNING:
Cigarettes are addictive.

300-QUIT-NOW

BRAND
20 Class A Cigarettes

The U.S. Food and Drug Administration has proposed that graphic warning images such as this one be placed on all cigarette packages and advertisements.

Source: U.S. Food and Drug Administration, "Proposed Cigarette Product Warning Labels," Accessed May 23, 2011, www.fda.gov/TobaccoProducts/Labeling/CigaretteWarningLabels/default.htm.

what do you think?

Is it fair to blame tobacco companies if smokers develop tobacco-related health problems?
● What is a tobacco company's ethical obligation to society?
● Should it be different from the ethical obligations of other industries?

Quitting

Smokers who want to quit must break both the physical addiction to nicotine and the psychological habit of lighting up at certain times or in certain situations. Approximately 70 percent of U.S. adult smokers want to quit smoking, and up to 44 percent make a serious attempt to quit each year. However, only 4 to 7 percent succeed.[69] Quitting is often a lengthy process involving several unsuccessful attempts before success is finally achieved. Even successful quitters suffer occasional slips.

what do you think?

Do you know anyone who has tried to quit smoking?
● Why did they do so?
● What was their experience like?
● Were they successful?
● If not, what will they do differently the next time?

Benefits of Quitting

Many body tissues damaged by smoking can repair themselves. As soon as smokers stop, the body begins the repair process. Within 8 hours, carbon monoxide and oxygen levels return to normal, and "smoker's breath" disappears. Often, within a month of quitting, the mucus that clogs airways is

START HERE

8 hours
- Carbon monoxide level in blood drops to normal.
- Oxygen level in blood increases to normal.

48 hours
- Nerve endings start regrowing.
- Ability to smell and taste is enhanced.

1 to 9 months
- Coughing, sinus congestion, fatigue, shortness of breath decrease.
- Cilia regrow in lungs, which increases ability to handle mucus, clean the lungs, reduce infection.
- Body's overall energy increases.

5 years
- Lung cancer death rate for average former smoker (one pack a day) decreases by almost half.

15 years
- Risk of coronary heart disease is the same as that of a nonsmoker.

20 minutes
- Blood pressure drops to normal.
- Pulse rate drops to normal.
- Body temperature of hands and feet increases to normal.

24 hours
- Chance of heart attack decreases.

2 weeks to 3 months
- Circulation improves.
- Walking becomes easier.
- Lung function increases up to 30%.

1 year
- Excess risk of coronary disease is half that of a smoker.

10 years
- Lung cancer death rate similar to that of nonsmokers.
- Precancerous cells are replaced.
- Risk of cancers of the mouth, throat, esophagus, bladder, kidney, and pancreas decreases.

FIGURE 12.6 **When Smokers Quit**
Within 20 minutes of smoking that last cigarette, the body begins a series of changes that continues for years. However, by smoking just one cigarette a day, the smoker loses all of these benefits of quitting smoking, according to the American Cancer Society.

Source: Data from Substance Abuse and Mental Health Services Administration, *Results from the 2010 National Survey on Drug Use and Health: National Findings*, NSDUH Series H-36, HHS Publication no. SMA 09-4434 (Rockville, MD: Office of Applied Studies, 2011), www.samhsa.gov/data/NSDUH/2k10NSDUH/2k10Results.htm.

broken up and eliminated. Circulation and the senses of taste and smell improve within weeks. Many ex-smokers say that they have more energy, sleep better, and feel more alert.

After 1 year, the risk for lung cancer and stroke decreases. The risk of developing cancer of the mouth, throat, esophagus, larynx, pancreas, bladder, or cervix is considerably reduced, as is the risk of peripheral artery disease, COPD, coronary heart disease, and ulcers. Women are less likely to bear babies of low birth weight. Within 2 years, the risk for heart attack drops to near normal. After 10 smoke-free years, ex-smokers can expect a normal life span. See Figure 12.6 for a time line of how the body recuperates after a smoker quits.

Another significant benefit of quitting smoking is the money saved. A single pack of cigarettes ranges from about $5.00 (including tax) to as much as $9.00 to $11.00 in the most expensive states. So a pack-a-day smoker who lives in an area where cigarettes cost $7.00 per pack spends $49.00 per week, or $2,548.00 per year.[70] That is money that could have gone toward school expenses, a down payment on a car, or a dreamed-about vacation. See the **Money & Health** box on page 371 for more on the cost of smoking vs. quitting.

How Can You Quit?

A person who wishes to quit smoking has several options. Most people who are successful quit "cold turkey"—that is, they simply decide not to smoke again. Others focus on gradual reduction in smoking levels, which can reduce risks over time. Some rely on short-term programs, such as those offered by the American Cancer Society, which are based on behavior modification and a system of self-rewards. Still others turn to treatment centers, community outreach programs, or a telephone helpline. Finally, some people work privately with their physicians to reach their goal. Programs that combine several approaches have shown the most promise. Financial considerations, personality, and level of addiction are all factors to consider in deciding on a method.

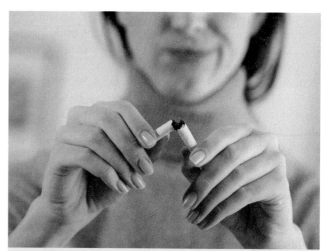

Quitting smoking is challenging, and you may be wondering whether the effort to quit will result in long-term health benefits. The answer is a definite Yes! Tobacco causes serious injury to your heart and lungs, but when you quit, your body immediately starts to recover and repair the damage. Over time, the body's repair processes reduce a former smoker's risk of heart disease and cancer; after 10 years, lung cancer risk is comparable to those of nonsmokers, and after 15 years, heart disease risk is the same.

Withdrawal Challenge	Estimated Length of Symptoms	Coping Strategies*
Anger, frustration, and irritability	Peaks in first week after quitting, but can last 2–4 weeks.	Avoid caffeine, which can amp up an already agitated mood. Get a massage, try deep breathing or exercise.
Anxiety	Builds over the first 3 days and may last up to 2 weeks.	Same strategies as above. Also remind yourself that the symptoms usually pass by themselves over time.
Mild depression	One month or less.	Be with supportive friends, increase physical activity, make a list of things that are upsetting you and write down possible solutions. If depression lasts longer than a month, seek medical advice.
Weight gain	Usually begins in the early weeks and continues through the first year after quitting.	Studies show nicotine replacement products such as gum and lozenges can help counter weight gain. You may also ask your doctor about the drug bupropion (brand names Wellbutrin or Zyban), which has also been shown to counter weight gain.

*Asking your doctor for nicotine replacement products or other medications is a valid coping strategy for any of the withdrawal challenges listed here.

Source: Adapted from "Handling Withdrawal Symptoms When You Decide to Quit," National Cancer Institute Fact Sheet, 2010, www.cancer.gov/cancertopics/factsheet/Tobacco/symptoms-triggers-quitting.

Breaking the Nicotine Addiction

Nicotine addiction may be one of the toughest addictions to overcome. Symptoms of **nicotine withdrawal** include irritability, restlessness, nausea, vomiting, and intense cravings for tobacco (see Table 12.3). The evidence is strong that consistent pharmacological treatments can help a smoker quit: An estimated 25 to 33 percent of people who have used nicotine replacement therapy or smoking-cessation medications continue to abstain from cigarettes for more than 6 months.[71]

Nicotine Replacement Products Nontobacco products that replace depleted levels of nicotine in the bloodstream have helped some people stop using tobacco. The two most common are nicotine chewing gum and the nicotine patch, both of which are available over the counter. The FDA has also approved nicotine lozenges, a nicotine nasal spray, and a nicotine inhaler. Another product called the e-cigarette is also available, though it comes with its own health concerns. See the **Tech & Health** box on page 372 for more information on e-cigarettes.

Nicotine gum is available without a prescription. The user chews up to 20 pieces of gum a day for 1 to 3 months. Nicotine gum delivers about the same amount of nicotine as a cigarette, but because it is absorbed through the mucous membrane of the mouth, it doesn't produce the same rush. Users experience no withdrawal symptoms and fewer cravings for nicotine as the dosage is reduced until they are completely weaned. Nicotine-containing lozenges are available in two strengths, and a 12-week program of use is recommended to allow users to taper off the drug.

The nicotine patch is generally used in conjunction with a com-prehensive smoking-cessation program. A small, thin patch placed on the smoker's upper body delivers a continuous flow of nicotine through the skin, helping to relieve cravings. Patches can be bought with or without a prescription and are available in different dosages. The FDA recommends using the patch for 3 to 5 months. During this time, the dose of nicotine is gradually reduced until the smoker is fully weaned from the drug. The patch costs less than a pack of cigarettes—about $4—and some insurance plans will pay for it.[72]

The nasal spray, which requires a prescription, is much more powerful and delivers nicotine to the bloodstream faster than gum, lozenges, or the patch. Patients are warned to be careful not to overdose; as little as 40 mg of nicotine taken at once could be lethal. The FDA has advised that the spray should be used for no more than 3 months and never for more than 6 months so that smokers don't find themselves as dependent on nicotine in spray form as they were on cigarettes. The FDA also advises that no one who experiences nasal or sinus problems, allergies, or asthma should use it.

The nicotine inhaler, which also requires a prescription, consists of a mouthpiece and cartridge. By puffing on the mouthpiece, the smoker inhales air saturated with nicotine, which is absorbed through the lining of the mouth, not the lungs, entering the body much more slowly than does the nicotine in cigarettes. Using the inhaler mimics the hand-to-mouth actions used in smoking and causes the back of the throat to feel as it would when inhaling tobacco smoke.

Smoking-Cessation Medications In 1997, the FDA approved bupropion, an antidepressant, for use as a smoking-cessation aid. The drug, sold under the brand name Zyban, is thought to work on dopamine and norepinephrine receptors in the brain to decrease craving and withdrawal symptoms. Chantix (varenicline), approved by the FDA in

nicotine withdrawal Symptoms including nausea, headaches, irritability, and intense tobacco cravings suffered by nicotine-addicted individuals who stop using tobacco.

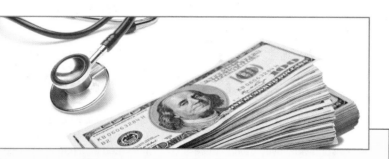

Money&Health
THE COST OF QUITTING VERSUS SMOKING

The cost of smoking cessation can add up, especially if you're going to rely on many stop-smoking aids, but there are many things to consider when comparing the cost of smoking to the cost of quitting.

THE COSTS OF QUITTING

Using a combination of aids such as the nicotine patch and gum can be pricey. Diane Massucci of the North Shore-LIJ Center for Tobacco Control in Great Neck, New York, says that a 12-week supply of the patches would cost approximately $180, and a 12-week supply of the gum would cost about $240, depending on frequency of us. The total for both aids would be estimated at $420 for less than 3 months of nicotine replacement treatment. This illustrates how quit-smoking strategies could get expensive.

However, smoking-cessation experts state that it's important to keep these stop-smoking costs in perspective. "In Michigan, where I live, the average cost of a pack of cigarettes is over $6.50," says Amanda L. Holm, MPH, manager of Tobacco Treatment Services at the Henry Ford Health System in Detroit. "That means that over the span of a year, a pack-a-day smoker will pay more than $2,372. That's more than enough savings to buy 3 or 6 month's worth of nicotine replacement or other medications, or to pay for a class or a few counseling sessions."

In other states, the costs of smoking are even higher. In Rhode Island, Alaska, Illinois, and Hawaii, a pack of cigarettes is over $9, and in New York it is almost $12 a pack. When comparing this to a supply of smoking-cessation aids, it is clear that quitting smoking is less costly than smoking.

In addition, these numbers don't take into account the potential future health care costs of continuing to smoke. "Smokers cost employers more to employ because smokers take more sick time, use more insurance dollars, and lose about 1 month of work time per year related to their smoking behaviors," Massucci says. "Quitting smoking or not smoking in the car or home can increase the resale value of the car or home. Nonsmokers have lower insurance premiums and increased wellness benefits, as some employers incentivize employees who do not smoke."

THE BOTTOM LINE

Add it all up, and the answer is evident. Even if you paid full price for all your smoking-cessation aids, it's still going to be less expensive in the long run than smoking. "Even if someone needed to take medications for longer than 6 months, the reduced health care costs down the road would likely result in substantial savings," Holm says.

Furthermore, people who want to quit smoking also have a number of resources at their disposal that can reduce the cost of quitting. There is a national smoking quit line, 1-800-QUIT-NOW, that can transfer you to your local quit-smoking hotline. The therapy and counseling sessions offered by these over-the-phone counselors are completely free, and in a number of studies, they have been shown to be very effective.

You can also ask your counselor if you can get free nicotine replacement products mailed to you. "Many quit lines offer a starter kit of nicotine replacement products, such as free patches, to help the smoker get their quit attempt started," Massucci says.

If you're looking for other ways to save on quitting, there are many generic versions of medication or the generic or store versions of nicotine replacement products. Holm says that "generic drugs are usually as good as brand-name forms."

Finally, many insurance companies now cover part of the cost of quitting smoking because they've realized that it is in their interest to do so. Therefore, if you have insurance, the first step is to find out if insurance will cover any costs. This makes it clear: It doesn't pay to continue to smoke.

Sources: W. Konrad, "For the New Year, Cost-Effective Options to Stop Smoking," 2010, *The New York Times*, www.nytimes.com/2010/01/09/health/09patient.html?_r=1; N. Hopper, "What a Pack of Cigarettes Costs, State by State," *The Awl*, 2011, www.theawl.com/2011/06/what-a-pack-of-cigarettes-costs-state-by-state; W. Myers, "Is It Cheaper to Smoke or Quit?" 2011, *Everyday Health*, www.everydayhealth.com/stop-smoking/is-it-cheaper-to-smoke-or-quit.aspx; J. Kritz, "Quitting Smoking Makes Economic Sense," *LA Times*, 2011, http://articles.latimes.com/2011/jan/03/health/la-he-quit-smoking-20110103.

March 2006, works in two ways: It reduces nicotine cravings and the urge to smoke, and it blocks the effects of nicotine at nicotine receptor sites in the brain. In July 2009, the FDA issued an advisory that the use of Chantix and Zyban had been associated with changes in behavior such as hostility, agitation, depressed mood, and suicidal thoughts or actions. People taking one of these drugs who experience any unusual changes in mood are advised to stop taking the drug immediately and contact their health care professional.[73]

A radical new way to help smokers quit is NicVAX, an antismoking vaccine currently under investigation in a series of large clinical trials. If the vaccine is proven effective, and the FDA approves it, it may become available in late 2012. The vaccine, administered in a series of shots, helps the body

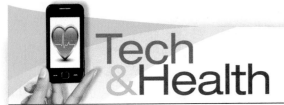
E-CIGARETTES: HEALTH RISKS AND CONCERNS

Electronic cigarettes, also called e-cigarettes, are increasingly used worldwide, even though there is limited information on their health effects. In the United States, they are readily available in shopping malls in most states and on the Internet.

E-cigarettes consist of a battery, a charger, a power cord, an atomizer, and a cartridge containing nicotine and propylene glycol. When a smoker draws air through an e-cigarette, an airflow sensor activates the battery that turns the tip of the cigarette red to simulate smoking and heats the atomizer to vaporize the propylene glycol and nicotine. Upon inhalation, the aerosol vapor delivers a dose of nicotine into the lungs of the smoker, after which, residual aerosol is exhaled into the environment. Nothing is known, however, about the chemicals present in the aerosolized vapors emanating from e-cigarettes.

Although manufacturers claim that electronic cigarettes are a safe alternative to conventional cigarettes, the U.S. Food and Drug Administration (FDA) analyzed samples of two popular brands and found variable amounts of nicotine and traces of toxic chemicals, including known cancer-causing substances (carcinogens). This prompted the FDA to issue a warning about potential health risks associated with electronic cigarettes. Furthermore, New York is pushing to become the first state to ban the devices. With various colors, fruity flavors, clever designs, and other options, e-cigarettes may hold too much appeal for young people, critics warn, offering an easy gateway to nicotine addiction.

Currently, e-cigarettes do not contain any health warnings comparable to FDA-approved nicotine replacement products or conventional cigarettes. They are often marketed as a method to quit smoking, but health professionals recommend using FDA-approved medications and aids that have been shown to be safe and effective for this purpose.

A study conducted at the University of California examined the design, accuracy and clarity of labeling, nicotine content, leakiness, defective parts and disposal, errors in filling orders, instruction manual quality, and advertising. The findings concluded the following:

* E-cigarettes lack important information regarding e-cigarette content, use, and essential warnings.
* E-cigarette cartridges leak, which could expose nicotine, an addictive and dangerous chemical, to children and adults, pets, and the environment.
* There are no methods for proper disposal of e-cigarette products and accessories, including cartridges, which could result in nicotine contamination from discarded cartridges entering water sources and soil and adversely impacting the environment.

* The manufacture, quality control, sales, and advertisement of e-cigarettes are unregulated.

As a result, health professionals continue to urge for more action to regulate these products.

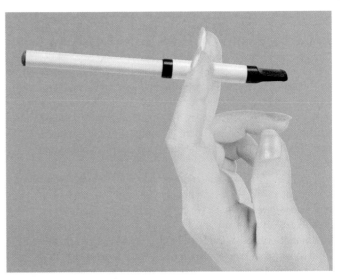

Electronic cigarette, or e-cigarette.

Sources: University of California, Riverside, "Electronic Cigarettes Are Unsafe and Pose Health Risks, UC Riverside Study Finds," 2010, http://newsroom.ucr.edu/news_item .html?action=page&id=2506; U.S. Food and Drug Administration, "FDA and Public Health Experts Warn About Electronic Cigarettes," 2010, www .fda.gov/newsevents/newsroom/pressannouncements/ucm173222.htm; L. Dale, Mayo Clinic, "Electronic Cigarettes: A Safe Way to Light Up?" 2011, www.mayoclinic.com/health/electronic-cigarettes/AN02025; E. Sohn, Discovery News, "How Safe are E-Cigarettes?" 2011, http://news.discovery.com/human/e-cigarettes-health-nicotine-tobacco-110127.html; A. Norton, "Are E-Cigarettes Bad for Health?" 2012, www .huffingtonpost.com/2012/01/05/study-finds-e-cigarettes-_n_1187166.html.

build antibodies to nicotine, essentially making nicotine less addictive.[74] One of the advantages of the vaccine over other cessation methods is that it will reduce relapses by making the cigarette much less enjoyable if the quitter smokes one again. Early clinical trial results report that twice as many people given the vaccine had quit smoking as those given the placebo.[75]

See **Table 12.4** for a summary of recommended smoking-cessation therapies. In addition to the medications and methods previously described, there are also a number of

Therapy	Duration
Buproprion (Zyban) A non–nicotine-based antidepressant that helps reduce nicotine withdrawal symptoms and the urge to smoke. Common side effects are dry mouth, difficulty sleeping, dizziness, and skin rash. Contraindicated if smoker has a history of seizures. *Availability:* Prescription only with a doctor consultation *Cost:* Approximately $2–$4 per day	7–12 weeks; maintenance up to 6 months; start 1–2 weeks before the quit date
Varenicline (Chantix) A non–nicotine-based prescription medicine developed for the sole purpose of helping people stop smoking. Interferes with nicotine receptors in the brain to lessen the pleasurable physical effects from smoking and to reduce symptoms of nicotine withdrawal. Usually well tolerated, but reported side effects have included headaches, nausea, vomiting, difficulty sleeping, flatulence, changes in taste, and depressed mood. *Availability:* Prescription only with a doctor consultation *Cost:* Approximately $2–$4 per day	12 weeks; maintenance of 12 weeks after successfully quitting; start 1–2 weeks in advance
Nicotine Gum A chewing gum that releases nicotine into the bloodstream through the lining of the mouth; might not be appropriate for people with temporomandibular joint disease or those with dentures or other dental work. Up to 2 mg dose if less than 25 cigarettes/day; 4 mg dose if more than 25 cigarettes/day. *Availability:* Over the counter (OTC) *Cost:* Varies upon usage, ranging from $5 to $10 a day	Up to 12 weeks
Nicotine Lozenges The lozenges are available in two strengths as part of a 12-week program. Doses can be regularly lowered as treatment progresses. Users should not eat or drink 15 minutes before using lozenges. *Availability:* OTC *Cost:* Depending on frequency of usage, ranges from $6 to $12 per day	The recommended dose is one lozenge every 1–2 hours for 6 weeks, then one lozenge every 2–4 hours for weeks 7–9, and one lozenge every 4–8 hours for weeks 10–12.
Nicotine Patch Patch supplies a steady amount of nicotine to the body through the skin. It is sold in varying strengths as an 8-week smoking-cessation treatment. Doses can be regularly lowered as treatment progresses or given as a steady dose during treatment. May not be a good choice for people with skin problems or allergies to adhesive tape. *Availability:* Either OTC or by prescription with a doctor consultation *Cost:* Approximately $4 per day.	4 weeks; then 2 weeks; then 2 weeks (8 weeks total)
Nicotine Nasal Spray Comes in a pump bottle containing nicotine that tobacco users can inhale when they have an urge to smoke. Not recommended for people with nasal or sinus conditions, allergies, or asthma, or for young tobacco users. *Availability:* Prescription only with a doctor consultation *Cost:* Approximately $5–$15 per day, depending on frequency of use	3–6 months
Nicotine Inhaler This device delivers a vaporized form of nicotine to the mouth through a mouthpiece attached to a plastic cartridge. Nicotine travels to the mouth and throat and is absorbed through the mucous membranes. Common side effects include throat and mouth irritation and coughing. Anyone with bronchial problems should use caution. *Availability:* Prescription only with a doctor consultation *Cost:* Ranges from $40 to $55 per package	Up to 6 months

Sources: ShopWiki.com, Smoking Cessation, 2012, www.shopwiki.com/wiki/Smoking-Cessation-Products; QuitSmokingSupport.com, Quit Smoking Using the Nicotrol Inhaler, 2012, www.quitsmokingsupport.com/inhaler.htm; Everyday Health, "Could Chantix or Zyban Help You to Stop Smoking?" 2011, www.everydayhealth.com/smoking-cessation/nicotine-free-smoking-cessation-aids.aspx.

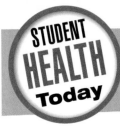

NONTRADITIONAL QUITTING METHODS: ARE THEY EFFECTIVE?

In addition to nicotine-replacement products and smoking-cessation drugs, there are many complementary and alternative methods that claim to help you quit smoking. But while the system for evaluating traditional drug therapies automatically involves studying them for safety and effectiveness, alternative quit-smoking methods suffer from a lack of hard data.

Often what studies are available for acupuncture, hypnosis, or aversive smoking therapies are small scale, may not be randomized or include a control group, and often contradict each other in terms of results. Alternative therapies can be expensive, costing hundreds of dollars per session. And unlike drug therapies, insurance may not cover alternative methods. How is a smoker to judge if the cost is worth it?

In 2012 *The American Journal of Medicine* (AJM) published a study that is more helpful for smokers hoping to evaluate these treatments. It conducted a meta-analysis of randomized controlled trials relating to alternative methods for quitting smoking. In meta-analysis, more than one study is examined to discover patterns in the overall data available.

Below is a description of popular nontraditional quitting methods, along with the AJM study's conclusion on effectiveness:

Acupuncture: For smoking cessation, acupuncture needles are generally

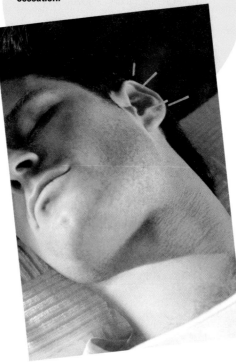

Acupuncture is one of several alternative therapies sometimes used to aid in smoking cessation.

placed along the ear. The AJM study found that people who used acupuncture were over 3.5 times more likely to quit smoking than those who quit "cold turkey." This is compared with current drug therapies, which are thought to increase smoking cessation by a factor of 2 to 2.5.

The study authors only used the best-quality studies in their analysis, but that meant the amount of data available was low, and they cautioned that this could throw results off. Still, study authors recommended that physicians promote acupuncture as a valid

option for patients to use when quitting smoking.

Hypnosis: This deep-relaxation and mental suggestion technique was judged to increase odds of successfully quitting smoking by a factor 4.26. Again, the lack of good studies available for the analysis made researchers caution the quality of these results. But there was enough evidence for the AJM study authors to suggest that doctors should bring this up as a viable quitting therapy for patients.

Smoking Aversion: In this technique, smokers rapidly take large numbers of puffs on a cigarette in a short period of time. This can make them feel sick—the goal being to remove the pleasure smokers feel when they light up, thereby making it easier for them to quit.

The AJM study found smoking aversion increased the success rate for quitting by a factor similar to hypnosis. However, there were very few recent studies on smoking aversion available, and that led the researchers to call for new and better research for this therapy, rather than endorsing it outright.

Sources: M. Tahiri, S. Mottillo, L. Joseph, and L. Pilote, "Alternative Smoking Cessation Aids: A Meta-Analysis of Randomized Controlled Trials," *American Journal of Medicine,* 125, no. 6 (2012): 576–84; and M. J. Eisenberg, "Pharmacotherapies for Smoking Cessation: A Meta-Analysis of Randomized Controlled Trials," *Canadian Medical Association Journal,* 179 (2008): 135–44.

alternative or nontraditional methods promoted as helpful in quitting smoking. Unlike the strategies previously discussed, these methods have not been scientifically proven to be effective. However, because anything that may help a smoker quit is beneficial, some additional options are discussed in the **Student Health Today** feature on the previous page.

Breaking the Smoking Habit

For some smokers, the road to quitting includes antismoking therapy. Two common techniques are operant conditioning and self-control therapy. Pairing the act of smoking with an external stimulus is a typical example of an operant strategy. For example, one technique requires smokers to carry a timer that sounds a buzzer at various intervals. When the buzzer sounds, the patient is required to smoke a cigarette. Once the smoker is conditioned to associate the sound of the buzzer with smoking, the buzzer is eliminated, and, one hopes, so is the smoking.

Self-control strategies view smoking as a learned habit associated with specific situations. Therapy aims to identify these situations and teach smokers the skills necessary to resist smoking. The **Skills for Behavior Change** box presents one of the American Cancer Society's approaches to quitting.

Tips for Quitting Smoking

Ready to quit tobacco? These strategies can help:

❭ Ask smokers who live with you to keep cigarettes out of sight and not offer you any.

❭ Use the four Ds: deep breaths, drink water, do something else, and delay (tell yourself you'll smoke in 10 minutes when the urge hits).

❭ Keep "mouth toys" handy: Hard candy, chewing gum, toothpicks, or carrot or celery sticks can help.

❭ Ask your doctor about nicotine gum, patches, nasal sprays, inhalers, or lozenges.

❭ Make an appointment with your dental hygienist to have your teeth cleaned.

❭ Examine those associations that trigger your urge to smoke.

❭ Spend your time in places that don't allow smoking.

❭ Take up a new sport, exercise program, hobby, or organizational commitment. This will help shake up your routine and distract you from smoking.

Tobacco: Are Your Habits Placing You at Risk?

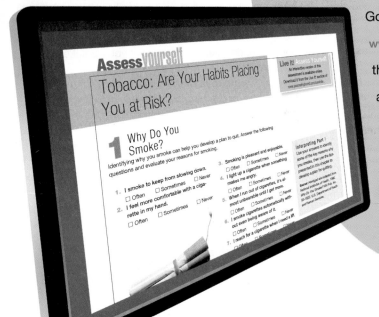

Go online to the **Live It!** section of www.pearsonhighered.com/donatelle to take the "Tobacco: Are Your Habits Placing You at Risk?" assessment.* Use the strategies outlined in the **YOUR PLAN FOR CHANGE** box to quit smoking.

*If your instructor so chooses, Assess Yourself Activities are available as a printed supplement or as assignable homework online at www.pearsonhighered.com/myhealthlab.

MyHealthLab®

YOUR PLAN FOR CHANGE

After completing the "Tobacco: Are Your Habits Placing You at Risk?" **Assess yourself**, tobacco users can use these steps to help cut down on their smoking and quit.

Today, you can:

○ Develop a plan to kick the tobacco habit. The first step is to identify why you want to quit. Write down your reasons and carry a copy with you. Every time you are tempted to smoke, go over your reasons for stopping.

○ Think about the times and places you usually smoke. What could you do instead of smoking at those times? Make a list of positive alternatives.

Within the next 2 weeks, you can:

○ Pick a day to stop smoking, and tell a family member or friend to gain support and accountability.

○ Throw away all your cigarettes, lighters, and ashtrays.

By the end of the semester, you can:

○ Focus on the positives. Now that you have stopped smoking, your mind and body will begin to feel better. Make a list of the good things about not smoking. Carry a copy with you, and look at it whenever you have the urge to smoke.

○ Reward yourself for stopping. Go to a movie, go out to dinner, or buy yourself a gift.

○ If you are having difficulty quitting, consult with your campus health center or your doctor to discuss medications or other therapies that may help you quit.

Summary

* Tobacco use involves many social and political issues, including advertising targeted at youth and women, the fastest-growing populations of smokers. Smoking costs the U.S. as much as $193 billion per year.

* Smoking delivers more than 7,000 chemicals to the lungs. Tobacco comes in smoking and smokeless forms; both contain nicotine, an addictive psychoactive substance.

* Health hazards include markedly higher rates of cancer, heart and circulatory disorders, respiratory diseases, sexual dysfunction, fertility problems, low birth-weight babies, and gum diseases. Smokeless tobacco increases risks for oral cancer and other oral problems.

* Environmental tobacco smoke puts nonsmokers at risk for cancer and heart disease.

* To quit, smokers must kick a chemical addiction and a behavioral habit. Nicotine-replacement products or drugs such as Zyban and Chantix can help wean smokers off nicotine. Various types of psychotherapy and alternative methods can also help.

Pop Quiz

1. What are bidis?
   a. A type of clove cigarette
   b. An Indian-made sweet-flavored cigarette
   c. A type of cigar made in India
   d. Tobacco rolled with marijuana

2. What is sidestream smoke?
   a. Smoke inhaled by a smoker
   b. Smoke released from the burning end of a cigarette
   c. Smoke from a low-tar cigarette
   d. None of the above

3. What effect does carbon monoxide have on a smoker's body?
   a. It accumulates on alveoli in lungs, making breathing difficult.
   b. It increases heart rate.
   c. It interferes with the ability of red blood cells to carry oxygen.
   d. It dulls taste and smell.

4. Which age group is most targeted by tobacco advertisers?
   a. Teenagers age 14 to 17
   b. Young adults age 18 to 24
   c. Adults age 25 to 30
   d. Married men age 31 to 35

5. What is the major psychoactive ingredient in tobacco products?
   a. Carbon monoxide
   b. Tar
   c. Formaldehyde
   d. Nicotine

6. What does nicotine do to cilia in the lungs?
   a. Instantly destroys them
   b. Thickens them
   c. Paralyzes them
   d. Accumulates on them

7. Which tobacco product contains eugenol, which allows smokers to inhale smoke more deeply?
   a. Bidis
   b. Cigars
   c. Snuff
   d. Clove cigarettes

8. Why do college students smoke?
   a. Stress reduction
   b. Social pressure
   c. Physical addiction
   d. All of the above

9. A major health risk of chewing tobacco is
   a. lung cancer.
   b. leukoplakia.
   c. heart disease.
   d. emphysema.

10. How quickly will an individual begin to see health benefits after quitting smoking?
    a. Within 8 hours
    b. Within a month
    c. Within a year
    d. Never

Answers to these questions can be found on page A-1.

Think about It!

1. Discuss the various ways that tobacco is used. Is any method less addictive or less hazardous to health than another?

2. Discuss the health hazards associated with tobacco. Who should be responsible for the medical expenses of smokers? Insurance companies? Smokers themselves?

3. Do you think restrictions on smoking are fair? Why or why not?

4. Describe the various methods of tobacco cessation. Which would be most effective for you? Why?

Accessing Your Health on the Internet

For links to the websites below, visit the Companion Website for *Access to Health*, 13th Edition, at www.pearsonhighered.com/donatelle.

1. *American Lung Association.* This site offers a wealth of information regarding smoking trends, environmental smoke, and advice on smoking cessation. www.lungusa.org

2. *Action on Smoking and Health (ASH).* The nation's oldest and largest antismoking organization, ASH works to fight smoking and protect nonsmokers' rights. www.ash.org

3. *Tobacco Information and Prevention Source (TIPS).* This site provides information regarding tobacco use in the United States, with specific information for young people. www.cdc.gov/tobacco

4. *The Tobacco Atlas.* This book and website, produced by the World Lung Foundation and the American Cancer Society, cover a range of topics including the history of tobacco use, prevalence of use, youth smoking, secondhand smoke, quitting, and more. www.tobaccoatlas.com

5. *Americans for Nonsmokers' Rights (ANR).* This site provides information about smoke-free communities across the United States and tips

for taking action to ban smoking in workplaces and other public areas.
www.no-smoke.org

References

1. Centers for Disease Control and Prevention, "Smoking & Tobacco Use: Fast Facts," Updated January 2012, www.cdc.gov/tobacco/data_statistics/fact_sheets/fast_facts.

2. American Cancer Society, "Cigarette Smoking," Revised November 2011, www.cancer.org/docroot/ped/content/ped_10_2x_cigarette_smoking.asp.

3. NIDA, "Landmark Collaboration Is the First Since the Passing of the 2009 Tobacco Control Act," October 2011, http://m.drugabuse.gov/news-events/news-releases/2011/10/fda-nih-announce-joint-study-tobacco-use-risk-perceptions.

4. CDC, Smoking & Tobacco, "Adult Cigarette Smoking in the United States: Current Estimate," January 2012, www.cdc.gov/tobacco/data_statistics/fact_sheets/adult_data/cig_smoking/index.htm.

5. SAMSHA, Results from the 2010 National Survey on Drug Use and Health Summary of National Findings, September 2011, http://oas.samhsa.gov/NSDUH/2k10NSDUH/2k10Results.htm#Ch4.

6. CDC, Smoking and Tobacco Use, "Fast Stats," 2012, www.cdc.gov/tobacco/data_statistics/fact_sheets/fast_facts/.

7. Centers for Disease Control and Prevention, Tobacco Control State Highlights, Last Reviewed 2012 (Atlanta: U.S. Department of Health and Human Services, Centers for Disease Control and Prevention, National Center for Chronic Disease Prevention and Health Promotion, Office on Smoking and Health, 2010), Available at www.cdc.gov/tobacco/data_statistics/state_data/state_highlights/2010/index.htm.

8. Campaign for Tobacco-Free Kids, "Tobacco Company Marketing to Kids," March 2012, Available at www.tobaccofreekids.org/research/factsheets.

9. American Lung Association, "General Smoking Facts," June 2011, www.lung.org/stop-smoking/about-smoking/facts-figures/general-smoking-facts.html.

10. Tobacco Free Providence, "Sweet Deceit Survey Results," January 2012, www.tobaccofreeprovidence.org/2012-01-27-sweet-deceit-survey-results/.

11. American Cancer Society, Cancer Facts & Figures 2012 (Atlanta: American Cancer Society, 2012), Available at www.cancer.org/acs/groups/content/@epidemiologysurveilance/documents/document/acspc-031941.pdf.

12. American Lung Association, "General Smoking Facts," 2011, www.lung.org/stop-smoking/about-smoking/facts-figures/general-smoking-facts.html.

13. Centers for Disease Control and Prevention, Tobacco Control State Highlights, 2010, 2010; Centers for Disease Control and Prevention, "Smoking-Attributable Mortality, Years of Potential Life Lost, and Productivity Losses, 2000–2004," Morbidity and Mortality Weekly Report 57, no. 45 (2008): 1226–28.

14. Campaign for Tobacco-Free Kids, "State Cigarette Excise Tax Rates & Rankings," December 2011, www.tobaccofreekids.org/research/factsheets/pdf/0097.pdf.

15. American Cancer Society, "Child and Teen Tobacco Use," 2011, www.cancer.org/Cancer/CancerCauses/TobaccoCancer/ChildandTeenTobaccoUse/child-and-teen-tobacco-use-facts-and-stats.

16. C. A. Wassenaar et al., "Relationship between CYP2A6 and CHRNA5-CHRNA3-CHRNB4 Variation and Smoking Behaviors and Lung Cancer Risk," JNCI Journal of the National Cancer Institute (2011), DOI: 10.1093/jnci/djr237; Francesca Ducci et al., "TTC12-ANKK1-DRD2 and CHRNA5-CHRNA3-CHRNB4 Influence Different Pathways Leading to Smoking Behavior from Adolescence to Mid-Adulthood," Biological Psychiatry 69, no. 7 (2011): 650; C. Amos, M. Spitz, and P. Cinciripini, "Chipping Away at the Genetics of Smoking Behavior," Nature Genetics 42 (2010): 366–68.

17. Francesca Ducci et al., TTC12-ANKK1-DRD2 and CHRNA5-CHRNA3-CHRNB4 Influence Different," 2011; C. Amos, M. Spitz, and P. Cinciripini, "Chipping Away at the Genetics of Smoking Behavior," 2010; T. Korhonen and J. Kaprio, "Genetic Epidemiology of Smoking Behaviour and Nicotine Dependence," 2011, eLS

18. T. Korhonen and J. Kaprio, "Genetic Epidemiology of Smoking Behaviour and Nicotine Dependence," 2011, eLS

19. C. Amos, M. Spitz, and P. Cinciripini, "Chipping Away at the Genetics of Smoking Behavior," 2010.

20. American College Health Association, American College Health Association–National College Health Assessment II : Reference Group Data Report, Spring 2011 (Baltimore, American College Health Association, 2012), Available at www.achancha.org/reports_ACHA-NCHAII.html.

21. Substance Abuse and Mental Health Services Administration, Results from the 2010 National Survey on Drug Use and Health: Summary of National Findings, NSDUH Series H-41, HHS Publication No. (SMA) 11-4658 (Rockville, MD: Substance Abuse and Mental Health Services Administration, 2011); American College Health Association, American College Health Association–National College Health Assessment II, 2012.

22. Ibid.

23. National Center on Addiction and Substance Abuse at Columbia University, Wasting the Best and the Brightest, Substance Abuse at America's Colleges and Universities (New York: National Center on Addiction and Substance Abuse at Columbia University, March 2007), Available at www.casacolumbia.org/templates/publications_reports.aspx.

24. Ibid.

25. C. Berg, "Smoker Self-Identification versus Recent Smoking among College Students," American Journal of Preventive Medicine 36, no. 4 (2009): 333–36.

26. L. Stoner et al., "Occasional Cigarette Smoking Chronically Affects Arterial Function," Ultrasound in Medicine and Biology 34, no. 12 (2008): 1885–92.

27. L. An et al., "Symptoms of Cough and Shortness of Breath among Occasional Young Adult Smokers," Nicotine & Tobacco Research 11, no. 2 (2009): 126–33.

28. Stop Smoking! "Smoking and Birth Control Pills Are Not Made for Each Other," Retrieved March 6, 2012, www.stop-smoking-updates.com/quitsmoking/smoking-factsheet/facts/smoking-and-birth-control-pills-are-not-made-for-each-other.htm.

29. National Center on Addiction and Substance Abuse at Columbia University, Wasting the Best and the Brightest, 2007.

30. U.S. Department of Health and Human Services, "How Tobacco Smoke Causes Disease: The Biology and Behavioral Basis for Smoking Attributable Disease: A Report of the Surgeon General," Office of the Surgeon General (2010), www.surgeongeneral.gov.

31. American Cancer Society, "Cigar Smoking: Who Smokes Cigars?" Revised November 2011, www.cancer.org/Cancer/CancerCauses/TobaccoCancer/CigarSmoking/cigar-smoking-who-smokes-cigars.

32. American Cancer Society, "Questions about Smoking, Tobacco, and Health: What about More Exotic Forms of Smoking Tobacco, Such as Clove Cigarettes, Bidis, and Hookahs?" Revised November 2011, www.cancer.org/Cancer/CancerCauses/TobaccoCancer/QuestionsaboutSmokingTobaccoandHealth/questions-about-smoking-tobacco-and-health-other-forms-of-smoking.

33. Centers for Disease Control and Prevention, "Smoking and Tobacco Use: Bidis and Kreteks," Updated June 2011, www.cdc.gov/tobacco/data_statistics/fact_sheets/tobacco_industry/bidis_kreteks.

34. Ibid.

35. W. Dunham, "Chewing Tobacco Use Surges among Boys," Reuters, March 25,

2009, www.reuters.com/article/idUSTRE5240WJ20090305.

36. Centers for Disease Control and Prevention, "Smoking-Attributable Mortality, Years of Potential Life Lost, and Productivity Losses, 2000–2004," 2008.

37. American Cancer Society, *Cancer Facts & Figures, 2012,* 2012, www.cancer.org/acs/groups/content/@epidemiologysurveilance/documents/document/acspc-031941.pdf.

38. Ibid.

39. Ibid.

40. Ibid.

41. American Heart Association, *Heart Disease and Stroke Statistics—2012 Update* (Dallas: American Heart Association, 2012), Available at http://circ.ahajournals.org/content/125/1/e2.

42. Ibid.

43. Ibid.

44. Ibid.

45. American Heart Association, "Stroke Risk Factors," 2012, www.strokeassociation.org/STROKEORG/AboutStroke/UnderstandingRisk/Understanding-Risk_UCM_308539_SubHomePage.jsp; CDC, "Health Effects of Cigarette Smoking," January 2012, www.cdc.gov/tobacco/data_statistics/fact_sheets/health_effects/effects_cig_smoking/.

46. American Lung Association, "Benefits of Quitting," March 2012, www.lungusa.org/stop-smoking/how-to-quit/why-quit/benefits-of-quitting.

47. American Cancer Society, *Cancer Facts & Figures, 2012,* 2012. www.cancer.org/acs/groups/content/@epidemiologysurveilance/documents/document/acspc-031941.pdf.

48. John Hopkins Health Alerts, "Emphysema: Symptoms and Remedies," Accessed March 2012, www.johnshopkinshealthalerts.com/symptoms_remedies/emphysema/96-1.html.

49. Health Canada, "Impotence and Smoking," 2009, www.hc-sc.gc.ca/hc-ps/tobac-tabac/body-corps/disease-maladie/infertilit-eng.php; National Kidney and Neurological Diseases Information Clearing House, "Erectile Dysfunction," NIH Publication no. 06-3923, 2010, http://kidney.niddk.nih.gov/kudiseases/pubs/ED/index.aspx.

50. Centers for Disease Control and Prevention, "Pregnant? Don't Smoke! Learn How and Why to Quit for Good," Updated November 2011, www.cdc.gov/Features/PregnantDontSmoke.

51. Centers for Disease Control and Prevention, "Tobacco Use and Pregnancy," Modified January 2012, www.cdc.gov/reproductivehealth/TobaccoUsePregnancy/index.htm.

52. American Academy of Periodontology, "Tobacco Use and Periodontal Disease," 2011, www.perio.org/consumer/smoking.htm.

53. J. Cataldo et al., "Cigarette Smoking Is a Risk Factor of Alzheimer's Disease: An Analysis Controlling for Tobacco Industry Affiliation," *Journal of Alzheimer's Disease* 19, no. 2 (2010): 465–80.

54. Centers for Disease Control and Prevention, "Smoking and Tobacco Use Facts: Estimates of Secondhand Smoke Exposure," Updated March 2012, www.cdc.gov/tobacco/data_statistics/fact_sheets/secondhand_smoke/general_facts/index.htm.

55. Centers for Disease Control and Prevention, "Smoking and Tobacco Use Fact Sheet: Secondhand Smoke," March 2012, www.cdc.gov/tobacco/data_statistics/fact_sheets/secondhand_smoke/general_facts/index.htm.

56. Ibid.

57. Ibid.

58. Centers for Disease Control and Prevention, "Secondhand Smoke (SHS) Facts," Updated March 21, 2012, www.cdc.gov/tobacco/data_statistics/fact_sheets/secondhand_smoke/general_facts/index.htm.

59. U.S. Department of Health and Human Services, *The Health Consequences of Involuntary Exposure to Tobacco Smoke, A Report of the Surgeon General* (Atlanta, GA: U.S. Department of Health and Human Services, Centers for Disease Control and Prevention, Coordinating Center for Health Promotion, National Center for Chronic Disease Prevention and Health Promotion, Office on Smoking and Health, 2006), Available at www.surgeongeneral.gov/library/secondhandsmoke; November 2011.

60. U.S. Department of Health and Human Services, *The Health Consequences of Involuntary Exposure to Tobacco Smoke,* November 2011; Centers for Disease Control and Prevention, "Smoking and Tobacco Use Fact Sheet," 2012, www.cancer.org/docroot/ped/content/ped_10_2x_secondhand_smoke-clean_indoor_air.asp.

61. U.S. Department of Health and Human Services, *The Health Consequences of Involuntary Exposure to Tobacco Smoke,* 2011.

62. S. Leatherdale et al., "Second-Hand Exposure in Homes and in Cars among Canadian Youth: Current Prevalence, Beliefs about Exposure, and Changes between 2004–2006," *Cancer Causes & Control* 20, no. 6 (2009): 1573–1625.

63. Z. Kabir, G. Connolly, and H. Alpert, "Secondhand Smoke Exposure and Neurobehavioral Disorders Among Children in the United States," *Pediatrics* (2011) DOI: 10.1542/peds.2011-00232011-0023.

64. Z. Kabir, G. Connolly, and H. Alpert, "Secondhand Smoke Exposure and Neurobehavioral Disorders, 2011.

65. O. Shafey, M. Eriksen, H. Ross, and J. Mackay, "Secondhand Smoking," in *The Tobacco Atlas,* 3d ed. (Atlanta: American Cancer Society, 2009), Available at www.cancer.org/aboutus/GlobalHealth/CancerandTobaccoControlResources/the-tobacco-atlas-3rd-edition.

66. Centers for Disease Control and Prevention, "CDC Health Disparities and Inequalities Report–United States, Supplement: Cigarette Smoking-United States, 1965–2008," *Morbidity and Mortality Weekly Report* 60, Supplement (2011): 109–113.

67. Tobacco-Free Kids, "1998 Tobacco Settlement: Decade of Broken Promises," 2011, www.tobaccofreekids.org/what_we_do/state_local/tobacco_settlement/.

68. *Family Smoking Prevention and Tobacco Control Act of 2009,* HR 1256, 111th Congress of the United States of America, Available at www.govtrack.us/congress/billtext.xpd?bill=h111-1256.

69. Centers for Disease Control and Prevention, "Tobacco Use: Smoking Cessation," Revised November 2011, www.cdc.gov/tobacco/data_statistics/fact_sheets/cessation/quitting/index.htm#quitting.

70. N. Hopper, "What a Pack of Cigarettes Costs, State By State," *The Awl* (2011), www.theawl.com/2011/06/what-a-pack-of-cigarettes-costs-state-by-state.

71. American Cancer Society, "Guide to Quitting Smoking: A Word about Quitting Success Rates," Revised February 2012, www.cancer.org/Healthy/StayAwayfromTobacco/GuidetoQuittingSmoking/guide-to-quitting-smoking-success-rates.

72. D. Thompson, "A Guide to Using the Nicotine Patch," *EveryDay Health,* www.everydayhealth.com/stop-smoking/smoking-cessation-aids-nicotine-patch.aspx.

73. U.S. Food and Drug Administration, "Public Health Advisory: FDA Requires New Boxed Warnings for the Smoking Cessation Drugs Chantix and Zyban," July 1, 2009, www.fda.gov/Drugs/DrugSafety/DrugSafetyPodcasts/ucm170906.htm.

74. National Institutes of Health, "NicVAX/Placebo as an Aid for Smoking Cessation," June 10, 2011, http://clinicaltrials.gov/ct2/show/NCT00836199.

75. J. Interlandi, "Are Vaccines the Answer to Addiction?" *Newsweek* CLI, no. 2 (January 14, 2008): 17.

Avoiding Drug Misuse and Abuse

13

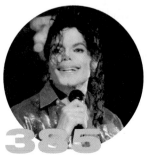

385

Why is prescription drug abuse on the rise?

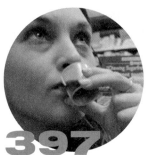

397

Why is it so hard to quit using heroin?

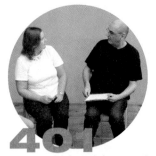

404

What works in helping people recover from drug addiction?

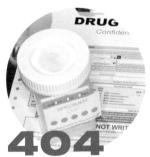

404

Is it legal for employers to require employees to take a drug test?

OBJECTIVES

* Discuss the six categories of drugs and their routes of administration.

* Discuss the use of illicit drugs among college students.

* Review problems relating to the misuse and abuse of prescription drugs.

* Discuss the use and abuse of controlled substances, including cocaine, amphetamines, marijuana, opioids, hallucinogens, club drugs, inhalants, and steroids.

* Profile illicit drug use in the United States, including who uses illicit drugs, financial impact, and impact on college campuses and the workplace.

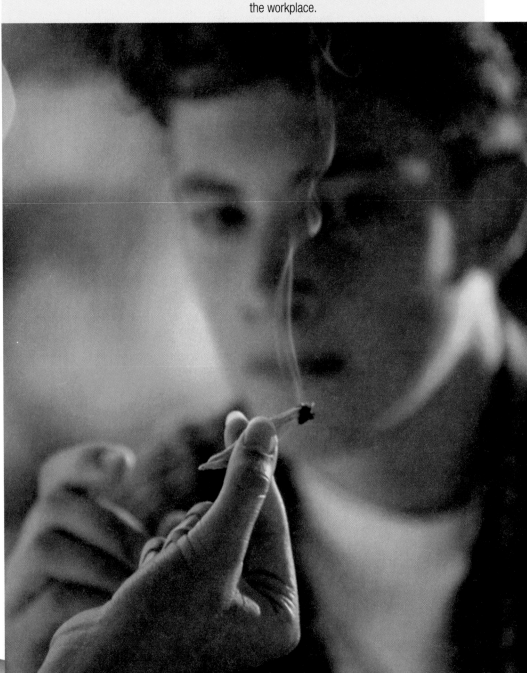

Drug misuse and abuse are enormous problems in our society. Whether it is the meth addict who has lost everything in a harrowing fall into dependence and crime or the high functioning executive who gets hooked on prescription drugs such as OxyContin or Vicodin to ease excruciating back pain, drug addiction wreaks havoc on individuals, families, businesses, and society. The use and abuse of drugs occurs at all income levels, among all ethnic groups, and at all ages. Forty-seven percent of Americans report using illicit drugs at some point in their lifetime.[1] Over 20 percent of high school students have taken prescription drugs without a doctor's permission.[2] Recently, the overall rate of drug use in the United States rose to its highest level in almost a decade, mostly driven by an increase in the use of marijuana.[3] Drug abuse costs taxpayers more than $467.7 billion annually in preventable health care costs, extra law enforcement, vehicle crashes, crime, and lost productivity.[4] It's impossible to put a dollar amount on the pain, suffering, and dysfunction that drugs cause in our everyday lives.

Why do people use drugs? Human beings appear to have a need to alter their consciousness, or mental state. We like to feel good, escape, and feel different. Sometimes we like to reduce pain or dull our senses. Consciousness can be altered in many ways: Children spinning until they become dizzy and adults enjoying the thrill of extreme sports are two examples. To change our awareness, some of us listen to music, ski, read, daydream, meditate, pray, or have sexual relations. Others turn to drugs to alter consciousness.

Drug Dynamics

Drugs work because they physically resemble the chemicals produced naturally within the body. Most bodily processes result from chemical reactions or from changes in electrical charge. Because drugs possess an electrical charge and chemical structure similar to those of chemicals that occur naturally in the body, they can affect physical functions in many different ways.

How Drugs Affect the Brain

Pleasure, which scientists call *reward,* is a powerful biological force for survival. If you do something that you experience as pleasurable, the brain is wired in such a way that you tend to do it again. Life-sustaining activities, such as eating, activate a circuit of specialized nerve cells devoted to producing and regulating pleasure. One important set of these nerve cells, which uses a chemical **neurotransmitter** called *dopamine,* sits at the very top of the brainstem in the *ventral tegmental area* (*VTA*). These dopamine-containing neurons relay messages about pleasure through their nerve fibers to nerve cells in the limbic system, structures in the brain regulating emotions. Still other fibers connect to a related part of the frontal region of the cerebral cortex, the area of the brain that plays a key role in memory, perception, thought, and consciousness. So, this "pleasure circuit," known as the *mesolimbic dopamine* system, spans the survival-oriented brainstem, the emotional limbic system, and the thinking frontal cerebral cortex.

All drugs that are addicting can activate the brain's pleasure circuit. Drug addiction is a biological, pathological process that alters the way in which the pleasure center, as well as other parts of the brain, functions. Almost all **psychoactive drugs** (those that change the way the brain works) do so by affecting chemical neurotransmission, either enhancing, suppressing, or interfering with it. Some drugs, such as heroin and lysergic acid diethylamide (LSD), mimic the effects of a natural neurotransmitter. Others, such as phencyclidine (PCP), block receptors and thereby prevent neuronal messages from getting through. Still others, such as cocaine, block the *reuptake* of neurotransmitters by neurons, thus increasing the concentration of the neurotransmitters in the synaptic gap, the space between individual neurons (**Figure 13.1** on page 382). Finally, some drugs, such as methamphetamine, cause neurotransmitters to be released in greater amounts than is normal.

neurotransmitter One of many chemical substances, such as acetylcholine or dopamine, that transmits nerve impulses between nerve fibers.

psychoactive drugs Drugs that have the potential to alter mood or behavior.

Types of Drugs

Scientists divide drugs into six categories: prescription, over-the-counter (OTC), recreational, herbal, illicit, and commercial drugs. Each category includes some drugs that stimulate the body, some that depress body functions, and others that produce hallucinations (images, auditory or visual, that are perceived but are not real). Each category also includes psychoactive drugs.

- **Prescription drugs.** These can be obtained only with a prescription from a licensed health practitioner. More than 10,000 types of prescription drugs are sold in the United States.
- **Over-the-counter (OTC) drugs.** These can be purchased without a prescription. More than 100,000 OTC products are available, and an estimated 3 out of 4 people routinely self-medicate with them.[5] Studies show that Americans are making more use of widely available OTC medicines each year.[6] (See **Chapter 18** for a discussion of the OTC label and common types of OTC drugs.)
- **Recreational drugs.** These belong to a somewhat vague category whose boundaries depend on how the term *recreation* is defined. Generally, recreational drugs contain chemicals used to help people relax or socialize. Most of them are legal even though they are psychoactive. Alcohol, tobacco, and caffeine products are included in this category.
- **Herbal preparations.** These encompass approximately 750 substances, including herbal teas and other products of botanical (plant) origin that are believed to have medicinal properties. (See **Chapter 18** for more on herbal preparations.)

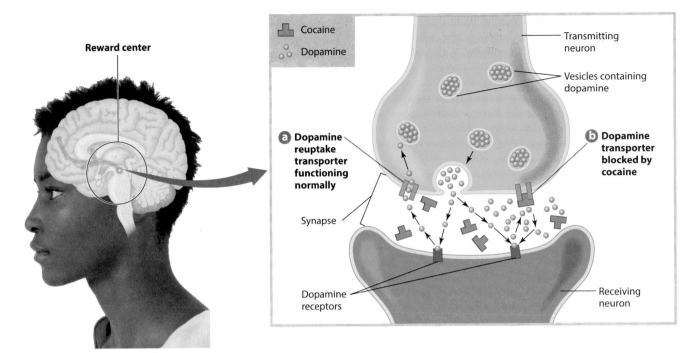

Reward center

Cocaine

Dopamine

ⓐ **Dopamine reuptake transporter functioning normally**

ⓑ **Dopamine transporter blocked by cocaine**

Transmitting neuron

Vesicles containing dopamine

Synapse

Receiving neuron

Dopamine receptors

FIGURE 13.1 **The Action of Cocaine at Dopamine Receptors in the Brain, an Example of Psychoactive Drug Action**
In normal neural communication, dopamine is released into the synapse between neurons. It binds temporarily to dopamine receptors on the receiving neuron and then is recycled back into the transmitting neuron by a transporter. When cocaine molecules are present, they attach to the dopamine transporter and block the recycling process. Excess dopamine remains active in the synaptic gaps between neurons, creating feelings of excitement and euphoria.

Source: Adapted from *NIDA Research Report—Cocaine Abuse and Addiction*, NIH Publication no. 09-4166, printed May 1999, revised May 2009, www.nida.nih.gov/PDF/RRCocaine.pdf.

Video Tutor: Psychoactive Drugs Acting on the Brain

oral ingestion Intake of drugs through the mouth.

inhalation The introduction of drugs through breathing into the lungs.

injection The introduction of drugs into the body via a hypodermic needle.

transdermal The introduction of drugs through the skin.

suppositories Mixtures of drugs and a waxy medium (designed to melt at body temperature) that are inserted into the anus or vagina.

● Illicit (illegal) drugs. These are the most notorious type of drug. Although laws governing their use, possession, cultivation, manufacture, and sale differ from state to state, illicit drugs are generally recognized as harmful. All of them are psychoactive.

● **Commercial preparations.** These are the most universally used yet least commonly recognized chemical substances. More than 1,000 of them exist, including seemingly benign items such as perfumes, cosmetics, household cleansers, paints, glues, inks, dyes, and pesticides.

Routes of Drug Administration

Route of administration refers to the way in which a drug is taken into the body. The route largely determines the rapidity of the drug's effect on the body (Figure 13.2 on page 383). The most common route is **oral ingestion**—swallowing a tablet, capsule, or liquid. Drugs taken by mouth don't reach the bloodstream as

Using a needle to inject drugs poses health threats beyond the effects of the drugs.

quickly as drugs introduced to the body by other means. A drug taken orally may not reach the bloodstream for 30 minutes.

Drugs can also enter the body through the respiratory tract via sniffing, smoking, or inhaling (**inhalation**). Drugs that are inhaled and absorbed by the lungs travel the most rapidly of all the routes of drug administration. Another rapid form of drug administration is by **injection** directly into the bloodstream (intravenously), muscles (intramuscularly), or just under the skin (subcutaneously). Intravenous injection, which involves inserting a hypodermic needle directly into a vein, is the most common method of injection for drug users due to the rapid speed (within seconds in most cases) in which a drug's effect is felt. It is also the most dangerous method of administration due to the risk of damaging blood vessels and contracting HIV (human immunodeficiency virus) and hepatitis (a severe liver disease). Drugs can also be absorbed through the skin or tissue lining (**transdermal**)—the nicotine patch is a common example of a drug that is administered in this manner—or through the mucous membranes, such as those in the nose (snorting) or in the vagina or anus (**suppositories**). Suppositories are typically mixed with a waxy medium that melts at body temperature, releasing the drug into the bloodstream.

However the drug enters the system, it eventually finds its way to the bloodstream and circulates throughout the

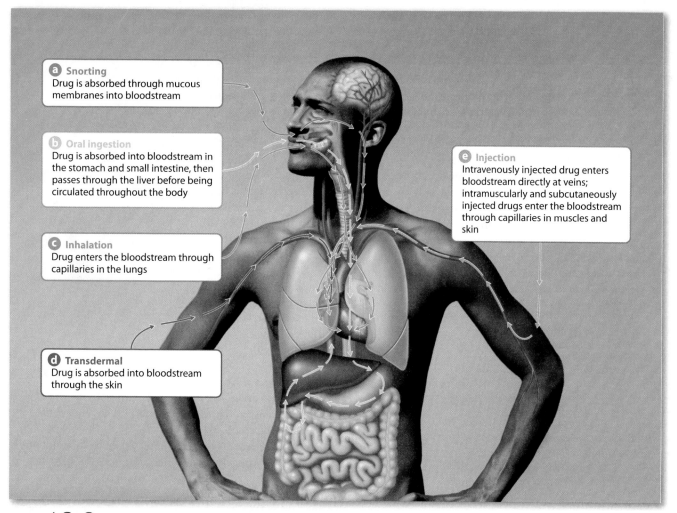

a Snorting
Drug is absorbed through mucous membranes into bloodstream

b Oral ingestion
Drug is absorbed into bloodstream in the stomach and small intestine, then passes through the liver before being circulated throughout the body

c Inhalation
Drug enters the bloodstream through capillaries in the lungs

d Transdermal
Drug is absorbed into bloodstream through the skin

e Injection
Intravenously injected drug enters bloodstream directly at veins; intramuscularly and subcutaneously injected drugs enter the bloodstream through capillaries in muscles and skin

FIGURE 13.2 **Routes of Drug Administration**
Drugs are most commonly swallowed, inhaled, or injected. They can also be absorbed through the skin or mucous membranes (as in snorting) and suppository use (not shown here).

body to various **receptor sites** where chemicals, enzymes, and other substances interact. Psychoactive drugs are able to cross the blood–brain barrier to reach receptor sites in the brain, where they can affect cognition, emotions, and physiological functioning. Once a drug reaches receptor sites in the brain and other body organs, it may remain active for several hours before it dissipates and is carried by the blood to the liver where it is metabolized (broken down by enzymes). The products of enzymatic breakdown, called *metabolites,* are then excreted, primarily through the kidneys (in urine) or the bowels (in feces), but also through the skin (in sweat) or through the lungs (in expired air).

Drug Interactions

Polydrug use—taking several medications, vitamins, recreational drugs, or illegal drugs simultaneously—can lead to dangerous health problems. Alcohol in particular frequently has dangerous interactions with other drugs. The most hazardous interactions are synergism, antagonism, inhibition, intolerance, and cross-tolerance. Some drug interactions occur as a result of the foods we eat or drink or other environmental exposures that might seem harmless. For instance, consuming grapefruit or grapefruit juice while taking a statin, a medication used for lowering blood pressure, allows too much of the drug to enter the bloodstream and can cause liver damage, and taking sulfa-based antibiotics when exposed to the sun can cause a skin rash or a severe sunburn.

Synergism, also called *potentiation,* is an interaction of two or more drugs in which the effects of the individual drugs are multiplied beyond what would normally be expected if they were taken alone. Think of synergism as 2 + 2 = 10. A synergistic reaction can be very dangerous and even deadly.

Antagonism, although usually less serious than synergism, can also produce unwanted and unpleasant effects. In an antagonistic reaction, drugs work at the

receptor sites Specialized areas of cells and organs where chemicals, enzymes, and other substances interact.

polydrug use Taking several medications, vitamins, recreational drugs, or illegal drugs simultaneously.

synergism The interaction of two or more drugs that produces more profound effects than would be expected if the drugs were taken separately; also called *potentiation.*

antagonism A drug interaction in which two drugs compete for the same available receptors, potentially blocking each other's actions.

inhibition A drug interaction in which the effects of one drug are eliminated or reduced by the presence of another drug at the same receptor site.

intolerance A drug interaction in which the combination of two or more drugs in the body produces extremely uncomfortable symptoms.

cross-tolerance Development of a physiological tolerance to one drug that reduces the effects of another, similar drug.

drug misuse Use of a drug for a purpose for which it was not intended.

drug abuse Excessive use of a drug.

same receptor site so that one drug blocks the action of the other. The blocking drug occupies the receptor site and prevents the other drug from attaching, thus altering its absorption and action.

With **inhibition,** the effects of one drug are eliminated or reduced by the presence of another drug at the receptor site.

Intolerance occurs when drugs combine in the body to produce extremely uncomfortable reactions. The drug Antabuse (disulfiram), used to help alcoholics give up alcohol, works by producing this type of interaction.

Cross-tolerance occurs when a person develops a physiological tolerance to one drug and shows a similar tolerance to certain other drugs as a result.

Using, Misusing, and Abusing Drugs

Although drug abuse is usually referred to in connection with illicit drugs, many people misuse or abuse prescription and OTC medications. **Drug misuse** involves using a drug for a purpose for which it was not intended. For example, taking a friend's high-powered prescription painkiller for your headache is a misuse of that drug. This is not too far removed from **drug abuse,** or the excessive use of any drug, and may cause serious harm. The misuse and abuse of any drug may lead to addiction, the habitual reliance on a substance or a behavior to produce a desired mood. (See **Chapter 10** for more on addiction).

Abuse of Over-the-Counter Drugs

OTC medications do not require a prescription and can simply be bought in drug stores, supermarkets, and the like. Although many people assume that no harm can come from legal nonprescription drugs, OTC medications can be abused, with resultant health complications and potential addiction. People who appear to be most vulnerable to abusing OTC drugs are teenagers, young adults, and people over age 65.

OTC drug abuse can involve taking more than the recommended dosage, combining it with other drugs, or taking it over a longer period of time than recommended.

Abuse of and addiction to OTC drugs can be accidental. A person may develop tolerance from continued use, creating an unintended dependence. Teenagers and young adults sometimes intentionally abuse OTC medications in search of a cheap high—by drinking large amounts of cough medicine, for instance. The following are a few types of OTC drugs that are subject to misuse and abuse:

Over-the-counter cough syrup is frequently abused by young people seeking a high from the ingredient DXM.

- **Sleep aids.** These drugs may be harmful in excess as they can cause problems with the sleep cycle, weaken areas of the body, or induce narcolepsy (a condition of excessive, intrusive sleepiness). Continued use can lead to tolerance and dependence.

- **Cold medicines (cough syrups and tablets).** There are many different ingredients in cough and cold medicines, but one of particular concern is dextromethorphan (DXM), which is present in about 125 different types of OTC medications. As many as 7 percent of high school seniors report taking drugs containing DXM to get high.[7] Large doses of products containing DXM can cause hallucinations, loss of motor control, and "out-of-body" (disassociative) sensations. Other possible side effects of DXM abuse include confusion, impaired judgment, blurred vision, dizziness, paranoia, excessive sweating, slurred speech, nausea, vomiting, abdominal pain, irregular heartbeat, high blood pressure, headache, lethargy, numb fingers and toes, facial redness, and dry and itchy skin. In extreme cases, DXM abuse can lead to loss of consciousness, seizures, brain damage, and even death. Some states have passed laws limiting the amount of products containing DXM a person can purchase or prohibiting sale to individuals under age 18.[8]

Pseudoephedrine is another cold and allergy medication ingredient that is frequently abused, most commonly in the illegal manufacture of methamphetamine (discussed later). United States law limits the number of products containing this drug that an individual may purchase in a month and requires that it be sold "behind the counter" (i.e., without a prescription, but only through a

"Why Should I Care?"

You may think drugs are helping you relax, improving your concentration, or enhancing your social enjoyment, but those effects are transient—and often illusory—and they are nothing compared to the many negative effects those same drugs can have on your life and health. Sooner or later, drug misuse and abuse is likely to catch up with you and cause problems—be they academic, social, career, legal, financial, or health related. Are a few moments of excitement really worth a lifetime of trouble?

pharmacist) and that photo identification be presented and recorded. Pharmacists are required to keep a record of purchasers for at least 2 years.[9]

● **Diet pills.** Some teens use diet pills as a way of getting high, whereas other people use these drugs in an attempt to lose weight. Diet pills often contain a stimulant such as caffeine (discussed later in the chapter) or an herbal ingredient claimed to promote weight loss, such as *Hoodia gordonii.* Many diet pills are marketed as "dietary supplements" and so are regulated by the U.S. Food and Drug Administration (FDA) as "food," not as "drugs."

Nonmedical Use or Abuse of Prescription Drugs

In the United States today, the abuse of prescription medications is at an all-time high. Only marijuana is more widely abused.[10] Individuals abuse these drugs because they are an easily accessible and inexpensive means of altering a user's mental and physical state. Some people also have the mistaken idea that prescription drugs are a "safer high."

The latest data available indicate that over 7 million Americans age 12 and older used prescription drugs for nonmedical reasons in the past month.[11] Prescription drug abuse is particularly common among teenagers and young adults. Every day, a significantly large number of people begin misusing prescription drugs; nearly 5,500 people start to misuse prescription painkillers. In 2010, 3 percent of teenagers age 12 to 17 and 6 percent of people 18 to 25 reported abusing prescription drugs in the past month.[12] The problem may be getting worse, with nearly one quarter of twelfth-graders reporting abuse of prescription drugs by the time they graduate from high school.[13]

The risks associated with prescription drug abuse vary depending on the drug. Abuse of opioids, narcotics, and pain relievers can result in life-threatening respiratory depression (reduced breathing). Overdoses involving prescription painkillers are at epidemic levels and now kill more Americans than heroine and cocaine combined.[14] Individuals who abuse depressants place themselves at risk of seizures, respiratory depression, and decreased heart rate. Stimulant abuse can cause elevated body temperature, irregular heart rate, cardiovascular system failure, and fatal seizures. It can also result in hostility or feelings of paranoia. Individuals who abuse prescription drugs by injecting them expose themselves to additional risks, including contracting HIV, hepatitis B and C, and other blood-borne viruses.

55.9%

of people who use pain relievers nonmedically get the drug from a friend or relative.

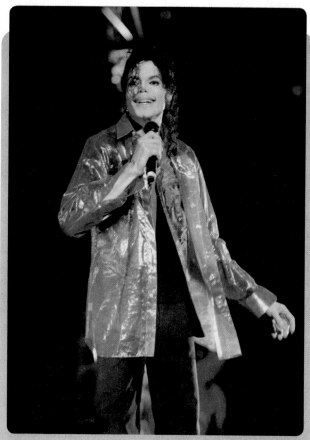

Why is prescription drug abuse on the rise?

Because there are legitimate, legal uses for prescription drugs, they are more readily available and easier to obtain than illicit drugs. As more people—especially students—turn to these medications to help them study or get high, the more socially acceptable their use becomes, and the rate of use continues to rise. In addition, the fact that prescription drugs are regulated and approved by the FDA leads to the impression that they are safer than illicit drugs. This is a fallacy, as tragically demonstrated by the 2010 death of singer Michael Jackson, whose death was ruled a homicide, but ultimately stemmed from his abuse of numerous prescription medications.

Unfortunately, prescription drugs are often easier to obtain than illegal ones. In some cases, unscrupulous pharmacists or other medical professionals either steal the drugs or sell fraudulent prescriptions. In a process called *doctor shopping,* abusers visit several doctors to obtain multiple prescriptions. Some may fake or exaggerate symptoms to persuade physicians to write prescriptions. Individuals may also call pharmacies with fraudulent prescriptions. Young people typically obtain prescription drugs from peers, friends, or family members. Some teenagers and college students who have legitimate prescriptions sell or give away their medications to other students or trade them for others. Some abusers order from Internet pharmacies where prescriptions are not always required. The **Student Health Today** box on page 386 discusses OxyContin and Vicodin abuse.

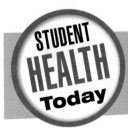

OxyContin and Vicodin Abuse

Since the mid-1990s there has been a sharp increase in prescription drug abuse among youth. The 2010 Monitoring the Future (MTF) study found that approximately 5 percent of college students had used Vicodin and 2 percent used OxyContin, both prescription painkillers, without a doctor's prescription in the past year.

As with most other drugs, some of the reasons college students use OxyContin and Vicodin are that they feel young and often invincible; they need to express their new-found independence; they like the excitement of risk-taking; or they feel pressure from their peers. Often, there is the perception that prescription drugs are safer than illicit drugs.

However, painkillers such as OxyContin, Percocet, Percodan, Vicodin, and others are highly addictive; if they are taken daily for several weeks, that is enough time for addiction to develop. OxyContin, in particular, can be a highly addictive and dangerous narcotic when abused. The "rush" is similar to that of heroin. In fact, it's common for people who are addicted to OxyContin to turn to heroin when they can't afford to buy OxyContin. Chronic use can also result in increasing tolerance, and more of the drug is needed to achieve the desired effect.

Many people who abuse prescription medications are simultaneously abusing illegal drugs. According to the MTF study, students who obtained prescription painkillers from peers reported higher levels of binge drinking and marijuana abuse than nonabusers or those who received painkillers from family. This poses another set of problems, as alcohol in combination with any one of these medications can make a dangerous cocktail. If someone you know seems unusually drunk, drowsy, slurs speech, has trouble moving, or passes out, call for help immediately.

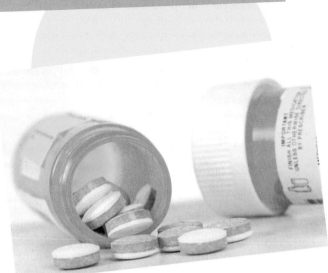

Sources: L. D. Johnston et al., *Monitoring the Future: National Survey Results on Drug Use, 1975–2010*, Volume 2, *College Students and Adults Ages 19–50* (Ann Arbor, MI: Institute for Social Research, The University of Michigan, 2011), Available at http://monitoringthefuture.org/new.html; Higher Education Center for Alcohol, Drug Abuse and Violence Prevention, "OxyContin & Oxycodone," 2010, www.higheredcenter.org/high-risk/drugs/prescription-drugs/oxycontin.

College Students and Prescription Drug Abuse

Prescription drug abuse among college students has increased dramatically over the past decade. Because they are prescribed by doctors and approved by the FDA, many college students seem to perceive prescription drugs as safer than illicit drugs. However, nothing could be further from the truth when these drugs are misused. Many students also perceive the misuse of prescription drugs to be more socially acceptable than other forms of drug use. Some students who abuse prescription drugs believe that such use will enhance their well-being or performance.

According to the 2011 *American College Health Association–National College Health Assessment,* the illicit use of prescription drugs is a growing trend on campuses. The report shows 15.3 percent of surveyed students reported illegally using prescription drugs in the last year, compared to 13.5 percent in 2008. Students who illegally use prescription drugs are also more likely to use other illegal drugs and binge drink.[15] Women, in particular, are also more likely to use prescription drugs as a method of self-medication for psychological distress.[16]

While much attention has focused on the illicit use of stimulant drugs such as Adderall and Ritalin on college campuses, the more commonly abused prescription drugs are pain killers (e.g., OxyContin and Vicodin). Approximately 9.5 percent of students report using pain killers that were not prescribed to them in the past 12 months. Of those reporting use, 11 percent were men and 8 percent women.[17]

Of particular concern on college campuses is the increased abuse of stimulant drugs such as Adderall and Ritalin, which are intended to treat attention-deficit/hyperactivity disorder (ADHD). Students primarily report using ADHD drugs for academic gain. A recent surveys conducted on colleges campuses find that approximately 7 percent of students have reported using stimulants that were not prescribed to them in the past 12 months.[18] An analysis of several studies found that between 16 and 29 percent of students with prescribed stimulant medications for ADHD reported having sold, traded, or been asked for their medications.[19] Users generally believed that the drugs were beneficial, despite frequent reports of adverse reactions. The most commonly reported adverse effects were sleeping difficulties, irritability, and reduced appetite.

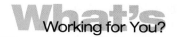

Illicit Drugs

The problem of illicit drug use touches us all. We may use illicit substances ourselves, watch someone we love struggle with drug abuse, or become the victim of a drug-related crime. At the very least, we are forced to pay increasing taxes for law enforcement and drug rehabilitation. When our coworkers use drugs, the effectiveness of our own work is diminished. If the car we drive was assembled by drug-using workers at the plant, we are in danger. A drug-using bus driver, train engineer, or pilot jeopardizes our safety.

Illicit drug users span all age groups, genders, ethnicities, occupations, and socioeconomic groups. Illicit drug use has a devastating effect on users and their families in the United States and in many other countries.

The good news is that the use of illicit drugs in the United States has leveled off and is not increasing for most groups of people. Use of most drugs peaked between 1979 and 1986 and declined until 1992, from which point it has not changed. In 2010, an estimated 22.6 million Americans were illicit drug users, about three quarters the 1979 peak level of 25 million users. Among youth, however, illicit drug use, notably of marijuana, has been rising in recent years.[20]

Illicit Drug Use on Campus Illicit drug use has seen a resurgence on college campuses. The percentage of college students nationwide who had tried any illicit drug in the previous year was about 19 percent; about 18 percent had smoked marijuana in the past year (see Table 13.1).[21] Cocaine use is down sharply, but LSD use has more than doubled. Daily use of marijuana is at its highest point since 1989.[22]

It is important to note that illicit drug use among college students is not the norm; however, the percentage of those who use drugs has increased dramatically in the past decade. For example, the proportion of students who use illicit drugs other than marijuana, such as cocaine, heroin, and Ecstasy, increased 52 percent—from 5 percent to 8 percent of all students—in the past decade.[23] College administrators, staff, and faculty are concerned about the link between substance abuse and poor academic performance, depression, anxiety, suicide, property damage, vandalism, fights, serious medical problems, and death.

Why Do Some College Students Use Drugs? Research has identified the following factors in a student's life that increase the risk of substance abuse. The more factors there are, the greater the risk:

● **Positive expectations.** The most common reason students give to explain why they drink, smoke, or use drugs is to relax,

TABLE 13.1 | **30-Day Drug Use Prevalence, Full-Time College Students vs. Respondents 1–4 Years beyond High School**

	Full-Time College (%)	Others (%)
Any illicit drug	19.2	21.9
Any illicit drug other than marijuana	8.1	10.1
Marijuana	17.5	18.9
Inhalants	0.5	0.1
Hallucinogens	1.4	1.0
LSD	0.7	0.3
Hallucinogens other than LSD	1.2	0.7
Ecstasy (methylene-dioxymeth-amphetamine, MDMA)	1.0	1.6
Cocaine	1.0	1.4
Crack	0.1	0.2
Other cocaine	1.0	1.4
Heroin	*	0.2
Narcotics other than heroin	2.3	5.4
Amphetamines, adjusted	4.1	3.3
Crystal methamphetamine	0.2	0.3
Sedatives (barbiturates)	0.6	1.6
Tranquilizers	1.3	2.2
Alcohol	65.0	54.8
Been drunk	43.6	29.4
Flavored alcoholic beverage	31.5	25.5
Cigarettes	16.4	29.2
Approximate weighted N =	1,260	730

*Indicates prevalence less than 0.05%.

Source: L. D. Johnston et al., *Monitoring the Future National Survey Results on Drug Use, 1975–2010*, Volume 2, *College Students and Adults Ages 19–50* (Ann Arbor, MI: Institute for Social Research, The University of Michigan, 2011), Available at http://monitoringthefuture.org/new.html.

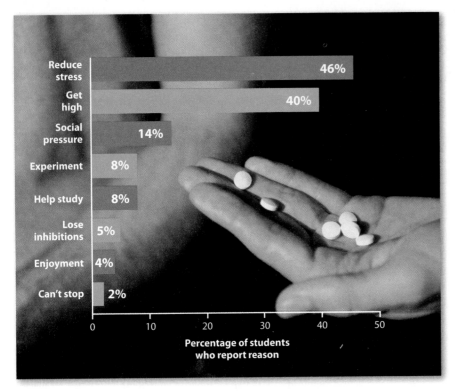

FIGURE 13.3 **Reasons College Students Use Illicit Drugs or Controlled Prescription Drugs**

Source: Adapted from *Wasting the Best and the Brightest: Substance Abuse at America's Colleges and Universities.* New York: National Center on Addiction and Substance Abuse at Columbia University, March 2007, page 47. Copyright © 2007. Used with permission. www.casacolumbia.org/templates/publications_reports.aspx.

stimulants Drugs that increase activity of the central nervous system.

reduce stress, or forget about problems (Figure 13.3). As noted previously, some students take drugs such as Adderall and Ritalin in the belief that the drugs will help them study.

● **Genetics and family history.** Genetics and family history play a significant role in the risk for developing an addiction.

● **Substance use in high school.** Two thirds of college students who use illicit drugs began doing so in high school.

● **Mental health problems.** Students who report being diagnosed with depression are more likely to have abused prescription drugs or to have used marijuana or other illicit drugs.

● **Sorority and fraternity membership.** Being a member of a sorority or fraternity increases the likelihood of using alcohol, marijuana, or cocaine and makes one twice as likely to abuse prescription drugs.

● **Stress.** For some students under academic and social stress, seemingly easy relief comes in the form of drugs or alcohol.

Why *Don't* Some College Students Use Drugs?

There can be many factors influencing a student to avoid drugs; some of the most commonly reported include the following:[24]

● **Parental attitudes and behavior.** Students who say they are more influenced by their parents' concerns or expectations

drink, use marijuana, and smoke significantly less than students less influenced by parents.

● **Religion and spirituality.** The greater the students' level of religiosity (hours in prayer, attendance at services), the less likely they are to drink, smoke, or use other drugs.

● **Student engagement.** The more students are involved in learning and in extracurricular activities, the less likely they are to binge drink, use marijuana, or abuse prescription drugs.

● **College athletics.** College athletes drink at higher rates than nonathletes but are less likely to use illicit drugs.

● **Healthy social network.** Having a wide range of friends and supports to help cope with the challenges of life is a well-known protective factor for many negative behaviors, including drug use.

To prepare yourself for a possible offer of drugs on campus, and to be ready to make the decision that is best for *you*, see the **Skills for Behavior Change** box on page 390.

Common Drugs of Abuse

Hundreds of drugs are subject to abuse—some are legal, such as recreational drugs and prescription medications, while others are illegal and classified as "controlled substances." For general purposes, drugs can be divided into the following categories: *stimulants, cannabis products (cannabinoids) including marijuana, narcotics and depressants, hallucinogens, inhalants,* and *anabolic steroids.* These categories are discussed in subsequent sections; Table 13.2 on the following page summarizes the categories, uses, and effects of various drugs of abuse, both legal and illicit.

Stimulants

A **stimulant** is a drug that increases activity of the central nervous system. Its effects usually involve increased activity, anxiety, and agitation; users often seem jittery or nervous while high. Commonly used stimulants include cocaine, amphetamines, methamphetamine, and caffeine. See **Chapter 12** for a discussion of nicotine, the addictive substance in tobacco products, which is another common stimulant.

what do you think?

How much caffeine do you consume regularly, and why?
● What is your pattern of caffeine consumption?
● Have you ever experienced any ill effects after going without caffeine for a period of time?

Drugs of Abuse: Uses and Effects

Category	Drugs	Trade or Street Names	Dependence	Usual Method	Possible Effects	Overdose Effects	Withdrawal Syndrome
Stimulants	Cocaine	Coke, Flake, Snow, Crack, *Coca, Blanca, Perico*	*Physical:* Possible *Psychological:* High *Tolerance:* Yes	Snorted, smoked, injected	Increased alertness, excitation, euphoria, increased pulse rate and blood pressure, insomnia, loss of appetite	Agitation, increased body temperature, hallucinations, convulsions, possible death	Apathy, long periods of sleep, irritability, depression, disorientation
	Amphetamine, methamphetamine	Crank, Ice, Cristal, Crystal Meth, Speed, Adderall, Dexedrine	*Physical:* Possible *Psychological:* High *Tolerance:* Yes	Oral, injected, smoked			
	Methylphenidate	Ritalin (Illys), Concerta, Focalin, Metadate	*Physical:* Possible *Psychological:* High *Tolerance:* Yes	Oral, injected, snorted, smoked			
Cannabis	Marijuana	Pot, Grass, Sinsemilla, Blunts, *Mota, Yerba, Grifa*	*Physical:* Possible *Psychological:* High *Tolerance:* Yes	Oral, smoked	Euphoria, relaxed inhibitions, increased appetite, disorientation	Fatigue, paranoia, possible psychosis	Hyperactivity, decreased appetite, insomnia
	Hashish, hashish oil	Hash, Hash oil	*Physical:* Unknown *Psychological:* Moderate *Tolerance:* Yes	Smoked, oral			
Narcotics	Heroin	Diamorphine, Horse, Smack, Black tar, *Chiva*	*Physical:* High *Psychological:* High *Tolerance:* Yes	Injected, snorted, smoked	Euphoria, drowsiness, respiratory depression, constricted pupils, nausea	Slow and shallow breathing, clammy skin, convulsions, coma, possible death	Watery eyes, runny nose, yawning, loss of appetite, irritability, tremors, panic, cramps, nausea, chills and sweating
	Morphine	MS-Contin, Roxanol	*Physical:* High *Psychological:* High *Tolerance:* Yes	Oral, injected			
	Hydrocodone, oxycodone	Vicodin, OxyContin, Percocet, Percodan	*Physical:* High *Psychological:* High *Tolerance:* Yes	Oral			
	Codeine	Acetaminophen w/Codeine, Tylenol w/Codeine	*Physical:* Moderate *Psychological:* Moderate *Tolerance:* Yes	Oral, injected			
Depressants	Gamma-hydroxybutyrate	GHB, Liquid Ecstasy, Liquid X	*Physical:* Moderate *Psychological:* Moderate *Tolerance:* Yes	Oral	Slurred speech, disorientation, drunken behavior without odor of alcohol, impaired memory of events, interacts with alcohol	Shallow respiration, clammy skin, dilated pupils, weak and rapid pulse, coma, possible death	Anxiety, insomnia, tremors, delirium, convulsions, possible death
	Benzodiazepines	Valium, Xanax, Halcion, Ativan, Rohypnol (Roofies, R-2), Klonopin	*Physical:* Moderate *Psychological:* Moderate *Tolerance:* Yes	Oral, injected			
	Other depressants	Ambien, Sonata, Barbiturates, Methaqualone (Quaalude)	*Physical:* Moderate *Psychological:* Moderate *Tolerance:* Yes	Oral			
Hallucinogens	Methylenedioxymethamphetamine (MDMA), analogs	Ecstasy, XTC, Adam, MDA (Love Drug), MDEA (Eve)	*Physical:* None *Psychological:* Moderate *Tolerance:* Yes	Oral, snorted, smoked	Heightened senses, teeth grinding, dehydration	Increased body temperature, electrolyte imbalance, cardiac arrest	Muscle aches, drowsiness, depression, acne
	LSD	Acid, Microdot, Sunshine, Boomers	*Physical:* None *Psychological:* Unknown *Tolerance:* Yes	Oral	Hallucinations, altered perception of time and distance	Longer, more intense "trips"	None
	Phencyclidine, analogs	PCP, Angel Dust, Hog, Ketamine (Special K)	*Physical:* Possible *Psychological:* High *Tolerance:* Yes	Smoked, oral, injected, snorted		Unable to direct movement, feel pain, or remember	Drug-seeking behavior
	Other hallucinogens	Psilocybe mushrooms, Mescaline, Peyote, Dextromethorphan	*Physical:* None *Psychological:* None *Tolerance:* Possible	Oral			
Inhalants	Amyl and butyl nitrite	Pearls, Poppers, Rush, Locker Room	*Physical:* Unknown *Psychological:* Unknown *Tolerance:* No	Inhaled	Flushing, hypotension, headache	Methemoglobinemia	Agitation
	Nitrous oxide	Laughing gas, Balloons, Whippets	*Physical:* Unknown *Psychological:* Low *Tolerance:* No	Inhaled	Impaired memory, slurred speech, drunken behavior, slow-onset vitamin deficiency, organ damage	Vomiting, respiratory depression, loss of consciousness, possible death	Trembling, anxiety, insomnia, vitamin deficiency, confusion, hallucinations, convulsions
	Other inhalants	Adhesives, spray paint, hairspray, lighter fluid	*Physical:* Unknown *Psychological:* High *Tolerance:* No	Inhaled			
Anabolic Steroids	Testosterone	Depo Testosterone, Sustanon, Sten, Cypt	*Physical:* Unknown *Psychological:* Unknown *Tolerance:* Unknown	Injected	Virilization, edema, testicular atrophy, gynecomastia, acne, aggressive behavior	Unknown	Possible depression
	Other anabolic steroids	Parabolan, Winstrol, Equipose, Anadrol, Dianabol	*Physical:* Unknown *Psychological:* Yes *Tolerance:* Unknown	Oral, injected			

Source: Adapted from U.S. Department of Justice Drug Enforcement Administration, "DEA Drug Fact Sheets," 2011, www.justice.gov/dea/pubs/all_fact_sheets.pdf

Responding to an Offer of Drugs

No matter what your experience has been up until now, it is likely that you will be invited to use drugs at some point in your life. Here are some questions to consider *before* you find yourself in a situation in which you have the opportunity or feel pressure to use illicit drugs:

❱ Why am I considering trying drugs? Am I trying to fit in or impress my friends? What does this say about my friends if I need to take drugs to impress them? Are my friends really looking out for what is best for me?

❱ Am I using this drug to cope or feel different? Am I depressed?

❱ What could taking drugs cost me? Will this cost me my career if I am caught using? Could using drugs prevent me from getting a job?

❱ What are the long-term consequences of using this drug?

❱ What will this cost me in terms of my friendships and family? How would my family and friends respond if they knew I was using drugs?

Even when you make the decision not to use drugs, it can be difficult to say no gracefully. Some good ways to turn down an offer:

❱ "Thanks, but I've got a big test (game, meeting) tomorrow morning."

❱ "I've already got a great buzz right now. I really don't need anything more."

❱ "I don't like how (insert drug name here) makes me feel."

❱ "I'm driving tonight. So I'm not using."

❱ "I want to go for a run in the morning."

❱ "No."

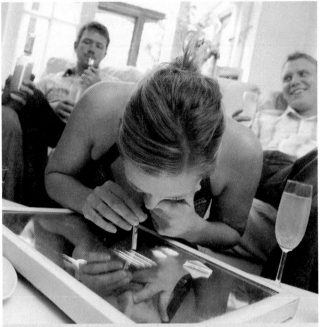

Although cocaine use has declined from its peak in the 1980s, it continues to be a commonly abused illicit drug.

Cocaine A white crystalline powder derived from the leaves of the South American coca shrub (not related to cocoa plants), *cocaine* ("coke") has been described as one of the most powerful naturally occurring stimulants.

Methods of Use and Physical Effects Cocaine can be taken in several ways, including snorting, smoking, and injecting. The powdered form is snorted through the nose, which can damage mucous membranes and cause sinusitis. It can destroy the user's sense of smell, and occasionally it even eats a hole through the septum. When snorted, the drug enters the bloodstream through the lungs in less than 1 minute and reaches the brain in less than 3 minutes. It binds at receptor sites in the central nervous system, producing an intense high that disappears quickly, leaving a powerful craving for more.

Cocaine alkaloid, or *freebase*, is obtained by removing the hydro-

amphetamines A large and varied group of synthetic agents that stimulate the central nervous system.

chloride salt from cocaine powder. *Freebasing* refers to smoking freebase by placing it at the end of a pipe and holding a flame near it to produce a vapor, which is then inhaled. *Crack* is identical pharmacologically to freebase, but the hydrochloride salt is still present and is processed with baking soda and water. It is a cheap, widely available drug that is smokable and very potent. Crack is commonly smoked in the same manner as freebase. Because crack is such a pure drug, it takes little time to achieve the desired high, and a crack user can become addicted quickly.

Some cocaine users inject the drug intravenously, which introduces large amounts into the body rapidly, creating a brief, intense high and subsequent crash. Injecting users place themselves at risk not only for contracting HIV and hepatitis (a serious liver disease) through shared needles, but also for skin infections, vein damage, inflamed arteries, and infection of the heart lining.

Cocaine is both an anesthetic and a central nervous system stimulant. In tiny doses, it can slow the heart rate. In larger doses, the physical effects are dramatic: increased heart rate and blood pressure, loss of appetite that can lead to dramatic weight loss, convulsions, muscle twitching, irregular heartbeat, and even death resulting from an overdose. Other effects of cocaine include temporary relief of depression, decreased fatigue, talkativeness, increased alertness, and heightened self-confidence. However, as the dose increases, users become irritable and apprehensive, and their behavior may turn paranoid or violent.

Amphetamines The **amphetamines** include a large and varied group of synthetic agents that stimulate the central nervous system. Small doses of amphetamines improve alertness, lessen fatigue, and generally elevate mood. With repeated use, however, physical and psychological dependencies develop. Sleep patterns are affected (insomnia); heart rate, breathing rate, and blood pressure increase; and restlessness, anxiety, appetite suppression, and vision problems are common. High doses over long time periods can produce hallucinations, delusions, and disorganized behavior.

Certain types of amphetamines or amphetamine-like drugs are used for medicinal purposes. As discussed earlier, drugs prescribed to treat ADHD are stimulants, which are increasingly abused on campus.

Methamphetamine An increasingly common form of amphetamine, *methamphetamine* (commonly called "meth") is a potent, long-acting, addictive drug that strongly activates the brain's reward center by producing a sense of euphoria. In 2010, 2.4 percent of high school seniors reported using methamphetamine in their lifetime. More than 1 million Americans have tried methamphetamine, and 353, 000 are current users.[25]

Methamphetamine can be snorted, smoked, injected, or orally ingested. When snorted, the effects can be felt in 3 to 5 minutes; if orally ingested, effects occur within 15 to 20 minutes. The pleasurable effects of methamphetamine are typically an intense rush lasting only a few minutes when snorted; in contrast, smoking the drug can produce a high lasting more than 8 hours.

Methamphetamine increases the release and blocks the reuptake of the neurotransmitter dopamine, leading to high levels of the chemical in the brain. Dopamine is involved in reward, motivation, the experience of pleasure, and motor function. Methamphetamine's ability to release dopamine rapidly in reward regions of the brain produces the intense euphoria, or "rush," that many users feel. However, over time, meth destroys dopamine receptors, making it impossible to feel pleasure. Researchers have now established that, due to the destruction of dopamine receptors, people who abuse methamphetamine or other amphetamine-like substances (cocaine) are more likely to develop Parkinson's disease than those who do not.[26]

Chronic methamphetamine abuse significantly changes how the brain functions. Noninvasive human brain imaging studies have shown alterations in the activity of the dopamine system that are associated with reduced motor skills and impaired verbal learning. Recent studies in chronic methamphetamine abusers have also revealed severe structural and functional changes in areas of the brain associated with emotion and memory, which may account for the emotional and cognitive problems observed in chronic methamphetamine abusers. Some of these changes persist after the methamphetamine abuse has stopped. Other changes reverse after sustained periods of abstinence from methamphetamine, lasting typically longer than a year, but problems often remain.

In the short term, methamphetamine produces increased physical activity, alertness, euphoria, rapid breathing, increased body temperature, insomnia, tremors, anxiety, confusion, and decreased appetite; however, the drug's effects quickly wear off. Users often experience tolerance after the first use, making methamphetamine highly addictive.

The long-term effects of methamphetamine can include severe weight loss, cardiovascular damage, increased risk of heart attack and stroke, hallucinations, extensive tooth decay and tooth loss ("meth mouth"), violence, paranoia, psychotic behavior, and even death.

It is believed that more than 13 million Americans have tried methamphetamine.[27] The rate of methamphetamine use may be increasing because it is relatively easy to make. Recipes often include common OTC ingredients such as ephedrine and pseudoephedrine.

"Bath salts" is the latest addition to the growing list of items people are using to get high. The new designer drug is synthetic powder sold legally online and in corner stores and truck stops. The powder substance is sold in a packet with a disclaimer "not for human consumption." It is not subject to FDA regulation. These packages contain various amphetamine or cocaine-like substances such as methylene-dioxypyrovalerone (MPDV), mephedrone, and pyrovalerone. The powder can be smoked, snorted, injected, and wrapped in pieces of paper and ingested or "bombed." These chemicals cannot be detected by routine drug screening, making them attractive for misuse.[28]

Effects include intense stimulation, alertness, euphoria, elevated mood, and pleasurable "rush." Users may describe feelings of closeness, sociability, and moderate sexual arousal. Other symptoms can include tremor, shortness of breath, and loss of appetite. Changes in body temperature regulation are accompanied by hot flashes and sweating, with bleeding from the nose and throat from ulcerations when snorted.[29]

This drug also can have significant effects on the cardiovascular system, resulting in rapid heart rate, increased blood pressure, and chest pain. Psychiatric effects at higher

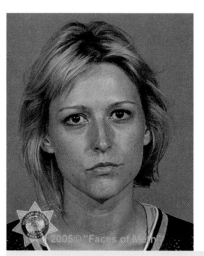
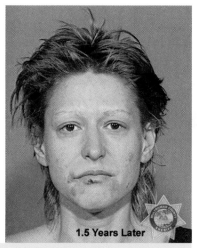

1.5 Years Later

The physical consequences of methamphetamine use are often dramatic. The photos above show a person before and 1.5 years after methamphetamine use.

doses consist of anxiety, agitation, hallucinations, paranoia, and erratic behavior. Depression and suicide have also been reported as a result of use. While withdrawal symptoms are reported as minimal, users often have described a strong craving for the drug.[30]

Caffeine What is the most popular and widely consumed drug in the United States? Caffeine. Almost half of all Americans drink coffee every day, and many others consume caffeine in some other form, mainly for its well-known "wake-up" effect. Drinking coffee, tea, soft drinks, and other caffeine-containing products is legal, even socially encouraged. Caffeine may seem harmless, but excessive consumption is associated with addiction and certain health problems.

Caffeine is derived from the chemical family called *xanthines,* which are found in plant products from which coffee, tea, and chocolate are made. The xanthines are mild, central nervous system stimulants that enhance mental alertness and reduce feelings of fatigue. Other stimulant effects include increased heart muscle contractions, oxygen consumption, metabolism, and urinary output. A person feels these effects within 15 to 45 minutes of ingesting a caffeinated product. It takes 4 to 6 hours for the body to metabolize half of the caffeine ingested, so, depending on the amount of caffeine taken in, it may continue to exert effects for a day or longer. **Figure 13.4** compares the caffeine content of various products.

Side effects of the xanthines include wakefulness, insomnia, irregular heartbeat, dizziness, nausea, indigestion, and sometimes mild delirium. Some people also experi-

marijuana Chopped leaves and flowers of *Cannabis indica* or *Cannabis sativa* plants (hemp); a psychoactive stimulant.

ence heartburn. As the effects of caffeine wear off, frequent users may feel let down—mentally or physically depressed, tired, and weak. To counteract this, they commonly choose to drink another cup of coffee. Habitually engaging in this practice leads to tolerance and psychological dependence. Symptoms of excessive caffeine consumption include chronic insomnia, jitters, irritability, nervousness, anxiety, and involuntary muscle twitches. Withdrawing from caffeine may compound the effects and produce headaches, fatigue, and nausea. Because caffeine meets the requirements for addiction—tolerance, psychological dependence, and withdrawal symptoms—it can be classified as addictive.

Long-term caffeine use has been suspected of being linked to several serious health problems. However, no strong evidence exists to suggest that moderate caffeine use (less than 300 mg daily, approximately 3 cups of regular coffee) produces harmful effects in healthy, nonpregnant people. Caffeine has not been linked to high blood pressure or strokes, nor is there any evidence of a relationship between caffeine and heart disease.[31] However, people who suffer from irregular heartbeat are cautioned against using caffeine because the resultant increase in heart rate might be life threatening.

Marijuana and Other Cannabinoids

Although archaeological evidence documents the use of **marijuana** ("grass," "weed," "pot") as far back as 6,000 years, the drug did not become popular in the United States until the 1960s. Today, marijuana is the most commonly used illicit drug in the United States. Approximately 41 percent of Americans over the age of 12 has tried marijuana at least once.[32] Some 29 million have reported using marijuana in the past

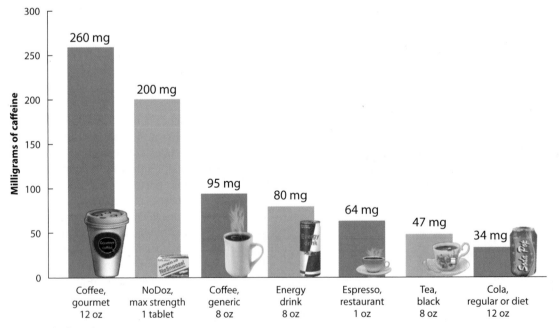

FIGURE 13.4 Caffeine Content Comparison

Source: Data are from *USDA National Nutrient Database for Standard Reference,* Release 22 (2009), www.ars.usda.gov/ba/bhnrc/ndl.

year, and more than 16.7 million have reported using marijuana within the past month. More than 1 million Americans over the age of 12 reported receiving treatment for marijuana use, more than any other illicit drug. Marijuana use is also on the rise on college campuses, following the trend of increased use in the general population.[33]

Methods of Use and Physical Effects

Marijuana is derived from either the *Cannabis sativa* or *Cannabis indica* (hemp) plant. Most of the time, marijuana is smoked, although it can also be ingested, as in brownies baked with marijuana in them. When marijuana is smoked, it is usually rolled into cigarettes (joints) or placed in a pipe or water pipe (bong).

Tetrahydrocannabinol (THC) is the psychoactive substance in marijuana and the key to determining how powerful a high it will produce. More potent forms of the drug can contain up to 27 percent THC, but most average 10 percent.[34] *Hashish,* a potent cannabis preparation derived mainly from the plant's thick, sticky resin, contains high THC concentrations. Hash oil, a substance produced by percolating a solvent such as ether through dried marijuana to extract the THC, is a tarlike liquid that may contain up to 300 mg of THC in a dose.

The effects of smoking marijuana are generally felt within 10 to 30 minutes and usually wear off within 3 hours. The most noticeable visible effect of THC is the dilation of the eyes' blood vessels, which gives the smoker bloodshot eyes. Marijuana smokers also exhibit coughing; dry mouth and throat ("cotton mouth"); increased thirst and appetite; lowered blood pressure; and mild muscular weakness, primarily exhibited in drooping eyelids. Users can also experience severe anxiety, panic, paranoia, and psychosis, and may have intensified reactions to various stimuli: Colors, sounds, and the speed at which things move may seem altered. High doses of hashish may produce vivid visual hallucinations.

Marijuana and Driving Marijuana use presents clear hazards for drivers of motor vehicles and others on the road with them. The drug substantially reduces a driver's ability to react and make quick decisions. Perceptual and other performance deficits resulting from marijuana use may persist for some time after the high subsides. Users who attempt to drive, fly, or operate heavy machinery often fail to recognize their impairment. Overall, marijuana is the most prevalent illegal drug detected in impaired drivers, fatally injured drivers, and motor vehicle crash victims.[35] Recent research has found that driving under the influence of marijuana is associated with a risk of having crash almost two times as high as driving unimpaired.[36] In many of these cases, alcohol is detected as well. Research by the National Highway Traffic Safety Administration indicates that a moderate dose of marijuana alone impairs driving performance; however, the effects of even a low dose of marijuana combined with alcohol are markedly greater than for either drug alone.[37]

One common way of smoking marijuana is to use a pipe.

Effects of Chronic Marijuana Use Because marijuana is illegal in most parts of the United States and has been widely used only since the 1960s, long-term studies of its effects have been difficult to conduct. Also, studies conducted in the 1960s involved marijuana with THC levels at only a fraction of today's levels, so their results may not apply to the stronger forms available today.

Marijuana smoke contains 50 to 70 percent more carcinogenic hydrocarbons than does tobacco smoke. Because marijuana smokers typically inhale more deeply and hold their breath longer than tobacco smokers, the lungs are exposed to more carcinogens. As well, effects from irritation (e.g., cough, excessive phlegm, and increased lung infections) similar to those experienced by tobacco smokers can occur.[38] Lung conditions such as chronic bronchitis, emphysema, and other lung disorders are also associated with smoking marijuana.

Inhaling marijuana smoke introduces carbon monoxide to the bloodstream. Because the blood has a greater affinity for carbon monoxide than it does for oxygen, its oxygen-carrying capacity is diminished, and the heart must work harder to pump oxygen to oxygen-starved tissues. Furthermore, the tar from cannabis contains higher levels of carcinogens than does tobacco smoke.

tetrahydrocannabinol (THC) The chemical name for the active ingredient in marijuana.

Frequent and/or long-term marijuana use may significantly increase a man's risk of developing testicular cancer. Researchers have found that being a marijuana smoker at

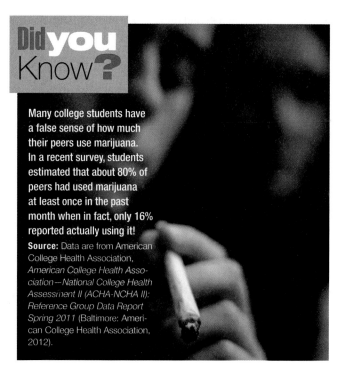

Did you Know?

Many college students have a false sense of how much their peers use marijuana. In a recent survey, students estimated that about 80% of peers had used marijuana at least once in the past month when in fact, only 16% reported actually using it!

Source: Data are from American College Health Association, *American College Health Association—National College Health Assessment II (ACHA-NCHA II): Reference Group Data Report Spring 2011* (Baltimore: American College Health Association, 2012).

the time of diagnosis was associated with a 70 percent higher risk of testicular cancer.[39] The risk was particularly elevated (about twice that of those who never smoked marijuana) for those who used marijuana at least weekly or who had long-term exposure to the substance beginning in adolescence. The results also suggested that the association with marijuana use might be limited to *nonseminoma,* an aggressive, fast-growing testicular malignancy that tends to strike early, between ages 20 and 35, and accounts for about 40 percent of all testicular cancer cases.[40]

depressants Drugs that slow down the activity of the central nervous system.

benzodiazepines A class of central nervous system depressant drugs with sedative, hypnotic, and muscle relaxant effects.

barbiturates Drugs that depress the central nervous system and have sedating, hypnotic, and anesthetic effects.

According to the National Survey on Drug Use and Health, teens and young adults who use marijuana are more likely to develop serious mental health problems. A number of studies have shown an association between marijuana use and increased rates of anxiety, depression, suicidal ideation, and schizophrenia.[41] Some of these studies have shown age at first use as an indicator of vulnerability to later problems. Among individuals 18 and older, those who used marijuana before age 12 were twice as likely to have a serious mental illness as those who first used marijuana at age 18 or older.[42]

Chronic use of marijuana can decrease the quality of sleep. Studies have found that chronic users of marijuana experience less rapid eye movement (REM) and slow-wave sleep (SWS), often referred to as deep sleep, both of which are important for the consolidation of memories. Not getting enough sleep interferes with the ability to think and remember, challenging students' ability to learn and perform well academically.[43]

Other risks associated with marijuana include suppression of the immune system, blood pressure changes, and impaired memory. Recent studies suggest that pregnant women who smoke marijuana are at a higher risk for stillbirth or miscarriage and for delivering low birth-weight babies and babies with abnormalities of the nervous system.[44]

Marijuana as Medicine Although recognized as a dangerous drug by the U.S. government, marijuana has several medical purposes. It helps control the severe nausea and vomiting produced by chemotherapy. It improves appetite and forestalls the loss of lean muscle mass associated with AIDS-wasting syndrome. Marijuana also reduces the muscle pain and spasticity caused by diseases such as multiple sclerosis. Marijuana's legal status for medicinal purposes continues to be hotly debated (see the **Points of View** box on the following page).

Synthetic Marijuana Also known as K2 or "Spice," synthetic marijuana is used to describe a diverse family of herbal blends marketed under many names, including K2, fake marijuana, Yucatan Fire, Skunk, Moon Rocks, and others. These products contain dried, shredded plant material and one or more synthetic cannabinoids, with results that mimic marijuana intoxication but with longer duration and poor detection on urine drug screens. K2 is sold legally as herbal blend incense. However, K2 is smoked by people to gain effects similar to marijuana, hashish, and other forms of cannabis.[45]

K2 is used by nearly 1 in 10 college students and is more commonly used by males and first- and second-year college students. Students who reported using K2 were more likely to have smoked cigarettes, marijuana, and hookahs. It is also gaining more attention among high school seniors, with reports that 1 in every 9, or 11.4 percent, of high school seniors are using this drug.[46]

The most common way of smoking K2 was in a "joint," followed by hookah use. People smoking K2 may experience several adverse health effects such as hallucinations, severe agitation, extremely elevated heart rate and blood pressure, coma, suicide attempts, and drug dependence, which is not common among cannabis users. Emergency departments are also reporting a significant increase in the numbers of people being treated for K2 use.[47]

Depressants and Narcotics

Whereas central nervous system stimulants increase muscular and nervous system activity, **depressants** have the opposite effect. These drugs slow down neuromuscular activity and cause sleepiness or calmness. If the dose is high enough, brain function can stop, causing death. Alcohol is the most widely used central nervous system depressant. (For details on alcohol's effect on the body see **Chapter 11**). Other forms include opioids, benzodiazepines, and barbiturates.

Benzodiazepines and Barbiturates A *sedative* drug promotes mental calmness and reduces anxiety, whereas a *hypnotic* drug promotes sleep or drowsiness. The most common sedative-hypnotic drugs are **benzodiazepines,** more commonly known as *tranquilizers.* These include prescription drugs such as Valium, Ativan, and Xanax. Benzodiazepines are most commonly prescribed for tension, muscular strain, sleep problems, anxiety, panic attacks, and alcohol withdrawal. **Barbiturates** are sedative-hypnotic drugs such as Amytal and Seconal. Today, benzodiazepines have largely replaced barbiturates, which were used medically in the past for relieving tension and inducing relaxation and sleep.

Sedative-hypnotics have a synergistic effect when combined with alcohol, another central nervous system depressant. Taken together, these drugs can lead to respiratory failure and death. All sedative or hypnotic drugs can produce physical and psychological dependence in several weeks. A complication specific to sedatives is cross-tolerance, which occurs when users develop tolerance for one sedative or become dependent on it and develop tolerance for others as well. Withdrawal from sedative or hypnotic drugs may range from mild discomfort to severe symptoms, depending on the degree of dependence.

Medical Marijuana:
TOO LEGAL OR NOT LEGAL ENOUGH?

For years, the use of medical marijuana has been hotly debated. Voters in 16 states (Alaska, Arizona, California, Colorado, Delaware, Hawaii, Maine, Michigan, Montana, New Mexico, New Jersey, Nevada, Oregon, Rhode Island, Vermont, and Washington) and the District of Columbia have chosen to legalize marijuana for medicinal use, and 18 other states have pending legislation.

These new state laws, however, conflict with federal laws against the possession of marijuana and have led to new, still unresolved, battles in court.

The arguments for and against the legalization of marijuana have been very strong over the past few decades. Below are some of the major points from both sides of the issue.

Arguments for Legalization

○ Marijuana is a safe and effective treatment for certain complications of dozens of conditions, such as cancer, AIDS, multiple sclerosis, pain, migraines, glaucoma, and epilepsy.

○ Legalizing marijuana and taxing its sale would bring in revenue for the government.

○ Legal government and U.S. Food and Drug Administration (FDA) oversight would allow for standardization of marijuana growth and production and promote more responsible cultivation methods.

Arguments against Legalization

○ It is not necessary to legalize marijuana for medical use because there are already FDA-approved drugs that are just as effective in treating the same conditions.

○ Marijuana use poses dangerous side effects including lung injury, immune system damage, and interference with fertility that make it inappropriate for FDA approval.

○ Marijuana is known to be addictive.

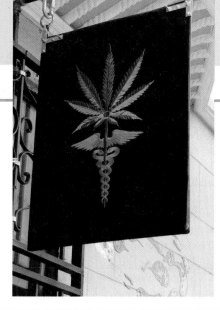

Where Do You Stand?

○ Do you think medical marijuana should be legalized by the federal government? What potential problems do you think this would create or solve?

○ Do you think marijuana use in general should be legalized?

○ What criteria do you think should be used to determine the legality of a particular substance? Who should make those determinations?

○ What are your feelings on drug laws in general—do you think they should be more or less prohibitive? What sort of policies would you propose to protect individuals and their rights?

Sources: ProCon.org, "Medical Marijuana," 2009, http://medicalmarijuana.procon.org; Marijuana Policy Project, "Medical Marijuana Overview," 2012, www.mpp.org/reports/medical-marijuana-overview.html.

Rohypnol One benzodiazepine of concern is Rohypnol, a potent tranquilizer similar in nature to Valium but many times stronger. The drug produces a sedative effect, amnesia, muscle relaxation, and slowed psychomotor responses. The most publicized "date rape" drug, Rohypnol has gained notoriety as a growing problem on college campuses. The drug has been added to punch and other drinks at parties, where it is reportedly given to women in hopes of lowering their inhibitions and facilitating potential sexual conquests. (See **Chapter 19** for more information about drug-facilitated rape.)

GHB *Gamma-hydroxybutyrate* (*GHB*) is a central nervous system depressant known to have euphoric, sedative, and anabolic (bodybuilding) effects. The FDA banned OTC sales of GHB in 1992, and it is now a Schedule I controlled substance.[48] Gamma-hydroxybutyrate is an odorless, tasteless fluid that can be made easily at home or in a chemistry lab. Like Rohypnol, GHB has been slipped into drinks without being detected, resulting in loss of memory, unconsciousness, amnesia, and even death. Other dangerous side effects include nausea, vomiting, seizures, hallucinations, coma, and respiratory distress.

Opioids (Narcotics) **Opioids** cause drowsiness, relieve pain, and produce euphoria. Also called *narcotics,* opioids are derived from the parent drug **opium,** a dark, resinous substance made from the milky juice of the opium poppy seedpod, and they are all highly addictive. Opium and heroin are both illegal in the United States, but some opioids are available by prescription for medical purposes: Morphine is sometimes prescribed for severe pain, and codeine is found in prescription cough syrups and other painkillers. Several prescription drugs, including Vicodin, Percodan, OxyContin, Demerol, and Dilaudid, contain synthetic opioids.

opioids Drugs that induce sleep and relieve pain, including derivatives of opium and synthetics with similar chemical properties; also called *narcotics.*

opium The parent drug of the opioids; made from the seedpod resin of the opium poppy.

endorphins Opioid-like hormones that are manufactured in the human body and contribute to natural feelings of well-being.

Physical Effects of Opioids Opioids are powerful depressants of the central nervous system. In addition to relieving pain, these drugs lower heart rate, respiration, and blood pressure. Side effects include weakness, dizziness, nausea, vomiting, euphoria, decreased sex drive, visual disturbances, and lack of coordination.

The human body's physiology could be said to encourage opioid addiction. Opioid-like hormones called **endorphins** are manufactured in the body and have multiple receptor sites, particularly in the central nervous system. When endorphins attach themselves at these points, they create feelings of painless well-being; medical researchers refer to them as "the body's own opioids." When endorphin levels are high, people feel euphoric. The same euphoria occurs when opioids or related chemicals are active at the endorphin receptor sites. The following section discusses heroin addiction; addiction to any opioid follows a similar path.

Heroin Use *Heroin* is a white powder derived from morphine. *Black tar heroin* is a sticky, dark brown, foul-smelling form of heroin that is relatively pure and inexpensive. Once considered a cure for morphine dependence, heroin was later discovered to be even more addictive and potent than morphine. Today, heroin has no medical use.

Heroin is a depressant that produces drowsiness and a dreamy, mentally slow feeling. It can cause drastic mood swings, with euphoric highs followed by depressive lows. Heroin slows respiration and urinary output and constricts the pupils of the eyes. Symptoms of tolerance and withdrawal can appear within 3 weeks of first use.

In 2010, 140,000 Americans reported using heroin for the first time, a considerably higher number than in previous years. The average age of first use was 21 years.[49] While heroin is usually injected, the contemporary version of heroin is so potent that users can get high by snorting or smoking the drug. This has attracted a more affluent group of users who may not want to inject because of the increased risk of contracting diseases such as HIV.

However, the most common route of administration for heroin addicts is "mainlining"—intravenous injection of powdered heroin mixed in a solution. Many users describe the "rush" they feel when injecting themselves as intensely pleasurable, whereas others report unpredictable and unpleasant side effects. The temporary nature of the rush contributes to the drug's high potential for addiction—many addicts shoot up four or five times a day. Mainlining can cause veins to scar and eventually collapse. Once a vein has collapsed, it can no longer be used to introduce heroin into the bloodstream. Addicts become expert at locating new veins to use: in the feet, the legs, the temples, under the tongue, or in the groin.

Treatment for Heroin Addiction Heroin addicts experience a distinct pattern of withdrawal. Symptoms include intense desire for the drug, sleep disturbance, dilated pupils, loss of appetite, irritability, goose bumps, and muscle tremors. The most difficult time in the withdrawal process occurs 24 to 72 hours following last use. All of the preceding symptoms continue, along with nausea, abdominal cramps, restlessness, insomnia, vomiting, diarrhea, extreme anxiety, hot and cold flashes, elevated blood pressure, and rapid heartbeat and respiration. Once the peak of withdrawal has passed, all these symptoms begin to subside. Still, the recovering addict has many hurdles to jump.

Methadone maintenance is one treatment available for people addicted to heroin or other opioids. Methadone is chemically similar enough to opioids to control the tremors, chills, vomiting, diarrhea, and severe abdominal pains of withdrawal. However, methadone maintenance is controversial because of the drug's own potential for addiction. Critics contend that the program merely substitutes one addiction for another. Proponents argue that people on methadone maintenance are less likely to engage in criminal activities to support their habits than heroin addicts are. For this reason, many methadone maintenance programs are financed by state or federal government and are available free of charge or at reduced cost.

A number of new drug therapies for opioid dependence are emerging. Naltrexone (Trexan), an opioid antagonist, has been approved as a treatment. While on naltrexone, recovering addicts do not have the compulsion to use heroin, and if they do use it, they don't get high, so there is no point in using the drug. More recently, researchers have reported promising results with buprenorphine (Temgesic), a mild, nonaddicting synthetic opioid that, like heroin and methadone, bonds to certain receptors in the brain, blocks pain messages, and persuades the brain that its craving for heroin has been satisfied.

Opium is extracted from opium poppy seedpods like this one.

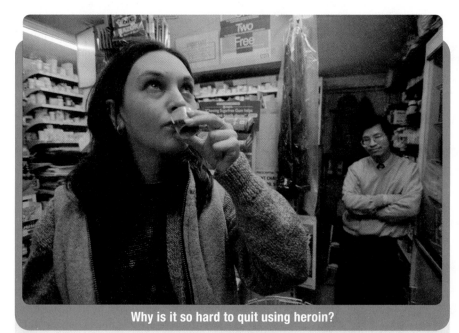

Why is it so hard to quit using heroin?

Heroin's effect on the body is similar to the painless well-being created by endorphins. Stopping heroin use causes withdrawal symptoms that can be very difficult to manage, which keeps many addicts from attempting to quit. Methadone is a synthetic narcotic that blocks the effects of withdrawal. Although it is still a narcotic and must be administered under the supervision of clinic or pharmacy staff, methadone allows many heroin addicts to lead somewhat normal lives.

Hallucinogens

Hallucinogens, or *psychedelics,* are substances that are capable of creating auditory or visual hallucinations and unusual changes in mood, thoughts, and feelings. The major receptor sites for most of these drugs are in the reticular formation (located in the brainstem at the upper end of the spinal cord), which is responsible for interpreting outside stimuli before allowing these signals to travel to other parts of the brain. When a hallucinogen is present at a reticular formation site, messages become scrambled, and the user may see wavy walls instead of straight ones or may "smell" colors and "hear" tastes. This mixing of sensory messages is known as *synesthesia.* Users may also become less inhibited or recall events long buried in the subconscious mind. The most widely recognized hallucinogens are LSD, Ecstasy, mescaline, psilocybin, PCP, and ketamine. All are illegal and carry severe penalties for manufacture, possession, transportation, or sale.

LSD Of all the psychedelics, *lysergic acid diethylamide* (*LSD*) is the most notorious. First synthesized in the late 1930s by Swiss chemist Albert Hoffman, LSD received media attention in the 1960s when young people used the drug to "turn on and tune out." In 1970, federal authorities placed LSD on the list of controlled substances (Schedule I).

Today, this dangerous psychedelic drug, known on the street as "acid," has been making a comeback. It is estimated that 6 percent of American age 18 to 25 have tried LSD.[50] A national survey of college students showed that 2 percent had used the drug in the past year.[51]

The most common and popular form of LSD is blotter acid—small squares of blotter-like paper that have been impregnated with a liquid LSD mixture. The blotter is swallowed or chewed briefly. LSD also comes in tiny thin squares of gelatin called *windowpane* and in tablets called *microdots,* which are less than an eighth of an inch across (it would take ten or more to equal the size of an aspirin tablet).

One of the most powerful drugs known to science, LSD can produce strong effects in doses as low as 20 micrograms (μg). (To give you an idea of how small a dose this is, the average postage stamp weighs approximately 60,000 μg.) The potency of a typical dose currently ranges from 20 to 80 μg, compared to 150 to 300 μg commonly used in the 1960s.

The psychological effects of LSD vary. Euphoria is the common psychological state produced by the drug, but dysphoria (a sense of evil and foreboding) may also be experienced. LSD also distorts ordinary perceptions, such as the movement of stationary objects, as well as auditory or visual hallucinations. In addition, the drug shortens attention span, causing the mind to wander. Thoughts may be interposed and juxtaposed, so the user experiences several different thoughts simultaneously. Users become introspective, and suppressed memories may surface, often taking on bizarre symbolism. Many more effects are possible, including decreased aggressiveness and enhanced sensory experiences.

> **hallucinogens** Substances capable of creating auditory or visual distortions and heightened states.

In addition to its psychedelic effects, LSD produces several physical effects, including increased heart rate, elevated blood pressure and temperature, gooseflesh (roughened skin), increased reflex speeds, muscle tremors and twitches, perspiration, increased salivation, chills, headaches, and mild nausea. Because the drug also stimulates uterine muscle contractions, it can lead to premature labor and miscarriage in pregnant women. Research into long-term effects has been inconclusive.

Although there is no evidence that LSD creates physical dependency, it may well create psychological dependence.

4.6%

of college students report having tried hallucinogens.

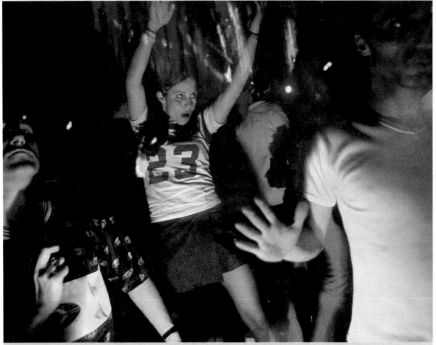

Just how risky are "club drugs"?
So-called club drugs are a varied group of synthetic drugs including Ecstasy, GHB, ketamine, Rohypnol, and meth that are often abused by teens and young adults at nightclubs, bars, or all-night dances. The sources and chemicals used to make these drugs vary, so dosages are unpredictable and drugs may not be "pure." Although users may think them harmless, research has shown that club drugs can produce hallucinations, paranoia, amnesia, dangerous increases in heart rate and blood pressure, coma, and, in some cases, death. Some club drugs work on the same brain mechanisms as alcohol and can be particularly dangerous when used in combination with alcohol. In addition, some club drugs can be easily slipped into unsuspecting partygoers' drinks, thus facilitating sexual assault and other crimes.

does not create visual hallucinations. Effects begin within 20 to 90 minutes and can last for 3 to 5 hours.

Some of the risks associated with Ecstasy use are similar to those of other stimulants. Because of the nature of the drug, Ecstasy users are at greater risk of inappropriate or unintended emotional bonding and have a tendency to say things they might feel uncomfortable about later. More physical consequences of Ecstasy use may include mild to extreme jaw clenching, tongue and cheek chewing, short-term memory loss or confusion, increased body temperature as a result of dehydration and heat stroke, and increased heart rate and blood pressure. Individuals with high blood pressure, heart disease, or liver trouble are at greatest danger when using this drug. Combined with alcohol, Ecstasy can be extremely dangerous and sometimes fatal. As the effects of Ecstasy wear off, the user can experience mild depression, fatigue, and a hangover that can last from days to weeks. Chronic use appears to damage the brain's ability to think and to regulate emotion, memory, sleep, and pain. Some studies indicate that the drug may cause long-lasting neurotoxic effects by damaging brain cells that produce serotonin.[52]

Many LSD users become depressed for 1 or 2 days following a trip and turn to the drug to relieve this depression. The result is a cycle of LSD use to relieve post-LSD depression, which can lead to psychological addiction.

Ecstasy *Ecstasy* is the most common street name for the drug *methylene-dioxymethamphetamine* (*MDMA*), a synthetic compound with both stimulant and mildly hallucinogenic effects. It is one of the most well-known **club drugs** or "designer drugs," terms applied to synthetic analogs of existing illicit drugs that tend to be popular among teens and young adults at nightclubs and all-night parties. Ecstasy creates feelings of extreme euphoria, openness, and warmth; an increased willingness to communicate; feelings of love and empathy; increased awareness; and heightened appreciation for music. Like other hallucinogenic drugs, Ecstasy can enhance the sensory experience and distort perceptions, but it

club drugs Synthetic analogs (drugs that produce similar effects) of existing illicit drugs.

Mescaline comes from "buttons" of the peyote cactus, like this one.

Mescaline *Mescaline* is one of hundreds of chemicals derived from the peyote cactus, a small, button-like plant that grows in the southwestern United States and in Latin America. Natives of these regions have long used the dried peyote "buttons" for religious purposes. It is both a powerful hallucinogen and a central nervous system stimulant.

Products sold on the street as mescaline are likely to be synthetic chemical relatives of the true drug. Street names of these products include DOM, STP, TMA, and MMDA. Any of these can be toxic in small quantities.

Users typically swallow 10 to 12 buttons. They taste bitter and generally induce immediate nausea or vomiting. Long-time users claim that the nausea becomes less noticeable with frequent use. Those who are able to keep the drug down begin to feel the effects within 30 to 90 minutes, when mescaline reaches maximum concentration in the brain. It may persist for 9 or 10 hours.

Psilocybin *Psilocybin* and *psilocin* are the active chemicals in a group of mushrooms sometimes called "magic mushrooms." Psilocybe mushrooms, which grow throughout the world, can be cultivated from spores or harvested wild. When consumed, these mushrooms can cause hallucinations. Because many mushrooms resemble the psilocybe variety, people who harvest wild mushrooms for any purpose should be certain of what they are doing. Mushroom varieties can be easily misidentified, and mistakes can be fatal. Psilocybin is similar to LSD in its physical effects, which generally wear off in 4 to 6 hours.

Psilocybe mushrooms produce hallucinogenic effects when ingested.

PCP The synthetic substance *phencyclidine* (*PCP*) was originally developed as a dissociative anesthetic—patients administered this drug could keep their eyes open, apparently remain conscious, and feel no pain during a medical procedure. Afterward, they would experience amnesia for the time that the drug was in their system. Such a drug had obvious advantages as an anesthetic, but its unpredictability and drastic effects (postoperative delirium, confusion, and agitation) caused it to be withdrawn from the legal market.

On the illegal market, PCP is a white, crystalline powder that users often sprinkle onto marijuana cigarettes. It is dangerous and unpredictable regardless of the method of administration. The effects of PCP depend on the dosage. A dose as small as 5 mg will produce effects similar to those of strong central nervous system depressants—slurred speech, impaired coordination, reduced sensitivity to pain, and reduced heart and respiratory rate. Doses between 5 and 10 mg cause fever, salivation, nausea, vomiting, and total loss of sensitivity to pain. Doses greater than 10 mg result in a drastic drop in blood pressure, coma, muscular rigidity, violent outbursts, and possible convulsions and death.

Psychologically, PCP may produce either euphoria or dysphoria. It is also known to produce hallucinations as well as delusions and overall delirium. Some users experience a prolonged state of "nothingness." The long-term effects of PCP use are unknown.

Ketamine The liquid form of *ketamine* ("Special K") is used as an anesthetic in some hospital and veterinary clinics. After stealing it from hospitals or medical suppliers, dealers typically dry the liquid (usually by cooking it) and grind the residue into powder. Special K causes hallucinations, as it inhibits the relay of sensory input; the brain fills the resulting void with visions, dreams, memories, and sensory distortions. The effects of ketamine are similar to those of PCP—confusion, agitation, aggression, and lack of coordination—but even less predictable. The aftereffects of Special K are less severe than those of Ecstasy, so it has grown in popularity as a club drug.

Inhalants

Inhalants are chemicals whose vapors, when inhaled, can cause hallucinations and create intoxicating and euphoric effects. Not commonly recognized as drugs, inhalants are legal to purchase and widely available, but dangerous. They generally appeal to young people who can't afford or obtain illicit substances. Some misused products include rubber cement, model glue, paint thinner, aerosol sprays, lighter fluid, varnish, wax, spot removers, and gasoline. Most of these substances are sniffed or "huffed" by users in search of a quick, cheap high.

Because they are inhaled, the volatile chemicals in these products reach the bloodstream and then the brain within seconds. This characteristic, along with the fact that dosages are extremely difficult to control because everyone has unique lung and breathing capacities, makes inhalants particularly dangerous. The effects of inhalants usually last for fewer than 15 minutes and resemble those of central nervous system depressants: dizziness, disorientation, impaired coordination, reduced judgment, and slowed reaction times. Combining inhalants with alcohol produces a synergistic effect and can cause severe and sometimes fatal liver damage. An overdose of fumes from inhalants can cause unconsciousness. If the user's oxygen intake is reduced during the inhaling process, death can result within 5 minutes. Sudden sniffing death (SSD) syndrome can be a fatal consequence, whether it's the user's first time or not. This syndrome can occur if a user inhales deeply and then participates in physical activity or is startled.

inhalants Products that are sniffed or inhaled in order to produce highs.

Amyl Nitrite Sometimes called "poppers" or "rush," *amyl nitrite* is packaged in small, cloth-covered glass capsules that can be crushed to release the active chemical for the user to inhale. The drug is often prescribed to alleviate chest pain in heart patients because it dilates small blood vessels and reduces blood pressure. Dilation of blood vessels in the genital area is

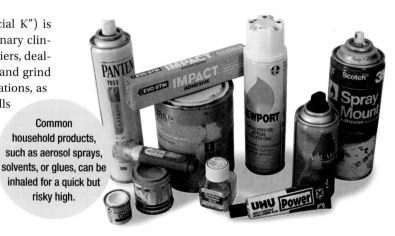

Common household products, such as aerosol sprays, solvents, or glues, can be inhaled for a quick but risky high.

thought to enhance sensations or perceptions of orgasm. It also produces fainting, dizziness, warmth, and skin flushing.

Nitrous Oxide *Nitrous oxide* is sometimes used as dental or minor surgical anesthesia. It is also a propellant chemical in aerosol products such as whipped toppings. Users who inhale nitrous oxide experience a state of euphoria, floating sensations, and illusions. Effects also include pain relief and a silly feeling (hence its nickname "laughing gas"). Regulating dosages of this drug can be difficult. Sustained inhalation can lead to unconsciousness, coma, and death.

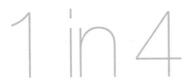

Americans who began using any addictive substance before age 18 are addicted, compared to 1 in 25 Americans who started using at age 21 or older.

Anabolic Steroids

Anabolic steroids are artificial forms of the male hormone testosterone that promote muscle growth and strength. Steroids are available in two forms: injectable solutions and pills. These **ergogenic drugs** are used primarily by people who believe the drugs will increase their strength, power, bulk (weight), speed, and athletic performance.

It was once estimated that approximately 17 to 20 percent of college athletes used steroids. Now that stricter drug-testing policies have been instituted by the National Collegiate Athletic Association (NCAA), reported use of anabolic steroids among intercollegiate athletes has decreased. Currently, less than half of 1 percent of college athletes surveyed report use of anabolic steroids within the past 12 months. Those who report using anabolic steroids use them less than once per week. Of those, half reported their first experience with anabolic steroids occurred after the age of 18.[53] The use of anabolic steroids on the college campus is very low; approximately 1 percent report using them within the past 30 days. However, the perception of anabolic steroid use on the college campus is much higher, with 32 percent of students perceiving their classmates had used anabolic steroids in the past 30 days.[54] Little data exist on the extent of steroid abuse by adults. It has been estimated that approximately 1 million adults have used anabolic steroids.[55] Among both adolescents and adults, steroid abuse is higher among men than it is among women. However, steroid abuse is growing most rapidly among young women.[56]

anabolic steroids Artificial forms of the hormone testosterone that promote muscle growth and strength.

ergogenic drug Substance believed to enhance athletic performance.

Physical Effects of Steroids Anabolic steroids produce a state of euphoria, diminished fatigue, and increased bulk and power in both sexes. These characteristics give steroids an addictive quality. When users stop, they can experience

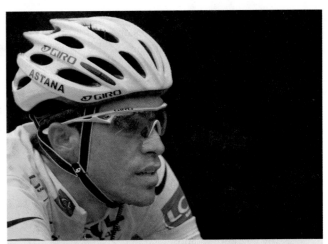

Cyclist Alberto Contador was suspended from the Tour de France for 2 years and stripped of 2010 victory after testing positive for performance-enhancing drug use.

psychological withdrawal and sometimes severe depression, in some cases leading to suicide attempts. If untreated, depression associated with steroid withdrawal has been known to last for a year or more after steroid use stops.

Men and women who use steroids experience a variety of adverse effects, including mood swings (aggression and violence, sometimes known as "roid rage"); acne; liver tumors; elevated cholesterol levels; hypertension; kidney disease; and immune system disturbances. There is also a danger of transmitting HIV and hepatitis through shared needles. In women, large doses of anabolic steroids may trigger the development of masculine attributes such as deeper voice, increased facial and body hair, and male pattern baldness; they may also result in an enlarged clitoris, smaller breasts, and changes in or absence of menstruation. When taken by healthy males, anabolic steroids shut down the body's production of testosterone, causing men's breasts to grow and testicles to atrophy.

Steroid Use and Society The Anabolic Steroids Control Act (ASCA) of 1990 makes it a crime to possess, prescribe, or distribute anabolic steroids for any use other than the treatment of specific diseases. Penalties for their illegal use include up to 5 years' imprisonment and a $250,000 fine for the first offense and up to 10 years' imprisonment and a $500,000 fine for subsequent offenses.

In recent years, high-profile athletes in sports such as cycling, track and field, swimming, and baseball have garnered media attention for suspected use of steroids or other banned performance-enhancing drugs.

what do you think?

Do you believe an athlete's admission of steroid use invalidates his or her athletic achievements?

● How do you think professional athletes who have used steroids or other performance enhancers should be disciplined?

● If you are an athlete, have you ever considered using some type of ergogenic aid to improve your performance?

Treatment and Recovery

An estimated 23.5 million Americans age 12 or older needed treatment for an illicit drug or alcohol use problem in 2010. Of these, only 2.6 million—approximately 11 percent—received treatment.[57] The most difficult step in the recovery process is for the substance abuser to admit that he or she is an addict. This can be difficult because of the power of *denial*—the inability to see the truth. Denial is the hallmark of addiction. It can be so powerful that a planned intervention is sometimes necessary to break down the addict's defenses against recognizing the problem.

Recovery from drug addiction is a long-term process and frequently requires multiple episodes of treatment. The first step generally begins with abstinence—refraining from using. **Detoxification** refers to the early abstinence period during which an addict adjusts physically and cognitively to being free from the substance's influence. It occurs in virtually every recovering addict. Detoxification is uncomfortable and can be dangerous. For some addicts, early abstinence may involve profound withdrawal that requires medical supervision. Because of this, most inpatient treatment programs provide a pretreatment component of supervised detoxification to achieve abstinence safely before further treatment begins.

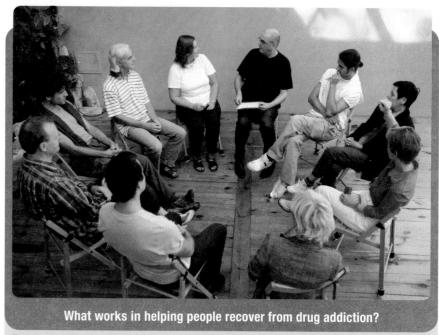

What works in helping people recover from drug addiction?

For most addicts, recovery is a long, difficult progress—for some people it can be a lifelong journey. Treatment and recovery for drug addiction usually begins with a period of detoxification, which may involve intense physical and psychological withdrawal symptoms. Once the body has adjusted to being without the drug, the addict usually enters behavioral or cognitive therapy to learn how to cope without the drug and avoid relapse. Therapy often takes the form of group meetings, such as those held by 12-step programs, for example Narcotics Anonymous.

Treatment Approaches

Outpatient behavioral treatment encompasses a variety of programs for addicts who visit a clinic at regular intervals. Most of the programs involve individual or group drug counseling. *Residential treatment programs* can also be very effective, especially for those with more severe problems. For example, therapeutic communities (TCs) are highly structured programs in which addicts remain at a residence, typically for 6 to 12 months. The focus of the TC is on the resocialization of the addict to a drug-free lifestyle.

12-Step Programs The first 12-step program was Alcoholics Anonymous (AA), begun in 1935 in Akron, Ohio. The 12-step program has since become the most widely used approach to dealing not only with alcoholism, but also with drug abuse and other dysfunctional behaviors. There are more than 200 different recovery programs based on the concept, including Narcotics Anonymous, Cocaine Anonymous, Crystal Meth Anonymous, Gamblers Anonymous, and Pills Anonymous.

The 12-step program is nonjudgmental and based on the idea that a program's only purpose is to work on personal recovery. Working the 12 steps involves admitting to having a serious problem, recognizing there is an outside power that could help, consciously relying on that power, admitting and listing character defects, seeking deliverance from defects, apologizing to those individuals one has harmed in the past, and helping others with the same problem. The 12-step meetings are held at a variety of times and locations in almost every city. There is no membership cost, and the meetings are open to anyone who wishes to attend.

Vaccines against Addictive Drugs A promising new cocaine vaccine is in development. The vaccine does not eliminate the desire for cocaine; instead, it keeps the user from getting high by stimulating the immune system to attack the drug when it's taken. Clinical human trials are expected to begin soon.

Vaccines against nicotine, heroin, and methamphetamine are also in development.

detoxification The early abstinence period during which an addict adjusts physically and cognitively to being free from the substance's influence.

College Students' Treatment and Recovery

For college students who have developed substance or behavioral addictions, early intervention increases the likelihood of successful treatment and completion of a college education. Depending on the severity of the problem, college students undergoing drug treatment may be required to spend time away from school in a residential drug rehabilitation (rehab) inpatient facility. The needs of college students seeking drug treatment in rehab do not differ greatly from other adult recovering addicts, but for best results, the community of addicts should include others of a similar age and educational background. Private therapy, group therapy, cognitive training, nutrition counseling, and health therapies can all help with recovery.

A growing number of colleges and universities offer "recovery communities" to students who are recovering from alcohol and other drug addiction and want to stay in school without being exposed to excessive drinking or drug use. Students can get specialized counseling and support that is not typically provided on a college campus.

For instance, at Kennesaw State's 4-year-old program, students first enter the Center for Young Adult Addiction and Recovery, where staff specializing in addiction treatment use clinical techniques such as motivational interviewing to support the social and academic success of students while they abstain from substance use. After students have been sober for 6 months, they enter the center's Collegiate Recovery Community, which includes weekly meetings and seminars on relapse prevention and community building and meetings with academic advisers.

A scholarship may be available for students who have a 3.0 grade point average and participate in the "peer community." Recovering students are trained to go back into the classroom and educate their peers who are most at risk of developing substance abuse problems, such as fraternity and sorority members and incoming freshmen.[58]

Another campus, Texas Tech University, received a federal grant to create a national model of its students-in-recovery program. The program offers scholarships to students in recovery, as well as on-campus 12-step meetings and academic support.[59]

Addressing Drug Misuse and Abuse in the United States

Stories of people who have tried illegal drugs may tempt you to try them yourself. You may convince yourself that one-time use is harmless. Given the dangers surrounding these substances, however, you should think twice. The

risks associated with drug use extend beyond the personal. The decision to try any illicit substance supports illicit drug manufacture and transport, thus contributing to the national drug problem.

Illegal drug use in the United States costs about $193 billion per year.[60] This estimate includes costs associated with treatment and prevention, health care, reduced job productivity and lost earnings, and social consequences such as crime and social welfare. In addition, roughly half of all expenditures to combat crime are related to illegal drugs. The burden of these costs is absorbed primarily by the government (46%), followed by people who abuse drugs and members of their households (44%).[61]

10 million

people reported driving under the influence of illicit drugs in the past year.

Drugs in the Workplace

According to the National Survey on Drug Use and Health, 50 percent of all U.S. workers who use illicit drugs are employed full time.[62] With such a large segment of drug users employed to some degree, the cost to American businesses soars into the billions of dollars. These costs reflect reduced work performance and efficiency, lost productivity, absenteeism, and turnover. Not surprisingly, it is estimated that the annual economic impact of illicit drug use is $128.6 billion in lost productivity alone.[63]

Many companies have instituted drug testing for their employees. Mandatory drug urinalysis is controversial. Critics argue that such testing violates Fourth Amendment rights of protection from unreasonable search and seizure. Proponents believe the personal inconvenience entailed in testing pales in comparison to the problems caused by drug use in the workplace.

Drug testing is expensive, with costs running as high as $100 per test. Moreover, some critics question the accuracy and reliability of the results. Both false positives and false negatives can occur. Despite the controversy, drug testing is becoming more common in the work environment. For more information on drug testing, see the **Tech & Health** box on the following page.

> **what do you think?**
> What do you believe are the moral and ethical issues surrounding drug testing of employees?
> ● Are you in favor of drug testing?
> ● Should employers have the right to conduct drug testing at the worksite?

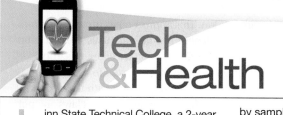

Tech & Health | TYPES OF DRUG TESTS

Linn State Technical College, a 2-year public institution, made the news in 2011 when it implemented a mandatory drug testing program for all students. The policy was later ruled to be a violation of students' right to privacy. But beyond the campus, drug testing is an ever-more-common condition of many employers.

There are many drug-test options. Each has strengths and weaknesses associated with it.

URINE TESTS

Urine tests are the least expensive test method, with costs varying between $7 and $50 for the home versions. They can be conducted anywhere, but labs must verify results. Urine tests are best at detecting drug use within the past week, although if someone uses a drug over a long period of time the ability of urine tests to detect it outside that effective window increases. There are some problems with this test: Many find giving a urine sample to be embarrassing and intrusive, and if drug users know the date of an upcoming urine test they can abstain for a short period of time to get a clean result and then go back to using afterward.

SALIVA TESTS

At $15 to $75 per test, saliva tests are easy to administer, and they are not seen by sample givers to be as much of a violation of privacy as urine tests often are. Like urine tests, they can be done at any location, but results must be verified by a lab. Saliva tests are growing in popularity and can detect more recent drug use than other testing methods, especially use in the past few days. They are good at detecting methamphetamine and opiates, but less reliable for THC and cannabinoids found in marijuana.

HAIR TESTS

Hair and follicle tests cost about $100 to $150 to perform. They cost more than saliva or urine tests, but they can give information on a person's drug use for the past 90 days rather than for just a few days or weeks. These tests have a positive result a little more than twice as often as urine tests. Hair tests also do not have as many false positives for certain substances, such as poppy seed ingestion versus opiate abuse. The tests are also difficult to "game," since shampoos and other follicle-cleansing products have not been shown to reliably remove drug metabolites from hair.

Opiates (codeine, morphine, heroin) lay down on the hair shaft very tightly and are shown not to migrate along the shaft; thus, if a long segment of hair is available, one can draw some "relative" conclusions about when the use occurred. However, cocaine, although very easy to detect, is able to migrate along the shaft, making it very difficult to determine when the drug was used and for how long.

A drawback to the test is that these tests are not good at detecting very recent use, such as in the past week. While hair tests are not considered to be as much of an intrusion of privacy as urine tests, the amount of hair required for a sample is about the diameter of a pencil and 1.5 inches long.

BLOOD TESTS

Blood tests are the most expensive type of testing, and they are therefore the type least frequently used. They are considered the most intrusive method of testing, but also the most accurate. The detection period is small—just hours or days, depending on the substance.

Sources: N. Koppel, "Suit Claims Public College's Drug Testing Policy is Unconstitutional," *The Wall Street Journal*, September 15, 2011, http://blogs.wsj.com/law/2011/09/15/suit-claims-public-colleges-drug-testing-policy-is-unconstitutional/; The Vaults of EROWID, "Drug Testing Basics," www.erowid.org/psychoactives/testing/testing_info1.shtml.

Preventing Drug Use and Abuse on Campus

Strategies that universities should consider to reduce the number of students who become involved in substance use include the following:

- Changing student expectations that college is a time to party and experiment with drugs
- Engaging parents about substance use on campus and encouraging them to continue open communication with their children
- Identifying high-risk students through early detection screening programs
- Providing services such as treatment programs specifically tailored for students

Most anti-drug programs have not been effective because they have focused on only one aspect of drug abuse rather than examining all factors that contribute to the problem. The pressure to take drugs is often tremendous, and the reasons for using them are complex. People who develop drug problems generally believe they can control their drug use when they start out. Initially, they view taking drugs as a fun and manageable pastime. However, since most illegal drugs and many prescription drugs produce physical and psychological dependency, it is unrealistic to think that a person can use them regularly without becoming addicted. Peer influence is

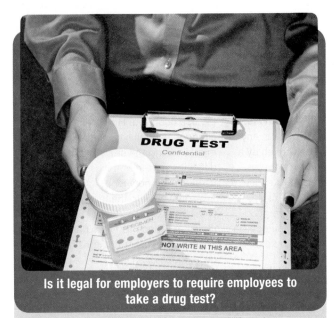

Is it legal for employers to require employees to take a drug test?

Several court decisions have affirmed the right of employers to test their employees for drug use. They contend that Fourth Amendment rights pertain only to employees of government agencies, not to those of private businesses. Most Americans apparently support drug testing for certain types of jobs.

also a strong motivator, especially among adolescents, who fear not being accepted as part of the group.

Possible Solutions to the Drug Problem

Americans are alarmed by the increasing use of illegal drugs. Respondents in public opinion polls feel that the most important strategy for fighting drug abuse is educating young people. They also endorse strategies such as the following:

- Stricter border surveillance to reduce drug trafficking
- Longer prison sentences for drug dealers
- Increased government spending on prevention
- Enforcing anti-drug laws
- Greater cooperation between government agencies and private groups and individuals providing treatment assistance

All of these approaches will probably help, but they do not offer a total solution to the problem. Drug abuse has been a part of human behavior for thousands of years, and it is not likely to disappear in the near future. For this reason, it is necessary to educate ourselves and develop the self-discipline necessary to avoid dangerous drug dependence.

For many years, the most popular anti-drug strategy

what do you think?

What is the attitude toward drug use on your campus?

- Are some substances considered more acceptable than others?
- Is drug use considered acceptable at certain times or occasions?

has been total prohibition. This approach has proved to be ineffective. Prohibition of alcohol during the 1920s created more problems than it solved, as did prohibition of opioids in 1914. A more recent campaign is commonly referred to as the "War on Drugs," undertaken by the U.S. government with the assistance of participating countries. This campaign includes laws and policies that are intended to reduce the illegal drug trade and discourage the production, distribution, and consumption of illicit substances.

In general, researchers in the field of drug education agree that a multimodal approach is best. Students should be taught the difference between drug use, misuse, and abuse. Factual information must be presented without scare tactics; lecturing and moralizing have proved not to work.

Harm Reduction Strategies Harm reduction is a set of practical approaches to reducing negative consequences of drug use, incorporating a spectrum of strategies from safer use to managed use to abstinence. For example, needle exchange programs for injection drug users provide clean needles and syringes and bleach for cleaning needles; these efforts help reduce the number of cases of HIV and hepatitis B. Harm reduction may involve changing the legal sanctions associated with drug use, increasing the availability of treatment services to drug abusers, and attempting to change drug users' behavior through education. Harm reduction strategies meet drug users "where they're at," addressing conditions of use along with the use itself. This strategy recognizes that people always have and always will use drugs and, therefore, attempts to minimize the potential hazards associated with drug use rather than the use itself.

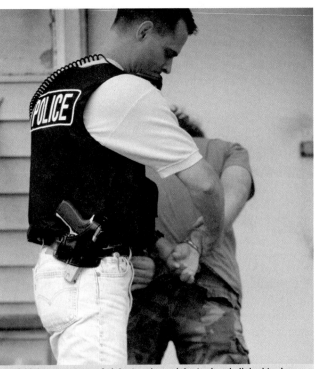

A high percentage of violent and nonviolent crime is linked to drug abuse, affecting not only the abuser, but also entire communities.

Learn to Recognize Drug Use and Potential Abuse

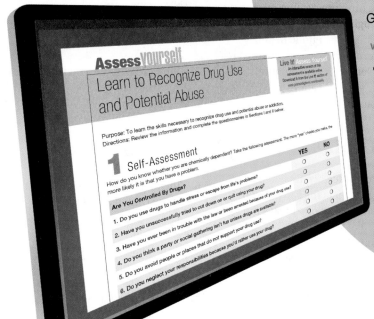

Assess Yourself

Learn to Recognize Drug Use and Potential Abuse

Live It! Assess Yourself
An interactive version of the assessment is available online. Download it from the Live It! section of www.pearsonhighered.com/donatelle.

Purpose: To learn the skills necessary to recognize drug use and potential abuse or addiction.
Directions: Review the information and complete the questionnaires in Sections I and I below.

1 Self-Assessment

	YES	NO
How do you know whether you are chemically dependent? Take the following assessment. The more "yes" checks you make, the more likely it is that you have a problem.		
Are You Controlled By Drugs?		
1. Do you use drugs to handle stress or escape from life's problems?	○	○
2. Have you unsuccessfully tried to cut down on or quit using your drug?	○	○
3. Have you ever been in trouble with the law or been arrested because of your drug use?	○	○
4. Do you think a party or social gathering isn't fun unless drugs are available?	○	○
5. Do you avoid people or places that do not support your drug use?	○	○
6. Do you neglect your responsibilities because you'd rather use your drug?	○	

Go online to the **Live It!** section of www.pearsonhighered.com/donatelle to take the "Learn to Recognize Drug Use and Potential Abuse" assessment.* Use the strategies outlined in the **YOUR PLAN FOR CHANGE** box to help you change your behavior.

*If your instructor so chooses, Assess Yourself Activities are available as a printed supplement or as assignable homework online at www.pearsonhighered.com/myhealthlab.

MyHealthLab®

YOUR PLAN FOR **CHANGE**

The **Assess Yourself** activity describes signs of being controlled by drugs or by a drug user. Depending on your results, you may need to change certain behaviors that may be detrimental to your health.

Today, you can:
○ Imagine a situation in which someone offers you a drug and think of several different ways of refusing. Rehearse these scenarios in your head.
○ Stop by your campus health center to find out about drug treatment programs or support groups they may have.

Within the next 2 weeks, you can:
○ Think about the drug use patterns among your social group. Are you ever uncomfortable with these people because of their drug use? Is it difficult to avoid using drugs when you are with them? If you answered yes, begin exploring ways to expand your social circle.
○ If you are concerned about your own drug use or the drug use of a close friend, make an appointment with a counselor to talk about the issue.

By the end of the semester, you can:
○ Participate in clubs, activities, and social groups that do not rely on substance abuse for their amusement.
○ If you have a drug problem, make a commitment to enter a treatment program. Acknowledge that you have a problem and that you need the assistance of others to help you overcome it.

Summary

∗ Mood-altering substances and experiences produce biochemical reactions that make the body feel good; when absent, the person feels the effects of withdrawal.

∗ The six categories of drugs are prescription drugs, over-the-counter (OTC) drugs, recreational drugs, herbal preparations, illicit drugs, and commercial preparations. Routes of administration include oral ingestion, inhalation, injection (intravenous, intramuscular, and subcutaneous), transdermal, and insertion of suppositories.

∗ Drugs of abuse (both legal and illegal) include stimulants, cannabis products including marijuana, narcotics/depressants, hallucinogens, inhalants, and anabolic steroids. Each has its own set of risks and effects.

∗ Over-the-counter medications do not require a prescription. Some OTC medications, including sleep aids, cold medicines, and diet pills, can be addictive.

∗ Prescription drug abuse is at an all-time high, particularly among college students. Only marijuana is more commonly abused. The most commonly abused prescription drugs are opioids/narcotics, depressants, and stimulants.

∗ People from all walks of life use illicit drugs, although college students report higher usage rates than do the general population. Drug use declined from the mid-1980s to the early 1990s but has remained steady since then. However, among young people, use of drugs has been rising in recent years.

∗ Treatment begins with abstinence from the drug or addictive behavior, usually instituted through intervention by close family, friends, or other loved ones. Treatment programs may include individual, group, or family therapy, as well as 12-step programs.

∗ The drug problem reaches everyone through crime and elevated health care costs. Public health and governmental approaches to the problem involve regulation, enforcement, education, and harm reduction.

Pop Quiz

1. Cross-tolerance occurs when
   a. drugs work at the same receptor site so that one blocks the action of the other.
   b. the effects of one drug are eliminated or reduced by the presence of another drug at the receptor site.
   c. a person develops a physiological tolerance to one drug and shows a similar tolerance to selected other drugs as a result.
   d. two or more drugs interact and the effects of the individual drugs are multiplied beyond what normally would be expected if they were taken alone.

2. Rebecca takes a number of medications for various conditions, including Prinivil (for high blood pressure), insulin (a diabetic medication), and Claritin (an antihistamine). This is an example of
   a. synergism.
   b. illegal drug use.
   c. polydrug use.
   d. antagonism.

3. The most commonly reported illicit drug used on college campus is
   a. Adderall.
   b. marijuana.
   c. Ecstasy.
   d. tranquilizers.

4. The most common method of injection among drug abusers is
   a. intramuscular.
   b. intravenous.
   c. subcutaneous.
   d. none of the above

5. The most common method for taking drugs is
   a. injection.
   b. inhalation.
   c. oral ingestion.
   d. transdermal.

6. The most widely used illegal drug in the United States is
   a. alcohol.
   b. heroin.
   c. marijuana.
   d. methamphetamine.

7. Which of the following is classified as a stimulant drug?
   a. Amphetamines
   b. Alcohol
   c. Marijuana
   d. LSD

8. *Freebasing* is
   a. mixing cocaine with heroin.
   b. burning heroin and inhaling the vapor.
   c. injecting a drug into the veins.
   d. burning cocaine and inhaling the vapor.

9. Heroin dependence can result in all of the following *except*
   a. blood veins scar and eventually collapse.
   b. HIV.
   c. enhanced sexual performance.
   d. severe symptoms of withdrawal.

10. The psychoactive drug mescaline is found in what plant?
    a. Mushrooms
    b. Peyote cactus
    c. Marijuana
    d. Belladona

Answers to these questions can be found on page A-1.

Think about It!

1. Explain the terms *synergism, antagonism,* and *inhibition.*

2. Do you think there is such a thing as responsible use of illicit drugs? Would you change any of the current laws governing drugs? How would you determine what is legitimate and illegitimate use?

3. What are the arguments for and against drug testing in the workplace? Would you apply for a job that had drug testing as an interview requirement? Why or why not?

4. Why do you think so many young people today are abusing prescription drugs? Do you perceive prescription drug abuse as being less dangerous or illegal than illicit drug use? Why? Do you think this is an accurate or biased perception?

5. What types of programs do you think would be effective in preventing drug abuse among high school and college students? How might programs for high school students differ from those for college students?

6. What could you do to help a friend who is fighting a substance abuse problem? What resources on your campus could help you?

Accessing Your Health on the Internet

The following websites explore further topics and issues related to personal health. For links to the websites below, visit the Companion Website for *Access to Health,* 13th Edition, at www.pearsonhighered.com/donatelle.

1. *Club Drugs.* The website provides science-based information about club drugs.
   www.drugabuse.gov/drugs-abuse/club-drugs

2. *Join Together.* This excellent site has the most current information related to substance abuse. It also includes information on alcohol and drug policy and provides advice on organizing and taking political action.
   www.drugfree.org/join-together

3. *National Institute on Drug Abuse (NIDA).* The home page of this U.S. government agency has information on the latest statistics and findings in drug research. www.nida.nih.gov

4. *Substance Abuse and Mental Health Services Administration (SAMHSA).* This website is an outstanding resource for information about national surveys, ongoing research, and national drug interventions.
   www.samhsa.gov

References

1. Substance Abuse and Mental Health Services Administration, *Results from the 2009 National Survey on Drug Use and Health: Volume I. Summary of National Findings,* Office of Applied Studies, NSDUH Series H-38A, HHS Publication No. SMA 10-4856 Findings, (Rockville, MD: Substance Abuse and Mental Health Services Administration, 2010).

2. National Drug Intelligence Center, "National Drug Threat Assessment 2010," 2010, www.justice.gov/ndic/pubs38/38661/drugImpact.htm; Centers for Disease Control and Prevention, "CDC Statement Regarding the Misuse of Prescription Drugs," June 2010, www.cdc.gov/media/pressrel/2010/s100603.htm.

3. National Institute of Drug Abuse, Drug Abuse at Highest Level in Nearly a Decade, NIDA Notes 23:3, 2010, www.nida.nih.gov/NIDA_notes/NNvol23N3/tearoff.html.

4. The National Center on Addiction and Substance Abuse at Columbia University, "Adolescent Substance Use: America's #1 Public Health Problem," June 2011, www.casacolumbia.org/upload/2011/2011062 9adolescentsubstanceuse.pdf.

5. U.S. Food and Drug Administration, "Drugs: Over-the Counter-Medications: What Is Right for You?" www.fda.gov/Drugs/ResourcesForYou/Consumers/BuyingUsingMedicineSafely/UnderstandingOver-the-CounterMedicines/Choosingtherightover-the-counter medicineOTCs/ucm150299.htm.

6. Consumer Healthcare Products Association, *OTC Medicines Serve an Important Health Care Need,* 2009, www.chpa-info.org/media/resources/r_4862.pdf.

7. L. D. Johnston et al., *Monitoring the Future National Survey Results on Drug Use, 1975–2010: Volume I, Secondary School Students* (Ann Arbor: Institute for Social Research, The University of Michigan, 2011).

8. Erowid, The DXM Vault, 2011, www.erowid.org/chemicals/dxm/dxm.shtml.

9. U.S. Food and Drug Administration, "Legal Requirements for the Sale and Purchase of Drug Products Containing Pseudoephedrine, Ephedrine, and Phenylpropanolamine," Updated July 2009, www.fda.gov/Drugs/DrugSafety/InformationbyDrugClass/ucm072423.htm.

10. National Youth Anti-Drug Media Campaign, "Prescription Drug (Rx) Abuse," 2010, www.theantidrug.com/drug-information/otc-prescription-drug-abuse/prescription-drug-rx-abuse/default.aspx.

11. Substance Abuse and Mental Health Services Administration, *Results from the 2010 National Survey on Drug Use and Health: Summary of National Findings,* NSDUH Series H-41, HHS Publication No. (SMA) 11-4658 (Rockville, MD: Substance Abuse and Mental Health Services Administration, 2011).

12. Centers for Disease Control and Prevention, "Prescription Pain Killer Overdoses at Epidemic Levels," Press Release, November 1, 2011, Atlanta, GA.

13. National Association of School Nurses, "Educational Campaigns: Drugs of Abuse," 2010, www.nasn.org/Default.aspx?tabid=506.

14. Centers for Disease Control and Prevention, "Prescription Pain Killer Overdoses at Epidemic Levels2011.

15. American College Health Association, *American College Health Association–National College Health Assessment Spring 2011* (Baltimore: American College Health Association, 2012), Available at www.achancha.org/docs/ACHA-NCHA-II_ReferenceGroup_ExecutiveSummary_Spring2011.pdf.

16. J. L. McCauley et al., "Non-medical Use of Prescription Drugs in a National Sample of Women," *Addictive Behaviors,* 36 (2011): 690–95.

17. American College Health Association, *American College Health Association–National College Health Assessment Spring 2011,* 2012.

18. Ibid.

19. T. E. Wilens et al. "Misuse and Diversion of Stimulants Prescribed for ADHD: A Systematic Review of the Literature," *Journal of*

the American Academy of Child and Adolescent Psychiatry 47, no. 1, (2008): 21–31.

20. Substance Abuse and Mental Health Services Administration, *Results from the 2010 National Survey on Drug Use and Health: Volume I,* 2011.

21. L. D. Johnston et al., *Monitoring the Future National Survey Results on Drug Use, 1975–2010, Volume II, College Students and Adults Ages 19–50* (Ann Arbor, MI: Institute for Social Research, The University of Michigan, 2011).

22. L. D. Johnston et al., *Monitoring the Future National Survey Results on Drug Use, 1975–2008, Volume II, College Students and Adults Ages 19–50,* NIH Publication no. 09-7403 (Bethesda, MD: National Institute on Drug Abuse, 2009), Available at monitoringthefuture.org/pubs .html.

23. National Center on Addiction and Substance Abuse at Columbia University, *Wasting the Best and the Brightest: Substance Abuse at America's Colleges and Universities* (New York: National Center on Addiction and Substance Abuse at Columbia University, 2007), Available at www.casacolumbia.org/templates/ publications_reports.aspx.

24. Ibid.

25. L. D. Johnston et al., *Monitoring the Future National Survey Results on Drug Use, 1975–2010: Volume I, Secondary School Students,* 2011; Substance Abuse and Mental Health Services Administration, *Results from the 2010 National Survey on Drug Use and Health,* 2011.

26. American College Health Association, *American College Health Association–National College Health Assessment Spring 2011,* 2012.

27. Substance Abuse and Mental Health Services Administration, *Results from the 2010 National Survey on Drug Use and Health: Volume I,* 2011.

28. N. Volkow, "Bath Salts: Emerging and Dangerous Products," *National Institute on Drug Abuse,* February 2011, www .drugabuse.gov/about-nida/directors-page/messages-director/2011/02/bath-salts-emerging-dangerous-products.

29. S. Melton, "Bath Salts: An 'Ivory Wave' Epidemic?" *Medscape,* August 26, 2011, www.medscape.com.

30. Ibid.

31. D. Schardt, "Caffeine: The Good, the Bad, and the Maybe," *Nutrition Action Healthletter* (March 2008): 1–7, Available at http://cspinet.org/nah/archives.html.

32. Office of National Drug Control Policy, "Marijuana Facts and Figures," 2010, www.whitehousedrugpolicy.gov/drug-fact/marijuana/marijuana_ff.html.

33. Ibid.

34. U.S. Department of Health and Human Services, *Marijuana: Facts for Teens,* 2010, http://teens.drugabuse.gov/facts/ facts_mj2.php.

35. National Institute on Drug Abuse, *Research Report: Marijuana Abuse,* NIH Publication no. 05-3859, 2005, Available at www.drugabuse.gov/ResearchReports/Marijuana; National Institute on Drug Abuse, "NIDA InfoFacts: Drugged Driving," 2009, www.nida.nih.gov/info-facts/driving.html.

36. M. Asbridge et al., "Acute Cannabis Consumption and Motor Vehicle Collision Risk: Systematic Review of Observational Studies and Meta-analysis," *British Medical Journal* 344 (2012): 1–9.

37. National Highway Traffic Safety Administration, "Traffic Safety Facts: Results of the 2007 National Roadside Survey of Alcohol and Drug Use by Drivers," July 2009, www.nhstsa.gov.

38. National Institute on Drug Abuse, "NIDA InfoFacts: Marijuana," Revised July 2009, http://drugabuse.gov/infofacts/ marijuana.html.

39. J. R. Daling et al., "Association of Marijuana Use and the Incidence of Testicular Germ Cell Tumors," *Cancer* 115, no. 6 (2009): 1215–23.

40. Ibid.

41. W. Hall and L. Degenhardt, "Adverse Health Effects of Non-Medical Cannabis Use," *The Lancet* 374, no. 9698 (2009): 1383–91.

42. Substance Abuse and Mental Health Services Administration, *Results from the 2008 National Survey on Drug Use and Health: National Findings,* NSDUH Series H-36, HHS Publication no. SMA 09-4434 (Rockville, MD: Office of Applied Studies, 2009), Available at www.oas.samhsa.gov/ nsduh/2k8nsduh/2k8Results.cfm.

43. A. Norton, "A Hidden Effect of Marijuana Use: Findings on Sleep Give Clinicians an Opportunity to Discuss Marijuana's Harms," *Addiction Professional* (2011), http://findarticles.com/p/articles/ mi_m0QTQ/is_4_6/ai_n27947952/.

44. H. Marroun et al., "Intrauterine Cannabis Exposure Affects Fetal Growth Trajectories: The Generation R Study," *Journal of Child & Adolescent Psychiatry* 48, no. 12 (2009): 1173–81.

45. National Institutes of Health, National Institute on Drug Abuse, "InfoFacts: Spice," 2011.

46. National Institutes of Health, "InfoFacts: Spice," 2011; L. D. Johnston et al., *Monitoring the Future National Survey Results on Drug Use, 1975–2010: Volume I, Secondary School Students,* 2011.

47. National Institutes of Health, "InfoFacts: Spice," 2011.

48. National Institute on Drug Abuse, "NIDA InfoFacts: Club Drugs (GHB, Ketamine, and Rohypnol)," Revised July 2010, www .drugabuse.gov/infofacts/clubdrugs .html.

49. Substance Abuse and Mental Health Services Administration, *Results from the 2010 National Survey on Drug Use and Health: Volume I. Summary of National Findings,* 2011.

50. Ibid.

51. L. D. Johnston et al., *Monitoring the Future National Survey Results on Drug Use, 1975–2010: Volume I, Secondary School Students,* 2011.

52. National Institute on Drug Abuse, "NIDA InfoFacts: MDMA (Ecstasy)," Revised March 2010, www.drugabuse.gov/ infofacts/ecstasy.html.

53. The National Collegiate Athletic Association, "Substance Use: National Study of Substance Use Trends Among NCAA College Student-Athletes," 2012, Available at www.ncaapublications.com/product-downloads/SAHS09.pdf.

54. American College Health Association, *American College Health Association–National College Health Assessment,* Spring 2011, 2012.

55. Office of National Drug Control Policy, "Steroids Facts & Figures," 2010, www .whitehousedrugpolicy.gov/drugfact/ steroids/steroids_ff.html.

56. National Institute on Drug Abuse, NIDA for Teens, "Anabolic Steroids," 2010, http://teens.drugabuse.gov/drnida/ drnida_ster1.php.

57. National Institutes of Health, "NIDA InfoFacts: Treatment Statistics," National Institute on Drug Abuse, March 2011, www.nida.nih.gov; Substance Abuse and Mental Health Services Administration, *Results from the 2010 National Survey on Drug Use and Health: Volume I,* 2011.

58. A. Grasgreen, "Students in Recovery," *Inside Higher Education,* July 13, 2011, www.insidehighered .com/news/2011/07/13/student_ addiction_recovery_centers_

communities_form_higher_education_
association#ixzz1oq13UApD.

59. Texas Tech University, "The Center for
the Study of Addiction and Recovery,"
www.depts.ttu.edu/hs/csa/.

60. U.S. Department of Justice, "The Eco-
nomic Impact of Illicit Drug Use on
American Society," National Intelligence
Center, product no. 2011-Q0317-002,

April 2011, www.justice.gov/ndic/
pubs44/44731/44731p.pdf.

61. National Drug Intelligence Center,
"National Drug Threat Assessment,"
DOJ 2010-Q0317-001 (Washington, DC:
National Drug Intelligence Center, 2010),
Available at www.justice.gove/ndic/
pubs38/38661/index.htm.

62. Substance Abuse and Mental Health
Services Administration, *Results from the
2010 National Survey on Drug Use and
Health: Volume I*, 2011.

63. Butler Center for Research, *Research
Update: Substance Use in the Workplace*
(Center City, MN: Hazelden Foundation,
2009), Available at www.hazelden.org/
web/public/researchupdates.page.

14

Protecting against Infectious Diseases and Sexually Transmitted Infections

OBJECTIVES

* Explain how your immune system works to protect you, and what you can do to boost its effectiveness.

* Discuss actions that you can take to protect yourself from the most common infectious diseases.

* Describe the most common pathogens infecting humans today, particularly young adults, and the typical diseases caused by each.

* Explain the major emerging and resurgent diseases affecting humans globally; discuss why they are on the rise and what actions can reduce risks.

* Discuss antimicrobial resistance, why it occurs, and what we can do to reduce the prevalence of resistant pathogens.

* Discuss the various sexually transmitted infections, means of transmission, and actions that can prevent their spread.

* Discuss human immunodeficiency virus (HIV) and acquired immunodeficiency syndrome (AIDS), trends in infection and treatment, and the impact of HIV/AIDS on special populations.

417

Why are vaccinations important?

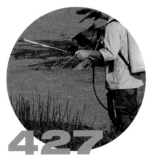

427

What can be done to prevent new diseases from emerging and spreading?

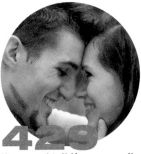

429

How can I tell if someone I'm dating has an STI?

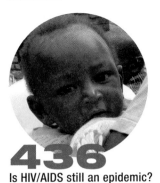

436

Is HIV/AIDS still an epidemic?

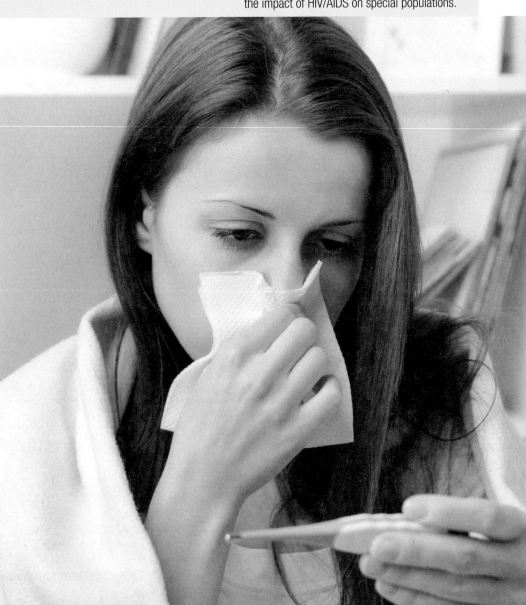

In 2009, when a new strain of killer flu, *H1N1,* became a global threat, healthy young adults seemed to be at greatest risk. Schools were closed, church services were canceled, and people feared the slightest cough or sneeze from others. At the same time, media reports of deaths in hospitals from a potent form of staph infection (methicillin-resistant *Staphylococcus aureus,* or MRSA) emerged. The effect of this media blitz about infectious disease caused people to fear for their safety in hospitals, wear masks in public, and avoid selected community settings. Today, worry over getting infected from others has prompted precautions such as elementary teachers sanitizing their students' hands after recess and grocery stores putting sanitary wipes next to their shopping carts. Is all of this anxiety over germs really necessary? What are the most ominous threats that we currently face? Who is at greatest risk? How can we protect ourselves and our loved ones? What policies, agencies, and programs are currently in place to protect us? The old adage is probably the best advice: "to be *forewarned* (knowledgeable) is to be *forearmed* (prepared)."

Disease-causing agents, called **pathogens,** are found in air and food and on nearly every object or person. We inhale them, swallow them, rub them in our eyes, and are constantly in a hidden, high-stakes battle with them, even as we sleep. Although many pathogens have existed as long as there has been life on the planet, new varieties of pathogens seem to be emerging daily. Historically, infectious diseases have always posed threats to life, wiping out whole groups of people through **epidemics** such as the Black Death, or bubonic plague, which killed up to one third of the population of Europe in the 1300s. A **pandemic,** or global epidemic, of influenza killed more than 20 million people in 1918, HIV and strains of tuberculosis and cholera continue to cause premature death throughout the world even today.

Despite constant bombardment by pathogens, our immune systems are remarkably adept at protecting us. Exposure to invading microorganisms actually helps us build resistance to various pathogens and teaches our immune systems to be more efficient. Millions of *endogenous micro-organisms* live in and on our bodies all the time, usually in a symbiotic, peaceful coexistence. These are generally harmless to someone in good health, but in sick people or those with weakened immune systems, these organisms can cause serious health problems.

Exogenous microorganisms are those that do not normally inhabit the body. When they do, they are apt to produce an infection or illness. The more easily these pathogens can gain a foothold in the body and sustain themselves, the more **virulent,** or aggressive, they may be in causing disease. By keeping your immune system strong, you increase your ability to resist and fight off even the most virulent pathogen.

The Process of Infection

Most diseases are **multifactorial:** They are caused by the interaction of several factors inside and outside the person.

For a disease to occur, the person, or *host,* must be *susceptible,* which means that the immune system must be in a weakened condition (**immunocompromised**); an *agent* capable of *transmitting* a disease must be present; and the *environment* must be *hospitable* to the pathogen in terms of temperature, light, moisture, and other requirements. Although all pathogens pose a threat if they gain entry and begin to grow in your body, the chances that they will do so are actually quite small.

Routes of Transmission

Pathogens enter the body in several ways. They may be transmitted by *direct contact* between infected persons, such as during sexual relations, kissing, or touching, or by *indirect contact,* such as by touching an object the infected person has had contact with. (**Table 14.1** lists common routes of transmission.) You may also **autoinoculate** yourself, or transmit a pathogen from one part of your body to another. For example, you may touch a herpes sore on your lip and transmit the virus to your eye when you scratch your itchy eyelid.

In addition to person-to-person transmission, your furry and feathered friends may also be sources of **zoonotic diseases**

pathogen A disease-causing agent.

epidemic Disease outbreak that affects many people in a community or region at the same time.

pandemic Global epidemic of a disease.

virulent Strong enough to overcome host resistance and cause disease.

multifactorial disease Disease caused by interactions of several factors.

immunocompromised Having an immune system that is impaired.

autoinoculate Transmit a pathogen from one part of your body to another part.

zoonotic diseases Diseases of animals that may be transmitted to humans.

TABLE

14.1 Routes of Disease Transmission

Mode of Transmission	Aspects of Transmission
Contact	Either *direct* (e.g., skin or sexual contact) or *indirect* (e.g., infected blood or body fluid)
Foodborne or waterborne	Eating or coming in contact with contaminated food or water, or products passed through them
Airborne	Inhalation; droplet-spread as through sneezing, coughing, or talking
Vectorborne	Vector-transmitted via secretions, biting, egg laying, as done by mosquitoes, ticks, snails, or birds
Perinatal	Similar to contact infection; happens in the uterus or as the baby passes through the birth canal, or through breast-feeding

or diseases of animals that may be transmitted to humans. Dogs, cats, livestock, and wild animals can spread numerous diseases through their body fluids, bites, or feces or by carrying infected insects or pathogens into living areas and transmitting diseases either directly or indirectly. Although *interspecies transmission* of diseases (diseases passed from humans to animals and vice versa) is rare, it does occur. The Centers for Disease Control and Prevention's (CDC's) National Center for Emerging and Zoonotic Infectious Diseases (www.cdc.gov/ncezid) provides an excellent up-to-date overview of these diseases.

Risk Factors You Can Control

With all these pathogens floating around, how can you be sure you don't get sick? Fortunately, there are some things you can avoid to reduce your risk. Too much stress, inadequate nutrition, a low fitness level, lack of sleep, misuse or abuse of legal and illegal drugs, poor personal hygiene, and high-risk behavior significantly increase the risk for many diseases. College students, in particular, often are at higher risk because of many of the above factors, in addition to the fact that alcohol and other drugs, increasing numbers of sexual experiences, and close living conditions all create higher risk for exposure to pathogens. There are things you can do to eliminate, reduce, or change your susceptibility to various pathogens. The **Skills for Behavior Change** box lists some actions you can take to keep your body's defenses in top form. There are also changes you can make in your community to clean up toxins, set policies on contaminant levels, and reduce the likelihood of being exposed to pathogens or toxins that could harm the immune system. The chain of infection between pathogen, environment, and host presents multiple opportunities for individuals and communities to intercede and "break the chain," preventing and controlling disease transmission; see **Figure 14.1** on page 413.

Risk Factors You Typically Cannot Control

Unfortunately, some of the factors that make you susceptible to a certain disease are either hard to control or completely beyond your control. The following are the most common:

- **Heredity.** Perhaps the single greatest factor influencing disease risk is genetics. It is often unclear whether hereditary diseases are due to inherited genetic traits or to inherited insufficiencies in the immune system. Some believe that we may inherit the quality of our immune system, so that some people are naturally "tougher" than others and more resistant to disease and infection.

- **Age.** People under age 5 and over age 65 are often more vulnerable to infectious diseases because body defenses that we take for granted are either not fully developed or

comorbidities The presence of one or more diseases at the same time.

opportunistic infections Infections that occur when the immune system is weakened or compromised.

Reduce Your Risk of Infectious Disease

❭ **Limit exposure to pathogens.** Don't drag yourself to classes or work and infect others when you are seriously ill. Also, don't share utensils or drinking glasses, and keep your toothbrush away from those of others. Wash your hands often and sneeze or cough into your arm or sleeve rather than your hands. Keep hands away from your mouth, nose, and eyes. Use disposable tissues rather than cloth, reusable handkerchiefs.

❭ **Exercise regularly.** Regular exercise raises core body temperature and kills pathogens. Sweat and oil make the skin a hostile environment for many bacteria. Avoid excessive exercise that could overtax the immune system.

❭ **Get enough sleep.** Sleep allows the body time to refresh itself, produce necessary cells, and reduce inflammation. Even a single night without sleep can increase inflammatory processes and delay wound healing.

❭ **Stress less.** Rest and relaxation, stress management practices, laughter, and calming music have all been shown to promote healthy cellular activity and bolster immune functioning.

❭ **Optimize eating.** Enjoy a healthy diet, including adequate amounts of water, protein, and complex carbohydrates. Eat more omega-3 fatty acids to reduce inflammation, and restrict saturated fats, replacing them with good fats such as olive oil. Antioxidants are believed to be important in immune functioning, so make sure you get your daily fruits and vegetables.

they are not as effective as they once were. Thinning of the skin, reduced sweating, and other physical changes can make the elderly more vulnerable to disease. In addition, as people age, certain **comorbidities** (diseases that occur at the same time) overwhelm the body's ability to ward off enemies and increase the risk of infection. In these situation, **opportunistic infections**, infections that normally cause disease only when the immune system is impaired, take over.

what do you think?

Do you have any risks for infectious disease that you were probably born with? Do you have any that are the result of your lifestyle?

● What actions can you take to reduce your risks?

● What behaviors do you or your friends engage in that might make you more susceptible to various infections?

● Are your risks greater today than before you entered college? Why or why not?

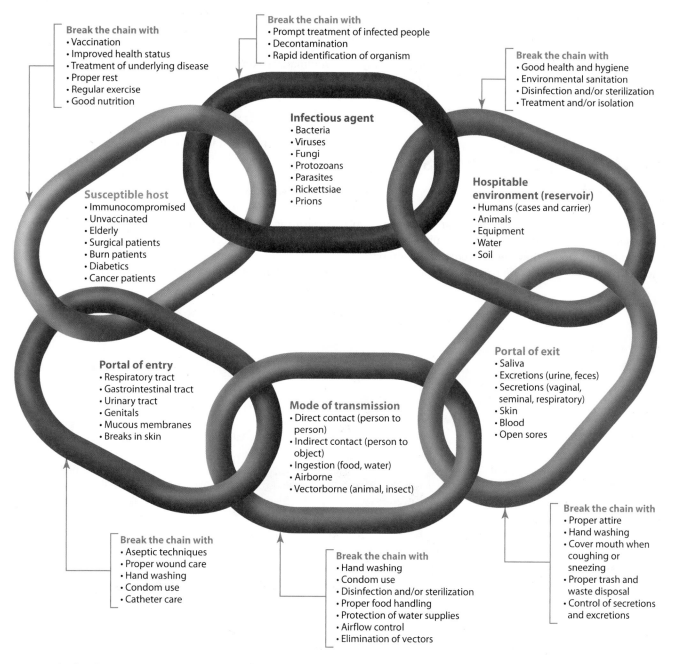

Break the chain with
• Vaccination
• Improved health status
• Treatment of underlying disease
• Proper rest
• Regular exercise
• Good nutrition

Break the chain with
• Prompt treatment of infected people
• Decontamination
• Rapid identification of organism

Break the chain with
• Good health and hygiene
• Environmental sanitation
• Disinfection and/or sterilization
• Treatment and/or isolation

Infectious agent
• Bacteria
• Viruses
• Fungi
• Protozoans
• Parasites
• Rickettsiae
• Prions

Susceptible host
• Immunocompromised
• Unvaccinated
• Elderly
• Surgical patients
• Burn patients
• Diabetics
• Cancer patients

Hospitable environment (reservoir)
• Humans (cases and carrier)
• Animals
• Equipment
• Water
• Soil

Portal of entry
• Respiratory tract
• Gastrointestinal tract
• Urinary tract
• Genitals
• Mucous membranes
• Breaks in skin

Mode of transmission
• Direct contact (person to person)
• Indirect contact (person to object)
• Ingestion (food, water)
• Airborne
• Vectorborne (animal, insect)

Portal of exit
• Saliva
• Excretions (urine, feces)
• Secretions (vaginal, seminal, respiratory)
• Skin
• Blood
• Open sores

Break the chain with
• Aseptic techniques
• Proper wound care
• Hand washing
• Condom use
• Catheter care

Break the chain with
• Hand washing
• Condom use
• Disinfection and/or sterilization
• Proper food handling
• Protection of water supplies
• Airflow control
• Elimination of vectors

Break the chain with
• Proper attire
• Hand washing
• Cover mouth when coughing or sneezing
• Proper trash and waste disposal
• Control of secretions and excretions

FIGURE 14.1 **The Chain of Infection**
The three key factors in transmission of an infectious disease are a susceptible host, an infectious agent, and a hospitable environment. Connecting these three factors are the portal of entry, mode of transmission, and portal of exit. Interfering with any of the links in the chain can prevent the transmission of infectious disease.

Video Tutor: Chain of Infection

● **Environmental conditions.** Unsanitary conditions and the presence of drugs, chemicals, and hazardous pollutants and wastes in food and water probably have a great effect on our immune systems. Also, a growing body of research points to climate change as a major contributor to infectious diseases. As temperatures rise, insect populations may increase; a rise in mosquito populations may increase the spread of malaria, for example. As water sources dry up in prolonged drought, those sources that remain are more likely to be contaminated. Birds and animals congregate more closely near scarce water sources, spreading diseases among themselves.[1] In addition, long-term exposure to toxic chemicals and catastrophic natural disasters such as earthquakes, floods, and tsunamis are believed to be significant contributors to increasing numbers of infectious diseases.[2]

● **Organism virulence and resistance.** Some organisms are particularly virulent, and even tiny amounts may make the most hardy of us ill. Other organisms have mutated and become resistant to the body's defenses and to medical treatments. Multidrug-resistant strains of tuberculosis, *Staphylococcus,* and other organisms are emerging in many parts of the world. See the **Be Healthy, Be Green** box on the next page for more on this topic.

Your Body's Defenses against Infection

Your body constantly protects against and defends from pathogens that could make you ill. For pathogens to gain entry into your body, they must overcome a number of effective safeguards: There are barriers that prevent pathogens from entering your body, mechanisms that weaken organisms that breach these barriers, and substances that counteract the threat that these organisms pose. Figure 14.2 summarizes some of the body's defenses that help protect against invasion and decrease susceptibility to disease.

Physical and Chemical Defenses

Our most critical first line of defense is also the largest organ in the body: the skin. Structured to provide an intricate web of physical and chemical barriers, the skin allows few pathogens to enter. When they do breech this barrier, *enzymes* in body secretions such as sweat provide additional protection, destroying microorganisms on skin surfaces by producing inhospitable pH levels.

In addition to early defenses, internal linings, structures, and secretions of the body provide another layer of protection.

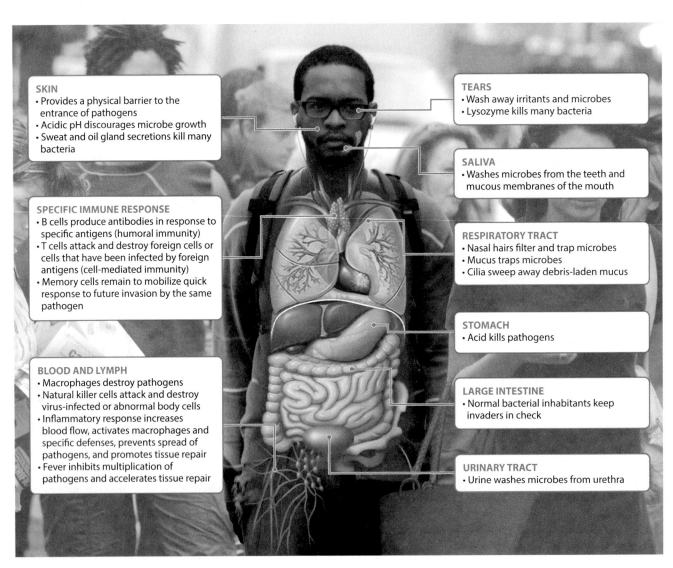

SKIN
- Provides a physical barrier to the entrance of pathogens
- Acidic pH discourages microbe growth
- Sweat and oil gland secretions kill many bacteria

SPECIFIC IMMUNE RESPONSE
- B cells produce antibodies in response to specific antigens (humoral immunity)
- T cells attack and destroy foreign cells or cells that have been infected by foreign antigens (cell-mediated immunity)
- Memory cells remain to mobilize quick response to future invasion by the same pathogen

BLOOD AND LYMPH
- Macrophages destroy pathogens
- Natural killer cells attack and destroy virus-infected or abnormal body cells
- Inflammatory response increases blood flow, activates macrophages and specific defenses, prevents spread of pathogens, and promotes tissue repair
- Fever inhibits multiplication of pathogens and accelerates tissue repair

TEARS
- Wash away irritants and microbes
- Lysozyme kills many bacteria

SALIVA
- Washes microbes from the teeth and mucous membranes of the mouth

RESPIRATORY TRACT
- Nasal hairs filter and trap microbes
- Mucus traps microbes
- Cilia sweep away debris-laden mucus

STOMACH
- Acid kills pathogens

LARGE INTESTINE
- Normal bacterial inhabitants keep invaders in check

URINARY TRACT
- Urine washes microbes from urethra

FIGURE 14.2 **The Body's Defenses against Disease-Causing Pathogens**
In addition to the defenses listed, many of the body's defensive secretions and fluids, such as earwax, tears, mucus, and blood, contain enzymes and other proteins that can kill some invading pathogens or prevent or slow their reproduction.

BE HEALTHY, BE GREEN

ANTIBIOTIC RESISTANCE: BUGS VERSUS DRUGS

Antibiotics are supposed to wipe out bacteria that are susceptible to them. However, many of our antibiotics are becoming ineffective against resistant strains. Bacteria and other microorganisms that cause infections and diseases evolve and develop ways to survive drugs that should kill or weaken them. This means that some of the bacteria and microorganisms are becoming "superbugs" that cannot be stopped with existing medications.

WHY IS ANTIBIOTIC RESISTANCE ON THE RISE?

✻ **Improper use of antibiotics and resulting growth of superbugs.** Bacteria adapt and mutate to bolster the traits that allow them to survive—in this case, drug resistance. But human negligence speeds the natural evolution of resistance greatly.

If patients stop taking a drug as soon as they start to feel better, rather than finishing the full course of antibiotics, then the surviving bacteria quickly build immunity to the drugs used to treat them. Doctors also overprescribe antibiotics: The Centers for Disease Control and Prevention (CDC) estimates that one third of the 150 million prescriptions written each year are unnecessary.

✻ **Overuse of antibiotics in food production.** About 70 percent of antibiotic production today is used to treat sick animals living in crowded feedlots and to encourage growth in livestock and poultry. Farmed fish may be given antibiotics to fight off disease in controlled water areas. Although research in this area is only in its infancy, many believe that ingesting meats, animal products, and fish full of antibiotics may contribute to antibiotic resistance in humans. In addition, water runoff and sewage from feedlots can contaminate the water in rivers and streams with antibiotics.

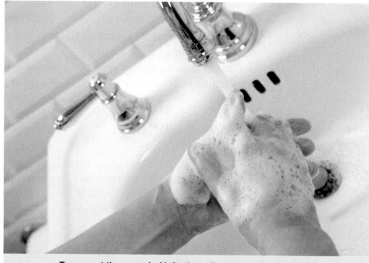

To prevent the spread of infectious disease, wash your hands!

✻ **Misuse and overuse of antibacterial soaps and other cleaning products.** Preying on the public's fear of germs and disease, the cleaning industry adds antibacterial ingredients to many of its dish soaps, hand cleaners, shower scrubs, surface scrubs, and most household products. Just how much these products contribute to overall resistance is difficult to assess; as with antibiotics, the germs these products do not kill may become stronger than before.

WHAT CAN YOU DO?

✻ **Be responsible with medications.** To help prevent antibiotic resistance, use antimicrobial drugs only for bacterial, not viral, infections. Take medications as prescribed and finish the full course. Consult with your health care provider if you feel it is necessary to stop your medication.

✻ **Use regular soap—not antibacterial soap—when washing your hands.** Some experts say that antibacterial cleaning products do more harm than good. Research suggests that antibacterial agents contained in soaps actually may kill normal bacteria, thus creating an environment for resistant, mutated bacteria that are impervious to antibacterial cleaners and antibiotics.

✻ **Avoid food treated with antibiotics.** Whenever possible buy meat from animals that were not dosed with antibiotics. (Look for that information on the label of meat products.)

Sources: Centers for Disease Control and Prevention, National Center for Emerging and Zoonotic Infectious Diseases, Division of Healthcare Quality Promotion, "Diseases/Pathogens Associated with Antimicrobial Resistance," Updated January, 2102, www.cdc.gov/drugresistance/Diseases ConnectedAR.html; Centers for DiseaseControl and Prevention, National Center for Immunization and Respiratory Diseases, Division of Bacterial Diseases, "Antibiotic Resistance Questions & Answers," Updated November 2011, www.cdc.gov/getsmart/antibiotic-use/anitbiotic-resistance-faqs.html; H. Boucher et al., "Bad Bugs, No Drugs: No ESKAPE! An Update from the Infectious Diseases Society of America," *Clinical Infectious Diseases* 48, no. 1 (2009): 1–12; Global Health Council, "The Impact of Infectious Diseases," 2010, www.globalhealth.org/infectious_diseases.

Sticky mucous membranes in the respiratory tract, for example, trap and engulf invading organisms. Cilia, hairlike projections in the lungs and respiratory tract, sweep invaders toward body openings, where they are expelled. Nose hairs trap airborne invaders with a sticky film. Tears, nasal secretions, earwax, and other secretions contain enzymes that destroy or neutralize pathogens. Pathogens that make it to the stomach are destroyed by stomach acids.

How the Immune System Works

As a second line of defense, the immune system is able to quickly identify "self" and recognize and destroy outside or foreign substances capable of causing disease known as **antigens.** *Immunity* is a condition of being able to resist a particular disease by counteracting the substance that produces the disease. An antigen can be a virus, a bacterium, a fungus, a parasite, a toxin, or a tissue or cell from another organism. The immune system has elaborate mechanisms for protecting you from invading microbes.

As soon as an antigen breaches the body's initial defenses, the body responds by forming substances called **antibodies** that are matched to that specific antigen, much as a key is matched to a lock. The body analyzes the antigen, considering the size and shape of the invader, verifies that the antigen is not part of the body itself, and then produces a specific antibody to destroy or weaken the antigen. This process, which is much more complex than described here, is part of a system called *humoral immune responses.* **Humoral immunity** is the body's major defense against many bacteria and the poisonous substances, called **toxins,** that they produce.

In **cell-mediated immunity,** specialized white blood cells called **lymphocytes** attack and destroy the foreign invader. Lymphocytes constitute the body's main defense against viruses, fungi, parasites, and some bacteria, and they are found in the blood, lymph nodes, bone marrow, and certain glands. Other key players

in this immune response are **macrophages** (a type of phagocytic, or cell-eating, white blood cell).

Two forms of lymphocytes in particular, the *B lymphocytes* (B cells) and *T lymphocytes* (T cells), are involved in the immune response. *Helper T cells* are essential for activating B cells to produce antibodies. They also activate other T cells and macrophages. Another form of T cell, known as the *killer T cell,* directly attacks infected or malignant cells. *Suppressor T cells* turn off or suppress the activity of B cells, killer T cells, and macrophages. After a successful attack on a pathogen, some of the attacker T and B cells are preserved as *memory T and B cells,* enabling the body to recognize and respond quickly to subsequent attacks by the same kind of organism at a later time.

Once people have survived certain infectious diseases, they become immune to those diseases, meaning that in all probability they will not develop them again. Upon subsequent attack by the same disease-causing microorganisms, their memory T and B cells are quickly activated to come to their defense. **Figure 14.3** provides a summary of the cell-mediated immune response.

When the Immune System Misfires: Autoimmune Diseases Although the immune response generally works in our favor, the body sometimes makes a mistake and targets

antigen Substance capable of triggering an immune response.

antibodies Substances produced by the body that are individually matched to specific antigens.

humoral immunity Aspect of immunity that is mediated by antibodies secreted by white blood cells.

toxins Poisonous substances produced by certain microorganisms that cause various diseases.

cell-mediated immunity Aspect of immunity that is mediated by specialized white blood cells that attack pathogens and antigens directly.

lymphocyte A type of white blood cell involved in the immune response.

macrophage A type of white blood cell that ingests foreign material.

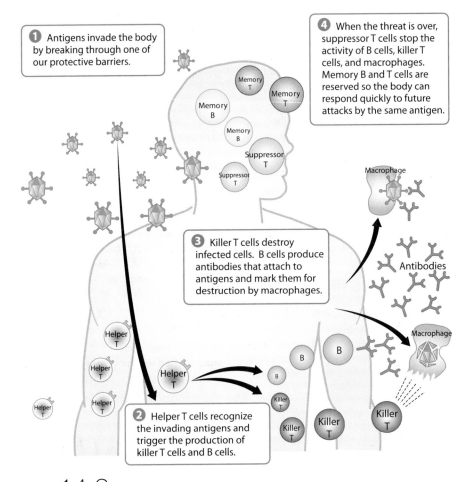

1. Antigens invade the body by breaking through one of our protective barriers.

2. Helper T cells recognize the invading antigens and trigger the production of killer T cells and B cells.

3. Killer T cells destroy infected cells. B cells produce antibodies that attach to antigens and mark them for destruction by macrophages.

4. When the threat is over, suppressor T cells stop the activity of B cells, killer T cells, and macrophages. Memory B and T cells are reserved so the body can respond quickly to future attacks by the same antigen.

FIGURE 14.3 **The Cell-Mediated Immune Response**

its own tissue as the enemy, builds up antibodies against that tissue, and attempts to destroy it. This is known as **autoimmune disease** (*auto* means "self"). The National Institutes of Health estimates that over 32 million Americans have autoantibodies, which are proteins made by the immune system that target the body's tissues. Their presence can indicate autoimmunity, in many cases well before the symptoms of autoimmune diseases such as type 1 diabetes, lupus, rheumatoid arthritis, and multiple sclerosis, actually begin.[3] Researchers estimate that there are between 80 and 140 different types of autoimmune disease, many of which are chronic, debilitating, and life threatening. (See Focus On: Minimizing Your Risk for Diabetes for more on these diseases.) Many people do not realize that autoimmune diseases are among the leading causes of death in female children and women under the age of 65.[4]

Inflammatory Response, Pain, and Fever If an infection is localized, pus formation, redness, swelling, and irritation often occur. These symptoms are components of the body's inflammatory response, and they indicate that the invading organisms are being fought systemically. The four cardinal signs of inflammation are *redness, swelling, pain,* and *heat.*

Pain is often one of the earliest signs that an injury or infection has occurred. Pathogens can kill or injure tissue at the site of infection, causing swelling that puts pressure on nerve endings in the area, causing pain. Pain plays a valuable, protective role in the body's response to injury or invasion by signaling to you that something is wrong and causing you to reduce or avoid activities that can aggravate the injury or site of infection. In addition to inflammation, another frequent indicator of infection is *fever,* or a body temperature above the average norm of 98.6°F. Fever is frequently caused by toxins secreted by pathogens that interfere with the control of body temperature. Although extremely elevated temperatures are harmful to the body, a mild fever is protective: Raising body temperature by 1 or 2 degrees provides an environment that destroys some disease-causing organisms. A fever also stimulates the body to produce more white blood cells, which destroy more invaders. As fevers increase beyond 101 or 102°F, risks to the patient outweigh any fever benefits. In these cases medical treatment should be obtained.

Vaccines: Bolstering Your Immunity

Recall that once people have been exposed to a specific pathogen, subsequent attacks will activate their memory T and B cells, thus giving them immunity. This is the principle on which **vaccination** is based.

A vaccine consists of killed or weakened versions of a disease-causing microorganism or an antigen that is similar to but less dangerous than the disease antigen. It is administered to stimulate the person's immune

autoimmune disease Disease caused by an overactive immune response against the body's own cells.

vaccination Inoculation with killed or weakened pathogens or similar, less dangerous antigens to prevent or lessen the effects of some disease.

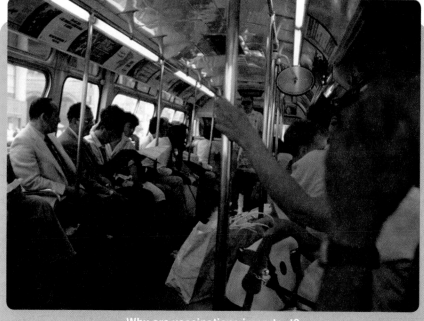

Why are vaccinations important?

Vaccinations can protect an individual from certain infectious diseases, and they are also important in controlling the prevalence of diseases in society at large. Certain diseases such as polio and diphtheria have become very rare as a result of immunizations, but until a disease is completely eradicated it is important to keep vaccinating people against it. Otherwise, there is nothing to stop the disease from making a comeback and causing an epidemic. People who spend time in crowded places, such as commuters or frequent air travelers, and people at particular risk, such as hospital workers or college students who often live in close quarters, should be especially certain to stay up-to-date on their vaccinations.

Recommended Vaccinations for Teens and College Students

- Tetanus-diphtheria-pertussis vaccine (Td/Tdap)
- HPV vaccine series
- Meningococcal vaccine*
- Influenza vaccine
- Hepatitis A vaccine series**
- Hepatitis B vaccine series
- Polio vaccine series
- Measles-mumps-rubella (MMR) vaccine series
- Varicella (chickenpox) vaccine series

*Booster at age 16
**For high-risk groups

Source: Centers for Disease Control and Prevention, "Recommendations and Guidelines: Vaccines Needed by Teens and College Students," Modified January 2012, www.cdc.gov/vaccines/recs/schedules/teen-schedule.htm.

system to produce antibodies against future attacks—without actually causing the disease (or by causing a very minor case of it). Vaccines typically are given orally or by injection, and this form of immunity is termed *artificially acquired*

active immunity, in contrast to *naturally acquired active immunity* (which is obtained by exposure to antigens in the normal course of daily life) or *naturally acquired passive immunity* (as occurs when a mother passes immunity to her fetus via their shared blood supply or to an infant via breast milk).

Specific schedules have been established for various population groups. See **Table 14.2** for recommended vaccines for one such group, teens and college students. **Figure 14.4** shows the recommended vaccination schedule for the general adult population. Childhood vaccine schedules are available at the CDC website. Concern about the safety of vaccines has caused an increase in the number of parents who refuse to vaccinate their children (see the **Health Headlines** box on page 419). As people refuse vaccinations, the likelihood of infectious diseases being spread to vulnerable populations increases.

Because of their close living quarters and frequent interactions with people, college students face a higher than average risk of infection from diseases that are largely preventable. Vaccines that should be a high priority among 20-somethings include *tetanus-diphtheria-pertussis vaccine (Tdap), meningococcal conjugate vaccine (MCV4), human papillomavirus (HPV)*, and the *influenza vaccine.*[5]

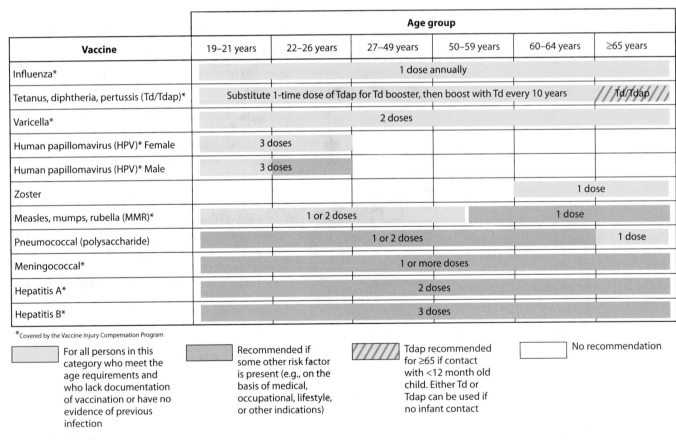

Vaccine	Age group					
	19–21 years	22–26 years	27–49 years	50–59 years	60–64 years	≥65 years
Influenza*	1 dose annually					
Tetanus, diphtheria, pertussis (Td/Tdap)*	Substitute 1-time dose of Tdap for Td booster, then boost with Td every 10 years					Td/Tdap
Varicella*	2 doses					
Human papillomavirus (HPV)* Female	3 doses					
Human papillomavirus (HPV)* Male	3 doses					
Zoster					1 dose	
Measles, mumps, rubella (MMR)*	1 or 2 doses			1 dose		
Pneumococcal (polysaccharide)	1 or 2 doses					1 dose
Meningococcal*	1 or more doses					
Hepatitis A*	2 doses					
Hepatitis B*	3 doses					

*Covered by the Vaccine Injury Compensation Program

For all persons in this category who meet the age requirements and who lack documentation of vaccination or have no evidence of previous infection

Recommended if some other risk factor is present (e.g., on the basis of medical, occupational, lifestyle, or other indications)

Tdap recommended for ≥65 if contact with <12 month old child. Either Td or Tdap can be used if no infant contact

No recommendation

FIGURE 14.4 **Recommended Adult Immunization Schedule, by Vaccine and Age Group, 2012**
Note there are important explanations and additions to these recommendations that should be consulted by checking the latest schedule at www.cdc.gov/vaccines/recs/schedules/adult-schedule.htm.
Source: Centers for Disease Control and Prevention, "Recommended Adult Immunization Schedule—United States, 2012," *MMWR Weekly* 61, no. 4 (2012).

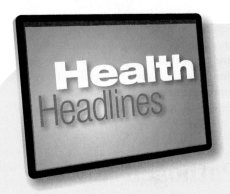

VACCINE BACKLASH: ARE THEY SAFE AND NECESSARY?

Immunizations against widespread infectious diseases are one of the greatest public health success stories of all time—so successful, in fact, that most people have never seen or heard of anyone having the diseases such as smallpox that once wiped out entire populations. Today, fear of the old "killer" diseases has waned and been replaced with distrust of the vaccines themselves.

How serious a problem is this? In some communities, such as Ashland, Oregon, up to 25 percent of kindergartners' parents opted their children out of at least one vaccine last year. In other U.S. school districts and counties, these rates are even higher, and a general trend of avoiding vaccinations is growing.

Undervaccination rates are particularly high in non-Hispanic, college-educated white families with incomes above $75,000 a year. Religious tenets, fear of vaccine safety, and worry about vaccine overload are among some of the more common reasons for parents' refusal to

vaccinate their children. Others object to mandatory vaccinations because they consider them to be a government intrusion into their individual rights.

The vaccine concerns receiving the most attention include fear that the measles, mumps, rubella (MMR) vaccine can lead to autism; fear that the hepatitis B vaccine is related to multiple sclerosis (MS); and fear that the combined tetanus-diphtheria-pertussis (Tdap) vaccine can cause sudden infant death syndrome (SIDS). Are these concerns valid?

Research is ongoing, but the Centers for Disease Control and Prevention (CDC) has found no evidence for any of these claims. Much of the initial anxiety over the MMR vaccine was fueled by an article in the medical journal *Lancet* in 1998 linking the vaccine to increased risk of autism and bowel disease. The article prompted many to refuse the vaccine in the United States and elsewhere, and the resulting drop-off in immunizations led to increased cases of measles in many parts of the world. Over 10 years later, after a thorough investigation of ethical and factual issues with the research, *Lancet* retracted the article as being false. The lead author of the paper was later fired from his research position and had his license to practice revoked.

Virtually all medical and public health organizations support vaccinations, pointing to stringent safety controls in the manufacturing and testing of vaccines, as well as ongoing safety monitoring, the long history of vaccines in wiping out killer diseases across the globe, and the fact that risks from the diseases themselves are almost always much greater than any risks associated with

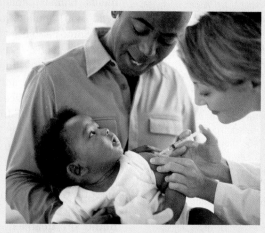

Some parents have expressed concern over the safety of vaccinations.

a vaccine. If large numbers of people were to avoid vaccinations, old killers would be likely to reemerge, and those people who were already sick or weak from other conditions would be extremely vulnerable. Today, the CDC's Immunization Safety Office monitors complaints and investigates potential problems with vaccines as they occur. The reasons for vaccination far outweigh any arguments against them. Local rashes and reactions at injection sites, low-grade fever, discomfort, and even allergic reactions can occur. But the danger of major complications from getting vaccinations is extremely low, and generally pales in comparison to the effects of contracting the diseases that the vaccinations protect against.

Sources: Centers for Disease Control and Prevention, "Vaccine Safety: Concerns about Autism," Modified March 2012, www.cdc.gov/vaccinesafety/Concerns/Autism/Index.html; The Editors of the *Lancet*. "Retraction—Ileal-lymphoid-nodular hyperplasia, non-specific colitis, and pervasive development disorder in Children," *Lancet* 375, no. 9713 (2010): 445; E. J. Gangarosa et al., "Impact of Anti-Vaccine Movements on Pertussis Control: The Untold Story," *Lancet* 351, no. 9099 (1998): 356–61.

Allergies: The Immune System Overreacts

An **allergy** occurs as part of the body's attempt to defend itself against a specific *antigen* or **allergen** by producing specific *antibodies*. Under normal conditions, the production of antibodies is a positive element in the body's defense system. However, for unknown reasons, in some people the body overreacts by developing an overly protective mechanism against relatively harmless substances. The resulting *hypersensitivity reaction* is fairly common, as anyone who has awakened with a runny nose or itchy eyes will testify. Most commonly, these hypersensitivity, or allergic, reactions occur as a response to

allergy Hypersensitive reaction to a specific antigen in which the body produces antibodies to a normally harmless substance.

allergen An antigen that induces a hypersensitive immune response.

histamine Chemical substance that dilates blood vessels, increases mucous secretions, and produces other symptoms of allergies.

immunotherapy Treatment strategies based on the concept of regulating the immune system by administering antibodies or desensitizing shots of allergens.

bacteria (singular: *bacterium*) Simple, single-celled microscopic organisms; about 100 known species of bacteria cause disease in humans.

antibiotics Medicines used to kill microorganisms, such as bacteria.

antibiotic resistance The ability of bacteria or other microbes to withstand the effects of an antibiotic.

environmental antigens such as molds, animal dander (hair and dead skin), pollen, ragweed, or dust. Some people are also allergic to certain foods. (See **Chapter 9** for more about food allergies.) Once excessive antibodies to allergens are produced, they trigger the release of **histamine,** a chemical that dilates blood vessels, increases mucous secretions, causes tissues to swell, and produces rashes, difficulty breathing, and other allergy symptoms. Many people have found that **immunotherapy** treatment, or "allergy shots," somewhat reduce the severity of their symptoms. In most cases, once the offending antigen has disappeared, allergy-prone people suffer few symptoms.

Hay Fever Hay fever, or *seasonal allergic rhinitis,* occurs throughout the world and is one of the most common chronic diseases in the United States, affecting nearly 10 percent of all adults in the last year and approximately 11 percent of all children.[6] It is usually considered a seasonal disease because it is most prevalent when pollen levels are high from ragweed, flowers, and grasses. Hay fever attacks are characterized by sneezing and itchy, watery eyes and nose; they make countless people miserable for weeks at a time every year. As with other allergies, hay fever results from an overzealous immune system that is hypersensitive to certain substances. You are more likely to have hay fever if you have a family history of allergies or asthma, are male, were exposed to cigarette smoke during your first year of life, or live or work in environments where allergens are constantly present, such as pet dander, dust mites, mold, or pollen. Avoiding the environmental triggers is the best way to pre-

vent hay fever. If you can't prevent it, shots or antihistamines often provide relief. Decongestants can reduce symptoms, as can air-conditioning and air purifiers. Over-the-counter nose sprays are usually of limited value, and their prolonged use may actually cause symptoms or make them worse. Inhaled steroids are often effective and may be prescribed, as are specific desensitizing injections.[7]

Types of Pathogens and the Diseases They Cause

We can categorize pathogens into six major types: bacteria, viruses, fungi, protozoans, parasitic worms, and prions. Figure 14.5 shows examples of several of these pathogens. Each has a particular route of transmission and characteristic elements that make it unique. In the following text, we discuss each of these categories and give an overview of some diseases they cause that have a significant impact on public health.

Bacteria

Bacteria (singular: *bacterium*) are simple, single-celled microscopic organisms. There are three major types of bacteria, which are classified by their shape: cocci, bacilli, and spirilla. Although there are several thousand known species of bacteria (and many thousands more that are unknown), just over 100 cause disease in humans. In many cases, it is not the bacteria themselves that cause disease but rather the toxins that they produce.

Antibiotics are among the potent groups of drugs designed to fight and kill specific bacteria. However, overuse and misuse of antibiotics has lead to **antibiotic resistance,** in which successive generations of bacteria change or adapt so that antibiotics are less effective in killing them. Many believe that antibiotic resistance is one of the world's greatest

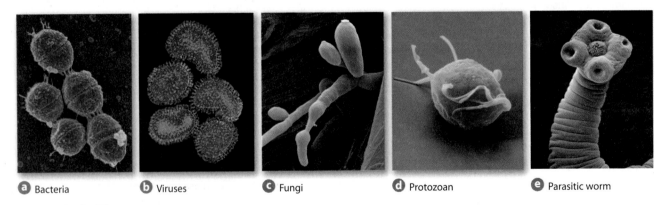

ⓐ Bacteria　ⓑ Viruses　ⓒ Fungi　ⓓ Protozoan　ⓔ Parasitic worm

FIGURE 14.5 **Examples of Five Major Types of Pathogens**
(a) Color-enhanced scanning electron micrograph (SEM) of *Streptococcus* bacteria, magnified 40,000×. (b) Colored transmission electron micrograph (TEM) of influenza (flu) viruses, magnified 32,000×. (c) Color SEM of *Candida albicans*, a yeast fungus, magnified 50,000×. (d) Color TEM of *Trichomonas vaginalis*, a protozoan, magnified 9,000×. (e) Color-enhanced SEM of a tapeworm, magnified 50×.

problems and that we may lose our ability to fight bacteria at rates that far exceed our ability to develop new, more powerful antibiotics. In fact, the percentage of bacteria that are resistant doubled between 2006 and 2008, and these percentages continue to increase.[8] For example, a deadly form of foodborne *Escherichia coli* bacteria in Europe left thousands infected and caused several deaths in 2011. Refer back to the **Be Healthy, Be Green** box on page 415 for more on the issues and concerns relating to antibiotic resistance.

Staphylococcal Infections **Staphylococci** are normally present on the skin or in the nostrils of 20 to 30 percent of us at any given time. Usually, they cause no problems for otherwise healthy persons. The presence of bacteria on or in a person without infection is called **colonization.** A person can be colonized and then spread the infection to others, yet never develop the disease. In contrast, when the pathogen is present and there is a cut or break in the *epidermis,* or outer layer of the skin, staphylococci may enter the system and cause an **infection.** If you have ever suffered from acne, boils, styes (infections of the eyelids), or infected wounds, you have probably had a "staph" infection.

Although most of these infections are readily defeated by the immune system, resistant forms of staph bacteria are on the rise. One of these resistant forms of staph, **methicillin-resistant *Staphylococcus aureus* (MRSA),** has come under intense international scrutiny as numerous cases have arisen around the world, especially in the United States.[9] Symptoms of MRSA infection often start with a rash or pimplelike skin irritation. Within hours, these early symptoms may progress to redness, inflammation, pain, and deeper wounds. If untreated, MRSA may invade the blood, bones, joints, surgical wounds, heart valves, and lungs, and can be fatal.[10]

In the past, most cases of MRSA were contracted in health care facilities such as hospitals, nursing homes, or clinics; these are known as health care–associated MRSA (HA-MRSA). However, growing numbers of cases are appearing among people who have not sought medical treatment. Known as community-acquired MRSA (CA-MRSA), this form of MRSA is a growing concern. Finally, linezolid-resistant *Staphylococcus aureus*, or LRSA, is a particularly potent bacterium that has evolved among patients using one of the last effective antibiotics, linezolid, as treatment for MRSA. Reports of deaths from LRSA in many regions of the world are on the rise. Questions about what happens when linezolid no longer works and the antibiotic "well" runs dry have raised red flags by health professionals everywhere. People recovering from surgery, those with weakened immune systems, and those with underlying respiratory problems may be at

tremendous risk if this resistant form of MRSA remains unchecked.

Streptococcal Infections

At least five types of the **Streptococcus** microorganism are known to cause infections. Group A streptococci (GAS) cause the most common diseases, such as streptococcal pharyngitis ("strep throat") and scarlet fever, which is often preceded by a sore throat or impetigo.[11] One particularly virulent group of GAS can lead to rare but serious diseases such as *toxic shock syndrome,* which can lead to dramatic drops in blood pressure and death, or *necrotizing fasciitis* (often referred to as "flesh-eating strep").[12] Rates of Group B streptococci infection are particularly high among newborns; however, it can affect adults of any age, with increasing risk after the age of 60. Currently, Group B strep is the leading cause of meningitis. It can lead to significant bloodstream infections or *sepsis,* as well as pneumonia and skin, soft tissue, and bone and joint infections. It also causes over 7 million cases of ear infections in the United States each year, many of which are resistant to penicillin, the primary drug used in treatment. About 25 percent of pregnant women carry Group B strep in their rectum or vagina, prompting CDC to recommend testing for it during the last weeks of pregnancy.[13]

Meningitis An infection and inflammation of the *meninges,* the membranes that surround the brain and spinal cord, is called **meningitis.** Some forms of bacterial meningitis are contagious and can be spread through contact with saliva, nasal discharge, feces, or respiratory and throat secretions.

staphylococci A group of round bacteria, usually found in clusters, that cause a variety of diseases in humans and other animals.

colonization The process of bacteria or some other infectious organisms establishing themselves in a host without causing infection.

infection The state of pathogens being established in or on a host and causing disease.

methicillin-resistant *Staphylococcus aureus* (MRSA) Highly resistant form of staph infection that is growing in international prevalence.

Streptococcus A round bacterium, usually found in chain formation.

meningitis An infection of the meninges, the membranes that surround the brain and spinal cord.

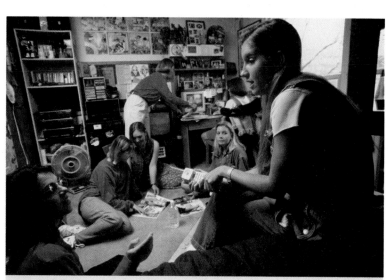

Close quarters, such as college dorms, are prime breeding grounds for contagious diseases such as meningitis.

Pneumococcal meningitis, the most common form of the disease, is also the most dangerous form of bacterial meningitis. Several thousand cases of meningitis are reported in the United States each year. *Meningococcal meningitis,* a virulent form of meningitis, has risen dramatically on college campuses in recent years.[14] Although meningitis can occur at any age, adolescents ages 16 to 21 have the highest rates of meningococcal disease, particularly those living in close living quarters such as dormitories.

The signs of meningitis are sudden fever, severe headache, and a stiff neck, particularly causing difficulty touching your chin to your chest. Persons who are suspected of having meningitis should receive immediate, aggressive medical treatment. Two types of vaccines are recommended for some types of meningitis on today's campuses. However, these vaccines are specific to the strain of the organism present at the time and may not work for strains in your area. Talk to the medical or health education staff at your local student health center to see if they have the vaccine most likely to protect you in your area.

Pneumonia A wide range of conditions can result in inflammation of the lungs and difficulty in breathing. These are generally referred to as **pneumonia**. It is characterized by chronic cough, chest pain, chills, high fever, fluid accumulation, and eventual respiratory failure. Although bacterial and viral pathogens are the most common cause of pneumonia, it can also be caused by fungi, yeast infections, occupational exposure, or trauma.

Bacterial pneumonia responds readily to antibiotic treatment in the early stages, but it can be deadly in more advanced stages. Other forms of pneumonia caused by viruses, fungi, chemicals, or other substances in the lungs are more difficult to treat. Although medical advances have reduced the overall incidence of pneumonia, it continues to be a major threat in the United States and throughout the world. Vulnerable populations include children; the poor; those displaced by war, famine, and natural disasters; older adults; those who have been occupationally exposed to chemicals and particulates that damage the lungs; and those already suffering from other illnesses.

Tuberculosis A major killer in the United States in the early twentieth century, **tuberculosis (TB)** was largely controlled by 1950 as a result of improved sanitation, isolation of infected persons, and treatment with drugs such as rifampin or isoniazid. Referred to as "consumption" in many parts of the world, this bacterial respiratory disease leads to wasting, chronic cough, fluid- and blood-filled lungs, and eventual spread throughout the body. Symptoms include persistent coughing, weight loss, fever, and spitting up blood. Coughing is the most common mode of transmitting TB. Infected people can be contagious without actually showing any symptoms. Those at highest risk for TB include the poor, especially children, and the chronically ill. People residing in poorly ventilated crowded prisons and homeless shelters who continuously inhale the same contaminated air are at higher risk. Persons with compromised immune systems are also at high risk, as are those in situations where comorbidity (suffering from more than one disease) exists.

Many health professionals assumed that TB was conquered in the United States, but that appears not to be the case. During the past 20 years, overcrowding and poor sanitation in some developing nations kept the disease alive. Failure to isolate active cases of TB and fully treat them, plus a migration of TB to the United States through immigration and international travel, as well as a weakened public health infrastructure that funded less screening, kept the disease from disappearing in North America. In 2010, there were about 11,200 cases of TB documented in the United States.[15]

Today about one third of the world's population is infected with TB. Over 60 percent of all TB cases and 88 percent of drug-resistant TB cases in the United States occurred among people born in other countries.[16] Treatments are available, but for the more resistant forms of TB, they are very costly. Most tuberculosis-related deaths occur in developing countries, where it accounts for 26 percent of all preventable deaths.[17] TB is the number one infectious killer of women of reproductive age worldwide, as well as the leading cause of death among HIV-positive patients.

As with many bacterial diseases, resistant forms of TB are increasing in the global population. **Multidrug-resistant TB (MDR-TB)** is a form of TB that is currently resistant to at least two of the best anti-TB drugs in use today. An even more dangerous form, **extensively drug-resistant TB (XDR-TB)**, is resistant to nearly all first- and second-line drug defenses against it and is extremely difficult to treat. These newer strains of tuberculosis are reaching epidemic proportions in many regions of the world, particularly among those whose immune systems are already compromised by HIV and other diseases.[18] In 2010, MDR-TB rates reached the highest rates ever, up 28 percent in some parts of the world.[19]

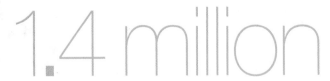

people die of tuberculosis each year.

Tickborne Bacterial Diseases In the past few decades, certain tickborne diseases have become major health threats in the United States. Those that are most noteworthy include two bacterially caused diseases, *Lyme disease* and *ehrlichiosis.* Both diseases spike in the summer months in many states, and both can cause significant disability and pose threats to humans and animals.

---

pneumonia Inflammatory disease of the lungs characterized by chronic cough, chest pain, chills, high fever, and fluid accumulation; may be caused by bacteria, viruses, fungi, chemicals, or other substances.

tuberculosis (TB) A disease caused by bacterial infiltration of the respiratory system.

multidrug-resistant TB (MDR-TB) Form of TB that is resistant to at least two of the best antibiotics available.

extensively drug-resistant TB (XDR-TB) Form of TB that is resistant to nearly all existing antibiotics.

Once believed to be closely related to viruses, **rickettsia** are now considered a small form of bacteria. They produce toxins and multiply within small blood vessels, causing vascular blockage and tissue death. Rickettsia require an insect vector (carrier) for transmission to humans. Two common forms of human rickettsial disease are *Rocky Mountain spotted fever* (*RMSF*), carried by a tick, and *typhus,* carried by a louse, flea, or tick. These diseases produce similar symptoms, including high fever, weakness, rash, and coma, and both can be life threatening.

Ticks are a vector for several devastating bacterial diseases.

For all insectborne diseases, the best protection is to stay indoors at dusk and early morning to avoid hours of high insect activity. If you must go out, wear protective clothing or use bug sprays containing natural oils, pyrethrins, or DEET (diethyltoluamide), all products regarded as generally safe. If you are traveling in areas where insectborne diseases are prevalent, bed nets and other protective measures may be necessary.

Viruses

Viruses are the smallest known pathogens, approximately 1/500th the size of bacteria. Essentially, a virus consists of a protein structure that contains either *ribonucleic acid* (*RNA*) or *deoxyribonucleic acid* (*DNA*). Viruses are incapable of carrying out any life processes on their own. To reproduce, they must invade and inject their own DNA and RNA into a host cell, take it over, and force it to make copies of themselves. The new viruses then erupt out of the host cell and seek other cells to invade. Hundreds of viruses are known to cause diseases in humans.

Viral diseases can be difficult to treat because many viruses can withstand heat, formaldehyde, and large doses of radiation with little effect on their structure. Some viruses have **incubation periods** (the length of time required to develop fully and cause symptoms in their hosts) that last for years, which delays diagnosis. Drug treatment for viral infections is also limited. Drugs powerful enough to kill viruses generally kill the host cells, too, although some medications block stages in viral reproduction without damaging the host cells.

The Common Cold Any given cold's most likely cause is the rhinovirus, which is responsible for up to 40 percent of all colds, followed by the coronavirus, which causes about 20 percent of all colds.[20] (Some experts believe there are at least 200 different viruses responsible for colds.) Colds are **endemic** (always present to some degree) throughout the world, with increasing prevalence as the weather turns colder and people spend more time indoors. Otherwise healthy people carry cold viruses in their noses and throats most of the time. These viruses are held in check until the host's resistance is lowered. It is possible to "catch" a cold from the airborne droplets of another person's sneeze or from skin-to-skin or mucous membrane contact, though the hands are the greatest avenue for transmitting colds and other viruses. Obviously, then, covering your nose and mouth with a tissue, handkerchief, or even the crook of your elbow when sneezing is better than using your bare hand. Contrary to popular belief, you cannot catch a cold from getting a chill, but the chill may lower your immune system's resistance to a pathogenic virus if one is present.

Influenza In otherwise healthy people, **influenza**, or flu, is usually not life threatening. However, for certain vulnerable populations, such as individuals with respiratory problems or heart disease, older adults (over age 65), or young children (under age 5), the flu can be very serious. Five to 20 percent of Americans get the flu each year, and of these, 200,000 will need hospitalization for treatment of the illness.[21] Once a person gets the flu, treatment is *palliative,* meaning that it is focused on relief of symptoms, rather than cure.

Determining whether you have a cold or the flu is a matter of assessing your symptoms: If you have bad body aches, fatigue, and fever, it is likely that you have the flu. In the absence of these symptoms, but the presence of a stuffy nose, sneezing, a sore throat, and often a cough, over-the-counter medicines targeting symptoms of the common cold may help.[22]

To date, three major varieties of flu virus have been discovered, with many different strains existing within each variety. The *A form* of the virus is generally the most virulent, followed by the *B and C varieties*. If you contract one form of influenza, you may develop immunity to it, but you will not necessarily be immune to other forms of the disease.

Strains of influenza are constantly changing, so flu vaccines are formulated each year that combine killed viruses from each of three main groups of influenza viruses. The viruses are selected based on forecasting of the strains likely to emerge in various regions of the world. Currently, national influenza centers in 101 countries conduct year-round studies to determine the flu viruses most likely to be circulating in

What's Working for You?

You probably already have habits or behaviors that help you avoid infection. Which of these habits do you have?

- [ ] I have soap for hand washing in the bathroom and kitchen and wash my hands regularly, particularly before preparing food and after using the bathroom.
- [ ] I make an effort to eat lots of fruits and vegetables and to exercise to help keep my immune system strong.
- [ ] I manage my stress and get enough sleep.
- [ ] When preparing food, I'm careful to make sure foods are cooked properly to avoid foodborne illnesses.

rickettsia A small form of bacteria that live inside other living cells.

viruses Pathogens that invade and inject their own DNA or RNA into a host cell, take it over, and force it to make copies of themselves.

incubation period The time between exposure to a disease and the appearance of symptoms.

endemic Describing a disease that is always present to some degree.

influenza A common viral disease of the respiratory tract.

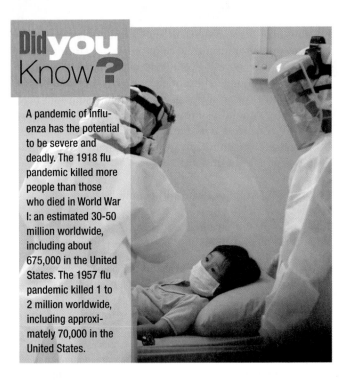
order to choose which to include in the upcoming flu vaccine. In a "good match" year, vaccines are between 70 and 90 percent effective in healthy adults.[23] In 2010, the CDC made sweeping changes in its influenza vaccine recommendations, stating that everyone 6 months and older should be vaccinated for the flu.[24] Children under the age of 5, particularly those under the age of 2, adults age 65 and over, pregnant women, American Indians and Alaskan Natives, people with respiratory ailments such as asthma, those with weakened immune systems, people living in nursing homes, health care workers, those with cardiovascular disease, and those who are morbidly obese, are among those who have high risks of complications if they get the flu and should be vaccinated. (See the complete list at www.cdc.gov/flu/keyfacts.htm.) If you have had a severe reaction to past flu shots, have a severe allergy to chicken eggs, are running a fever, or have other issues, consult with your doctor before having a shot. An optional nasal spray flu vaccine is available for healthy people age 1 to 49 who are not pregnant. Flu shots take 2 to 3 weeks to become effective, so people at risk should get these shots in the fall before the flu season begins.

Most campus health services offer flu vaccines for $20 or less. Other options for low- or no-cost vaccines are local

mononucleosis A viral disease that causes pervasive fatigue and other long-lasting symptoms.

hepatitis A viral disease in which the liver becomes inflamed, producing symptoms such as fever, headache, and possibly jaundice.

36,000
Americans die of the flu each year.

public health departments, local pharmacies and big box stores, and community centers. Compared to the high cost of lost days of work or missed classes, possible hospitalization, and expensive medicines to treat symptoms, the flu vaccine is a sound investment.

Infectious Mononucleosis Caused primarily by the Epstein-Barr virus, **mononucleosis** is most widespread among people between the ages of 15 and 24, with college students or those living in close quarters among those at highest risk. By adulthood, 90 to 95 percent of people have been infected, many without ever showing symptoms.[25] Because saliva seems to be a key route of transmission, "mono" has often referred to as the "kissing disease." However, kissing isn't the only means of spreading this infection. Sharing eating utensils, drinking out of someone else's glass or cup, sharing towels or cosmetics such as lipstick, or even coughing can spread the virus. Body fluids, including blood, genital secretions, and mucus can also spread the disease. Common symptoms include bone-crushing fatigue, headache, fever, aches and pains, sore throat, rashes, and swollen lymph nodes. Pain in the area of the spleen may indicate spleen enlargement, a potentially dangerous risk for those involved in exercise or athletics where contact with the ground or others is common. Anything that weakens the immune system, such as having another illness, high stress, lack of sleep, poor diet, or too much alcohol or drug use, can increase risk. A simple blood test can determine whether you have mono. Rest, balanced nutrition, stress management, and healthy lifestyle are the best treatments.

Hepatitis One of the most highly publicized viral diseases is **hepatitis**, a virally caused inflammation of the liver. Hepatitis symptoms include fever, headache, nausea, loss of appetite, skin rashes, pain in the upper right abdomen, dark yellow (with brownish tinge) urine, and jaundice. Internationally, viral hepatitis is a major contributor to liver disease and accounts for much illness and many deaths. Currently, there are several known forms (A, B, C, D, and E), with hepatitis A, B, and C having the highest rates of incidence.

Hepatitis A (HAV) is contracted by eating food or drinking water contaminated with human feces. Since vaccinations became available, HAV rates have declined by nearly 92 percent in the United States. However, over 21,000 people per year are still infected.[26] Handlers of infected food, children at day care centers, those who have sexual contact with HAV-positive individuals, or those who travel to regions where HAV is endemic are at higher risk. In addition, those who ingest seafood from contaminated water and people who use contaminated needles are also at risk. Fortunately, individuals infected with hepatitis A do not become chronic carriers, and vaccines for the disease are available. Many who contract HAV are asymptomatic (symptom-free).

Hepatitis B (HBV) is spread through body fluid exchange during unprotected sex; sharing needles when injecting drugs; through accidental needlesticks on the job; or, in the case of a baby, from an infected mother. Hepatitis B can lead to chronic liver disease or liver cancer. Since vaccines became available in 1981, numbers of HBV cases have declined rapidly. However, there are still nearly 40,000 new cases reported each year and over 1.2 million people in the United States who are chronically infected with HBV. The highest rates of infection are among males ages 25 to 44.[27] Needle exchange programs have helped reduce risks of HBV infection in some populations. Globally, HBV infections are on the decline, but they continue to be a major health problem affecting over 350 million people, with the highest rates in Asia and Africa.[28] Because the hepatitis B virus is 50 to 1,000 times more infectious than HIV, efforts to increase global vaccination rates have become a major priority.[29] Hepatitis C (HCV) infections are on an epidemic rise in many regions of the world as resistant forms of the virus are emerging. Some cases can be traced to blood transfusions or organ transplants. Currently, an estimated 17,000 new cases of HCV are diagnosed in the United States each year, with over 3.2 million people chronically infected.[30] Over 85 percent of those infected develop chronic infections; if the infection is left untreated, the person may develop cirrhosis of the liver, liver cancer, or liver failure. Liver failure resulting from chronic hepatitis C is the leading reason for liver transplants in the United States.[31] Although there is no vaccine for HCV, there are new drugs available with high levels of success in treating the disease. The problem is that millions of people, primarily "baby boomers," do not know that they are infected and are not seeking these treatments. Educating these individuals about potential risks and getting them tested and treated is a top priority.

To prevent the spread of HBV and HCV, follow these precautions: use latex condoms correctly every time you have sex; don't share personal-care items that might have blood on them, such as razors or toothbrushes; get a blood test for HBV so you know your status; never share needles; if you are having body art done, go only to reputable artists or piercers who follow established sterilization and infection-control protocols.

Mumps When a vaccine was introduced in 1968, reported cases of **mumps** declined from 80 per 100,000 people to less than 2 per 100,000 people in 1984. However, an epidemic in 2006 among college students infected thousands of people in Iowa and the central United States.[32] No one knows how this outbreak started, but it is suspected that many did not receive their second mumps vaccination, making them susceptible. An outbreak of over 1,500 cases in 2009, triggered by an 11-year-old boy who had just returned from the United Kingdom, was a grim reminder that even though mumps is largely controlled in the United States, many countries of the world have continued problems, and outbreaks here may be just a plane ride away.[33]

Approximately one half of all mumps infections produce only minor symptoms. The most common symptom is the swelling of the parotid (salivary) glands; however, about one third of all infected people never have this symptom. One of the greatest dangers associated with mumps is the potential for sterility in men who contract the disease in young adulthood. Some victims also suffer hearing loss.

Herpes Viruses: Chickenpox, Shingles, and Herpes Gladiatorum

From the annoying cold sore to the painful marks of chickenpox, herpes-caused diseases are known for painful, blistering rashes and are easily transmitted via physical contact. They can become chronic problems for the person infected. (Note that genital herpes is covered in this chapter's section on sexually transmitted infections.)

Caused by the *herpes varicella zoster virus (HVZV)*, **chickenpox** produces characteristic symptoms of fever and fatigue 13 to 17 days after exposure, followed by skin eruptions that itch, blister, and produce a clear fluid. The virus is present in these blisters for approximately 1 week. Although a vaccine for chickenpox is available, and all children should receive it, many parents incorrectly assume that the vaccine is not necessary and that if a child gets the disease, it will ensure lifelong immunity. Failure to vaccinate means many children still contract the disease.

For a small segment of the population, the chickenpox virus reactivates later in life during times of high stress or when the immune system is taxed by other diseases. This painful, blistering rash and extreme pain at the nerve site where the blisters occur, with other possible complications, is called **shingles.** Shingles affects over 1 million people in the United States, most of whom are over the age of 60. A vaccine for those over 60 is now recommended.[34]

Another form of herpes-caused disease that is increasing on college campuses is **herpes gladiatorum** (Figure 14.6), which shows itself as a blistered rash on the face, neck, or torso. It is caused by the herpes simplex type 1

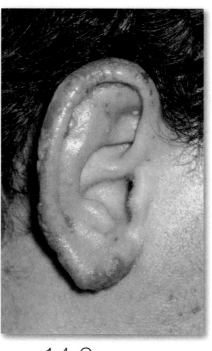

FIGURE 14.6 **Herpes Gladiatorum**
A series of fluid-filled blisters on the face, neck, or torso can be a sign of this form of herpes, which is easily spread, especially among athletes.

virus. Highly contagious via mats used by many people, for example, in a yoga studio or a gym, or body-to-body contact, herpes gladiatorum is also referred to as "mat pox" or "wrestler's herpes."

Measles and Rubella

Measles is a viral disorder that often affects young children, but it is increasing among young adults today, particularly on college campuses where vaccinations are not required or monitored. Many young adults today may not have been vaccinated in their youth, as their parents may have thought the disease was no longer a problem in the United States. Symptoms, appearing about 10 days after exposure, include an itchy rash and a high fever.

Rubella (German measles) is a milder viral infection that causes rashes, usually on upper extremities, and is believed to be spread by inhalation. Mild in most adults, rubella is a threat to the very young and unborn, as it is known to cause blindness, deafness, heart defects, and cognitive impairments in fetuses and newborns. Immunization has reduced the incidence of both measles and rubella. Infections in children not immunized against measles can lead to fever-induced problems such as rheumatic heart disease, kidney damage, and neurological disorders.

measles A viral disease that produces symptoms such as an itchy rash and a high fever.

rubella (German measles) A milder form of measles that causes a rash and mild fever in children and may damage a fetus or a newborn baby.

rabies A viral disease of the central nervous system; often transmitted through animal bites.

fungi A group of multicellular and unicellular organisms that obtain their food by infiltrating the bodies of other organisms, both living and dead; several microscopic varieties are pathogenic.

protozoans Microscopic single-celled organisms that can be pathogenic.

parasitic worms The largest of the pathogens, most of which are more a nuisance than they are a threat.

prion A recently identified self-replicating protein-based pathogen.

Rabies

The **rabies** virus infects many warm-blooded animals. Bats are believed to be asymptomatic carriers. Their urine, which they spray when flying, contains the virus, so even the air of densely populated bat caves may be infectious. In most other hosts, the disease is extremely virulent and usually fatal. The most obvious symptoms of the disease are extreme activity in the cerebral region of the brain, rage, increased salivation, spasms in the throat muscles, extreme drive to find water, and the inability to swallow. Rabid animals may attempt to bite other animals and people. Not only does this behavior cause injury, but it also spreads the virus through saliva.

The incubation period for rabies is usually 1 to 3 months. The disease may be fatal if not treated immediately with the rabies vaccine. Anyone bitten by an animal that might be carrying rabies should seek immediate medical attention and try to bring the animal along for testing. If you are wondering whether you should spring for the cost of rabies shots for your

Bats infected with rabies do not exhibit symptoms of the disease and easily spread it.

pets, do it. Pets that bite and are not current on their rabies vaccinations are routinely euthanized.

Other Pathogens

Bacteria and viruses account for many, but not all, of the common diseases in both adults and children. Other very small or microscopic organisms can also infect and cause disease symptoms in a host. Among these are fungi, protozoans, parasitic worms, and prions.

Fungi Our environment is inhabited by hundreds of species of **fungi**, multi- or unicellular organisms that obtain their food by infiltrating the bodies of other organisms, both living and dead. Many fungi, such as edible mushrooms, penicillin, and the yeast used in making bread, are useful to humans, but some species can produce infections. *Candidiasis* (as in a vaginal yeast infection, discussed later), athlete's foot, ringworm, jock itch, and toenail fungus are examples of some of the most common fungal diseases. With most fungal diseases, keeping the affected area clean and dry and treating it promptly with appropriate medications (often available over the counter), will generally bring relief. Fungal diseases are transmitted via physical contact, so avoid going barefoot in public showers, hotel rooms, and other areas where fungus may be present. Also use care when having pedicures and other foot treatment where you may come in contact with infected instruments, floors, or foot baths.

Protozoans **Protozoans** are microscopic single-celled organisms that are generally associated with tropical diseases such as African sleeping sickness and malaria. Although these pathogens are prevalent in nonindustrialized countries, they are largely controlled in the United States. The most common protozoan disease in the United States is *trichomoniasis* (discussed in this chapter's section on sexually transmitted infections). A common waterborne protozoan disease in many regions of the country is *giardiasis*. Persons who are exposed to the *giardia* pathogen may suffer intestinal pain and discomfort weeks after infection. Protection of water supplies is the key to prevention.

Parasitic Worms **Parasitic worms** are the largest of the pathogens. Ranging in size from small pinworms typically found in children to the large tapeworms found in warm-blooded animals, including humans, most parasitic worms are more a nuisance than they are a threat. Of special note today are worm infestations associated with eating raw fish such as sushi. You can prevent worm infestations by cooking fish and other foods to temperatures sufficient to kill the worms and their eggs. Other preventive measures you can take include getting your pets checked for worms and wearing shoes in parks or public places where animal feces are present.

Prions A **prion** is a self-replicating, protein-based agent that can infect humans and animals. One such prion is believed to be the underlying cause of spongiform diseases such as *bovine spongiform encephalopathy* (*BSE*) or "mad cow disease." Evidence indicates that there is a relationship between outbreaks of BSE in Europe and a disease in humans called *variant Creutzfeldt-Jakob disease*.[35] Both disorders are fatal brain diseases with unusually long incubation periods (measured in years), and both are caused by prions. To date, there have been no confirmed human infections from U.S. beef; however, infected cattle have been found.

Emerging and Resurgent Diseases

Within the past decade, rates for infectious diseases have rapidly increased. This trend can be attributed to a combination of overpopulation, inadequate health care systems, increasing poverty, extreme environmental degradation, and drug resistance.[36] At the same time that world travel has become increasingly fast and easy, drug-resistant pathogens—those that are not killed or inhibited by antibiotics and antimicrobial compounds—have been on the rise globally.

West Nile Virus Spread by infected mosquitoes, several thousand active cases of West Nile virus surface in the United States every year, resulting in chronic disability or even death for some victims. The elderly and those with impaired immune systems bear the brunt of the disease burden.[37] Today, only Alaska and Hawaii remain free of the disease.

Most infected people have very mild symptoms, but rarely it can result in severe or fatal illness. Symptoms include fever, headache and body aches, often with skin rash and swollen lymph glands, and a form of encephalitis (inflammation of the brain). Avoiding mosquito bites is the best way to prevent it: using EPA-registered insect repellents such as those with DEET or eucalyptus; wearing long-sleeved clothing and long pants when outdoors; staying indoors during dawn, dusk, and other peak mosquito feeding times; and removing any standing water sources around the home.[38]

Avian (Bird) Flu Avian influenza is an infectious disease of birds. There has been considerable media flurry in the past few years over a strain of avian (bird) flu, H5N1, which is highly pathogenic and is capable of crossing the species barrier to cause severe illness in humans. This virulent flu strain began to emerge in bird populations throughout Asia, including domestic birds such as chickens and ducks, as early as 1997. By 2007, bird flu had spread to birds in parts of western Europe, eastern Europe, Russia, and northern Africa.[39] Although the virus has yet to mutate into a form highly infectious to humans, outbreaks in which people contract the disease from birds in rural areas of the world (where people often live in close proximity to poultry and other animals) have occurred. As of March 2012, the World Health Organization (WHO) had recorded 503 cases of bird flu in humans, with 346 deaths.[40]

Many health experts suggest that if this virus becomes transmissible between humans, it is virulent enough to surpass the lethality of the influenza epidemics of 1918 and 1919,

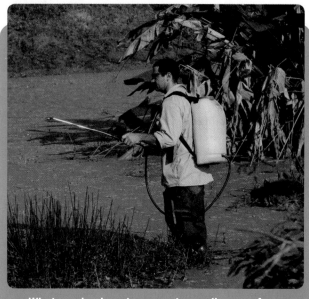

What can be done to prevent new diseases from emerging and spreading?

Poor control of pests, such as disease-spreading mosquitoes, is a symptom of larger problems such as infrastructure overload, pesticide misuse, lack of government funding, poverty, and environmental degradation. Attention to these issues is essential in preventing new and more virulent forms of disease from emerging and spreading.

which caused millions of deaths. This type of pandemic flu or global epidemic could decimate the world's population.

Escherichia Ecoli O157:H7 *Escherichia coli* O157:H7 is one of over 170 types of *E. coli* bacteria that can infect humans. Most *E. coli* organisms are harmless and live in the intestines of healthy animals and humans. *E. coli* O157:H7, however, produces a lethal toxin and can cause severe illness or death. It can live in the intestines of healthy cattle and then contaminate food products at slaughterhouses. Eating ground beef that is rare or undercooked, drinking unpasteurized milk or juice, or swimming in sewage-contaminated water or public pools can also cause infection via ingestion of infected fecal matter.

A symptom of infection is nonbloody diarrhea, usually 2 to 8 days after exposure; however, asymptomatic cases have been noted. Children, older adults, and people with weakened immune systems are particularly vulnerable to serious side effects such as kidney failure.

Strengthened regulations on the cooking of meat and regulation of chlorine levels in pools have helped reduce rates of *E. coli* infection nationally. However, a newer, drug-resistant form of the pathogen has emerged. Scientists are studying the potential threat and developing strategies to prevent its spread.

Listeriosis Luncheon meats or deli foods are particularly susceptible to transmitting the bacterium responsible for listeriosis, a disease that has proved fatal in many cases in recent years. Early symptoms begin with mild fever and progress to headache and inflammation of the brain. Those who are immuno-compromised and pregnant women are at greatest risk. New regulations that require strict monitoring of food-processing plants should help reduce the risk of listeria infection.

Malaria Today approximately 50 percent of the world's population, mostly those living in the poorest countries, are at risk for malaria. The disease is transmitted by mosquitoes carrying a parasite. There were 216 million cases of malaria and an estimated 780,00 deaths in 2010, even though mortality rates have dropped by over 25 percent in the last decade.[41] Most deaths occur among poor and vulnerable children and pregnant women in sub-Saharan Africa, Latin America, the Middle East, and parts of Europe.[42]

Travelers from malaria-free regions entering areas where there is malaria transmission are highly vulnerable, as they have little or no immunity and often receive a delayed or wrong malaria diagnosis when they return home.[43] Mosquito nets and use of insect repellents are particularly important to prevention, as is removal of standing water in yards. Natural disasters that leave standing water in which mosquitoes can flourish pose increased risks. Resistance to chloroquine, once a widely used and highly effective treatment, is now found in most regions of the world, and other treatments are losing their effectiveness at alarming rates.

Sexually Transmitted Infections

Sexually transmitted infections (STIs) have been with us since our earliest days on Earth. There are more than 20 known types of STIs. More virulent strains and antibiotic-resistant forms spell trouble in the days ahead.

Every year, there are at least 19 million new cases of STIs, only some of which are curable. Almost half of the newly diagnosed cases of STIs are in the adolescent/young adult population. Sexually transmitted infections affect men and women of all backgrounds and socioeconomic levels. However, they disproportionately affect women, minorities, and infants. In addition, STIs are most prevalent in teens and young adults.[44]

Early symptoms of an STI are often mild and unrecognizable

sexually transmitted infections (STIs) Infections transmitted through some form of intimate, usually sexual, contact.

Men only
• A drip or drainage from penis

Men and Women
• Sore bumps or blisters near sex organs or mouth
• Burning or pain when urinating
• Swelling or redness in throat
• Fever, chills, aches
• Swelling of lymph nodes near genitals or swelling of genitals
• Feeling the need to urinate frequently

Women only
• Vaginal discharge or odor from the vagina
• Pain in the lower pelvis or deep in the vagina during sex
• Burning or itching around the vagina
• Bleeding from the vagina at times other than the regular menstrual periods

FIGURE 14.7 **Signs or Symptoms of Sexually Transmitted Infections (STIs)** In their early stages, many STIs may be asymptomatic or have such mild symptoms that they are easy to overlook.

(see Figure 14.7). Left untreated, some of these infections can have grave consequences, such as sterility, blindness, central nervous system destruction, disfigurement, and even death. Infants born to mothers carrying the organisms for these infections are at risk for a variety of health problems.

What's Your Risk?

Several reasons have been proposed to explain the present high rates of STIs. The first relates to the moral and social stigmas associated with these infections. Shame and embarrassment often keep infected people from seeking treatment. Unfortunately, they usually continue to be sexually active, thereby infecting unsuspecting partners. People who are uncomfortable discussing sexual issues may also be less likely to use and ask their partners to use condoms to protect against STIs and pregnancy.

Another reason proposed for the STI epidemic is our casual attitude about sex. Bombarded

"Why Should I Care?"

Getting an STI can be painful, and you can infect your current partner with it. In the long term it could affect your health, the health of your children—even your ability to have children.

by a media that glamorizes sex, many people take sexual partners without considering the consequences. Others are pressured into sexual relationships they don't really want. Generally, the more sexual partners a person has, the greater the risk for contracting an STI.

Ignorance—about the infections, their symptoms, and the fact that someone can be asymptomatic but still infected—is also a factor. A person who is infected but asymptomatic can unknowingly spread an STI to an unsuspecting partner, who may in turn ignore or misinterpret any symptoms. By the time either partner seeks medical help, he or she may have infected several others. In addition, many people mistakenly believe that certain sexual practices—oral sex, for example—carry no risk for STIs. In fact, oral sex practices among young adults may be responsible for increases in herpes and other STIs. Figure 14.8 shows the continuum of risk for various sexual behaviors, and the Skills for Behavior Change box on page 431 offers tips for ways to practice safer sex.

Routes of Transmission

Sexually transmitted infections are generally spread through some form of intimate sexual contact. Vaginal intercourse, oral–genital contact, hand–genital contact, and anal intercourse are the most common modes of transmission. Less likely, but still possible, modes of transmission include mouth-to-mouth contact or contact with fluids from body sores that may be spread by the hands. Although each STI is

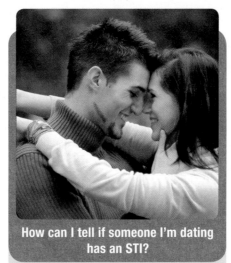

How can I tell if someone I'm dating has an STI?

You can't tell if someone has an STI just by looking at them; it isn't something broadcast on a person's face, and many people with STIs are themselves unaware of the infection because it could be asymptomatic. The only way to know for sure is to go to a clinic and get tested. In addition, partners need to be open and honest with each other about their sexual histories and practice safer sex.

a different infection caused by a different pathogen, all STI pathogens prefer dark, moist places, especially the mucous membranes lining the reproductive organs. Most of them are susceptible to light and excess heat, cold, and dryness, and many die quickly on exposure to air. Like other communicable infections, STIs have both pathogen-specific incubation periods and periods of time during which transmission is most likely, called *periods of communicability*.

Chlamydia

Chlamydia, an infection caused by the bacterium *Chlamydia trachomatis* that often presents no symptoms, is the most commonly reported STI in the United States. Chlamydia infects an estimated 2.8 million Americans annually, the majority of them women.[45] Public health officials believe that this estimate could be higher, because many cases go unreported.

Signs and Symptoms In men, early symptoms may include painful and difficult urination; frequent urination; and a watery, puslike discharge from the penis. Symptoms in women may include a yellowish discharge, spotting between periods, and occasional spotting after intercourse. However, many chlamydia victims display no symptoms and therefore do not seek help until the disease has done secondary damage. Women are especially likely to be asymptomatic; over 70 percent do not realize they have the disease, which can put them at risk for secondary damage.[46]

chlamydia Bacterially caused STI of the urogenital tract.

High-risk behaviors	Moderate-risk behaviors	Low-risk behaviors	No-risk behaviors
Unprotected vaginal, anal, and oral sex—any activity that involves direct contact with bodily fluids, such as ejaculate, vaginal secretions, or blood—are high-risk behaviors.	Vaginal, anal, or oral sex with a latex or polyurethane condom and a water-based lubricant used properly and consistently can greatly reduce the risk of STI transmission. Dental dams used during oral sex can also greatly reduce the risk of STI transmission.	Mutual masturbation, if there are no cuts on the hand, penis, or vagina, is very low risk. Rubbing, kissing, and massaging carry low risk, but herpes can be spread by skin-to-skin contact from an infected partner.	Abstinence, phone sex, talking, and fantasy are all no-risk behaviors.

FIGURE 14.8 **Continuum of Risk for Various Sexual Behaviors**
There are different levels of risk for various behaviors and various sexually transmitted infections (STIs); however, no matter what, any sexual activity involving direct contact with blood, semen, or vaginal secretions is high risk.

Complications The secondary damage resulting from chlamydia is serious in both men and women. Men can suffer injury to the prostate gland, seminal vesicles, and bulbourethral glands, and they can suffer from arthritis-like symptoms and inflammatory damage to the blood vessels and heart. Men can also experience epididymitis, inflammation of the area near the testicles. In women, chlamydia-related inflammation can injure the cervix or fallopian tubes, causing sterility, and it can damage the inner pelvic structure, leading to **pelvic inflammatory disease (PID)**. If an infected woman becomes pregnant, she has a high risk for miscarriage and stillbirth. Symptoms of PID vary but generally include lower abdominal pain, fever, unusual vaginal discharge, painful intercourse, painful urination, and irregular menstrual bleeding. The vague symptoms associated with PID cause 85 percent of women to delay seeking medical care, thereby increasing the risk of permanent damage and scarring that can lead to infertility and ectopic pregnancy.

Women are also at greater risk than men for developing a general **urinary tract infection (UTI)**. Urinary tract infections can be caused by various factors, including untreated STIs. Women are disproportionately affected by UTIs because a woman's urethra is much shorter than a man's, making it easier for bacteria to enter the bladder. In addition, a woman's urethra is closer to her anus than is a man's, allowing bacteria to spread into her urethra and cause an infection. Symptoms of a UTI in women include a burning sensation during urination and lower abdominal pain. A UTI can be diagnosed through a urine test and treated by antibiotics. If left untreated, UTIs can cause kidney damage.

Note that men can also get UTIs, although they are rarer than UTIs in women. One form is nongonoccocol urethritis, which is most commonly caused by *Chlamydia trachomatis*. Infections should be taken seriously—if you have a milky penile discharge and/or burning during urination, contact your health care provider.[47]

Chlamydia may also be responsible for one type of *conjunctivitis*, an eye infection that affects not only adults but also infants, who can contract the disease from an infected mother during delivery (Figure 14.9). Untreated conjunctivitis can cause blindness.[48]

Diagnosis and Treatment Diagnosis of chlamydia is determined through a laboratory test. A sample of urine or fluid from the vagina or penis is collected to identify the presence of the bacteria. Unfortunately, chlamydia tests are not a routine part of many health clinics' testing procedures. Usually a person must specifically request it. If detected early, chlamydia is easily treatable with antibiotics such as tetracycline, doxycycline, or erythromycin.

Gonorrhea

Gonorrhea is one of the most common STIs in the United States, surpassed only by chlamydia in number of cases. The CDC estimates that there are over 700,000 cases per year, plus numbers that go unreported.[49] Caused by the bacterial pathogen *Neisseria gonorrhoeae*, gonorrhea primarily infects the linings of the urethra, genital tract, pharynx, and rectum. It may spread to the eyes or other body regions by the hands or through body fluids, typically during vaginal, oral, or anal sex. Most cases occur in individuals between the ages of 20 and 24.[50]

Signs and Symptoms In men, a typical symptom is a white, milky discharge from the penis accompanied by painful, burning urination 2 to 9 days after contact (Figure 14.10).

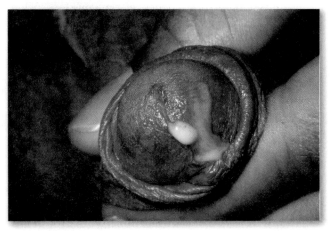

FIGURE 14.10 **Gonorrhea**
One common symptom of gonorrhea in men is a milky discharge from the penis, accompanied by burning sensations during urination. Whereas these symptoms will cause most men to seek diagnosis and treatment, women with gonorrhea are often asymptomatic, so they may not be aware they are infected.

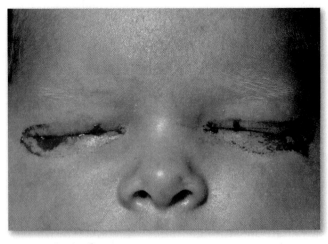

FIGURE 14.9 **Conjunctivitis in a Newborn's Eyes**
Untreated chlamydia and gonorrhea in a pregnant woman can be passed to her child during delivery, causing the eye infection conjunctivitis.

Safe Is Sexy

Practicing the following behaviors will help you reduce your risk of contracting a sexually transmitted infection (STI):

❱ Avoid casual sexual partners. All sexually active adults who are not in a lifelong monogamous relationship should practice safer sex.

❱ Use latex condoms consistently and correctly. Remember that condoms do not provide 100 percent protection against all STIs.

❱ Postpone sexual involvement until you are assured that your partner is not infected; discuss past sexual history and, if necessary, get tested for any potential STIs.

❱ Avoid injury to body tissue during sexual activity. Some pathogens can enter the bloodstream through microscopic tears in anal or vaginal tissues.

❱ Avoid unprotected oral, anal, or vaginal sexual activity in which semen, blood, or vaginal secretions could penetrate mucous membranes or enter through breaks in the skin.

❱ Always use a condom or a dental dam (a sensitive latex sheet, about the size of a tissue, that can be placed over the female genitals to form a protective layer) during vaginal, oral, or anal sex.

❱ Avoid using drugs and alcohol, which can dull your senses and affect your ability to take responsible precautions with potential sex partners.

❱ Wash your hands before and after sexual encounters. Urinate after sexual relations and, if possible, wash your genitals.

❱ Total abstinence is the only absolute way to prevent the transmission of STIs, but abstinence can be a difficult choice to make. If you have any doubt about the potential risks of having sex, consider other means of intimacy (at least until you can assure your safety)— massage, dry kissing, hugging, holding and touching, and masturbation (alone or with a partner).

❱ Think about situations ahead of time to avoid risky behaviors, including settings with alcohol and drug use.

❱ If you are worried about your own HIV or STI status, get tested. Don't risk infecting others.

❱ If you contract an STI, ask your health care provider for advice on notifying past or potential partners.

Sources: American College of Obstetricians and Gynecologists, *How to Prevent Sexually Transmitted Diseases*, ACOG Education Pamphlet AP009 (Washington, DC: American College of Obstetricians and Gynecologists, 2011), Available at www.acog.org/~/media/For%20 Patients/faq009.pdf?dmc=1&ts=20120215T1334311398; American Social Health Association, "Sexual Health: Reduce Your Risk," 2012, www.ashastd.org/std-sti/reduce-your-risk.html; Idaho Department of Health and Welfare, "How Do I Find Out If I Have an STD?" 2011, www.nakedtruth.idaho.gov/do-I-have-an-std.aspx; Nemours Foundation, "Telling Your Partner You Have an STD," 2012, http://kidshealth.org/teen/sexual_health/stds/stds_talk.html.

Epididymitis can also occur as a symptom of infection. However, some men with gonorrhea are asymptomatic.

In women, the situation is just the opposite: Most women do not experience any symptoms, but if a woman does experience symptoms, it can include vaginal discharge or a burning sensation on urinating.[51] The organism can remain in the woman's vagina, cervix, uterus, or fallopian tubes for long periods with no apparent symptoms other than an occasional slight fever. Thus a woman can be unaware that she has been infected and that she is infecting her sexual partners.

Complications In a man, untreated gonorrhea may spread to the prostate, testicles, urinary tract, kidney, and bladder. Blockage of the vasa deferentia due to scar tissue may cause sterility. In some cases, the penis develops a painful curvature during erection. If the infection goes undetected in a woman, it can spread to the fallopian tubes and ovaries, causing sterility or, at the very least, severe inflammation and PID. The bacteria can also spread up the reproductive tract or, more rarely, through the blood and infect the joints, heart valves, or brain. If an infected woman becomes pregnant, the infection can be transmitted to her baby during delivery, potentially causing blindness, joint infection, or a life-threatening blood infection.

Diagnosis and Treatment Diagnosis of gonorrhea is similar to that of chlamydia, requiring a sample of either urine or fluid from the vagina or penis to detect the presence of the bacteria. If detected early, gonorrhea is treatable with antibiotics, but the *Neisseria gonorrhoeae* bacterium has begun to develop resistance to some antibiotics. It is also important to recognize that chlamydia and gonorrhea often occur at the same time, but different antibiotics are needed to treat each infection separately.[52]

65 million

people are currently living with an incurable STI.

Syphilis

Syphilis is caused by a bacterium, the spirochete called *Treponema pallidum*. The incidence of syphilis is highest in adults aged 20 to 39 and is particularly high among African Americans and men who have sex with men. Because it is extremely delicate and dies readily on exposure to air, dryness, or cold, the organism is generally transferred only through direct sexual contact or from mother to fetus. The incidence of syphilis in newborns has continued to increase in the United States.[53]

syphilis One of the most widespread bacterial STIs; characterized by distinct phases and potentially serious results.

Signs and Symptoms Syphilis is known as the "great imitator," because its symptoms resemble those of several other infections. It should be noted, however, that some people experience no symptoms at all. Syphilis can occur in four distinct stages:[54]

● **Primary syphilis.** The first stage of syphilis, particularly for men, is often characterized by the development of a **chancre** (pronounced "shank-er"), a sore located most frequently at the site of initial infection that usually appears 3 to 4 weeks after initial infection (see **Figure 14.11**).

chancre Sore often found at the site of syphilis infection.

In men, the site of the chancre tends to be the penis or scrotum; in women, the site of infection is often internal, on the vaginal wall or high on the cervix where the chancre is not readily apparent and the likelihood of detection is not great. Whether or not it is detected, the chancre is oozing with bacteria, ready to infect an unsuspecting partner. In both men and women, the chancre will disappear in 3 to 6 weeks.

● **Secondary syphilis.** If the infection is left untreated, a month to a year after the chancre disappears secondary symptoms may appear, including a rash or white patches on the skin or on the mucous membranes of the mouth, throat, or genitals. Hair loss may occur, lymph nodes may enlarge, and the victim may develop a slight fever or headache. In rare cases, sores develop around the mouth or genitals. As during the active chancre phase, these sores contain infectious bacteria, and contact with them can spread the infection.

● **Latent syphilis.** After the secondary stage, if the infection is left untreated, the syphilis spirochetes begin to invade body organs, causing lesions called *gummas*. The infection now is rarely transmitted to others, except during pregnancy, when it can be passed to the fetus.

● **Tertiary/late syphilis.** Years after syphilis has entered the body, its effects become all too evident if still untreated. Late-stage syphilis indications include heart and central nervous system damage, blindness, deafness, paralysis, premature senility, and, ultimately, dementia.

Complications Pregnant women with syphilis can experience complications, including premature births, miscarriages, and stillbirths. An infected pregnant woman may transmit the syphilis to her unborn child. The infant will then be born with *congenital syphilis,* which can cause death; severe birth defects such as blindness, deafness, or disfigurement; developmental delays; seizures; and other health problems. Because in most cases the fetus does not become infected until after the first trimester, treatment of the mother during this time will usually prevent infection of the fetus.

Diagnosis and Treatment There are two methods that can be used to diagnose syphilis. In the primary stage, a sample from the chancre is collected to identify the bacteria. Another method of diagnosing syphilis is through a blood test. Syphilis can easily be treated with antibiotics, usually penicillin, for all stages except the late stage.

Herpes

As mentioned previously in this chapter text, *herpes* is a general term for a family of infections characterized by sores or eruptions on the skin and caused by the herpes simplex virus. The herpes family of diseases is not transmitted exclusively

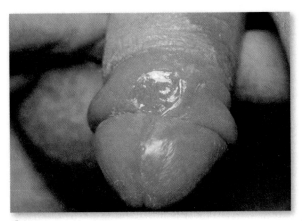

ⓐ Primary syphilis

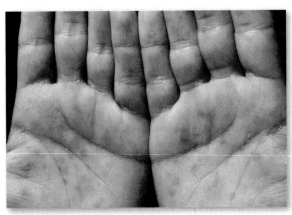

ⓑ Secondary syphilis

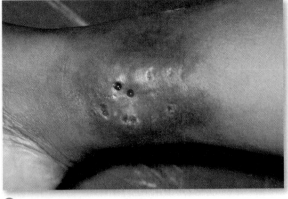

ⓒ Latent syphilis

FIGURE 14.11 **Syphilis**
A chancre on the site of the initial infection is a symptom of primary syphilis (a). A rash is characteristic of secondary syphilis (b). Lesions called "gummas" are often present in latent syphilis (c).

by sexual contact. Kissing or sharing eating utensils can also exchange saliva and transmit the infection. Herpes infections range from mildly uncomfortable to extremely serious. **Genital herpes** affects approximately 16.2 percent of the population aged 14 to 49 in the United States.[55]

There are two types of herpes simplex virus. Only about 1 in 5 Americans currently has HSV-2; however, 50 percent of adults have HSV-1, usually appearing as cold sores on their mouths.[56] Both herpes simplex types 1 and 2 can infect any area of the body, producing lesions (sores) in and around the vaginal area; on the penis; and around the anal opening, buttocks, thighs, or mouth (see Figure 14.12). Whether you contract HSV-1 or HSV-2 on your genitals, the net results may be just as painful, just as long term, and just as infectious for future partners. Herpes simplex virus remains in certain nerve cells for life and can flare up when the body's ability to maintain itself is weakened.

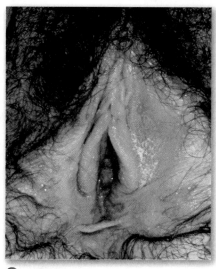

(a) Genital herpes is a highly contagious and incurable STI. It is characterized by recurring cycles of painful blisters on the genitalia.

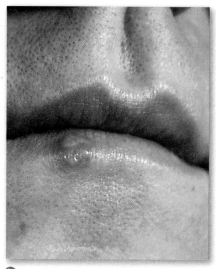

(b) Oral herpes, caused by the same virus as genital herpes, is extremely contagious and can cause painful sores and blisters around the mouth.

FIGURE 14.12 **Herpes**
Both genital and oral herpes can be caused by either herpes simplex virus type 1 or 2. Genital herpes is highly contagious and incurable (a). Oral herpes is the same virus as genital herpes, but occurs in and around the mouth (b).

Signs and Symptoms The precursor phase of a herpes infection is characterized by a burning sensation and redness at the site of infection. During this time, prescription medicines such as acyclovir and over-the-counter medications such as Abreva will often keep the disease from spreading. However, this phase of the disease is quickly followed by the second phase, in which a blister filled with a clear fluid containing the virus forms. If you pick at this blister or otherwise touch the site and spread this fluid with fingers, lipstick, lip balm, or other products, you can autoinoculate other body parts. Particularly dangerous is the possibility of spreading the infection to your eyes, for a herpes lesion on the eye can cause blindness.

Over a period of days, the unsightly blister will crust over, dry up, and disappear, and the virus will travel to the base of an affected nerve supplying the area and become dormant. Only when the victim becomes overly stressed, when diet and sleep are inadequate, when the immune system is overworked, or when excessive exposure to sunlight or other stressors occur will the virus become reactivated (at the same site every time) and begin the blistering cycle all over again. Each time a sore develops, it casts off (sheds) viruses that can be highly infectious. However, it is important to note that a herpes site can shed the virus even when no overt sore is present, particularly during the interval between the earliest symptoms and blistering. People may get genital herpes by having sexual contact with others who don't know they are infected or who are having outbreaks of herpes without any sores. A person with genital herpes can also infect a sexual partner during oral sex. The virus is spread only rarely, if at all, by touching objects such as a toilet seat or hot tub seat.

Complications Genital herpes is especially serious in pregnant women because the baby can be infected as it passes through the vagina during birth. Many physicians recommend cesarean deliveries for infected women. Additionally, women with a history of genital herpes appear to have a greater risk of developing cervical cancer.

Diagnosis and Treatment Diagnosis of herpes can be determined by collecting a sample from the suspected sore or by performing a blood test to identify an HSV-1 or HSV-2 infection. Although there is no cure for herpes at present, certain drugs can be used to treat symptoms. Unfortunately, they seem to work only if the infection is confirmed during the first few hours after contact. The effectiveness of other treatments, such as L-lysine, is largely unsubstantiated. Over-the-counter medications may reduce the length of time you have sores/symptoms. Other drugs, such as famciclovir (FAMVIR), may reduce viral shedding between outbreaks. This means that if you have outbreaks, you may reduce risks to your sexual partners.[57]

genital herpes STI caused by the herpes simplex virus.

genital warts Warts that appear in the genital area or the anus; caused by the human papillomavirus (HPV).

human papillomavirus (HPV) A group of viruses, many of which are transmitted sexually; some types of HPV can cause genital warts or cervical cancer.

Human Papillomavirus (HPV) and Genital Warts

Genital warts (also known as *venereal warts* or *condylomas*) are caused by a group of viruses known as **human papillomavirus (HPV)**. There are over 100 different types of HPV;

more than 30 types are sexually transmitted and are classified as either low risk or high risk. A person becomes infected when certain types of HPV penetrate the skin and mucous membranes of the genitals or anus. This is among the most common forms of STI, with 20 million Americans currently infected with genital HPV and approximately 6 million new cases each year.[58]

Signs and Symptoms Genital HPV appears to be relatively easy to catch. The typical incubation period is 6 to 8 weeks after contact. People infected with low-risk types of HPV may develop genital warts, a series of bumps or growths on the genitals, ranging in size from small pinheads to large cauliflower-like growths (see Figure 14.13).

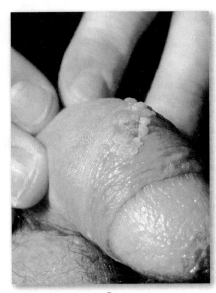
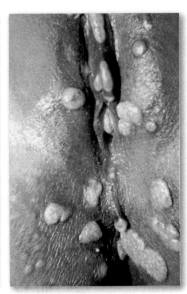

FIGURE 14.13 **Genital Warts**
Genital warts are caused by certain types of the human papillomavirus.

Complications Infection with high-risk types of HPV poses a significant risk for cervical cancer in women. It may lead to *dysplasia*, or changes in cells that may lead to a precancerous condition. Exactly how high-risk HPV infection leads to cervical cancer is uncertain. It is known that 6 out of 10 cervical cancers occur in women who have never received a Pap test or have not been tested for HPV in the past 5 years.[59]

Of those cases that become precancerous and are left untreated, 70 percent will eventually result in actual cancer. In addition, HPV may pose a threat to a fetus that is exposed to the virus during birth. Cesarean deliveries may be considered in serious cases. New research has also implicated HPV as a possible risk factor for coronary artery disease. It is hypothesized that HPV causes an inflammatory response in the artery walls, which leads to cholesterol and plaque buildup (see **Chapter 15**).

> **candidiasis** Yeastlike fungal infection often transmitted sexually; also called *moniliasis* or *yeast infection*.
>
> **trichomoniasis** Protozoan STI characterized by foamy, yellowish discharge and unpleasant odor.

Diagnosis and Treatment Diagnosis of genital warts from low-risk types of HPV is determined through a visual examination by a health care provider. High-risk types can be diagnosed in women through microscopic analysis of cells from a Pap smear or by collecting a sample from the cervix to test for HPV DNA. There is currently no HPV DNA test for men.

Treatment is available only for the low-risk forms of HPV that cause genital warts. The warts can be treated with topical medication or can be frozen with liquid nitrogen and then removed. Large warts may require surgical removal. There are currently two HPV vaccines that are licensed by the U.S. Food and Drug Administration (FDA) and recommended by the CDC. See the **Student Health Today** box on the next page for more information about these vaccines.

Candidiasis (Moniliasis)

Most STIs are caused by pathogens that come from outside the body; however, the yeastlike fungus *Candida albicans* is a normal inhabitant of the vaginal tract in most women. (See Figure 14.5c on page 420 for a micrograph of this fungus.) Only when the normal chemical balance of the vagina is disturbed will these organisms multiply and cause the fungal disease **candidiasis**, also sometimes called *moniliasis* or a *yeast infection*.

Signs and Symptoms Symptoms of candidiasis include severe itching and burning of the vagina and vulva and a white, cottage cheese–like vaginal discharge.[60] When this microbe infects the mouth, whitish patches form, and the condition is referred to as *thrush*. Thrush infection can also occur in men and is easily transmitted between sexual partners. Symptoms of candidiasis can be aggravated by contact with soaps, douches, perfumed toilet paper, chlorinated water, and spermicides.

Diagnosis and Treatment Diagnosis of candidiasis is usually made by collecting a vaginal sample and analyzing it to identify the pathogen. Antifungal drugs applied on the surface or by suppository usually cure candidiasis in just a few days.

Trichomoniasis

Unlike many STIs, **trichomoniasis** is caused by a protozoan, *Trichomonas vaginalis*. (See Figure 14.5d on page 420 for a micrograph of this organism.) An estimated 3.8 million Americans have the infection, but only 30 percent experience symptoms.[61]

Signs and Symptoms Symptoms among women include a foamy, yellowish, unpleasant-smelling discharge accompanied by a burning sensation, itching, and painful urination. Most men with trichomoniasis do not have any

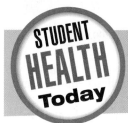

STUDENT HEALTH Today

Q&A ON HPV VACCINES

Most sexually active people will contract some form of human papillomarvirus (HPV) at some time in their lives, though they may never even know it. There are about 40 types of sexually transmitted HPV, most of which cause no symptoms and go away on their own. Low-risk types can cause genital warts, but some high-risk types can cause cervical and other cancers. Every year in the United States, about 12,000 women are diagnosed with cervical cancer, and almost 4,000 die from this disease. There are currently two HPV vaccines that can help prevent women from becoming infected with HPV and subsequently developing cervical cancer.

✻ Who should get the HPV vaccine?
There are two vaccines currently available—Cervarix and Gardasil. HPV vaccines are recommended for 11- and 12-year-old girls, but can be given to girls as young as 9 years old. It is also recommended for girls and women ages 13 through 26 who have not yet been vaccinated or completed the vaccine series. Ideally, females should get a vaccine before they become sexually active. Females who are sexually active may get less benefit from it because they may have already contracted an HPV type targeted by the vaccines.

One of the HPV vaccines, Gardasil, is also licensed, safe, and effective for males ages 9 through 26 years. The CDC recommends Gardasil for all boys 11 or 12 years old and for males ages 13 through 21 years who did not get any or all of the three recommended doses when they were younger. All men may receive the vaccine through the age of 26, but it is recommended that they should speak with their doctor to find out if getting vaccinated is right for them.

✻ How are the two HPV vaccines, Cervarix and Gardasil, similar and different? Both vaccines are very effective against high-risk HPV types 16 and 18, which cause 70 percent of cervical cancer cases. Both vaccines are given as shots and require three doses. But only Gardasil protects against low-risk HPV types 6 and 11. These HPV types cause 90 percent of cases of genital warts in females and males, so Gardasil is approved for use with males as well as females.

✻ What do the two vaccines *not* protect against? The vaccines do not protect against all types of HPV, so about 30 percent of cervical cancers will not be prevented by the vaccines. It will be important for women to continue getting screened for cervical cancer through regular Pap tests. Also, the vaccines do not prevent other sexually transmitted infections (STIs).

✻ How safe are the HPV vaccines? The vaccines are licensed by the FDA and approved by the CDC as safe and effective. They have been studied in thousands of females (ages 9 through 26) around the world, and their safety continues to be monitored by the CDC and the FDA. Studies have found no serious side effects.

Because the HPV vaccine is relatively new, some first-year college students who are eligible for the vaccination have not yet received it. Many state health departments and college campuses offer free or low-cost vaccines for those whose insurance does not cover the cost.

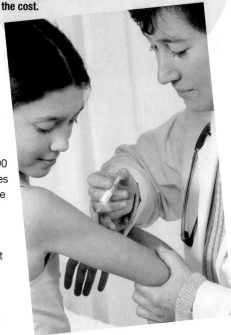

Sources: Centers for Disease Control and Prevention, "Vaccines and Preventable Diseases: HPV Vaccine—Questions & Answers," Reviewed January 2011, www.cdc.gov/vaccines/vpd-vac/hpv/vac-faqs.htm; American Cancer Society, 2010, "Human Papillomavirus (HPV), Cancer and HPV Vaccines—Frequently Asked Questions," Revised October 2010, www.cancer.org/Cancer/CancerCauses/OtherCarcinogens/InfectiousAgents/HPV/HumanPapillomaVirusandHPVVaccinesFAQ/index.

symptoms, though some men experience irritation inside the penis, mild discharge, and a slight burning after urinating.[62] Although usually transmitted by sexual contact, the "trich" organism can also be spread by toilet seats, wet towels, or other items that have discharged fluids on them.

Diagnosis and Treatment Diagnosis of trichomoniasis is determined by collecting fluid samples from the penis or vagina to test for the presence of the protozoan. Treatment includes oral metronidazole, usually given to both sexual partners to avoid the possible "ping-pong" effect of repeated cross-infection typical of STIs.

Pubic Lice

pubic lice Parasitic insects that can inhabit various body areas, especially the genitals.

Pubic lice, often called "crabs," are small parasitic insects that are usually transmitted during sexual contact (see **Figure 14.14** on page 436). More annoying than dangerous, they move easily from partner to partner during sex. They have an affinity for pubic hair and attach themselves to the

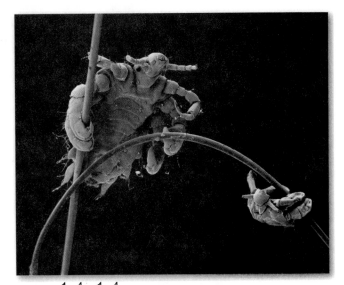

FIGURE **14.14** **Pubic Lice**
Pubic lice, also known as "crabs," are small, parasitic insects that attach themselves to pubic hair.

base of these hairs, where they deposit their **eggs** (nits). One to 2 weeks later, these nits develop into adults that lay **eggs** and migrate to other body parts, thus perpetuating the cycle.

Signs and Symptoms Symptoms of pubic lice infestation include itchiness in the area covered by pubic hair, bluish-gray skin color in the pubic region, and sores in the genital area.

Diagnosis and Treatment Diagnosis of pubic lice involves an examination by a health care provider to identify the eggs in the genital area. Treatment includes washing clothing, furniture, and linens that may harbor the eggs. It usually takes 2 to 3 weeks to kill all larval forms. Although sexual contact is the most common mode of transmission, you can "catch" pubic lice from lying on sheets or sitting on a toilet seat that an infected person has used.

HIV/AIDS

Acquired immunodeficiency syndrome (AIDS) is a significant global health threat. Since 1981, when AIDS was first recognized, approximately 65 million people in the world have become infected with **human immunodeficiency virus (HIV)**, the virus that causes AIDS. At the end of 2010, there were approximately 34 million people worldwide living with HIV.[63]

There are 1.2 million HIV-infected people in the United States. In 2010, about 47,000 people were diagnosed with HIV infection in the 46 states with long-term, confidential, name-based HIV infection reporting.[64]

acquired immunodeficiency syndrome (AIDS) A disease caused by a retrovirus, the human immunodeficiency virus (HIV), that attacks the immune system, reducing the number of helper T cells and leaving the victim vulnerable to infections, malignancies, and neurological disorders.

human immunodeficiency virus (HIV) The virus that causes AIDS by infecting helper T cells.

About 17,000 people died from HIV/AIDS in 2009 (the last year for which data are available).[65]

Initially, people with HIV were diagnosed as having AIDS only when they developed blood infections, the cancer known as Kaposi's sarcoma, or any of 21 other indicator diseases, most of which were common in male AIDS patients. The CDC has expanded the indicator list to include pulmonary tuberculosis, recurrent pneumonia, and invasive cervical cancer. Perhaps the most significant indicator today is a drop in the level of the body's master immune cells, CD4 cells (also called helper T cells), to one fifth the level in a healthy person.

AIDS cases have been reported state by state throughout the United States since the early 1980s. Today, the CDC recommends that all states report HIV infections as well as AIDS. Because of medical advances in treatment and increasing numbers of HIV-infected persons who do not progress to AIDS, it is believed that AIDS incidence statistics may not provide a true picture of the epidemic, the long-term costs of treating HIV-infected individuals, and other key information.

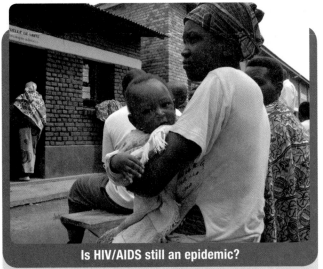

Is HIV/AIDS still an epidemic?

Yes! With swine flu and other emerging diseases dominating the news, it may seem as if HIV/AIDS is no longer a problem; however, nothing could be further from the truth. In North America, 1.4 million people are living with HIV, and HIV and AIDS are still at epidemic levels all over the world, especially in developing nations. Sub-Saharan Africa has been hit hardest: 22.4 million people in the region are living with the disease. Another 3.8 million in south/southeast Asia are infected and 2 million in Latin America. The epidemic is spreading most rapidly in eastern Europe and central Asia, where 1.5 million people currently have HIV.

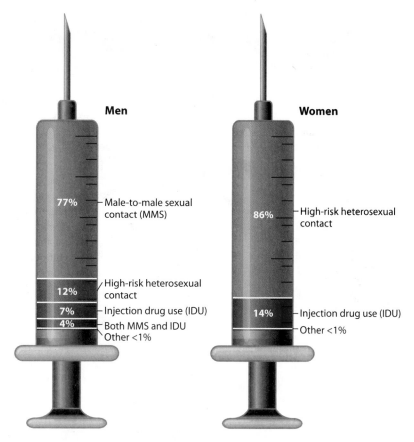

FIGURE 14.15 **Sources of HIV Infection among Adults and Adolescents in the United States, 2010**

Source: Data are from Centers for Disease Control and Prevention, *HIV Surveillance: Epidemiology of HIV Infection (through 2010)*, March 2012, www.cdc.gov/hiv/topics/surveillance.

How HIV Is Transmitted

HIV typically enters one person's body when another person's infected body fluids (e.g., semen, vaginal secretions, blood) gain entry through a breach in body defenses. Mucous membranes of the genital organs and the anus provide the easiest route of entry. If there is a break in the mucous membranes (as can occur during sexual intercourse, particularly anal intercourse), the virus enters and begins to multiply. After initial infection, HIV multiplies rapidly, invading the bloodstream and cerebrospinal fluid. It progressively destroys helper T cells (recall that these cells call the rest of the immune response to action), weakening the body's resistance to disease.

It is important to know that HIV/AIDS is not highly contagious. HIV cannot reproduce outside its living host, except in a controlled laboratory environment, and does not survive well in open air. As a result, HIV cannot be transmitted through casual contact, including sharing glasses, cutlery, or musical instruments. Transmission also cannot occur through swimming pools, showers, or by sharing washing facilities or toilet seats.[66] Research also provides overwhelming evidence that insect bites do not transmit HIV.[67]

Engaging in High-Risk Behaviors AIDS is not a disease of gay people or minority groups. Although during the early days of the epidemic it appeared that HIV infected only homosexuals, it quickly became apparent that the disease was not confined to groups of people, but rather was related to high-risk behaviors such as having unprotected sexual intercourse and sharing needles.

People who engage in high-risk behaviors increase their risk for the disease; people who do not engage in these behaviors have minimal risk. Figure 14.15 shows the breakdown of sources of HIV infection among U.S. men and women.

The majority of HIV infections arise from the following high-risk behaviors:

- **Exchange of body fluids.** The greatest risk factor is the exchange of HIV-infected body fluids during vaginal or anal intercourse. Substantial research indicates that blood, semen, and vaginal secretions are the major fluids of concern. In rare instances, the virus has been found in saliva, but most health officials state that saliva is a less significant risk than other shared body fluids.
- **Injecting drugs.** A significant percentage of AIDS cases in the United States result from sharing or using HIV-contaminated needles and syringes. Although users of illegal drugs are

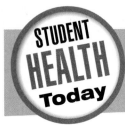
BODY PIERCING AND TATTOOING: POTENTIAL RISKS

A look around any college campus reveals many examples of body piercings and tattoos. The practice can be done safely, but health professionals cite several concerns, most commonly skin reactions, infections, allergic reactions, and scarring. More serious is the potential transmission of dangerous pathogens that can occur with any puncture of the skin. Unsterile needles can spread serious infections such as staph, HIV, hepatitis B and C, and tetanus.

Laws and policies regulating body piercing and tattooing vary greatly by state. Because of the lack of universal regulatory standards and the potential for transmission of dangerous pathogens, anyone who receives a tattoo, body piercing, or permanent makeup tattoo cannot donate blood for 1 year. Finding a safe and reputable body artist for a tattoo or piercing should be the priority. The following tips can help reduce risks:

✳ Look for clean, well-lighted work areas, and inquire about sterilization procedures. Be wary of establishments that won't answer questions or show you their sterilization equipment.

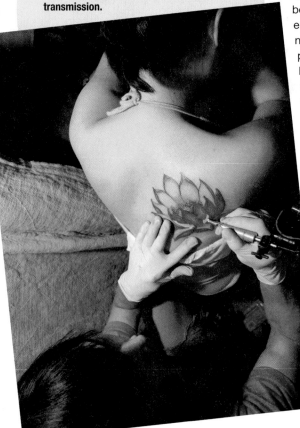

Like any activity that involves bodily fluids, tattooing carries some risk of disease transmission.

✳ Packaged, sterilized needles should be used only once and then discarded. A piercing gun should not be used, because it cannot be sterilized properly. Watch that the artist uses new needles and tubes from a sterile package before your procedure begins. Ask to see the sterile confirmation logo on the bag itself.

✳ Immediately before piercing or tattooing, the body area should be carefully sterilized. The artist should wash his or her hands and put on new latex gloves for each procedure. Make sure the artist changes gloves if he or she touches anything else, such as the telephone, while working.

✳ Leftover tattoo ink should be discarded after each procedure. Do not allow the artist to reuse ink that has been used for other customers. Used needles should be disposed of in a "sharps" container, a plastic container with the biohazard symbol clearly marked on it.

Source: Mayo Clinic Staff, "Tattoos: Understand Risks and Precautions," March 2012, www.mayoclinic.com/health/tattoos-and-piercings/MC00020.

---

commonly considered the only members of this category, others may also share needles—for example, people with diabetes who inject insulin or athletes who inject steroids. People who share needles and also engage in sexual activities with members of high-risk groups, such as those who exchange sex for drugs, increase their risks dramatically. Tattooing and piercing can also be risky (see the **Student Health Today** box).

95%

of people with HIV worldwide live in developing nations.

Mother-to-Child (Perinatal) Transmission

Mother-to-child transmission occurs when an HIV-positive woman passes the virus to her baby. This can occur during pregnancy, during labor and delivery, or through breast-feeding. Without antiretroviral treatment, approximately 25 percent of HIV-positive pregnant women will transmit the virus to their infant.[68]

Symptoms of HIV/AIDS

A person may go for months or years after infection by HIV before any significant symptoms appear. The incubation time varies greatly from person to person. For adults who receive no medical treatment, it takes an average of 8 to 10 years for the virus to cause the slow, degenerative changes in the immune system that are characteristic of AIDS. During this time, the person may experience *opportunistic infections* (infections that gain a foothold when the immune system is not functioning effectively). Colds, sore throats, fever, tiredness, nausea, night sweats, and other generally non–life-threatening conditions commonly appear and are described as pre-AIDS symptoms. Other symptoms of progressing HIV infection include wasting syndrome, swollen lymph nodes, and neurological problems. As the immune system continues to decline, the body becomes more vulnerable to infection. A diagnosis of AIDS, the final stage of HIV infection, is made when the infected person has either a dangerously low CD4 (helper T) cell count (below 200 cells per cubic milliliter of blood) or has contracted one or more opportunistic infections characteristic of the disease (such as Kaposi's sarcoma or *Pneumocystis carinii* pneumonia).

Testing for HIV Antibodies

Once antibodies have formed in reaction to HIV, a blood test known as the *ELISA* (enzyme-linked immunosorbent assay) may detect their presence. It can take 3 to 6 months after initial infection for sufficient antibodies to develop in the body to show a positive test result. Therefore, individuals with negative test results should be retested within 6 months. If sufficient antibodies are present, the test will be positive. When a person who previously tested *negative* (no HIV antibodies present) has a subsequent test that is *positive,* seroconversion is said to have occurred. In such a situation, the person would typically take another ELISA test, followed by a more precise test known as the *Western blot,* to confirm the presence of HIV antibodies.

It should be noted that these tests are not AIDS tests per se. Rather, they detect antibodies for HIV, indicating the presence of the virus in the person's system. Whether the person will develop AIDS depends to some extent on the strength of the immune system.

Health officials distinguish between *reported* and *actual* cases of HIV infection because it is believed that many HIV-positive people avoid being tested. One reason is fear of knowing the truth. Another is the fear of recrimination from employers, insurance companies, and medical staff. However, early detection and reporting are important because immediate treatment for someone in the early stages of HIV disease is critical. See the **Points of View** box on page 440 for more on the issue of HIV testing.

New Hope and Treatments

Drugs have slowed the progression from HIV to AIDS and have prolonged life expectancies for most AIDS patients. Current treatments combine selected drugs, especially protease inhibitors and reverse transcriptase inhibitors. *Protease inhibitors* (e.g., amprenavir, ritonavir, and saquinavir) act to prevent the production of the virus in chronically infected cells that HIV has already invaded. Other drugs, such as AZT, Riplivirine (RPV), ddI, ddC, d4T, and 3TC, inhibit the HIV enzyme *reverse transcriptase* before the virus has invaded the cell, thereby preventing the virus from infecting new cells. These drugs are categorized as either non-nucleoside reverse transcriptase inhibitors or nucleoside reverse transcriptase inhibitors, based on their mechanism to inhibit the enzyme. All of the protease drugs seem to work best in combination with other therapies. The FDA has approved several fixed-dose combinations of drugs from two or more classes, most recently, Complera, which combines nucleoside reverse transcriptase inhibitors with non-nucleoside reverse transcriptase inhibitors.[69]

Although these drugs provide new hope and longer survival rates for people living with HIV, it is important to maintain caution. We are still a long way from a cure. Apathy and carelessness may abound if too much confidence is placed in these treatments. Newer drugs that held much promise are becoming less effective as HIV develops resistance to them. Costs of taking multiple drugs are prohibitive, and they can cause serious damage to the liver if they are not carefully monitored (see the **Tech & Health** box on page 441 for more on efforts to make these drug regimens safer). Furthermore, the number of people becoming HIV infected each year has increased in some communities, meaning that we are still a long way from beating this disease.

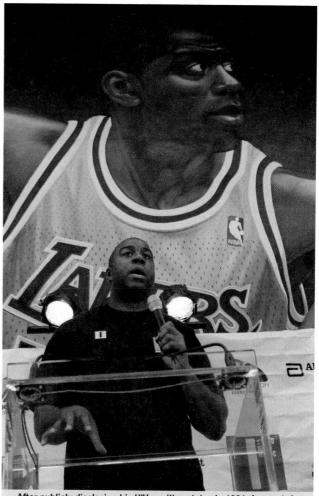

After publicly disclosing his HIV-positive status in 1991, former L.A. Laker star Earvin "Magic" Johnson became the first openly HIV-positive basketball player in the NBA.

POINTS OF VIEW

HIV Testing:
SHOULD IT BE MANDATORY?

Should there be mandatory testing and reporting of HIV status? The debate concerning this issue is heated and complicated. In a nutshell, the idea is that in order to combat the epidemic of HIV, health care providers need to know who carries the virus. For multiple reasons, however, people in all populations in the United States don't want to be tested. The epidemic continues in part because people who don't know they are infected continue to spread the disease.

Arguments for Mandatory Testing and Reporting

○ If health care providers know who is infected, they can treat those who are ill.
○ If governments know the true scope of the problem, they can allocate resources to respond to it properly.
○ Studies show that if those who have HIV know that they have it, they are more likely to use protection in order to avoid spreading it.
○ Given that HIV/AIDS is life threatening, mandatory testing and reporting is a matter of protecting society from disease and death.

Arguments against Mandatory Testing and Reporting

○ Mandatory testing and reporting constitute an invasion of privacy.
○ Once mandatory testing and reporting are in place, forced treatment may follow.
○ Testing is expensive. Funding for HIV/AIDS should focus on prevention efforts instead.
○ Some fear violence at home or discrimination in the workplace as a result of a positive test.

Where Do You Stand?

○ Should governments gather this information and use it to help combat the epidemic, or is that an invasion of privacy?
○ What sort of limits, if any, might you put on mandatory testing? Should anyone be exempt?
○ If the information is gathered, what limits should there be on how it can be used and who has access to it?

Sources: Centers for Disease Control and Prevention, "HIV Testing among Adolescents," Updated July 2011, Available at www.cdc.gov/healthyyouth/sexualbehaviors; L. Bisaillon, "Human Rights Consequences of Mandatory HIV Screening Policy of Newcomers to Canada," *Health and Human Rights* 12, no 2 (2010): 119–34; K. Morris and D. R. Wessner, "Compulsory HIV Testing," 2010, http://the-aids-pandemic.blogspot.com/2010/10/compulsory-hiv-testing.html.

Preventing HIV Infection

Although scientists have been working on a variety of HIV vaccine trials, none is currently available. The only way to prevent HIV infection is through the choices you make in sexual behaviors and drug use and by taking responsibility for your own health and the health of your loved ones. You can't determine the presence of HIV by looking at a person; you can't tell by questioning the person, unless he or she has been tested recently, if that person is HIV-negative and is giving an honest answer. So what should you do?

Of course, the simplest answer is abstinence. If you don't exchange body fluids, you won't get the disease. As a second line of defense, if you decide to be intimate, the next best option is to use a condom. However, in spite of all the educational campaigns, surveys consistently indicate that most college students throw caution to the wind if they think they "know" someone—and they have unprotected sex.

Where to Go for Help If you are concerned about your own risk or that of a close friend, arrange a confidential meeting with the health educator or other health professional at your college health service. He or she will provide you with the information that you need to decide whether you should be tested for HIV antibodies. If the student health service is not an option for you, seek assistance through your local public health department or community STI clinic.

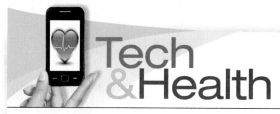

Tech & Health

SIMPLER TESTS CAN IMPROVE TREATMENT OUTCOMES FOR HIV AND TB PATIENTS

One of the side effects of AIDS antiviral therapy and tuberculosis treatment is liver failure due to the toxicity of the medication used to treat those diseases. In Africa that's been especially difficult to combat, as the tests routinely used to monitor liver function for signs of trouble require tubes of blood, laboratory facilities, time for processing results, as well as money for all of the above. In a place where poverty and patients are widespread but skilled health care workers and equipment are scarce, liver function often goes unmonitored in those who are at greatest risk. It is esti-

mated that in resource-poor countries, approximately 25 percent of HIV/AIDS patients lack access to diagnostic tools and die as a result of liver complications related to treatment. But a new cheap and simple test that determines liver function could change that.

The new test is a piece of specially treated paper the size of a stamp that costs around 10 cents. A small amount of blood or urine is applied, and then chemicals in the paper change color to show the result. As with diabetes or pregnancy home testing kits, the test is designed to be simple enough so the person reading

it doesn't need to be a trained medical professional to understand the results and it doesn't need any external power or equipment. This test improves the odds for patients with tuberculosis or HIV/AIDS that they will be able to withstand the side effects of their treatments successfully.

Source: Diagnostics For All, "Liver Function Test," 2011, http://dfa.org/projects/liverfunction .html; D. McNeil, "Far from Any Lab, Paper Bits Find Illness," September 27, 2011, *The New York Times,* p D1; A. Maloney, "AlterNet's Top 20 Big Ideas that Don't Cost the Earth," 2011, www.trust .org/alertnet/news/alertnets-top-20-big-ideas- that-dont-cost-the-earth.

Assess yourself

STIs: Do You Really Know What You Think You Know?

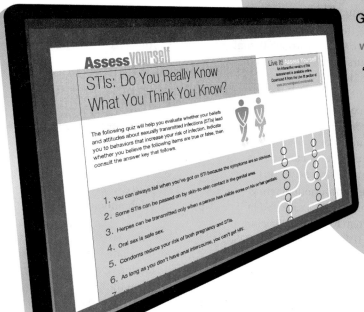

Go online to the **Live It!** section of www.pearsonhighered.com/donatelle to take the "STIs: Do You Really Know What You Think You Know?" assessment.* Use the strategies outlined in the **YOUR PLAN FOR CHANGE** box to change behaviors that may be putting you at risk.

*If your instructor so chooses, Assess Yourself Activities are available as a printed supplement or as assignable homework online at www.pearsonhighered.com/myhealthlab.

MyHealthLab®

YOUR PLAN FOR CHANGE

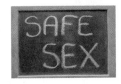

After completing the "STIs: Do You Really Know What You Think You Know?" **Assessyourself**, you can begin to change behaviors that may be putting you at risk for STIs and for infection in general.

Today, you can:

○ Put together an "emergency" supply of condoms. Outside of abstinence, condoms are your best protection against an STI. If you don't have a supply on hand, visit your local drugstore or health clinic. Remember that both men and women are responsible for preventing the transmission of STIs.

○ To prevent infections in general, get in the habit of washing your hands regularly. After you cough, sneeze, blow your nose, use the bathroom, or prepare food, find a sink, wet your hands with warm water, and lather up with soap. Scrub your hands for about 20 seconds (count to 20 or recite the alphabet), rinse well, and dry your hands.

Within the next 2 weeks, you can:

○ Talk with your significant other honestly about your sexual history. Make appointments to get tested if either of you think you may have been exposed to an STI.

○ Adjust your sleep schedule so that you're getting an adequate amount of rest every night. Being well rested is one key aspect of maintaining a healthy immune system.

By the end of the semester, you can:

○ Check your immunization schedule and make sure you're current with all recommended vaccinations. Make an appointment with your health care provider if you need a booster or vaccine.

○ If you are due for an annual pelvic exam, make an appointment. Ask your partner if he or she has had an annual exam and encourage him or her to make an appointment if not.

Summary

* Your body uses several defense systems to keep pathogens from invading. The skin is the body's major protection, helped by enzymes. The immune system creates antibodies to destroy antigens. Fever and pain play a role in defending the body. Vaccines bolster the body's immune system against specific diseases. Allergies are an overreaction of the immune system.

* The major classes of pathogens are bacteria, viruses, fungi, protozoans, parasitic worms, and prions. Bacterial infections include staphylococcal infections, streptococcal infections, meningitis, pneumonia, tuberculosis, and tickborne diseases. Major viral infections include the common cold; influenza; mononucleosis; hepatitis; mumps; the herpes viruses, including chickenpox, shingles, and herpes gladiatorum; measles and rubella; and rabies.

* Emerging and resurgent diseases such as avian flu or West Nile virus pose significant threats for future generations. Many factors contribute to these risks. Possible solutions focus on a public health approach to prevention.

* Sexually transmitted infections (STIs) are spread through sexual intercourse, oral–genital contact, anal sex, hand–genital contact, and sometimes through mouth-to-mouth contact. Major STIs include chlamydia, gonorrhea, syphilis, herpes, human papillomavirus (HPV) and genital warts, candidiasis, trichomoniasis, and pubic lice.

* Acquired immunodeficiency syndrome (AIDS) is caused by the human immunodeficiency virus (HIV). Globally, HIV/AIDS has become a major threat to the world's population. Anyone can get HIV by engaging in high-risk sexual activities that include exchange of body fluids or by injecting drugs (or by having sex with someone who does). You can reduce your risk for contracting HIV significantly by not engaging in risky sexual activities or IV drug use.

Pop Quiz

1. Which of the following do not assist the body in fighting disease?
   a. Antigens
   b. Antibodies
   c. Lymphocytes
   d. Macrophages

2. Which of the following diseases is caused by a prion?
   a. Shingles
   b. Listeria
   c. Mad cow disease
   d. Trichomoniasis

3. An example of passive immunity is
   a. inoculation with a vaccine containing weakened antigens.
   b. when the body makes its own antibodies to a pathogen.
   c. the antibody-containing part of the vaccine that came from someone else.
   d. None of the above

4. One of the best ways to prevent contagious viruses from spreading is to
   a. wash your hands frequently.
   b. cover your mouth with your arm when sneezing, and dispose of your tissues.
   c. keep your hands away from your mouth and eyes.
   d. All of the above

5. Which of the following is a *viral* disease?
   a. Measles
   b. Pneumonia
   c. Malaria
   d. Streptococcal infection

6. Which of the following STIs cannot be treated with antibiotics?
   a. Chlamydia
   b. Gonorrhea
   c. Syphilis
   d. Herpes

7. Pelvic inflammatory disease (PID) is
   a. a sexually transmitted infection.
   b. a type of urinary tract infection.
   c. an infection of a woman's fallopian tubes or uterus.
   d. a disease that both men and women can get.

8. The most widespread sexually transmitted bacterium is
   a. gonorrhea.
   b. chlamydia.
   c. syphilis.
   d. chancroid.

9. Jennifer touched her viral herpes sore on her lip and then touched her eye. She ended up with the herpes virus in her eye as well. This is an example of
   a. acquired immunity.
   b. passive spread.
   c. autoinoculation.
   d. self-vaccination.

10. Which of the following is *not* a true statement about HIV?

a. You can tell if a potential sex partner has the virus by looking at him or her.
b. The virus can be spread through semen or vaginal fluids.
c. You cannot get HIV from a public restroom toilet seat.
d. Unprotected anal sex increases risk of exposure to HIV.

Answers to these questions can be found on page A-1.

Think about It!

1. What are three lifestyle changes you could make right now that would reduce your risk of developing an infectious disease? What could you do to help protect your friends and family members? Partner? How can you help reduce antibiotic resistance in the world today?
2. What is a pathogen? What does it mean if someone says a pathogen is particularly *virulent*? What are *antigens*? *Antibodies*? Discuss uncontrollable and controllable risk factors that can make you more or less susceptible to infectious pathogens in your immediate surroundings.
3. Explain why it is important to wash your hands often when you have a cold.
4. What is the difference between active and passive immunity? How do they compare to natural and acquired immunity?
5. Discuss the importance of vaccinations in reducing societal risks for infectious diseases.
6. Identify five STIs and their symptoms. How do they develop? What are their potential long-term effects?
7. Why are women more susceptible to HIV infection than men? What implication does this have for prevention, treatment, and research?

Accessing Your Health on the Internet

The following websites explore further topics and issues related to personal health. For links to the websites below, visit the Companion Website for *Access to Health*, 13th Edition, at www.pearsonhighered.com/donatelle.

1. *Centers for Disease Control and Prevention (CDC).* This is the home page for the government agency dedicated to disease intervention and prevention, with links to all the latest data and publications put out by the CDC—including the *Morbidity and Mortality Weekly Report* (*MMWR*), *HIV/AIDS Surveillance Report,* and the *Journal of Emerging Infectious Diseases*—and access to the CDC research database, Wonder. www.cdc.gov
2. *American Social Health Association.* This site provides facts, support, resources, and referrals about sexually transmitted infections and diseases. www.ashastd.org
3. *San Francisco AIDS Foundation.* This community-based AIDS service organization focuses on ending the HIV/AIDS pandemic through education, services for AIDS patients, advocacy and public policy efforts, and global programs. www.sfaf.org
4. *World Health Organization (WHO).* You'll gain access to the latest information on world health issues and direct access to publications and fact sheets at WHO's site. www.who.int
5. *Specialized CDC sites.* These sites focus on infectious diseases:
   - National Center for Immunization and Respiratory Diseases. www.cdc.gov/ncird/index.html
   - National Center for Emerging and Zoonotic Infectious Diseases. www.cdc.gov/ncezid
   - National Center for HIV/AIDS, Viral Hepatitis, STD and TB Prevention. www.cdc.gov/nchhstp

- National Center for Preparedness, Detection and Control of Infectious Diseases. www.cdc.gov/ncpdcid

6. *AVERT*. This is an international site with information on HIV/AIDS, global STI statistics, interactive quizzes, and graphics displaying current statistics for vulnerable populations. www.avert.org

References

1. Environmental Protection Agency, "Climate Change—Health and Environmental Effects," Updated November 2011, www.epa.gov/climatechange/effects/health.html; A. Greer et al., "Climate Change and Infectious Diseases in North America: The Road Ahead," *Canadian Medical Association Journal* 178, no. 6 (2008): 715–22; E. Shuman, "Global Climate Change and Infectious Diseases," *New England Journal of Medicine* 362 (2010): 1061–63.

2. B. Feingold et al., "A Niche for Infectious Disease in Environmental Health: Rethinking the Toxicological Paradigm," *Environmental Health Perspectives* 118, no. 8 (2010): 1165–72; L. Martin et al., "The Effects of Anthropogenic Global Changes on Immune Functions and Disease Resistance," *Annals of the New York Academy of Sciences* 1195, no. 1 (2010): 129–48.

3. National Institute of Environmental Health Sciences, "NIH News—New Study Shows 32 Million Americans Have Autoantibodies That Target Their Own Tissues," 2012, www.nih.gov/news/health/jan2012/niehs-13.htm.

4. American Autoimmune Related Diseases Association, "Autoimmune Statistics," 2012, www.aarda.org/autoimmune_statistics.php.

5. Centers for Disease Control and Prevention, " "Figure 2, Recommended Immunization Schedule for Persons Aged 7–18 Years, United States," 2012, www.cdc.gov/vaccines/recs/schedules/downloads/child/7-18yrs-schedule-pr.pdf[0].

6. Centers for Disease Control and Prevention, "Vital and Health Statistics for U.S. Adults: National Health Interview Survey, 2010," 2012, www.cdc.gov/nchs/data/series/sr_10/sr10_252.pdf; Centers for Disease Control and Prevention "Vital and Health Statistics for U.S. Children: National Health Interview Survey, 2010," December 2011, www.cdc.gov/nchs/data/series/sr_10/sr10_250.pdf.

7. R. deShazo, S. Kemp, and J. Corren, "Patient Information: Allergic Rhinitis (Seasonal Allergies—Beyond the Basics," 2012, www.uptodate.com/contents/patient-information-allergic-rhinitis-seasonal-allergies-beyond-the-basics.

8. Centers for Disease Control and Prevention, "Antibiotics: Will They Work When You Really Need Them?" Uploaded March 2012, www.cdc.gov/getsmart/healthcare/learn-from-others/factsheets/antibiotics.html.

9. M. R. Klevens et al., "Invasive Methicillin-Resistant *Staphylococcus aureus* Infections in the United States," *Journal of the American Medical Association* 298, no. 15 (2007): 1763–71.

10. W. Jarvis, "Prevention and Control of Methicillin-Resistant *Staphylococcus aureus*: Dealing with Reality, Resistance, and Resistance to Reality," *Clinical Infectious Diseases* 50, no. 2 (2010): 218–20.

11. Centers for Disease Control and Prevention, "Group A Streptococcal (GAS)—Disease," 2010 Provisional Data, Uploaded March 2012, www.cdc.gov/ncidod/dbmd/diseaseinfo/groupastreptococcal_g.htm.

12. Ibid.

13. Centers for Disease Control and Prevention, "Fast Facts: Group B Strep (GBS)," 2010, www.cdc.gov/groupbstrep/about/fast-facts.html.

14. Centers for Disease Control and Prevention, "Meningitis Questions and Answers," Updated November 2011, www.cdc.gov/meningitis/about/faq.html.

15. Centers for Disease Control and Prevention, "Tuberculosis: Data and Statistics," December 2011, www.cdc.gov./tb/statistics/default.htm; Centers for Disease Control and Prevention, "Trends in Tuberculosis, 2010," October 2011, www.cdc.gov/tb/publications/factsheets/statistics/TBTrends.htm.

16. Centers for Disease Control and Prevention, "Global Tuberculosis (TB)," October 2011, www.cdc.gov/tb/topic/globaltb/default.htm; Centers for Disease Control and Prevention, "Fact Sheet: Trends in Tuberculosis, 2010," October 2011, www.cdc.gov/tb/publications/factsheets/statistics/TBTrends.htm.

17. World Health Organization, *WHO Report 2009—Global Tuberculosis Control: Epidemiology, Strategy, Financing* (Geneva: World Health Organization, 2009), Available at www.who.int/tb/publications/global_report/2009/en.

18. World Health Organization, "Global Tuberculosis Control 2010," 2010.

19. Ibid.

20. WebMD, "Cold Guide: Understanding Common Cold—Basics," 2011, www.webmd.com/cold-and-flu/cold-guide/understanding-common-cold-basics.

21. Centers for Disease Control and Prevention, "Seasonal Influenza: Key Facts about Influenza (Flu) and Flu Vaccine," Updated October 2011, www.cdc.gov/flu/keyfacts.htm.

22. National Institute of Allergy and Infectious Diseases, "Is It a Cold or the Flu?" 2008, www.niaid.nih.gov/topics/flu/documents/sick.pdf.

23. Centers for Disease Control and Prevention, "Selecting the Viruses in the Seasonal Influenza (Flu) Vaccine," 2011, www.cdc.gov/flu/professionals/vaccination/virusqa.htm.

24. Centers for Disease Control and Prevention, "CDC's Advisory Committee on Immunization Practices Recommends Universal Annual Influenza Vaccination," 2010, www.cdc.gov/media/pressrel/2010/r100224.htm.

25. S. Doerr, "Mononucleosis," 2012, www.emedicinehealth.com/script/main/art.asp?articlekey=58850&pf=3; Centers for Disease Control and Prevention, "Epstein-Barr Virus and Infectious Mononucleosis," 2012, www.cdc.gov/ncidod/diseases/ebv.htm.

26. Centers for Disease Control and Prevention, "Hepatitis A FAQs for Health Professionals," Updated April 2011, www.cdc.gov/hepatitis/HAV/HAVfaq.htm.

27. Centers for Disease Control and Prevention, "Hepatitis B Fact Sheet," 2010, www.cdc.gov/hepatitis/HBV/PDFs/HepBGeneralFactSheet.pdf.

28. Centers for Disease Control and Prevention, "Hepatitis B: A Global Perspective," 2012, www.cdc.gov/Features/dsHepatitisAwareness.

29. Ibid.

30. Centers for Disease Control and Prevention, "Hepatitis C FAQs for Health Professionals," Updated June 2010, www.cdc.gov/hepatitis/HCV/HCVfaq.htm.

31. S. Rajaguru and M. Nettleman, "Hepatitis C," MedicineNet.com, 2010, www.medicinenet.com/hepatitis_c/article.htm.

32. Centers for Disease Control and Prevention, "Mumps Outbreaks," Updated May 2010, www.cdc.gov/mumps/outbreaks.html.

33. A. E. Barskey et al., "Mumps Resurgences in the United States: A Historical Perspective on Unexpected Elements," *Vaccine* 27, no. 44 (2009): 6186–95.

34. Centers for Disease Control and Prevention, "Prevention of Herpes Zoster: Recommendations of the Advisory Committee on Immunization Practices (ACIP)," *MMWR Recommendations and Reports* 57, no. 5 (2008): 1–30; Centers for Disease Control and Prevention, "Shingles Vaccinations: What You Need to Know," 2012, www.cdc.gov/vaccines/vpd-vac/shingles/vacc-need-know.htm.

35. Centers for Disease Control and Prevention, "About vCJD (Variant Creutzfeldt-Jakob Disease)," 2010, www.cdc.gov/ncidod/dvrd/cjd.

36. Centers for Disease Control and Prevention, "Get Smart: Know When Antibiotics Work: Fast Facts," Updated March 2010, www.cdc.gov/getsmart/antibiotic-use/fast-facts.html; J. Ritterman, "Preventing Antibiotic Resistance: The Next Step," *Permanente Journal* 10, no. 3 (2006): 22–24.

37. Centers for Disease Control and Prevention, "West Nile virus (WNV) Activity Reported to ArboNET, by State, United States, 2011," 2012, www.cdc.gov/ncidod/dvbid/westnile/Mapsactivity/surv&control11MapsAnybyState.htm.

38. Centers for Disease Control and Prevention, Division of Vector-Borne Diseases, "West Nile Virus: Fight the Bite," Updated January 2012, www.cdc.gov/ncidod/dvbid/westnile/.

39. World Health Organization, "Confirmed Human Cases of Avian Influenza A (H5N1)," 2012, www.who.int/influenza/human_animal_interface/H5N1_cumulative_table_archives/en/index.html.

40. Ibid.

41. World Health Organization, "Malaria, Fact Sheet no. 94," 2012, www.who.int/mediacentre/factsheets/fs094/en.

42. Ibid; Global Program on Malaria, "Malaria FAQ Factsheet," 2012, www.malariafreefuture.org/resource-type/fact-sheets.

43. World Health Organization, "Malaria," 2012.

44. Centers for Disease Control and Prevention, "Sexually Transmitted Disease Surveillance, 2010," 2011, www.cdc.gov/std/stats10/default.htm.

45. Centers for Disease Control and Prevention, "Chlamydia Fact Sheet," Updated February 2012, www.cdc.gov/std/chlamydia/STDFact-Chlamydia.htm.

46. Center for Young Women's Health, "Chlamydia," Updated January 2010, www.youngwomenshealth.org/chlamydia.html.

47. MedlinePlus, "Pelvic Inflammatory Disease (PID)," Updated September 2011, www.nlm.nih.gov/medlineplus/ency/article/000888.htm; Mayo Clinic Staff, "Urinary Tract Infection: Risk Factors," 2010, www.mayoclinic.com/health/urinary-tract-infection/DS00286/DSECTION=risk-factors.

48. National Institute of Allergy and Infectious Diseases, "Chlamydia: Complications," Updated March 2009, www.niaid.nih.gov/topics/chlamydia/understanding/pages/complications.aspx.

49. Centers for Disease Control and Prevention, "Gonorrhea Fact Sheet," April 2011, www.cdc.gov/std/gonorrhea/stdfact-gonorrhea.htm.

50. Centers for Disease Control and Prevention, "Sexually Transmitted Diseases Surveillance, 2010," 2011.

51. Centers for Disease Control and Prevention, "Gonorrhea Fact Sheet," 2011.

52. National Institute of Allergy and Infectious Diseases, "Gonorrhea: Treatment," Updated 2011, www.niaid.nih.gov/topics/gonorrhea/understanding/Pages/treatment.aspx.

53. Centers for Disease Control and Prevention, "Syphilis Fact Sheet," September 2010, www.cdc.gov/std/syphilis/STDFact-Syphilis.htm.

54. National Institute of Allergy and Infectious Diseases, "Syphilis: Symptoms," Updated 2010, www.niaid.nih.gov/topics/syphilis/understanding/Pages/symptoms.aspx.

55. Centers for Disease Control and Prevention, "Genital Herpes—CDC Fact Sheet," Modified January 2012, www.cdc.gov/std/herpes/stdfact-herpes.htm.

56. American Social Health Association, "Learn about Herpes: Fast Facts," 2012, www.ashastd.org/std-sti/Herpes/learn-about-herpes.html.

57. Ibid.

58. Centers for Disease Control and Prevention, "Genital HPV Infection—CDC Fact Sheet," Modified November 2011, www.cdc.gov/std/HPV/STDFact-HPV.htm.

59. National Women's Law Center, 2010, http://hrc.nwlc.org/status-indicators/pap-smears; Centers for Disease Control and Prevention, "Cervical Cancer," Updated 2011, www.cdc.gov/cancer/cervical.

60. Centers for Disease Control and Prevention, January 2012, "Genital/Vulvovaginal Candidiasis," www.cdc.gov/fungal/Candidiasis/genital.

61. Centers for Disease Control and Prevention, "Trichomoniasis: CDC Fact Sheet," Modified November 2011, www.cdc.gov/std/trichomonas/STDFact-Trichomoniasis.htm.

62. Ibid.

63. Joint United Nations Programme on HIV/AIDS (UNAIDS) and World Health Organization (WHO), *2011 UNAIDS World AIDS Day Report* (Geneva: UNAIDS, 2012), Available at www.unaids.org/en.

64. Centers for Disease Control and Prevention, "HIV Surveillance Report, 2010," vol. 22, March 2012, http://www.cdc.gov/hiv/topics/surveillance/resources/factsheets/us_overview.htm.

65. Centers for Disease Control and Prevention, "HIV in the United States: At a Glance," March 2012, http://www.cdc.gov/hiv/resources/factsheets/us.htm.

66. AVERT, "Can You Get HIV From …?" Updated 2011, www.avert.org/can-you-get-hiv-aids.htm.

67. Ibid.

68. AVERT, "Preventing Mother-to-Child Transmission," Updated 2011, www.avert.org/motherchild.htm.

69. U.S. Department of Health and Human Services, "FSA-Approved Anti-HIV Medications," November 2011, http://aidsinfo.nih.gov/contentfiles/ApprovedMedstoTreatHIV_FS_en.pdf.

Understanding Your Health Inheritance

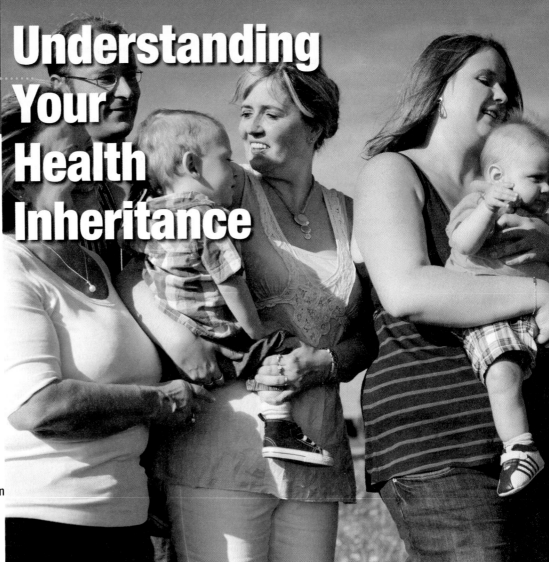

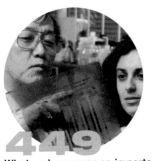

449

What makes genes so important to health?

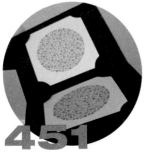

451

Why is color blindness common in males—and rare in females?

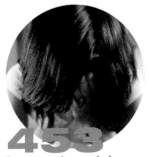

453

Do genes play a role in any psychiatric disorders?

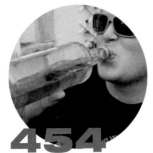

454

Are certain addictive tendencies predetermined by heredity?

It was spring break, and most of Ben's classmates were off to the beach. Although Ben had tickets to fly to Cancun, he had to make a quick change of plans and head to Minneapolis to be with his family. His older brother Nathan, age 29, had just had a major heart attack.

As the minutes dragged by on his 3-hour flight, Ben had flashbacks of being at the hospital just 5 years earlier when he had witnessed his father die at age 46 of a heart attack. He remembered his father's doctor talking about how some aspects of heart disease risk were hereditary and how in one long-term study some families had no males live into their forties. It had all been just mumbo jumbo to him at the time. However, terms such as *high cholesterol, stroke,* and *increased risk for family members* now flashed before him. The doctor had also spoken of the need for Ben and his brother to get regular checkups, maintain a healthy weight, watch their diet, and avoid smoking. He knew that, like their late father, Nathan had a pack-a-day habit. But who worries about developing heart disease when you're in your twenties?

We seldom think of young adults dying of heart disease or other chronic illnesses, and statistically such situations are rare.

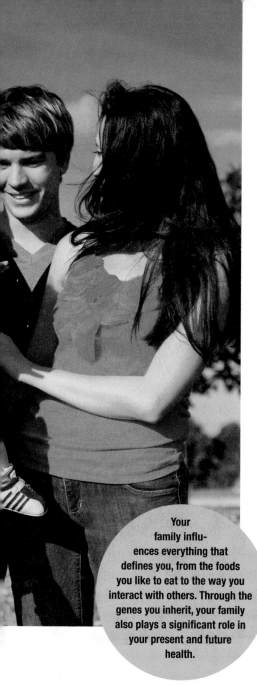

However, research such as the study that Ben's father's doctor described points to a clear hereditary risk for certain conditions in some families.[1] Not only do we inherit our tendency to be short or tall or have blue or brown eyes, we also inherit a tendency for increased risk for certain conditions. Are we "doomed" by our genetic predispositions? Are some conditions inevitable? If so, why do we hear so much about prevention and risk reduction? What about all those other determinants, such as we talked about in Chapter 1: our personal behaviors, aspects of our social and physical environment, public policies and interventions, and access to health care? Where do they fit in?

We do have an increased risk of developing inherited diseases that have been experienced by other members of our family. However, inheritance is just one determinant of health—it doesn't dictate anyone's destiny! Throughout this book we have shown you how your health choices and behaviors—from what you eat and how much you exercise to whether you smoke or misuse alcohol—can affect your quality of life and your risk of major disease and disability. If that's the case, then why should you bother to find out your family health history? There are three reasons. First, if you know that certain diseases run in your family, you can change your behaviors to reduce your risk. Second, you can share your family health portrait with your health care providers so that they can provide better care, for instance, by looking for early warning signs of a condition in your family. Third, compiling a family health history is important if you are planning to have children. That's because a handful of disorders are indeed controlled by inheritance. These are known collectively as *genetic disorders,* and we'll discuss them later in this chapter. If your research were to reveal a family history of any of these genetic disorders, you could then talk to your health care provider about genetic testing and counseling.

If you're adopted, or your parents and grandparents are already deceased, it may be more challenging for you to determine your family health history. But undertaking the investigation is important, because it has become increasingly evident that your genetic background plays a role in your future health. Before you set out to gather your family health history, you need to understand the basic substances, structures, and processes involved in human inheritance.

What Role Do Genes Play in Inheritance?

Inheritance is the process by which physical and biological characteristics—called *traits*—are transmitted from parents to their offspring. For instance, you may have inherited your dad's curly hair, but your mom's blood type. To appreciate how this transmission of traits occurs, let's look at the key players in the process.

Genes Are Coding Regions of DNA

You probably know that all of the structures of your body—from your skin to your bones—are composed of functional units called *cells.* Within each cell is a small, dark sac called the *nucleus.* It's dark because it's densely packed with **DNA (deoxyribonucleic acid),** a complex molecule that stores all of the programming code that your body uses for its initial assembly, growth from infancy to adulthood, and functioning throughout life. DNA is an extraordinarily long molecule that's shaped like a twisted rope ladder (commonly known as a *double helix*) with two long side strands

---

inheritance Process by which physical and biological characteristics—called traits—are transmitted from parents to their offspring.

DNA (deoxyribonucleic acid) Compound residing in the nucleus of body cells that stores in its sequence of chemical subunits the instructions for assembling body proteins.

Your family influences everything that defines you, from the foods you like to eat to the way you interact with others. Through the genes you inherit, your family also plays a significant role in your present and future health.

"Why Should I Care?"

You may have inherited traits or characteristics that affect your health every day, such as color blindness or a tendency toward depression. Knowing your family's health history, and sharing it with your health care provider, may help you treat symptoms or head off conditions that you might otherwise overlook or ignore.

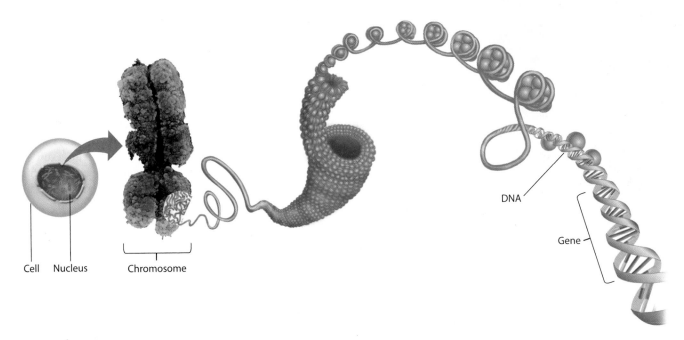

FIGURE 1 Chromosomes, DNA, and Genes
Almost every cell of the human body contains genetic information densely packed into the cell nucleus, which organizes itself into 46 chromosomes when the cell is preparing to divide. Chromosomes are bundles composed of DNA, a weak acid that forms long strands of a characteristic double-helix shape. DNA consists of noncoding regions as well as regions called *genes* that code for the assembly of body proteins.

Source: Adapted from Michael D. Johnson, *Human Biology: Concepts and Current Issues*, 5th ed., © 2010. Printed and electronically reproduced by permission of Pearson Education, Inc., Upper Saddle River, New Jersey.

connected by short "rungs." For much of the life of a cell, its DNA exists as tangled masses dispersed within the nucleus. But when a cell gets ready to divide, its DNA becomes organized into 46 distinct bundles called **chromosomes** (see Figure 1). These 46 chromosomes exist as two sets of 23; you get one full set of 23 chromosomes from each parent.

The long rope ladder of DNA that makes up each chromosome contains hundreds of unique regions called **genes,** which store the code for assembling particular body proteins. Genes occupy about 1 percent of the total DNA in human chromosomes.[2] The rest of your DNA has noncoding functions, such as assisting in regulating the quantity of proteins made or maintaining the structure of the chro-

mosome.[3] Your full complement of DNA—including genes and non-coding regions—is your **genome.** The branch of human biology that studies the human genome, genetic variation, and inheritance is known as *genetics.*

Genes Are Expressed as Proteins

Genes can be likened to particular "pages" in the code book of DNA, in that they contain the instructions for assembling—or *expressing*—specific body proteins. But what makes proteins so important? Essentially all cells and tissues of the human body are composed of proteins. In addition, proteins include a vast array of molecules

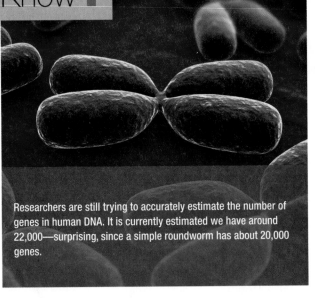

Did you Know?

Researchers are still trying to accurately estimate the number of genes in human DNA. It is currently estimated we have around 22,000—surprising, since a simple roundworm has about 20,000 genes.

that participate in the physiological processes that enable you to function. Therefore, by controlling the expression of proteins, genes control your body's appearance and structure as well as its functioning.

---

chromosome Discrete bundle of DNA, 46 of which are present in the nucleus of almost all cells of the human body.

gene Discrete segment of DNA in a chromosome that stores the code for assembling a particular body protein.

genome All of the genetic information an organism possesses.

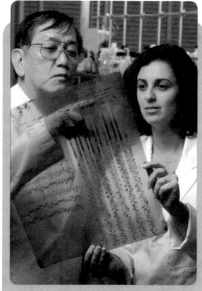

What makes genes so important to health?

Genes contain the code for assembling proteins necessary for your body's structures and functions. The way these proteins are put together can affect whether you are more at risk for certain conditions or have particular traits that can influence your health.

To understand how genes express proteins, it's important to recall that proteins are made up of subunits called *amino acids.* Just as a vast quantity of 20 different Lego parts could be assembled in various combinations into thousands of different toys, a vast quantity of the 20 amino acids in your body can be assembled into an estimated 10,000 to 50,000 unique body proteins.[4] For the instructions indicating how to make each of these proteins, the cell turns to DNA: Each gene on the DNA is a sequence of chemical instructions for combining amino acids into a specific protein.

Proteins Express Traits

Minute differences in proteins from one person to another result in the unique physical and physiological characteristics each of us possesses. For instance, pigments are proteins, and they account for variations in the color of people's skin, hair, and eyes. But proteins also account for traits that

are not visible, such as aspects of our functioning. For example, certain proteins contribute to three different types of cone cells in the eye. Cone cells allow us to distinguish colors, and if we don't have the genes to code for all three types of cone cells, we will have some form of color blindness.

How Are Traits Inherited?

You may have inherited your father's height or your mother's hazel eyes, or even a grandparent's jawline or big nose. Just as people can inherit aspects of their appearance from family members, people can inherit genetic disorders or susceptibility to chronic diseases experienced by others in their family. But precisely how are such traits passed down?

Traits Are Inherited via Chromosomes

We said earlier that your body cells have two sets of 23 chromosomes, one set from each parent. In other words, chromosomes exist as pairs that are alike in size and appearance. Geneticists can arrange chromosomes by pair in a configuration called a *karyotype* (Figure 2), with pair 1 being the largest and pair 22 the smallest. These are the 22 pairs of body chromosomes, called *autosomes.*

Pair 23 is your solitary pair of *sex chromosomes,* called XX or XY, which determines whether you are female or male, respectively. That is, every female gets one X chromosome from each parent to make up her twenty-third pair. The one she gets from her mother is one of the two Xs that make up her mother's twenty-third pair. The one she gets from her father

99.9% of the DNA sequence in humans is identical; the remaining 0.1% is what makes each person unique.

is the only X he has to give—because the other chromosome in his twenty-third pair is a Y. Every male gets his father's only Y chromosome, but he could get either one of his mother's two Xs. Notice that, for this reason, it is the father's genetic contribution that determines the baby's sex.

Because you have two copies of each chromosome, you have two copies of each gene. Again, one copy comes from your father, and one from your mother. Your two gene copies may be similar, or they may be different. Different forms of the same gene are known as **alleles.**

For example, do you have freckles? Researchers believe that the presence or absence of freckles is coded by just one gene. However, that gene has two alleles—two forms. If you have freckles, you may have inherited the allele for freckles from both of your parents. But even if you inherited the freckle

alleles One of potentially several variants of the same gene.

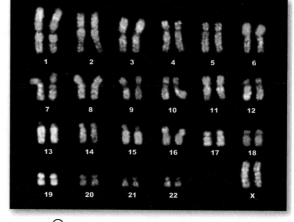

FIGURE 2 **Human Karyotype**
A karyotype is a complete set of chromosomes arranged into pairs by size. This karyotype is from a female. You can tell because the chromosomes making up the last pair (pair 23) look almost identical (XX). In contrast, the male's XY chromosomes look different (the Y chromosome is shorter).

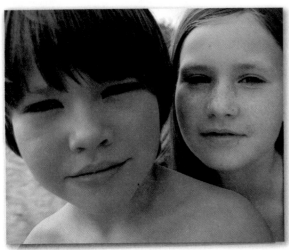

FIGURE 3 **Effect of Dominant versus Recessive Alleles**
Freckles are coded for by a single gene with two forms, or alleles. The allele that codes for freckles is dominant, whereas the allele that results in absence of freckles is recessive. If you inherit the dominant allele from both parents, or even from just one parent, you'll have freckles (right). If you inherit the recessive gene from both parents, you won't have freckles (left).

dominant Term describing an allele that is expressed even if there is only one copy in the pair.

recessive Term describing an allele that is expressed only in the absence of a dominant allele, that is, if both alleles are recessive or if the recessive gene is on the X chromosome of the twenty-third pair.

single-gene disorder A disorder characterized by structural and/or functional impairments resulting from a defect involving only one gene.

allele from just one parent, you'll still have freckles! Why? Because the allele for freckles is **dominant,** whereas the allele for absence of freckles is **recessive**. A dominant allele always "dominates"; that is, it always expresses the trait it codes for. In contrast, a recessive allele "recedes" in the presence of a dominant allele. When there is no dominant allele around, for instance, when you inherit two recessive alleles, then you express that recessive trait (Figure 3).

So if you *don't* have freckles, you must have inherited the recessive allele from both of your parents. Is it possible for you to have freckle-free skin even if both of your parents have freckles? The answer is yes. If both parents have one dominant and one recessive allele, they will both have freckles. Yet they could both have transmitted to you their recessive allele, in which case you would not have freckles.

Just as humans can pass on physical traits—like freckles—that are the expressions of proteins, they can also pass on genetic disorders. That's because any genetic defect, at its most fundamental level, is either the production of a defective form of a body protein or a failure to produce a body protein at all. *Geneticists*—scientists who specialize in genetics—recognize three types of genetic disease: single-gene disorders, multifactorial disorders, and chromosome disorders.

Single-Gene Disorders

Single-gene disorders occur as a result of a defect, called a *mutation,* involving just one gene. For example, the disease *cystic fibrosis* occurs because of a defect on the *CFTR* gene on chromosome 7. Without the protein normally coded by this gene, a person with cystic fibrosis develops thick, sticky mucus that clogs his or her airways and gastrointestinal tract, interfering with breathing and digestion and absorption of food. Although many single-gene disorders, like cystic fibrosis, show up in childhood, a few manifest only in adulthood.

There are four common types of single-gene disorders (Figure 4). These are classified according to the type of

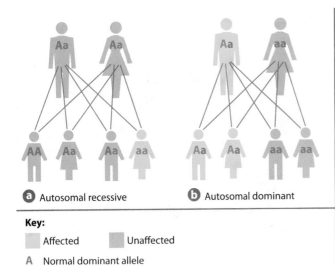
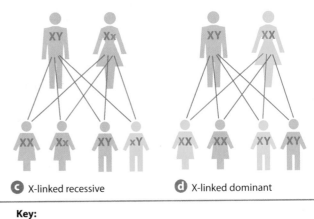

a Autosomal recessive **b** Autosomal dominant **c** X-linked recessive **d** X-linked dominant

Key:

☐ Affected ☐ Unaffected

A Normal dominant allele
A Abnormal dominant allele
a Normal recessive allele
a Abnormal recessive allele

Key:

☐ Affected ☐ Unaffected

X X chromosome with normal allele
X X chromosome with abnormal dominant allele
x X chromosome with abnormal recessive allele
Y Y chromosome

FIGURE 4 **Inheritance Patterns of Single-Gene Disorders**

Video Tutor: Inheritance Pattern of Single-Gene Disorders

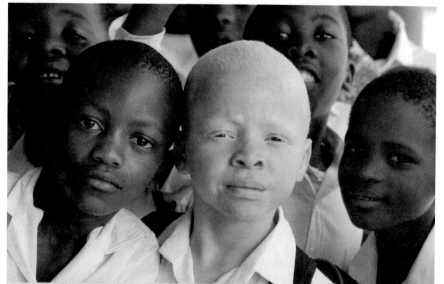

Albinism—a partial or total lack of pigmentation of the skin, hair, and eyes—is an autosomal recessive disorder: It occurs only if the defective allele is passed on from both parents.

chromosome affected (autosome or sex chromosome) and type of allele (recessive or dominant).

Autosomal Recessive Disorders

Cystic fibrosis is classified as an **autosomal recessive disorder** because it occurs on an autosome (recall that all body chromosomes, 1 through 22, are autosomes) and the allele responsible is recessive (see Figure 4a). Autosomal recessive disorders are rare because very few people inherit the recessive allele for the disorder from both parents. However, many more people are "silent carriers" of the responsible recessive gene. A **carrier** is a person who has one dominant normal allele and one recessive abnormal allele. Carriers thus do not develop the disorder and may have no idea that they carry the recessive gene. In fact, grandparents and even great-grandparents may unknowingly also be carriers.

In addition to cystic fibrosis, common autosomal recessive disorders include the following:

- *Albinism* is a partial or complete lack of pigmentation of the skin, hair, and eyes.
- *Tay-Sachs disease* is a neurological disorder that causes a progressive deterioration of mental and physical abilities that begins around 6 months of age and is typically fatal before age 4.

Autosomal Dominant Disorders

An **autosomal dominant disorder** will occur even if an individual inherits just one defective allele because the defective allele is dominant (see Figure 4b). This is the case, for example, with *Huntington's disease,* in which a defective gene on chromosome 4 causes cells to synthesize a flawed protein. This flaw eventually causes nerve cells in the brain and spinal cord to deteriorate, so the person begins to experience involuntary movements, memory loss, and changes in personality. The disease typically begins to manifest around middle age and, although its progression varies according to the extent of the genetic defect, most patients die within 20 years of initial symptoms.

Recall that with autosomal recessive disorders, it's entirely possible that neither parent of the affected child has the disease—both may be "silent carriers" of the recessive gene. In contrast, in autosomal dominant disorders, a parent does have the disease, and offspring have a 50/50 chance of inheriting it. Thus, affected families are more likely to be aware of their health history and seek genetic counseling.

X-Linked Recessive Disorders

Some single-gene disorders are carried on the twenty-third chromosome pair—the sex chromosomes. The most common are **X-linked recessive disorders** (see Figure 4c). An example of X-linked inheritance is color blindness, which, as we mentioned earlier, is a failure of the normal assembly of proteins involving the cone cells of the eye. This condition is coded by a recessive

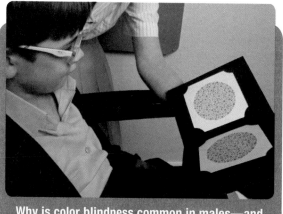

Why is color blindness common in males—and rare in females?

One out of every 10 American males is color blind. The most common color blindness is the inability to distinguish between red and green. It is more common in males because the trait is carried by a gene on the X chromosome. Although it is a recessive trait, there is no comparable gene on the male's Y chromosome; thus, a man needs only one copy of the recessive allele to be color blind. Females inherit two X chromosomes and so will be color blind only if they inherit two copies of the recessive allele.

allele, so if a dominant, normal gene is present, the child will not be color blind. However, it is carried on the X chromosome of pair 23—the sex chromosomes, which determine gender. Recall that, whereas females inherit an X chromosome each from their father and their mother, males inherit an X chromosome from their mother but a Y chromosome from their father. The Y chromosome has different genes from those of the X chromosome. So if the X chromosome a male inherits from his mother has a defective gene, even if it's recessive, it won't have any competition from a dominant, normal gene from his father. Thus, the male child will inherit the disorder.

Notice, too, that a man who is color blind will never pass on the problem to his son, since the son will get his Y gene. However, he will always pass on the trait to his daughter, who will be a carrier. The only instance in which a female will be color blind is when she inherits the recessive allele from both her father and her mother.

Other commonly known X-linked recessive disorders include the following:

- *Hemophilia* is a rare bleeding disorder caused by a genetic defect that results in the absence of a protein that assists blood to clot (called a clotting factor). Fortunately, the missing clotting factor is now produced in laboratories and can be injected into the bloodstream.
- *Duchenne muscular dystrophy* is a disorder that causes muscle weakness that progresses throughout childhood until, by about age 12, the child is usually unable to walk. It is caused by a defective gene for dystrophin, a muscle protein.

X-Linked Dominant Disorders
X-linked dominant disorders are extremely rare (see Figure 4d). The most common affect the bones or the kidneys, and in males are often fatal.

X-linked dominant disorder Single-gene disorder that occurs in individuals who have inherited at least one copy of an X chromosome with the affected dominant allele.

multifactorial disorder A disorder attributable to more than one of a variety of factors.

Even though the responsible allele is dominant, when females inherit it, the single copy of the recessive, normal allele can mitigate somewhat the disorder's effects.

In Multifactorial Disorders, Genes Interact with Other Factors

Genes operate in a complex network, interacting and overlapping with one another in ways that can promote health or lead to disease. Moreover, genes interact with aspects of the environment, including diet, exposure to cigarette smoke and other toxins, viruses, radiation, and probably many

other factors. These factors can act like a switch, turning on or off genes so that the proteins they code for are, or are not, assembled. Disorders in which genes play a role—but not the only role—are called **multifactorial disorders** (Figure 5). They are known to include obesity, heart disease, type 2 diabetes, Alzheimer's disease, and certain types of cancer; however, some researchers contend that nearly all conditions and diseases have a genetic component.[5]

In addition, genes are known to play at least some role in certain psychiatric disorders. These include the following:

- *Schizophrenia* is a complex disorder in which the person interprets reality in an abnormal way. In addition to genetic factors, exposure to malnutrition

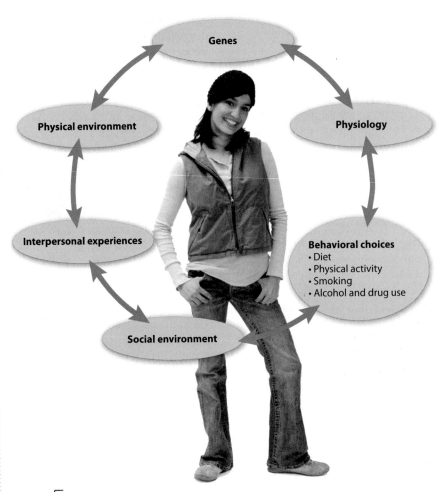

FIGURE 5 Multifactorial Disorders
Whereas single-gene disorders are determined entirely by genes, multifactorial disorders result from the influence of multiple genes on a vast number of physiological processes, all interacting with behavioral choices, interpersonal experiences, and a variety of factors in the social and physical environment.

or viruses during fetal development is linked to schizophrenia, as are stress and the use of certain psychoactive drugs.

- *Bipolar disorder,* which formerly was known as manic-depression, is characterized by periods of excitability and exuberance alternating with periods of depression. Although researchers have not identified specific genes involved, bipolar disorder is more common in people who have a family member with the disorder. However, many other structural and chemical differences in the body, as well as stress and drug or alcohol abuse, may contribute.

- *Clinical depression* (also called *major depressive disorder*) is characterized by persistent feelings of sadness, hopelessness, and/or irritability. As with bipolar disorder, no specific "depression" genes have yet been identified, and many other factors are also thought to be involved.

In short, although genes do play a role in multifactorial disorders, they are just one determinant of anyone's health. If a multifactorial disorder runs in your family, you should learn about the other factors influencing development of the disorder and make healthy choices to reduce your risk.

Some Disorders Involve Missing, Extra, or Damaged Chromosomes

Chromosome disorders are caused by errors in an entire chromosome or part of a chromosome, rather than in one or a few genes.[6] For example, an entire chromosome may be missing, or an extra chromosome may be present, or a chromosome may be broken. Such problems sometimes arise while the mother's egg or the father's sperm is developing. After the egg and sperm unite at conception, the chromosomal defect is repeated with every cell division as the embryo grows to become a fetus and then an infant. The additional or missing genetic code can then be expressed as a wide

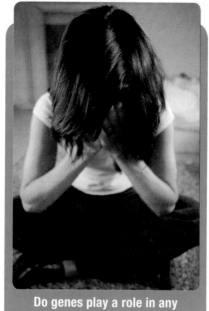

Do genes play a role in any psychiatric disorders?

Genetic factors probably play some role in the development of psychiatric disorders such as depression, schizophrenia, and bipolar disorder. However, other aspects of the individual's environment and development are also critical. Factors such as stress, use of psychoactive drugs, imbalances in body chemicals, and childhood trauma are thought to contribute to the risk of certain psychiatric disorders.

range of abnormalities, including heart defects, kidney disorders, and mental retardation. With severe defects, the child may not survive.

One of the most common chromosome disorders is *Down syndrome,* a pattern of mental retardation and physical abnormalities, including heart defects and characteristic facial features such as a somewhat flattened profile. Down syndrome occurs when the child inherits an extra copy of chromosome 21, a defect that occurs at conception. Although researchers do not understand why, the chance of having a child with Down syndrome increases significantly as the mother ages: In their

1,200 genetic tests are currently available.

chromosome disorder A disorder arising from a missing or extra chromosome or damage to part of a chromosome.

twenties, women have about a 1 in 1,230 chance of having a child with Down syndrome. By age 35, the risk increases to 1 in 270, and at age 45, the risk is 1 in 22.[7]

Ethnicity Plays a Role in Many Genetic Disorders

Some genetic disorders tend to occur more frequently among people who trace their ancestry to a particular geographic area.[8] People in an ethnic group often share certain versions of their genes, which have been passed down from common ancestors. If one of these genes contains a disease-causing mutation, a particular genetic disorder may be more frequently seen in this group.

For example, Tay-Sachs disease, mentioned earlier, is more common among Jewish people of eastern and central Europe, French Canadians, and Cajuns. About 1 in 27 American Jews carries the recessive allele for Tay-Sachs disease, whereas only about 1 in 250 are carriers in the population at large.[9] In addition, both cystic fibrosis and Huntington's disease are more common among Americans of European descent.[10]

Ethnicity is also believed to play at least some role in many multifactorial diseases. For example, hypertension, heart attack, and stroke are all more common among African Americans. Type 2 diabetes is more common among African Americans, Hispanic Americans, Native Americans, and Asian Americans than among Caucasian Americans. Whether developing type 2 diabetes is due to ethnic background, lifestyle, or environmental factors, or it is caused by a combination of these factors, remains in question. Also, although it's not clear why, African Americans are more likely to develop cancer than are Caucasian Americans, whereas Hispanic and Asian Americans are less likely to develop most cancers.[11] Still to be determined is how large a role genetics plays in these trends and how much is a result of

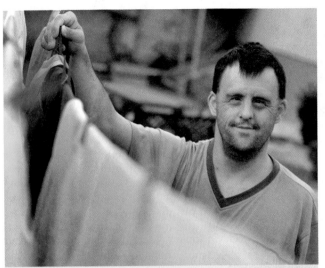
Some children born with Down syndrome have severe health problems, though the majority have mild to moderate mental retardation and physical challenges, as well as unique gifts and talents.

environmental factors shared by people of a certain ethnicity.

Genetic Counseling Helps Families Evaluate Options

If you were to discover a family history of a genetic or multifactorial disease, one smart response would be to see a genetic counselor. Most genetic counselors have graduate degrees and experience in medical genetics and work within health care organizations to provide information and support to families. For instance, they help couples identify their risk for giving birth to a baby with a genetic disorder, investigate disorders already present within a family, review available options, and provide supportive counseling.[12]

Some people who consult a genetic counselor decide to undergo testing. A DNA sample can be obtained from any tissue. Gene tests can tell you whether or not you are a carrier of a genetic disorder. They can also be used for prenatal diagnosis, newborn screening, or to predict the presence of an adult-onset genetic disorder prior to symptom development. Testing is also available to estimate the risk of a very rare form of

behavioral genetics The science that studies the role of inheritance in human behavior.

breast cancer associated with certain genes, as well as a particularly severe form of Alzheimer's disease linked to certain genes. Genetic testing can also confirm a diagnosis of specific disorders in individuals with symptoms.[13] There are significant ethical issues connected with genetic testing, especially with direct-to-consumer testing; see the **Tech & Health** box on the next page.

Do Genes Influence Behavior?

Animal breeders have long recognized that certain species of domestic and farm animals have a higher prevalence of certain desirable behavioral traits than others. For instance, border collies are famous for their herding behavior and belted Galloways (a Scottish breed of cattle) are known for their docility. Recently, a relatively new field of **behavioral genetics** has begun to study how genetic factors might contribute to variations in human behaviors as well. One tool commonly used in behavioral genetics is *twin studies* involving identical twins. Because identical twins have the same DNA, differences between them are assigned to variations in their environment—whether during fetal life, growing up in the same family, or growing up apart.

Even in studies involving twins, teasing out genetics from environment is not an easy task for several reasons.[14] First, in order to study a behavior, researchers have to be able to define and measure it precisely. It's easy to define, say, short stature in a child as being below the fifth percentile for height, and then measure each child in the study. But what would

constitute a valid scientific definition of shyness? And how would you measure it? Finally, because behaviors, like most disorders, involve multiple genes and many factors within the environment, any claim we make about the hereditary nature of a behavior tells us only about the precise population studied. We can't readily extrapolate from there to the general population.

With these limitations in mind, let's look at what the research has to say about the heritability of the following behaviors.

- **Personality.** Human personality traits that can be reliably measured by rating scales do show a considerable heritable component.[15] In some cases, the effect of genes appears to be expressed as variations in the production of certain neurotransmitters. Researchers have asserted claims for a genetic basis of impulsivity, novelty seeking, aggression, and nurturing.

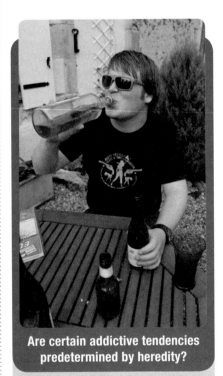
Are certain addictive tendencies predetermined by heredity?
No one is destined to engage in addictive behaviors. Genes only affect body processes that interact with one another and with your life experiences to influence your susceptibility. Many other factors, including environment, physiology, and behavioral choices contribute to the development of an addiction.

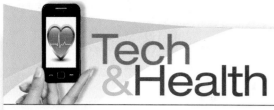

Tech & Health

AT-HOME GENETIC TESTING: DUBIOUS AT BEST

Do Alzheimer's disease, depression, cancer, or alcoholism "run in your family"? If you saw an ad promoting a test you could take at home to find out whether or not you have "the gene" associated with such disorders, would you be tempted? As more Americans seek genetic testing, many are purchasing tests they can conduct without anyone—including their physician—getting involved.

Typically, so-called direct-to-consumer (DTC) tests are purchased online or in drugstores, and cost upwards of several hundred dollars. The consumer mails a swab from inside the cheek or a very small blood sample to a laboratory for analysis. Results are sent back via mail or posted online with a confidential code.

It sounds simple, but the tests raise a number of ethical concerns, including the following:

✳ Validity. The Federal Trade Commission (FTC) warns that some DTC testing companies are making unwarranted claims about the validity of their tests. For example, they may claim that the test can measure a consumer's risk for multifactorial diseases such as type 2 diabetes or cancer, or even for "susceptibility to substance abuse." It's hard for consumers to distinguish between tests widely used by qualified health care providers—such as for single-gene disorders like cystic fibrosis—and tests whose validity is unproven.

✳ Ambiguity. Even for disorders known to be linked to specific genes, the results of most genetic tests are not black-and-white. They require evaluation and interpretation by a qualified health care provider. DTC testing can prompt consumers to make major life decisions, including whether to have children, on unreliable data.

✳ Fraud. As mentioned, these tests are costly. And some companies also make huge profits by selling worthless dietary supplements they claim will reduce the consumer's genetic vulnerability to specific disorders. A company might offer, for example, an "oxidative stress supplement" for clients with a genetic profile suggestive of cancer or a "circulatory supplement" for those at risk for cardiovascular disease.

✳ Potential for harm. Without genetic counseling, consumers are left on their own to respond to the results of a DTC test. What happens when a young woman finds out via a form letter that she has "the breast cancer gene," or a young man types his code into an online site and learns that he has "the genetic profile indicating high risk for Alzheimer's disease"? When genetic tests are conducted by qualified health care providers, results are interpreted and explained by a clinician with training in genetics,

and follow-up support is encouraged, not only from a professional counselor, but also from others who have faced similar diagnoses.

Although all states have laws protecting consumers from false advertising, none has laws specific to genetic testing. The U.S. Food and Drug Administration is currently researching federal regulatory oversight of companies offering DTC testing, but no home genetic test has yet been reviewed by the FDA. In the meantime, the FTC, FDA, and the U.S. Centers for Disease Control, along with the National Society of Genetic Counselors, advise that all genetic tests be performed in a specialized laboratory and that results be interpreted by a physician or trained genetic counselor who understands the value of genetic testing for the particular situation. The bottom line? If you're considering genetic testing, see your doctor.

Sources: K. Drabiak-Syed, *Direct-to-Consumer Genetic Testing: PredictER La w and Policy Update,* Indiana University Center for Bioethics, September 8, 2010, http://bioethics.iu.edu/programs/predicter/legal-updates/dtcgenetics; Federal Trade Commission, "At-Home Genetic Tests: A Healthy Dose of Skepticism May Be the Best Prescription," 2006, *FTC Facts for Consumers,* www.ftc.gov/bcp/edu/pubs/consumer/health/hea02.pdf; The National Society of Genetic Counselors, "Position Statement: Direct-to-Consumer Genetic Testing," 2011, www.nsgc.org/Media/PositionStatements/tabid/330/Default.aspx#DTC.

However, environmental factors significantly modify gene effects.

● **Intelligence.** The controversy over the relative contributions of "nature versus nurture" to human intelligence has raged for over a century. The available research evidence does suggest that an adult's general cognitive ability is about 50 percent attributable to inheritance.[16] Nonetheless, no individual "intelligence" genes have yet been identified. This also means that other, non-genetic factors are equally responsible for intelligence. These are thought to include, for example, nutrition, socioeconomic status, and aspects of the fetal environment such as fetal exposure to alcohol. Moreover, both genetics and environment appear to influence ability to develop intellectual potential.[17]

● **Abuse and addiction.** Variation in genes related to impulse control and sensitivity to reward may partially explain people's vulnerability to addictive behaviors.[18] For example, research over many decades has identified at least a dozen genes that influence susceptibility to alcohol dependence.[19] Still, alcohol dependence is not entirely genetic: Genes affect processes in the body, including the brain, that interact with one another and with an individual's life experiences to produce either protection or susceptibility.[20] Similar gene–environment interactions may be at work in addictions to tobacco, illegal drugs, and even prescription drugs.

What's Your Family Health History?

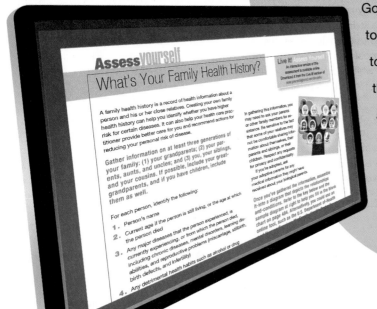

Go online to www.pearsonhighered.com/donatelle to fill out the "What's Your Family Health History" assessment.* Use the steps outlined in the **YOUR PLAN FOR CHANGE** box to take action on the information uncovered by the Assess Yourself.

*If your instructor so chooses, Assess Yourself Activities are available as a printed supplement or as assignable homework online at www.pearsonhighered.com/myhealthlab.

MyHealthLab®

YOUR PLAN FOR CHANGE

The **Assess Yourself** activity gave you the chance to create your own family health history and identify the health risks present in your family. Now you can take steps to make sure you stay in control of your destiny!

Today, you can:

◯ List the disorders that occur within your family. For each, identify the environmental factors and/or lifestyle choices most strongly associated with development of the disorder.

◯ Jot down one small step you can take to positively influence your risk. For example, let's say that two close relatives have experienced lung cancer. You identify smoking as a lifestyle factor in each case. Maybe you don't smoke—but your roommate does. Today, you can share with your roommate your family history of lung cancer and ask your roommate to smoke outside from now on.

Within the next 2 weeks, you can:

◯ Share your health history—and the patterns it reveals—with other members of your family. Invite them to fill in any gaps, and talk to them about the healthy choices you're making.

By the end of the semester, you can:

◯ Share your health history with your primary health care provider. Ask him or her for more advice about choices you can make to take charge of your health.

◯ If there is a multifactorial disorder in your family history, commit to behavior changes that reduce your risk of developing the disorder, such as getting your cholesterol checked or beginning an exercise program.

References

1. Framingham Heart Study, "About the Framingham Heart Study," 2010, www.framinghamheartstudy.org/about/index.html.
2. Genetics Home Reference, "Cells and DNA," February 27, 2012, http://ghr.nlm.nih.gov/handbook/basics.
3. Genetic Alliance and the New England Public Health Genetics Education Collaborative, *Understanding Genetics: A New England Guide for Patients and Health Professionals* (Washington, DC: Genetic Alliance, 2010), www.geneticalliance.org/understanding.genetics.
4. J. L. Thompson, M. M. Manore, and L. A. Vaughan, *The Science of Nutrition*, 3rd ed. (San Francisco: Benjamin Cummings, 2014).
5. Genetics Home Reference, "Mutations and Health," 2012, http://ghr.nlm.nih.gov/handbook/mutationsanddisorders.
6. March of Dimes, "Birth Defects: Chromosomal Abnormalities," December 2009, www.marchofdimes.com/Baby/birthdefects_chromosomal.html.
7. Ibid.
8. Genetics Home Reference, "Inheriting Genetic Conditions," 2012, http://ghr.nlm.nih.gov/handbook/inheritance.
9. National Human Genome Research Institute, "Learning about Tay-Sachs Disease," 2011, www.genome.gov/page.cfm?pageID=10001220.
10. Genetics Home Reference, "Genetic Conditions," 2012, http://ghr.nlm.nih.gov/condition.
11. American Cancer Society, *Cancer Facts & Figures 2012* (Atlanta: American Cancer Society, 2012), www.cancer.org/Research/CancerFactsFigures.
12. National Society of Genetic Counselors, "FAQs about Genetic Counselors and the NSGC," http://www.nsgc.org/About/FAQsaboutGeneticCounselorsandtheNSGC/tabid/143/Default.aspx.
13. Ibid.
14. Human Genome Project, "Behavioral Genetics," 2008, www.ornl.gov/sci/techresources/Human_Genome/else/behavior.shtml.
15. V. McKusick et al., "Novelty Seeking Personality Trait," 2010, www.ncbi.nlm.nih.gov/omim/601696.
16. I. J. Deary, W. Johnson, and L. M. Houlihan "Genetic Foundations of Human Intelligence," *Human Genetics* 126, no. 1 (2009): 215–32.
17. F. Grasso, "I.Q.—Genetics or Environment," 2004, http://allpsych.com/journal/iq.html.
18. S. F. Stoltenberg et al., "Associations among Types of Impulsivity, Substance Use Problems and Neurexin-3 Polymorphisms," *Drug Alcohol Depend* 119, no. 3 (2011): e31–38; M. M. Sweltzer, E. C. Donny, and A. R. Hariri, "Imaging Genetics and the Neurobiological Basis of Individual Differences in Vulnerability to Addiction," *Drug Alcohol Depend*, February 16, 2012,
19. V. McKusick et al., "Alcohol Dependence," 2010, www.ncbi.nlm.nih.gov/omim/103780.
20. J. I. Nurnberger Jr. and L. J. Bierut, "Seeking the Connections: Alcoholism and Our Genes," *Scientific American* 296, no. 4 (2007): 46–53.

Preventing Cardiovascular Disease

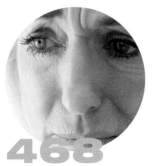

468
Can you die from a broken heart?

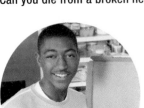

470
Is there anything I can do to improve my cholesterol level?

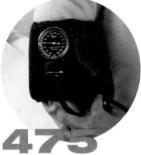

475
Is heart disease hereditary?

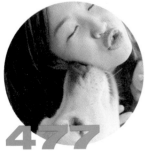

477
What are things that can help you recover from a cardiac event?

OBJECTIVES

✳ Describe the anatomy and physiology of the heart and circulatory system and the importance of healthy heart function.

✳ Discuss the incidence, prevalence, and outcomes of cardiovascular disease in the United States, including its impact on society.

✳ Review major types of cardiovascular disease.

✳ Discuss modifiable and nonmodifiable risk factors, methods of prevention, and current strategies for diagnosis and treatment of cardiovascular disease.

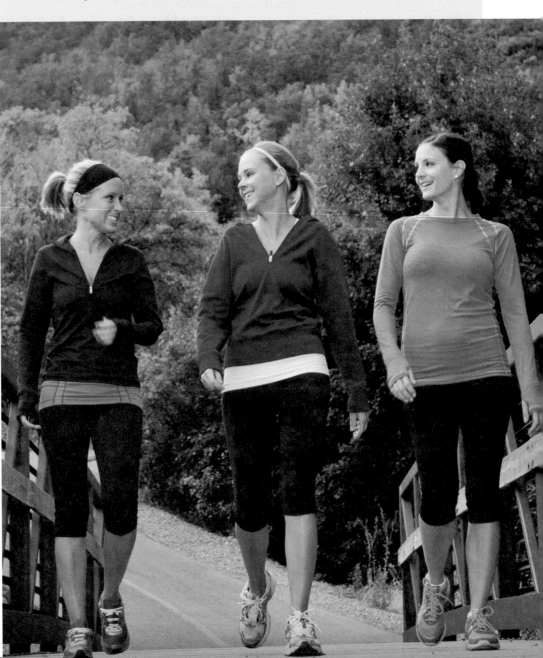

Over 82.6 million Americans—1 out of every 3 adults—suffer from one or more types of **cardiovascular disease (CVD)**, the broad term used to describe diseases of the heart and blood vessels.[1] Cardiovascular disease is not a new problem. It has been the leading killer of U.S. adults every year since 1900, except in 1918, when a pandemic flu killed more people. We spend billions on research for prevention strategies, treatments, and cures, and we have the most sophisticated media warnings and educational programs telling us how to avoid risks. Nevertheless, Americans are more obese and spending more on treatment of cardiovascular disease than ever before, even though the rates of mortality from CVD continues to decline.[2] When seven key risk factors (weight, smoking, cholesterol, hypertension, fasting glucose levels, poor diet, and lack of physical activity) are considered, U.S. CVD profiles look rather grim. Only 6 percent of U.S. adults are free of risk factors in these seven areas and nearly 40 percent score in the "poor" range with over three significant CVD risks.[3] This chapter describes a healthy cardiovascular system, the factors that put your system at risk, and what happens when various diseases occur. It provides an epidemiological overview of CVD in the United States, as well as why your actions right now can predispose you to premature problems, regardless of your age. There are things you can do today to reduce your own long-term risks for CVD and optimize your cardiovascular health.

Understanding the Cardiovascular System

Before we can talk about cardiovascular disease, it's helpful to understand how the system normally functions. The **cardiovascular system** is the network of organs and vessels through which blood flows as it carries oxygen and nutrients to all parts of the body. It includes the heart, arteries, arterioles (small arteries), veins, venules (small veins), and capillaries (minute blood vessels).

The Heart: A Mighty Machine

The heart is a muscular, four-chambered pump, roughly the size of your fist. It is a highly efficient, extremely flexible organ that contracts 100,000 times each day and pumps the equivalent of 2,000 gallons of blood to all areas of the body. In a 70-year lifetime, an average human heart beats 2.5 billion times.

Under normal circumstances, the human body contains approximately 6 quarts of blood, which transports nutrients, oxygen, waste products, hormones, and enzymes throughout the body. Blood also aids in regulating body temperature, cellular water levels, and acidity levels of body components, and it helps defend the body against toxins and harmful microorganisms. An adequate blood supply is essential to health and well-being.

The heart's four chambers work together to circulate blood constantly throughout the body. The two upper chambers of the heart, called **atria,** are large collecting chambers that receive blood from the rest of the body. The two lower chambers, known as **ventricles,** pump the blood out again. Small valves regulate the steady, rhythmic flow of blood between chambers and prevent leakage or backflow between them.

Heart Function Heart activity depends on a complex interaction of biochemical, physical, and neurological signals. **Figure 15.1** (see page 460) shows blood flow through the heart:

1. Deoxygenated blood enters the right atrium after having been circulated through the body.
2. From the right atrium, blood moves to the right ventricle and is pumped through the pulmonary artery to the lungs, where it receives oxygen.
3. Oxygenated blood from the lungs then returns to the left atrium of the heart.
4. Blood from the left atrium moves into the left ventricle. The left ventricle pumps blood through the aorta to all body parts.

Various types of blood vessels are required for different parts of this process. **Arteries** carry blood away from the heart; all arteries carry oxygenated blood, *except* for pulmonary arteries, which carry deoxygenated blood to the lungs, where the blood picks up oxygen and gives up carbon dioxide. After the arteries branch off from the heart, they branch into smaller blood vessels called **arterioles**, and then into even smaller blood vessels known as **capillaries.** Capillaries have thin walls that permit the exchange of oxygen, carbon dioxide, nutrients, and waste products with body cells. Carbon dioxide and other waste products are transported to the lungs and kidneys through **veins** and **venules** (small veins).

For the heart to function properly, the four chambers must beat in an organized manner. Your heartbeat is governed by an electrical impulse that directs the heart muscle to move when the impulse travels across it, which results in a sequential contraction of the chambers. This signal starts in a small bundle of highly specialized cells in the right atrium, called the **sinoatrial node (SA node).** The SA

cardiovascular disease (CVD) Diseases of the heart and blood vessels.
cardiovascular system Organ system, consisting of the heart and blood vessels, that transports nutrients, oxygen, hormones, metabolic wastes, and enzymes throughout the body.
atria (singular: *atrium*) The heart's two upper chambers, which receive blood.
ventricles The heart's two lower chambers, which pump blood through the blood vessels.
arteries Vessels that carry blood away from the heart to other regions of the body.
arterioles Branches of the arteries.
capillaries Minute blood vessels that branch out from the arterioles and venules; their thin walls permit exchange of oxygen, carbon dioxide, nutrients, and waste products among body cells.
veins Vessels that transport waste and carry blood back to the heart from other regions of the body.
venules Branches of the veins.
sinoatrial node (SA node) Cluster of electric pulse-generating cells that serves as a natural pacemaker for the heart.

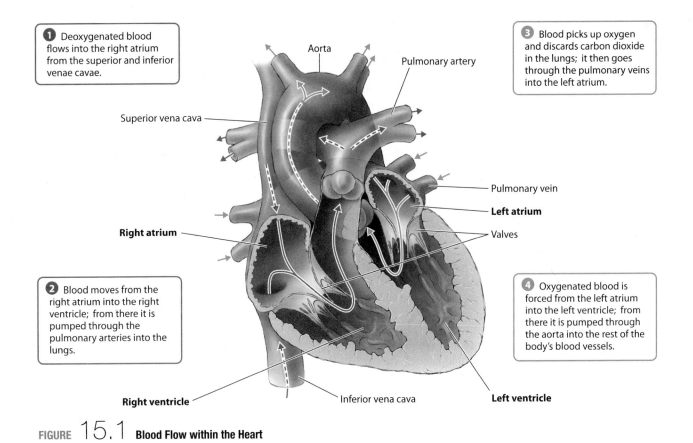

① Deoxygenated blood flows into the right atrium from the superior and inferior venae cavae.

③ Blood picks up oxygen and discards carbon dioxide in the lungs; it then goes through the pulmonary veins into the left atrium.

Aorta

Pulmonary artery

Superior vena cava

Pulmonary vein

Left atrium

Right atrium

Valves

② Blood moves from the right atrium into the right ventricle; from there it is pumped through the pulmonary arteries into the lungs.

④ Oxygenated blood is forced from the left atrium into the left ventricle; from there it is pumped through the aorta into the rest of the body's blood vessels.

Right ventricle

Inferior vena cava

Left ventricle

FIGURE 15.1 **Blood Flow within the Heart**

node serves as a natural pacemaker for the heart. People with a damaged SA node must often have a mechanical pacemaker implanted to make the heart beat.

The average adult heart at rest beats 70 to 80 times per minute, although a well-conditioned heart may beat only 50 to 60 times per minute to achieve the same results. If your resting heart rate is routinely in the high 80s or 90s, it may indicate that you are out of shape, carrying too much weight, or suffering from some underlying illness. When overly stressed, a heart may beat more than 200 times per minute. A healthy heart functions more efficiently and is less likely to suffer damage from overwork.

Cardiovascular Disease: An Epidemiological Overview

Every year about 785,000 Americans have a first coronary attack, and 470,000 others who have already had one or more coronary attacks have another attack (Figure 15.2).[4] Cardiovascular disease claims more lives each year than the next three leading causes of death combined(cancer, chronic lower respiratory diseases, and accidents), accounting for 32.8 percent of all deaths in the United States.[5]

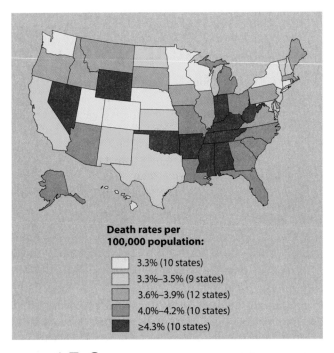

Death rates per 100,000 population:

☐	3.3% (10 states)
☐	3.3%–3.5% (9 states)
☐	3.6%–3.9% (12 states)
☐	4.0%–4.2% (10 states)
☐	≥4.3% (10 states)

FIGURE 15.2 **Prevalence of Heart Attacks Among U.S. Adults** 2009 prevalence of acute myocardial infarction (heart attack) among U.S. adults (18+).

Source: Division for Heart Disease and Stroke Prevention: Data Trends & Maps website. U.S. Department of Health and Human Services, Centers for Disease Control and Prevention (CDC), National Center for Chronic Disease Prevention and Health Promotion, Atlanta, GA, 2010. Available at www.cdc.gov/dhdsp/.

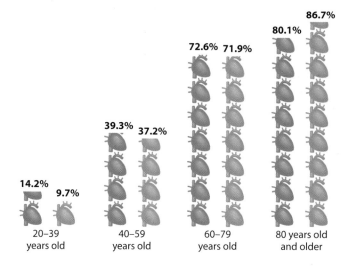

86.7%

80.1%

72.6% 71.9%

39.3% 37.2%

14.2%
9.7%

| 20–39 years old | 40–59 years old | 60–79 years old | 80 years old and older |

 Men with CVD; each heart = 10% of the population

Women with CVD; each heart = 10% of the population

FIGURE 15.3 **Prevalence of Cardiovascular Disease (CVD) in U.S. Adults Aged 20 and Older by Age and Sex**

Source: Data are from American Heart Association Writing Group, V. Roger et al., "Heart Disease and Stroke Statistics—2012 Update: A Report from the American Heart Association," *Circulation* 125, no. 1 (2012): e2–220, Available at http://circ.ahajournals.org/content/125/1/e2.full.

Consider the following facts:[6]

● More than 2,200 Americans die each day from CVD—an average of 1 death every 39 seconds. There are nearly 1.4 million deaths annually, nearly 55 percent of all deaths in the United States, for which CVD is listed as an underlying or contributing cause. Many of these fatalities are **sudden cardiac deaths,** meaning an abrupt, profound loss of heart function (cardiac arrest) that causes death either instantly or shortly after symptoms occur.

● It may surprise you to know that in terms of total deaths, CVD has claimed the lives of more women than men every year since 1984. Only among those people ages 20 to 39 is CVD significantly more prevalent among men than it is among women (Figure 15.3). Women also have a higher lifetime prevalence of stroke, having over 55,000 more strokes per year than men.[7]

● African Americans have the highest rates of CVD deaths of any group in the United States, with rates of nearly 302 per 100,000 for African American men and 201 per 100,000 people for African American women. In contrast, non-Hispanic white men and women have rates of nearly 236 and 150 deaths per 100,000 people, respectively. Overall, African Americans are 40 percent more likely to have high blood pressure and 10 percent less likely to have it under control than the rest of the population.[8]

● Among men age 20 to 39, 20.3 percent have metabolic syndrome (MetS), a dangerous grouping of key risk factors for CVD. This compares to 15.6 percent of women in the 20 to 39 age group. Among those age 40 to 59, rates jumped to a whopping 40.8 percent and for women, 37 percent.[9]

sudden cardiac death Death that occurs as a result of abrupt, profound loss of heart function.

Of the millions of Americans who currently live with one of the major categories of CVD, many lack health insurance and fail to receive appropriate screening and diagnostic tests. Others fail to recognize subtle symptoms until they result in a major cardiovascular event. Still others live in rural or remote areas where emergency transportation and care are not available. In spite of major improvements in medication, surgery, and other health care procedures, the prognosis for many of these individuals is not good:[10] Twenty-five percent of men and 38 percent of women will die within 1 year after having an initial heart attack. The older the age at first heart attack, the greater the risk of dying.

The economic burden of cardiovascular disease on our society is huge—more than $297 billion in direct and indirect costs.[11] This figure includes the direct cost of physicians and other professionals, hospital services, prescribed medication, and home health care, as well as lost productivity resulting from illness, disability and death, but not the cost of nursing home care. As Americans live longer with chronic diseases, costs will continue to increase, resulting in a tremendous burden on the health care system. While economic concerns are huge, the effects of CVD on patients, their families, communities, the health care system, and society may be even greater.

Cardiovascular disease is not a uniquely American health problem. With an international trend toward obesity, more and more countries face epidemic CVD rates. In fact, according to the most recent World Health Organization (WHO) estimates, CVD accounts for 30 percent of all deaths globally. Many have the mistaken idea that CVD is only a "developed" nation problem. Unfortunately, over 80 percent of the world's deaths from CVD occur in low- and middle-income countries, places where people have more risks and fewer options for prevention and treatment. People with CVD in these countries die at younger ages, often during their most productive years.[12]

what do you think?

Why are certain populations within the United States especially at risk for CVD?

● Why are developing regions of the world experiencing major increases in CVD rates?

● With all of the media focus on reducing risks for CVD, why do you think we aren't seeing more dramatic reductions in CVD deaths?

Key Cardiovascular Diseases

There are several types of cardiovascular disease, including atherosclerosis, coronary heart disease (CHD), stroke, hypertension, angina pectoris, arrhythmia, congestive heart failure

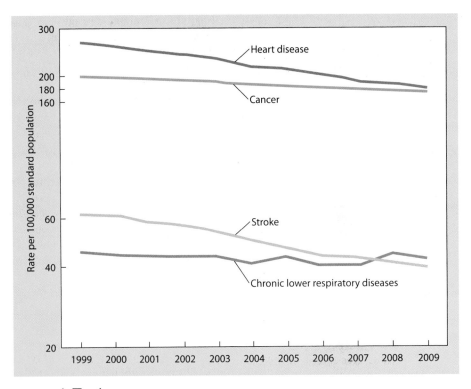

FIGURE 15.4 **Heart Disease and Stroke Death Rates**

Heart disease and stroke have long ranked among the leading causes of death in the United States. This graph shows age-adjusted death rates for leading causes of death 1999–2007, with preliminary data for 2008 and 2009. Rates are plotted on a logarithmic scale.

Source: National Centers for Health Statistics Data Brief number 64, July 2011, "Death in the United States, 2009," Arialdi M. Miniño, M.P.H. U.S. Department of Health and Human Services, Centers for Disease Control and Prevention, National Center for Health Statistics. Available at www.cdc.gov/nchs/data/databriefs/db64.pdf.

atherosclerosis Condition characterized by deposits of fatty substances (plaque) on the inner lining of an artery.

plaque Buildup of deposits in the arteries.

coronary artery disease (CAD) A narrowing or blockage of coronary arteries, usually caused by atherosclerotic plaque buildup.

(CHF), and congenital cardiovascular defects. **Figure 15.4** presents a breakdown of deaths from common diseases in the United States.

Many of these forms of CVD are potentially fatal; many can also cause significant physical and psychological disability. Although death rates are relatively easy to calculate, the short- and long-term psychological problems that occur after a person has a heart attack are harder to measure. Imagine wondering each time you exercise if your heart will fail you or fearing that sexual activity might cause another heart attack. Getting a grip on the anxieties that follow a cardiac event can be challenging. Knowing more about your specific CVD risks and what you can do about them is key to taking healthy action.

Atherosclerosis and Coronary Artery Disease

Atherosclerosis comes from the Greek words *athero* (meaning gruel or paste) and *sclerosis* (hardness). In this condition,

fatty substances, cholesterol, cellular waste products, calcium, and fibrin (a clotting material in the blood) build up in the inner lining of an artery. *Hyperlipidemia* (an abnormally high blood lipid level) is a key factor in this process, and the resulting buildup is called **plaque.** It is a condition that underlies many cardiovascular health problems and is believed to be the biggest contributor to disease burden globally.

As plaque accumulates, vessel walls become narrow and may eventually block blood flow or cause vessels to rupture (**Figure 15.5**). The pressure buildup is similar to putting your thumb over the end of a hose while water is on. Pressure builds within arteries just as pressure builds in the hose. If vessels are weakened and pressure persists, they may burst or the plaque itself may break away from the walls of the vessels and obstruct blood flow. In addition, fluctuation in the blood pressure levels within arteries can damage their internal walls, making it even more likely that plaque will stick to injured wall surfaces and accumulate.

Atherosclerosis is often called **coronary artery disease (CAD)** because of the damage to the body's main coronary arteries on the outer surface of the heart. These are the arteries that provide blood supply to the heart muscle itself. Most

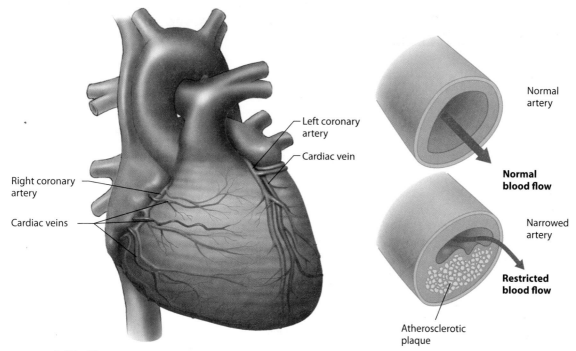

Normal artery

Normal blood flow

Narrowed artery

Restricted blood flow

Atherosclerotic plaque

Left coronary artery

Cardiac vein

Right coronary artery

Cardiac veins

FIGURE 15.5 **Atherosclerosis and Coronary Artery Disease**

The coronary arteries are located on the exterior of the heart and supply blood and oxygen to the heart muscle itself. In atherosclerosis, arteries become clogged by a buildup of plaque. When atherosclerosis occurs in coronary arteries, blood flow to the heart muscle is restricted and a heart attack may occur.

Sources: Adapted from Joan Salge Blake, *Nutrition & You*, 2nd ed., MyPlate edition, and Michael D. Johnson, *Human: Biology: Concepts and Current Issues*, 6th ed. Both copyright © 2012 Pearson Education, Inc. Reprinted by permission.

Video Tutor: Atherosclerosis and Coronary Artery Disease

heart attacks result from blockage of these arteries. Atherosclerosis and other circulatory impairments also often reduce blood flow and limit the heart's blood and oxygen supply, a condition known as **ischemia.**

Peripheral Artery Disease

When atherosclerosis occurs in the upper or lower extremities, such as in the arms, feet, calves, or legs, and causes narrowing or complete blockage of arteries, it is often called **peripheral artery disease (PAD)**. Over 8 million people—20 percent of adults 65 and older in the United States—have symptoms, and many are not receiving treatment.[13] PAD is most often characterized by pain and aching in the legs, calves, or feet upon walking or exercise and is relieved by rest (known as *intermittent claudication*). PAD can be disabling at best and lead to fatalities at its worst. While both men and women develop PAD in equal numbers, research and treatment of women has lagged behind that of men.[14] In recent years, increased attention has been drawn to PAD's role in subsequent blood clots and resultant heart attacks. Sometimes PAD in the arms can be caused by trauma, certain diseases, radiation therapy, or repetitive motion syndrome, or the combined risks of these factors and atherosclerosis.

Damage to vessels and threats to health can be severe, with a two- to three-times greater risk of stroke and heart attack among those who have PAD.[15] According to current thinking, four factors discussed later in this chapter are responsible for this damage: inflammation, elevated levels of cholesterol and triglycerides in the blood, high blood pressure, and tobacco use.

Coronary Heart Disease

Of all the major cardiovascular diseases, **coronary heart disease (CHD)** is the greatest killer, accounting for nearly 1 in 6 deaths in the United States. Approximately 785,000 new heart attacks and 470,000 recurrent attacks occur each year. Another 195,000 people have *silent heart attacks*, which don't produce the usual signs or symptoms.[16] A **myocardial infarction (MI), or heart attack,** involves an area of the heart that suffers permanent damage because its normal blood supply has been blocked. This condition is often brought on by a **coronary thrombosis** (clot) or an atherosclerotic narrowing that blocks a coronary artery (an artery supplying the heart muscle with blood; refer to **Figure 15.5**). When a clot, or **thrombus,** becomes dislodged

ischemia Reduced oxygen supply to a body part or organ.

peripheral artery disease (PAD) Atherosclerosis occurring in the lower extremities, such as in the feet, calves, or legs, or in the arms.

coronary heart disease (CHD) A narrowing of the small blood vessels that supply blood to the heart.

myocardial infarction (MI) or heart attack A blockage of normal blood supply to an area in the heart.

coronary thrombosis A blood clot occurring in a coronary artery.

thrombus Blood clot attached to a blood vessel's wall.

WOMEN AND HEART ATTACKS

"Having a heart attack" usually brings to mind an older man gasping for breath, clutching his chest, and toppling over in the middle of a workout. So the story of comedienne and former talk show host Rosie O'Donnell's heart attack doesn't seem to fit the mold: O'Donnell, 50, didn't even know she'd had one at first. She reported on her blog that "my body hurt, I had an ache in my chest, both my arms were sore; everything felt bruised." At first, she wondered if she might have strained a muscle. Later she felt hot, clammy, and vomited. Fortunately, she took an aspirin and eventually went to the doctor, despite initially doubting a serious problem. It turned out O'Donnell had an almost complete blockage of a heart artery that required a stent.

Rosie isn't alone. According to a recent study, women who suffer heart attacks under the age of 55 are not only less likely to have classic chest pain or pressure, but also they tend to delay going to the doctor. When they do seek medical attention, they often report more atypical symptoms, such as shortness of breath or pain in the neck, shoulder, arms, and stomach. Many women chalk up heart symptoms to stress, flu, or lack of exercise. Because of treatment delays, women are more likely to have heart damage and to die from a heart attack than men of the same age.

So how can a woman tell if she is having a heart attack? In addition to the symptoms already mentioned, women may experience chest pressure or pain; radiating pains in the arms, shoulder, neck, jaw, or back; dizziness; abdominal pain; and unexplained feelings of fatigue, anxiety, or weakness—especially during exertion. But the real answer to the question of how to tell if a woman is having a heart attack is this: *let a doctor* determine that. If you or someone you know has even a few of these symptoms, don't delay. Crush or chew a full strength aspirin and swallow it with water. In addition to being a pain killer, aspirin has blood-thinning properties, so taking one can prevent fatal blood clots from forming. Then have someone drive you to a health care facility for evaluation, or call 9-1-1 to get an ambulance.

Sources: J. Canto, W. Rogers, R. Goldberg, et al., "Association of Age and Sex with Myocardial Infarction Symptom Presentation and In-Hospital Mortality." *JAMA*, 2012, 307(8): 813–822; National Coalition for Women with Heart Disease, Women Heart, "Are You Having a Heart Attack?," 2012, www.womenheart.org.

---

embolus A blood clot that becomes dislodged from a blood vessel wall and moves through the circulatory system.

collateral circulation Adaptation of the heart to partial damage accomplished by rerouting needed blood through unused or underused blood vessels while the damaged heart muscle heals.

stroke A condition occurring when the brain is damaged by disrupted blood supply; also called *cerebrovascular accident.*

aneurysm A weakened blood vessel that may bulge under pressure and, in severe cases, burst.

40%
of heart attack victims die within the first hour following the heart attack.

and moves through the circulatory system, it is called an **embolus.** Whenever blood does not flow readily, there is a corresponding decrease in oxygen flow to tissue below the blockage. If the blockage is extremely minor, an otherwise healthy heart will adapt over time by enlarging existing blood vessels and growing new ones to reroute needed blood through other areas. This system, called **collateral circulation,** is a form of self-preservation that allows an affected heart muscle to cope with damage.

When a heart blockage is more severe, however, the body is unable to adapt on its own, and outside lifesaving support is critical. The hour following a heart attack is the most crucial period—with the events of the first hour after an attack being critical to survival. See the **Health in a Diverse World** box above, the **Skills for Behavior Change** box on page 467, and **Table 15.1** on page 465 to learn common signs and symptoms as well as what to do in case of a heart attack.

Stroke

Like heart muscle cells, brain cells must have a continuous and adequate supply of oxygen in order to survive. A **stroke** (also called a *cerebrovascular accident*) occurs when the blood supply to the brain is interrupted. Strokes may be either *ischemic,* caused by plaque formation or a clot that reduces blood flow, or *hemorrhagic,* meaning a blood vessel weakens and either bulges or ruptures. **Figure 15.6** illustrates some of the blood vessel disorders that can lead to a stroke. An **aneurysm** is the most well known and most life-threatening of the hemorrhagic strokes. When any of these events occur, oxygen deprivation kills brain cells.

Some strokes are mild and cause only temporary dizziness or slight weakness or numbness. More serious interruptions in blood flow may impair speech, memory, or motor

TABLE 15.1 Common Heart Attack Symptoms and Signs	
Sign or Symptom	Gender Who Most Commonly Experiences It
Crushing or squeezing chest pain	More common in men
Pain radiating down arm, neck, or jaw	More common in men
Chest discomfort or pressure with shortness of breath, nausea/vomiting, or lightheadedness	Women more likely to feel pressure than pain. Shortness of breath and nausea, and lightheadedness common in both women and men
Shortness of breath without chest pain, discomfort in back, neck, or jaw or in one or both arms	More common in women
Unusual weakness	More common in women
Unusual fatigue	More common in women
Sleep disturbances	More common in women
Indigestion, flulike symptoms	More common in women

Sources: J. Canto et al., "Symptom Presentation of Women with Acute Coronary Syndromes: Myth vs. Reality," *Archives of Internal Medicine* 167, no. 22 (2007): 2405–13; American Heart Association, "Symptoms of Heart Attack in Women," 2012, www.heart.org/HEARTORG/Conditions/HeartAttack/WarningSignsofaHeartAttack/Heart-Attack-Symptoms-in-Women_UCM_436448_Article.jsp.

control. Other strokes affect the parts of the brain that regulate heart and lung function and kill within minutes. According to the American Heart Association's latest statistics, every year more than 7 million Americans suffer strokes, 136,000 of whom die as a result. Hypertension is a leading risk factor for stroke. Men have more strokes in their younger years; women suffer more strokes in their later years, accounting for over 60 percent of stroke cases in the United States. (The **Health Headlines** box on page 466 gives more information on strokes and young people.) Strokes cause much disability and suffering and account for 1 in 18 deaths each year, surpassed only by CHD and cancer.[17]

Many strokes are preceded days, weeks, or months earlier by **transient ischemic attacks (TIAs),** brief interruptions of the blood supply to the brain that cause temporary impairment.[18] Symptoms of TIAs include dizziness, particularly when first rising in the morning, weakness, temporary paralysis or numbness in the face or other regions, temporary memory loss, blurred vision, nausea, headache, slurred speech or difficulty in speaking, or other unusual physiological reactions. Some people may actually experience unexpected falls or have blackouts; others may have no obvious symptoms. Transient ischemic attacks often indicate an impending major stroke. The earlier a stroke is recognized and treatment started, the more effective that treatment will be. See the **Skills for Behavior Change** box on page 468 for tips on recognizing a stroke.

One of the great medical successes in recent years has been the decline in the death rate from strokes, which has dropped by over one third in the United States since the 1980s and continues to fall.[19] Improved diagnostic procedures, better surgical options, clot-busting drugs injected soon after a stroke has occurred, and acute care centers specializing in stroke treatment and rehabilitation have all been factors. Unfortunately, like many victims of other forms of CVD, stroke survivors do

transient ischemic attack (TIA) Brief interruption of the blood supply to the brain that causes only temporary impairment; often an indicator of impending major stroke.

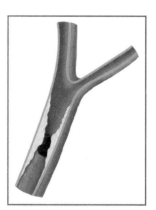

a A thrombus is a blood clot that forms inside a blood vessel and blocks the flow of blood at its origin. A thrombus in a cerebral artery can lead to an ischemic stroke.

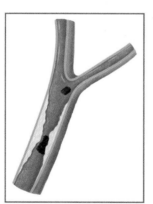

b An embolus is a blood clot that breaks off from its point of formation and travels in the bloodstream until it lodges in a narrowed vessel and blocks blood flow. Emboli in brain blood vessels can cause ischemic strokes.

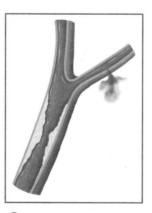

c A hemorrhage occurs when a blood vessel bursts, allowing blood to flow into the surrounding tissue or between tissues. There are two types of hemorrhagic strokes: subarachnoid, in which a vessel on the brain's surface bursts, and intracerebral, in which a vessel within the brain bursts.

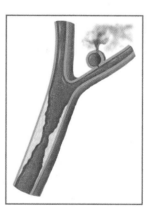

d An aneurysm is the bulging of a weakened blood vessel wall. Aneurysms in the brain can cause hemorrhagic strokes if they burst.

FIGURE 15.6 **Blood Vessel Disorders That Can Lead to Stroke**

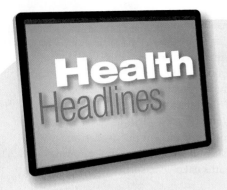

Health Headlines

YOUNG MEN AND WOMEN: STROKE ALERT!

Stroke: It only happens to those older, gray-haired folks or hyperanxious, go-go-go people, right? Not necessarily. In a surprising announcement, researchers from the Centers for Disease Control and Prevention analyzed hospitalizations for stroke between 1995 and 2007 and discovered that stroke rates increased the most (up a dramatic 51 percent) among young men age 15 to 34! Stroke rates rose among women in this age group, too, but at a slower rate of 17 percent during the same time frame. Why is this happening? Although the growing prevalence of obesity, high-fat diets, increased sodium consumption, and sedentary lifestyle are mentioned as likely contributors, trends went in the opposite direction among older adults, with stroke rates dropping 25 percent in men aged 65 and older and down 28 percent among women in the same age group. Better awareness of stroke risks among older adults and increased use of antihypertensive medicines are among the possible reasons for these declines. More research is needed to find out why young adults seem to be having more strokes.

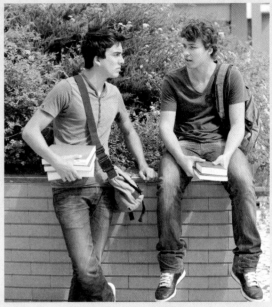

Young men, in particular, are at an elevated risk for stroke.

Source: M. George et al., "Trends in Stroke Hospitalizations and Associated Risk Factors among Children and Young Adults," *Annals of Neurology* 70, no. 5 (2011): 713–21.

---

hypertension Sustained elevated blood pressure.
systolic pressure The upper number in the fraction that measures blood pressure, indicating pressure on arterial walls when the heart contracts.
diastolic pressure The lower number in the fraction that measures blood pressure, indicating pressure on arterial walls during the relaxation phase of heart activity.

Hypertension

Hypertension refers to sustained high blood pressure. It is known as the "silent killer" because it often has few overt symptoms. Its prevalence has increased by over 30 percent in the past 10 years; today 1 in 3 adult Americans has a higher-than-optimal blood pressure, and the incidence among teens and young adults is on the rise.[20] Prevalence among African Americans is among the highest in the world. High blood pressure is also two to three times more common in women who take oral contraceptives than in women who do not take them.[21]

not always make a full recovery. Problems with speech, memory, swallowing, and activities of daily living and other consequences can persist, even with physical therapy and medications. Depression is also an issue for many post-stroke survivors.

"Why Should I Care?"

Hypertension is becoming more common among college students. You can't tell whether you have it by how you feel or how you look in the mirror, but it poses a major potential threat to your quality of life. Get your blood pressure checked. It's easy to do, and it could save your life!

Blood pressure is measured by two numbers, for example, 110/80 mm Hg, stated as "110 over 80 millimeters of mercury." The top number, **systolic blood pressure,** refers to the pressure of blood in the arteries when the heart muscle contracts, sending blood to the rest of the body. The bottom number, **diastolic blood pressure,** refers to the pressure of blood on the arteries when the heart muscle relaxes, as blood is reentering the heart chambers. Normal blood pressure varies depending on age, weight, and physical condition. Systolic blood pressure tends to increase with age, whereas diastolic blood pressure typically increases until age 55 and then declines. Women are about as likely as men to develop high blood pressure during their lifetimes. However, for people under 45 years old, the condition affects more men than women. For people 65 years and older, it affects more women than men.[22]

High blood pressure is usually diagnosed when systolic pressure is 140 or above. When only systolic pressure is high, the condition is known as *isolated systolic hypertension* (*ISH*), the most common form of high blood pressure in older Americans. See Table 15.2 for a summary of blood pressure values.

TABLE

15.2 Blood Pressure Classifications

Classification	Systolic Reading (mm Hg)		Diastolic Reading (mm Hg)
Normal	Less than 120	and	Less than 80
Prehypertension	120–139	or	80–89
Hypertension			
Stage 1	140–159	or	90–99
Stage 2	Greater than or equal to 160	or	Greater than or equal to 100

Note: If systolic and diastolic readings fall into different categories, treatment is determined by the highest category. Readings are based on the average of two or more properly measured, seated readings on each of two or more health care provider visits.

Source: National Heart, Lung, and Blood Institute, *The Seventh Report of the Joint National Committee on Prevention, Detection, Evaluation, and Treatment of High Blood Pressure,* NIH Publication no. 03-5233 (Bethesda, MD: National Institutes of Health, 2003).

Angina Pectoris

Angina pectoris occurs when there is not enough oxygen to supply the heart muscle, resulting in chest pain or pres-

What to Do When a Heart Attack Hits

People often miss the signs of a heart attack, or they wait too long to seek help, which can have deadly consequences. Knowing what to do in an emergency could save your life or somebody else's. (See Table 15.1 on page 465 for information on signs and symptoms.)

❱ Keep a list of emergency rescue service numbers next to your telephone and in your pocket, wallet, or purse. Be aware of whether your local area has a 9-1-1 emergency service.

❱ Expect the person to deny the possibility of anything as serious as a heart attack, particularly if that person is young and appears to be in good health. If you're with someone who appears to be having a heart attack, don't take no for an answer; insist on taking prompt action.

❱ If you are with someone who suddenly collapses, perform cardiopulmonary resuscitation (CPR). See www .heart.org for information on the new chest-compression-only techniques recommended by the American Heart Association. If you're trained and willing, use conventional CPR methods.

Sources: Adapted from American Heart Association, "Warning Signs of Heart Attack, Stroke, and Cardiac Arrest," 2012, www.heart.org/ HEARTORG/Conditions/Conditions_UCM_305346_SubHomePage .jsp.

sure. Approximately 2 percent of the U.S. population between the ages of 25 and 45 experience angina pectoris, with over 13 percent of men and nearly 11 percent of women experiencing mild to moderate symptoms by the age of 65. For some, the pain is similar to a mild case of indigestion; for others, the pain is crushing, with heart-attack-like symptoms that may require powerful medications to control.[23] Generally, the more serious the oxygen deprivation, the more severe the pain. Although angina pectoris is not a heart attack, it does indicate underlying heart disease.

Currently, there are several methods of treating angina. Mild cases may be treated simply with rest. Drugs such as *nitroglycerin* can dilate veins and provide pain relief. Other medications, such as *calcium channel blockers*, can relieve cardiac spasms and arrhythmias, lower blood pressure, and slow heart rate. *Beta-blockers,* the other major type of drugs used to treat angina, control potential overactivity of the heart muscle.

Arrhythmias

Over the course of a lifetime, most people experience some type of **arrhythmia,** an irregularity in heart rhythm that occurs when the electrical impulses in your heart that coordinate heartbeat don't work properly. **Fibrillation** is known as asporadic, quivering pattern of heartbeat that results in extreme inefficiency in moving blood through the cardiovascular system.

angina pectoris Chest pain occurring as a result of reduced oxygen flow to the heart.

arrhythmia An irregularity in heartbeat.

fibrillation A sporadic, quivering pattern of heartbeat that results in extreme inefficiency in moving blood through the cardiovascular system.

Often described as a heart "fluttering" or racing, these irregularities send many people to the emergency room, only to find that they are fine. A person with a racing heart in the absence of exercise or anxiety may be experiencing *tachycardia,* the medical term for abnormally fast heartbeat. On the other end of the continuum is *bradycardia,* or abnormally slow heartbeat. When a heart goes into fibrillation, it beats in a sporadic, quivering pattern, resulting in extreme inefficiency in moving blood through the cardiovascular system. If untreated, fibrillation may be fatal.

Not all arrhythmias are life-threatening. In many instances, excessive caffeine or nicotine consumption can trigger an arrhythmia episode. However, severe cases may require drug therapy or external electrical stimulus to prevent serious complications. When in doubt, it is always best to check with your doctor.

400,000

new cases of angina are diagnosed each year.

Heart Failure

When the heart muscle is damaged and can't pump enough blood to supply body tissues, fluids may begin to accumulate in various parts of the body, most notably, the lungs, feet, ankles, and legs. Acute shortness of breath and fatigue are often key additional symptoms. Known as **heart failure (HF)** or **congestive heart failure (CHF)** this condition is increasingly common, particularly among those with a history of other heart problems. Currently, nearly 6.6 million adults age 20 and over in the United States have HF. By 2030, estimates are that there will be nearly 10 million cases.[24]

> **congestive heart failure (CHF)** or **heart failure (HF)** An abnormal cardiovascular condition that reflects impaired cardiac pumping and blood flow; pooling blood leads to congestion in body tissues.

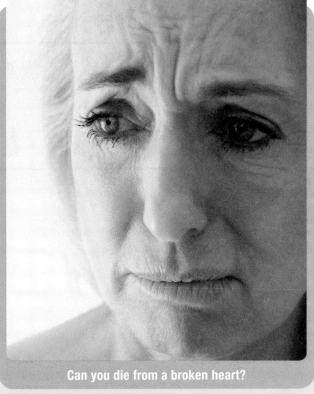

Can you die from a broken heart?

As first described in a 2005 article in the *New England Journal of Medicine*, researchers reported "broken heart syndrome," which has come to be known as *stress cardiomyopathy*. In this phenomenon, the heart is so stressed by traumatic emotional events that it receives a "concussion," a type of heart attack triggered by extreme, overwhelming stress, grief, horror, or anger. This is believed to affect about 6 percent of women who have an apparent heart attack.

Underlying causes of HF may include heart injury from uncontrolled high blood pressure, rheumatic fever, pneumonia, heart attack and damage to the heart, heart valve issues, and general coronary artery diseases. Certain prescription drugs such as NSAIDS and diabetes medications also increase risks, as do chronic drug and alcohol abuse. In some cases, the damage is due to cancer radiation or chemotherapy treatments. Untreated, HF can be fatal. However, most cases respond well to treatment that includes *diuretics* ("water pills") to relieve fluid accumulation; drugs, such as *digitalis,* that increase the pumping action of the heart; and drugs called *vasodilators,* which expand blood vessels and decrease resistance, allowing blood to flow more freely and making the heart's work easier. Prevention of underlying CVD risks, such as reducing sodium intake and following a heart smart diet, are the best ways to reduce your risks of HF.

Congenital Cardiovascular Defects

Approximately 32,000 infants are expected to be born in the United States each year with some form of

---

Skills for Behavior Change

A Simple Test for Stroke

People often ignore, minimize, or misunderstand stroke symptoms. Starting treatment within just a few hours is crucial for the best recovery outcomes. So if you suspect someone is having a stroke, use the Cincinnati Prehospital Stroke Scale to clarify what may be happening. Many emergency medical teams have adopted this tool to evaluate patients. Anyone with three abnormal signs has an over 70 percent likelihood of stroke.

1. Facial Droop: Ask the person to smile. It is normal for both sides of the face to move equally, and it is abnormal if one side moves less easily.
2. Arm Drift: Ask the person to raise both arms. It is normal if both arms move equally (or not at all). It is abnormal if one arm drifts or cannot be raised as high as the other.
3. Speech: Have the patient restate a sentence such as, "You can't teach an old dog new tricks." It is normal if they can say the sentence correctly, and it is abnormal if they use inappropriate words, slur, or cannot speak.

Source: Cincinnati Prehospital Stroke Scale, adapted from the Uniform Document for Georgia EMS Providers, Department of Public Health, State of Georgia. Available at ems.ga.gov/programs/ems/emsdocs/Georgia%20Stroke%20Assessment%20Form%20-%20v.1%20-%2011-02-2011.pdf.

congenital cardiovascular defect (*congenital* means the problem is present at birth).[25] These forms may be relatively minor, such as slight *murmurs* (low-pitched sounds caused by turbulent blood flow through the heart) caused by valve irregularities that some children outgrow. About 25 percent of those born with congenital heart defects must undergo invasive procedures to correct problems within the first year of life.[26] The underlying causes of these defects are unknown, but they may be related to hereditary factors; maternal diseases, such as rubella, that occurred during fetal development; or the mother's chemical intake (particularly alcohol or methamphetamine) during pregnancy. Because of advances in pediatric cardiology, the prognosis for children with congenital heart defects is better than ever before.

Rheumatic heart disease can cause similar heart problems in children. It is attributed to rheumatic fever, an inflammatory disease caused by an unresolved *streptococcal infection* of the throat (strep throat). Over time, this strep infection can affect many connective tissues of the body, especially those of the heart, joints, brain, or skin. In some cases, this infection can lead to an immune response in which antibodies attack the heart as well as the bacteria. Many of the thousands of operations on heart valves performed per year in the United States are related to rheumatic heart disease.

Reducing Your Risks

Scientific evidence has shown a large cluster of factors related to a person's being at a higher risk for developing cardiovascular diseases over the life span. Obesity and overweight, smoking and exposure to secondhand smoke, high levels of cholesterol and other lipids, physical inactivity, high blood pressure, diabetes mellitus, metabolic syndrome, and genetics and family history are all associated with increased risk of CVD development.[27] Interestingly, although selected factors increase risks specific to CVD, the combination of these and other risk factors appears also to increase risks for insulin resistance and type 2 diabetes.[28] It may also increase risk for Alzheimer's disease.[29] The term **cardiometabolic risks** refers to these combined risks, which indicate physical and biochemical changes that can lead to diseases. Some risks result from choices and behaviors and so are modifiable, whereas others are inherited or are intrinsic (such as your age and gender) and cannot be changed.

Metabolic Syndrome: Quick Risk Profile

Over the past decade, different health professionals have attempted to establish diagnostic cutoff points for a cluster of combined cardiometabolic risks, variably labeled as *syndrome X, insulin resistance syndrome,* and most recently, **metabolic syndrome (MetS)**. Historically, metabolic syndrome is believed to increase the risk for atherosclerotic heart disease by as much as three times the normal rates. It has captured international attention because over 20 percent of people age 20 to 39, 41 percent of people age 40 to 59, and nearly 52 percent of those over the age of 60 meet the criteria for MetS.[30] Although different professional organizations have slightly different criteria for MetS, that of the National Cholesterol Education Program's Adult Treatment Panel (NCEP/ATPIII) is most commonly used. According to these criteria, for a diagnosis of metabolic syndrome a person would have three or more of the following risks:[31]

● Abdominal obesity (waist measurement of more than 40 inches in men or 35 inches in women)
● Elevated blood fat (triglycerides greater than 150)
● Low levels of HDL ("good") cholesterol (less than 40 in men and less than 50 in women)
● Elevated blood pressure greater than 135/85 mm Hg
● Elevated fasting glucose greater than 100 mg/dL (a sign of insulin resistance or glucose intolerance)

Other professional groups may add high levels of *C-reactive proteins* as a part of the criteria for MetS. High levels of these proteins in the blood may indicate high inflammatory processes in the body that increase CVD risks.

The use of the metabolic syndrome classification and other, similar terms has been important in highlighting the relationship between the number of risks a person possesses and that person's likelihood of developing CVD and diabetes. However, critics have indicated that it is impossible to tell how important each of these factors is—either individually or in combination—or which ones should be prioritized when taking action to reduce risks. Overall lifestyle changes targeting these factors are important.

Although the link between MetS and the risks of CVD is still being researched, it is clear that having several of the characteristics of MetS can affect your daily life even without a diagnosis of CVD (see Figure 15.7).

congenital cardiovascular defect Cardiovascular problem that is present at birth.

rheumatic heart disease A heart disease caused by untreated streptococcal infection of the throat.

cardiometabolic risks Physical and biochemical changes that are risk factors for the development of cardiovascular disease and type 2 diabetes.

metabolic syndrome (MetS) A group of metabolic conditions occurring together that increase a person's risk of heart disease, stroke, and diabetes.

Modifiable Risks

It may surprise you to realize that younger adults are not invulnerable to CVD risks. The reality is that from the first

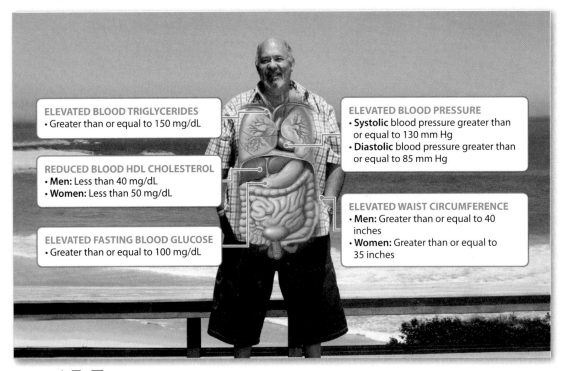

FIGURE 15.7 **Risk Factors Associated with Metabolic Syndrome**

ELEVATED BLOOD TRIGLYCERIDES
• Greater than or equal to 150 mg/dL

REDUCED BLOOD HDL CHOLESTEROL
• **Men:** Less than 40 mg/dL
• **Women:** Less than 50 mg/dL

ELEVATED FASTING BLOOD GLUCOSE
• Greater than or equal to 100 mg/dL

ELEVATED BLOOD PRESSURE
• **Systolic** blood pressure greater than or equal to 130 mm Hg
• **Diastolic** blood pressure greater than or equal to 85 mm Hg

ELEVATED WAIST CIRCUMFERENCE
• **Men:** Greater than or equal to 40 inches
• **Women:** Greater than or equal to 35 inches

moments of your life, you begin to accumulate increasing numbers of risks. Your past and current lifestyle choices may haunt you as you enter your middle and later years of life. Behaviors you choose today and over the coming decades can actively reduce or promote your risk for CVD.

Avoid Tobacco Although smoking rates declined by over 50 percent between 1965 and 2007, about 21 percent of U.S. adults age 18 and over are still regular smokers.[32] In spite of massive campaigns to educate us about the dangers of smoking and increasing numbers of states and municipalities enacting "smoke free" zones and policies, tobacco use remains the leading cause of preventable death in the United States, accounting for around 1 of every 5 deaths. Likewise, nonsmokers regularly exposed to second-hand smoke have a 25

Is there anything I can do to improve my cholesterol level?

About 25 percent of your blood cholesterol level comes from foods you eat, and this is where you can make real improvements.

to 30 percent increased risk of heart disease, with over 35,000 deaths per year.

Just how great a risk is smoking when it comes to CVD? Consider these statistics:[33]

● Cigarette smokers are two to four times more likely to develop coronary heart disease than are nonsmokers.
● Cigarette smoking doubles a person's risk of stroke.
● Smokers are more than 10 times more likely than non-smokers to develop peripheral vascular diseases.

Smoking is thought to damage the heart in several ways. Nicotine increases heart rate, blood pressure, and oxygen use by heart muscles, which over time forces the organ to work harder. The other explanation for smoking's link to heart disease is that chemicals in smoke may damage and inflame coronary arteries, allowing cholesterol and plaque to accumulate more easily and increasing blood pressure.

The good news is that if you stop smoking, your heart appears able to mend itself. A former smoker's risk of heart disease drops by 50 percent 1 year after quitting. Between 5 to 15 years after quitting, the risk of stroke and CHD becomes similar to that of nonsmokers.[34] College-age students, take note: Studies show quitting by age 30 reduces chances of dying prematurely from tobacco-related diseases by more than 90 percent. Those who already have been diagnosed with early stage lung cancer fare much better after quitting. [35]

Cut Back on Saturated Fat and Cholesterol
Cholesterol is a type of soft, waxy fat-like substance found in your bloodstream and in your body cells. Cholesterol plays an important role in the production of cell membranes and

hormones (estrogen and testosterone), and it helps process vitamin D. However, when levels of it in the blood get too high, your risk for CVD increases. Much of your blood cholesterol level is predetermined: About 75 percent of it is produced by your body, and the rest comes from foods in your diet. The good news is that changing your diet can make real improvements in your overall cholesterol level, even if yours is naturally high.

Diets high in saturated fat and *trans* fats are known to raise cholesterol levels, send the body's blood-clotting system into high gear, and make the blood more viscous in just a few hours, thereby increasing the risk of heart attack or stroke. High levels of cholesterol in the blood also contribute to atherosclerosis.

The *type* of cholesterol is just as important as total cholesterol. **Low-density lipoprotein (LDL)**, often referred to as "bad" cholesterol, is believed to build up on artery walls. In contrast, **high-density lipoprotein (HDL)**, or "good" cholesterol, appears to remove cholesterol from artery walls. In theory, if LDL levels get too high or HDL levels too low, cholesterol will accumulate inside arteries and lead to cardiovascular problems. **Triglycerides** are also gaining increasing attention as a key factor in CVD risk. When you consume extra calories, the body converts the extra to triglycerides, which are stored in fat cells. Hormones release triglycerides throughout the day to provide energy. High counts of blood triglycerides are often found in people who are obese and overweight and have high cholesterol levels, heart problems, or diabetes. As they age, particularly if they gain weight, people's triglyceride and cholesterol levels tend to rise. It is recommended that a baseline cholesterol test (known as a lipid panel or lipid profile) be taken at age 20, with follow-ups every 5 years. Men over the age of 35 and women over the age of 45 should have their lipid profile checked annually, with more frequent tests for those at high risk. See Table 15.3 for recommended levels of cholesterol and triglycerides.

Perhaps the best method of evaluating cholesterol-level risk is to examine the ratio of HDL to total cholesterol, or the percentage of HDL in total cholesterol. If the HDL level is lower than 35 mg/dL, the risk increases. A person with an at-risk ratio can try to lower LDL and raise HDL. Regular exercise and a healthy diet low in saturated fat continue to be the best methods for maintaining healthy ratios.

In spite of all of the education on the dangers of high cholesterol and the importance of lowering dietary fat and cholesterol in the diet, Americans continue to have higher-than-recommended levels. Nearly 46 percent of adults age 20 and over have cholesterol levels at or above 200 mg/dL, and another 16 percent have levels in excess of 240 mg/dL.[36] Forty-five percent of all adults age 60 and over in the United States are on cholesterol-lowering drugs. Add to that the nearly 20 percent on diuretics for high blood pressure and CVD and the over 26 percent on beta-blockers for high blood pressure and heart disease, and it becomes clear that pharmaceutical treatments for CVD risks are on the rise.[37]

TABLE 15.3 — Recommended Cholesterol Levels for Lower/Moderate-Risk Adults

Total Cholesterol Level (lower numbers are better)	
Less than 200 mg/dL	Desirable
200 to 239 mg/dL	Borderline high
240 mg/dL and above	High
HDL Cholesterol Level (higher numbers are better)	
Less than 40 mg/dL (for men)	Low
60 mg/dL and above	Desirable
LDL Cholesterol Level (lower numbers are better)	
Less than 100 mg/dL	Optimal
100 to 129 mg/dL	Near or above optimal
130 to 159 mg/dL	Borderline high
160 to 189 mg/dL	High
190 mg/dL and above	Very high
Triglyceride Level (lower numbers are better)	
Less than 150 mg/dL	Normal
150–199 mg/dL	Borderline high
200–499 mg/dL	High
500 mg/dL and above	Very high

Source: Adapted from ATP III Guidelines At-a-Glance Quick Desk Reference, National Heart, Lung, and Blood Institute, National Institutes of Health. Update on Cholesterol Guidelines, 2004.

Strive for a Heart-Healthy Diet Research continues into other dietary modifications that may affect heart health. An overall approach, such as the DASH (Dietary Approaches to Stop Hypertension) eating plan from the National Heart, Lung, and Blood Institute (Figure 15.8), has strong evidence to back up its recommendations. The guidelines include the following dietary changes to reduce CVD risk:

- Consume 5 to 10 milligrams per day of soluble fiber from sources such as oat bran, fruits, vegetables, legumes, and psyllium seeds. Even this small dietary modification may result in a 5 percent drop in LDL levels.
- Consume about 2 grams per day of **plant sterols,** which are naturally present in small quantities in many fruits, vegetables, nuts, seeds, and other plant sources. Sterols are also used to enrich products such as Benecol and Take Control margarine. Intake of plant sterols can reduce LDL by another 5 percent.
- Eat less sodium. Excess sodium has been linked to high blood pressure, which can in turn affect CVD risk.

low-density lipoproteins (LDLs) Compounds that facilitate the transport of cholesterol in the blood to the body's cells and cause the cholesterol to build up on artery walls.

high-density lipoproteins (HDLs) Compounds that facilitate the transport of cholesterol in the blood to the liver for metabolism and elimination from the body.

triglycerides The most common form of lipid in the body; excess calories are converted into triglycerides and stored as body fat.

plant sterols Essential components of plant membranes that, when consumed in the diet, appear to help lower cholesterol levels.

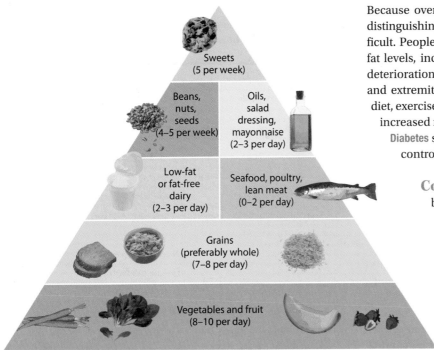

FIGURE 15.8 **The DASH Eating Plan**

Source: Data adapted from U.S. Department of Health and Human Services, National Institutes of Health, National Heart, Lung, and Blood Institute, *Your Guide to Lowering Your Blood Pressure with DASH*, NIH Publication no. 06-4082, Revised April, 2006 (Bethesda, MD: National Institutes of Health, 2006).

See the **Health Headlines** box on page 473 for more information on foods that may be heart protective.

Maintain a Healthy Weight No question about it—body weight plays a role in CVD. Researchers are not sure whether high-fat, high-sugar, high-calorie diets are a direct risk for CVD or whether they invite risk by causing obesity, which strains the heart, forcing it to push blood through the many miles of capillaries that supply each pound of fat. A heart that has to continuously move blood through an overabundance of vessels may become damaged. Overweight people are more likely to develop heart disease and stroke even if they have no other risk factors. If you're heavy, losing even 5 to 10 pounds can make a significant difference.[38] This is especially true if you're an "apple" (thicker around your upper body and waist) rather than a "pear" (thicker around your hips and thighs).

Exercise Regularly Inactivity is a definite risk factor for CVD.[39] The good news is that you do not have to be an exercise fanatic to reduce your risk. Even modest levels of low-intensity physical activity—walking, gardening, housework, dancing—are beneficial if done regularly and over the long term. Exercise can increase HDL, lower triglycerides, and reduce coronary risks in several ways.

Control Diabetes Heart disease death rates among adults with diabetes are two to four times higher than the rates for adults without diabetes. At least 65 percent of people with diabetes die of some form of heart disease or stroke.[40]

Because overweight people have a higher risk for diabetes, distinguishing between the effects of the two conditions is difficult. People with diabetes also tend to have elevated blood fat levels, increased atherosclerosis, and a tendency toward deterioration of small blood vessels, particularly in the eyes and extremities. However, through a prescribed regimen of diet, exercise, and medication, they can control much of their increased risk for CVD. (See Focus On: Minimizing Your Risk for Diabetes starting on page 482 for more on preventing and controlling diabetes.)

Control Your Blood Pressure Although blood pressure typically creeps up with aging, lifestyle changes can dramatically reduce risks. Among the most beneficial actions you can take are losing weight, cutting back sodium in your diet, exercising more, reducing alcohol intake, quitting smoking, and reducing your caffeine intake.

Manage Stress Some scientists have noted a relationship between CVD risk and a person's stress level. Stress may influence established risk factors. For example, people under stress may start smoking or smoke more than they otherwise would. A large, landmark study found that impatience and hostility, two key components of the Type A behavior pattern, increase young adults' risk of developing high blood pressure. Other related factors, such as competitiveness, depression, and anxiety, did not appear to increase risk.[41] In recent years, scientists have tended to agree that unresolved stress appears to increase risk for hypertension, heart disease, and stroke. Although the exact mechanism is unknown, scientists are closer to discovering why stress can affect us so negatively. Newer studies indicate that chronic stress may result in three times the risk of hypertension, CHD, and sudden cardiac death and that there is a link between anxiety, depression, and negative cardiovascular effects.[42]

Nonmodifiable Risks

Unfortunately not all risk factors for CVD can be prevented or controlled. The most important are the following:

● **Race and ethnicity.** Although Caucasians tend to have more heart disease, African Americans are 40 percent more likely to have hypertension and 10 percent less likely to have it under control and have a stroke. The rate of high blood pressure in African Americans is among the highest in the world. CVD risks are also higher among Hispanic/Latino Americans. Importantly, racial and ethnic minorities have a significantly greater risk of dying from CVD-related diseases.[43] See Figure 15.9 for a summary of the percentages of total deaths for various ethnic groups by heart disease and stroke.

See It! Videos

Is good cholesterol even better than we thought? Watch **Tips to Raise Good Cholesterol** at www.pearsonhighered.com/donatelle.

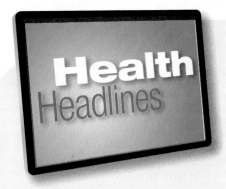

Health Headlines

HEART-HEALTHY SUPER FOODS

The foods you eat play a major role in your CVD risk. While many foods can increase your risk, several have been shown to reduce the chances that cholesterol will be absorbed in the cells, reduce levels of LDL cholesterol, or enhance the protective effects of HDL cholesterol. To protect your heart, include the following in your diet:

✻ **Fish high in omega-3 fatty acids.** Consumption of fish such as salmon, sardines, and herring helps reduce blood pressure and the risk associated with blood clots as well as lower cholesterol.

✻ **Olive oil.** Using any of a number of monounsaturated fats in cooking, particularly extra virgin olive oil, helps lower total cholesterol and raise your HDL levels. Canola oil; margarine labeled "*trans* fat free"; and cholesterol-lowering margarines such as Benecol, Promise Activ, or Smart Balance are also excellent choices.

✻ **Whole grains and fiber.** Getting enough fiber each day in the form of 100 percent whole wheat, steel cut oats, oat bran, flaxseed, fruits, and vegetables helps lower

LDL or "bad" cholesterol. Soluble fiber, in particular, seems to keep cholesterol from being absorbed in the intestines.

✻ **Plant sterols and stanols.** These are essential components of plant membranes and are found naturally in vegetables, fruits, and legumes. In addition, many food products, including juices and yogurt, are now fortified with them. These compounds are believed to benefit your heart health by blocking cholesterol absorption in the bloodstream, thus reducing LDL levels.

✻ **Nuts.** Long maligned for being high in calories, walnuts, almonds, and other nuts are naturally high in omega-3 fatty acids, which are important in lowering cholesterol and good for the blood vessels themselves.

✻ **Green tea.** Over the past decade, several studies have indicated that green tea may reduce LDL cholesterol. The flavonoids in it act as powerful antioxidants that protect the cells of the heart and blood vessels.

✻ **Red wine.** In recent years, many observational studies have indicated that one glass of red wine may be protective and reduce your risk of CHD. Theories explaining this include possible antioxidant protective factors, increases in HDL (good) cholesterol levels, and anticlotting properties in the wine itself. Critics of these studies argue that the research is often confounded by lifestyle, diet, and cultural factors. Although the research is promising, the American Heart Association is slow to endorse drinking alcohol to reduce CVD risk and instead recommends tried and true behaviors such as dietary modification, exercise, and stress reduction, while supporting addi-

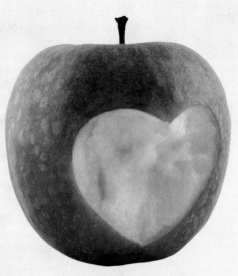

tional research. What is clear is that while one drink of red wine might be protective, adding additional "doses" of wine won't help and, in fact, is likely to be harmful.

Sources: L. Hooper et al., "Effects of Chocolate, Cocoa, and Flavan-3-ols on Cardiovascular Health: A Systematic Review and Meta-analysis of Randomized Trials," *American Journal of Clinical Nutrition* 95, no. 3 (2012): 740–51; American Heart Association, "Alcoholic Beverages and Cardiovascular Disease," 2011, Available at www.heart.org/HEARTORG/Getting Healthy/NutritionCenter/Alcoholic-Beverages-and-Cardiovascular-Disease_UCM_305864_Article.jsp; A. Mente, L. deKoning, M. Shannon, and S. Anand, "A Systematic Review of the Evidence Supporting a Causal Link between Dietary Factors and Coronary Heart Disease," *Archives of Internal Medicine* 169, no. 7 (2009): 659–69; P. Ronksley et al., "Association of Alcohol Consumption with Selected Cardiovascular Disease Outcomes: A Systematic Review and Meta-analysis." *British Medical Journal* 342 (2011): 671–81; Z. Wang et al., "Black and Green Tea Consumption and the Risk of Coronary Artery Disease: A Meta Analysis." *American Journal of Clinical Nutrition* 93, no. 3 (2011): 506–15.

● **Heredity.** A family history of heart disease increases risk of CVD significantly. As stated previously, the amount of cholesterol you produce, tendencies to form plaque, and a host of other factors seem to have genetic links. If you have close relatives with CVD, your risk may be double that of others. The difficulty comes in sorting out genetic influences from the modifiable factors shared by family members, such as environment, stress, dietary habits, and so on. Newer research has focused on studying the interactions between nutrition and genes (nutrigenetics) and the role that diet may play in increasing or decreasing risks among certain genetic profiles.[44]

● **Age.** Although cardiovascular disease can affect all ages, 75 percent of heart attacks occur in people over age 65. Increasing age ups the risk for CVD for all.

● **Gender.** Men are at greater risk for CVD until about age 60, when women catch up and then surpass them. Otherwise healthy women under age 35 have a fairly low risk, although oral contraceptive use and smoking increase the risk. After menopause, or after estrogen levels are otherwise reduced (for example, because of hysterectomy), women's LDL levels tend to go up, which increases the chance for CVD.

Other Risk Factors

Several other factors and indicators have been linked to CVD risk, including inflammation and homocysteine levels.

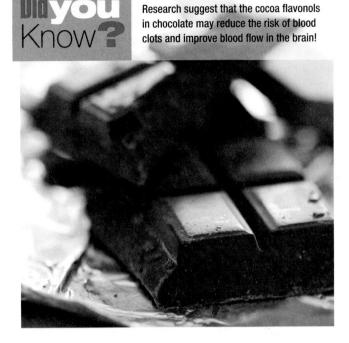

Did **you** Know?

Research suggest that the cocoa flavonols in chocolate may reduce the risk of blood clots and improve blood flow in the brain!

Inflammation and C-Reactive Protein Many experts believe inflammation plays a major role in atherosclerosis development. It occurs when bacteria, trauma, toxins, or heat injure blood vessel walls, making them more prone to plaque formation. Cigarette smoke, high blood pressure, high LDL cholesterol, diabetes, certain forms of arthritis, and exposure to toxins have all been linked to increased risk of inflammation. However, the greatest risk appears to be from certain infectious disease pathogens, most notably *Chlamydia pneumoniae,* a common cause of respiratory infections; *Helicobacter pylori,* a bacterium that causes ulcers; herpes simplex virus; and *Cytomegalovirus,* another herpes virus infecting most Americans before the age of 40. During an inflammatory reaction, C-reactive proteins (CRPs) tend to be present at high levels. Many scientists believe the presence of these proteins in the blood may signal elevated risk for angina and heart attack. Doctors can test patients, and if CRP levels are high, action could be taken to prevent progression to a heart attack or other coronary event. More research is necessary to determine the actual role that inflammation plays in increased risk of CVD or if there is something unique about inflammation that may actually play a greater role.[45]

Homocysteine Over the last decade, there was mounting evidence that homocysteine, an amino acid normally present in the blood, increased the risk of CVD. Early studies indicated that at high levels homocysteine was a prelude to coronary heart disease, peripheral artery disease (PAD), and increased risk of stroke. Scientists hypothesized that homocysteine works in much the same way as CRPs, inflaming the inner lining of the arterial walls and promoting fat deposits on the damaged walls and development of blood clots.[46] Other research suggested that high homocysteine levels are implicated in declining cognitive functioning, Alzheimer's, and other conditions.[47] When early studies indicated that folic acid and other B vitamins may help break down homocysteine in the body, food manufacturers responded by adding folic acids to a number of foods and touting the CVD benefits. However, over time, and with conflicting research, the connection between homocysteine, folic

What's Working for You?

Maybe you're already managing the modifiable risks to your heart's health. Which of the things below are you already incorporating into your life?

☐ I don't smoke.

☐ I eat a balanced diet.

☐ My family has a history of hypertension, so I monitor my blood pressure and control salt in my diet.

☐ I'm trying to get organized to reduce my stress levels.

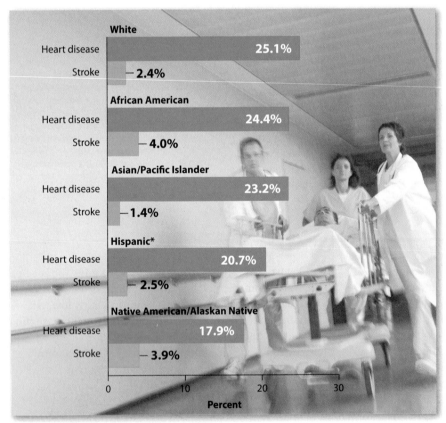

	White
Heart disease	25.1%
Stroke	2.4%
	African American
Heart disease	24.4%
Stroke	4.0%
	Asian/Pacific Islander
Heart disease	23.2%
Stroke	1.4%
	Hispanic*
Heart disease	20.7%
Stroke	2.5%
	Native American/Alaskan Native
Heart disease	17.9%
Stroke	3.9%

Percent

FIGURE 15.9 Deaths from Heart Disease and Stroke in the United States by Ethnicity

Source: Data are from A.M. Minifino et al., "Deaths: Final Data for 2008," *National Vital Statistics Reports* 59, no. 10 (Hyattsville, MD: National Center for Health Statistics, 2011).

*Persons of Hispanic origin may be of any race.

acid, and cardiovascular disease is slowly unraveling.[48] Professional groups such as the American Heart Association do not currently recommend taking folic acid supplements to lower homocysteine levels and prevent CVD.[49] Instead, they recommend a healthy diet as the best way to reduce risk.

Lipoprotein(a) Scientists now believe that there are other blood lipid factors that may also increase CVD risk, such as *lipoprotein-associated phospholipase A*2 (*Lp-PLA*2), an enzyme that circulates in the blood and attaches to LDL. Lp-PLA2 plays an important role in plaque accumulation and increased risk for stroke and coronary events, particularly in men. Studies suggest that the higher the Lp-PLA2 level, the higher the risk of developing CVD.[50] Another relatively new consideration is the presence of apolipoprotein B (apo B), a primary component of LDL that is essential for cholesterol delivery to cells. Although the mechanism is unclear, some researchers believe that apo B levels may be more important to heart disease risk than total cholesterol or LDL levels.[51]

Diagnosing and Treating Cardiovascular Disease

There many diagnostic, treatment, prevention, and rehabilitation options. Medications can strengthen heartbeat, control arrhythmias, remove fluids, reduce blood pressure, and improve heart function. *Statins* can be used to lower blood

cholesterol levels, *ACE inhibitors* can lower blood pressure by causing the muscles surrounding blood vessels to contract, and *beta-blockers* can reduce blood pressure by blocking the effects of the hormone epinephrine. Long-standing methods of cardiopulmonary resuscitation (CPR) have also changed recently to focus primarily on chest compressions rather than mouth-to-mouth procedures. The thinking behind this is that people will be more likely to do CPR if the risk for exchange of body fluids is reduced, and any effort to save a person in trouble is better than inaction.

Electrocardiogram, angiography, and positron emission tomography scans are some techniques for diagnosing CVD. An **electrocardiogram (ECG)** is a record of the heart's electrical activity. Patients may undergo a *stress test*—standard exercise on a stationary bike or treadmill with an electrocardiogram and no injections—or a *nuclear stress test,* which involves injecting a radioactive dye and taking images of the heart to reveal problems with blood flow. Although these tests provide a good indicator of potential heart

electrocardiogram (ECG) A record of the electrical activity of the heart; may be measured during a stress test.

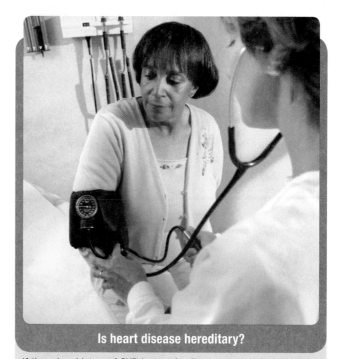

Is heart disease hereditary?

If there is a history of CVD in your family or your racial or ethnic background indicates a propensity for CVD, it is all the more important for you to have regular blood pressure and blood cholesterol screenings and for you to avoid lifestyle risks, including tobacco use, physical inactivity, and poor nutrition.

blockage or blood flow abnormalities, a more accurate method of testing for heart disease is **angiography** (also referred to as *cardiac catheterization*), in which a needle-thin tube called a *catheter* is threaded through heart arteries, a dye is injected, and an X ray is taken to discover which areas are blocked. A more recent and even more effective method of measuring heart activity is a *positron emission tomography (PET) scan,* which produces 3D images of the heart as blood flows through it. Other common tests include the following:

- Magnetic resonance imaging (*MRI*) involves using powerful magnets to look inside the body. Computer-generated pictures can show the heart muscle and help physicians identify damage from a heart attack, diagnose congenital heart defects, and evaluate disease of larger blood vessels such as the aorta.
- Ultrafast computed tomography (*CT*), an especially fast form of heart X ray, can be used to evaluate bypass grafts, diagnose ventricular function, and identify other heart irregularities.
- Coronary calcium score is derived from another type of ultrafast CT used to diagnose levels of calcium in heart vessels. Calcium accumulations on vessel walls provide an indication of plaque formation and heart attack risks; however, most people will show some level of calcium accumulation.

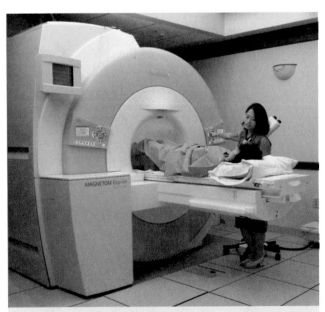

Magnetic resonance imaging is one of several methods used to detect heart damage, abnormalities, or defects.

Surgical Options: Bypass Surgery, Angioplasty, and Stents

Coronary bypass surgery has helped many patients who suffered coronary blockages or heart attacks. In a coronary artery bypass graft (CABG, referred to as a "cabbage"), a blood vessel is taken from another site in the patient's body (usually the saphenous vein in the leg or the internal thoracic artery, or ITA, in the chest) and implanted to "bypass" blocked coronary arteries and transport blood to heart tissue. Increasing numbers of heart surgeries are done using a minimally invasive bypass surgery in which the chest is not cracked; the surgeon enters the body through a series of ports and performs the surgery with cameras.

Another procedure, **angioplasty** (sometimes called *balloon angioplasty*), carries fewer risks and may be more effective than bypass surgery in selected cases. As in angiography, a thin catheter is threaded through blocked heart arteries. The catheter has a balloon at the tip, which is inflated to flatten fatty deposits against the arterial walls, allowing blood to flow more freely. Today, many people with heart blockage undergo angioplasty and have a **stent** inserted to hold the vessel open after the procedure. A stent is a stainless steel mesh-like tube that is inserted to prop open the artery. Although stents are highly effective, inflammation and tissue growth in the area may actually increase after the procedure, leading to another blockage. In about 30 percent of patients, the treated arteries become clogged again within 6 months. Newer stents are usually medicated to reduce this risk. Nonetheless, some surgeons argue that given this high rate of recurrence, bypass may be a more effective treatment. Today, newer forms of laser angioplasty and *atherectomy*, a procedure that removes plaque, are being done in several clinics.

Aspirin and Other Drug Therapies

Research is ongoing into drugs that may offer some hope for heart attack prevention and reduction of harm from heart attack. Aspirin has been touted for its blood-thinning qualities, although even its proponents recommend that only people of certain ages take it regularly because of its possible side effects. Furthermore, once a patient has taken aspirin regularly for possible protection against CHD, stopping this regimen may, in fact, increase his or her risk.[52]

When a coronary artery is blocked, the heart muscle doesn't die immediately. Time determines how much damage occurs, and prompt action is vital. If a victim reaches an emergency room and is diagnosed fast enough, a form of clot-busting therapy called **thrombolysis** can be performed. Thrombolysis involves injecting an agent such as *tissue plasminogen activator* (*tPA*) to dissolve the clot and restore some blood flow, thereby reducing the amount of tissue that dies from ischemia.[53] These drugs must be administered within 1 to 3 hours after a heart attack for best results.

Cardiac Rehabilitation and Recovery

Every year, more than 1 million Americans survive heart attacks. Over 7 million more have unstable angina, approximately 1.43 million have angioplasty, 448,000 have bypass procedures, 1.2 million have diagnostic angiograms, nearly 100,000 receive implantable defibrillators, and nearly 200,000 have pacemakers implanted to keep their hearts working properly.[54] Many patients leave the hospital with varying degrees of heart failure and fear of future cardiac problems. Although most of these patients are eligible for cardiac rehabilitation (including exercise training and health education classes on good nutrition and CVD risk management) and need only a doctor's prescription for these services, many will not attend these programs. Either they lack insurance, lack transportation, lack facilities close to their home, or face other barriers. Perhaps the biggest deterrent is fear of having another attack due to exercise. The benefits of cardiac rehabilitation (including increased stamina and strength and faster recovery), however, far outweigh the risks when these programs are run by certified health professionals.

People who suspect they have cardiovascular disease are often overwhelmed and frightened. Where should they go for diagnosis? What are the best treatments? Should they stay closer to home for ease of treatment and family assistance, or should they travel to a top-notch facility in another city or state? What are their options? Answering these questions becomes even more difficult if they are upset, scared, or tend to listen unquestioningly to doctors' orders. Usually, it is a son or daughter (particularly those in college and computer savvy) who is called on to be a personal advocate, do the behind-the-scenes research, and help with decision making and follow-up. If you are called on to help, having the information in this

The American Heart Association recommends certain people with increased risk of heart attack or stroke take aspirin daily for its blood-thinning properties.

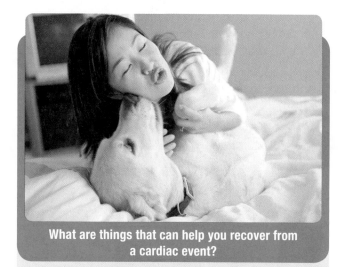

What are things that can help you recover from a cardiac event?

The path to recovery after a heart attack, stroke, or other cardiac problem can be a challenging one, possibly involving medication, physical therapy, and diet modifications. Another important element is stress reduction. Having a pet is one way to focus on something other than your medical condition.

chapter will help. In addition, the information in **Chapter 18** focusing on maneuvering in an increasingly complex health care system will be invaluable.

We still have much to learn about CVD and its causes, treatments, and risk factors. Staying informed is an important part of staying healthy. Good dietary habits, regular exercise, stress management, prompt attention to suspicious symptoms, and other healthy behaviors will greatly enhance your chances of remaining CVD free. Other factors that influence risk include how much emphasis our health care systems place on access to health care for all underserved populations, education about risk, and other community-based interventions. Action on both community and individual levels can help address the challenge of CVD.

What's Your Personal CVD Risk?

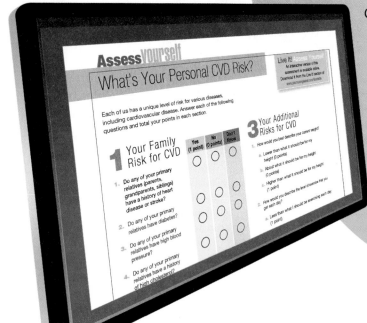

Go online to the **Live It!** section of

www.pearsonhighered.com/donatelle to take the

"What's Your Personal CVD Risk?" assess-

ment.* Use the strategies outlined in the Your

Plan for Change box to change behaviors that

may be putting you at risk.

*If your instructor so chooses, Assess Yourself Activities are
available as a printed supplement or as assignable homework
online at www.pearsonhighered.com/myhealthlab.

MyHealthLab®

YOUR PLAN FOR CHANGE

An **Assess yourself** activity for evaluating your risk of heart disease is found at
www.pearsonhighered.com/donatelle. Based on your results and the advice of your
physician, you may need to take steps to reduce your risk of CVD.

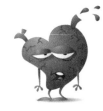

Today, you can:

○ Get up and move! Take a walk in the evening, use the stairs instead of the escalator, or ride your bike to class. Start thinking of ways you can incorporate more physical activity into your daily routine.

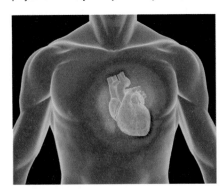

○ Begin improving your dietary habits by eating a healthier dinner. Replace the meat and processed foods you might normally eat with a serving of fresh fruit or soy-based protein and green leafy vegetables. Think about the amounts of saturated and *trans* fats you consume— which foods contain them and how can you reduce consumption of these items.

Within the next 2 weeks, you can:

○ Begin a regular exercise program, even if you start slowly. Set small goals and try to meet them. (See **Chapter 9** for ideas.)

○ Practice a new stress management technique. For example, learn how to

meditate. (See **Chapter 3** for other ideas for managing stress.)

○ Get enough rest. Make sure you get at least 8 hours of sleep per night.

By the end of the semester, you can:

○ Find out your hereditary risk for CVD. Call your parents and find out if your grandparents or aunts or uncles developed CVD. Ask if they know their latest cholesterol LDL/HDL levels. Do you have a family history of diabetes?

○ Have your own cholesterol and blood pressure levels checked. Once you know your levels, you'll have a better sense of what risk factors to address. If your levels are high, talk to your doctor about how to reduce them.

Summary

* The cardiovascular system consists of the heart and circulatory system and is a carefully regulated, integrated network of vessels that supplies the body with the nutrients and oxygen necessary to perform daily functions.
* Cardiovascular diseases include atherosclerosis, coronary artery disease, peripheral artery disease, coronary heart disease, stroke, hypertension, angina pectoris, arrhythmias, congestive heart failure, and congenital and rheumatic heart disease. These combine to make CVD the leading cause of death in the United States today.
* *Cardiometabolic risks* refer to combined factors that increase a person's chances of CVD and diabetes. A person who possesses three or more cardiometabolic risk factors may have metabolic syndrome.
* Many risk factors for cardiovascular disease can be modified, such as cigarette smoking, high blood cholesterol and triglyceride levels, hypertension, lack of exercise, a diet high in saturated fat, obesity, diabetes, and emotional stress. Some risk factors, such as age, gender, and heredity, cannot be modified. Many of these factors have a compounded effect when combined.
* New methods developed for treating heart blockages include coronary bypass surgery and angioplasty with the use of stents. Drug therapies can be used to prevent and treat CVD.

Pop Quiz

1. The heart's upper chambers are called the
   a. valves.
   b. ventricles.
   c. atria.
   d. sinoatrial node.

2. Which of the following is *not* correct about aspirin?
   a. It can cause gastrointestinal tract bleeding, increased surgical risks, and ulcers.
   b. It is recommended for all college students who are overweight.
   c. It has been shown to reduce risks of stroke in older women.
   d. It seems to reduce risks by "thinning" the blood.

3. What does a person's cholesterol level indicate?
   a. The formation of fatty substances, called *plaque,* which can clog the arteries
   b. The level of triglycerides in the blood, which can increase risk of coronary disease
   c. Hypertension, which leads to thickening and hardening of the arteries
   d. None of the above

4. CVD kills more Americans every year than which of the following?
   a. Breast cancer
   b. Respiratory diseases
   c. Lung cancer
   d. All of the above

5. A stroke results
   a. when a heart stops beating.
   b. when cardiopulmonary resuscitation has failed to revive the stopped heart.
   c. when blood flow in the brain has been compromised, either due to blockage or hemorrhage.
   d. when blood pressure rises above 120/80 mm Hg.

6. An irregularity in the heartbeat is called a(n)
   a. fibrillation.
   b. bradycardia.
   c. tachycardia.
   d. arrhythmia.

7. The "bad" type of cholesterol found in the bloodstream is known as
   a. high-density lipoprotein (HDL).
   b. low-density lipoprotein (LDL).
   c. total cholesterol.
   d. triglyceride.

8. Ken's physician informed him that he has hypertension and must work at lowering it to avoid a possible heart attack. Possible strategies include
   a. decreasing sodium.
   b. increasing levels of exercise.
   c. practicing stress management/control.
   d. All of the above

9. Severe chest pain due to reduced oxygen flow to the heart is called
   a. angina pectoris.
   b. arrhythmias.
   c. myocardial infarction.
   d. congestive heart failure.

10. Which of the following is *correct* about metabolic syndrome?
    a. It is decreasing among the general population both in the United States and globally.
    b. It lowers your risk of cardiovascular disease.
    c. High fasting blood glucose, obesity, high triglyceride levels, hypertension, and other risks are part of the symptoms often experienced.
    d. All of the above

Answers to these questions can be found on page A-1.

Think about It!

1. Which risk factors for CVD are modifiable? Which ones are *not*? What are your risks right now for CVD? How are these affected by your family medical history? How might you lower your risks in the next year?
2. List the different types of CVD. Compare and contrast their symptoms, risk factors, prevention, and treatment.
3. Why do you think hypertension rates are rising among today's college students?

4. Discuss the role that exercise, stress management, dietary changes, medical checkups, sodium reduction, and other factors can play in reducing risk for CVD. What role might chronic infections play in CVD risk?

5. Discuss why age is an important factor in women's risk for CVD. Do men face the same age-related risks? Why or why not? What can be done to decrease women's risk in later life?

6. Describe some of the diagnostic, preventive, and treatment alternatives for CVD. Who should be taking a low-dose aspirin each day? Why? If you had a heart attack today, which treatment would you prefer? Explain why.

Accessing Your Health on the Internet

The following websites explore further topics and issues related to personal health. For links to the websites below, visit the Companion Website for *Access to Health*, 13th Edition, at www.pearsonhighered.com/donatelle.

1. *American Heart Association.* This is the home page of the leading private organization dedicated to heart health. This site provides information, statistics, and resources regarding cardiovascular care, including an opportunity to test your risk for CVD. www.heart.org

2. *National Heart, Lung, and Blood Institute.* This valuable resource provides information on all aspects of cardiovascular health and wellness. www.nhlbi.nih.gov

3. *Global Cardiovascular Infobase.* This site contains epidemiological data and statistics for cardiovascular diseases for countries throughout the world, with a focus on developing nations. www.cvdinfobase.ca

References

1. American Heart Association Writing Group, V. Roger, et al., "Heart Disease and Stroke Statistics—2012 Update: A Report from the American Heart Association," *Circulation* 125, no. 1 (2012): e2–220, http://circ.ahajournals.org/content/125/1/e2.full.

2. Ibid.

3. Ibid.

4. Roger VL, Go AS, Lloyd-Jones DM, et al. "Heart Disease and Stroke Statistics—2012 Update: A Report from the American Heart Association," *Circulation.* Epub 2011 Dec 15.

5. Ibid.

6. Ibid.

7. Ibid.

8. Centers for Disease Control and Prevention, "Table 17," *National Vital Statistics Report* 59, no.10 (2011), Available at www.cdc.gov/nchs/data/nvsr/nvsr59/nvsr59_10.pdf.

9. American Heart Association, Roger et al., "Heart Disease and Stroke Statistics—2012 Update," 2012.

10. Ibid.

11. Ibid.

12. World Health Organization, "Cardiovascular Diseases (CVDs)—Key Facts," September 2011, www.who.int/mediacentre/factsheets/fs317/en/index.html.

13. American Heart Association, Roger et al., "Heart Disease and Stroke Statistics—2012 Update," 2012.

14. American Heart Association, "Peripheral Artery Disease: Undertreated and Understudied in Women," 2012, http://newsroom.heart.org/pr/aha/peripheral-artery-disease-undertreated-228645.aspx.

15. Ibid.

16. American Heart Association, Roger et al., "Heart Disease and Stroke Statistics—2012 Update," 2012.

17. Ibid.

18. Ibid.

19. Ibid.

20. Ibid.

21. Centers for Disease Control and Prevention, "High Blood Pressure Facts, 2012," www.cdc.gov/bloodpressure/facts.htm.

22. Ibid; American Heart Association, Roger et al., "Heart Disease and Stroke Statistics—2012 Update," 2012.

23. National Heart, Blood, and Lung Institute, "Angina: What Is Angina?" Revised March 2010, www.nhlbi.nih.gov/health/dci/Diseases/Angina/Angina_WhatIs.html.

24. American Heart Association, Roger et al., "Heart Disease and Stroke Statistics—2012 Update," 2012.

25. Ibid.

26. Ibid.

27. Ibid.; S. Haffner, "Epidemiology of Cardiometabolic Diseases," *Mechanisms and Syndromes of Cardiometabolic Disease: Emerging Science in Atherosclerosis Hypertension and Diabetes*, 2009, Medscape CME, http://cme.medscape.com.

28. S. Grundy, "Pre-Diabetes, Metabolic Syndrome, and Cardiovascular Risk," *Journal of the American College of Cardiology* 59, no. 7 (2012): 635–43; D. Lee, S. Xuemiei, and T. Church et al., "Changes in Fitness and Fatness on the Development of Cardiovascular Risk Factors Hypertension, Metabolic Syndrome, and Hypercholesterolemia," *Journal of the American College of Cardiology* 59, no. 7 (2012): 665–72; T. Horwich and G. Fonarow, "Glucose, Obesity, Metabolic Syndrome, and Diabetes Relevance to Incidence of Heart Failure," *Journal of the American College of Cardiology* 55, no. 4 (2010): 283–93.

29. S. Sharp, D. Aarland, and S. Day et al., "Hypertension Is a Potential Risk Factor for Vascular Dementia: Systematic Review," *International Journal of Geriatric Psychiatry* 26, no. 7 (2011): 661–69; F. Testai, and P. Gorelick, "Vascular Cognitive Impairment and Alzheimer's Disease: Are These Disorders Linked to Hypertension and Other Cardiovascular Risk Factors?" *Clinical Hypertension and Vascular Diseases*, Part 4 (2011): 195–210.

30. American Heart Association, Roger et al., "Heart Disease and Stroke Statistics—2012 Update," 2012.

31. S. Grundy, H. Brewer, J. Cheeman, S. Smith, and C. Lenfant, "Definition of Metabolic Syndrome. Report of the National Heart, Lung, and Blood Institute/American Heart Association Conference on Scientific Issues Related to Definition," *Circulation* 109, no. 2 (2011): 433–39.

32. American Heart Association, Roger et al., "Heart Disease and Stroke Statistics—2012 Update," 2012.

33. Ibid.

34. National Cancer Institute, "Fact Sheet: Harms of Smoking and Benefits of Quitting," January 2011, www.cancer.gov/cancertopics/factsheet/tobacco/cessation.

35. A. Parsons, A. Daley, R. Begh, and P. Aveyard, "Influence of Smoking Cessation After Diagnosis of Early Stage Lung Cancer on Prognosis: Systematic Review of Observational Studies with Meta-analysis," *British Medical Journal* 340 (2010): b5569.

36. American Heart Association, Roger et al., "Heart Disease and Stroke Statistics—2012 Update," 2012

37. Centers for Disease Control and Prevention, "Data Brief #42: Prescription Drug Use Continues to Increase: U.S. Prescription Drug Data for 2007–2008," 2010, www.cdc.gov/nchs/data/databriefs/db42.htm.

38. Mayo Clinic, "Top 5 Lifestyle Changes to Reduce Cholesterol," 2011, www.mayoclinic.com/health/reducecholesterol/CL00012.

39. American Heart Association, Roger et al., "Heart Disease and Stroke Statistics—2012 Update," 2012.

40. Ibid.

41. L. Yan, K. Liu, K. Matthews et al., "Psychological Factors and Risk of Hypertension: The Coronary Artery Risk Development in Young Adults (CARDIA) Study," *Journal of the American Medical Association* 290, no. 16 (2003): 2138–48; C. Vlachopoulous, P. Xaplanteris, and C. Stefanadis, Editorial, "Mental Stress, Arterial Stiffness, Central Pressures and Cardiovascular Risk," *Hypertension* 56, no. 3 (2010): e28–e30.

42. Y. Chida and A. Steptoe, "Response to Mental Stress, Arterial Stiffness, Central Pressures, and Cardiovascular Disease," *Hypertension* 56, no. 3 (2010): e29–e34; G. Lambert et al., "Stress Reactivity and Its Association with Increased Cardiovascular Risk: A Role for the Sympathetic Nervous System," *Hypertension* 55 (2010): e20–e23; A. Flaa, I. Eide, S. Kjeldsen, and M. Rostrup, "Sympathoadrenal Stress Reactivity Is a Predictor of Future Blood Pressure. An 18 Year Follow-Up Study," *Hypertension* 52 (2008): 336–41.

43. American Heart Association, Roger et al., "Heart Disease and Stroke Statistics—2012 Update," 2012.

44. T. Ong and L. Perusse, "Impact of Nutritional Epigenomics on Disease Risk and Prevention: Introduction." *Journal of Nutrigenetics and Nutrigenomics* 4, no. 5 (2011): 245–47; D. Corella et al., "Saturated Fat Intake and Alcohol Consumption Modulate the Association between the *APOE* Polymorphism and Risk of Future Coronary Heart Disease: A Nested Case-Control Study in the Spanish EPIC Cohort," *The Journal of Nutritional Biodiversity* 22, no. 5 (2011): 487–94; A. Angelakopoulou et al. "Comparative Analysis of Genome-wide Association Studies Signals for Lipids, Diabetes, and Coronary Heart Disease: Cardiovascular Biomarker Genetics Collaboration," *European Heart Journal* 33, no. 3 (2012): 393–407; G. Thanassoulis et al., "A Genetic Risk Score Is Associated with Incident Cardiovascular Disease and Coronary Artery Calcium,"

Circulation: Cardiovascular Genetics, no. 5 (2012): 11321; C. Chow et al., "Parental History and Myocardial Infarction Risk Across the World: The Interheart Study," *Journal of the American College of Cardiology* 57 (2011): 619–27.

45. B. Keavney, "C reactive Protein and the Risk for Cardiovascular Disease," *British Medical Journal* 342 (2011): d144; The Emerging Risk Factors Collaboration, "C-reactive Protein Concentration and Risk of Coronary Heart Disease, Stroke, and Mortality: An Individual Participant Meta-analysis," *Lancet* 375, no. 9709 (2010): 132–40.

46. D. Wald, J. Morris, and N. Wald, "Reconciling the Evidence on Serum Homocysteine and Ischemic Heart Disease: A Meta-Analysis," *PLoS ONE* 6, no. 2 (2011): e16473; J. Abraham and L. Cho, "The Homocysteine Hypothesis: Still Relevant to the Prevention and Treatment of Cardiovascular Disease?" *Cleveland Clinic Journal of Medicine* 77, no. 12 (2010): 911–18.

47. B. Hooshmand, et al., "Associations between Serum Homocysteine, Holotranscobalamin, Folate, and Cognition in the Elderly: A Longitudinal Study," *Journal of Internal Medicine* 271, no. 2 (2012): 204–12; R. Clarke, et al., "Effects of Lowering Homocysteine Levels with B Vitamins on Cardiovascular Disease, Cancer, and Cause-Specific Mortality: Meta-Analysis of 8 Randomized Trials Involving 37485 Individuals," *Archives of Internal Medicine* 170, no. 18 (2010): 1622–68; M. Lee, K. Hong, S. Chang, and J. Saver, "Efficacy of Homocysteine-Lowering Therapy with Folic Acid in Stroke Prevention: A Meta-Analysis," *Stroke* 41 (2010): 1205–08.

48. A. H. Ford et al., "Homocysteine, Grey Matter and Cognitive Function in Adults with Cardiovascular Disease," *PLoS ONE* 7, no. 3 (2012): e33345; R. Clarke et al., "Homocysteine and Coronary Heart Disease: Meta-analysis of *MTHFR* Case-Control Studies, Avoiding Publication Bias," *PLoS Med* 9, no. 2 (2012): e1001177.

49. American Heart Association, "Homocysteine, Folic Acid, and Cardiovascular Disease," January 2012, www.heart.org/HEARTORG/GettingHealthy/NutritionCenter/Homocysteine-Folic-Acid-and-Cardiovascular-Disease_UCM_305997_article.jsp.

50. C. A. Garza et al., "The Association between Lipoprotein-Associated Phospholipse A2 and Cardiovascular Disease: A Systematic Review," *Mayo Clinic Proceedings* 82, no. 2 (2007): 159–65.

51. C. Cannon et al., "Current Use of Aspirin and Antithrombotic Agents in the United States among Outpatients with Atherothrombotic Disease (from the REduction of Atherothrombosis for Continued Health [REACH] Registry)," *American Journal of Cardiology* 105, no. 4 (2010): 445–52; G. Biondi-Zoccai et al., "A Systematic Review and Meta-Analysis on the Hazards of Discontinuing or Not Adhering to Aspirin among 50,279 Patients at Risk for Coronary Artery Disease," *European Heart Journal* 27, no. 22 (2006): 2667–74; C. Campbell et al., "Aspirin Dose for the Prevention of Cardiovascular Disease: A Systematic Review," *Journal of the American Medical Association* 297, no. 18 (2007): 2018–24; A. Mathews, "The Danger of Daily Aspirin," *Wall Street Journal,* February 23, 2010, http://online.wsj.com/article/SB10001424052748704511304575075701363436686.html.

52. American Heart Association, "Heart Attack Prevention and Treatment," 2011, http://www.heart.org/HEARTORG/Conditions/HeartAttack/PreventionTreatmentofHeartAttack/Prevention-and-Treatment-of-Heart-Attack_UCM_002042_Article.jsp.

53. American Heart Association, "Heart Disease and Stroke Statistics—2010 Update: A Report from the American Heart Association," *Circulation* 121, no. 7 (2010): e46–e215, Available at http://circ.ahajournals.org/cgi/content/full/121/.7/e46.

FOCUS ON Minimizing Your Risk for Diabetes

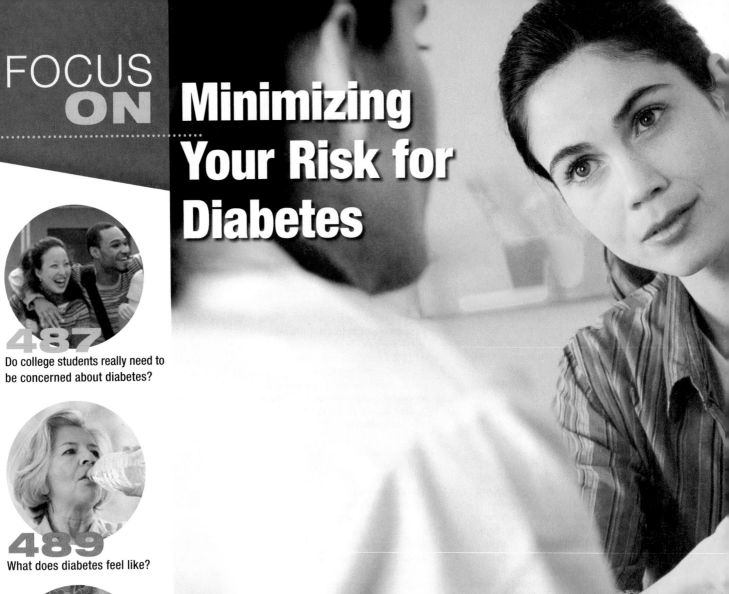

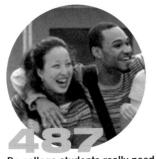

487

Do college students really need to be concerned about diabetes?

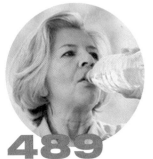

489

What does diabetes feel like?

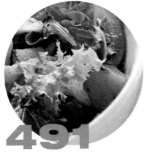

491

Must people with diabetes avoid sweets?

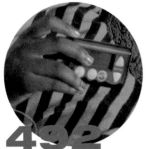

492

Do people with diabetes have to give themselves injections?

Like many college students and American adults, Nora is overweight. She used to figure it was no big deal and that she'd go on a strict diet and exercise program as soon as she graduated with her engineering degree and started to live "a normal life." But last week, her mom called with some bad news. She told Nora that she'd just been diagnosed with type 2 diabetes. Her voice sounded shaky as she told Nora about her own mother's death from kidney failure—a complication of diabetes—at age 52, a few months before Nora was born. When Nora got off the phone, she searched online for information about diabetes. What she

discovered made her feel scared, too: Her Hispanic ethnicity, family history, high stress level and lack of sleep, excessive weight, and sedentary lifestyle all increased her own risk for diabetes.

Nora made an appointment for a diabetes screening. She was instructed to fast the night before and was scheduled for an appointment first thing in the morning. At her visit, the nurse practitioner took a blood sample. A few days later, she called with the news: Nora has pre-diabetes, and needs to make changes to reduce her risk for developing type 2 diabetes like her mom.

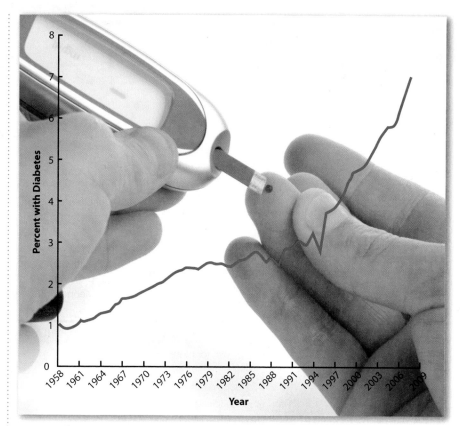

FIGURE 1 Percentage of U.S. Population with Diagnosed Diabetes, 1958–2009.

Source: Data from Centers for Disease Control and Prevention, Division of Diabetes Translation, "National Diabetes Surveillance System," 2010, www.cdc.gov/diabetes/statistics.

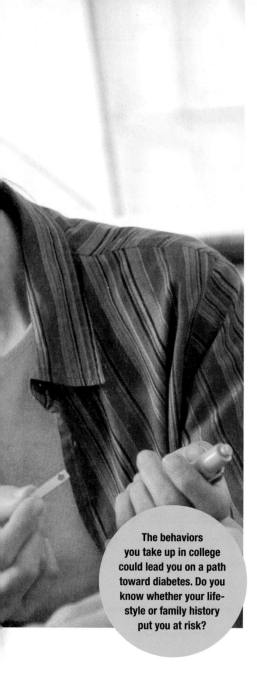

The behaviors you take up in college could lead you on a path toward diabetes. Do you know whether your lifestyle or family history put you at risk?

7.8%

of the U.S. population has some form of diabetes.

Diabetes is one of the fastest growing health threats in the world today, with over 366 million people classified as diabetic in 2011 and estimates of 552 million cases by 2030.[1] While rates of diabetes have increased in all societies where obesity, lack of physical exercise, and smoking rates are high, 80 percent of diabetes deaths occur in lower- and middle-income countries, places where access to prevention and treatment are less than desirable.[2] According to the experts, diabetes has been called the "noninfectious epidemic of our time."[3] The United States isn't immune to epidemic rates of diabetes. In fact, the Centers for Disease Control and Prevention (CDC) estimates that 26 million people—8.3 percent of the U.S. population—have diabetes. Based on rapid increases in rates since the 1950s, estimates are that by 2050, more than 1 in 3 Americans will have diabetes.[4] (See Figure 1.)

Diabetes rates climb with age. While they aren't as high for college-age adults, overall rates have increased, even among the youngest populations. Prevalence among Americans age 20 to 44 is 3.7 percent, and over 215,000 people under the age of 20 have type 1 or type 2 diabetes.[5] Approximately 225,000 people die each year of diabetes-related complications, making diabetes the seventh leading cause of death in the United States today.[6]

Millions have no idea that they are barreling down the road toward diabetes or that there are important actions such as weight loss and increased exercise that they can take now to prevent or delay diabetes onset. By the time they realize it, significant damage may already have occurred.

For an explanation of the financial toll that goes along with the damage to the body with diabetes, read the **Money & Health** box on page 484.

What Is Diabetes?

Diabetes mellitus is a disease characterized by a persistently high level of glucose, a type of sugar, in the blood. One sign of diabetes is the production of an unusually high volume of glucose-laden urine, a fact reflected in

diabetes mellitus A group of diseases characterized by elevated blood glucose levels.

Money&Health

DIABETES: AT WHAT COST?

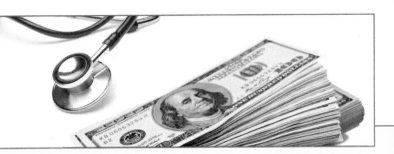

One in every 5 health care dollars is being spent on diabetes care today. Fees for doctor visits, testing supplies, laboratory results, and other necessities are often only partially covered, even for those who have insurance. If you are underinsured or uninsured, the *diabetes drain* on your bank account could be major. Today, nearly 50 million Americans are uninsured and millions more are underinsured.

To give you an idea of what it might cost someone who is diagnosed with type 2 diabetes and who doesn't have insurance, consider these very conservative monthly estimates.

These numbers are consistent with American Diabetes estimates of $350–$900 per month for the typical type 2 diabetic. Insulin-dependent diabetics may have costs that are two to three times higher.

The monthly individual cost of diabetes adds up to the equivalent of a car loan or home mortgage payment. The annual health care costs for an individual with diabetes are approximately $13,000, compared to approximately $2,600 for someone without diabetes.

Diabetic Health Care Need	Estimated Monthly Cost
Doctor visit for monitoring and testing	$200
Lab tests: A1C	$30–$50
Glucose tolerance	$75
Glucose meter test strips	$100
Lancets and lancing devices	$5–$10
Oral medications (metformin)	$13–$15

its name: *Diabetes* derives from a Greek word meaning "to flow through," and *mellitus* is the Latin word for "sweet." The high blood glucose levels—or **hyperglycemia**—seen in diabetes can lead to many serious health problems and even premature death.

Diabetes is actually a group of diseases, each with its own mechanism. Before we describe what goes wrong to cause the different types of diabetes, let's look at how the body regulates blood glucose in a healthy person. The digestive system breaks down the carbohydrates we eat into glucose, which it releases into the bloodstream for use by all body cells. Glucose is one

---

hyperglycemia Elevated blood glucose level.

pancreas Organ that secretes digestive enzymes into the small intestine and hormones, including insulin, into the bloodstream.

insulin Hormone secreted by the pancreas and required by body cells for the uptake and storage of glucose.

---

of the main sources of energy for living organisms. Our red blood cells can only use glucose to fuel functioning, and brain and other nerve cells prefer glucose over other fuels. When glucose levels drop below normal, you may feel unable to concentrate, and certain mental functions may be impaired. Many other cells within the body use glucose to fuel metabolism, movement, and other activities. When there is more glucose available than required to meet your body's immediate needs, the excess glucose is stored as glycogen in the liver and muscles for later use. The average adult has about 5 to 6 grams of glucose in the blood at any given time, enough to provide energy for about 15 minutes under normal activity levels. Once that circulating glucose is used, the body begins to draw upon its glycogen reserves.

Glucose can't simply cross cell membranes on its own. Instead, cells have structures that transport glucose

7 million

people in the U.S. are undiagnosed diabetics.

across in response to a signal that is generated by the **pancreas,** an organ located just beneath the stomach. Whenever a surge of glucose enters the bloodstream, the pancreas secretes a hormone called **insulin.** Insulin stimulates cells to take up glucose from the bloodstream and carry it into the cell, where it's used for immediate energy. Conversion of glucose to glycogen for storage in the liver and muscles is also assisted by insulin. These actions lower the blood level of glucose, and in response, the pancreas stops secreting insulin—until the next influx of glucose arrives.

Type 1 Diabetes Is an Immune Disorder

The more serious and less prevalent form of diabetes, called **type 1 diabetes** (or insulin-dependent diabetes), is an autoimmune disease in which the individual's immune system attacks and destroys the insulin-making cells in the pancreas. Destruction of these cells causes a dramatic reduction, or total cessation, of insulin production. Without insulin, cells cannot take up glucose, and blood glucose levels become permanently elevated. Too much glucose in the bloodstream can wreak havoc with tissue and organs in the body, damaging the kidneys and the nerves in the hands and feet and causing a wide range of other serious health consequences. The higher the blood glucose and the more sustained the high level, the greater the risk.

---

what do you think?

Why do you think type 2 diabetes is increasing in the United States?

● Why is it increasing among young people?

● Do you think young people are generally aware of what diabetes is and their own susceptibility for it?

This form of diabetes used to be called *juvenile diabetes* because it most often appears during childhood or adolescence; however, it can begin at any age. European ancestry, a genetic predisposition, and certain viral infections all increase the risk.[7]

People with type 1 diabetes require daily insulin injections or infusions and must carefully monitor their diet and exercise levels. Often they face unique challenges as the "lesser known" diabetic type, with fewer funds available for research and fewer options for treatment.

Type 2 Diabetes Is a Metabolic Disorder

Type 2 diabetes (non–insulin-dependent diabetes) accounts for 90 to 95 percent of all cases.[8] In type 2, either the pancreas does not make sufficient insulin, or body cells are resistant to its effects and thus don't efficiently use the insulin that is available **(Figure 2)**. This latter condition is generally referred to as **insulin resistance.**

Development of the Disease

Unlike type 1 diabetes, which can appear suddenly, type 2 usually develops slowly. In early stages, cells throughout the body begin to resist the effects of insulin. One culprit known to contribute to insulin resistance is an overabundance of free fatty acids concentrated in

type 1 diabetes Form of diabetes mellitus in which the pancreas is not able to make insulin, and therefore blood glucose cannot enter the cells to be used for energy.

type 2 diabetes Form of diabetes mellitus in which the pancreas does not make enough insulin or the body is unable to use insulin correctly.

insulin resistance State in which body cells fail to respond to the effects of insulin; obesity increases the risk that cells will become insulin resistant.

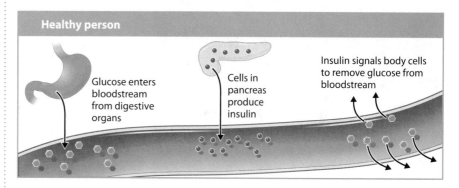

Healthy person

Glucose enters bloodstream from digestive organs

Cells in pancreas produce insulin

Insulin signals body cells to remove glucose from bloodstream

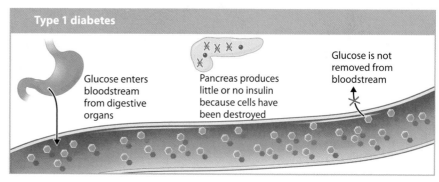

Type 1 diabetes

Glucose enters bloodstream from digestive organs

Pancreas produces little or no insulin because cells have been destroyed

Glucose is not removed from bloodstream

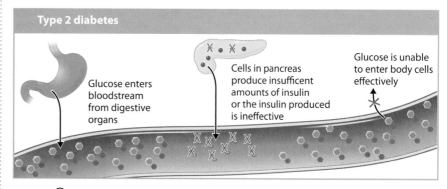

Type 2 diabetes

Glucose enters bloodstream from digestive organs

Cells in pancreas produce insufficent amounts of insulin or the insulin produced is ineffective

Glucose is unable to enter body cells effectively

FIGURE 2 **Diabetes: What It Is and How It Develops**

In a healthy person, a sufficient amount of insulin is produced and released by the pancreas and used efficiently by the cells. In type 1 diabetes, the pancreas makes little or no insulin. In type 2 diabetes, either the pancreas does not make sufficient insulin, or cells are resistant to insulin and are not able to use it efficiently.

Video Tutor: How Diabetes Develops

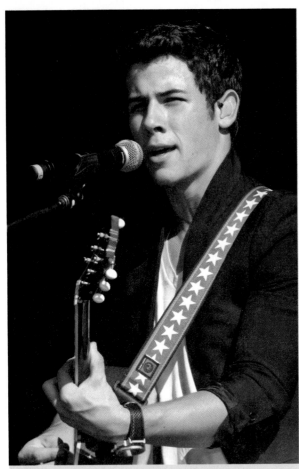

Singer and pop star Nick Jonas is one of the 5 to 10 percent of diabetics diagnosed with type 1.

a person's fat cells (as may be the case in an obese individual). These free fatty acids directly inhibit glucose uptake by body cells. They also suppress the liver's sensitivity to insulin, so its ability to self-regulate its conversion of glucose into glycogen begins to fail. As a consequence of both problems, blood levels of glucose gradually rise. Detecting this elevated blood glucose, the pancreas attempts to compensate by producing more insulin.

The pancreas cannot maintain its hyperproduction of insulin indefinitely. As the progression to type 2 diabetes continues, more and more pancreatic insulin-producing cells sustain physical damage and become nonfunctional. Insulin output declines, and blood glucose levels rise high enough to warrant a diagnosis of type 2 diabetes.

Nonmodifiable Risk Factors

Type 2 diabetes is associated with a cluster of nonmodifiable risk factors, that is, factors over which you have no control. These include increased age, certain ethnicities, genetic factors, and biological factors.

One in 4 adults over age 65 has the disease.[9] In fact, type 2 diabetes used to be referred to as *adult-onset diabetes*; now, however, it is being diagnosed at younger ages, even among children and teens. In the United States, prior to the year 2000, only 1 to 2 percent of patients below age 18 diagnosed with diabetes had type 2. Adolescents who develop type 2 diabetes are typically overweight or obese and have a family history of the disease. Most are Native American, black, Asian, or Hispanic/Latino. In fact, Native Americans and blacks are nearly twice as likely to develop diabetes as non-Hispanic white youth.[10]

Having a close relative with type 2 diabetes is another significant risk factor. In fact, most experts support the theory that type 2 diabetes is caused by the complex interaction between environmental factors, lifestyle, and genetic susceptibility. However, although numerous potential genes have been identified as likely culprits in increased risk, the mechanisms by which they may lead to actual inherited diabetes remains poorly understood.[11]

Modifiable Risk Factors Body weight, dietary choices, and your level of physical activity, as well as sleep patterns and your level of stress, are all diabetes-related factors people have more control over. In both children and adults, type 2 diabetes is linked to overweight and obesity. In adults, a body mass index (BMI) of 25 or greater increases the risk.[12] In particular, excess weight carried around the waistline—a condition called *central adiposity*—and measured by waist circumference is a significant risk factor for older women.[13]

A sedentary lifestyle also increases the risk, not only because inactivity fails to burn calories, but also because activity itself, and buildup of muscle tissue, improves insulin uptake by cells.[14] People with type 2 diabetes who lose weight and increase their physical activity can significantly improve their blood glucose levels.

Several recent studies suggest that sleep contributes to healthy metabolism, including healthy glucose control, while inadequate sleep may contribute to the development of both obesity and type 2 diabetes. There seems to be a link between the body clock hormone *melatonin* and type 2 diabetes. Because the release of insulin, which adjusts blood sugar levels, is regulated by melatonin, body clock disruptions may lead to disruptions in insulin and issues with blood sugar control. People who have genetic defects in receptors for melatonin and have disrupted sleep may increase their risk of type 2 diabetes by six times.[15] Other studies have shown than even pulling an "all nighter" during exams may induce insulin resistance, particularly in young, healthy subjects. For pre-diabetes and those at high risk, sleep deprivation could pose significant risks

"Why Should I Care?"

You may think you are too young to worry about developing diabetes, but the statistics say otherwise. Type 2 diabetes used to be almost nonexistent in young people, but in the past decade, cases of type 2 diabetes in people under the age of 20 have risen to the tens of thousands. Each year, 3,700 people under 20 are diagnosed with type 2 diabetes. Overall, the risk of death among people with diabetes is about twice that of people of similar age but without diabetes.

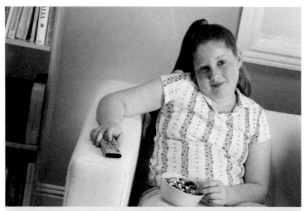

Unhealthy eating habits and a sedentary lifestyle can lead to type 2 diabetes, even among children.

of diabetes development.[16] For example, people who routinely fail to get enough sleep have been shown to be at higher risk for *metabolic syndrome* (discussed shortly), a cluster of risk factors that include poor glucose metabolism.[17]

Recent data from large epidemiological studies provide evidence of a link between diabetes and psychological or physical stress; however, a recent analysis of studies focused on the role of work-related stress on type 2 diabetes development failed to show a strong association between the two.[18] More research is necessary. However a recent study of young adults experiencing significant financial stressors and who had impaired fasting glucose showed that physical activity played a key role in reducing stress and blood sugar levels.[19] Research on the effect of chronic stress and lack of sleep on insulin production and diabetes development is in its infancy. The best rule of thumb appears to be to manage stress and sleep more if you want to reduce your risks.[20]

Pre-Diabetes Can Lead to Type 2 Diabetes

An estimated 79 million Americans age 20 or older have an ominous set of symptoms known as **pre-diabetes,** a condition in which blood glucose levels are higher than normal, but not high enough to be classified as diabetes.

See It! Videos

How will we care for ballooning numbers of diabetes patients? Watch **Will Diabetes Double in 25 Years?** at www.pearsonhighered.com/donatelle.

Having a fasting blood glucose level between 100 and 125 mg/dL is the typical guideline for diagnosing pre-diabetes. An estimated 35 percent of all adults in the United States today would meet this classification.[21] This translates into more than 35 percent of the adult population. Current rates of pre-diabetes in college students are unknown; however, based on increased rates of obesity, sedentary lifestyle, and metabolic risks, it is reasonable to assume that pre-diabetic rates on campus are on the rise.[22]

Although pre-diabetes doesn't cause overt symptoms, the condition is, in a sense, like a ticking time bomb: If it's not "defused," diabetes eventually strikes. On the upside, a diagnosis of pre-diabetes represents a tremendous opportunity to take actions that could prevent diabetes or at least delay its onset.

Often, pre-diabetes is one of the risk factors linked to overweight and obesity that together constitute a dangerous health risk known as *metabolic syndrome.* You would be labeled as having metabolic syndrome if you have three of the following factors:

- Abdominal obesity
- Triglyceride level of 150 milligrams per deciliter of blood (mg/dL) or greater
- HDL cholesterol of less than 40 mg/dL in men or less than 50 mg/ dL in women
- Systolic blood pressure (top number) of 130 millimeters of mercury (mm Hg) or greater
- Diastolic blood pressure (bottom number) of 85 mm Hg or greater

pre-diabetes Condition in which blood glucose levels are higher than normal, but not high enough to be classified as diabetes.

- Fasting glucose of 100 mg/dL or greater
- Insulin resistance or glucose intolerance (the body can't properly use insulin or blood sugar)

In fact, of the six conditions, pre-diabetes and central adiposity appear to be the dominant factors for metabolic syndrome.[23] As we discussed in the chapter on cardiovascular disease, this syndrome dramatically increases an individual's risk for heart disease. In addition, a person who has it is five times more likely to develop type 2 diabetes than is a person without the syndrome.[24]

If you have already been diagnosed with pre-diabetes or type 2 diabetes, you can follow the tips in the **Skills for Behavior Change** box on page 488 to halt or slow the progression of your condition. But what if you've never had your blood glucose tested? Are there steps you could take right now to reduce your risk? Absolutely.

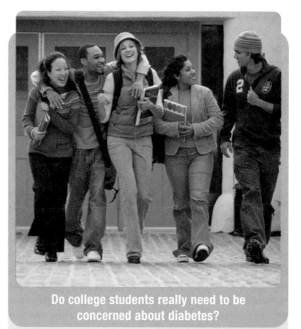

Do college students really need to be concerned about diabetes?

About 215,000 people younger than 20 have type 1 or type 2 diabetes, with thousands more estimated to have pre-diabetes.

Source: Data from Centers for Disease Control and Prevention, "National Diabetes Fact Sheet: National Estimates and General Information on Diabetes and Prediabetes in the United States, 2011" (Atlanta, GA: U.S. Department of Health and Human Services, Centers for Disease Control and Prevention, 2012).

Six Steps to Begin Reducing Your Risk for Diabetes

❱ Maintain a healthy weight. (For tips, see the chapter on achieving and maintaining a sensible weight.)

❱ Eat smaller portions and choose foods with less fat, salt, and added sugars.

❱ Get your body moving. At least 30 minutes of moderate activity 5 days a week is a minimum recommendation.

❱ Quit smoking; in addition to cancer and heart disease, smoking increases blood glucose levels.

❱ Reduce or eliminate alcohol consumption. It's high in calories and can interfere with blood glucose regulation.

❱ Get enough sleep. Inadequate sleep may contribute to the development of type 2 diabetes.

Sources: Adapted from National Diabetes Education Program, *Small Steps, Big Rewards: Your GAME PLAN to Prevent Type 2 Diabetes* (Bethesda, MD: National Institutes of Health, 2006); American Diabetes Association, "Diabetes Basics: Smoking," 2010, www.diabetes.org/diabetes-basics/prevention/checkup-america/smoking.html.

---

gestational diabetes Form of diabetes mellitus in which women who have never had diabetes have high blood sugar (glucose) levels during pregnancy.

The first step is to consider your risk factors. Use the **Assess Yourself** activity on this book's website (see the box at the end of this chapter for the Web address) to find out whether your risk for diabetes is higher than average. If it is, make an appointment to talk with your heath care provider about diabetes screening.

Gestational Diabetes

A third type of diabetes, **gestational diabetes,** is a state of high blood glucose level during pregnancy. It is thought to be associated with metabolic stresses that occur in response to changing hormonal levels. Gestational diabetes occurs in 4 percent of all pregnancies.[25] Studies show that between 50 and 70 percent of gestational diabetics may develop type 2 diabetes within about a decade of their initial diagnosis of gestational diabetes in the absence of risk-reducing behaviors such as weight control, improved diet, and physical exercise.[26]

In addition, women who are overweight and have high blood sugar or those with gestational diabetes have been shown to have increased risks of birth-related complications such as a difficult labor, high blood pressure, high blood acidity, increased infections, and death. One of the adverse outcomes for these women is to give birth to large babies, a result of excess fat accumulation that is often a hallmark sign of gestational diabetes. The large size of these babies increases the risk of injury to the baby during normal delivery and often result in caesarean sections, which increase risks to both mother and infant. If a pregnant woman has higher blood sugar along with excess weight, it can trigger higher insulin levels and blood sugar fluctuations in the newborn. This may increase the risks of obesity and diabetes in childhood. In addition, babies born to women with gestational diabetes have other risks. These include malformations of the heart, nervous system, and bones; respiratory distress; and fetal death.[27]

Results from a small, preliminary investigation of other potential risks to the fetus raise the specter of a new threat. Children raised by mothers with gestational diabetes were shown to have twice the risk of developing attention deficit/hyperactivity disorder (ADHD) by the age of 6 than did their peers, particularly among low-income families.[28] More rigorous research is necessary to confirm this association; however, it does raise the very real possibility of other threats from gestational diabetes.

What Are the Symptoms of Diabetes?

The symptoms of diabetes are similar for both type 1 and type 2. The following are among the most common:

● **Thirst.** The kidneys filter excessive glucose from the blood. When they do, they dilute it with water so that it can be excreted in urine. This pulls too

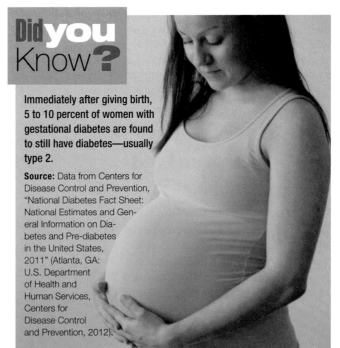

Did you Know?

Immediately after giving birth, 5 to 10 percent of women with gestational diabetes are found to still have diabetes—usually type 2.

Source: Data from Centers for Disease Control and Prevention, "National Diabetes Fact Sheet: National Estimates and General Information on Diabetes and Pre-diabetes in the United States, 2011" (Atlanta, GA: U.S. Department of Health and Human Services, Centers for Disease Control and Prevention, 2012).

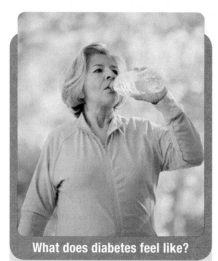

What does diabetes feel like?

People with undiagnosed or uncontrolled diabetes may experience blurred vision, tingling in the hands or feet, and fatigue. One of the most common symptoms is unusual thirst.

much water from the body and leaves the person dehydrated and thirsty.

● **Excessive urination.** For the same reason, diabetics need to urinate much more frequently than usual.

● **Weight loss.** Because so many calories are lost in the glucose that passes into urine, the person with diabetes often feels hungry. Despite eating more, he or she typically loses weight.

● **Fatigue.** When glucose cannot enter cells, fatigue and weakness occur.

● **Nerve damage.** A high glucose concentration damages the smallest blood vessels of the body, including those supplying nerves in the hands and feet. This can cause numbness and tingling.

● **Blurred vision.** Too much glucose causes body tissues to dry out. When this happens to the eye lens, vision deteriorates.

● **Poor wound healing and increased infections.** High levels of glucose can affect the body's ability to ward off infections and may affect overall immune system functioning.

Complications of Diabetes

Poorly controlled diabetes leads to a variety of significant prob-

lems. The main complications include the following:[29]

● **Diabetic coma.** A coma from high blood acidity known as *diabetic ketoacidosis* can occur when, in the absence of glucose, body cells break down stored fat for energy. The process produces acidic molecules called *ketones*. Although essential to provide fuel to the brain in the absence of glucose, ketones released in excessive amounts into the blood raise its acid level dangerously high. The diabetic person slips into a coma and, without medical intervention, will die.

● **Cardiovascular disease.** More than 68 percent of diabetics have hypertension, increasing risk of heart attack and stroke by two to four times. Blood vessels become damaged as the glucose-laden blood flows more sluggishly and essential nutrients and other substances are not transported as effectively.

● **Kidney disease.** The kidneys become scarred by overwork and the high blood pressure in their vessels. Each year, over 48,000 diabetics develop kidney failure, and more than 202,000 are in treatment for this condition.

● **Amputations.** More than 60 percent of nontraumatic amputations of legs, feet, and toes are due to diabetes (see Figure 3a). The problem may begin with a minor infection, but impaired immune response combined with damaged blood vessels enable the

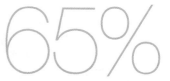

of diabetics die from heart disease or stroke.

infection to spread and resist treatment. Often, the damage to nerves in feet and other areas make it difficult for the diabetic to notice a blister or feel pain in the area. By the time they do, the problem is often difficult to treat. Once infections progress and tissue death is significant, the body part must be amputated.

● **Eye disease and blindness.** Diabetes is the leading cause of new blindness in the United States. Nearly 35 percent of those over the age of 40 have early-stage retinopathy, which could lead to blindness without treatment (Figure 3b).

● **Infectious diseases.** Persons with diabetes have increased risk of poor wound healing and greater susceptibility to infectious diseases, particularly influenza and pneumonia. Once infection occurs, it is more difficult to treat.

● **Other complications.** Diabetics may have gum and tooth disease, foot neuropathy, and chronic pain that makes walking, driving, and simple tasks more difficult. In addition, persons with diabetes are more likely to suffer from depression, making intervention and treatment more difficult. Those

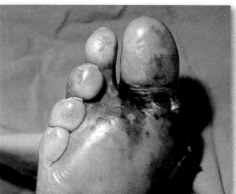

ⓐ Infections in the feet and legs are common in people with diabetes, and healing is impaired; thus, amputations are often necessary.

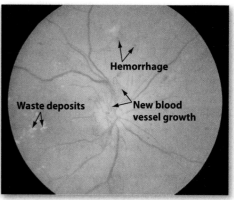

Hemorrhage

Waste deposits

New blood vessel growth

ⓑ Uncontrolled diabetes can damage the eye, causing swelling, leaking, and rupture of blood vessels; growth of new blood vessels; deposits of wastes; and scarring. All of these can progress to blindness.

FIGURE 3 **Complications of Uncontrolled Diabetes: Amputation and Eye Disease**

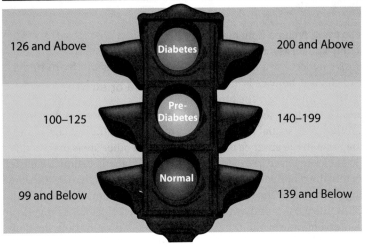

FPG Levels	Diagnosis	OGTT Levels
126 and Above	Diabetes	200 and Above
100–125	Pre-Diabetes	140–199
99 and Below	Normal	139 and Below

FIGURE 4 **Blood Glucose Levels in Pre-Diabetes and Untreated Diabetes**
The fasting plasma glucose (FPG) test measures levels of blood glucose after a person fasts overnight. The oral glucose tolerance test (OGTT) measures levels of blood glucose after a person consumes a concentrated amount of glucose.

Source: Data for FPG and OGTT levels taken from Table 1 (FPG Test) and Table 2 (OGTT) of "Diagnosis of Diabetes," National Diabetes Information Clearinghouse (NDIC), a service of the National Institute of Diabetes and Digestive and Kidney Diseases (NIDDK), National Institutes of Health (NIH), http://diabetes.niddk.nih.gov/dm/pubs/diagnosis/.

who are depressed are 60 percent more likely to develop type 2 diabetes.

Blood Tests Diagnose and Monitor Diabetes

Diabetes and pre-diabetes are diagnosed when a blood test reveals elevated blood glucose levels. Generally, a physician orders either of two blood tests to diagnose pre-diabetes or diabetes:

● The *fasting plasma glucose* (*FPG*) *test* requires the patient to fast for 8 to 10 hours prior to the test. Then, a small sample of blood is tested for glucose concentration. As you can see in Figure 4, an FPG level greater than or equal to 100 mg/dL indicates pre-diabetes, and a level greater than or equal to 126 mg/dL indicates diabetes.
● The *oral glucose tolerance test* (*OGTT*) requires the patient to drink concentrated glucose. A sample of blood is drawn for testing 2 hours after the patient drinks the solution. As

shown in Figure 4, a reading greater than or equal to 140 mg/dL indicates pre-diabetes, whereas a reading greater than or equal to 200 mg/dL indicates diabetes.

Diagnosed diabetics typically have their blood glucose levels monitored by their physicians every 3 to 6 months with the *hemoglobin A1C test*. Previously, A1C results were given to patients using a percentage, but a new method for reporting A1C results is a number called the *estimated average glucose* (eAG). This number indicates the average blood glucose level over the A1C testing period, using the same units (mg/dL) that patients are used to seeing in regular blood glucose tests. This makes it easier for them to understand the importance of their A1C levels. People with diabetes also need to check their blood glucose level several times throughout each day to make sure they stay within their own target range. To check you must prick a finger to obtain a drop of blood and evaluate the sample with a handheld glucose meter.

Treating Diabetes

Treatment options for people with pre-diabetes and type 1 and type 2 diabetes vary according to the type that they have and how far the disease has progressed. Numerous pharmaceutical options are available to treat diabetes. In addition, there are several lifestyle changes that can help lower glucose levels and reduce the risks of diabetes complications.

Lifestyle Changes

For people like Nora (mentioned in the chapter introduction) who have been diagnosed with pre-diabetes, it's important to initiate lifestyle changes immediately to prevent progression of the condition. In fact, studies have shown that people with pre-diabetes can prevent or delay the development of type 2 diabetes by up to 58 percent through changes to their lifestyle that include modest weight loss and regular exercise.[30] Even for people who have already been diagnosed with type 2 diabetes, lifestyle changes can sometimes prevent or delay the need for medication or insulin injections. As discussed here, weight loss, exercise, and a high-quality diet are all parts of the lifestyle formula.

Weight Loss The key to preventing type 2 diabetes in people with pre-diabetes is weight loss. Results of a landmark multicenter clinical trial over a decade ago provided the basis for our current intervention strategies focused on weight loss, exercise, and dietary change or the diabetes drug metformin in preventing or delaying type 2 diabetes. According to the study, known as the *Diabetes Prevention Program (DPP)*, losing huge amounts of weight wasn't necessary in order to have a significant impact on whether or not a person developed diabetes; in

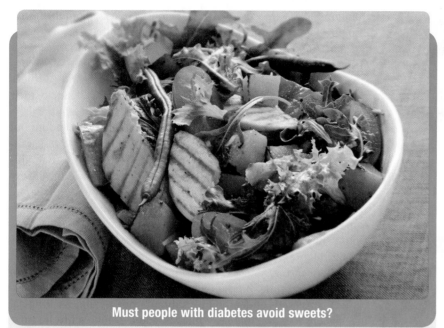

Must people with diabetes avoid sweets?

People with diabetes can occasionally indulge in sweets, but meals low in saturated and *trans* fats and high in fiber, like this salad of salmon and fresh vegetables, are recommended for helping to control blood glucose and body weight.

fact, as little as 5 to 7 percent of current body weight significantly lowered the risk of progressing to diabetes.[31] Today, national recommendations for weight loss often focus on initial weight losses of 5 to 10 percent of total body weight in order to fight diabetes progression.[32]

Adopting a Healthy Diet The DPP recommends people lose weight by adopting a low-fat, reduced-calorie eating plan. In addition, diabetes researchers have studied a variety of specific foods for their effect on blood glucose levels. Here is a brief summary of some intriguing findings:

- **Whole grains.** A recent review of studies over many years suggests that a diet high in whole grains reduces a person's risk of developing type 2 diabetes.[33]
- **High-fiber foods.** Eating foods high in fiber may reduce the risk of diabetes by improving blood sugar levels.[34] High-fiber foods include fruits, vegetables, beans, nuts, and seeds.
- **Fatty fish.** An impressive body of evidence links the consumption of fatty fish such as salmon, which is high in omega-3 fatty acids, with

decreased progression of insulin resistance.[35]

It is also important for people with diabetes to prevent surges in blood sugar after they eat. The glycemic index compares the potential of foods containing the same amount of carbohydrate to raise blood glucose. A food's glycemic load is defined as its glycemic index multiplied by the number of grams of carbohydrate it provides, divided by 100. The concept of glycemic load was developed by scientists to simultaneously describe the quality (glycemic index) and quantity of carbohydrate in a meal.[36] By learning to combine high and low glycemic index foods to avoid surges in blood glucose, diabetics can help control their average blood glucose levels throughout the day. Paying attention to the amount of food consumed is also critical.

Increasing Physical Fitness The DPP recommends 30 minutes of physical activity 5 days a week to reduce your risk of type 2 diabetes.[37] Exercise increases sensitivity to insulin. The more muscle you have and the more you use your muscles, the more

efficiently cells use glucose for fuel, meaning there will be less glucose circulating in the bloodstream. For most people, activity of moderate intensity can help keep blood glucose levels under control.

Oral Medications and Weight Loss Surgery

When lifestyle changes fail to provide adequate control of type 2 diabetes, oral medications may be prescribed. Some medications reduce glucose production by the liver, whereas others slow the absorption of carbohydrates from the small intestine. Other medications increase insulin production by the pancreas, whereas still others work to increase the insulin sensitivity of cells.

Of tremendous interest to the scientific community are recent findings that people who have undergone gastric bypass surgery appear to have high rates of diabetes cure, even before their weight was lost. The American Heart Association recently reversed their position on bariatric surgery, stating that "it can result in long-term weight loss and significant reductions in cardiac and other risk factors for some severely obese adults."[38] Gastric bypass surgeries are not without risks, however, and can include death and serious complications. (See **Chapter 8** for more on gastric bypass surgeries.)

Insulin Injections May Be Necessary

Recall that with type 1 diabetes, the pancreas can no longer produce adequate amounts of insulin. Thus, insulin injections are absolutely essential for those with type 1 diabetes. In addition, people with type 2 diabetes whose blood glucose levels cannot be adequately controlled with other treatment options require insulin injections. Incidentally, insulin cannot be taken in pill form because it's a protein and thus would be digested in the gastrointestinal tract. It must

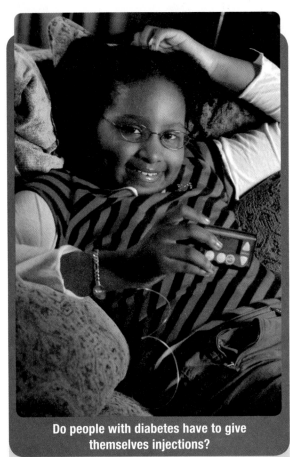

Do people with diabetes have to give themselves injections?

Some type 2 diabetics can control their condition with changes in diet and lifestyle habits or with oral medications. However, some type 2 diabetics and all type 1 diabetics require insulin injections or infusions.

therefore be injected into the fat layer under the skin, from which it is absorbed into the bloodstream.

People with diabetes used to need two or more insulin injections each day. Now, many diabetics use an insulin infusion pump. The external portion is only about the size of an MP3 player and can easily be hidden by clothes. It delivers insulin in minute amounts throughout the day through a thin tube and catheter inserted under the patient's skin. This infusion is more effective than delivering a few larger doses of insulin and obviously is less painful. Insulin inhalers, another form of insulin delivery, although available in the past, were taken off the market due to safety concerns. Ongoing research and advances in the technology may lead to their being available again in the future.

To overcome the limitations of current insulin therapy, researchers are currently working to link glucose monitoring and insulin delivery by developing an artificial pancreas. An artificial pancreas would be a system that would mimic, as closely as possible, the way a healthy pancreas detects changes in blood glucose levels and responds automatically to secrete appropriate amounts of insulin. Although not a cure, an artificial pancreas could significantly improve diabetes care and management and could reduce the burden of monitoring and managing blood glucose.[39]

Are You at Risk for Diabetes?

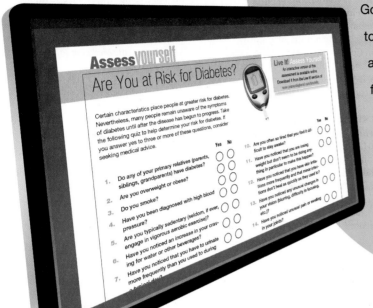

Go online to www.pearsonhighered.com/donatelle to fill out the "Are You at Risk for Diabetes?" assessment.* If you need to make some changes, follow the strategies outlined in the **YOUR PLAN FOR CHANGE** box.

*If your instructor so chooses, Assess Yourself Activities are available as a printed supplement or as assignable homework online at www.pearsonhighered.com/myhealth.

MyHealthLab®

YOUR PLAN FOR CHANGE

If the results of the **Assess yourself** activity, "Are You at Risk for Diabetes?," indicate you need to take further steps to decrease your risks, then follow this plan.

Today, you can:

◯ Call your parents and ask them if there is a history of diabetes mellitus in your family. If there is, ask which type (type 1, 2, or gestational) the family member(s) had.

◯ Take stock of other risk factors you may have for diabetes—do you exercise regularly and watch your weight? Do you eat healthfully? Make a list of small steps you can take in the immediate future to address any of these potential risk factors.

Within the next 2 weeks, you can:

◯ If you are at high risk for diabetes, make an appointment with your health care provider to have your blood glucose levels tested.

◯ If you smoke, begin devising a plan to quit. Look at the suggestions in **Chapter 12** to give you ideas about how to go about this. You may want to consult your doctor about medications or nicotine replacement therapies that could help.

By the end of the semester, you can:

◯ Make the lifestyle changes that will reduce your risk. Pay attention to what you eat; increase your intake of whole grains, fruits, and vegetables; and decrease your consumption of saturated fats, *trans* fats, and sugar.

◯ Make physical activity and exercise part of your daily routine.

References

1. The International Diabetes Federation, *Diabetes Atlas.* 5th ed., 2012, Available at www.idf.org/diabetesatlas/5e/the-global-burden.
2. The World Health Organization, "Diabetes," Fact sheet 312, November 2009, www.who.int/mediacentre/factsheets/fs312/en/index.html.
3. M. Konrad, "Protecting Yourself from the Cost of Type 2 Diabetes," *New York Times Health*, 2010, www.nytimes.com/2010/11/13/health/13patient.html.
4. Centers for Disease Control and Prevention (CDC), "National Diabetes Fact Sheet: National Estimates and General Information on Diabetes and Prediabetes in the United States, 2011" (Atlanta, GA: U.S. Department of Health and Human Services, Centers for Disease Control and Prevention, 2012).
5. Ibid.
6. S. Murphy, J. Xu, and K. Kochanek, "National Vital Statistics Reports—Deaths: Preliminary Data for 2010," *National Center for Health Statistics* 60, no. 4 (2012).
7. American Diabetes Association, "Diabetes Basics: Type 1," 2010, www.diabetes.org/diabetes-basics/type-1.
8. The National Institute of Diabetes and Digestive and Kidney Diseases (NIDDK) National Diabetes Information Clearinghouse (NDIC), "National Diabetes Statistics," 2011, Updated December 11, 2011, http://diabetes.niddk.nih.gov/dm/pubs/statistics/#fast.
9. CDC, "National Diabetes Fact Sheet, 2011," 2012.
10. American Heart Association, Statistical Fact Sheet, 2012, "Diabetes," 2012, www.heart.org/idc/groups/heart-public/@wcm/@sop/@smd/documents/downloadable/ucm_319585.pdf.
11. R. Mihaescu et al., "Genetic Risk Profiling for Prediction of Type 2 Diabetes," *PLoS Currents* 3(2011): DOI: 10.1371/currents.RRN1208, www.ncbi.nlm.nih.gov/pmc/articles/PMC3024707; E. Ntzani, K. Evangelia, and F. Kavvoura, "Genetic Risk Factors for Type 2 Diabetes: Insights from the Emerging Genomic Evidence," *Current Vascular Pharmacology* 10, no. 2 (2012): 147–55.
12. S. Wannamethee et al., "Assessing Prediction of Diabetes in Older Adults Using Different Adiposity Measures: A 7-Year Prospective Study in 6,923 Older Men and Women," *Diabetologia* 53 (2010): 890–98.
13. Ibid.; M. Schulze et al., "Body Adiposity Index, Body Fat Content and Incidence of Type 2 Diabetes," *Diabetologia* (2012), DOI. 10.1007/s00125-012-2499-z.
14. American Diabetes Association, "Top 10 Benefits of Being Active," 2010, www.diabetes.org/food-nutrition-lifestyle/fitness/fitness-management/top-10-benefits-being-active.jsp.
15. A. Bonnefond et al., "Rare MTNRIB Variants Impairing Melatonin Receptor 1B Function Contribute to Type 2 Diabetes," *Nature Genetics* (2012), DOI: 10.1038/ng.1053; E. Donga et al. "A Single Night of Practical Sleep Deprivation Induces Insulin Resistance in Multiple Metabolic Pathways in Healthy Subjects," *Journal of Clinical Endocrinology and Metabolism* 95, no. 6 (2010): 2963–68; F. Cappuccio et al., "Quantity and Quality of Sleep and Incidence of Type 2 Diabetes: A Systematic Review and Meta-Analysis," *Diabetes Care* 33, no. 2 (2010): 414–20; R. Aronsohn et al., "Diabetes, Sleep Apnea, and Glucose Control," *American Journal of Respiratory and Critical Care Medicine* 182, no. 2 (2010): 287–89; R. Hancox and C. Landlus, "Association Between Sleep Duration and Haemoglobin A1c in Young Adults," *Journal of Epidemiology & Community Health,* Published online first, November 7, 2011, DOI: 10.1136/jech-2011-200217.
16. E. Donga et al., "A Single Night of Partial Sleep Deprivation Induces Insulin Resistance," 2010; A. Nedeltcheva, L. Kessler, J. Imperial, and P. Penev, "Exposure to Recurrent Sleep Restriction in the Setting of High Caloric Intake and Physical Inactivity Results in Increased Insulin Resistance and Reduced Glucose Tolerance," *Journal of Clinical Endocrinology and Metabolism* 94, no. 9 (2009): 3242–50; R. Hancox and C. Landlus, "Associations between Sleep Duration and Haemoglobin," 2011.
17. R. Hancox and C. Landlus, "Associations between Sleep Duration and Haemoglobin," 2011; A. Nedeltcheva, "Exposure to Recurrent Sleep Restriction in the Settings of High Caloric Intake and Physical Inactivity Results in Increased Insulin Resistance and Reduce Glucose Tolerance," *Journal of Clinical Endocrinology and Metabolism* 94, no. 9 (2009): 3242–50.
18. M. Cosgrove, L. Sargeant, R. Caleyachetty and S. Griffin, "Work Related Stress and Type 2 Diabetes: A Systematic Review and Meta-Analysis," *Occupational Medicine* (2012) DOI: 10.1093/occmed/kqs002; F. Pouwer et al., "Does Emotional Stress Cause Type 2 Diabetes Mellitus? A Review from the European Depression In Diabetes (EDID) Research Consortium," *Discovery Medicine* 9, no. 45 (2010) 112–18; Y. Fan et al., "Dynamic Changes in Salivary Cortisol and Secretory Immu-

noglobulin a Response to Acute Stress," *Stress and Health* 25, no. 2 (2009): 189–94.
19. E. Puterman, N. Adler, K., Matthews and E. Epel, "Financial Strain and Impaired Fasting Glucose: The Moderating Role of Physical Activity in the Coronary Artery Ris development in Young Adults Study," *Psychosomatic Medicine* 74, no. 2 (2012): 187–92.
20. P. Puustinen et al., "Psychological Distress Predicts the Development of Metabolic Syndrome: A Prospective Population-Based Study," *Psychosomatic Medicine* 73 (2011): 158–65.
21. CDC, "National Diabetes Fact Sheet, 2011," 2012.
22. J. M. Schilter and L. C. Dalleck, "Fitness and Fatness: Indicators of Metabolic Syndrome and Cardiovascular Disease Risk Factors in College Students?" *Journal of Exercise Physiology Online* 13, no. 4 (2010): 29–39.
23. American Heart Association, "Metabolic Syndrome," 2012, www.americanheart.org/presenter.jhtml?identifier=4756.
24. National Heart Lung and Blood Institute, "What Is Metabolic Syndrome?" Revised January 2010, www.nhlbi.nih.gov/health/dci/Diseases/ms/ms_whatis.html.
25. American Diabetes Association, "Diabetes Basics: What Is Gestational Diabetes?" 2012, www.diabetes.org/diabetes-basics/gestational/what-is-gestational-diabetes.html.
26. Ibid.; C. Kim et al., "Gestational Diabetes and the Incidence of Type 2 Diabetes: A Systematic Review," *Diabetes Care* 25, no. 10 (2002): 1862–68.
27. P. M. Catalano et al., "The Hyperglycemia and Adverse Pregnancy Outcome Study: Associations of GDM and Obesity with Pregnancy Outcomes," *Diabetes Care* 35, no. 4 (2012): 780: DOI: 10.2337/dc11-1790.
28. Y. Nomura et al., "Exposure to Gestational Diabetes Mellitus and Low Socioeconomic Status: Effects on Neurocognitive Development and Risk of Attention-Deficit/Hyperactivity Disorder in Offspring," *Archives of Pediatrics and Adolescent Medicine* 166, no. 4 (2012): 337–43.
29. American Diabetes Association, "Diabetes Basics: Pre-Diabetes FAQs," 2010, www.diabetes.org/diabetes-basics/prevention/pre-diabetes/pre-diabetes-faqs.html.
30. Ibid.
31. Diabetes Prevention Program Research Group, "Reduction in the Incidence of Type 2 Diabetes in the Incidence of Type 2 Diabetes with Lifestyle Intervention or Metformin," *New England Journal of Medicine* 345 (2002): 393–403.

32. National Diabetes Education Program, *Small Steps, Big Rewards: Your GAME PLAN to Prevent Type 2 Diabetes* (Bethesda, MD: National Institutes of Health, 2006); W. Knowles et al., "10 Year Follow-Up of Diabetes Incidence and Weight Loss in the DPP Outcomes Study," *Lancet* 374, no. 9702 (2009): 1677–86.

33. S. Jonnalagadda et al., "Putting the Whole Grain Puzzle Together: Health Benefits Associated with Whole Grains— Summary of American Society for Nutrition 2010 Satellite Symposium," *Journal of Nutrition* 41, no. 5 (2011): 10115–25.

34. R. Post et al., "Dietary Fiber for the Treatment of Type 2 Diabetes Mellitus: A Meta Analysis," *Journal of the American Board of Family Medicine* 25, no. 1 (2012): 16–23; J. Tuomilehto., P. Schwarz, and J. Lindstrom, "Long Term Benefits from Lifestyle Intervention for Type 2 Diabetes Prevention," *Diabetes Care*, 34 (2011): 5210S–14S; J. Anderson et al., "Health Benefits of Dietary Fiber," *Nutrition Reviews* 67, no. 4 (2009): 188–205.

35. A. Wallin, D. Giuseppe, N. Orsini, et al. "Fish Consumption, Dietary Long-Chain N-3 Fatty Acids, and the Risk of Type 2 Diabetes: Systematic review and Meta Analysis of Prospective Studies," *Diabetes Care*, 35, no. 4 (2012): 918-929; L. Djousse et al., "Dietary Omega-3 Fatty Acids and Fish Consumption and Risk of Type 2 Diabetes," *American Journal of Clinical Nutrition* 93, no. 1 (2011): 113–50.

36. Linus Pauling Institute, "Glycemic Index and Glycemic Load," Updated April 2010, http://lpi.oregonstate.edu/infocenter/foods/grains/gigl.html.

37. National Institute of Diabetes and Digestive and Kidney Diseases, "Diabetes-Prevention Program," 2008.

38. P. Poirier et al. on Behalf of the American Heart Association Obesity Committee of the Council on Nutrition, Physical Activity, and Metabolism, "Bariatric Surgery and Cardiovascular Risk Factors: A Scientific Statement from the American Heart Association," *Circulation,* March (2011): DOI:10.1161/CIR.0b013e3182149099.

39. National Diabetes Information Clearinghouse, National Institute of Diabetes and Digestive and Kidney Diseases, "Alternative Devices for Taking Insulin," NIH Publication no. 09–4643, May 2009, Available at http://diabetes.niddk.nih.gov/dm/pubs/insulin/index.htm.

Reducing Your Cancer Risk

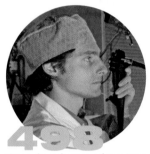

498

What does it mean for a tumor to be malignant?

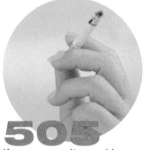

503

Are there chemicals in our food that may be linked to cancer?

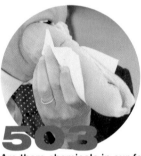

505

If my mom quits smoking now, will it reduce her risk of lung cancer or is it too late?

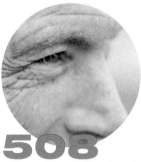

508

Is there any safe way to get a tan?

OBJECTIVES

✳ Understand what cancer is, how it develops, and its causes.

✳ Discuss ways to prevent cancer and the implications of behavioral risks.

✳ Describe the different types of cancer and the risks they pose to people at different ages and stages of life.

✳ Explain the importance of early detection, self-exams, and medical exams, and understand the symptoms related to different types of cancer.

✳ Discuss cancer diagnosis and treatment, including radiotherapy and chemotherapy and other common methods of detection and treatment.

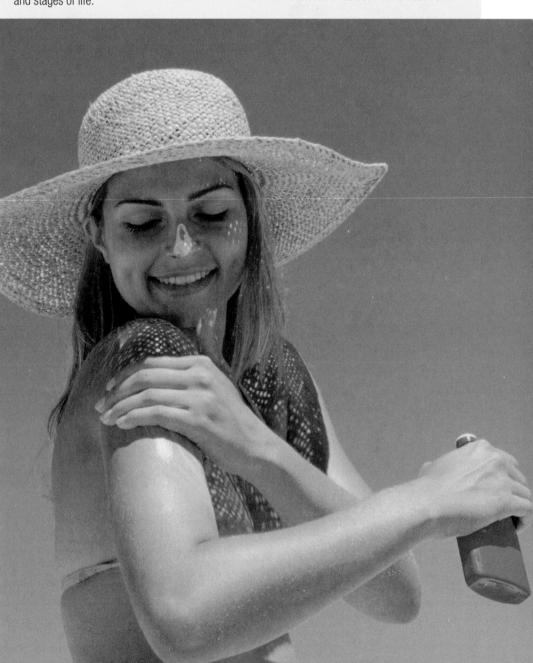

As recently as 50 years ago, a cancer diagnosis was typically a death sentence. Health professionals could only guess at the cause, and treatments were often as deadly as the disease itself. Because we didn't understand the disease process, fears about "catching cancer" from those who had it led to ostracism and bigotry—much like people with HIV were treated in the early days of the AIDS epidemic. Fortunately, we've come a long way in our understanding of cancer, our willingness to talk about the disease openly, and our ability to treat cancer successfully.

Knowledge of risks and symptoms, early detection, and significant developments in technology and treatment have dramatically improved the prognosis for most cancer patients, particularly those who are diagnosed in the earliest stages of disease. We have also learned that there are many actions we can take individually and as a society to prevent cancer. Understanding the facts about cancer, recognizing your own risk, and taking action to reduce your risk are important steps in the battle.

An Overview of Cancer

Cancer is the second most common cause of death in the United States, exceeded only by heart disease.[1] Although there were over 1.6 million *new* cancer diagnoses and over 577,000 deaths in 2012, the good news is that death rates have been declining by over 2 percent per year in the last decades. Increased emphasis on education and awareness, greater emphasis on prevention and early intervention, advancements in diagnosis and treatment, and policies and programs designed to decrease environmental risks are among key factors that have contributed to declining rates and increasing survival rates.[2]

The **5-year survival rates** (the relative rates for survival in persons who are living 5 years after diagnosis) have increased greatly from the 50 percent survival rates of past generations (**Figure 16.1**). Today, about 67 percent of people diagnosed with cancer each year will be alive 5 years after their diagnosis.[3] Survival rates for people with many cancers caught in their earliest stages approach 100 percent. Of those treated for cancer, many will be considered "cured," meaning that they have no new cancer in their bodies 5 years after their original diagnosis and can expect to live a long and productive life. Among the most amazing improvements in outlook are acute lymphocytic leukemia,

Hodgkin's disease, Burkitt's lymphoma, Ewing's sarcoma (a form of bone cancer), Wilms' tumor (a kidney cancer in children), testicular cancer, and osteogenic (bone) sarcoma.

Although treatments and survival statistics have improved, nearly half of all American males and one third of American females will still develop cancer at some point in their life.[4] What factors increase our risk and which are preventable? In the following sections, we provide an overview of factors that increase risk of cancer and discuss ways to reduce those risks.

5-year survival rates The percentage of people in a study or treatment group who are alive 5 years after they were diagnosed with or treated for a disease such as cancer.

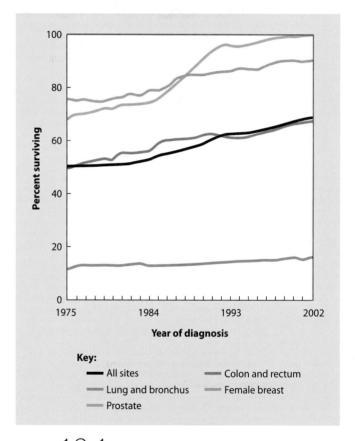

FIGURE 16.1 **Trends in 5-Year Survival Cancer Rates by Site** Since the 1970s, survival rates have increased steadily for nearly all types of cancer. The exception to this trend has been lung cancer survivorship. Its survival rates remain both relatively steady and low, mostly likely due to the late stage at which most lung cancer cases are detected.

Source: Data from SEER program, National Cancer Institute, *Cancer Trends Progress Report–2009/2010 Update*, Available at http://progressreport.cancer.gov/; Incidence data are from all nine SEER areas, http://seer.cancer.gov/registries/terms.html. Data are not age-adjusted. See also http://progressreport.cancer.gov/doc_detail.asp?pid=1&did=2009&chid=95&coid=927&mid=#estimate.

25%

of all deaths that occur on a given day are from some form of cancer.

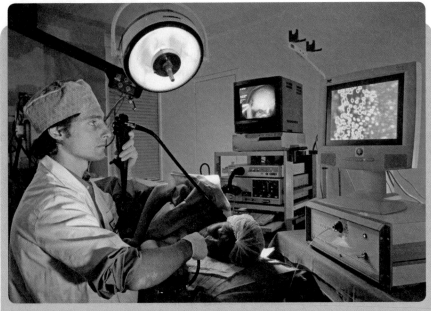

What does it mean for a tumor to be malignant?

A malignant tumor is one whose cells are cancerous. Malignant tumors are generally more dangerous than benign tumors because cancer cells divide quickly and can spread, or metastasize, from the original tumor to other parts of the body. Physicians usually order biopsies of tumors, in which sample cells are taken from the tumor and studied under a microscope to determine whether they are cancerous. Newer techniques, such as the minimally invasive "optical biopsy" shown here, allow microscopic examination of tissue without doing a physical biopsy.

What Is Cancer?

Cancer is the general term for a large group of diseases characterized by the uncontrolled growth and spread of abnormal cells. Unchecked, cancer cells impair vital functions of the body and lead to death. When something interrupts normal cell programming, uncontrolled growth and abnormal cellular development result in a **neoplasm,** a new growth of tissue serving no physiological function. This neoplasmic mass often forms a clump of cells known as a **tumor.**

Not all tumors are **malignant** (cancerous). In fact, most are **benign** (noncancerous). Benign tumors are generally harmless unless they grow to obstruct or crowd out normal tissues. A benign tumor of the brain, for instance, becomes life threatening when it grows enough to restrict blood flow and cause a stroke. The only way to determine whether a tumor is malignant is through

cancer A large group of diseases characterized by the uncontrolled growth and spread of abnormal cells.

neoplasm A new growth of tissue that serves no physiological function and results from uncontrolled, abnormal cellular development.

tumor A neoplasmic mass that grows more rapidly than surrounding tissue.

malignant Very dangerous or harmful; refers to a cancerous tumor.

benign Harmless; refers to a noncancerous tumor.

biopsy Removal and examination of a tissue sample to determine if a cancer is present.

metastasis Process by which cancer spreads from one area to different areas of the body.

mutant cells Cells that differ in form, quality, or function from normal cells.

cancer staging A classification system that describes how far a person's disease has advanced.

biopsy, the removal and microscopic examination of a sample of cells.

Benign tumors generally consist of ordinary-looking cells enclosed in a fibrous shell or capsule that prevents their spreading to other body areas. Malignant tumors are usually not enclosed in a protective capsule and can therefore spread to other organs (Figure 16.2 on page 499). This process, known as **metastasis,** makes some forms of cancer particularly aggressive in their ability to overwhelm bodily defenses. By the time they are diagnosed, malignant tumors have frequently metastasized throughout the body, making treatment extremely difficult. Unlike benign tumors, which merely expand to take over a given space, malignant cells invade surrounding tissue, emitting clawlike protrusions that disturb the RNA and DNA within normal cells. Disrupting these substances, which control cellular metabolism and reproduction, produces **mutant cells** that differ in form, quality, and function from normal cells.

Cancer staging is a classification system that describes how far a person's disease has advanced. Usually, either through surgery or clinical or pathological analysis, it is possible to determine the size of the tumor and how deeply it has penetrated, the number of lymph nodes that are affected, and the degree of metastasis or spread, known as the *TNM* (for tumor, node, and metastasis) system, of the disease. Cancers are staged based on these variables. The most commonly known staging system assigns the numbers zero to four to the disease (see Table 16.1). Staging is important because it helps doctors and patients decide on appropriate treatments and estimate a person's life expectancy.[5]

TABLE 16.1 Cancer Stages

Stage	Definition
0	Early cancer, when abnormal cells remain only in the place they originated.
I	Higher numbers indicate more extensive disease: Larger tumor size and/or spread of the cancer beyond the organ in which it first developed to nearby lymph nodes and/or organs adjacent to the location of the primary tumor.
II	
III	
IV	Cancer has spread to other organs

Source: National Cancer Institute, National Institutes of Health, "Fact Sheet, Cancer Staging," 2010, www.cancer.gov/cancertopics/factsheet/detection/staging.

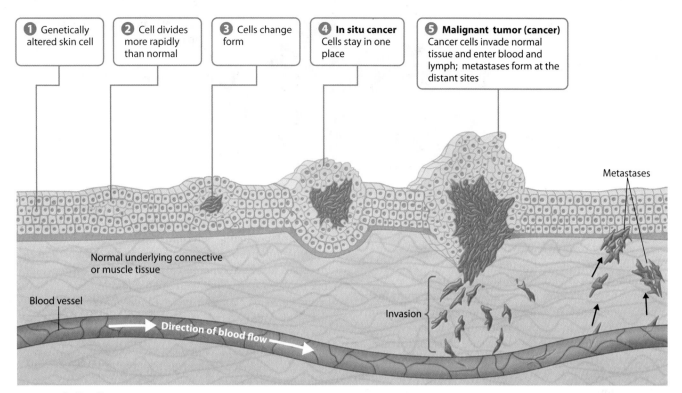

Legend boxes:

1 Genetically altered skin cell

2 Cell divides more rapidly than normal

3 Cells change form

4 **In situ cancer** Cells stay in one place

5 **Malignant tumor (cancer)** Cancer cells invade normal tissue and enter blood and lymph; metastases form at the distant sites

Metastases

Normal underlying connective or muscle tissue

Blood vessel

Direction of blood flow

Invasion

FIGURE 16.2 **Metastasis**
A mutation to the genetic material of a skin cell triggers abnormal cell division and changes cell formation, resulting in a cancerous tumor. If the tumor remains localized, it is considered in situ cancer. If the tumor spreads, it is considered a malignant cancer.

Video Tutor: Metastasis

What Causes Cancer?

Causes are generally divided into two categories of risk factors: *hereditary* and *acquired* (environmental). Heredity factors cannot be changed, but environmental factors are potentially modifiable. Environmental factors include the physical environment and personal lifestyle habits and conditions such as tobacco use; quality of nutrition; physical inactivity; obesity; certain infectious agents; certain medical treatments; drug and alcohol consumption; excessive sun exposure; and exposure to **carcinogens** (cancer-causing agents), such as pollutants in the food, water, and air. Hereditary and environmental factors may interact to make cancer more likely, accelerate cancer progression, or increase susceptibility during certain periods of life. The mechanisms underlying cancer development are not fully understood. Two people with seemingly identical risk factors may end up with very different experiences when it comes to developing cancer, and at present, why that is remains a mystery.

Lifestyle Risks for Cancer

Cancer occurs in all age groups, but the older you get, the greater your risk. Nearly 77 percent of all cancers are diagnosed in adults over age 55.[6] Cancer researchers refer to one's cancer risk when they assess risk factors. *Lifetime risk* refers to the probability that an individual, over the course of a lifetime, will develop cancer. In the United States, men have a lifetime risk of about 1 in 2; women have a lower risk, at 1 in 3.[7] Risks also vary by race, socioeconomic status, occupation, geographic location, and several other factors.

Relative risk is a measure of the strength of the relationship between risk factors and a particular cancer. Basically, it compares your risk of cancer if you engage in certain known risk behaviors with that of someone who does not engage in such behaviors. For example, if you are a man and smoke, your relative risk of getting lung cancer is about twice that of a male nonsmoker.[8]

carcinogens Cancer-causing agents.

Over the years, researchers have found that diet, a sedentary lifestyle (and resultant obesity), overconsumption of alcohol, tobacco use, stress, and other lifestyle factors play a key role in the incidence (number of new cases) of cancer. Keep in mind that a high relative risk does not guarantee cause and effect. It merely indicates the likelihood of a particular risk factor being related to a particular outcome.

Tobacco Use Of all the risk factors for cancer, smoking is among the greatest. In the United States, tobacco is responsible for nearly 1 in 5 deaths, or about 443,000 premature deaths each year. In addition, nearly 9 million more people suffer from smoking-related diseases, such as chronic bronchitis, emphysema, and cardiovascular disease (CVD).[9] Smoking remains the major cause of preventable death worldwide and accounts for at least 30 percent of all cancer deaths and 80 percent of all lung cancer deaths in the United States alone.[10] Smoking is associated with increased risk of at least 15 different cancers, including nasopharynx, nasal cavity, paranasal sinuses, lip, oral cavity, pharynx, larynx, lung, esophagus, pancreas, uterine cervix, ovary, kidney, bladder, stomach, colorectal, and acute myeloid leukemia. Chances of developing cancer are 23 times higher among male smokers and 13 times higher among female smokers, compared to nonsmokers. Coincidence? Not likely. In fact, new research has implicated smoking in the development of breast cancer and gastric ulcers as well as a host of additional respiratory problems.[11] In the past 20 years, British and U.S. lung cancer rates have declined. However, lung cancer rates among men are still increasing in most developing countries and in eastern Europe, where smoking rates remain high and are still increasing in some areas.[12]

Of the several lifestyle risk factors for cancer, tobacco use is the most significant—and the most preventable.

Alcohol and Cancer Risk Over the past decade, countless studies have implicated alcohol as a risk factor for cancer. The cumulative amount of alcohol a woman consumes during adulthood is the best predictor of her breast cancer risk. Even low levels of alcohol consumption (as few as three drinks a week) are associated with increased risk of breast cancer, and binge drinkers significantly increase their risk.[13] Moderate alcohol intake (above one drink per day) in women also appears to increase the risk of cancers of the oral cavity and pharynx, esophagus, and larynx, and binge drinking may increase gastric and pancreatic cancer risk as well. Similar to breast cancer, the more women drink, the greater their risk of all these types of cancers, along with likely increased risk of gastric cancer and pancreatic cancer in binge drinkers.[14]

The risk is also increased for men who drink. In a Canadian study of over 3,500 men aged 35 to 70, regular heavy consumption of alcohol increased the risk of esophageal and liver cancers more than sevenfold. The risk of colon, stomach, and prostate cancers was about 80 percent higher among heavy drinkers, while lung cancer risk rose by almost 60 percent compared to nondrinkers.[15]

Poor Nutrition, Physical Inactivity, and Obesity

Mounting evidence suggests that about one third of cancer deaths in the United States each year may be due to lifestyle factors such as overweight or obesity, physical inactivity, and poor nutrition.[16] Aside from choosing not to use tobacco, dietary choices and physical activity are the most important modifiable determinants of cancer risk. Cancer is more common among people who are overweight, and risk increases as obesity increases. There is clear evidence of a link between overweight and obesity and increased risks of breast cancer; colon and rectal cancer; and esophageal, kidney, and pancreatic cancers.[17] Women who gain 55 pounds or more after age 18 have almost a 50 percent greater risk of breast cancer compared to those who maintain their weight.[18]

Body mass index (BMI) plays a role in male cancer as well. The relative risk of colon cancer in men is 40 percent higher for obese men than it is for nonobese men. The relative risk of gallbladder cancer is five times higher in obese individuals than in individuals of healthy weight. Numerous other studies support the link between various forms of cancer and obesity.[19]

"Why Should I Care?"

Lifestyle, tobacco use, nutrition, and activity are things you control, and areas where you can start good habits now to reduce your chances of developing cancer.

Stress and Psychosocial Risks Stress has been implicated in increased susceptibility to several types of cancers. Although medical personnel are skeptical of overly simplistic solutions, we cannot rule out the possibility that negative emotional states contribute to illness. People who are under chronic, severe stress or who suffer from depression or other persistent emotional problems show higher rates of cancer than their healthy counterparts. Several newer studies appear to support the premise that stress can play a role in cancer development.[20] Sleep disturbances, unhealthy diet, and emotional or physical trauma may weaken the body's immune system, increasing susceptibility to cancer.

Other possible contributors to cancer are poverty and the health disparities associated with low socioeconomic status. To reduce your risks of cancer, see the **Skills for Behavior Change** box.

what do you think?

How should we determine whether a behavior or substance is a risk factor for a disease and whether programs should be enacted to reduce the risk or stop a behavior?

● Do you think that a clear, undeniable causal link must be shown between smoking and lung cancer before smoking bans should be enacted in all 50 states?

Genetic and Physiological Risks

If one of your close family members develops cancer, does it mean that you have a genetic predisposition for it? Scientists believe that about 5 percent of all cancers are strongly hereditary. It seems that some people may be more predisposed to the malfunctioning of genes that ultimately cause cancer.[21]

Suspected cancer-causing genes are called **oncogenes.** Although these genes are typically dormant, certain conditions such as age; stress; and exposure to carcinogens, viruses, and radiation may activate them. Once activated, oncogenes cause cells to grow and reproduce uncontrollably. Scientists are uncertain whether only people who develop cancer have oncogenes, or whether we all have genes that can become oncogenes under certain conditions.

Certain cancers, particularly those of the breast, stomach, colon, prostate, uterus, ovaries, and lungs, appear to run in families. For example, a woman runs a much higher risk of breast cancer if her mother or sisters have had the disease, particularly at a young age. Hodgkin's disease and certain leukemias show similar familial patterns. Can we attribute these familial patterns to genetic susceptibility or to the fact that people in the same families experience similar environmental risks? To date, the research in this area is inconclusive.

Some forms of cancer have strong genetic bases; daughters of women with breast cancer have an increased risk of the disease.

It is possible that we can inherit a tendency toward a cancer-prone, weak immune system, or conversely, that we can inherit a cancer-fighting potential. But the complex interaction of heredity, lifestyle, and environment on the development of cancer makes it a challenge to determine a single cause. Even among those predisposed to mutations, avoiding risks may decrease chances of cancer development.

oncogenes Suspected cancer-causing genes present on chromosomes.

Reproductive and Hormonal Factors The effects of reproductive factors on breast and cervical cancers have been well documented. Increased numbers of fertile or menstrual cycle years (early menarche, late menopause), not having children or having them later in life, recent use of birth control pills or hormone replacement therapy, and opting not to breast-feed, all appear to increase risks of breast cancer.[22] However, while the above factors appear to play a significant role in increased risk for non-Hispanic white women, they do not appear to have as strong an influence on Hispanic women.[23] Studies also suggest that women on hormone supplements or hormone replacement therapy have a slightly increased risk of lung cancer.[24]

Occupational and Environmental Risks

Overall, workplace hazards account for only a small percentage of all cancers. However, various substances are known to cause cancer when exposure levels are high or prolonged. One is asbestos, a fibrous material once widely used in the construction, insulation, and automobile industries. Nickel; chromate; and chemicals such as benzene, arsenic, and vinyl chloride have been shown definitively to be carcinogens. Also, people who routinely work with certain dyes and radioactive substances may have increased risks for cancer. Working with coal tars, as in the mining profession, or with inhalants, as in the auto-painting business, is hazardous. So is working with herbicides and pesticides, although the evidence is inconclusive for low-dose exposures. Several federal and state agencies are responsible for monitoring such exposures and ensuring that businesses comply with standards designed to protect workers.

You don't have to work in one of these industries to come in contact with environmental carcinogens. See the **Be Healthy, Be Green** box on the following page to explore some ways you can avoid carcinogens in the products you buy and use every day.

Radiation Ionizing radiation (IR)—radiation from X rays, radon, cosmic rays, and ultraviolet radiation (primarily UVB radiation)—is the only form of radiation proven to cause human cancer. Evidence that high-dose IR causes cancer comes from studies of atomic bomb survivors, patients receiving radiotherapy, and

BE HEALTHY, BE GREEN

GO GREEN AGAINST CANCER

There are many things you can do to help reduce the number of carcinogens in the environment and limit your exposure to them. Here are just a few ideas:

1. Leave the car at home. Commute by bicycle or on foot instead of driving. This will reduce your carbon footprint and your risk for cancer by increasing your physical activity.

2. Eat less processed, packaged food and more whole fruits and vegetables. Avoid consuming chemicals and pesticides that may elevate our risk for cancer.

Don't risk your health for beauty! Read the labels on your cosmetics and avoid products containing potentially carcinogenic chemicals such as phthalates and parabens.

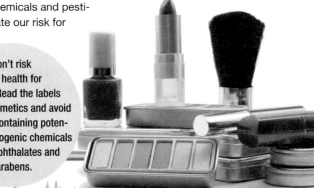

3. Shop for flooring and other furnishings made from bamboo, cork, reclaimed wood, recycled glass, and metal tiles. This ensures the best possible indoor air quality and minimizes carcinogenic exposure.

4. Use paper products that are bleach free, whose production reduces the amount of carcinogenic dioxins released into the atmosphere.

5. Many hygiene products contain petroleum and plastics, agents that are not good for your skin or the environment. Avoid products containing the following confirmed or suspected carcinogens:

✳ Diethanolamine (DEA), commonly found in shampoos
✳ Formaldehyde, commonly found in eye shadows
✳ Phthalates, found in many nail polishes and perfumes
✳ Parabens, used as preservatives in food and makeup, lotion, shampoo, and soap

6. Avoid dry cleaning. Conventional dry cleaning uses a chemical called *perchloroethylene (PERC)*, an agent known to increase the risk for cancer and harm the environment. If dry cleaning is unavoidable, explore local dry cleaners using eco-friendly alternatives such as "wet cleaning," which includes biodegradable soaps or silicone-based solvents and special machinery used to reduce shrinkage.

---

certain occupational groups, such as uranium miners. Virtually any part of the body can be affected by IR, but bone marrow and the thyroid are particularly susceptible. Radon exposure in homes can increase lung cancer risk, especially in cigarette smokers. To reduce the risk of harmful effects, diagnostic medical and dental X rays are set at the lowest dose levels possible.

Nonionizing radiation produced by radio waves, cell phones, microwaves, computer screens, televisions, electric blankets, and other products has been a topic of great concern in recent years, but research has not proven excess risk to date. Although highly controversial, some suggest that cell phones beam radio frequency energy that can penetrate the brain, particularly in small children, raising concerns about cancers of the head and neck, brain tumors, or leukemia. Although a wide range of studies has been conducted, and although brain cancer deaths are on the rise among younger adults, these studies have not shown a consistent link between cell phone use and cancers of the brain, nerves, or other tissues of the head or neck. More research is needed because cell phone technology and how people use cell phones have been changing rapidly.[25] (See **Chapter 20** for more on the potential hazards of both ionizing and nonionizing radiation.)

Chemicals in Foods Much of the concern about chemicals in food centers on the possible harm caused by pesticide and herbicide residues. Whereas some of these chemicals cause cancer at high doses in experimental animals, the government considers the very low concentrations found in some foods to be safe. Continued research regarding pesticide and herbicide use is essential, and scientists and consumer groups stress the importance of a balance between chemical use and the production of high-quality food products.

Infectious Diseases and Cancer Risks

According to experts, over 10 percent of all cancers in the United States are caused by infectious agents such as viruses, bacteria, or parasites.[26] Worldwide, approximately 20 percent of human cancers have been traced to infectious agents, primarily viruses.[27] Infections are thought to influence cancer development in several ways, most commonly through chronic inflammation, suppression of the immune system, or chronic stimulation. Some of the pathogens that are linked to cancers are discussed on the following page.

Hepatitis B, Hepatitis C, and Liver Cancer Viruses that cause chronic forms of hepatitis B (HBV) and C (HCV) are believed to stimulate growth of cancer cells in the liver because they chronically inflame liver tissue This may prime the liver for cancer or make it more hospitable for cancer development. Global increases in hepatitis B and C rates and concurrent rises in liver cancer rates seem to provide evidence of such an association. Vaccines that prevent hepatitis B may reduce the risk of liver damage as well as cancer.

Human Papillomavirus and Cervical Cancer Nearly 100 percent of women with cervical cancer have evidence of human papillomavirus (HPV) infection, which is believed to be a major cause of cervical cancer. Fortunately, only a small percentage of HPV cases progresses to cervical cancer.[28] Today, a vaccine is available to help protect people from becoming infected with HPV. (For more information on this controversial vaccine, see the discussion of HPV in **Chapter 14.**)

Helicobacter pylori and Stomach Cancer *Helicobacter pylori* is a potent bacterium found in the stomach lining of approximately 30 to 40 percent of Americans. It causes inflammation, scarring, and ulcers, damaging the lining of the stomach and leading to cellular changes that may lead to cancer. More than half of all cases of stomach cancer are thought to be linked to *H. pylori* infection, even though most infected people don't develop cancer.[29] Treatment with antibiotics often cures the ulcers, which appears to reduce risk of new stomach cancer.[30]

Medical Factors

Some medical treatments can increase a person's risk for cancer. One example is the use of estrogen and progesterone for relieving women's menopausal symptoms. Estrogen use is now recognized to contribute to multiple cancer risks and provides fewer benefits than originally believed. Prescriptions for estrogen therapy have declined dramatically, and many women

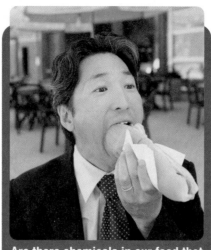

Are there chemicals in our food that may be linked to cancer?

Food additives, particularly sodium nitrate, are used to preserve and give color to red meat and protect against pathogens, particularly *Clostridium botulinum*, the bacterium that causes botulism. Concern about the carcinogenic properties of nitrates, which are often used in hot dogs, hams, and luncheon meats, has led to the introduction of meats that are nitrate-free or contain reduced levels of the substance.

What's Working for You?

You may already be taking actions to lessen your cancer risk. Which of the following are true for you?

☐ I don't smoke or I have committed to quitting and joined a group to do this.

☐ I apply sunscreen before I leave the house every day.

☐ I am aware of what "normal" looks like for my breasts or testicles and watch for any changes that may signal a problem.

are trying to reduce or eliminate their use of the hormone.

Ironically, medicines used to treat cancers, such as selected chemotherapy drugs, have been shown to increase risks for other cancers. Weighing the benefits versus harms of these treatments is always necessary.

Types of Cancers

As mentioned earlier, *cancer* refers not to a single disease, but to hundreds of different diseases. They are grouped into four broad categories based on the type of tissue from which the cancer arises:

- **Carcinomas.** Epithelial tissues (tissues covering body surfaces and lining most body cavities) are the most common sites for cancers; cancers occurring in epithelial tissue are called *carcinomas*. These cancers affect the outer layer of the skin and mouth as well as the mucous membranes. They metastasize through the circulatory or lymphatic system initially and form solid tumors.
- **Sarcomas.** Sarcomas occur in the mesodermal, or middle, layers of tissue—for example, in bones, muscles, and general connective tissue. In early stages, they metastasize primarily via the blood. Sarcomas are less common but generally more virulent than carcinomas. They also form solid tumors.
- **Lymphomas.** Lymphomas develop in the lymphatic system—the infection-fighting regions of the body—and metastasize through the lymphatic system. Hodgkin's disease is an example. Lymphomas also form solid tumors.
- **Leukemias.** Cancer of the blood-forming parts of the body, particularly the bone marrow and spleen, is called leukemia. A nonsolid tumor, leukemia is characterized by an abnormal increase in the number of white blood cells that the body produces.

Figure 16.3 on page 504 shows the most common sites of cancer and the number of new cases and deaths from each type that were estimated to have occurred in 2012. A comprehensive discussion of the many different forms of cancer is beyond the scope of this book, but we will discuss the most common types in the next sections.

Lung Cancer

Lung cancer is the leading cause of cancer deaths for both men and women in the United States. It killed an estimated 160,340 Americans in 2012, accounting for nearly 28 percent of all cancer deaths, even though rates have decreased in

Estimated New Cases of Cancer*		Estimated Deaths from Cancer*	
Female	Male	Female	Male
Breast 226,870 (29%)	**Prostate** 241,740 (29%)	**Lung & bronchus** 72,590 (26%)	**Lung & bronchus** 87,750 (29%)
Lung & bronchus 109,690 (14%)	**Lung & bronchus** 116,470 (14%)	**Breast** 39,510 (14%)	**Prostate** 28,170 (9%)
Colon & rectum 70,040 (9%)	**Colon & rectum** 73,420 (9%)	**Colon & rectum** 25,220 (9%)	**Colon & rectum** 26,470 (9%)
Uterine corpus 47,130 (6%)	**Urinary bladder** 55,600 (7%)	**Pancreas** 18,540 (7%)	**Pancreas** 18,850 (6%)
Thyroid 43,210 (5%)	**Melanoma of the skin** 44,250 (5%)	**Ovary** 15,500 (6%)	**Liver & intrahepatic bile duct** 13,980 (5%)
Melanoma of the skin 32,000 (4%)	**Kidney & renal pelvis** 40,250 (5%)	**Leukemia** 10,040 (4%)	**Leukemia** 13,500 (4%)
Non-Hodgkin lymphoma 31,970 (4%)	**Non-Hodgkin lymphoma** 38,160 (4%)	**Non-Hodgkin lymphoma** 8,620 (3%)	**Esophagus** 12,040 (4%)
Kidney & renal pelvis 24,520 (3%)	**Oral cavity & pharynx** 28,540 (3%)	**Uterine corpus** 8,010 (3%)	**Urinary bladder** 10,510 (3%)
Ovary 22,280 (3%)	**Leukemia** 26,830 (3%)	**Liver & intrahepatic bile duct** 6,570 (2%)	**Non-Hodgkin lymphoma** 10,320 (3%)
Pancreas 21,830 (3%)	**Pancreas** 22,090 (3%)	**Brain & other nervous system** 5,980 (2%)	**Kidney & renal pelvis** 8,650 (3%)
All Sites 790,740 (100%)	**All Sites** 848,170 (100%)	**All Sites** 275,370 (100%)	**All Sites** 301,820 (100%)

*Excludes basal and squamous cell skin cancers and in situ carcinoma except urinary bladder. Percentages may not total 100% due to rounding.

FIGURE 16.3 **Leading Sites of New Cancer Cases and Deaths, 2012 Estimates**

Source: Data from Table on page 4, American Cancer Society, *Cancer Facts & Figures 2012* (Atlanta: American Cancer Society, Inc.). Note that percentages do not add up to 100 due to omissions of certain rare cancers as well as rounding of statistics.

recent decades due to declines in smoking and policies that prohibit smoking in public places.[31] The lifetime risks for males and females getting lung cancer is 1 in 13 and 1 in 16, respectively. Risks begin to rise around age 40 and continue to climb through all age groups thereafter. The average risk of developing lung cancer for men and women ages 40 to 59 is 1 in 109 and 1 in 132, respectively.[32]

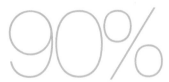

90%

of all lung cancers could be avoided if people simply did not smoke.

Since 1987, more women have died each year from lung cancer than from breast cancer, which over the previous 40 years had been the major cause of cancer deaths in women. Although past reductions in smoking rates have boded well for cancer statistics, there is growing concern about the number of young people, particularly young women and persons of low income and low educational levels, who continue to pick up the habit.

There is also growing concern about the increase in lung cancers among lifelong *never smokers*—a group of people who, as the name suggests, have never smoked, but nevertheless now have as much as 15 percent of all lung cancers. Never smokers' lung cancer is believed to be related to exposure to secondhand smoke, radon gas, asbestos, indoor wood-burning stoves, and aerosolized oils caused by cooking with oil and deep fat frying.[33] Unfortunately, because doctors often don't think of lung cancer when a never smoker presents with a cough, patients are often put on antibiotics or cough suppressants as therapy. By the time they recognize that it's really lung cancer, the prognosis is bleak.[34]

Detection, Symptoms, and Treatment Symptoms of lung cancer include a persistent cough, blood-streaked sputum, voice change, chest pain or back pain, and recurrent attacks of pneumonia or bronchitis. Newer computerized tomography (CT) scans, molecular markers in saliva, and newer biopsy techniques have improved screening accuracy for lung cancer but have a long way to go. Treatment depends on the type (large or small scale) and stage of the cancer. Surgery, radiation therapy, chemotherapy, and targeted biological therapies are all options.[35] If the cancer is localized, surgery is usually the treatment of choice. If it has spread, surgery is combined with radiation and chemotherapy. Unfortunately, despite advances in medical technology, survival rates 1 year after diagnosis are low, at 52 percent for cases diagnosed early, but only 16 percent overall when all stages are combined, and the 5-year survival rate for all stages combined is only 16 percent.[36]

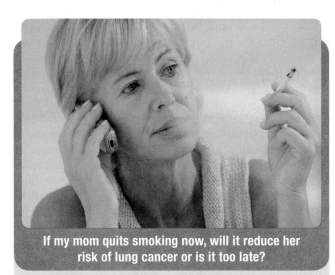

If my mom quits smoking now, will it reduce her risk of lung cancer or is it too late?

It's never too late to quit. Stopping smoking at any time will reduce your risk of lung cancer, in addition to the numerous other health benefits that are gained. Studies of women show that within 5 years of quitting, their risk of death from lung cancer decreases by 21 percent, compared to people who continue smoking.

Risk Factors and Prevention Risks for cancer increase dramatically based on the quantity of cigarettes smoked and the number of years smoked, often referred to as *pack years*. The greater the number of pack years smoked, the greater the risk of developing cancer. Quitting smoking does reduce the risk of developing lung cancer.[37] People who have been exposed to industrial substances such as arsenic and asbestos or to radiation are at the highest risk for lung cancer. Exposure to both secondhand cigarette smoke and radon gas (a gas that leaks into houses from naturally occurring uranium in the soil) is believed to play an important role in lung cancer development for smokers, past smokers, and people who have never been smokers.[38]

Breast Cancer

Breast cancer is a group of diseases that cause uncontrolled cell growth in breast tissue, particularly in the glands that produce milk and the ducts that connect those glands to the nipple. Cancers can also form in the connective and lymphatic tissues of the breast. In 2012, approximately 226,870 women and 2,190 men in the United States were diagnosed with invasive breast cancer for the first time. In addition, 63,300 new cases of in situ breast cancer, a

more localized cancer, were diagnosed. About 39,510 women (and 410 men) died, making breast cancer the second leading cause of cancer death for women.[39] Although incidence rates of breast cancer declined by about 7 percent between 2002 and 2003, newer research indicates that these declines did not continue between 2003 and 2007, even though hormone use declined significantly. In fact, although there was little change in rates for most groups, incidence rates increased for certain types of breast cancer in those age 40 to 49,[40] although further study is necessary. Generally speaking, women have a 1 in 8 lifetime risk of being diagnosed with breast cancer. From birth to age 39, the risk is 1 in 203, but between the ages of 40 and 59, the chance for breast cancer falls becomes 1 in 27.[41] This is why most health groups have advocated screening for breast cancer more thoroughly after age 40.

Detection The earliest signs of breast cancer are usually observable on mammograms, often before lumps can be felt. However, mammograms are not foolproof, and there is debate regarding the optimal age at which women should start regularly receiving them (see the **Points of View** box on the following page). Hence, regular breast self-examination (BSE) is also important (see **Figure 16.4**). Mammograms detect 80 to 90 percent of breast cancers in women without symptoms. A newer form of magnetic resonance imaging (MRI) appears to be even more accurate, particularly in women with genetic risks for tumors.[42]

Breast Awareness and Self-Exam Breast self-exam has been recommended by major health organizations as a form of early breast cancer screening for the last two decades. However, a 2009 "study of studies" done by the U.S. Preventive Services Task Force determined that breast self-exams did not decrease suffering and death and, in fact, often lead to

See It! Videos

When should women start getting mammograms? Watch **Mammogram Controversy** at www.peasonhighered.com/donatelle.

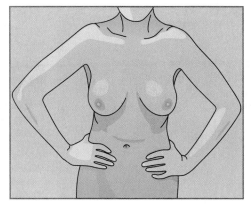

❶ Face a mirror and check for changes in symmetry.

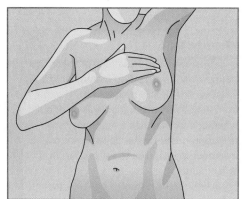

❷ Either standing or lying down, use the pads of the three middle fingers to check for lumps. Follow an up and down pattern on the breast to ensure all tissue gets inspected.

FIGURE 16.4 Breast Awareness and Self-Exam

Source: Adapted from Breast Self-Exam Illustration Series, National Cancer Institute Visuals Online Collection, U.S. National Institutes of Health.

Mammography for Women under Age 50:
TO SCREEN OR NOT TO SCREEN?

In 2009, the U.S. Preventive Services Task Force (USPSTF), made up of experts from across the country, suggested that women should not have a mammogram until they are 50 and then have one only every other year. Why? While evidence shows that women aged 50 to 74 seem to benefit from mammograms, similar benefits for women under age 40 appeared to be much less apparent. This recommendation caused a furor in the general public and prompted groups such as the National Cancer Institute, the American Cancer Society, and Susan G. Komen for the Cure to publicly disagree. Critics argued that the USPSTF recommendations were politically and economically motivated and did not consider all of the facts.

Consider the following arguments for and against routine mammography screening for women between the ages of 40 and 50.

Arguments for Mammograms for Women Aged 40 to 50

◯ The causes of breast cancer are not well understood and no reliable method of prevention is currently available. Most research to date shows the probability of successful treatment is greatest when it is found at an earlier stage, when cancer tumors have not spread. Early detection offers a woman the best chance for a cure, and mammography is essential for early detection of breast cancer.

◯ Digital mammography significantly improves the detection of cancer in younger women and in women with dense breast tissue.

◯ Women who are screened with mammography between the ages of 39 and 49 experience a 15 percent reduction in breast cancer deaths.

◯ New research indicates that the recommendations for women in their forties failed to consider key benefits. Some researchers argue that by only assessing numbers of lives saved, short- and long-term benefits of less aggressive treatments for cases screened earlier in the disease course were not factored into the harm/benefit equation.

◯ The United States has one of the highest breast cancer rates in the world. About 40 percent of the deaths and 56 percent of the years of women's lives lost come from cancers that emerge between the years of 40 and 59. This is when mammograms may reduce the potential for pain and suffering and even death. This action would be regressive and is based primarily on cost estimates and financial considerations, not preventive medicine.

Arguments against Mammograms for Women Aged 40 to 50

◯ There is insufficient evidence indicating that screening mammograms are beneficial in women under the age of 40.

◯ High cumulative doses of low-energy radiation may actually lead to more cancers in younger women, particularly those with the *BRCA1* or *BRCA2* gene. Although inconclusive, there are studies that show slightly increased risks of eye, lung, and breast cancers in those who have had an annual mammogram over many years.

◯ Some studies indicate that there is significant added anxiety, stress, and other psychological problems that result from mammograms.

◯ Those who receive an abnormal mammogram often have to go back for more screenings, even though there may be a false-positive result. Radiation exposure in these instances may increase overall risks of breast cancer.

◯ Costs for some of the procedures, such as biopsy, may be high.

Where Do You Stand?

◯ What are the implications of the recommendations regarding mammograms for you? Your family members?

◯ Who should make the decision about whether a woman has a mammogram? Is it appropriate for the government or insurance companies to set policies in these matters?

◯ What are the potential benefits and risks—to individuals or to a society—from such a policy?

◯ When it comes to cancer prevention, do you think more screening is always better? Why or why not?

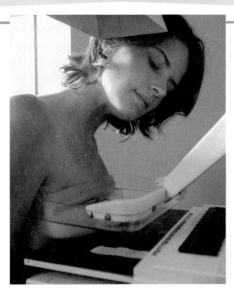

Sources: J. Malmgren, M. Atwood, and H. Kaplan, "Breast Cancer Detection Method Among 20–49 Year Old Patients at a Community Based Cancer Center: 1990–2008," *The Breast Journal*, April 5, 2012, DOI: 10.111/j.1524-4741.2012.01231.x; M. Yaffe, "The Pros and Cons of Mammography: Report Card on Canada—2011–2012," www.canceradvocacy.ca/reportcard/2012/The%20Pros%20and%20Cons%20of%20Screening%20Mammography.pdf; Agency for Healthcare Research and Quality, Recommendations of the U.S. Preventive Services Task Force, "Screening for Breast Cancer: Recommendation Statement," Updated December 2009, www.uspreventiveservices taskforce.org/uspstf/uspsbrca.htm; Carol Milgard Breast Center, "Breast Screening Guidelines Position Statement," Uploaded March 2010, www.carolmilgardbreastcenter.org/index.php/news/35/breast_screening_guidelines; American Cancer Society, "Response to Changes to USPSTF Mammography Guidelines," 2009, http://pressroom.cancer.org/index.php?s=43&item=201.

unnecessary worry, unnecessary tests, and increased health care costs. As a result of this research, several groups have downgraded the recommendation about breast self-exams from "do them and do them regularly" to "learn how to do them, and if you desire, do them to know your body and be able to recognize changes."

To do a breast self-exam, begin by standing in front of a mirror to inspect the breasts, looking for their usual symmetry. Some breasts are not symmetrical, and if this is not a change, it is okay. Raise and lower both arms while checking that the breasts move evenly and freely. Next, inspect the skin, looking for areas of redness, thickening, or dimpling, which might have the appearance of an orange peel. Look for any scaling on the nipple.

To feel for lumps, raise one arm above your head while either standing or lying. This will flatten out the breast, making it easier to feel the tissue. Using the index, middle, and fourth fingers of your opposite hand, gently push down on the breast tissue and move the fingers in small circular motions, varying pressure from light to more firm. Start at one edge of the breast and move upward and then downward, working your way across the breast until all of the breast tissue has been covered. Often breast tissue will feel dense and irregular, and this is usually normal. It helps to do regular self-exams to become familiar with what your breast tissue feels like; then, if there is a change, you will notice. Cancers usually feel like a dense or firm little rock and are very different from the normal breast tissue.

Next, lower the arm and reach into the top of the underarm and pull downward with gentle pressure feeling for any enlarged lymph nodes. To complete the exam, squeeze the tissue around the nipple. If you notice discharge from the nipple and you have not recently been breastfeeding, consult your doctor. Likewise, if you notice any asymmetry, skin changes, scaling on the nipple, or new lumps in the breast, you should see your doctor for evaluation.

Symptoms and Treatment If breast cancer grows large enough, it can produce the following symptoms: a lump in the breast or surrounding lymph nodes, thickening, dimpling, skin irritation, distortion, retraction or scaliness of the nipple, nipple discharge, or tenderness.

Treatments range from a lumpectomy to radical mastectomy to various combinations of radiation or chemotherapy. Among nonsurgical options, promising results have been noted among women using *selective estrogen-receptor modulators* (*SERMs*) such as tamoxifen and raloxifene, particularly among women whose cancers appear to grow in response to estrogen. These drugs, as well as new *aromatase inhibitors*, work by blocking estrogen. The

5-year survival rate for people with localized breast cancer (which includes all people living 5 years after diagnosis, whether they are in remission, disease free, or under treatment) has risen from 80 percent in the 1950s to 98 percent today.[43] However, these statistics vary dramatically, based on the stage of the cancer when it is first detected and whether it has spread. If the cancer has spread to the lymph nodes or other organs, the 5-year survival rate drops to as low as 27 percent.[44]

Risk Factors and Prevention The incidence of breast cancer increases with age. Although there are many possible risk factors, those that are well supported by research include family history of breast cancer, menstrual periods that started early and ended late in life, obesity after menopause, recent use of oral contraceptives or postmenopausal hormone therapy, never bearing children or bearing a first child after age 30, consuming two or more drinks of alcohol per day, and physical inactivity.[45] Having *BRCA1* and *BRCA2* gene mutations appears to account for approximately 5 to 10 percent of all cases of breast cancer, and women who possess these genes have a 60 to 80 percent risk of developing breast cancer by age 70 as compared to a 7 percent risk in women without the mutations. Because these genes are rare, routine screening for them is not recommended unless there is a strong family history of breast cancer.[46]

International differences in breast cancer incidence correlate with variations in diet, especially fat intake, although a causal role for these dietary factors has not been firmly established. Sudden weight gain has also been implicated. Research also shows that regular exercise, even some forms of recreational exercise, can reduce risk.[47] In particular, two large meta-analyses of studies focused on the role of dietary fiber indicate strong inverse relationships between dietary fiber and breast cancer. In short, if you eat more fiber, breast cancer rates seem to go down, and if you eat less, rates seem to increase.[48]

Colon and Rectal Cancers

Colorectal cancers (cancers of the colon and rectum) continue to be the third most commonly diagnosed cancer in both men and women and the second leading cause of cancer deaths, even though death rates are declining. Most cases occur in people age 50 and over, but new cases can occur at any age.[49] In 2012, there were 103,170 cases of colon and 40,290 cases of rectal cancer diagnosed in the United States and nearly 52,000 deaths.[50] Men age 40 to 59 have a 1 in 109 risk of developing it, and a lifetime risk of 1 in 19. Women age 40 to 59 have a 1 in 137 chance of developing colorectal cancer, and a 1 in 20 lifetime risk.[51]

See It! Videos
What does a family do when breast cancer hits almost all the women? Watch **Breast Cancer Hits Four of Five Sisters** at www.pearsonhighered.com/donatelle.

"Why Should I Care?"

Breast cancer accounts for 1 in every 3 cancer diagnoses in women in the United States. You can take action to reduce your risk by keeping your weight within a healthy range, drinking less than one alcoholic drink a day, and exercising regularly. Starting now is your best means of prevention.

Detection, Symptoms, and Treatment Because colorectal cancer tends to spread slowly, the prognosis is quite good if caught in early stages; in fact, when caught at an early, localized stage, 5-year survival rates are over 90 percent. However, the bad news is that in its early stages, colorectal cancer typically has no symptoms and only 39 percent of cases are caught in the earliest stage. Those without insurance, or who avoid testing even with insurance, often are diagnosed at later stages when 5-year survival rates are much less. As the disease progresses, bleeding from the rectum, blood in the stool, and changes in bowel habits are the major warning signals. Only 10 percent of all Americans over age 50 have had the most basic screening test—the at-home *fecal occult blood* test (FBOT)—in the past year, and slightly over 50 percent have had an endoscopy test.[52] Although these rates are low, it should be noted that rates are even lower among people age 50 to 64 and especially lower among those who are non-white, have fewer years of education, lack health insurance, and are recent immigrants.[53] Interesting regional differences in screening occur, with Delaware having the highest overall screening rates at 72 percent and Oklahoma having the lowest rates at 52 percent. No state meets the American Cancer Society (ACS) 2015 goals of 75 percent screened.[54] Colonoscopies and other screening tests should begin at age 50 for most people. Virtual colonoscopies and fecal DNA testing are newer diagnostic techniques that have shown promise. Treatment often consists of radiation or surgery. Chemotherapy, although not used extensively in the past, is today a possibility.

> **malignant melanoma** A virulent cancer of the melanocytes (pigment-producing cells) of the skin.

Risk Factors and Prevention The older you are, the greater your chances of colorectal cancer. Although anyone can develop it, people who are over age 50, who are obese, who have a family history of colon and rectal cancer, who have a personal or family history of polyps (benign growths) in the colon or rectum, or who have inflammatory bowel problems such as colitis run an increased risk. A history of diabetes also seems to increase risk. Other possible risk factors include diets high in fat or low in fiber, high consumption of red and processed meats, smoking, sedentary lifestyle, high alcohol consumption, and low intake of fruits and vegetables. Regular exercise, a diet with lots of fruits and other plant foods, a healthy weight, and moderation in alcohol consumption appear to be among the most promising prevention strategies. Consumption of milk and calcium and higher blood levels of vitamin D decrease risks. New research suggests that non-steroidal anti-inflammatory drugs (NSAIDs) such as aspirin, postmenopausal hormones, folic acid, calcium supplements, selenium, and vitamin E may also help.[55] However, drugs are not recommended as a preventive measure as these each have other risks that might outweigh any benefit.

Skin Cancer

The exact number of basal and squamous cell skin cancers is unknown as these cases are not required to be reported to cancer registries. It is widely accepted, however, that skin cancer is the most common form of cancer in the United States today, with over 3.5 million diagnosed cases in 2012. Millions more remain undiagnosed and untreated, and 1 in 5 people in the United States will be diagnosed in their lifetime! In 2012, an estimated 12,190 deaths from skin cancer will occur, 9,180 from melanoma and 3,010 from other skin cancers.[56] The two most common types of skin cancer—basal cell and squamous cell carcinomas—are highly curable. **Malignant melanoma,** the third most common form of skin cancer, is the most deadly. The majority of these deaths are in men over the age of 50; however, rates have increased among all age groups. Between 65 percent and 90 percent of melanomas are caused by exposure to ultraviolet (UV) light or sunlight. Even though the incidence of many of the common cancers has been steadily declining, it is important to note that the incidence of melanoma continues to rise at a rate faster than that of any of the seven most common cancers.[57] Men age 40 to 59 have a 1 in 158 chance of developing it, with a 1 in 36 lifetime risk. Women age 40 to 59 have a 1 in 180 chance of developing it, with a 1 in 55 lifetime risk.[58]

Detection, Symptoms, and Treatment Basal and squamous cell carcinomas show up most commonly on the face, ears, neck, arms, hands, and legs as warty bumps, colored spots, or scaly patches. Bleed-

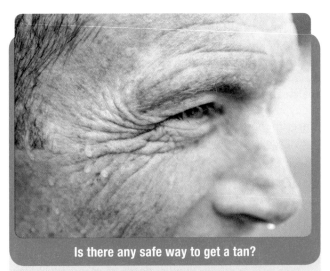

Is there any safe way to get a tan?

Unfortunately, no. There is no such thing as a "safe" tan, because a tan is visible evidence of UV-induced skin damage. The injury accumulated through years of tanning contributes to premature aging and increases your risk for disfiguring skin cancer, eye problems, and possible death from melanoma. According to the American Cancer Society, tanned skin provides only the equivalent of sun protection factor (SPF) 4 sunscreen—much too weak to be protective. It isn't possible or practical to avoid sunlight completely, but wearing sunscreen of SPF 15 or higher every day can prevent further damage and diminish the cumulative effects of sun exposure.

ing, itching, pain, or oozing are other symptoms that warrant attention. Surgery may be necessary to remove them, but they are seldom life threatening.

In striking contrast is melanoma, an invasive killer that may appear as a skin lesion. Typically, the lesion's size, shape, or color changes, and it spreads to regional organs and throughout the body. Malignant melanomas account for over 75 percent of all skin cancer deaths. Like other cancers, survival is largely dependent on how advanced the cancer is when diagnosed. If melanoma has not yet penetrated the underlying layers of skin, chances of survival are over 90 percent. However, if it is diagnosed after deeper layers of skin are penetrated and it has spread to other organs, the survival rate falls to 15 percent.[59] Figure 16.5 compares melanoma with basal cell and squamous cell carcinomas. The *ABCD* rule can help you remember the warning signs of melanoma:

- **Asymmetry.** One half of the mole or lesion does not match the other half.
- **Border irregularity.** The edges are uneven, notched, or scalloped.
- **Color.** Pigmentation is not uniform. Melanomas may vary in color from tan to deeper brown, reddish black, black, or deep bluish black.
- **Diameter.** Diameter is greater than 6 millimeters (about the size of a pea).

Treatment of skin cancer depends on the type of cancer, its stage, and its location. Surgery, laser treatments, topical chemical agents, *electrodesiccation* (tissue destruction by heat), and *cryosurgery* (tissue destruction by freezing) are all common forms of treatment. For melanoma, treatment may involve surgical removal of the regional lymph nodes, radiation, or chemotherapy.

Risk Factors and Prevention Anyone who overexposes himself or herself to ultraviolet (UV) radiation without adequate protection is at risk for skin cancer. The risk is greatest for people who:

- Have fair skin; blonde, red, or light brown hair; blue, green, or gray eyes
- Always burn before tanning or burn easily and peel readily
- Don't tan easily but spend lots of time outdoors
- Use no or low–sun protection factor (SPF) sunscreens or expired suntan lotions
- Have had skin cancer or a family history of skin cancer
- Experienced severe sunburns during childhood. Contrary to popular thinking, there is no such thing as getting a base tan that protects against damage. The greater the exposure dose and the longer the time periods of exposure, the greater the risk.

Preventing skin cancer is a matter of limiting exposure to harmful UV rays, whether in natural sunlight or tanning beds. What happens when you expose yourself to sunlight? The skin responds to photodamage by increasing its thickness and the number of pigment cells (melanocytes), which produce the "tan" look. (A tan is actually the body's way of trying to protect itself or defend against UV attack. It can fight the onslaught only for a short time before damage begins to accrue.) Ultraviolet light damages the skin's immune cells, lowering the normal immune protection of the skin and priming it for cancer. Photodamage also causes wrinkling by impairing the elastic substances (collagens) that keep skin soft and pliable. See the **Skills for Behavior Change** box on the following page for tips on staying safe in the sun.

In spite of the risks, many Americans are still "working on a tan," either outdoors or in tanning salons. There is increasing interest in determining *why* so many people continue tanning despite overwhelming evidence of potential harm. Some have suggested that tanning may have addictive qualities that actually keep people coming back even when they know better.[60] Perhaps there is a link between high levels of UV light and increases in "feel good" endorphins. This little tanning high may make it harder for tanners to stop. Stay tuned! Research in this area is in its infancy. For information

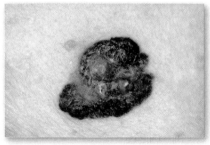
(a) Malignant melanoma

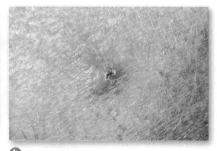
(b) Basal cell carcinoma

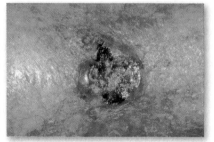
(c) Squamous cell carcinoma

FIGURE 16.5 **Types of Skin Cancers**
Preventing skin cancer includes keeping a careful watch for any new pigmented growths and for changes to any moles. The ABCD warning signs of melanoma (a) include *a symmetrical* shapes, irregular *borders*, *color* variation, and an increase in *diameter*. Basal cell carcinoma (b) and squamous cell carcinoma (c) should be brought to your physician's attention, but they are not as deadly as melanoma.

Tips for Protecting Your Skin in the Sun

❭ Seek shade from 10 AM to 4 PM, when the sun's rays are strongest. Even on a cloudy day, up to 80 percent of the sun's rays can get through.

❭ Apply a sunscreen with SPF 15 or higher evenly to all uncovered skin before going outside. Look for a "broad-spectrum" sunscreen that protects against both UVA and UVB radiation. If the sunscreen label does not specify otherwise, assume you need to apply it 15 minutes before going outside.

❭ Check the expiration date on your sunscreen. Sunscreens lose effectiveness over time. Often those sunscreen sales are on dated products. Beware! It's not a bargain if it doesn't work!

❭ Put sunscreen on your lips, nose, ears, neck, hands, and feet. If you don't have much hair, apply sunscreen to the top of your head, too.

❭ Reapply sunscreen at least every 2 hours. The label will tell you how often you need to do this. If it isn't waterproof, reapply after swimming or if you are sweating.

❭ Wear loose-fitting, light-colored clothing. You can now purchase clothing that has SPF protection in most sporting goods stores. A wide-brimmed hat will protect your head and face.

❭ Use sunglasses with 99 to 100 percent UV protection to protect your eyes. Look for polarized lenses.

❭ Check your skin for cancer, keeping an eye out for changes in birthmarks, moles, or sunspots.

Source: U.S. Food and Drug Administration, "Sun Safety: Save Your Skin!" Updated December 2012, www.fda.gov/ForConsumers/ConsumerUpdates/ucm049090.htm.

on the risks of tanning salons, see the **Student Health Today** box on page 511.

Prostate Cancer

After skin cancer, prostate cancer is the most frequently diagnosed cancer in American males today. Importantly, it is the second leading cause of cancer deaths in men after lung cancer. In 2012, about 241,740 new cases of prostate cancer were diagnosed in the United States. About 1 in 6 men will be diagnosed with prostate cancer during his lifetime. The older a man is, the greater the chance of developing it. However, with improved screening and early diagnosis, 5-year survival rates are 100 percent for all but the most advanced cases.[61]

prostate-specific antigen (PSA) An antigen found in prostate cancer patients.

Detection, Symptoms, and Treatment The prostate is a muscular, walnut-sized gland that surrounds part of a man's urethra, the tube that transports urine and sperm out of the body. A part of the reproductive system, its primary function is to produce seminal fluid. Symptoms of prostate cancer may include weak or interrupted urine flow; difficulty starting or stopping urination; feeling the urge to urinate frequently; pain on urination; blood in the urine; or pain in the low back, pelvis, or thighs. Many men have no symptoms in the early stages.

Men over age 40 should have an annual digital rectal prostate examination. Another screening method for prostate cancer is the **prostate-specific antigen (PSA)** test, a blood test that screens for an indicator of prostate cancer. However, much as they did for breast self-exam recommendations in 2011, the United States Preventive Services Task Force recommended that otherwise asymptomatic men no longer receive the routine PSA test because, overall, it does not save lives and may in fact lead to painful, unnecessary cancer treatments. If you have a family history or other symptoms, consult with your physician.

Fortunately, prostate cancers tend to progress slowly, and most prostate cancers are detected while they are still in the local or regional stages. Over the past 20 years, the 5-year survival rate for all stages combined has increased from 67 percent to almost 99 percent, and the 15-year survival rate is over 76 percent.[62]

Risk Factors and Prevention Chances of developing prostate cancer increase dramatically with age. Almost 2 out of every 3 prostate cancers are diagnosed in men over age 65.[63] Sometimes the disease has progressed to the point of displaying symptoms, or more likely, men are seeing a doctor for other problems and get a screening test or PSA test.

Race is also a risk factor in prostate cancer: African American men and Jamaican men of African descent have the

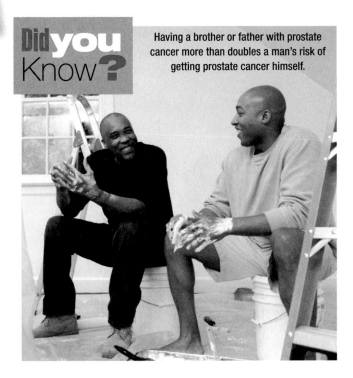

Did you Know?

Having a brother or father with prostate cancer more than doubles a man's risk of getting prostate cancer himself.

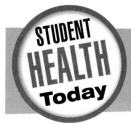
Indoor Tanning: Sacrificing Health for Beauty

In our culture, being tan is equated with being healthy, chic, and attractive. In a study of nearly 3,000 adults, over 18 percent of women and nearly 6.5 percent of men report tanning in the last 12 months. Teens and 20-somethings are the most likely to be users of indoor tanning overall. Indoor tanning is a multi-billion-dollar industry. But users should know that their "glow" comes with a greatly increased cancer risk.

Many people believe—incorrectly—that tanning booths are safer than sitting in the sun. But all tanning lamps emit UVA rays, and most emit UVB rays as well. Both types of light rays cause long-term skin damage and can contribute to cancer. Consider the following:

✳ A 2010 study that looked specifically at indoor tanning found it significantly increased risk of melanoma, regardless of age and for virtually all types of tanning bed exposure. The evidence was so compelling that tanning devices have been listed as carcinogenic for humans.
✳ People who use tanning beds are 2.5 times more likely to develop squamous cell carcinoma and 1.5 times more likely to develop basal cell carcinoma.
✳ New high-pressure sunlamps used in some salons emit doses of UV radiation that can be as much as 12 times that of the sun.
✳ People who tan regularly end up with older-looking skin. Up to 90 percent of visible skin changes commonly blamed on aging are caused by the sun.

Because of the many salons that are springing up across the country, the artificial tanning industry is difficult to monitor and regulate. Some tanning facilities do not calibrate the UV output of their tanning bulbs or ensure sufficient rotation of newer and older bulbs, which can lead to more or less exposure than you paid for. And unlike most beachgoers, tanning facility patrons often try for a total body tan. This is a problem because the buttocks and genitalia are particularly sensitive to UV radiation and are prone to developing skin cancer.

Finally, shared tanning booths and beds pose significant hygiene risks. Anytime you come in contact with body secretions from others, you run the risk of an infectious disease. Don't assume that those little colored water sprayers used to "clean" the inside of the beds are sufficient to kill organisms. The busier the facility, the more likely you are to come into contact with germs that could make you ill.

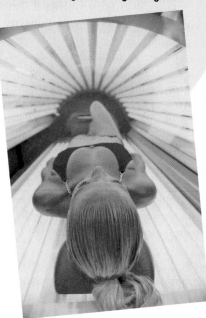

Indoor tanning—greatly increased risk of melanoma comes along with the "golden glow."

Sources: K. Hoerster et al., "Density of Indoor Tanning Facilities in 116 Large U.S. Cities," 2009. *American Journal of Preventive Medicine* 36, no. 3 (2009): 243–6; D. Lazovich et al., "Indoor Tanning and Risk of Melanoma: A Case-Control Study in a Highly Exposed Population," *Cancer Epidemiology Biomarkers and Prevention* 19, no. 6 (2010): 1557-68, DOI:10.1158/1055-9965.EPI-09-1249; National Cancer Institute, "Tanning Bed Study Shows Strongest Evidence Yet of Increased Melanaoma Risk," *NCI Cancer Bulletin*, 2010, www.cancer.gov/ncicancerbulletin/060110/page2; Skin Cancer Foundation, "Skin Cancer Facts," 2012, www.skincancer.org/skin-cancer-information/skin-cancer-facts.

highest documented prostate cancer incidence rates in the world and are more likely to be diagnosed at more advanced stages than other racial groups.[64]

Having a father or brother with prostate cancer more than doubles a man's risk of getting prostate cancer himself. Interestingly, the risk is higher for men with an affected brother than it is for those with an affected father. Men who have had several relatives with prostate cancer, especially those with relatives who developed prostate cancer at younger ages, are also at higher risk.[65]

Eating more fruits and vegetables, particularly those containing lycopene, a pigment found in tomatoes and other red fruits, may lower the risk of prostate cancer. Diets high in processed meats or dairy and obesity also appear to increase risks.[66] Some studies have suggested that vitamin E or selenium may be beneficial, but in a major clinical trial of more than 35,000 men conducted over 5 years neither supplement was found to lower prostate cancer risk.[67] The best advice is to follow the dietary recommendations (Dietary Guidelines for Americans) of the U.S. Department of Agriculture discussed in **Chapter 7** and maintain a healthy weight.

There is some evidence that risk for prostate cancer is elevated in firefighters. In addition, men who have had a history of sexually transmitted diseases and other inflammation of the prostate may have an increased risk.[68]

Ovarian Cancer

Ovarian cancer is the fifth leading cause of cancer deaths for women, with about 22,800 being diagnosed with this form of

Pap test A procedure in which cells taken from the cervical region are examined for abnormal cellular activity.

cancer in 2012 and 15,500 dying from it.[69] Ovarian cancer causes more deaths than any other cancer of the reproductive system because women tend not to discover it until the cancer is at an advanced stage. Overall, 1-year survival rates are 75 percent, and 5-year survival rates are 44 percent.[70]

Detection, Symptoms, and Treatment Unfortunately, early ovarian cancer usually has no obvious symptoms. The most common symptom is enlargement of the abdomen. In some women, there may be a vague feeling of bloating, pelvic or abdominal pain, gas, fatigue, weight loss, difficulty eating or feeling full, and/or bowel or bladder irregularity. Women over age 40 may experience persistent digestive disturbances as well. Abnormal vaginal bleeding or discharge is rarely a symptom until the disease is advanced.[71]

Treatment for early-stage ovarian cancer typically includes surgery, chemotherapy, and occasionally radiation therapy. Depending on the patient's age and her desire to bear children in the future, one or both ovaries, fallopian tubes, and the uterus may be removed. Chemotherapy and radiation are also sometimes used in addition to surgery.

Risk Factors and Prevention Primary relatives (mother, daughter, sister) of a woman who has had ovarian cancer are at increased risk. A family or personal history of breast or colon cancer is also associated with increased risk. Women who have never been pregnant are more likely to develop ovarian cancer than those who have given birth, and the more children a woman has had, the less risk she faces. The use of estrogen alone as postmenopausal therapy may increase a woman's risk, as well as smoking and obesity.[72]

Research shows that long-term use of oral contraceptives, adhering to a low-fat diet, having multiple children, breast-feeding, and tubal ligation may reduce your risk of ovarian cancer.[73] So, should you get pregnant or start taking birth control pills to reduce risk? No. General prevention strategies such as focusing on diet, exercise, sleep, stress management, and weight control are good ideas for combating the risk of ovarian and any of the other cancers discussed in this text.

To protect yourself, get a complete annual pelvic examination. Women over 40 should have a cancer-related checkup every year. Uterine ultrasound or a blood test is recommended for those with risk factors or unexplained symptoms.

Cervical and Endometrial (Uterine) Cancer

Most uterine cancers develop in the body of the uterus, usually in the endometrium. The rest develop in the cervix, located at the base of the uterus. In 2012, an estimated 12,170 new cases of cervical cancer and 47,130 cases of endometrial cancer were diagnosed in the United States.[74] The overall incidence of cervical and uterine cancer has been declining steadily over the past decade. This decline may be due to more regular screenings of younger women using the **Pap test,** a procedure in which cells taken from the cervical region are examined for abnormal cellular activity. Although Pap tests are very effective for detecting early-stage cervical cancer, they are less effective for detecting cancers of the uterine lining. Women have a lifetime risk of 1 in 147 for being diagnosed with cervical cancer and a 1 in 38 risk of being diagnosed with uterine corpus cancer.[75] Early warning signs of uterine cancer include bleeding outside the normal menstrual period or after menopause or persistent unusual vaginal discharge.

Risk factors for cervical cancer include early age at first intercourse, multiple sex partners, cigarette smoking, and certain sexually transmitted infections, including HPV (the cause of genital warts) and herpes. For endometrial cancer, age is a risk factor; however, estrogen and obesity are also strong risk factors. In addition, risks are increased by treatment with tamoxifen for breast cancer, metabolic syndrome, late menopause, never bearing children, a history of polyps in the uterus or ovaries, a history of other cancers, and race (white women are at higher risk).[76]

Testicular Cancer

Testicular cancer is one of the most common types of solid tumors found in young adult men, affecting nearly 8,590 young men in 2012.[77] Those between the ages of 15 and 35 are at greatest risk. There has been a steady increase in testicular cancer frequency over the past several years in this age group.[78] However, with a 96 percent 5-year survival rate, it is one of the most curable forms of cancer. Although the cause of testicular cancer is unknown, several risk factors have been identified. Men with undescended testicles appear to be at greatest risk, and some studies indicate a genetic influence.

Testicular Self-Exam

In general, testicular tumors first appear as an enlargement of the testis or thickening in testicular tissue. Because this enlargement is often painless, the first indication young men have of a problem often comes from a testicular self-examination (see Figure 16.6).

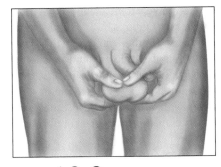

FIGURE 16.6 **Testicular Self-Exam**

Source: From Michael Johnson, *Human Biology: Concepts and Current Issues*. 3rd ed. Copyright © 2006. Reprinted with permission of Pearson Education, Inc.

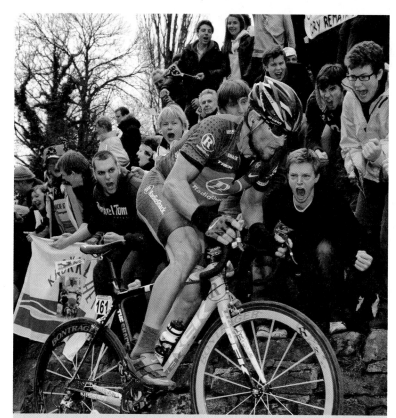

One of the most remarkable testicular cancer stories is the survival of cyclist Lance Armstrong. After recovering from an invasive form of testicular cancer that spread to several parts of his body, including his brain, Armstrong went on to win the Tour de France seven consecutive times and to create a foundation dedicated to cancer education, research, and advocacy.

Testicular self-exams have long been recommended for teen boys and young men to perform monthly as a means of detecting testicular cancer. However, recent studies have found that they are not cost-effective because the incidence of testicular cancer is low and most findings from self-exams result in testing what ultimately ends up being a noncancerous condition. For this reason, the U.S. Preventive Services Task Force has dropped their recommendation for monthly testicular exams. Regardless, most cases of testicular cancer are discovered through self-exam, and there is currently no other screening test for the disease.

The testicular self-exam is best done after a hot shower, which will relax the scrotum and make the exam easier. Inspect the scrotum for any changes in color or in the size of each testicle. It is common for one testicle to be larger than the other, and if this is not a change, it is okay.

Hold a testicle using the three middle fingers of one hand. Using small circular motions and light pressure, move the index and middle fingers of the second hand over the testicle until the whole surface has been covered. Feel for changes in texture or small nodules that may feel like a pea or a grain of rice. Also note if there are areas where touch produces pain. Along the back of each testicle is the epididymis, which contains the spermatic cord and the blood vessels serving the testicle. Feel this area with the index finger and the thumb, again looking for painful areas, changes in texture, or small lumps. Repeat the process for the second testicle. If you notice any of the above, consult your doctor for further evaluation.

Leukemia

Leukemia is a cancer of the blood-forming tissues that leads to proliferation of millions of immature white blood cells. These abnormal cells crowd out normal white blood cells (which fight infection); platelets (which control hemorrhaging); and red blood cells (which carry oxygen to body cells). Resulting symptoms include fatigue, paleness, weight loss, easy bruising, repeated infections, nosebleeds, and other forms of hemorrhaging.

Leukemia can be acute or chronic and can strike both sexes and all age groups. An estimated 47,150 new cases were diagnosed in the United States in 2012.[79] Chronic leukemia can develop over several months and have few symptoms. It is usually treated with radiation and chemotherapy. Other treatments include bone marrow and stem cell transplants.

Lymphoma

Just a few short years ago, not many people had heard much about lymphomas, a group of cancers of the lymphatic system that include Hodgkin's disease and non-Hodgkin lymphoma. Today, however, lymphomas are among the fastest growing cancers, with an estimated 70,130 new cases in 2012.[80] Much of this increase has occurred in women. The cause is unknown; however, a weakened immune system is suspected—particularly one that has been exposed to viruses such as HIV, hepatitis C, Epstein-Barr virus (EBV), and others. Treatment for lymphoma varies by type and stage; however, chemotherapy and radiotherapy are commonly used.

Facing Cancer

There is much you can do to reduce your own risk of cancer. Make a realistic assessment of your own risk factors, avoid behaviors that put you at risk, and increase healthy behaviors. Even if you have significant risks, those are factors you can control. Follow the recommendations for self-exams and medical checkups in Table 16.2. on page 514. The earlier cancer is diagnosed, the better the prognosis will be.

Detecting Cancer

If you are at high risk for developing cancer, or if you notice potential cancer symptoms, your health care provider might use one or more tests to diagnose or rule out cancer.

Cancer Site	Screening Procedure	Age and Frequency of Test
Breast	Mammograms	The NCI recommends that women in their forties and older have mammograms every 1 to 2 years. Women who are at higher-than-average risk of breast cancer should talk with their health care provider about whether to have mammograms before age 40 and how often to have them.
Cervix	Pap test (Pap smear)	Women should begin having Pap tests 3 years after they begin having sexual intercourse or when they reach age 21 (whichever comes first). Most women should have a Pap test at least once every 3 years.
Colon and rectum	**Fecal occult blood test:** Sometimes cancer or polyps bleed. This test can detect tiny amounts of blood in the stool. **Sigmoidoscopy:** Checks the rectum and lower part of the colon for polyps. **Colonoscopy:** Checks the rectum and entire colon for polyps and cancer.	People aged 50 and older should be screened. People who have a higher-than-average risk of cancer of the colon or rectum should talk with their doctor about whether to have screening tests before age 50 and how often to have them.
Prostate	Prostate-specific antigen (PSA) test	Some groups encourage yearly screening for men over age 50, and some advise men who are at a higher risk for prostate cancer to begin screening at age 40 or 45. Others caution against routine screening. Currently, Medicare provides coverage for an annual PSA test for all men age 50 and older.

NCI, National Cancer Institute.

Sources: National Cancer Institute, National Institutes of Health, "What You Need to Know About Cancer Screening," www.cancer.gov/cancertopics/wyntk/cancer/page4; National Cancer Institute, "Fact Sheet, Prostate-Specific Antigen (PSA) Test," www.cancer.gov/cancertopics/factsheet/detection/PSA.

Magnetic resonance imaging (MRI) uses a huge electromagnet to detect tumors by mapping the vibrations of the atoms in the body on a computer screen. The **computerized axial tomography (CAT) scan** uses X rays to examine parts of the body. In both of these painless, noninvasive procedures, cross-sectioned pictures can reveal a tumor's shape and location more accurately than can conventional X rays. *Prostatic ultrasound* (a rectal probe using ultrasonic waves to produce an image of the prostate) is being investigated as a means to increase the early detection of prostate cancer. In 2011 the FDA approved the first 3D mammogram machines, which offer significant improvements in imaging and breast cancer detection but deliver nearly double the radiation risk of conventional mammograms.

magnetic resonance imaging (MRI) A device that uses magnetic fields, radio waves, and computers to generate an image of internal tissues of the body for diagnostic purposes without the use of radiation.

computerized axial tomography (CAT) scan A scan by a machine that uses radiation to view internal organs not normally visible in X rays.

radiotherapy The use of radiation to kill cancerous cells.

chemotherapy The use of drugs to kill cancerous cells.

Cancer Treatments

Cancer treatments vary according to the type and stage of cancer. Surgery, in which the tumor and surrounding tissue are removed, is one common strategy. It may be performed alone or in combination with other treatments. The surgeon may operate using traditional surgical instruments such as a scalpel, or by using a laser, laparoscope, or other tools for less invasive results. Pain and infection are the most common problems after surgery.

Radiotherapy (the use of radiation) or **chemotherapy** (the use of drugs) to kill cancerous cells are also used. Radia-

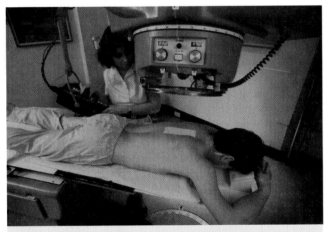

Radiation therapy is often used to target and destroy cancerous tumors. The machine in this photograph emits gamma rays, which are typically used to treat localized secondary cancers and also provide pain relief for otherwise untreatable cancers. Gamma rays are less powerful than the X rays emitted from linear accelerators, another machine frequently used in radiation therapy.

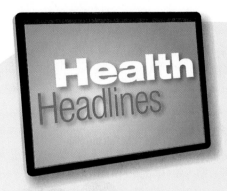

NEW TREATMENTS FOR CANCER

Surgery, chemotherapy, and radiation therapy remain the most common treatments for all types of cancer. However, newer techniques are constantly being investigated that may be more effective for certain cancers or certain patients:

✳ **Immunotherapy.** The goal of immunotherapy is to enhance the body's own disease-fighting systems. Biological response modifiers such as interferon and interleukin-2 are under study. Immunotherapies have been particularly effective against melanomas and certain kidney cancers.

✳ **Biological therapies.** One of the most exciting new approaches for spurring the immune system to ward off cancer is the use of *cancer-fighting vaccines*. These alert the body's immune defenses to good cells that have gone bad. Rather than preventing disease as other vaccines do, they help people who are already ill.

✳ **Gene therapies.** Research on the effectiveness of *gene therapy* has moved into early clinical trials. Scientists have found signs of a virus carrying genetic information that makes the cells it infects (such as cancer cells) susceptible to an antiviral drug. Scientists are also looking at ways to transfer genes that increase the patient's immune response to the cancerous tumor or that confer drug resistance to the bone marrow to allow higher doses of chemotherapeutic drugs.

✳ **Angiogenesis inhibitors.** Researchers are testing compounds that may stop tumors from forming new blood vessels, a process called *angiogenesis*. Without adequate blood supply, tumors either die or grow very slowly, giving other chemotherapeutic agents a better chance to fight them.

✳ **Disrupting cancer pathways.** In recent years, scientists have identified various steps in what is termed the *cancer pathway*. These include oncogene actions, hormone receptors, growth factors, metastasis, and angiogenesis. Preliminary studies are under way to design compounds that inhibit actions at these various steps.

✳ **Smart drugs.** Drugs such as Herceptin, Gleevec, and Avastin are new forms of *targeted smart-drug therapies* that attack only the cancer cells and do not hit the entire body.

✳ **Enzyme inhibitors.** A powerful enzyme inhibitor, *TIMP2*, shows promise for slowing the metastasis of tumor cells. A metastasis suppressor gene, *NM23*, has also been identified. Both of these therapies are aimed at disrupting cancer pathways.

✳ **Neoadjuvant chemotherapy.** This method (which uses chemotherapy to shrink the tumor and then surgically removing it) has been tried against various types of cancers.

✳ **Stem cell research.** When a patient's bone marrow has been destroyed by disease, chemotherapy, or radiation, transplants of stem cells from donor bone marrow may successfully restore blood stem cells (the cells that divide to produce blood cells).

---

tion destroys malignant cells or stops cell growth. It is most effective in treating localized cancer masses because it can be targeted to a particular area of the body. Over the course of several weeks, patients are treated by a machine that exposes the designated part of the body to high-energy rays. Radiotherapy usually takes place on an outpatient basis. Side effects include fatigue, changes to the skin in the affected area, and a small increase in the chance of developing another type of cancer.

Chemotherapy may be used to shrink a tumor before surgery or radiation therapy, after surgery or radiation therapy to kill remaining cancer cells, or on its own. Powerful drugs are administered, usually in on-and-off cycles so the body can recover from their effects. Side effects may include nausea, hair loss, fatigue, increased chance of bleeding, bruising, infection, and anemia, and go away as the drugs leave the body after treatment. Other possible effects, such as the loss of fertility, may be permanent.

In the process of killing malignant cells, some healthy cells are also destroyed, and long-term damage to the cardiovascular system and other body systems from radiotherapy and chemotherapy can be significant.

Participation in clinical trials (people-based studies of new drugs or procedures) has provided a new source of hope for many patients undergoing cancer treatment. Because of the many unknown variables, deciding whether to participate in a clinical trial can be a difficult decision. Despite the risks, which should be carefully considered, thousands of clinical trial participants have benefited from treatments that would otherwise be unavailable to them.

Several newer treatments described in the **Health Headlines** box are either being used in clinical trials or have become available in selected cancer centers throughout the country. In addition, psychosocial and behavioral research has become increasingly important as health professionals learn more about lifestyle factors that influence risk and survivability. Health practitioners have become more aware of the psychological needs of patients and families and have begun to tailor treatment programs to meet their diverse needs.

Before beginning any form of cancer therapy, it is imperative to be a vigilant and vocal consumer. Read and seek

See It! Videos

Studies show that some surprising drugs may help treat cancer. Watch **Treating Cancer with Bone Drugs** at www.pearsonhighered.com/donatelle.

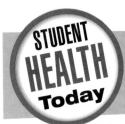

STUDENT HEALTH Today

BEING A HEALTH ADVOCATE FOR YOURSELF OR SOMEONE YOU LOVE

Any time cancer is diagnosed, people react with anxiety, fear, and anger. Emotional distress is sometimes so intense that patients and their loved ones are unable to make critical health care decisions. Of course you want to remain calm and check out all your options, but that is easier said than done. If you or a loved one are diagnosed with cancer, the following actions may help:

✳ **Pair up for doctor appointments.** Even suspecting cancer can cause fear and shock, and that can prevent a patient from asking important questions or from hearing key details. Bring a trusted friend or relative with you to the doctor, and talk together about what you heard later.

✳ **Find out as much as possible about the cancer.** Ask the doctor to explain the type and stage of cancer, the treatment plan, the other options available, and the potential risks and benefits. Read about your cancer on reliable websites such as the American Cancer Society, the National Cancer Institute, or Susan G. Komen for the Cure. If your doctor recommends that you participate in a clinical drug trial, request a copy of the documents outlining potential risks and benefits.

✳ **Get a second opinion.** Request a copy of the diagnostic test results, and get an "out of group" physician (someone unaffiliated with your original doctor) to review them. Find an oncologist (cancer specialist) at a

big teaching hospital where they see a large number of patients with your type of cancer. Don't worry about hurting the original doctor's feelings. It's your life!

✳ **Check out the credentials of the hospital, surgeon, and treatment specialist.** If surgery is recommended, find out about the patient-to-caregiver ratio in the hospital and the plan for aftercare, and ask for recommendations from patients who've had the procedures that are planned for you.

✳ **Find local resources and support groups.** It can be helpful to talk with someone who isn't emotionally involved in your personal situation. Survivor support groups can provide information you can get only from people who have lived through cancer. Talking with a counselor is another good way to keep the focus on getting well.

✳ **Get your personal ducks in a row.** Write down financial information, where to find important papers, and other relevant information. Find someone to take care of your home if you will be hospitalized.

✳ **Know what insurance does and doesn't cover.** Call your insurer ahead of time and know what procedures require permission. Find out what percentage of the bill is the

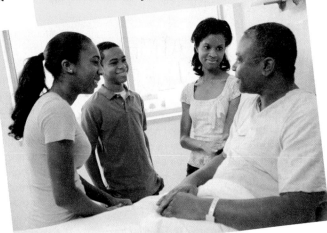

If you or someone you love is diagnosed with cancer, it is important to seek out all the help and information that you can find.

patient's responsibility and how this may change if you need to see specialists. If you do not have insurance, talk with social service agencies, your student health center financial director, or others who can help you come up with a plan for payment.

✳ **Mobilize family and friends to help.** If you or your loved one will be bedridden, ask friends to make and deliver dinners, do errands, or help around the house. Don't be afraid to ask for the help you need. Friends and family usually want to have some concrete way to help in times of crisis.

---

information from cancer support groups. Check the skills of your surgeon, your radiation therapist, and your doctor in terms of clinical experience and interpersonal interactions. Look at Oncolink and other websites supported by the National Cancer Institute and the American Cancer Society (ACS), and check out clinical trials, reports on effectiveness of various treatments, new experimental therapies, and other options. Also, although you may like and trust your family doctor, it is always a good idea to seek advice or consultation from large cancer facilities that see many patients and are well equipped to deal with all situations. See the **Student Health Today** box for more on being your own advocate or an advocate for someone you love.

Cancer Survivors

The number of people surviving cancer is at an all time high in the United States, at nearly 12 million survivors. Importantly, they are surviving better than any previous generation, largely due to heightened public awareness, less stigma, and a much greater level of support for cancer patients. Cancer patients are much less likely to face cancer alone or make decisions about treatment in isolation. Cancer support groups, cancer information workshops, and low-cost medical consultation are more widely available than ever. The Internet has helped educate individuals about treatment options and where to go for assistance. Groups such as the

Susan G. Koman for the Cure Foundation have provided support for survivors and their families and have helped people realize that cancer is not a death sentence—not something to be hidden from others. Coping with cancer can be difficult, but there are ways to ease the burden and make surviving less challenging for all concerned.[81]

Although survival used to be measured almost exclusively by whether a person had gone 5 years without cancer symptoms, **survivorship** is now viewed much more broadly in terms of both years and the quality of life that a person experiences after diagnosis. Today, survivorship comprises the unique ways in which people survive and thrive after cancer has been diagnosed. The National Cancer Institute defines this term as the "physical, psychological, emotional, and economic issues of cancer from diagnosis until the end of life."[82]

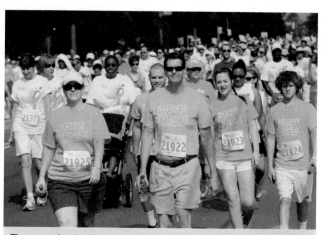

14%

of the estimated 10.8 million cancer survivors in the U.S. today were diagnosed more than 20 years ago.

Accumulating evidence makes clear that breast cancer survivorship, for example, is influenced by a constellation of important factors, including age, socioeconomic status, availability of support services, education level, relationship status, social support, sexual identity, race, stress level, coping style, spirituality, and depression. Some suggest that psychosocial factors such as quality of life, including spiritual, social, and emotional well-being, are among the most significant and the most in need of study for understanding their influence in breast cancer survivorship.[83]

Rather than looking only at the number of years people survive, quality of the survival experience is becoming increasingly important. In fact, quality-of-life measures may influence whether a person actually reaches the 5-year survivor milestone.

There may be physical and emotional issues as well as financial issues related to health insurance and cost of care to cope with for years after cancer diagnosis and treatment. Survivors also have to live with the possibility of a recurrence. However, cancer survivors can and do live active, productive lives despite these challenges. Many survivors and their relatives find it emotionally satisfying to participate in cancer research fund-raiser walks and other events.

survivorship Physical, psychological, emotional, and economic issues of cancer from diagnosis until the end of life.

What's Your Personal Risk for Cancer?

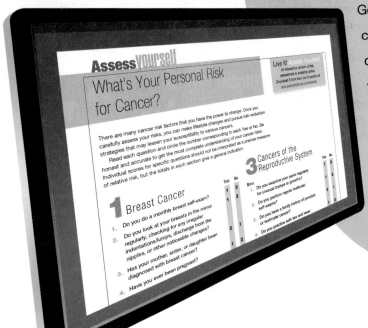

Go online to www.pearsonhighered.com/donatelle to complete the "What's Your Personal Risk for Cancer?" assessment.* Once you carefully assess your risks, you can make lifestyle changes and pursue risk-reduction strategies that may lessen your susceptibility to various cancers. See the **YOUR PLAN FOR CHANGE** box for ways to implement those risk-reduction strategies.

*If your instructor so chooses, Assess Yourself Activities are available as a printed supplement or as assignable homework online at www.pearsonhighered.com/myhealthlab.

MyHealthLab®

YOUR PLAN FOR CHANGE

If the **Assess yourself** activity identified particular risky behaviors you want to change, follow these steps:

Today, you can:

○ Assess your personal risks for specific cancers, looking at lifestyle, as well as your genetic risks. For which cancers might you be most at risk?

○ Take advantage of the salad bar in your dining hall for lunch or dinner and load up on greens, or request veggies such as steamed broccoli or sautéed spinach.

Within the next 2 weeks, you can:

○ Buy a bottle of sunscreen (with SPF 15 or higher) and begin applying it as part of your daily routine. (Be sure to check the expiration date, particularly on sale items!) Also, stay in the shade from 10 AM to 2 PM, as this is when the sun is strongest.

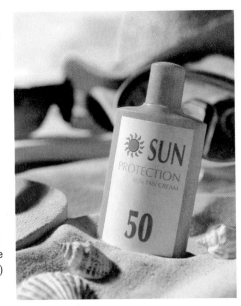

○ Find out your family health history. Talk to your parents, grandparents, or an aunt or uncle to find out if family members have developed cancer. This will help you assess your own genetic risk.

By the end of the semester, you can:

○ Work toward achieving a healthy weight. If you aren't already engaged in a regular exercise program, begin one now. Maintaining a healthy body weight and exercising regularly will lower your risk for cancer.

○ Stop smoking, avoid secondhand smoke, and limit your alcohol intake.

Summary

* Cancer is a group of diseases characterized by uncontrolled growth and spread of abnormal cells. These cells may create tumors. Benign (noncancerous) tumors grow in size but do not spread; malignant (cancerous) tumors spread to other parts of the body.
* Lifestyle factors for cancer include smoking and obesity as well as poor diet, lack of exercise, stress, and other factors. Biological factors include inherited genes, age, and gender. Potential environmental carcinogens include asbestos, radiation, preservatives, and pesticides. Infectious agents may increase your risks for cancer; those that appear most likely to cause cancer are chronic hepatitis B and C, human papillomavirus, and genital herpes. Medical factors may elevate the chance of cancer.
* There are many different types of cancer, each of which poses different risks, depending on several factors. Common cancers include that of the lung, breast, colon and rectum, skin, prostate, testis, ovary, and uterus; leukemia; and lymphomas.
* The most common treatments for cancer are surgery, chemotherapy, and radiation; however, newer therapies, including biological, smart drugs, immunotherapy, and others, show promising results and should always be considered.
* Early diagnosis improves survival rate. Self-exams for breast, testicular, and skin cancer aid early diagnosis.

Pop Quiz

1. When cancer cells have *metastasized*,
   a. they have grown into a malignant tumor.
   b. they have spread to other parts of the body, including vital organs.
   c. the cancer is retreating and cancer cells are dying off.
   d. None of the above

2. A cancerous *neoplasm* is
   a. a type of biopsy.
   b. a form of benign tumor.
   c. a type of treatment for a tumor.
   d. a malignant group of cells or tumor.

3. Who is at a higher risk for developing skin cancer?
   a. People who have fair skin
   b. People who freckle and burn more when in the sun
   c. People who have a history of bad sunburn as a child
   d. All of the above

4. "If you are male and smoke, your chances of getting lung cancer are 23 times greater than those of a nonsmoker." This statement refers to a type of risk assessed statistically, known as
   a. relative risk.
   b. comparable risk.
   c. cancer risk.
   d. genetic predisposition.

5. The leading type of cancer-related deaths for men and women in the United States is
   a. colorectal cancer.
   b. pancreatic cancer.
   c. lung cancer.
   d. stomach cancer.

6. The most common type of cancer in men and women in the United States is
   a. lung.
   b. bladder.
   c. oral.
   d. skin.

7. One of the biggest factors in increased risk for cancer is
   a. increasing age.
   b. presence of another disease.
   c. being of long-lived parents.
   d. increased consumption of fruits and vegetables.

8. One of the best ways to reduce a person's risk of developing cancer is to
   a. quit smoking now if currently smoking.
   b. eat a very healthy diet with more fruits and vegetables.
   c. maintain a healthy weight (avoiding overweight and obesity).
   d. All of the above

9. Which of the following is correct?
   a. Certain infectious diseases can cause inflammation and increase cancer risks.
   b. Carcinoma in situ of the breast is one of the most lethal forms of breast cancer.
   c. Your risk of dying of breast cancer as a 20-year-old female is approximately 1 in 8.
   d. All of the above

10. The most serious and life-threatening type of skin cancer is
    a. basal cell carcinoma.
    b. squamous cell carcinoma.
    c. melanoma.
    d. lymphoma.

Answers to these questions can be found on page A-1.

Think about It!

1. What is cancer? How does it spread? What is the difference between a benign tumor and a malignant tumor?
2. List the likely causes of cancer. Which of these causes would be a risk for you, in particular? What can you do to reduce these risks? What risk factors do you share with family members? Friends?
3. What are the symptoms of lung, breast, prostate, and testicular cancers? How can you reduce your risk of developing these cancers or increase your chances of surviving them?
4. What are the differences between carcinomas, sarcomas, lymphomas, and leukemia? Which is the most common? Least common?

Why is it important that you know the stage of your cancer?

5. Why are breast and testicular self-exams especially important for college students? What factors keep you from doing your own self-exams? What could you do to make sure you do regular self-exams?

Accessing Your Health on the Internet

The following websites explore further topics and issues related to personal health. For links to the websites below, visit the Companion Website for *Access to Health,* 13th Edition, at www.pearsonhighered.com/donatelle.

1. *American Cancer Society.* This private organization is dedicated to cancer prevention. Here you'll find information, statistics, and resources regarding cancer. www.cancer.org

2. *National Cancer Institute.* On this site you will find valuable information on cancer facts, results of research, new and ongoing clinical trials, and the Physician Data Query (PDQ), a comprehensive database of cancer treatment information. www.cancer.gov

3. *National Women's Health Information Center (NWHIC).* A wealth of information about cancer in women is presented on this site, which is cosponsored by the National Cancer Institute. http://womenshealth.gov

4. *Oncolink.* Sponsored by the University of Pennsylvania Cancer Center, this site educates cancer patients and their families by offering information on support services, cancer causes, screening, prevention, and common questions. www.oncolink.com

5. *Susan G. Komen for the Cure.* Up-to-date information about breast cancer, issues in treatment, and support groups are presented here; there is also a wealth of videos and information. This site is especially useful for diagnosed patients looking for additional support and advice. www.komen.org

6. *National Coalition for Cancer Survivorship.* Cancer survivors share their experiences advocating for themselves during and after cancer treatment. www.canceradvocacy.org

References

1. American Cancer Society, *Cancer Facts and Figures, 2012* (Atlanta: American Cancer Society, 2012), www.cancer.org/acs/groups/content/@epidemiology surveilance/documents/document/acspc-031941.pdf.
2. Ibid.
3. Ibid.
4. Ibid.
5. National Cancer Institute at the National Institutes of Health, "Fact Sheet, Cancer Staging," 2010, www.cancer.gov/cancer topics/factsheet/detection/staging.
6. American Cancer Society, *Cancer Facts and Figures,* 2012.
7. Ibid.
8. Ibid.
9. Ibid.
10. American Cancer Society, *Cancer Facts and Figures,* 2012; Centers for Disease Control and Prevention, *Tobacco Use: Targeting the Nation's Leading Killer—At-a-Glance 2010* (Atlanta: Centers for Disease Control and Prevention, National Center for Chronic Disease Prevention and Health Promotion, 2010), Available at www.cdc.gov/chronicdisease/resources/publications/AAG/osh.htm.
11. American Cancer Society, *Cancer Facts and Figures,* 2012; National Cancer Institute, "Harms of Smoking and Health Benefits of Quitting—Fact Sheet," 2011, www.cancer.gov/cancertopics/factsheet/Tobacco/cessation.
12. World Health Organization, *WHO Report on Global Tobacco Epidemic, 2008: The MPOWER Package* (Geneva, Switzerland: World Health Organization, 2008), Available at www.who.int/tobacco/mpower/2008/en/index.html.
13. W. Chen et al., "Moderate Alcohol Consumption During the Adult Life, Drinking Patterns and Breast Cancer Risk," *Journal of the American Medical Association* 306, no. 17 (2011): 1884–90.
14. American Cancer Society, *Cancer Facts and Figures,* 2012; D. Parkin, "Cancers Attributable to Consumption of Alcohol in the UK in 2010," *British Journal of Cancer* 105 (2011): S14–S18, DOI:10:10.1038/bjc.2011.476; N. Allen et al., "Moderate Alcohol Intake and Cancer Incidence in Women," *Journal of the National Cancer Institute* 101, no. 5 (2009): 296–305; I. Tramacere et al., "A Meta-Analysis on Alcohol Drinking and Gastric Cancer Risk." *Annals of Oncology* 23, no. 1 (2012): 28–36; S. Gupta et al., "Risk of Pancreatic Cancer by Alcohol Dose, Duration, and Pattern of Consumption, Including Binge Drinking: A Population-Based Study," *Cancer Causes & Control* 21, no. 7 (2010): 1047–59.
15. A. Benedetti et al., "Lifetime Consumption of Alcoholic Beverages and Risk of 13 Types of Cancer in Men: Results from a Case-Control Study in Montreal," *Cancer Epidemiology* 32, no. 5 (2009): 352–62.
16. American Cancer Society, *Cancer Facts and Figures,* 2012.
17. D. Guh et al., "The Incidence of Co-Morbidities Related to Obesity and Overweight: A Systematic Review and Meta-Analysis," *BMC Public Health* 9, no. 88 (2009); American Cancer Society, *Cancer Facts and Figures,* 2012.
18. H. R. Harris, W. Willett, K. Terry, and K. Michels, "Body Fat Distribution and Risk of Premenopausal Breast Cancer in the Nurses' Health Study II," *Journal of the National Cancer Institute* 103, no. 3 (2011): 373–78.
19. T. Kay, E. Spencer, and G. Reeves, "Overnutrition: Consequences and Solutions—Obesity and Cancer Risks," *Proceedings of the Nutrition Society* 69 (2010): 86–90.
20. E. Reiche, H. Morimoto, and S. Nunes, "Stress and Depression-Induced Immune Dysfunction: Implications for the Development and Progression of Cancer," *International Review of Psychiatry* 17, no. 6 (2005): 515–27; K. Ross, "Mapping Pathways from Stress to Cancer Progression," *Journal of the National Cancer Institute* 100, no. 13 (2008): 914–915, 917; Tel Aviv University, "Stress and Fear Can Affect Cancer's Recurrence," *Science Daily,* February 29, 2008, www.sciencedaily.com/releases/2008/02/080227142656.htm.
21. American Cancer Society, *Cancer Facts and Figures,* 2012.
22. American Cancer Society, "Breast Cancer Overview: What Causes Breast Cancer?" Revised July 2012, www.cancer.org/Cancer/BreastCancer/DetailedGuide/breast-cancer-what-causes.
23. L. Hines et al., "Comparative Analysis of Breast Cancer Risk Factors among Hispanic and Non-Hispanic White Women," *Cancer* 116, no. 13 (2010): 3215–23.
24. American Cancer Society, "Menopausal Hormone Therapy and Cancer Risk," 2012, www.cancer.org/Cancer/CancerCauses/OtherCarcinogens/MedicalTreatments/menopausal-hormone-replacement-therapy-and-cancer-risk; R. T. Chlebowski et al., "Lung Cancer Among Postmenopausal Women Treated with Estrogen Alone in the Women's Health Initiative Randomized

Trial," *Journal of the National Cancer Institute* 102, no. 18 (2010): 1413–21.

25. National Cancer Institute, "Fact Sheet—Cell Phones and Cancer Risk," October 2011, www.cancer.gov/cancertopics/factsheet/Risk/cellphones.

26. American Cancer Society, "Infectious Agents and Cancer," 2012, www.cancer.org/Cancer/CancerCauses/OtherCarcinogens/InfectiousAgents/InfectiousAgentsandCancer/infectious-agents-and-cancer-intro.

27. National Institute of Allergy and Infectious Diseases, "Viral Infections: Treating Cancer as an Infectious Disease," Updated March 2009, www.niaid.nih.gov/topics/viral/pages/cancerinfectiousdisease.aspx; American Cancer Society, *Cancer Facts and Figures,* 2012.

28. American Cancer Society, *Cancer Facts and Figures* 2012; National Cancer Institute, "Fact Sheet–HPV and Cancer," 2012, www.cancer.gov/cancertopics/factsheet/Risk/HPV.

29. American Cancer Society, *Cancer Facts and Figures,* 2012.

30. American Cancer Society, "Infectious Agents and Cancer," 2012.

31. American Cancer Society, *Cancer Facts and Figures,* 2012.

32. Ibid.

33. American Cancer Society, "Lung Cancer Also Affects Nonsmokers," 2011, www.cancer.org/Cancer/news/News/lung-cancer-also-affects-nonsmokers; J. Samet et al., "Lung Cancer in Never Smokers: Clinical Epidemiology and Environmental Risk Factors," *Clinical Cancer Research* 15, no. 18 (2009): 5626–45; C. Rudin et al., "Lung Cancer in Never Smokers: A Call to Action," *Clinical Cancer Research* 15, no. 18 (2009): 5622–25.

34. J. Samet et al., "Lung Cancer in Never Smokers," 2009.

35. American Cancer Society, *Cancer Facts and Figures,* 2012.

36. Ibid.

37. American Lung Association, "Benefits of Quitting," 2012, www.lung.org/stop-smoking/how-to-quit/why-quit/benefits-of-quitting/.

38. American Cancer Society, *Cancer Facts and Figures,* 2012.

39. Ibid.

40. C. DeSantis, N. Howlader, K. Cronin, and A. Jemal, "Breast Cancer Incidence Rates in U.S. Women Are No Longer Declining," *Cancer Epidemiology, Biomarkers & Prevention* 20 (2011): 733–39.

41. American Cancer Society, *Cancer Facts & Figures,* 2012.

42. American Cancer Society, *Cancer Facts & Figures,* 2010.

43. Ibid.

44. Ibid.

45. T. M. Peters et al., "Physical Activity and Postmenopausal Breast Cancer Risk in the NIH-AARP Diet and Health Study," *Cancer Epidemiology, Biomarkers, and Prevention* 18, no. 1 (2009): 289–96; American Cancer Society, *Cancer Facts and Figures 2010.*

46. Susan G. Komen for the Cure, "Table 11: *BRCA1* and *BRCA2* Gene Mutations and Cancer Risk," 2009, ww5.komen.org/BreastCancer/Table11BRCA1or2genemutationsandcancerrisk.html.

47. R. Patterson, L. Cadmus, and T. Emond, "Physical Activity, Diet, Adiposity and Female Breast Cancer Prognosis: A Review of Epidemiological Literature," *Maturitas* 66 (2010): 5–15.

48. J. Dong et al., "Dietary Fiber Intake and Risk of Breast Cancer: A Meta-Analysis of Prospective Cohort Studies," *American Journal of Clinical Nutrition* 94, no. 3 (2011): 900–905; D. Aune et al. "Dietary Fiber and Breast Cancer Risks: A Systematic Review and Meta Analysis of Prospective Studies," *Annals of Oncology,* 2012: DOI:10.1093/annuls/mdr589.

49. American Cancer Society, *Colorectal Cancer Facts and Figures 2011–2013* (Atlanta: American Cancer Society, 2011), Available at www.cancer.org/Research/CancerFactsFigures/ColorectalCancerFactsFigures/colorectal-cancer-facts-figures-2011-2013; American Cancer Society, *Cancer Facts and Figures,* 2012.

50. American Cancer Society, *Cancer Facts and Figures* 2012.

51. Ibid.

52. American Cancer Society, *Colorectal Cancer Facts and Figures,* 2011; American Cancer Society, *Cancer Facts and Figures,* 2012.

53. American Cancer Society, *Colorectal Cancer Facts and Figures,* 2011.

54. Ibid.

55. American Cancer Society, *Cancer Facts and Figures,* 2012; American Cancer Society, *Colorectal Cancer Facts and Figures,* 2011.

56. American Cancer Society, *Cancer Facts and Figures,* 2012.

57. Skin Cancer Foundation, "Skin Cancer Facts," 2012, www.skincancer.org/skin-cancer-informatino/skin-cancer-facts.

58. American Cancer Society, *Cancer Facts and Figures,* 2012.

59. Skin Cancer Foundation, "Skin Cancer Facts," 2012.

60. C. Mosher and S. Danoff-Burg, "Addiction to Indoor Tanning," *Archives of Dermatology* 146, no. 4 (2010): 412–17; A. Shal. et al., "Thriving Dependence: Is Tanning an Addiction?" in *Shedding Light on Indoor Tanning,* eds. C. Heckman and S. Manne (New York, Springer Publishing, 2012, pp 107–120), DOI: 10.1007/978-94-007-2048-0-7.hg.

61. American Cancer Society, *Cancer Facts and Figures,* 2012.

62. American Cancer Society, *Colorectal Cancer Facts and Figures,* 2011; American Cancer Society, *Cancer Facts and Figures,* 2012.

63. American Cancer Society, "Prostate Cancer: What Causes Prostate Cancer?" 2012, www.cancer.org/Cancer/ProstateCancer/OverviewGuide/prostate-cancer-overview-what-causes.

64. American Cancer Society, *Cancer Facts and Figures,* 2012.

65. American Cancer Society, "Prostate Cancer: Risk Factors, Causes and Prevention," 2012, www.cancer.org/Cancer/ProstateCancer/DetailedGuide/prostate-cancer-risk-factors.

66. American Cancer Society, *Cancer Facts and Figures,* 2012.

67. S. M. Lippman et al., "Effect of Selenium and Vitamin E on Risk of Prostate Cancer and Other Cancers: The Selenium and Vitamin E Cancer Prevention Trial (SELECT)," *Journal of the American Medical Association* 301, no. 1 (2009): 39–51.

68. American Cancer Society, "Prostate Cancer: Risk Factors, Causes and Prevention," 2012.

69. American Cancer Society, *Cancer Facts and Figures,* 2012.

70. Ibid.

71. Ibid.

72. American Cancer Society, *Cancer Facts and Figures,* 2012.

73. Ibid.

74. Ibid.

75. Ibid.

76. National Cancer Institute, "Endometrial Cancer," 2012, www.cancer.gov/cancertopics/types/endometrial.

77. American Cancer Society, *Cancer Facts and Figures,* 2012.

78. National Cancer Institute, "Testicular Cancer," 2012, www.cancer.gov/cancertopics/types/testicular.

79. American Cancer Society, *Cancer Facts and Figures,* 2012.

80. Ibid.

81. Centers for Disease Control and Prevention, "Cancer Survivors—United States, 2007," 2012, www.cdc.gov/cancer/survivorship/what_cdc_is_doing/research/survivors_article.htm; National Cancer Survivors Day Foundation, "Cancer Survivorship Issues," 2010, www.ncsdf.org/Pages/Issues.html.

82. National Cancer Institute, "Dictionary of Cancer Terms," 2012, www.cancer.gov/dictionary.

83. J. Jabson, *Breast Cancer Survivorship: Factors Influencing Ability to Thrive,* doctoral dissertation, Oregon State University, Corvallis, OR, April 2010.

Reducing Risks and Coping with Chronic Conditions

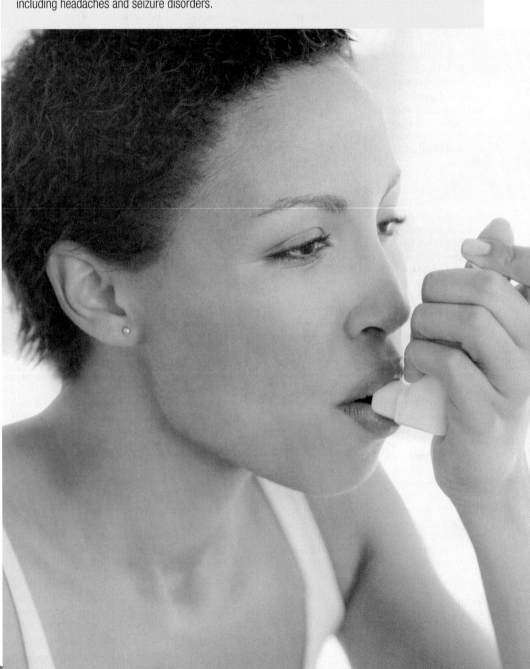

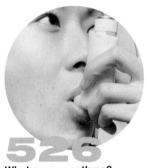

526
What causes asthma?

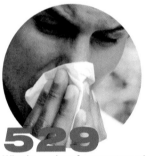

529
Why is my hay fever worse at certain times of the year?

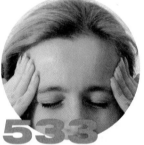

533
What triggers a migraine headache?

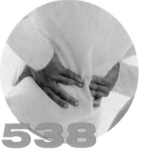

538
What is the major cause of disability among young adults?

OBJECTIVES

✷ Discuss key chronic respiratory diseases, including bronchitis, emphysema, and asthma.

✷ Describe the allergic response and complications associated with allergies.

✷ Explain common neurological disorders, including headaches and seizure disorders.

✷ Understand the major digestive disorders affecting adults in the United States today.

✷ Discuss the effects of various musculoskeletal diseases, including arthritis and low back pain.

Typically, when we think of major noninfectious ailments, we think of "killer" diseases such as cancer and heart disease. Although these diseases do make up the major portion of life-threatening diseases, other chronic conditions can also cause pain, suffering, and disability. Fortunately, many of them can be prevented and their symptoms delayed or relieved.

Chronic diseases and conditions often develop over a long period of time, cause progressive damage to human tissues, and are not easily cured. Lifestyle and personal health habits are often implicated as underlying causes, although some "newer" chronic maladies seem to defy conventional wisdom about causation. For those for which the underlying cause is known, actions to prevent these causes are presented. An increasing number of diseases are **idiopathic** (of unknown cause). In these cases, health professionals often use **palliative treatments,** those designed to treat or ease symptoms but not cure the disease. In general, prevention or intervention for chronic diseases requires investment in education about risks where they are known, lifestyle changes, environmental risk reduction, and assistance via pharmaceuticals and other medical interventions. Public support in the form of targeted research is also key to reducing illness and deaths.

In this chapter, we discuss some of the leading chronic diseases, other than cardiovascular disease (CVD) and cancer, that affect millions of Americans at all ages and stages of life. (The **Health in a Diverse World** box on page 524 describes shortcomings in chronic disease treatment internationally, while the **Health in a Diverse World** box on page 539 discusses maladies specific to women.) Whether you or a loved one currently have one of these diseases or are at risk for one, knowledge is a key weapon in reducing risks, preventing disease, and controlling threats to health now and in the future (see **Figure 17.1**).

Coping with Respiratory Problems

The average person takes 20,000 breaths each day.[1] Our respiratory systems move fresh air into the body and waste gases out. Breath really is *life*, but the respiratory system does much more than push air in and out. It protects you

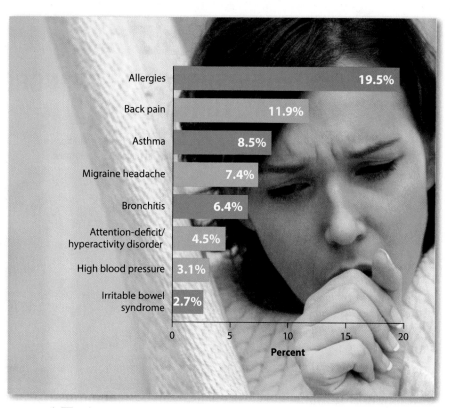

FIGURE 17.1 **Proportion of College Students Diagnosed with or Treated for Chronic Conditions in the Past 12 Months**

Do you think chronic diseases and health problems are a concern only for older Americans? Think again. College students are affected by chronic health issues, too.

Source: Data are from American College Health Association, *American College Health Association—National College Health Assessment II (ACHA-NCHA II): Reference Group Data Report Spring 2011* (Baltimore: American College Health Association, 2012).

from invaders by trapping and expelling harmful particles that you inhale with a cough or a sneeze. It also filters the air you breathe and is a finely tuned machine when it is healthy.

Unfortunately, several respiratory diseases are on the rise. **Chronic lower respiratory disease (CLRD)** (including bronchitis, emphysema, and asthma) is the number three killer in the United States (right after heart disease, cancer, and stroke) and is responsible for 1 in 6 deaths, or over 400,000 people each year. Thousands die from CLRD, but over 35 million Americans currently have some form of lung disease and suffer from varying degrees of disability.[2]

Virtually any disease or disorder in which lung function is impaired is considered a lung disease. The lungs can be damaged by a single exposure to a toxic chemical or severe heat or be impaired from years of inhaling the tar and chemicals in tobacco smoke. Occupational or home exposure to toxic environmental substances such as asbestos, silica dust, paint fumes and lacquers, or pesticides can cause lung deterioration. Of course, cancers, infections, and degenerative changes can

idiopathic Of unknown cause.

palliative treatment Those treatments designed to treat or ease symptoms but not cure the disease.

chronic lower respiratory disease (CLRD) Lung diseases such as emphysema, asthma, and some forms of bronchitis that are long-term in nature.

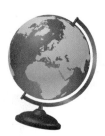

CHRONIC DISEASES: AN INCREASING GLOBAL THREAT

The balance between infectious and non-communicable diseases is shifting. The WHO [World Health Organization] predicts that leading infectious diseases will soon kill fewer people globally, and by 2030, three-quarters of all deaths in the world will be due to chronic non-communicable diseases like heart disease and some cancers.

—Colin Mathers, "Better Statistics Key to Tackling Chronic Diseases"

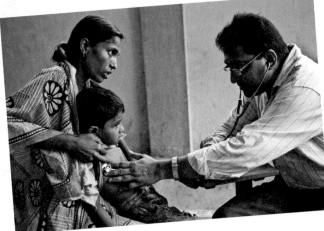

Resources to treat chronic conditions are often lacking in developing countries.

The statement above may surprise you. After all, we've long thought of the developing regions of the world as being plagued by killer infectious diseases such as HIV/AIDS, tuberculosis, and malaria. Although these diseases are still present and still cause premature death and disability at alarming rates, the numbers pale in comparison to chronic diseases.

For example, cancer kills more people annually than HIV/AIDS, malaria, and tuberculosis combined. Yet the WHO spends only $0.50 per person on chronic diseases compared to $7.50 per person for major infectious diseases. Other big philanthropic organizations such as

the Bill and Melinda Gates Foundation spend very little on chronic conditions in comparison to their spending for infectious diseases.

Why? One reason is that only about a third of the world's population is covered by national death registration systems that list causes of death. Although such coverage is over 95 percent in Europe, it is lower than 5 percent in Africa, and when surveillance and death registries exist, they often cover children rather than adults. Statistics about deaths provide the rationale for help in controlling certain diseases.

Faulty perceptions are another factor. Many people think that chronic diseases primarily affect the elderly in wealthy countries. Poorer nations believe they'll have a better chance of getting money for research and treatment through their established networks and are less skilled in seeking funds for chronic diseases.

Because many international leaders continue to see chronic diseases as "lifestyle choices," they believe that these poor outcomes are outside their range of responsibilities. They are not yet geared up to manage chronic conditions that require long-term and complex treatments. Prevention programs for most chronic diseases are not in place.

What is true is that the growing pandemic of chronic diseases can no longer be ignored. International organizations, leaders, and communities will need to tackle these problems soon.

Sources: P. Shetty, "Chronic Disease—A Neglected Priority," 2008, www.scidev.net/en/south-east-asia/editorials/chronic-disease-a-neglected-priority.html; C. Mathers, "Better Statistics Key to Tackling Chronic Diseases," 2008, www.scidev.net/en/middle-east-and-north-africa/opinions/better-statistics-key-to-tackling-chronic-diseases.html.

---

also wreak havoc with lung function. When the lungs are impaired, a condition known as **dyspnea,** a choking type of breathlessness, can occur, even with mild exertion. As the body is deprived of oxygen, the heart is forced to work harder, and over time, cardiovascular problems, suffocation, and death can occur. Compromised lungs show symptoms of distress, including prolonged coughing, shortness of breath, excess mucous production, wheezing, pain, and coughing up phlegm or blood. Fatigue, increased heart rate, and a host

dyspnea Shortness of breath, usually associated with disease of the heart or lungs.

chronic obstructive pulmonary disease (COPD) The chronic lung diseases of emphysema and chronic bronchitis.

of other problems may occur. Keeping your lungs healthy is an important part of an overall healthy lifestyle.

Chronic Obstructive Pulmonary Disease

Chronic obstructive pulmonary disease (COPD) is a progressive respiratory disease that may begin with shortness of breath after small exertion, but may eventually leave patients gasping for air and needing onboard oxygen to perform even the simplest tasks. In the United States, the term COPD refers

BE HEALTHY, BE GREEN

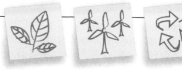

BE ECO-CLEAN AND ALLERGEN FREE

Exposure to household chemicals, dust, and pet dander may exacerbate asthma, allergies, and other respiratory problems. You can reduce exposure to noxious household chemicals and create a clean, comfortable home by using cleaning supplies and household products that are less toxic to the home environment. Because some companies may want you to believe their product is greener than it actually is, read the labels carefully and look for independent certifications such as the Green Seal and the Environmental Protection Agency's (EPA's) Design for the Environment program.

✳ For a handy glass and surface cleaner, mix 1/2 cup of white vinegar with 4 cups of water. Pour the solution into a spray bottle and keep the remainder for a quick and cheap refill. You can make another surface cleaner by combining 2 tablespoons of lemon juice with 4 cups of water.
✳ Baking soda is a great deodorizer and cleaner. Use it to remove carpet

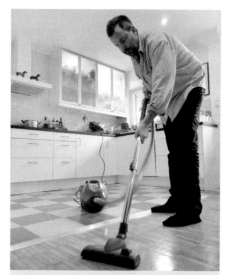

Making your own cleansers ensures that they are not harmful to your health.

odors and to scour sinks, toilets, and bathtubs.
✳ Because chlorine can damage lungs, skin, and eyes, and chlorine production

adds toxic chemicals such as carcinogenic dioxins to our environment, use a chlorine bleach alternative. For example, use 1/2 cup of hydrogen peroxide in your laundry or try oxygen-based bleaches.
✳ An all-purpose cleaner can be made of 1/2 cup of borax (found in the laundry aisle) and 1 gallon of hot water.
✳ For green air fresheners, use essential oils, such as lemon or lavender. Many store-bought air fresheners contain phthalates, often called "fragrance," that are related to respiratory problems and other noninfectious conditions. Place a few drops of essential oils on a piece of tissue paper, in a bowl of warm water, or in a store-bought diffuser.

As you transition to green cleaning, do not just throw old products in the trash, as these can wind up polluting landfills and leaching into water supplies. Instead, take them to a hazardous chemical recycling facility.

---

to two specific diseases, *chronic bronchitis* and *emphysema,* which often occur together and can lead to issues with emptying the lungs or exhaling. About 24 million U.S. adults have impaired lung function overall, with over 9.9 million diagnosed with chronic bronchitis and 4.3 million diagnosed with emphysema.[3]

what do you think?

Have you or any of your friends or family experienced any of the conditions discussed in this section?
● Why do you think the incidence of COPD is increasing?
● What actions can you or the people in your community take to reduce risks and problems from these diseases on campus? In your homes? In your communities?

Throughout all age groups up to age 75, women have more COPD than men; after age 75, men have higher rates. Up to 90 percent of persons with COPD have a history of smoking.[4] Other risk factors include exposure to air pollution, secondhand smoke, occupational and industrial dusts and chemicals, heredity, and other lung irritants, including childhood respiratory infections. Usually,

COPD develops over time; however, one big dose of superheated air or another lung-damaging event can cause it.

There is no cure for COPD; however, there is much that can be done to prevent it, including quitting smoking and avoiding secondhand smoke. In addition, be sure to read labels when spraying chemicals and cleaning products and wear protective masks and equipment to avoid toxic exposure. If you have symptoms, don't wait. See a doctor for advice on what options are available to prevent further damage. For instance, the **Be Healthy, Be Green** box describes ways to minimize exposure to household chemicals.

Bronchitis Bronchitis involves inflammation and eventual scarring of the lining of the bronchial tubes (*bronchi*) that connect the windpipe to the lungs. When the bronchi become inflamed or infected with bacteria, less air is able to flow from the lungs and heavy mucus begins to form. Although some mucus is normal and necessary, bronchitis sufferers typically have numerous coughing spasms in a day as they try to rid their bodies of phlegm. Frequent

bronchitis Inflammation of the lining of the bronchial tubes.

emphysema A respiratory disease in which the alveoli become distended or ruptured and are no longer functional.

alveoli Tiny air sacs of the lungs where gas exchange occurs (oxygen enters the body and carbon dioxide is removed).

asthma A chronic respiratory disease characterized by attacks of wheezing, shortness of breath, and coughing spasms.

clearing of the throat, a sensation of tightness in the chest, back pain, and shortness of breath are other bronchitis symptoms.

Inhaling certain chemicals, cigarette smoke, and fumes from hairsprays and many other substances can trigger bronchitis. The more common *acute bronchitis* is often caused by other infectious diseases. Symptoms often begin to go away in a week or two once the sources are removed and any inflammation and infections are treated.

When the symptoms of bronchitis last for at least 3 months of the year for 2 consecutive years, the condition is considered *chronic bronchitis*. In some cases, this chronic inflammation and irritation goes undiagnosed for years, particularly in smokers who feel it's a normal part of their lives. By the time these individuals receive medical care, the damage to their lungs is severe and may lead to heart and respiratory failure or to a chronic need to carry oxygen to aid in breathing. Coal miners, grain handlers, metalworkers, painters, and others exposed to fumes, dusts, and hazards are particularly susceptible. Nearly 10 million Americans suffer from chronic bronchitis; 33 percent are under age 45.[5]

To help prevent the problems associated with bronchitis, stop smoking, avoid particulates that trigger bronchitis attacks, and see a doctor promptly if you have recurrent symptoms. Prescription drugs can reduce inflammation, prevent mucus buildup, and stop secondary bacterial infections from setting in. Avoid smoke-filled bars or other settings where you could make your situation worse. If the pollution index is high, stay indoors, make sure windows and doors are closed, and use air filtration systems.

Emphysema Over 4.3 million Americans suffer from **emphysema**. Emphysema was historically a "man's disease," but today more women than men are diagnosed with emphysema.[6] Emphysema involves the gradual, irreversible destruction of the **alveoli** (tiny air sacs through which gas exchange occurs) of the lungs. Destruction of the alveoli walls impairs the transfer of oxygen and carbon dioxide into and out of the blood and makes the lungs less elastic, which makes it harder to breathe. As the alveoli are destroyed, the affected person finds it more and more difficult to exhale.

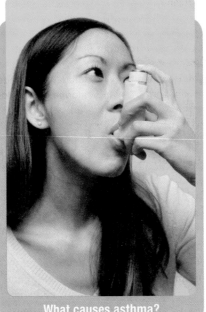

What causes asthma?

Asthma is caused by inflammation of the airways in the lungs, restricting them and leading to wheezing, chest tightness, shortness of breath, and coughing. In most people, asthma is brought on by contact with allergens or irritants in the air; some people also have exercise-induced asthma. People with asthma can generally control their symptoms through the use of inhaled medications, and most asthmatics keep a "rescue" inhaler of bronchodilating medication on hand to use in case of a flare-up.

People with emphysema liken this experience to engaging in heavy exercise while breathing through a straw. What most of us take for granted—the easy, rhythmic flow of air in and out of the lungs—becomes a continuous, anxious, and life-threatening struggle.

The cause of emphysema is uncertain. There is, however, a strong relationship between emphysema and long-term cigarette smoking and exposure to air pollution. (See **Chapter 12** for more on the connection between smoking and emphysema.) To avoid emphysema, don't smoke. If you smoke, quit. If you can't quit, reduce consumption and keep trying to quit. Avoid occupational exposure that involves inhaling chemicals and fumes. If you must take a job that involves inhaling toxins, use appropriate protection.

Whether you have emphysema, or have a family member or loved one who does, a key to coping is to make sure the patient complies with doctor's orders. Prescribed medications must be taken. Healthy meals, exercise, stress management, and adequate rest are imperative to keep the body functioning at maximum capacity, not to mention keeping depression at bay. Many persons on oxygen supplementation become depressed and irritable. You may need to suggest counseling or help from social services. Support groups can be very helpful, as well as respite care for the caregiver.

Although it is easy to blame the victim, particularly someone who has smoked for decades, remember that this is not a time for blame. Ensuring quality of life is imperative.

Asthma

Asthma is a long-term, chronic inflammatory disorder that blocks airflow into and out of the lungs. Asthma causes tiny airways in the lung to overreact with spasms in response to certain triggers (**Figure 17.2** on page 527). Symptoms include wheezing, difficulty breathing, shortness of breath, and coughing spasms. Although most asthma attacks are mild, severe attacks can trigger bronchospasms (contractions of the bronchial tubes in the lungs) that are so severe that, without rapid treatment, death may occur. Between attacks, most people have few symptoms. Approximately 28 million people in the United States have asthma. It is the most common chronic disease of childhood, affecting nearly 10 percent of all children in the United States today.[7]

Asthma falls into two distinctly different types. The more common form, *extrinsic* or *allergic asthma*, is typically associated with allergic triggers; it tends to run in families and develop in childhood. Often by adulthood, a person has few episodes, or the disorder completely goes away. The less common form of asthma, *intrinsic* or *nonallergic asthma,* may be triggered by anything except an allergy.

Several factors, including medical conditions, foods and medicines, animal dander and saliva, mold, pests in the home or school/work environment, exercise, smoke, food allergies, weather, pollen, and air pollution trigger asthma flare-ups. In fact, even emotions such as anger, fear, or stress can result in an asthma attack.[8] Genetics may play a role in asthma development. If your mom or dad has asthma, or if family members have a history of allergies, asthma is more likely. If you had respiratory infections when you were younger, such as colds, the flu, or sinus infections, or if you are exposed to environmental allergens and irritants, you are more likely to develop asthma.[9] In some individuals, stress, exercise, certain medications, cold air, and or sulfites are also potential triggers. Interestingly, 1 in 5 asthmatics can suffer an attack from taking aspirin, leading to the terminology, "aspirin-induced asthma." Certain fever reducers or anti-inflammatory drugs may also be triggers. Some people may have asthma attacks triggered by strong odors, such as perfumes or cleaning agents.[10]

Asthma can occur at any age but is most likely to appear between infancy and age 5 and in adults before age 40. In childhood, asthma strikes more boys than girls; in adulthood, it strikes more women than men. The asthma rate is 50 percent higher among African Americans than whites, and four times as many African Americans die of asthma as do whites.[11] Asthma rates have increased over 30 percent in the last 20 years. Even with advances in treatment, asthma deaths have continued to rise, with nearly 3,500 deaths last year in the United States.[12] Many believe that today's homes contain more triggers (such as dust mites in mattresses, chemicals in carpets and furniture, and air-tight buildings for efficient cooling and heating).

25%

of all school absences are due to asthma.

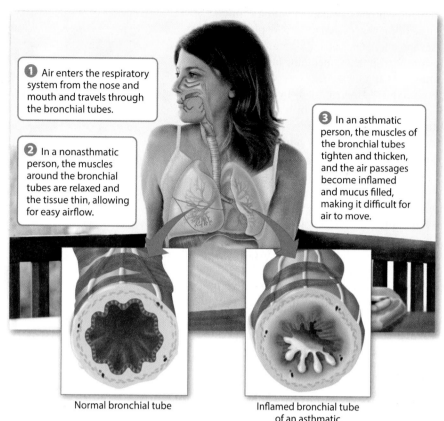

① Air enters the respiratory system from the nose and mouth and travels through the bronchial tubes.

② In a nonasthmatic person, the muscles around the bronchial tubes are relaxed and the tissue thin, allowing for easy airflow.

③ In an asthmatic person, the muscles of the bronchial tubes tighten and thicken, and the air passages become inflamed and mucus filled, making it difficult for air to move.

Normal bronchial tube

Inflamed bronchial tube of an asthmatic

FIGURE 17.2 Asthma Is an Inflammation of the Airways within the Lungs

Video Tutor: Lungs During an Asthma Attack

The **Skills for Behavior Change** box on page 529 suggests ways to reduce potential asthma and allergy triggers. In addition to avoiding triggers, finding the most effective medications can help asthmatics cope with their condition and avoid severe attacks.

Coping with Allergies

Allergies are diseases characterized by an overreaction of the immune system to a foreign protein substance (*allergen* or *antigen*) that is swallowed, breathed into the lungs, injected, or touched.[13] When foreign pathogens such as bacteria or viruses enter the body, the body responds by producing antibodies to destroy these invaders. Normally, antibody production is a positive element in the body's defense system. However, for unknown reasons, sometimes the body develops an overly elaborate protective mechanism against relatively harmless substances. The resulting *hypersensitivity reaction* to specific allergens or antigens in the environment is fairly common, as

allergies Hypersensitivity reactions in which the body produces antibodies to a normally harmless substance in the environment.

anyone who has awakened with a runny nose or itchy eyes can attest. People with severe allergies can suffer much more extreme responses, including hives, vomiting, and anaphylaxis.

Allergies are grouped by the kind of trigger, time of year, or where symptoms appear on the body into *outdoor* or *indoor allergies, food and drug allergies, latex allergies, insect allergies, skin allergies,* and *eye allergies.*[14] Environmental triggers can include molds, animal dander, pollen, grasses, ragweed, or dust. Other triggers include foods such as peanuts, shellfish, or milk; insect bites; and medicines (both over-the-counter [OTC] and prescription drugs). Once excessive antibodies to these antigens are produced, they, in turn, trigger the release of **histamine,** a chemical substance that dilates blood vessels, increases mucous secretions, swells tissues, and produces other allergy symptoms, particularly in the respiratory system (Figure 17.3). Many people have found that **immunotherapy** treatment, or "allergy shots," somewhat reduce the severity of their symptoms. In most cases, once the offending antigen is removed, allergy-prone people suffer few symptoms.

More than half (54.6 %) of all Americans test positive for one or more allergens, and at least 50 percent of homes have at least six allergens present. Allergic disease affects as many as 40 to 50 million people in the United States. Asthma (discussed above) is a unique disease in that it is typically considered to be both a key respiratory disease, as well as one of the major allergic diseases.[15] Prevention of allergies usually is focused on preventing exposure to things that cause you to react. If you are exposed, treatments may be as simple as quickly washing off the substance you came in contact with, taking antihistamines or getting shots to avoid serious reactions, and working with your doctor to come up with a treatment regimen that will work best for you.

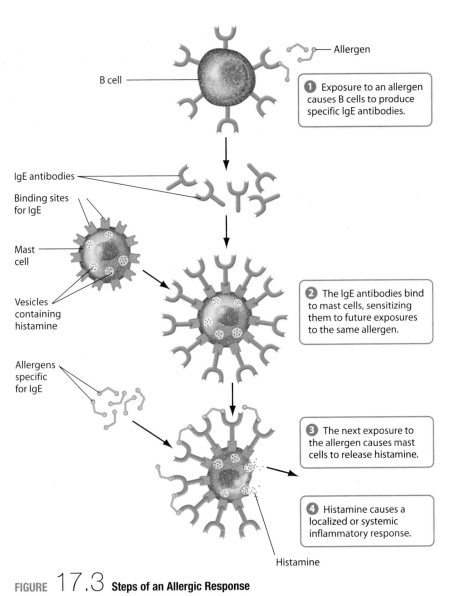

1 Exposure to an allergen causes B cells to produce specific IgE antibodies.

2 The IgE antibodies bind to mast cells, sensitizing them to future exposures to the same allergen.

3 The next exposure to the allergen causes mast cells to release histamine.

4 Histamine causes a localized or systemic inflammatory response.

FIGURE 17.3 **Steps of an Allergic Response**

Source: Adapted from Johnson, Michael D., *Human Biology: Concepts and Current Issues,* 5th, © 2010. Printed and electronically reproduced by permission of Pearson Education, Inc., Upper Saddle River, New Jersey.

histamine Chemical substance that dilates blood vessels, increases mucus secretions, and triggers other allergy symptoms.

immunotherapy Treatment strategies based on the concept of regulating the immune system, as by administering antibodies or desensitization shots of allergens.

hay fever A chronic allergy-related respiratory disorder that is most prevalent when ragweed and flowers bloom.

Hay Fever

Hay fever, or *pollen allergy,* occurs throughout the world and is one of the most common chronic diseases in the United States, affecting nearly 18 million

adults and over 7 million children each year.[16] It is usually considered a seasonal disease because it is most prevalent when ragweed and flowers are blooming. Hay fever attacks are characterized by sneezing and itchy, watery eyes and nose, and they make countless people miserable for weeks at a time every year. As with other allergies, hay fever results from an overzealous immune system that is hypersensitive to certain substances. You are more likely to have hay fever if you have a family history of allergies, are male, were born during pollen season, are a firstborn child, were exposed to cigarette smoke during your first year of life, or are exposed to dust mites.

The best way to prevent hay fever is to avoid its environmental triggers. If you can't prevent it, there are numerous treatments available, including *nasal corticosteroid sprays* that reduce inflammation; *antihistamines* that help with itching, sneezing, and runny nose, but may not work when you are "stuffed up"; *decongestants,* available in a variety of

Preventing Asthma Attacks

Although asthma rates continue to increase around the world, there is much that individuals and communities can do to reduce risk:

〉 Purchase a good air filter for your home, and clean furnace filters regularly. If you have a fireplace or wood-burning stove, check it regularly to make sure that it is not spewing smoke and particulate matter.

〉 Wash pillows and sheets regularly. Use pillow protectors and mattress protectors. Don't purchase used mattresses, which may be teeming with mites.

〉 If you're a pet lover but animal dander bothers you, try a nonshedding breed of dog or cat. Keep pets off your bed, and wash them and their bedding weekly. Vacuum up their shed hair regularly.

〉 Keep your home clean and pest free; cockroaches and other vermin have enzymes in their saliva or particles on their bodies that may trigger allergic reactions. Use a high-suction vacuum rather than a broom to reduce dust particles suspended in the air.

〉 Use anti-mold cleaners or run a dehumidifier to keep moisture levels down and reduce the growth of mold.

〉 Avoid mowing the lawn or other activities leading to excessive outdoor exposure to pollen during high-pollen times. If you must be outdoors, wear a pollen mask.

〉 Exercise regularly to keep your lungs functioning well.

〉 Avoid cigarette, cigar, and pipe smoke.

〉 Keep asthma medications handy. Let people close to you know that you are asthmatic, and educate them about what to do if you have an asthma attack.

〉 Investigate local regulations on the burning of household and yard trash, field burning, wood-burning stoves, and secondhand smoke from cigarettes—all known triggers for asthma attacks—and work to revise them as necessary.

forms and prescriptions; and *desensitizing injections* that provide more powerful relief of symptoms. Many of these aids come with side effects and should be carefully monitored, particularly in long-term use. More simple treatments include reducing exposure to allergens by using air purifiers and air filters on furnaces and air conditioners, wearing masks during high-pollen-count days, or using neti pots or similar devices to rinse your nose and clear nasal passages, can also be helpful.

Food Allergies

A **food allergy** is an immune response to food. It should not be confused with **food intolerance,** which is the inability to digest a particular food due to problems with the physical, hormonal, or biochemical systems in your digestive tract. While 1 in 3 people thinks that a family member has food allergies and changes the family's diet because of it, only about 5 percent of children and 4 to 5 percent of teens and adults really have one! Instead of having food allergies, they may lack specific enzymes necessary to digest certain foods, such as lactose (see the section on digestion-related disorders later in this chapter). Others may think they have an allergy when they are reacting to specific pathogens in the food and really have a foodborne illness. True allergies for adults are most often triggered by milk, eggs, peanuts and other nuts, soybeans, wheat, fish, and shellfish. Children are more likely to have allergies to eggs, milk, and peanuts, and while children may outgrow their allergies, adults usually do not.[17]

Symptoms of a food allergy are similar to other allergies and may include swelling in the mouth or esophagus, difficulty breathing, itching, stomach pain, diarrhea, dizziness, or nausea. The reaction can be so severe that the victim goes into *anaphylactic shock,* with a rapid heart rate, changes in blood pressure, swelling of the tongue or throat, breathing difficulties, and death. Over 200 Americans die each year from food allergies, and another 30,000 or more end up in the emergency room because of their symptoms. Millions more suffer from allergies without knowing why they don't feel well or have a bit of itching after eating.[18]

Although some food allergies can be outgrown, there is no cure. If you do have an allergy, you can avoid many reactions by reading labels, asking questions in restaurants, and knowing exactly what you are eating. Wear a medical alert bracelet or necklace that says you have food allergies, and let your friends, family members, and instructors know that

food allergy An immune response against a specific food that the majority of people can eat without problem.

food intolerance Difficulty or inability to digest certain foods due to problems with the physical, hormonal, or biochemical systems in your digestive tract. Dairy (lactose) and gluten (wheat protein) are common food intolerances.

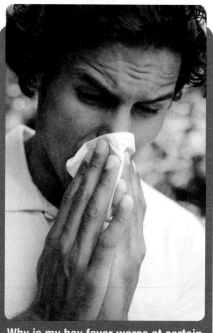

Why is my hay fever worse at certain times of the year?

Hay fever is triggered by the pollen from ragweed, a plant most common in the Northeast, Midwest, and South. It produces most of its pollen in the fall, making this the hardest time of year for many allergy sufferers. Steps you can take to minimize your exposure include keeping windows closed, staying indoors when pollen counts are highest (typically 10 AM to 4 PM), and changing clothes after spending time outdoors.

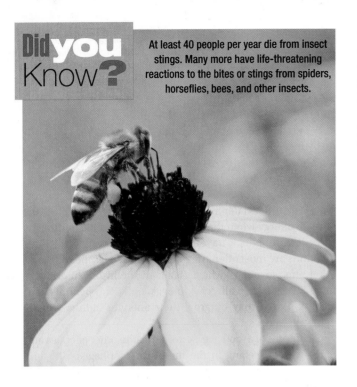
you react to certain foods. Carry antihistamines or auto-injector devices containing epinephrine (adrenaline) so that you can quickly respond in the event of accidental exposure.

Coping with Neurological Disorders

More than 600 disorders can affect the nervous system, and an estimated 50 million Americans are afflicted with them each year.[19] Some of these disorders, such as migraine headaches and epilepsy, are well known, but there are others known only to those who suffer from them and still others that elude diagnosis. (See the **Health Headlines** box on page 532 for pain treatment options).

Headaches

Millions of people see their doctors for headaches each year, and millions more silently put up with the pain or take pain relievers to blunt their symptoms. The good news is that most of the time headaches are not the sign of a serious disease and go away fairly quickly. Most headaches are tension-type headaches or migraines, whereas some are specific to certain underlying causes; see **Table 17.1** for a summary of the latter.

migraine A condition characterized by localized headaches that possibly result from alternating dilation and constriction of blood vessels.

Tension-Type Headaches
Nearly 80 percent of adults have the most common type of headache, *tension-type headache,* during their lives, with women having slightly more than men. Most cases occur after the age of 40.[20] Symptoms include dull, aching head pain; a sensation of tightness or pressure across the forehead, sides, and back of your head; tenderness on the scalp, neck, and shoulder muscles; and, occasionally, loss of appetite.[21]

The cause(s) of tension headaches remain unknown. Tension-type headaches were typically thought to be caused by tension in the neck, face or head; however, that theory remains in question. Today, a more widely accepted theory is that tension headaches are caused by some type of faulty or overactive pain receptors in the brain. There is a wide range in the frequency and severity of symptoms, with occurrences categorized as episodic (occurring less than once a month and triggered by stress, anxiety, fatigue, or anger); frequent (occurring 1 to 15 days per month along with migraines); and chronic (occurring more than 15 days per month, with varying pain). Possible triggers include stress, depression and anxiety, jaw clenching, poor posture, working in an awkward position or holding a position. Red wine, lack of sleep, extreme fasting, hormonal changes, and certain food additives or preservatives have also been implicated.[22]

Tension-type headaches are most often prevented by reducing triggers. If stress is a trigger, try to relax with a hot bath, relaxing music, hot compresses, massage, or other relaxation techniques. Exercise can relieve some types of tension headaches, while aspirin, ibuprofen, acetaminophen, and naproxen sodium remain the standby forms of pain relief. If headaches occur more frequently and are difficult to treat with OTC medications, they are probably *chronic tension headaches*—the result of physical or psychological problems or depression. These more difficult forms of tension headaches warrant a visit to the doctor to assess the underlying cause.

Migraine Headaches
Nearly 30 million Americans—three times more women than men—suffer from **migraines,** a type of headache that often has debilitating symptoms. Symptoms include moderate to severe pain on one or both sides of the head, head pain with a pulsating or throbbing quality, pain that worsens with physical activity or interferes with regular activity, nausea with or without vomiting, and sensitivity to light and sound.[23] In fact, 1 out of 4 households has a migraine sufferer. Usually, migraine incidence peaks in young adulthood (between ages 20 and 45).[24]

Migraine appears to run in families: If both your parents experience migraines, you have a 75 percent chance of experiencing them, too; if only one parent has them, you have a 50 percent chance. If any of your relatives have them, you have a 20 percent risk.[25]

Whereas all headaches can be painful, migraines can be disabling. Symptoms vary greatly by individual, and attacks can last anywhere from 4 to 72 hours, with distinct phases of symptoms. In about 25 percent of cases, migraines are preceded by a sensory warning sign called an *aura,* which includes flashes of light, flickering vision, blind spots, tingling in arms or legs, or a

what do you think?

Have you ever experienced a migraine or tension-type headache? How did you alleviate the pain?
● What actions can you take to reduce your risks of severe headaches in the future?

Type	Symptoms	Precipitating Factors	Treatment	Prevention
Allergy	Generalized headache. Nasal congestion, watery eyes.	Seasonal allergens such as pollen, molds. Allergies to food are not usually a factor.	Antihistamine medication; topical, nasal cortisone-related sprays, or desensitization injections.	None.
Caffeine-withdrawal	Throbbing headache caused by rebound dilation of the blood vessels, occurring multiple days after consumption of large quantities of caffeine.	Caffeine.	In extreme cases, treat by terminating caffeine consumption.	Avoid excess caffeine.
Cluster	Excruciating pain in vicinity of eye. Tearing of eye, nose congestion, flushing of face. Pain frequently develops during sleep and may last for several hours. Attacks occur every day for weeks/months, then disappear for up to a year. 80% of cluster patients are male, most ages 20–50.	Alcoholic beverages, excessive smoking.	Oxygen, ergotamine, sumatriptan, or intranasal application of local anesthetic agent.	Use of steroids, ergotamine, calcium channel blockers, and lithium.
Exertion	Generalized head pain of short duration (minutes to 1 hour) during or following physical exertion (running, jumping, or sexual intercourse) or passive exertion (sneezing, coughing, moving one's bowels, etc.).	10% caused by organic diseases (aneurysms, tumors, or blood vessel malformation). 90% are related to migraine or cluster headaches.	Cause must be accurately determined. Most commonly treated with aspirin, indomethacin, or propranolol. Extensive testing is necessary to determine the headache cause. Surgery to correct organic disease is occasionally indicated.	Alternative forms of exercise. Avoid jarring exercises.
Eyestrain	Usually frontal, bilateral pain, directly related to eyestrain. Rare cause of headache.	Muscle imbalance. Uncorrected vision, astigmatism.	Correction of vision.	Same as treatment.
Hangover	Migraine-like symptoms of throbbing pain and nausea not localized to one side.	Alcohol, which causes dilation and irritation of the blood vessels of the brain and surrounding tissue.	Liquids (including broth). Consumption of fructose (honey, tomato juice are good sources) to help burn alcohol.	Drink alcohol only in moderation.
Hunger	Pain strikes just before mealtime. Caused by muscle tension, low blood sugar, and rebound dilation of the blood vessels, oversleeping, or missing a meal.	Strenuous dieting or skipping meals.	Regular, nourishing meals containing adequate protein and complex carbohydrates.	Same as treatment.
New daily persistent headache (NDPH)	This headache can best be described as the rapid development (less than 3 days) of unrelenting headache, and typically presents in a person with no past history of a headache.	Typically NDPH does not evolve from migraine or episodic tension-type headache. NDPH begins as a new headache. It may be the result of a viral infection.	In some cases, NPDH can resolve on its own within several months. Other cases persist and are more refractory.	Does not respond to traditional options. However, antiseizure medications, topiramate, or gabapentin can be used.
Sinus	Gnawing pain over nasal area, often increasing in severity throughout the day. Caused by acute infection, usually with fever, producing blockage of sinus ducts and preventing normal drainage. Sinus headaches are rare. Migraine and cluster headaches are often misdiagnosed as sinus in origin.	Infection, nasal polyps, anatomical deformities, such as a deviated septum, that block the sinus ducts.	Treat with antibiotics, decongestants, surgical drainage if necessary.	None

Source: Adapted from "The Complete Headache Chart," 2010, www.headaches.org. Reprinted by permission of the National Headache Foundation.

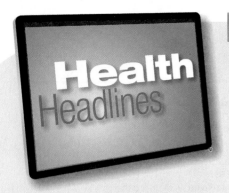
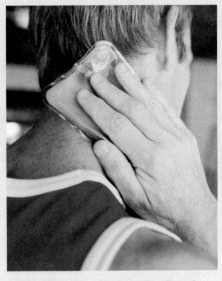
epilepsy A neurological disorder caused by abnormal electrical brain activity; can be accompanied by altered consciousness or convulsions.

sensation of odor or taste.[26] The triggers of a migraine vary widely from one person to the next. Although vascular abnormalities in the brain have long been thought to be underlying causes, experts are beginning to believe that migraines may be triggered within the brain itself as a result of a complex biochemical and inflammatory process.[27]

When true migraines occur, relaxation is only minimally effective as a treatment. Often, prescription pain relievers are necessary. See your doctor for more information or go to the National Headache Foundation website (www.headaches.org) for the latest information on treatments.

Cluster Headaches The severe pain of a cluster headache has been described as "killer" or "suicidal" headache Usually these headaches cause excruciating, stabbing pain on one side of the head, behind the eye, or in one defined spot. Fortunately, cluster headaches are relatively rare, affecting less than 1 percent of people, usually men. Young adults in their twenties tend to be particularly susceptible.[28]

Cluster headaches can last for weeks and disappear quickly. However, more commonly, they last for 40 to 90 minutes and often occur in the middle of the night, usually during rapid eye movement (REM) sleep. Oxygen therapy, drugs, and even surgery have been used to treat severe cases.

Seizure Disorders

Approximately 3 million people in the United States suffer from **epilepsy** or some other seizure-related disorder (the word *epilepsy* derives from the Greek *epilepsia,* meaning "seizure"). Each year, some 300,000 people in the United States will have a seizure for the first time, and an estimated 5 to 10 percent of the population will experience at least one seizure in their lives. Over a third of all new seizures this year will occur in people under age 18, with males having a slightly greater risk than females.[29]

Seizure disorders are generally caused by abnormal electrical activ-

70%

of people with epilepsy who take medication remain seizure-free for 5 years or more.

ity in the brain and are characterized by loss of control of muscular activity and unconsciousness. Risk factors include taking certain drugs, withdrawing from drugs, having a high fever and abnormal blood levels of sodium or glucose, or experiencing physical, chemical, or temperature trauma. Symptoms vary widely and can range from temporary confusion to major seizure activity.

Although causes of nearly half of seizure disorders are unknown, likely contributors include stroke, head injury, congenital abnormalities, injury or illness resulting in inflammation of the brain or spinal column, high fever, drug reactions, tumors, nutritional deficiency, and heredity. See the appendix at the end of this book for information on providing first aid to someone experiencing a seizure.

In most cases, people with seizure disorders can lead normal, seizure-free lives as a result of advancements in diagnosis

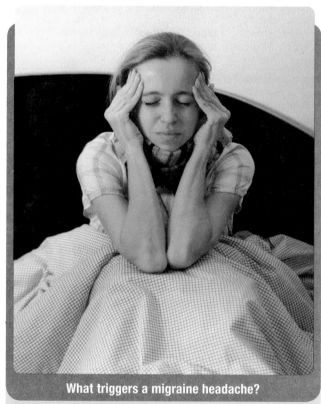

What triggers a migraine headache?

Patients report that migraines can be triggered by emotional stress, fatigue, too much or not enough sleep, fasting, caffeine, chocolate, alcohol, menses, hormone changes, altitude, weather, certain foods, and a litany of other causes. There is tremendous variability in these. What triggers a migraine in one person may relieve it in another.

and treatment. Public ignorance and stigma associated with having these disorders can have a significant impact on sufferers and their families as they cope with the challenges of treatment and daily living.

Coping with Digestion-Related Disorders

Digestive disorders are on the increase in the United States, with more than 95 million people suffering from one or more of these ailments.[30] Unfortunately, the causes of digestive disorders are often complex, symptoms are often subtle, and there is great variability in type of treatment and effectiveness. Two of the most common disorders are *lactose intolerance* and *celiac disease* (gluten intolerance), discussed in **Chapter 7;** disorders that are not related to a specific nutrient are described below. See Table 17.2 on the following page for discussion of gallbladder disease, another common digestive disorder, as well as several other modern maladies.

Inflammatory Bowel Disease

Inflammatory bowel disease (IBD) is an umbrella term for a group of disorders in which the intestines become inflamed. The cause is not known, but the symptoms tend to come and go. Typically, they are severe, with stomach cramping, bloating, pain, and bloody bouts of diarrhea present. People with severe cases may have as many as 20 bouts of bloody diarrhea a day. About 25 percent of those with IBD develop it before age 20, with the majority of additional cases in the 15 to 35 age groups, especially those who have a family history of the disease. Whites and African Americans tend to have similar rates, but Asian Americans have lower rates. More than 1 million people in the United States have been diagnosed, with the majority of cases being whites, particularly persons of Jewish descent. Numbers of cases in African Americans and Latinos are increasing without clear patterns by geographical region.[31] The most common types of IBD are **ulcerative colitis (UC),** which affects the colon and large intestine, and **Crohn's disease,** which can affect any part of the digestive tract from the mouth to the anus.

inflammatory bowel disease (IBD) A group of disorders in which the intestines become inflamed.

ulcerative colitis (UC) An inflammatory disorder that affects the mucous membranes of the large intestine, producing bloody diarrhea.

Crohn's disease An autoimmune inflammatory disease of the gastrointestinal tract characterized by cramping and diarrhea.

Although some experts believe that colitis occurs more frequently in people with high stress levels, this theory is controversial. Smokers have a higher risk of UC, as do those who have had measles and certain bacterial infections. Hypersensitive reactions to certain foods are also a possible cause. Determining the cause of colitis is difficult because the disease can go into remission and then recur without apparent reason. This pattern often continues over periods of years and may be related to the later development of colorectal cancer.

TABLE
17.2 | **Other Modern Maladies**

Disease	Who's Affected?	Causes and Risk Factors	Symptoms	Treatment	Prevention
Fibromyalgia Extreme fatigue; painful, aching joints and muscles.	Affects 3%–7% of population. Rates increase with age.	Unknown. Affects primarily women in their 30s and 40s.	Numbness, tingling, pain, headache, dizziness.	Pain medications, anti-inflammatories, rest, stress management.	Rest, dietary adjustments. Avoid extreme temperatures.
Gallbladder diseases Most common are cholecystitis (inflammation) and cholelithiasis (gallstones).	50% of women and 80% of men by age 75. Highest in Mexican Americans and Native Americans.	Chemical exposure, infections, traumatic injury, obesity, cirrhosis of liver, rapid weight loss, diabetes, cholesterol-lowering drugs.	Acute pain in the upper right quadrant of abdomen, particularly after eating fatty food; nausea, vomiting. Often asymptomatic.	Medications to relieve inflammation or cause of inflammation; removal of gallstones through lithotripsy or surgery.	Reduce dietary fat; avoid alcohol, fried foods, whole grains.
Multiple sclerosis Degenerative, autoimmune neurological disease caused by breakdown of protective sheath around nerves.	Over 400,000 cases, most between ages of 20 and 40. Overall risk for general population is 1 in 800.	Suspected causes include genetics, viruses, allergies, and environmental toxins. Caucasians are at greatest risk.	From minor numbness, blurred vision, fatigue, balance issues to severe disability. Intermittent course for some.	No cure, but drug therapy, climate change, and lifestyle choices can reduce symptoms and increase healthy years.	Flare up prevention possible with healthy lifestyle, adequate sleep, healthy diet, stress management, and avoidance of temperature extremes.
Parkinson's disease Chronic, progressive, neurological disease that affects motor function.	50,000–60,000 new cases/year. Nearly 2 million total, mostly over age 50.	Cause currently unknown.	Tremors of limbs and head; rigidity, postural instability, slowness, balance issues, shuffling gait; speech difficulties.	No cure, but medications can relieve symptoms. Deep brain stimulation and gamma knife surgery may help.	None obvious. Healthy lifestyle may help slow progression.
Raynaud's syndrome Exaggerated constriction of small arteries in the extremities.	5%–10% of adults, primarily women.	Unknown.	Fingers and toes become numb, turn white or purple; throbbing pain.	Topical medications to reduce symptoms.	More common in those exposed to extreme cold repeatedly, so avoid frostbite or medications that affect blood flow.
Rosacea Inflammatory skin condition causing redness and small red bumps or pustules on the face.	Affects over 14 million Americans; more common in menopausal women and people with fair skin/sensitive skin.	Still unknown, many suspects, ranging from genetic predisposition to blushing, skin mites, bacteria. None conclusive.	Can progress from flushing and spider veins on face to lumps and bumps. Skin thickening, red itchy eyes, bulbous nose in later stages.	No cure, but controls include prescription medications and lotions, less irritating soaps, surgery, laser treatments, freezing.	Unknown.
Systemic lupus erythematosus Autoimmune disease in which antibodies destroy or injure organs such as kidneys, brain, and heart.	1 in 700 Caucasians, 1 in 250 African Americans. 90% of patients are women between ages 18 and 45. Ratio of females to males is 10:1.	Cause unknown. Possible genetic predisposition combined with environment and hormones.	Sensitivity to light, arthritis, swelling, tendency toward increased infections, butterfly-shaped rash across nose and cheeks.	Medications such as steroids to reduce symptoms and complications.	Healthy lifestyle; other possible preventive measures unknown.

Sources: Data are from National Fibromyalgia Association, "About Fibromyalgia," www.fmaware.org/site/PageServer?pagename=fibromyalgia; A. Assumpção et al., "Prevalence of Fibromyalgia in a Low Socioeconomic Status Population," *BMC Musculoskeletal Disorders* 10 (2009): 64–67; K. Maurer, M. Carey, and J. Fox, "Roles of Infection, Inflammation, and Immune System in Cholesterol Gallstone Formation," *Gastroenterology* 136, no. 2 (2009): 425–40; eMedicineHealth, "Gallstones," www.emedicinehealth.com/gallstones/article_em.htm; WebMD, "Cholecystitis: Overview," www.webmd.com/digestive-disorders/tc/cholecystitis-overview; National Multiple Sclerosis Society, "Who Gets MS?," www.nationalmssociety.org/about-multiple-sclerosis/what-we-know-about-ms/who-gets-ms/index.aspx; P. Sweeney, Cleveland Clinic, Center for Continuing Education, "Parkinson's Disease," www.clevelandclinicmeded.com/medicalpubs/diseasemanagement/neurology/parkinsons-disease; The National Rosacea Society, "The Many Faces of Rosacea," http://rosacea.org/patients/faces.php; What Health?, "Rosacea Statistics," www.whathealth.com/rosacea/incidence.html; P. Schur and B. Hahn, "Epidemiology and Pathogenesis of Systemic Lupus Erythematosus," www.uptodate.com/patients/content/topic.do?topicKey=~/3ljrinen9.

Because the cause is unknown, it is important to treat symptoms and avoid substances that may trigger attacks. Treatment focuses on relieving the symptoms by decreasing foods that are hard to digest (raw vegetables, seeds, nuts, and high-fiber foods); taking probiotics; and taking anti-inflammatory drugs, steroids, and other medications to reduce inflammation and soothe irritated intestinal walls.

Crohn's disease is an inflammatory bowel disease usually diagnosed in men and women in their twenties and thirties. It can affect any part of the digestive system but most commonly occurs in the small intestine. It is characterized by intense stomach pain, often in the lower right area, fever, weight loss, joint pain, mouth ulcers, and watery diarrhea. Bleeding may also occur and can be serious enough to cause anemia, fatigue, and immune system dysfunction. The most common complication is actually bowel obstruction due to swelling and scar tissue and ulcers that erode and form little infection-prone out-pouches known as fistula. Those diagnosed with this disease must carefully monitor their diet to ensure adequate nutrition, be "tuned in" to their body and changes that may occur, see their doctors if symptoms develop, and take medications to reduce inflammation and prevent infection.[32]

Irritable Bowel Syndrome (IBS)

Inflammatory bowel disease (IBD) and **irritable bowel syndrome (IBS)** are not the same condition, although they may sound as if they were. Irritable bowel syndrome is a functional bowel disorder (affecting how the bowel works, hence the term *spastic colon*). The exact cause is unknown, but in individuals with IBS, the normal muscular contractions in the intestines don't work properly and food isn't processed or eliminated as it should be.[33]

IBD is used to describe a wide range of conditions where the intestinal tract is chronically inflamed. A unique aspect of both diseases is that they tend to be diseases of early adulthood, occurring most often in people between the ages of 18 and 35 years.[34]

Irritable bowel syndrome may begin after an infection, a stressful life event, or onset of maturity without any other medical indicators. Characterized by nausea, pain, gas, diarrhea, bloating, or cramps after eating certain foods or during unusual stress, IBS can be uncomfortable, but usually does not permanently harm the intestines unless symptoms are severe. Symptoms may vary from week to week and can fade for long periods of time, only to return. Researchers suspect that people with IBS have digestive systems that are overly sensitive to what they eat and drink, to stress, and to certain hormonal changes. Often, because symptoms are so similar to other gastrointestinal tract diseases, IBS is only diagnosed after all the other gastrointestinal diseases have been ruled out. It occurs more often in women than in men, and it is a disease of younger adults, often occurring before the age of 35.[35]

Although there is no cure for IBS, treatments to attempt to relieve symptoms, stress management, relaxation techniques, regular activity, and diet changes can control it in the vast majority of cases. Problems with diarrhea can be reduced by cutting down on fat and avoiding caffeine and sorbitol, a sweetener found in diet foods and chewing gum. Constipation can be relieved by a gradual increase in fiber and increased fluid consumption. Some sufferers benefit from drugs that relax the intestinal muscle or from antidepressant drugs and counseling to reduce stress.

irritable bowel syndrome (IBS) Nausea, pain, gas, or diarrhea caused by certain foods or stress.
gastroesophageal reflux disease (GERD) Chronic condition in which stomach acid backflows into the esophagus, causing heartburn and potential damage to the esophagus.

Gastroesophageal Reflux Disease

Gastroesophageal reflux disease (GERD), commonly referred to as *heartburn* or *acid reflux*, affects millions of people throughout the world. Risk factors include age, diet, alcohol use, obesity, pregnancy, and smoking. At any given time, people of all ages and stages of life suffer from a sensation of heartburn, or backflow of stomach acid into the esophagus, characterized by discomfort or a burning sensation behind the breastbone. Symptoms usually occur after a meal and can include coughing, choking, heartburn, or vomiting. When these symptoms are severe and occur more than two to three times per week, GERD is often the diagnosis.

Prevention of GERD focuses on determining which foods or beverages trigger symptoms (coffee, sodas, high-acid food and juices, and alcohol are the big culprits) and avoiding spicy or fried foods. Dietary control is often a key in reducing heartburn symptoms. Also, it is important to find out whether there are mechanical causes of reflux, such as sleeping or sitting in positions that exacerbate symptoms. It may be helpful to elevate your upper body if acid rushes into the esophagus when you lie down. If repositioning doesn't work, taking medications to reduce stomach acids can help. If heartburn persists, see your doctor.

Coping with Musculoskeletal Diseases

Musculoskeletal diseases—including back pain, arthritis, bodily injuries, and osteoporosis—are more common than any other health condition in the United States.[36] In the past year, over 108 million adults, or 1 in every 2 age 18 or over, suffered from a musculoskeletal condition lasting 3 months or longer. These conditions cost over $850 billion annually in treatment and lost wages. More than half of all days of work missed due to a major medical condition result from musculoskeletal problems such as joint pain, arthritis, and back/neck pain (**Figure 17.4** on page 536). Because of musculoskeletal diseases, over 15 million adults are unable to perform at least one activity of daily living, such as self-care, walking, or getting out of a chair or bed, on a regular basis.[37] With each decade, these numbers have gotten worse. Sedentary lifestyle and obesity are listed as major contributors to this growing epidemic.[38]

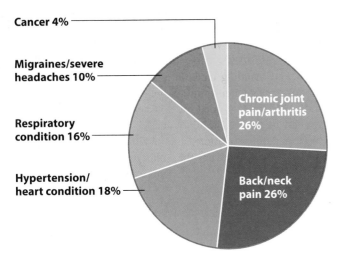

Cancer 4%

Migraines/severe headaches 10%

Respiratory condition 16%

Hypertension/ heart condition 18%

Chronic joint pain/arthritis 26%

Back/neck pain 26%

FIGURE 17.4 **Proportion of Lost Work Days for Persons Age 18 and Older by Major Medical Condition**

Source: © 2008, American Academy of Orthopaedic Surgeons, Modified with permission from The Burden of Musculoskeletal Diseases in the United States. Source of data: National Center for Health Statistics, National Health Interview Survey, Adult Sample, 2005.

Arthritis and Related Conditions

Called "the nation's primary crippler," **arthritis** strikes 1 in 5 Americans, or over 47 million people.[39] Symptoms range from the occasional tendinitis of the weekend athlete to the horrific pain of rheumatoid arthritis. There are over 100 types of arthritis diagnosed today, the most common of which are osteoarthritis and rheumatoid arthritis. Each year arthritis accounts for over 30 million lost workdays and costs the U.S. economy over $282 billion in treatments.[40] Add in the cost of lost wages and productivity, prescriptions, and OTC pain relief medications and the numbers skyrocket. Unfortunately, as epidemic rates of obesity and sedentary lifestyle contribute to the development of arthritis, by 2030 over 67 million Americans age 18 and over will be diagnosed with the disease, a number that will have staggering consequences for our health care system.[41]

arthritis Painful inflammatory disease of the joints.

osteoarthritis (OA) Progressive deterioration of bones and joints that has been associated with the wear-and-tear theory of aging.

rheumatoid arthritis An autoimmune inflammatory joint disease.

Osteoarthritis Also called *degenerative joint disease,* **osteoarthritis (OA)** is the most common form of arthritis. If you notice that your parents or grandparents are slow to get up or walk stiffly after getting out of bed, they may be showing the early signs of OA. Over 27 million adults in the United States have this disease, most of whom are women.[42] This progressive deterioration of cartilage, bones, and joints has been associated with the "wear-and-tear" theory of aging.

Although age and injury are undoubtedly factors in osteoarthritis, heredity, abnormal joint use, diet, abnormalities in joint structure, and impaired blood supply to the joint may also contribute. For most people, anti-inflammatory drugs and pain relievers such as aspirin and cortisone-related agents ease discomfort. In some sufferers, applications of heat, mild exercise, and massage also relieve the pain. When joints become so distorted that they impair activity, surgical intervention is often necessary. Joint replacement and bone fusion are increasingly common.

Rheumatoid Arthritis The most crippling form of arthritis, **rheumatoid arthritis** is an autoimmune disease involving chronic inflammation. It is most common in young adults, particularly those between the ages of 20 and 45, and affects more than 2.1 million Americans.[43] Symptoms include stiffness, pain, redness, and swelling of multiple joints, particularly those of the hands and wrists, and can be gradually progressive or sporadic, with occasional unexplained remissions. Although the cause of rheumatoid arthritis is unknown, some theorists believe that invading microorganisms take over the joint and cause the immune system to begin attacking the body's own tissues. Exposure to toxic chemicals and stress are also possible triggers. Genetic markers that seem to increase risk have also been identified. Regardless of the cause, treat-

what do you think?

Do you know anyone who currently has problems with arthritis?

● Which joints seem to be most affected?

● What factors do you think might have contributed to their problems?

● What could they have done to reduce their risks?

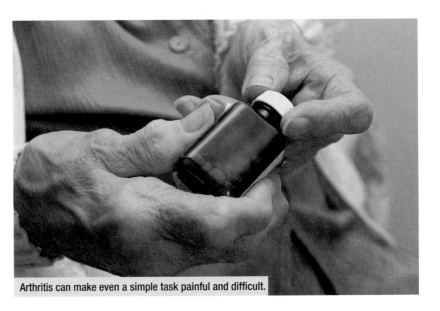

Arthritis can make even a simple task painful and difficult.

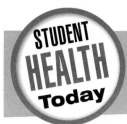

STUDENT HEALTH Today

COLLEGE STUDENTS AND LOW BACK PAIN: OH, MY ACHING BACKPACK?

Did you know that more than half of your college peers suffer from back problems? Why are there so many issues with the back? Although athletics, exercise regimens, sitting for hours while studying, and other normal activities can cause problems, modern conveniences may also be a huge factor. Look no further than the backpacks, messenger bags, and supersized purses in vogue today. Laptops, books, bottled water, wallets, MP3 players, smartphones, headphones, cell phones, snacks, and a change of shoes or a T-shirt are but a few of the items that can be found in the typical "portable locker" students tote on their backs. Not surprisingly, lugging such an assortment around each day can inflame muscles and other soft tissues. According to one study, 85 percent of college students report neck or back pain attributable to carrying heavy backpacks or laptops.

Whereas hikers have long recognized the importance of internal frames and heavy-duty hip straps to displace the weight of heavy packs, most college students carry less supportive (and cheaper) daypacks that contain as much as 30 to 40 pounds of stuff, supported with only a shoulder strap. Over time, this weight can wreak havoc on even the most fit and healthy backs and shoulders. And college students are not alone; even elementary schoolchildren are toting heavy backpacks—sometimes carrying amounts that are 10 to 15 percent of their total body weight. Because such repetitive strain on the back can result in a lifetime of pain and disability, prevention is imperative. If you

must carry a pack all day, protect your back by following this advice:

✳ Opt for the lightest pack available and make sure that it has a heavy-duty hip strap so that you are not carrying the bulk of the weight around your back and shoulders. Adjust the strap so the weight is primarily on your hips.
✳ If you can afford a small internal-frame pack, buy one. There are many excellent packs available from outdoor recreation supply companies, or consider a rolling computer case.
✳ Use and carry the lightest computer possible. Although big screens are nice, they add weight. Remember that a laptop is meant to be portable. Larger devices are often designed for business travelers who use wheeled suitcases.
✳ Keep extras to a minimum when loading your pack. Don't bring your books to class unless your instructor asks you to. Plan ahead and bring only those study materials to campus that you can complete while you're there; carry a smaller notepad; store files on a jump drive and upload to a campus computer to do work.
✳ Limit the amount of personal items you carry each day. Wallets, makeup, hair products, and so on should be kept to a minimum.
✳ When lifting your pack to put it on your back, stand with both feet on the ground, knees slightly flexed, and your back straight. Twisting the back while swinging up the load can cause back injuries.
✳ Pack heavy items on the bottom and as close to your back as possible.

Overstuffed backpacks can lead to a lifetime of back pain.

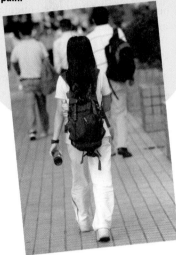

✳ Once you're ready to go, weigh the pack. If it's over 15 pounds, reassess what is necessary and ditch the rest.

Sources: L. Hestbaek et al., "The Course of Low Back Pain from Adolescence to Adulthood: Eight-Year Follow-Up of 9,600 Twins," *Spine* 31, no. 4 (2006): 468–72; American Occupational Therapy Association, "Study: Most University Students Self-Report Discomfort, Pain Due to Backpack Usage," Press release, September 3, 2008, www.prlog .org/10113114-study-most-university-students-self-report-discomfort-pain-due-to-backpack-usage .html; D. Gilkey et al., "Risk Factors Associated with Back Pain: A Cross-Sectional Study of College Students," *Journal of Manipulative and Physiological Therapeutics* 33, no. 2 (2010): 88–95; American College Health Association, *American College Health Association—National College Health Assessment II (ACHA-NCHA II): Reference Group Executive Summary Fall 2009* (Baltimore: American College Health Association, 2010), Available at www.achancha.org/reports_ACHA-NCHAII.html.

ment of rheumatoid arthritis is similar to that for osteoarthritis, emphasizing pain relief and improved functional mobility. In some instances, immunosuppressant drugs can reduce the inflammatory response, and in advanced cases, surgery may be necessary. Advanced rheumatoid arthritis often involves destruction of the bony ends of joints. The remedy for this condition is typically bone fusion, which leaves the joint immobile. In some instances, joint replacement may be a viable alternative.

Osteoporosis

Osteoporosis is a disease in which bones become brittle and weak and break easily. Most commonly, bones in the spine fracture, resulting in back pain, loss of height over time, and a stooped posture. Ultimately, bones in other parts of the body fracture easily, too, including the hands, wrists, and hip.

Osteoporosis affects men and women of all races. But white and Asian women—especially those who are past

low back pain (LBP) Pain or discomfort in the lumbosacral region of the back.

menopause—are at highest risk. Medications, dietary supplements, and weight-bearing exercise can help strengthen bones.

The good news is that recent research has shown significant decreases in osteoporosis in persons 50 and over in recent years. Rates are still high (10% of women and 2% of men had osteoporosis, and 49% of women and 30% of men had low bone mineral density [osteopenia] in a recent study), but they are much better than rates of even 10 years ago.[44]

Low Back Pain

If you're like 85 percent of the population, at some point you will injure your back. The resulting pain may be mild, involving short-lived muscle spasms, or it may be more severe, involving damage to discs, dislocation, a fracture, or another form of spinal trauma. Treatment may involve surgery, rehabilitation, and medications.

Low back pain (LBP), in particular, is increasingly common, especially among young adults (see the **Student Health**

Today box on the previous page for one possible cause).[45] Back injuries are the most frequently mentioned complaints in injury-related lawsuits and result in high medical and rehabilitation bills; in the United States, direct and indirect costs (such as lost wages) relating to spinal injuries cost over $200 billion annually.[46] As a result, employers throughout the country have become increasingly interested in preventing these injuries.

The following factors contribute to LBP:

- **Age.** People between the ages of 20 and 45 run the greatest risk of LBP. At age 50, the condition becomes less common. After age 65, the incidence again rises, apparently because of bone and joint deterioration. For college students, heavy purses or backpacks can be major precipitators of back problems, particularly among those who are primarily sedentary or who have weak core muscles.
- **Body type.** Many studies indicate that people who are very tall, have a high body mass index (BMI), or have a lanky body type run an increased risk of LBP. However, much of this research is controversial.
- **Posture.** Poor posture may be one of the greatest contributors to LBP. If you routinely slouch, you run an increased risk.
- **Strength and fitness.** People with LBP tend to have less overall trunk strength (core strength) than other people. The total level of fitness and conditioning is also a factor—the more fit you are, the better. Sedentary people who suddenly decide to "get fit" often are among those most at risk for LBP. They engage in strenuous activity without first strengthening supporting muscles.
- **Psychological factors.** Numerous psychological factors appear to increase risk for LBP. Depression, apathy, inattentiveness, boredom, emotional upsets, drug abuse, and family and financial problems all heighten risk.
- **Occupational risk.** The type of work you do and the conditions you do it in greatly affect risk. For example, truck drivers, who must endure the bumps and jolts of the road while in a sitting position, frequently suffer from back pain.

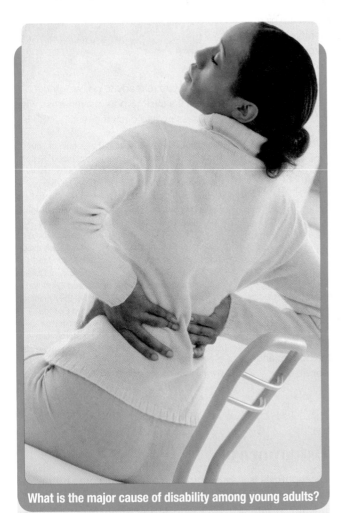

What is the major cause of disability among young adults?

In the United States, low back pain is the major cause of disability for people age 20 to 45, who suffer more frequently and severely from this problem than older people do. It is one of the most common chronic ailments among college students.

437 million

days of work are missed annually due to musculoskeletal conditions.

Repetitive Motion Disorders

It's the end of the term, and you have finished the last of several papers. After hours of nonstop typing, your hands are numb and you feel an intense, burning pain that makes the thought of

MALADIES SPECIFIC TO WOMEN

Because of their different anatomies and lifestyles, men and women frequently experience different rates of chronic conditions. In addition, there are some conditions that are specific to one gender or the other because they affect body structures and organs associated with reproductive functions.

FIBROCYSTIC BREAST CONDITION

About 90 percent of all women in the United States, particularly those over the age of 30, have a noncancerous condition called *fibrocystic breast condition.* Indeed, it is so common that many experts have taken it out of the disease category and refer to it as *benign breast changes*.

Symptoms range from one small, palpable lump to large masses of irregular tissue found in both breasts. Although most cysts consist of fibrous tissue, some are filled with fluid. The underlying causes of the condition are unknown; it may relate to an imbalance between estrogen and progesterone or to hormonal changes that occur during the normal menstrual cycle. Some experts believe that caffeine raises hormone levels, which can increase susceptibility to fibrous tissue buildup. Women with certain types of fibrocystic tissue may have a slightly higher risk of breast cancer, but this may be because fibrous tissue makes it more difficult to notice an abnormal lump. Treatment,

This image, created by computerized analysis of the light absorption of tissues, shows a fibrocystic breast.

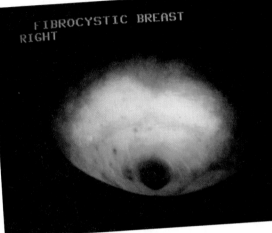

if needed, often involves removing fluid from the affected area or surgically removing the cyst.

ENDOMETRIOSIS

Endometriosis is a hormonal and immune system disease affecting at least 6.3 million women and girls in the United States, and more than 89 million worldwide Endometriosis is characterized by abnormal growth and development of endometrial tissue (the tissue lining the uterus) in regions of the body other than the uterus. It is most likely to appear between ages 20 to 40. Symptoms of endometriosis include severe cramping during and between menstrual cycles, irregular periods, unusually heavy or light menstrual flow, abdominal bloating, fatigue, painful bowel movements with periods, painful

intercourse, constipation, diarrhea, infertility, and low back pain. Among the most widely accepted theories concerning the causes of endometriosis are the transmission of endometrial tissue to other regions of the body during surgery or through the birthing process, the movement of menstrual fluid backward through the fallopian tubes during menstruation, and abnormal cell migration through body-fluid movement. Women with cycles shorter than 27 days or flows longer than a week are at increased risk. The more aerobic exercise a woman engages in and the earlier she starts it, the less likely she is to develop endometriosis.

Treatment for endometriosis ranges from bed rest and stress reduction to *hysterectomy* (surgical removal of the uterus) or surgical removal of one or both ovaries and the fallopian tubes. More conservative treatments involve dilation and curettage, surgically scraping endometrial tissue off the fallopian tubes and other reproductive organs. Combinations of hormone therapy have also become more acceptable.

Sources: M. Conrad-Stoppler, "Fibrocystic Breast Condition," 2012, www.medicinenet.com/fibrocystic_breast_condition/page3.htm; Endometriosis Association, "What Is Endometriosis?" May 2012, www.endometriosisassn.org/endo.html; National Institutes of Health, Medline Plus, "Endometriosis," Updated September 2010, www.nlm.nih.gov/medlineplus/endometriosis.html; The Endometriosis Association, "Treatment Options," Accessed May 2012, www.endometriosisassn.org/treatment.html.

---

typing one more word almost unbearable. If this happens, you may be suffering from a repetitive motion disorder (RMD). Repetitive motion disorders include carpal tunnel syndrome, bursitis, tendonitis, ganglion cysts, and others.[47] Twisting of the arm or wrist, overexertion, and incorrect posture or position are usually contributors. The areas most likely to be affected are the hands, wrists, elbows, and shoulders, but the neck, back, hips, knees,

feet, ankles, and legs can be affected, too. Over time, repetitive motion can cause permanent damage to nerves, soft tissue, and joints.

One of the most common RMDs is carpal tunnel syndrome, a product of spending hours gaming, texting, typing, or using the latest media device. RMDs are not limited to leisure or office job activities. Motions such as flipping

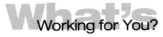
groceries through computerized scanners or other tasks requiring repeated hand and wrist movements can irritate the median nerve in the wrist, causing numbness, tingling, and pain in the fingers and hands. Although carpal tunnel syndrome risk can be reduced by proper placement of the keyboard, mouse, wrist pads, and other techniques, it is often overlooked until significant damage has been done. Better education and ergonomic workplace designs can eliminate many injuries of this nature. Physical and occupational therapy is an important part of treatment and eventual recovery.

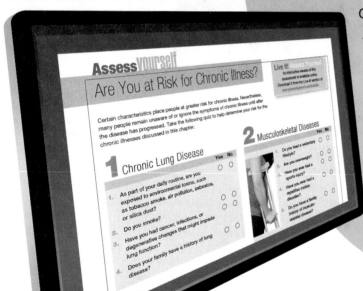

Now that you have completed the **Assess yourself** activity and considered your results, you may need to take further steps to understand and address your risks.

Today, you can:

○ Make an appointment with your doctor to find out more about any symptoms you've been having or discuss your potential risk factors.

○ Call your parents and find out if they have ever had similar problems or if they know of anyone in your family who has had these problems.

○ Weigh your full backpack, and if it's more than 10 percent of your body weight, unpack it and decide what you can leave at home.

Within the next 2 weeks, you can:

○ Find out more about your family history of chronic illness and what you can do to cut down your risk. Ask your parents what sorts of illnesses your family members have had and use that information for your health. For example, if your parent has lung disease, find out ways to cut down on environmental exposure to smoke and other toxins yourself.

○ If you suffer from migraines, pay attention to what triggers them for you and then work on creating a routine that keeps you out of harm's way.

○ If you suffer from heartburn, identify the foods or situations (such as sleeping postures) that bring it on. Make an effort to eliminate problematic foods or positions.

By the end of the semester, you can:

○ Adjust your routine to avoid environmental toxins. Avoid going to parties where people smoke, for example.

○ Keep track of allergy-related symptoms to see if you can identify any likely triggers.

○ Replace all of your cleaning products for your house, apartment, or dorm room with less toxic ones made from vinegar, lemon juice, and other natural ingredients (see the **Be Healthy, Be Green** box on page 525 for tips on how to make these yourself. Find out how to safely dispose of the chemical-intensive products that you previously used.

Summary

* Chronic lower respiratory disease (CLRD) (including bronchitis, emphysema, and asthma) is the third leading cause of death in the United States (right after heart disease and cancer).

* Allergies occur as the immune system responds to allergens. They can be triggered by pollens, foods, or other substances.

* Neurological conditions include headaches and seizure disorders such as epilepsy. The most common types of headache are tension and migraine.

* Inflammatory bowel disease includes ulcerative colitis and Crohn's disease. Irritable bowel syndrome (IBS) and other digestive problems affect increasing numbers of adults.

* Musculoskeletal problems such as arthritis, repetitive motion disorders, low back pain, and osteoporosis cause significant pain and disability in millions of people. Many of these problems are preventable.

* Modern maladies specific to women include fibrocystic breast disease and endometriosis, both of which cause discomfort or pain and problems for women, particularly in early adulthood.

Pop Quiz

1. Diseases and health conditions for which the cause(s) are unknown are referred to as
   a. homeopathic.
   b. iatrogenic.
   c. idiopathic.
   d. psychotic.

2. Which of the following is *not* correct?
   a. Women have more migraine headaches; men have more cluster headaches.
   b. Inflammatory bowel disease and irritable bowel syndrome are the same thing.
   c. An asthma attack can be fatal.
   d. Osteoarthritis is also referred to as "wear-and tear-arthritis."

3. The gradual destruction of the alveoli in a smoker's lung usually causes which COPD characterized by difficulty in exhaling?
   a. Dyspnea
   b. Bronchitis
   c. Emphysema
   d. Asthma

4. The leading chronic disease in school-aged children today is
   a. bronchitis.
   b. common cold.
   c. attention-deficit disorder.
   d. asthma.

5. Julie has found that she cannot eat nuts without suffering from itching and nausea. What condition is she likely to be suffering from?
   a. Irritable bowel syndrome
   b. Ulcerative colitis
   c. Food allergy
   d. Diabetes mellitus

6. Which of the following conditions is the leading cause of employee sick time and lost productivity in the United States?
   a. Low back pain
   b. Upper respiratory infections
   c. Asthma
   d. On-the-job injuries

7. If you experience an aura, a sensory warning sign that may include flickering vision or blind spots, you are likely to
   a. have an asthma attack.
   b. have a migraine headache.
   c. be suffering from an allergic reaction.
   d. be showing symptoms of glaucoma.

8. Margaret experiences occasional wheezing, shortness of breath, and coughing spasms. What chronic respiratory disorder is she likely suffering from?
   a. Sleep apnea
   b. Bronchitis
   c. Asthma
   d. COPD

9. Which of the following statements is *not* correct?
   a. Many people who think they have food allergies may have problems with digestion or may be experiencing foodborne illnesses.
   b. Food allergies and food intolerance are the same thing.
   c. Children are more likely than adults to outgrow allergies to foods.
   d. Food allergies appear to be on the increase in the United States.

10. Which of the following is *not* correct?
    a. Endometriosis is an infectious disease of the female reproductive system.
    b. Fibrocystic breast problems usually decrease after a woman goes through menopause.
    c. Women with fibrocystic breast condition often find it more difficult to detect cancerous changes in their breasts.
    d. Younger adult women tend to have the greatest risk of fibrocystic breast condition and endometriosis.

Answers to these questions can be found on page A-1.

Think about It!

1. What are some of the major noninfectious chronic diseases affecting Americans today? Do you think there is a pattern in the types of diseases that we get? What are the common risk factors?
2. List common respiratory diseases affecting Americans. Which of these has a genetic basis? An environmental basis? An individual basis?
3. Compare and contrast the different types of headaches.
4. Compare the symptoms of ulcerative colitis, gastroesophageal reflux disease, and Crohn's disease. How can you tell whether your stomach is reacting to final exams or telling you that you have a serious medical condition?
5. What is the difference between a food allergy and food intolerance?
6. What are the major disorders of the musculoskeletal system? Describe the difference between osteoarthritis and rheumatoid arthritis.

Accessing Your Health on the Internet

The following websites explore further topics and issues related to personal health. For links to the websites below, visit the Companion Website for *Access to Health*, 13th Edition, at www.pearsonhighered.com/donatelle.

1. *American Academy of Allergy, Asthma, and Immunology.* This site presents an overview of asthma information, particularly as it applies to children with allergies. It also offers interactive quizzes to test your knowledge and an ask-the-expert section. www.aaaai.org
2. *American Lung Association.* The latest news on asthma and lung disease is available here. www.lungusa.org
3. *National Center for Chronic Disease Prevention and Health Promotion.* A wide range of information is available from this organization, which is dedicated to chronic diseases and health promotion. The organization is linked to the Centers for Disease Control and Prevention. www.cdc.gov/chronicdisease
4. *National Institute of Neurological Disorders and Stroke.* This site contains up-to-date information to help individuals cope with pain-related difficulties. www.ninds.nih.gov
5. *National Institute for Diabetes and Digestive and Kidney Diseases (NIDDK).* This valuable resource provides key information about diabetes and the major digestive and kidney diseases, as well as resources for prevention and treatment options. www2.niddk.nih.gov/

References

1. American Lung Association. "How the Lungs Work," 2012, www.lung.org/your-lungs/how-lungs-work/.
2. American Lung Association, "Lung Disease," 2012, www.lungusa.org/lung-disease.
3. Centers for Disease Control and Prevention, "Chronic Obstructive Pulmonary Disease (COPD) Includes: Chronic Bronchitis and Emphysema," Data from Summary Health Statistics for U.S. Adults: National Health Interview Survey, 2010, FastStats, 2012, www.cdc.gov/nchs/fastats/copd.htm.
4. American Lung Association, "Chronic Obstructive Pulmonary Disease Fact Sheet," February 2011, www.lungusa.org/lung-disease/copd/resources/facts-figures/COPD-Fact-Sheet.html.
5. Ibid.
6. American Lung Association, "Lung Disease," 2011, www.lungusa.org/lung-disease.
7. National Center for Health Statistics, "FastStats Asthma," Updated January, 2012, www.cdc.gov/nchs/fastats/asthma.htm; American Lung Association, "Asthma," 2012, www.lung.org/lung-disease/asthma/; J. S. Schiller, J. W. Lucas, B. W. Ward, and J. A. Peregoy, "Summary Health Statistics for U.S. Adults: National Health

Interview Survey, 2010," National Center for Health Statistics, *Vital and Health Statistics* 10, no. 252(2012); B. Bloom, R. A. Cohen, and G. Freeman, "Summary Health Statistics for U.S. Children: National Health Interview Survey, 2010," National Center for Health Statistics, *Vital Health and Statistics* 10, no. 250 (2011).

8. American Lung Association, "Reduce Asthma Triggers," 2012, www.lung.org/lung-disease/asthma/taking-control-of-asthma/reduce-asthma-triggers.html.

9. Ibid.

10. American Lung Association, "Asthma," 2012; U. Gohil, A. Modan, and P. Gohil, "Aspirin-Induced Asthma–A Review," *Global Journal of Pharmacology* 4, no. 1 (2011): 19–30.

11. Centers for Disease Control and Prevention, "Asthma in the U.S. Growing Every Year," *Vital Signs*, May 2011, www.cdc.gov/VitalSigns/Asthma/index.html.

12. National Center for Health Statistics, "FastStats Asthma," 2012; Schiller et al., "Summary Health Statistics for U.S. Adults," 2012; Bloom et al., "Summary Health Statistics for U.S. Children," 2012.

13. Asthma and Allergy Foundation of America, "Allergy Facts and Figures," 2012, www.asfa.org/display.cfm?id=9&sub=30.

14. Asthma and Allergy Foundation of America, "Allergy Overview," April 2012, www.aafa.org/display.cfm?id=9.

15. American Academy of Allergy, Asthma, and Immunology, "Allergy Statistics," 2012, www.aaaai.org/media/statistics/allergy-statistics.asp.

16. Centers for Disease Control and Prevention, "FastStats–Allergies and Hay Fever"; Schiller et al., "Summary Health Statistics for U.S. Adults," 2012.

17. A. H. Liu et al., "National Prevalence and Risk Factors for Food Allergy and Relationship to Asthma: Results from the National Health and Nutrition Examination Survey 2005–2006," *Journal of Allergy and Clinical Immunology* 126, no. 4 (2010): 798–806 e13; WebMD, Allergies Health Center, "Food Allergies and Food Intolerance," 2012, www.webmd.com/allergies/guide/food-allergy-intolerances?print=true.

18. U.S. Food and Drug Administration, "Food Allergies: What You Need to Know–Food Facts," 2012, www.fda.gov/food/resourcesforyou/consumer.

19. National Institute of Neurological Disorders and Stroke, "NINDS Overview," February 2009, www.ninds.nih.gov/about_ninds/ninds_overview.htm.

20. National Headache Foundation, "Press Kits: Categories of Headache," 2010, www.headaches.org/press/NHF_Press_Kits/Press_Kits_-_Categories_of_Headache.

21. Mayo Clinic, "Tension Headache: Symptoms," February 2009, www.mayoclinic.com/health/tension-headache/ds00304/dsection=symptoms.

22. Mayo Clinic, "Tension Headaches Risk Factors," 2011, www.mayoclinic.com/health/tension-headache.

23. National Headache Foundation, "Migraine," 2011, www.headaches.org/education/Headache_Topic_Sheets/Migraine.

24. National Headache Foundation, "The Complete Guide to Headache: Migraine," April 2012, www.headaches.org/educational_modules/completeguide/migrindex.html.

25. Ibid.

26. Ibid.

27. Ibid.

28. National Headache Foundation, "Headache Topic Sheets: Cluster Headaches," 2011, www.headaches.org/education/Headache_Topic_Sheets/Cluster_Headaches.

29. Epilepsy Foundation, "Epilepsy and Seizure Statistics," April 2012, www.epilepsyfoundation.org/about/statistics.cfm.

30. American College of Gastroenterology, "Common GI Problems, Volume 1," 2010, www.acg.gi.org/patients/cgp/cgpvol1.asp.

31. S. Kane, "Inflammatory Bowel Disease Defined," IBD Support Foundation, Accessed July 2010, www.ibdsf.com; M. Basson and J. Katz, "Ulcerative Colitis," Medscape Reference, 2012, http://emedicine.medscape.com/article/183084-overview.

32. National Digestive Diseases Information Clearinghouse (NDDIC), "Crohn's Disease," 2011, http://ddigiestve.niddk.nih.gov/ddiseases.pubs.com; Centers for Disease Control and Prevention, "Inflammatory Bowel Disease–About Crohn's Disease," 2012, www.cdc.gov/ibd/.

33. E. Roberts, "IBD and IBS Are Not the Same Thing," April 2009, www.healthcentral.com/ibd/c/2623/66985/ibd-ibs-thing.

34. CDC, "Inflammatory Bowel Disease," 2012, www.cdc.gov/ibd/.

35. National Digestive Diseases Information Clearinghouse (NDDIC), "Irritable Bowel Syndrome," May 2012.

36. U.S. Bone and Joint Decade, *The Burden of Musculoskeletal Diseases in the United States: Prevalence, Societal and Economic Costs* (Rosemont, IL: American Academy of Orthopaedic Surgeons, 2008), Available at www.boneandjointburden.org.

37. Ibid.

38. R. Shiri et al., "The Association Between Obesity and Low Back Pain: A Meta-Analysis," *American Journal of Epidemiology* 171, no. 2 (2010): 135–54.

39. Brigham and Women's Hospital, "Arthritis and Other Rheumatic Diseases Statistics," Modified March 2009, http://healthlibrary.brighamandwomens.org/RelatedItems/85,P00068; U.S. Bone and Joint Decade, *The Burden of Musculoskeletal Diseases in the United States*, 2008.

40. U.S. Bone and Joint Decade, *The Burden of Musculoskeletal Diseases in the United States*, 2008.

41. J. M. Hootman and C. G. Helmick, "Projections of U.S. Prevalence of Arthritis and Associated Activity Limitations," *Arthritis & Rheumatism* 54, no. 1 (2006): 226–29.

42. Arthritis Foundation, "Disease Center: Osteoarthritis: What Is It?" 2010, www.arthritis.org/disease-center.php?disease_id=32.

43. Ibid.

44. A. C. Looker et al., "Prevalence and Trends in Low Femur Bone Density Among Older US Adults: NHANES 2005–2006 Compared With NHANES III," *Journal of Bone and Mineral Research* 25, no. 1 (2010):64–71.

45. National Institute of Neurological Disorders and Stroke, "Low Back Pain Fact Sheet," NIH Publication no. 03-5161, Updated June 2011, www.ninds.nih.gov/disorders/backpain/detail_backpain.htm.

46. U.S. Bone and Joint Decade, *The Burden of Musculoskeletal Diseases in the United States*, 2008.

47. Centers for Disease Control and Prevention, National Institute of Neurological Disorders, "NINDS Repetitive Motion Disorders Information Page," Updated October.

18 Choosing Conventional and Complementary Health Care

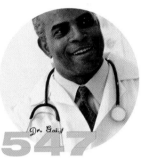

547

What questions should I ask my health care provider about proposed tests, treatments, or medications?

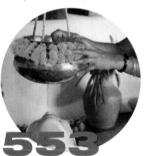

553

Why are so many people using alternative medicine?

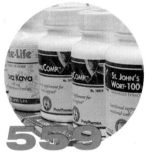

559

Do herbal remedies have any risks or side effects?

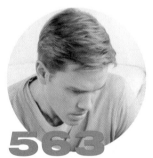

563

What should I consider when choosing health insurance?

OBJECTIVES

✱ Explain why it is important to be a responsible health care consumer and how to encourage health care consumers to take action.

✱ Identify several factors to consider when making health care decisions.

✱ Describe and discuss conventional and complementary and alternative health care.

✱ Discuss types of health care products and treatments available in conventional and complementary care and their potential benefits and risks.

✱ Describe the U.S. health care system in terms of types of insurance; the changing structure of the system; and issues concerning cost, quality, and access to services.

✱ Discuss issues facing our health care system today.

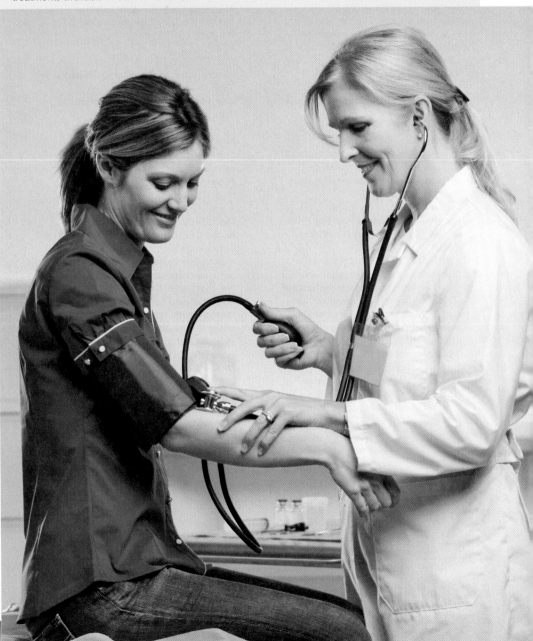

Have there been times when you wondered whether you were sick enough to go to your campus health clinic? Have you left visits with your health care provider feeling that the doctor didn't give you a thorough exam or that you had more questions than you did when you arrived? Do you engage in risky behaviors, such as riding your bike without a helmet, and don't know where or how you would be treated if you were injured? Are you one of the 20 percent of college students without health insurance? Have you ever had to help a family member or loved one make health care decisions? If the answer to any of these questions is yes, then you will find the information in this chapter valuable in helping you become a better health care consumer. Learning how to navigate the health care system is an important part of taking charge of your health.

35 million

Americans are admitted to the hospital each year.

Taking Responsibility for Your Health Care

Acting responsibly in times of illness can be difficult. If you are not feeling well, you must first decide whether you really need to seek medical advice. Not seeking treatment, whether because of high costs or limited coverage, or trying to medicate yourself when a professional diagnosis and treatment are needed, is potentially dangerous. Being knowledgeable about the benefits and limits of self-care is critical for responsible consumerism.

Self-Care

Individuals can practice behaviors that promote health and reduce the risk of disease. We can also treat minor afflictions without seeking professional help. Self-care consists of knowing your body, paying attention to its signals, and taking appropriate action to stop the progression of illness or injury. Common forms of self-care include the following:

- Diagnosing symptoms or conditions that occur frequently but may not require physician visits (e.g., the common cold, minor abrasions)
- Using over-the-counter remedies to treat mild, infrequent, and unambiguous pain and other symptoms
- Performing first aid for common, uncomplicated injuries and conditions
- Checking blood pressure, pulse, and temperature

- Performing monthly breast or testicular self-examinations
- Doing periodic checks for blood glucose, cholesterol, or other levels as prescribed by a physician
- Learning from reliable self-help books, websites, and DVDs
- Performing meditation and other relaxation techniques
- Maintaining a healthful diet, getting adequate rest, and exercising

In addition, a vast array of at-home diagnostic kits are now available to test for pregnancy, allergies, HIV, genetic disorders, and many other conditions. Caution is in order here: Although many of these devices are valuable for making an initial diagnosis, others are not valid or reliable. Moreover, home health tests are not substitutes for regular, complete examinations by a trained practitioner.

Many people also use self-care treatment methods inappropriately. Taking prescription drugs used for a previous illness to treat your current illness, using unproven self-treatment, or using other people's medications are examples of inappropriate self-care. Using self-care methods appropriately takes education and effort.

When to Seek Help

Monitoring your symptoms and deciding which warrant professional attention is not always easy. Generally, you should consult a physician if you experience *any* of the following:

- A serious accident or injury
- Sudden or severe chest pains, especially if they cause breathing difficulties

Hear It! Podcasts

Want study podcasts for this chapter? Download **Consumerism: Selecting Health Care Products and Services** and **Complementary** and **Alternative Medicine** from www.pearsonhighered.com/donatelle.

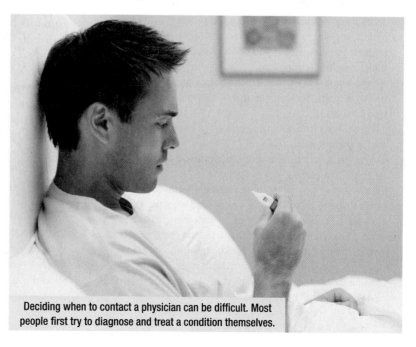

Deciding when to contact a physician can be difficult. Most people first try to diagnose and treat a condition themselves.

- Trauma to the head or spine accompanied by persistent headache, blurred vision, loss of consciousness, vomiting, convulsions, or paralysis
- Sudden high fever or recurring high temperature (over 102°F for children and 103°F for adults) and/or sweats
- Tingling sensation in the arm accompanied by slurred speech or impaired thought processes
- Adverse reactions to a drug or insect bite (shortness of breath, severe swelling, dizziness)
- Unexplained sudden weight loss
- Persistent or recurrent diarrhea or vomiting
- Blue-colored lips, eyelids, or nail beds
- Any lump, swelling, thickness, or sore that does not subside or that grows for over a month
- Any blood in the stool or urine, or significant pain or marked, persistent change in bowel or bladder habits
- Yellowing of the skin or the whites of the eyes
- Any symptom that is unusual and recurs over time
- Pregnancy

See the **Skills for Behavior Change** box for information on taking an active role in your own health care.

Assessing Health Professionals

Suppose you decide that you do need medical help. How should you go about assessing the qualifications of a health care provider? Numerous studies document the importance of good communication skills: The most satisfied patients are those who feel their health care provider explains diagnosis and treatment options thoroughly and involves them in decisions regarding their own care.[1]

When evaluating health care providers, consider the following questions:

- Do they listen to you, respect you as an individual, and give you time to ask questions? Do they return your calls, and are they available to answer questions between visits?
- What professional education and training have they had? What license or board certification(s) do they hold? Note that there is a difference between "board certified" and "board eligible" physicians. *Board certified* indicates that the physician has passed the national board examination for his or her specialty (e.g., pediatrics) and has been certified as competent in that specialty. In contrast, *board eligible* merely means that the physician is eligible to take the specialty board's exam, but not necessarily that he or she has passed it.
- Are they affiliated with an accredited medical facility or institution? The Joint Commission is an independent nonprofit organization that evaluates and accredits more than 15,000 health care organizations and programs in the United States. Accreditation requires that these institutions verify all education, licensing, and training claims of their affiliated practitioners.
- Are they open to complementary or alternative strategies? Would they refer you for different treatments if appropriate?
- Do they indicate clearly how long a given treatment may last, what side effects you might expect, and what problems you should watch for?
- Who will be responsible for your care when your physician is on vacation or off call?
- Are there professional reviews and information on any lawsuits against them available online?

Questions to ask yourself about the quality of care you are receiving include the following:

- Did your health care provider take a thorough health history and ask for any recent updates to your health history? Was your examination thorough?
- Did your health care provider listen to you?
- Did you feel comfortable asking questions? Did your health care provider answer thoroughly,

Skills for Behavior Change

Be Proactive in Your Health Care

The more you know about your body and the factors that can affect your health, the better you will be at communicating with health care providers. The following points can help:

❭ Know your own and your family's medical history.

❭ Research your condition—causes, physiological effects, possible treatments, and prognosis. Don't rely on the health care provider for this information.

❭ If you're concerned about an upcoming medical visit, bring a friend or relative along to help you review what the doctor says. If you go alone, take notes.

❭ Ask the practitioner to explain the problem and possible tests, treatments, and medications in a clear and understandable way. If you don't understand something, ask for clarification.

❭ If the health care provider prescribes any medications, ask whether you can take generic equivalents that cost less.

❭ Ask for a written summary of the results of your visit and any lab tests.

❭ If you have any doubt about recommended tests or treatments, seek a second opinion.

❭ After seeing a health care professional, write down an accurate account of what happened and what was said. Be sure to include the names of the provider and all other people involved in your care, the date, and the place.

❭ When filling prescriptions, make sure the pharmacist provides you with a drug information sheet that lists medical considerations and details about potential drug and food interactions.

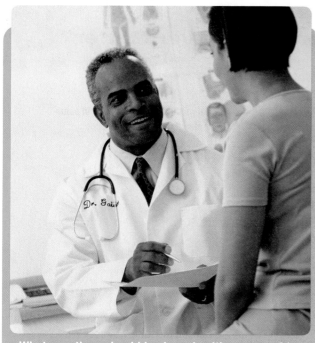

What questions should I ask my health care provider about proposed tests, treatments, or medications?

It's important to understand recommendations that your health care provider makes. Questions to ask include how often the practitioner has performed a procedure, the proportion of successful outcomes for the treatment or procedure, any side effects and whether they can be treated or reduced, whether a hospital stay will be required, and why a test has been ordered.

in a way that was easy to understand? Did he or she admit to not knowing an answer to your question when appropriate?
● Would you feel comfortable seeing the health care provider again?

Asking the right questions at the right time may save you personal suffering and expense. Many patients find that writing their questions down before an appointment helps them get all the answers they need. You don't need to accept a defensive or hostile response; asking questions is your right as a patient.

Active participation in your treatment is the only sensible course in a health care environment that encourages **defensive medicine,** an approach to health care in which the practitioner orders tests or treatments, or avoids high-risk patients or procedures, largely to reduce their liability to malpractice suits. Unwarranted tests and treatments to protect against malpractice exposure are two significant factors driving up the cost of medicine. It is estimated that between $250 and $325 billion per year are spent on medical tests and procedures that do not improve health outcomes.[2]

Your Rights as a Patient

In addition to asking the suggested questions above, being proactive in your health care also means that you should be aware of your rights as a patient, as follows:[3]

1. The right of informed consent means that before receiving any care, you should be fully informed of what is being planned; the risks and potential benefits; and possible alternative forms of treatment, including the option to refuse treatment. Your consent must be voluntary and without any form of coercion. It is critical that you read any consent forms carefully and amend them as necessary before signing.

2. You are entitled to know whether the treatment you are receiving is standard or experimental. In experimental conditions, you have the legal and ethical right to know if any drug is being used in the research project for a purpose not approved by the Food and Drug Administration (FDA) and whether the study is one in which some people receive treatment whereas others receive a placebo. (See the **Student Health Today** box on the following page for more on placebos and the placebo effect.)

3. You have the right to privacy. This means that you do not have an obligation to reveal the source of payment for your treatment. It also means you have the right to make personal decisions concerning all reproductive matters.

4. You have the right to receive care, as well as to refuse treatment and to cease treatment at any time.

5. You are entitled to have access to all of your medical records and to have those records remain confidential.

6. You have the right to seek the opinions of other health care professionals regarding your condition.

Conventional Health Care

Conventional health care, also called **allopathic medicine,** mainstream medicine, or traditional Western medical practice, is the dominant type of health care delivered in the United States, Canada, Europe, and much of the developed world. Among U.S. health care providers, the majority currently receives conventional medical training and treats patients using conventional medicine. Allopathic medicine is based on the premise that illness is a result of exposure to pathogens, such as bacteria and viruses, or organic changes in the body. The prevention of disease and the restoration of health involve vaccines, drugs, surgery, and other treatments.

Be aware, however, that not all allopathic treatments have had the benefit of the extensive clinical trials and long-term studies of outcomes

What's Working for You?

Maybe you already have your health care under control. Below is a list of some things you can do to manage your health care successfully:

☐ I research conditions I may have using newspapers, magazines, textbooks, research articles, and reliable websites.

☐ I discuss all of my health care decisions with my care provider.

☐ I try to weigh risks and benefits before starting any treatment.

☐ I have health insurance, and I understand what it covers.

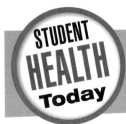
The Placebo Effect: Mind Over Matter?

The *placebo effect* is an apparent cure or improved state of health brought about by a substance, product, or procedure that has no generally recognized therapeutic value. Patients often report improvements in a condition based on what they expect, desire, or were told would happen after receiving a treatment, even though the treatment was, for example, simple sugar pills instead of powerful drugs.

Researchers are investigating how and why placebos work on some people. One theory is that expecting a positive outcome activates the same natural pathways in the brain as some medications do. One study involved patients with Parkinson's disease. The patients who thought that they were receiving the real treatment but actually received a placebo had the same changes in their brains on positron-emission tomography (PET) scans as those who received the medication. Similar chemical changes on brain imaging tests were seen with placebos in studies of pain and depression.

In a recent trial, a sample of alcohol-dependent patients received either the drugs naltrexone or acamprosate, or a placebo, for a period of 12 weeks. They were also asked whether they thought they were receiving an active medication or a placebo. Those who believed they had been taking medication consumed fewer alcoholic drinks and reported less alcohol dependence and cravings, regardless of whether they really were receiving the drug.

Placebos are also used in clinical research studies. Patients with a particular condition are given either the treatment that is being tested or a placebo. If a significantly greater number of patients receiving the treatment have a significantly more beneficial outcome than the patients receiving the placebo, then the treatment can be considered effective. Most such studies are double-blinded; that is, neither the patients nor the doctors involved in the study are told until the study ends who had the real treatment and who had the placebo.

Incidentally, there is also a *nocebo* effect, in which a practitioner's negative assessment of a patient's symptoms leads to a worsening of the condition. Ethical considerations make the nocebo effect

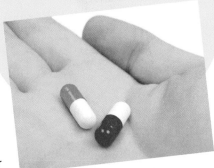

Is it a real medicine or a placebo? In some cases, it may not make a difference.

difficult to study; however, available experimental evidence links negative expectations with increased anxiety and pain.

Sources: J. Friedman and R. Dubinsky, "The Placebo Effect," *Neurology* 71, no. 9 (2008): e25–e26; R. de la Fuente-Fernandez et al., "Expectation and Dopamine Release: Mechanism of the Placebo Effect in Parkinson's Disease," *Science* 293 (2001): 1164–66; N. Diedrich and C. Goetz, "The Placebo Treatments in Neurosciences: New Insights from Clinical and Neuroimaging Studies," *Neurology* 71 (2008): 677–84; F. Benedetti, M. Lanotte, L. Lopiano, and L. Colloca, "When Words Are Painful: Unraveling the Mechanisms of the Nocebo Effect," *Neuroscience* 147, no. 2 (2007), pages 260–71.

that would be necessary to conclusively prove effectiveness in different populations. Even when studies appear to support the health benefits of a particular treatment or product, other studies with equal or better scientific validity often refute these claims. Also, today's recommended treatment may change dramatically in the future as new technologies and medical advances replace older practices. Like other professionals, medical doctors are only as good as their training, continued acquisition of knowledge, and resources.

Health care providers strive to ensure the quality of care they provide to their patients, and one of the ways they do this is by using **evidence-based medicine.** Decisions regarding patient care are based on clinical expertise, patient values, and current best scientific evidence. Clinical expertise refers to the clinician's cumulative experience, education, and clinical skills. The patient brings his or her own personal and unique concerns, expectations, and values. The best evidence is usually found in clinically relevant research that has been conducted using sound methodology.

Conventional Health Care Practitioners

Selecting a **primary care practitioner (PCP)**—a medical practitioner whom you can visit for routine ailments, preventive care, general medical advice, and appropriate referrals—is not an easy task. The PCP for most people is a family practitioner, an internist, or for women, an obstetrician-gynecologist (ob-gyn). Many people routinely see nurse practitioners or physician assistants who work for an individual doctor or a medical group, and others use nontraditional providers as their primary source of care. As a college student, you may opt to visit a PCP at your campus health center. The reputation of health care providers on college campuses is excellent. In national surveys, students have indicated that

evidence-based practice Decisions regarding patient care based on clinical expertise, patient values, and current best scientific evidence.

primary care practitioner (PCP) A medical practitioner who treats routine ailments, advises on preventive care, gives general medical advice, and makes appropriate referrals when necessary.

the health center medical staff is their most trusted source of health information.[4]

91%

of U.S. physicians admitted that they sometimes order unnecessary medical tests because they are concerned about being sued for malpractice.

Doctors undergo rigorous training before they can begin practicing. After 4 years of undergraduate work, students typically spend 4 years studying for their medical degree (MD). After this general training, some students choose a specialty, such as pediatrics, cardiology, cancer, radiology, or surgery, and spend 1 year in an internship and several years doing a residency. Some doctors receive additional training in order to specialize in certain elective surgeries (see the **Student Health Today** box on page 550). Some specialties also require a fellowship; in all, the time spent in additional training after receiving a medical degree can be up to 8 years.

Osteopaths are general practitioners who receive training similar to that of a medical doctor but place special emphasis on the skeletal and muscular systems. Their treatments may involve manipulation of the muscles and joints. Osteopaths receive the degree of doctor of osteopathy (DO) rather than MD.

Eye care specialists can be either ophthalmologists or optometrists. An **ophthalmologist** holds a medical degree and can perform surgery and prescribe medications. An **optometrist** typically evaluates visual problems and fits glasses but is not a trained physician. If you have an eye infection, glaucoma, or other eye condition needing diagnosis and treatment, you need to see an ophthalmologist.

Dentists are specialists who diagnose and treat diseases of the teeth, gums, and oral cavity. They attend dental school for 4 years and receive the title of doctor of dental surgery (DDS) or doctor of medical dentistry (DMD). They must also pass both state and national board examinations before receiving a license to practice. The field of dentistry includes many specialties. For example, *orthodontists* specialize in the alignment of teeth. *Oral surgeons* perform surgical procedures to correct problems of the mouth, face, and jaw.

Nurses are trained health care professionals who provide a wide range of services for patients and their families, including patient education, counseling, community health and disease prevention information, and administration of medications. They may choose from several training options. Registered nurses (RNs) in the United States complete either a 4-year program leading to a bachelor of science in nursing (BSN) degree or a 2-year associate degree program. They must then pass a national certification exam. Lower-level licensed practical or vocational nurses (LPN or LVN) complete a 1- to 2-year training program, which may be based in either a community college or a hospital, and take a licensing exam.

Nurse practitioners (NPs) are nurses with advanced training obtained through either a master's degree program or a specialized nurse practitioner program. Nurse practitioners have the training and authority to conduct diagnostic tests and prescribe medications (in some states). They work in a variety of settings, particularly in HMOs (health maintenance organizations), clinics, and student health centers. Nurses and nurse practitioners may also earn the clinical doctor of nursing degree (ND), doctor of nursing science (DNS and DNSc degrees), or a research-based PhD in nursing.

Physician assistants (PAs) are licensed to examine and diagnose patients, offer treatment, and write prescriptions under a physician's supervision. An important difference between a PA and a NP is that the PA must practice under a physician's supervision. Like other health care providers, PAs are licensed by state boards of medicine.

Conventional Health Products

Recall from **Chapter 13** that prescription drugs can be obtained only with a written prescription from a physician, whereas over-the-counter drugs can be purchased without a prescription. Just as making wise decisions about providers is an important aspect of responsible health care, so is making wise decisions about medications.

Prescription Drugs In about two thirds of doctor visits, the physician administers or prescribes at least one medication. In fact, prescription drug use has risen by 25 percent over the past decade. Even though these drugs are administered under medical supervision, the wise consumer still takes precautions. Adverse effects and complications arising from the use of prescription drugs are common, as is failure to respond to a medication.

Consumers have a variety of resources available to determine the risks of various prescription medicines and to make educated decisions about whether to take a certain drug. One of the best resources is the FDA's Center for Drug Evaluation and Research website (www.fda.gov/drugs). This consumer-specific section of the FDA website provides current information on risks and benefits of prescription drugs. Being knowledgeable about what you are taking or thinking about taking is a sound strategy to ensure safety.

osteopath General practitioner who receives training similar to a medical doctor's but with an emphasis on the skeletal and muscular systems; often uses spinal manipulation as part of treatment.

ophthalmologist Physician who specializes in the medical and surgical care of the eyes, including prescriptions for glasses.

optometrist Eye specialist whose practice is limited to prescribing and fitting lenses.

dentist Specialist who diagnoses and treats diseases of the teeth, gums, and oral cavity.

nurse Health professional who provides many services for patients and who may work in a variety of settings.

nurse practitioner (NP) Professional nurse with advanced training obtained through either a master's degree program or a specialized nurse practitioner program.

physician assistant (PA) A midlevel practitioner trained to handle most standard cases of care under the supervision of a physician.

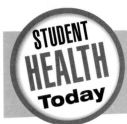
CHOOSING SURGERY: ELECTIVE PROCEDURES

The National Center for Health Statistics states that over 40 million elective medical procedures—surgeries and treatments that are planned, nonemergency procedures—are performed every year, and that number seems to be growing. Although not considered medically necessary, many types of elective procedures, from musculoskeletal to weight loss surgeries, greatly improve people's health and functioning, and some can reduce the patient's risk for chronic disease. Even purely cosmetic surgeries can enhance the patient's self-esteem.

If a procedure is considered not medically necessary, it may not be covered by insurance. In some cases, insurance companies may require a second opinion before approving payment on elective surgical procedures. If you are considering elective surgery, review your coverage requirements with your health insurance carrier before scheduling the procedure.

An elective surgical procedure is typically performed by a surgeon or qualified physician in either a hospital or an ambulatory center. Some simple, minimally invasive procedures may even be performed in a doctor's office. The type of surgery will mandate the qualifications and background of the surgeon or physician who performs it. The following are some of the more common elective surgeries.

LASIK

Millions of Americans have had surgery to reduce their dependence on contact lenses or glasses. The most common technique is called Lasik (laser-assisted in situ keratomileusis), in which a surgeon uses a razorlike instrument or laser to cut a flap in the cornea, the clear covering on the front of the eye, and then reshapes the exposed area using a laser. The surgery alters the way the eye focuses light, correcting nearsightedness, farsightedness, and some astigmatism. However, Lasik is not effective at treating close-up vision problems in middle-aged adults.

The procedure usually takes less than 5 minutes, is painless, and the patient is awake the entire time. Postoperative complications can include infection or night glare—starbursts or halos that appear when you are viewing lights at night.

COSMETIC SURGERY

Cosmetic surgery is performed to enhance appearance. Approximately 1.5 million cosmetic surgeries are performed every year. The most common include:

* Breast augmentation, the surgical placement of an implant behind each breast to increase breast volume and enhance shape
* Liposuction, the removal of pockets of fatty tissue with a vacuumlike device, to slim the hips, thighs, abdomen, or other areas
* Rhinoplasty, correction and reconstruction of the nose
* Dermabrasion, a surgical scraping of the top layers of the skin to remove fine wrinkles, acne scars, and skin growths

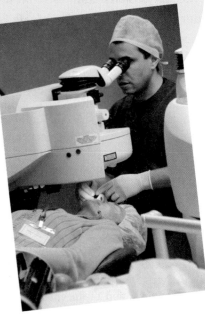

If you have imperfect vision and want to ditch your glasses or contact lenses for good, you may want to consider Lasik laser eye surgery.

* Rhytidectomy, commonly called a facelift, to improve signs of aging such as sagging skin in the face and neck

Risks and complications of cosmetic surgery include infection, bruising, numbness, bleeding, and poor healing.

Sources: U.S. Food and Drug Administration, "LASIK," 2011, December 9, www.fda.gov/Medical-Devices/ProductsandMedicalProcedures/Surgery-andLifeSupport/LASIK/default.htm; American Society for Aesthetic Plastic Surgery, "Quick Facts," 2010, www.surgery.org/media/statistics; American Society of Plastic Surgeons, "Plastic Surgery Information for Patients and Consumers," 2010, www.plasticsurgery.org/Patients_and_Consumers.html.

Common types of prescription drugs discussed in this text include antidepressants and antianxiety drugs (**Chapter 2**), hormonal contraceptives (**Chapter 6**), weight-loss aids (**Chapter 8**), smoking-cessation aids (**Chapter 12**), stimulants and sedatives (**Chapter 13**), antibiotics (**Chapter 14**), and statins and other cholesterol-lowering drugs (**Chapter 15**).

Generic drugs, medications sold under a chemical name rather than a brand name, contain the same active ingredients as brand-name drugs but are less expensive. Not all drugs are available as generics. If your doctor prescribes a drug, always ask if a generic equivalent exists and if it would be safe and effective for you to try.

Be aware, though, that there is some controversy about the effectiveness of generic drugs, because substitutions sometimes are made in minor ingredients that can affect the way the drug is absorbed, potentially causing discomfort or even allergic reactions in some patients. Always note any reactions you have to medications and tell your doctor about them.

Many consumers choose to have prescriptions filled online. Although many websites are operating legally and

generic drugs Medications marketed by chemical names rather than brand names.

observe the safeguards of traditional procedures for dispensing drugs, some sell counterfeit drugs of inconsistent quality or sidestep required consumer protections. If you buy medications online, buy only from state-licensed pharmacy sites based in the United States. Look for sites with the Verified Internet Pharmacy Practice Sites (VIPPS) seal, awarded by the National Association of Boards of Pharmacy (NABP) to Internet pharmacy sites that meet their criteria. Don't provide any personal health or financial information, including a Social Security number, unless you are sure the website will keep your information safe and private.[5]

Over-the-Counter (OTC) Drugs Medications available without a prescription are referred to as over-the-counter (OTC) drugs. Although physicians often recommend OTC remedies to patients for common conditions such as muscle pain or constipation, OTC drugs are also used in the course of self-diagnosis and self-treatment. American consumers spend billions of dollars yearly on OTC preparations for relief of everything from runny noses to ingrown toenails. Those most commonly used are pain relievers; cold, cough, allergy, and asthma medications; stimulants; sleeping aids and relaxants; and dieting aids (Table 18.1).

TABLE
18.1
Common Over-the-Counter Drugs, Their Uses, and Potential Side Effects

Type/Name of Drug	Use	Examples	Potential Hazards/Common Side Effects
Acetaminophen	Pain reliever, fever reducer.	Tylenol	Bloody urine, painful urination; skin rash; bleeding and bruising; yellowing of the eyes or skin; difficulty in diagnosing overdose because reaction may be delayed up to a week; liver damage from chronic low-level use.
Antacids	Relieve "heartburn."	Tums Maalox	Reduced mineral absorption from food; possible concealment of ulcer; reduced effectiveness of anticlotting medications; interference with the function of certain antibiotics (for antacids that contain aluminum); worsened high blood pressure (for antacids that contain sodium); aggravated kidney problems.
Anticholinergics	Often added to cold preparations to reduce nasal secretions and tears.	atropine scopolamine	None of the preparations tested by the FDA have been found to be Generally Recognized as Effective (GRAE) or Generally Recognized as Safe (GRAS). Some cold compounds contain alcohol in concentrations greater than 40%.
Antihistamines	Central nervous system depressants that dry runny noses, clear postnasal drip and sinus congestion, and reduce tears.	Claritin Benadryl Xyzal	Drowsiness, sedation, dizziness, disturbed coordination.
Aspirin	Pain reliever; reduces fever and inflammation.	Bayer Bufferin	Stomach upset and vomiting; stomach bleeding; worsening of ulcers; enhancement of the action of anticlotting medications; hearing damage from loud noise; severe allergic reaction; association with Reye's syndrome in children and teenagers; prolonged bleeding when combined with alcohol.
Decongestants	Reduce nasal stuffiness due to colds.	Sudafed DayQuil Allermed	Nervousness, restlessness, excitability, dizziness, drowsiness, headache, nausea, weakness, sleep problems.
Diet pills, caffeine	Aid to weight loss.	Dexatrim	Organ damage or death from cerebral hemorrhage; nervousness; irritability; dehydration.
Expectorants	Loosen phlegm, which allows the user to cough it up and clear congested respiratory passages.	Mucinex	Safety issues may arise when combined with other medications, particularly in frail or very ill individuals. Effectiveness is sometimes in question.
Ibuprofen	Pain reliever; reduces fever and inflammation.	Advil Motrin	Allergic reaction in some people with aspirin allergy; fluid retention or swelling (edema); liver damage similar to that from acetaminophen; enhancement of anticlotting medications; digestive disturbances.
Laxatives	Relieve constipation.	ex-lax Citrucel	Reduced absorption of minerals from food; dehydration; dependency.
Naproxen sodium	Pain reliever; reduces fever and inflammation.	Aleve Naprosyn	Potential bleeding in the digestive tract; possible stomach cramps or ulcers.
Sleep aids and relaxants	Help relieve occasional sleeplessness.	Nytol Sleep-Eze Sominex	Drowsiness the next day; dizziness; lack of coordination; reduced mental alertness; constipation; dry mouth and throat; dependency.

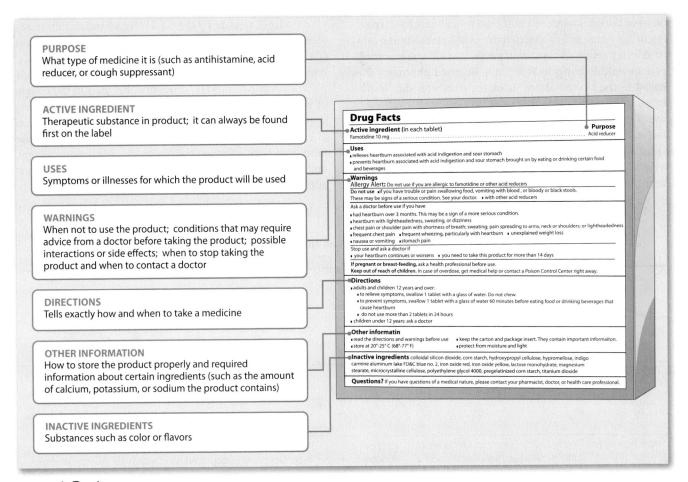

PURPOSE
What type of medicine it is (such as antihistamine, acid reducer, or cough suppressant)

ACTIVE INGREDIENT
Therapeutic substance in product; it can always be found first on the label

USES
Symptoms or illnesses for which the product will be used

WARNINGS
When not to use the product; conditions that may require advice from a doctor before taking the product; possible interactions or side effects; when to stop taking the product and when to contact a doctor

DIRECTIONS
Tells exactly how and when to take a medicine

OTHER INFORMATION
How to store the product properly and required information about certain ingredients (such as the amount of calcium, potassium, or sodium the product contains)

INACTIVE INGREDIENTS
Substances such as color or flavors

Drug Facts

Active ingredient (in each tablet) — **Purpose**
Famotidine 10 mg . . . . Acid reducer

Uses
- relieves heartburn associated with acid indigestion and sour stomach
- prevents heartburn associated with acid indigestion and sour stomach brought on by eating or drinking certain food and beverages

Warnings
Allergy Alert: Do not use if you are allergic to famotidine or other acid reducers
Do not use ■ if you have trouble or pain swallowing food, vomiting with blood , or bloody or black stools. These may be signs of a serious condition. See your doctor. ■ with other acid reducers
Ask a doctor before use if you have
- had heartburn over 3 months. This may be a sign of a more serious condition.
- heartburn with lightheadedness, sweating, or dizziness
- chest pain or shoulder pain with shortness of breath; sweating; pain spreading to arms, neck or shoulders; or lightheadedness
- frequent chest pain ■ frequent wheezing, particularly with heartburn ■ unexplained weight loss
- nausea or vomiting ■ stomach pain
Stop use and ask a doctor if
- your heartburn continues or worsens ■ you need to take this product for more than 14 days
If pregnant or breast-feeding, ask a health professional before use.
Keep out of reach of children. In case of overdose, get medical help or contact a Poison Control Center right away.

Directions
- adults and children 12 years and over:
    - to relieve symptoms, swallow 1 tablet with a glass of water. Do not chew.
    - to prevent symptoms, swallow 1 tablet with a glass of water 60 minutes before eating food or drinking beverages that cause heartburn
    - do not use more than 2 tablets in 24 hours
- children under 12 years: ask a doctor

Other informatin
- read the directions and warnings before use   ■ keep the carton and package insert. They contain important informaiton.
- store at 20°-25° C (68°-77° F)   ■ protect from moisture and light

Inactive ingredients colloidal silicon dioxide, corn starch, hydroxypropyl cellulose, hypromellose, indigo carmine aluminum lake FD&C blue no. 2, iron oxide red, iron oxide yellow, lactose monohydrate, magnesium stearate, microcrystalline cellulose, polyethylene glycol 4000, pregelatinized corn starch, titanium dioxide

Questions? If you have questions of a medical nature, please contact your pharmacist, doctor, or health care professional.

FIGURE 18.1   **The Over-the-Counter Medicine Label**
Source: Consumer Healthcare Products Association, OTC Label, www.otcsafety.org. Used with permission.

Despite a common belief that OTC products are safe and effective, indiscriminate use and abuse can occur with these drugs as with all others. For example, people who frequently drop medication into their eyes to "get the red out" or pop antacids after every meal are likely to become dependent. Many people also experience adverse side effects because they ignore the warnings on the labels or simply do not read them.

complementary medicine Treatment used in conjunction with conventional medicine.

alternative medicine Treatment used in place of conventional medicine.

The FDA has developed a standard label that appears on most OTC products **(Figure 18.1)**. It includes directions for use, active and inactive ingredients, warnings, and other useful information.

Complementary and Alternative Medicine (CAM)

Although the terms *complementary* and *alternative* are often used interchangeably when referring to therapies, there is a distinction between them. **Complementary medicine** is used *together with* conventional medicine, as part of the modern integrative-medicine approach.[6] An example of complementary medicine is to use massage therapy along with prescription medicine to treat anxiety. **Alternative medicine** has traditionally been used *in place of* conventional medicine, such as following a special diet or herbal remedy to treat cancer instead of using radiation, surgery, or other conventional treatments.

The National Center for Complementary and Alternative Medicine (NCCAM), part of the National Institutes of Health (NIH), provides a mechanism for reliable information about CAM practices. The NCCAM serves as a clearinghouse for CAM information and a focal point for research initiatives, policy development, and general recommendations. A survey conducted by the NCCAM and the National Center for Health Statistics (NCHS; part of the Centers for Disease Control and Prevention) revealed that 38 percent of adults use some form of CAM.[7] The following groups are more likely to have used CAM:

- More women than men
- People with higher educational levels
- People who have been hospitalized in the past year

- Former smokers (compared with current smokers or those who have never smoked)
- People with back, neck, head, or joint aches or other painful conditions
- People with gastrointestinal disorders or sleeping problems

Figure 18.2 summarizes the conditions for which respondents to the NCCAM/NCHS survey used CAM.

As with traditional Western medicine, practitioners of most complementary and alternative therapies spend years learning their practice. In addition, various forms of CAM are increasingly being taught in U.S. medical schools. However, there is no national training, certification, or licensure standard for CAM practitioners, and state regulations differ (this is also true for conventional medicine). Whereas practitioners of conventional medicine have graduated from U.S.-sanctioned schools of medicine or are licensed medical practitioners recognized by the American Medical

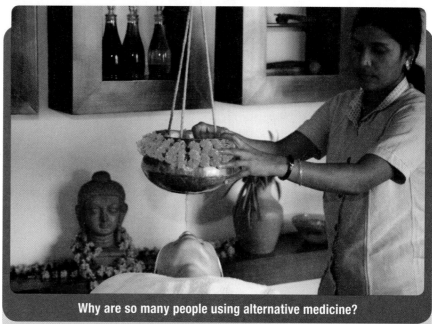

Why are so many people using alternative medicine?

People use alternative medicine for multiple reasons, and many treatments can benefit a variety of physical and mental ailments. For example, *shirodhara*—a traditional Ayurvedic treatment in which warm herbalized oil is poured over the forehead in guided rhythmic patterns—is said to relieve stress and anxiety, treat insomnia and chronic headaches, and improve memory.

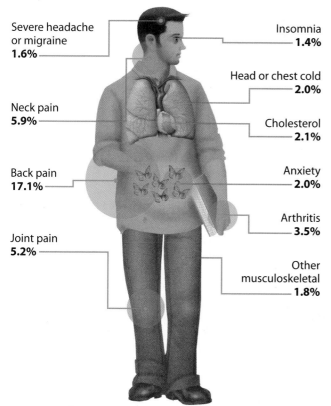

Severe headache or migraine
1.6%

Neck pain
5.9%

Back pain
17.1%

Joint pain
5.2%

Insomnia
1.4%

Head or chest cold
2.0%

Cholesterol
2.1%

Anxiety
2.0%

Arthritis
3.5%

Other musculoskeletal
1.8%

FIGURE 18.2 **Diseases and Conditions for Which CAM Is Most Frequently Used among Adults, 2007**

Source: Data are from P. M. Barnes, B. Bloom, and R. Nahin, "Complementary and Alternative Medicine Use among Adults and Children: United States, 2007," *CDC National Health Statistics Report*, no. 12 (December 2008).

Association (AMA)—the governing body for all physicians—each CAM domain has a different set of training standards, guidelines for practice, and licensure procedures.

Types and Domains of Complementary and Alternative Medicine

Many people seek CAM therapies as alternatives to the conventional Western system of medicine, which some people regard as too invasive, too high-tech, and too toxic in terms of laboratory-produced medications. In contrast, complementary and alternative medical therapies incorporate a **holistic** approach to medicine that focuses on treating the whole person, rather than just an isolated part of the body. Some CAM patients believe that alternative practices will give them greater control over their health care.

holistic Relating to or concerned with the whole body and the interactions of systems, rather than treatment of individual parts.

Nearly all health insurance providers cover at least one form of CAM, with acupuncture, chiropractic, and massage therapy being the most common. However, people who choose CAM often must pay the full cost of services themselves.

The ten most common CAM therapies are identified in Figure 18.3 on the following page. CAM therapies vary widely in terms of the nature and extent of the treatment and the types of problems for which they offer help. They also vary in effectiveness. Research has shown some to be ineffective, whereas others simply have not been studied, and others have limited research evidence supporting their effectiveness. A search of the NCCAM website reveals

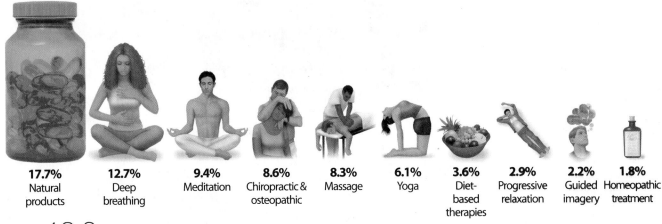

| 17.7% | 12.7% | 9.4% | 8.6% | 8.3% | 6.1% | 3.6% | 2.9% | 2.2% | 1.8% |
| Natural products | Deep breathing | Meditation | Chiropractic & osteopathic | Massage | Yoga | Diet-based therapies | Progressive relaxation | Guided imagery | Homeopathic treatment |

FIGURE 18.3 **The 10 Most Common CAM Therapies among U.S. Adults**

Source: Data are from P. M. Barnes, B. Bloom, and R. Nahin, "Complementary and Alternative Medicine Use among Adults and Children: United States, 2007," *CDC National Health Statistics Report*, no. 12 (December 2008).

alternative (whole) medical systems Complete systems of theory and practice that involve several CAM domains.

traditional Chinese medicine (TCM) Ancient comprehensive system of healing that uses herbs, acupuncture, and massage to bring the body into balance and to remove blockages of vital energy flow that lead to disease.

ayurveda (ayurvedic medicine) A comprehensive system of medicine, derived largely from ancient India, that places equal emphasis on the body, mind, and spirit, and strives to restore the body's innate harmony through diet, exercise, meditation, herbs, massage, exposure to sunlight, and controlled breathing.

that, even for some of the most mainstream CAM therapies, such as acupuncture, massage therapy, and yoga, the studies of effectiveness for pain and other conditions are, as yet, inconclusive.[8]

Before considering any treatments, consult reliable resources to thoroughly evaluate risks, the scientific basis of claimed benefits, and any contraindications to using the product or service. Avoid practitioners who promote their treatments as a cure-all for every health problem or who seem to promise remedies for ailments that have thus far defied the best scientific efforts of mainstream medicine. In short, apply the same strategies to researching CAM as you would to choosing allopathic care.

The NCCAM has grouped the many varieties of CAM into five general domains of practice, recognizing that the domains may overlap (Figure 18.4).

Alternative Medical Systems

Alternative (whole) medical systems are therapies reflecting specific philosophies of health and balance. Many have been practiced by various cultures throughout the world for centuries.

Traditional Chinese Medicine The concept of *qi* (pronounced "chee"), or vital energy, is foundational to **traditional Chinese medicine (TCM).** When *qi* is in balance, the person is in a state of health; imbalance of *qi* results in disease. Diagnosis is based on personal history, observation of the body (especially the tongue), palpation, and pulse diagnosis, an elaborate procedure requiring considerable skill and experience by the practitioner. Techniques such as acupuncture, herbal medicine, massage, and *qigong* (a form of energy therapy) are among the TCM approaches to health and healing.

Traditional Chinese medicine practitioners within the United States must complete a graduate program at a college or university approved by the Accreditation Commission for Acupuncture and Oriental Medicine (ACAOM). Graduate programs vary based on the specific area of concentration within TCM but usually involve an extensive 3- or 4-year clinical internship. In addition, an examination by the National Commission for the Certification of Acupuncture and Oriental Medicine, a standard for licensing in the United States, must be completed. Specific practices incorporated in TCM are discussed later in the chapter under the different CAM domains.

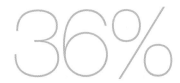

of 18- to 29-year-olds report having used some form of CAM.

Ayurveda The "science of life," **ayurveda (ayurvedic medicine)** is an alternative medical system that has evolved over thousands of years in India . Ayurveda seeks to integrate and balance the body, mind, and spirit and to restore harmony in the individual.[9] Ayurvedic practitioners use various techniques, including questioning, observation, and pulse palpation, to determine which of three vital energies, or *doshas,* is dominant in the particular patient. They then establish a treatment plan, the goal of which is not to cure a specific disorder, but to bring the doshas into balance, thereby reducing the patient's symptoms. Dietary modification and herbal remedies drawn from the botanical wealth of the Indian subcontinent are common. Treatments may also include certain yoga postures, meditation, massage, steam baths, changes in sleep patterns and sun exposure, and controlled breathing.

Training of Ayurvedic practitioners varies. There is no national standard for certification, although professional groups are working toward creating licensing guidelines.

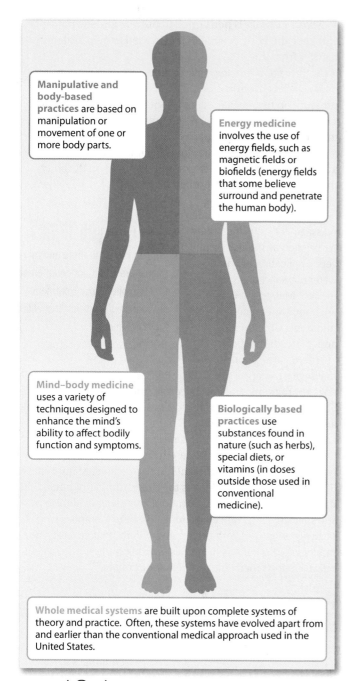

Manipulative and body-based practices are based on manipulation or movement of one or more body parts.

Energy medicine involves the use of energy fields, such as magnetic fields or biofields (energy fields that some believe surround and penetrate the human body).

Mind–body medicine uses a variety of techniques designed to enhance the mind's ability to affect bodily function and symptoms.

Biologically based practices use substances found in nature (such as herbs), special diets, or vitamins (in doses outside those used in conventional medicine).

Whole medical systems are built upon complete systems of theory and practice. Often, these systems have evolved apart from and earlier than the conventional medical approach used in the United States.

FIGURE 18.4 The Domains of Complementary and Alternative Medicine (CAM)

NCCAM groups CAM practices into five domains, recognizing that there can be some overlap. In particular, CAM whole medical systems cut across all domains.

Source: National Center for Complementary and Alternative Medicine, "The Use of Complementary and Alternative Medicine in the United States," NCCAM Publication no. D434, 2009.

Homeopathy **Homeopathic medicine** is an unconventional Western system based on the principle that "like cures like." In other words, the same substance that in large doses produces the symptoms of an illness will in highly diluted doses prompt the body's own defenses to cure the illness. It was developed in the late 1700s by Samuel Hahnemann, a Ger-

man physician, as an approach to medicine that was not as harsh as other treatments of the time, such as bloodletting and blistering.[10] Although homeopathic physicians do use certain standard remedies for certain conditions, they also classify patients by type and work within each patient's type to heal ever-deeper layers of disturbance.

Homeopathic training varies considerably and is offered through diploma programs, certificate programs, short courses, and correspondence courses. Laws that detail requirements to practice vary from state to state.

Naturopathy **Naturopathic medicine** views disease as a manifestation of an alteration in the processes by which the body naturally heals itself. Disease results from the body's effort to ward off impurities and harmful substances from the environment. Naturopathic physicians emphasize restoring health rather than curing disease. They employ an array of healing practices, including diet and clinical nutrition; homeopathy; acupuncture; herbal medicine; hydrotherapy (the use of water in a range of temperatures and methods of application); spinal and soft-tissue manipulation; physical therapies involving electric currents, ultrasound, and light therapy; therapeutic counseling; and pharmacology.

Several major naturopathic schools in the United States and Canada provide training, conferring the *naturopathic doctor* (*ND*) degree on students who have completed a 4-year graduate program that emphasizes humanistically oriented family medicine.

homeopathic medicine Unconventional Western system of medicine based on the principle that "like cures like."

naturopathic medicine System of medicine originating from Europe that views disease as a manifestation of alterations in the body's natural self-healing processes and that emphasizes health restoration as well as disease treatment.

manipulative and body-based practices Treatments involving manipulation or movement of one or more body parts.

"Why Should I Care?"

The ultimate choice about health care remains with you. In order to make sound decisions about what is best for your health, you need to understand as much as you can about your options.

Other Alternative Medical Systems Native American, Aboriginal, African, Middle Eastern, and South American cultures also have their own unique alternative systems. As the number of alternative therapists grows and systems become intertwined, so do the number of options available to consumers.

Manipulative and Body-Based Practices

The CAM domain of **manipulative and body-based practices** includes methods that are based on manipulation or movement of the body.

Chiropractic Medicine **Chiropractic medicine** has been practiced for more than 100 years and focuses on manipulation of the spine and other neuromuscular structures.[11]

chiropractic medicine Manipulation of the spine to allow proper energy flow.

A century ago, allopathic medicine and chiropractic medicine were in direct competition. Today, however, many health care organizations work closely with chiropractors, and many insurance companies will pay for chiropractic treatment, particularly if it is recommended by a medical doctor.

Chiropractic medicine is based on the idea that a life-giving energy flows through the nervous system, including the spinal cord. If the spine is partly misaligned or dislocated, that force is disrupted. Chiropractors use a variety of techniques to manipulate the spine back into proper alignment so the energy can flow unimpeded. It has been established that their treatment can be effective for back pain, neck pain, and headaches.

The average chiropractic training program includes intensive courses in biochemistry, anatomy, physiology, diagnostics, pathology, nutrition, and related topics, combined with hands-on clinical training. Many chiropractors continue their training to obtain specialized certification, for instance, in neurology, geriatrics, or pediatrics. Most state licensing boards require a 4-year course of study after completing at least a 3-year undergraduate program. Although states vary, increasing numbers require a 4-year undergraduate degree prior to entrance into chiropractic colleges. After completion of these requirements, applicants must pass an extensive examination given by the National Board of Chiropractic Examiners to obtain a license. The practice of chiropractic is licensed and regulated in all 50 states.[12]

Massage Therapy *Massage therapy* is soft tissue manipulation by trained therapists for relaxation and healing. References to massage have been found in ancient writings from many cultures, including those of ancient Greece, ancient Rome, Japan, China, Egypt, and the Indian subcontinent.[13] Today, massage therapy is used as a means of treating painful conditions, relaxing tired and overworked muscles, reducing stress and anxiety, rehabilitating sports injuries, and promoting general health. This is accomplished by manipulating the muscles and connective tissues to loosen the fibers and break up adhesions, improve the body's circulation, and remove waste products. There are many different types of massage therapy; the following are some of the more popular:

- *Swedish massage* uses long strokes, kneading, and friction on the muscles and moves the joints to aid flexibility.
- *Deep tissue massage* uses patterns of strokes and deep finger pressure on parts of the body where muscles are tight or knotted, focusing on layers of muscle deep under the skin.

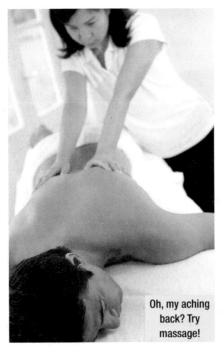

Oh, my aching back? Try massage!

- *Sports massage* is performed to prevent athletic injury and keep the body flexible. It is also used to help athletes recover from injuries.
- *Trigger point massage* (also called *pressure point massage*) uses a variety of strokes but applies deeper, more focused pressure on myofascial trigger points—"knots" that can form in the muscles, are painful when pressed, and cause symptoms elsewhere in the body as well.
- *Shiatsu massage* is a traditional healing art from Japan that applies firm finger pressure to specified points on the body that are believed to be important for the flow of vital energy.

Other varieties include massage of specific body parts, such as the feet or fingers, application of hot rocks, water massage, or other techniques. Massage techniques are important aspects of both traditional Chinese medicine and Ayurvedic medicine.

There are about 1,500 massage therapy schools, college programs, and training programs in the United States.[14] The course of study typically covers subjects such as anatomy and physiology; kinesiology; therapeutic evaluation; massage techniques; first aid; business, ethical, and legal issues; and hands-on practice. These educational programs vary in length, quality, and whether they are accredited. Many require 500 hours of training, which is the same number of hours that many states require for certification. Some therapists also pursue specialty or advanced training. Massage therapists work in an array of settings both private and public: medical and chiropractic offices, studios, hospitals, nursing homes, fitness centers, and sports medicine facilities, for example.[15]

what do you think?

Why do you think more and more people are opting for complementary and alternative treatments?
- What are the potential benefits of these treatments?
- What are the potential risks?

Bodywork Several body-centered modalities fall into the category of bodywork, including the following:

- The *Alexander Technique* is a movement education method designed to release harmful tension in the body to improve ease of movement, balance, and coordination.
- The *Feldenkrais Method* is a system of gentle movements and exercises. It is designed to improve movement, flexibility, coordination, and overall functioning through techniques that enhance awareness and retrain the nervous system.
- *Rolfing Structural Integration* is a form of bodywork that reorganizes the connective tissues to release tension, balance the body, and alleviate pain. The therapist applies firm—sometimes

painful—pressure to different areas; this process can release repressed emotions as well as dissipate muscle tension.

- *Pilates* is a popular exercise method focused on improving flexibility, strength, and body awareness. It involves a series of controlled movements, some of which are performed using special equipment.
- The *Trager Approach* is also known as psychophysical integration or mind/body integration. One aspect employs gentle, shaking motions of the patient's limbs in a rhythmic fashion to induce states of deep, pleasant relaxation.[16]

Energy Medicine

Energy medicine is a general term for therapies that focus either on energy fields thought to originate within the body (biofields) or on fields from other sources (electromagnetic fields). The existence of these fields has not been experimentally proven. Most forms of energy therapy manipulate biofields by applying pressure and/or manipulating the body by placing the hands in, or through, these fields.[17] Popular examples of biofield therapy include qigong, Reiki, therapeutic touch, acupuncture, and acupressure.

- *Qigong,* a component of traditional Chinese medicine, combines movement, meditation, and regulation of breathing to enhance the flow of vital energy (*qi*), improve blood circulation, and enhance immune function.
- *Reiki,* whose name derives from the Japanese words representing "universal" and "vital energy," or *ki,* is based on the belief that by channeling *ki* to the patient, the practitioner facilitates healing.
- *Therapeutic touch* is based on the premise that the therapist has the ability to perceive, through his or her hands held just above the patient's body, imbalances in the patient's energy. The therapist promotes healing by increasing the flow of the body's energies and bringing them into balance.

361

points along 14 meridians exist on the human body, according to classic acupuncture theory.

- **Acupuncture,** one of the oldest and most popular TCM therapies, is used to relieve a wide variety of health conditions, from musculoskeletal dysfunction to depression. The therapist stimulates various points on the body with a series of precisely placed and extremely fine needles. The stimulation of these acupuncture points is thought to increase the flow of *qi* through the *meridians,* or energy pathways, in the body (Figure 18.5). Following acupuncture, most participants in clinical studies report high levels of satisfaction with the treatment, improved quality of life, improvement in or cure of the condition, and reduced reliance on prescription drugs

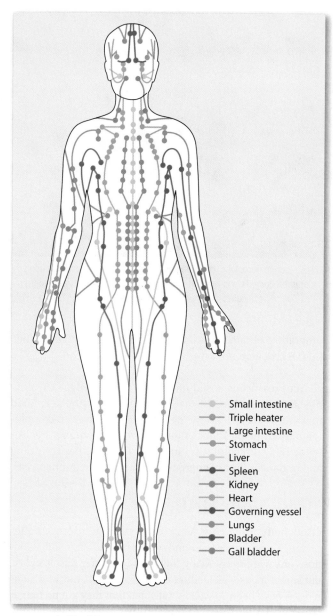

FIGURE 18.5 **The Main Meridian Channels**
Acupuncture and acupressure are two therapies within traditional Chinese medicine based on the belief that vital energy flows through meridian channels in the body.

Source: Courtesy of the Association for Energy and Meridian Therapies (The AMT), East Sussex, UK, http://theamt.com.

and surgery. In particular, results have been promising in the treatment of nausea associated with chemotherapy, headaches, fibromyalgia, and low back pain.[18] Some Western researchers are looking at potential biomechanisms to understand how acupuncture may work to relieve pain, such as activating opioids in the brain.[19] U.S. acupuncturists are state licensed, and most have completed a 2- to 3-year postgraduate

energy medicine Therapies using energy fields, such as magnetic fields or biofields.

acupuncture Branch of traditional Chinese medicine that uses the insertion of long, thin needles to affect flow of energy (*qi*) along pathways (meridians) within the body.

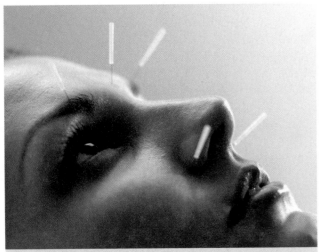

In acupuncture, long, thin needles are inserted into specific points along the body. This is thought to increase the flow of life-force energy, providing many physical and mental benefits.

program to obtain a master of traditional Oriental medicine (MTOM) degree.

Acupressure is based on the same knowledge of energy flow as acupuncture. Instead of needles, pressure is applied to points critical to balancing *yin* and *yang*, the two complementary principles that influence overall harmony (health) of the body. Practitioners must have the same basic training and understanding of energy pathways as do acupuncturists.

Mind–Body Medicine

Mind–body medicine employs a variety of techniques designed to enhance the mind's capacity to affect bodily functions and symptoms. Many therapies fall under this category, but some, such as biofeedback and cognitive-behavioral techniques, have been so well investigated that they are no longer considered alternative. At present, meditation, yoga, tai chi, certain uses of hypnosis, dance, music and art therapies, and prayer are still categorized as CAM. (See **Chapter 9** for more on yoga and tai chi and **Chapters 2** and **3** and Focus On: Cultivating Your Spiritual Health for more on the mind–body connection.)

As discussed in Chapter 3, *psychoneuroimmunology* (*PNI*) is a relatively new field of study. The PNI Research Society defines it as the "study of interrelationships among behavioral, neural, endocrine, and immune processes."[20] Many researchers have postulated that excessive stress and maladaptive coping can lead to immune system dysfunction and increase the risk of disease. Scientists are exploring ways in which relaxation, biofeedback, meditation, yoga, tai chi, and activities that involve either conscious or unconscious mind "quieting" may counteract negative stressors. For example, a recent review study of PNI found that psychological support—including relaxation therapies—can improve wound healing,[21] whereas inflammatory molecules such as C-reactive protein, which is a risk factor for heart disease, were found to be reduced in older adults after 16 weeks of tai chi.[22] Studies have also shown promising positive effects of mind–body techniques that encourage relaxation and other stress-reduction strategies for people with cancer.[23]

Dietary Products

Dietary products, including specially formulated foods and dietary supplements, are perhaps the most controversial domain of CAM therapies because of the sheer number of options available and the many claims that are made about their effects. Many of these claims have not been thoroughly investigated, and many of the products are not currently regulated.

Functional Foods Changes to the diet are often part of CAM therapies, and such changes commonly involve increased intake of certain *functional foods*—foods said to improve some specific aspect of physical or mental functioning beyond the contribution of their specific nutrients. Both whole foods, such as broccoli and nuts, and modified foods, such as an energy bar said to enhance memory, are classified as functional foods.[24] Food producers sometimes referred to their functional foods as **nutraceuticals** to emphasize their combined nutritional and pharmaceutical benefits. For example, the label on a bar of dark chocolate may state that modest consumption helps to reduce the risk of heart disease. The claim is backed up by research: Plant compounds called flavonoids found in chocolate improve several risk factors for heart disease.[25] The FDA regulates claims made on food labels; however, the FDA does not test functional foods prior to their coming to market and can only remove a product from the market if it is found to be unsafe.

In recent years, the most commonly advertised functional foods have been those containing *antioxidants*. Antioxidants are chemicals that combat free radicals and oxidative damage in cells. They include vitamins C and E, the mineral selenium, and a variety of phytochemicals, naturally occurring compounds present in many whole and processed plant foods, from fruits and vegetables to coffee and tea.

Other common functional foods and their purported benefits include the following:

- **Plant stanols/sterols.** Can lower "bad" (low-density lipoprotein [LDL]) cholesterol.
- **Oat fiber.** Can lower LDL cholesterol; serves as a natural soother of nerves; stabilizes blood sugar levels.
- **Sunflower seeds and oil.** Can lower risk of heart disease; may prevent angina.
- **Soy protein.** May lower heart disease risk by reducing LDL cholesterol and triglycerides.
- **Garlic.** Lowers cholesterol and reduces clotting tendency of blood; lowers blood pressure; may serve as form of antibiotic.

acupressure Branch of traditional Chinese medicine related to acupuncture. Uses application of pressure to selected body points to balance energy.

mind–body medicine Techniques designed to enhance the mind's ability to affect bodily functions and symptoms.

nutraceuticals Term often used interchangeably with *functional foods;* refers to the combined nutritional and pharmaceutical benefit derived through use of foods or food supplements.

- **Ginger.** May prevent motion sickness, stomach pain, and stomach upset; discourages blood clots; may relieve rheumatism.
- **Yogurt.** Yogurt that is labeled "Live and Active Cultures" contains active, friendly bacteria that can fight infections.

Herbal Remedies and Other Dietary Supplements The Office of Dietary Supplements, part of the National Institutes of Health, defines a dietary supplement as a "product (other than tobacco) that is intended to supplement or add to the diet; contains one or more dietary ingredients (including vitamins, minerals, herbs or other botanicals, amino acids, and other substances) or their constituents; is intended to be taken by mouth as a pill, capsule, tablet, or liquid; and is labeled on the front panel as being a dietary supplement."[26] Typically, people take dietary supplements—often without guidance from any CAM practitioner—to improve health, prevent disease, or enhance mood.

Other than vitamin/mineral supplements, herbal remedies, often referred to as botanicals, are among the most common dietary supplements sold. People have been using herbal remedies for thousands of years. Herbs were the original sources for compounds found in approximately 25 percent of the pharmaceutical drugs we use today, including aspirin (white willow bark), the heart medication digitalis (foxglove), and the cancer treatment Taxol (Pacific yew tree). In addition, scientists continue to make pharmacological advances by studying the herbal remedies used in cultures throughout the world. With conventional scientists now recognizing the benefits of herbs, it is no wonder that more and more consumers are turning to herbal products.

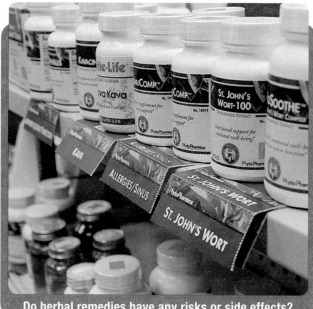

Do herbal remedies have any risks or side effects?

Herbs do have the potential to cause negative side effects. St. John's wort, for example, has potentially dangerous interactions with some prescription antidepressants and should never be taken with them. Other herbs, such as kava, can have negative effects even when taken alone.

However, herbal remedies are not to be taken lightly. Just because something is natural does not necessarily mean that it is safe. For example, in recent years, the NCCAM has warned that certain herbal products containing kava may be associated with severe liver damage.[27] Even rigorously tested products can be risky. Many plants are poisonous, and some can be toxic if ingested in high doses. Others may be dangerous when combined with prescription or over-the-counter drugs, could disrupt the normal action of the drugs, or could cause unusual side effects.[28]

Herbal remedies come in several different forms. Tinctures (extracts of fresh or dried plants) usually contain a high percentage of grain alcohol to prevent spoilage and are among the best herbal options. Freeze-dried extracts are very stable and offer good value for your money. Standardized extracts, often available in pill or capsule form, are also among the more reliable forms of herbal preparations.

Video Tutor: CAM: Risks vs. Benefits

In general, herbal medicines tend to be milder than chemical drugs and produce their effects more slowly; they also are much less likely to cause toxicity because they are diluted rather than concentrated forms of drugs. But diluted or not, and no matter how natural they are, herbs still contain many of the same chemicals as synthetic prescription drugs. Too much of any herb, particularly one from nonstandardized extracts, can cause problems. Table 18.2 on page 560 gives an overview of some of the most common herbal supplements on the market.

Not all the supplements on the market today are directly derived from plant sources. In recent years, there have been increasing reports in the media on the health benefits of various hormones, amino acids, and other biological compounds. Table 18.3 on page 561 lists popular nonherbal supplements and their risks and benefits.

Consumer Protection The burgeoning popularity of functional foods and dietary supplements concerns many scientists and consumers. Although particular products, such as chocolate or zinc lozenges, have been widely studied, there is little quality research to support the claims of many others. It is important to gather whatever information you can on both the safety and efficacy of any CAM treatment you are considering. In the case of functional foods and dietary supplements, start your own research with NCCAM (www.nccam.nih.gov) and the Cochrane Collaboration's review on complementary and alternative medicine (www.cochrane.org).

Dietary supplements can currently be sold without FDA approval. This raises issues of consumer safety. Even when products are dispensed by CAM practitioners, the situation can be risky. Some homeopaths and herbalists who mix their own tonics may not use standardized measures. Lack of standard regulation means that some unskilled and untrained people may be treating patients without fully understanding the potential chemical interactions of their preparations. Products sold in "health food" stores and over

TABLE
18.2

Common Herbs and Herbal Supplements: Benefits, Research, and Risks

	Herb	Claims of Benefits	Research Findings	Potential Risks
	Echinacea (purple coneflower, *Echinacea purpurea*, *E. angustifolia*, *E. pallida*)	Stimulates the immune system and increases the effectiveness of white blood cells that attack bacteria and viruses. Useful in preventing and treating colds or the flu.	Many studies in Europe have provided preliminary evidence of its effectiveness, but a recent controlled study in the United States indicated that it is no more effective than a placebo in preventing or treating a cold.	Allergic reactions, including rashes, increased asthma, gastrointestinal problems, and anaphylaxis (a life-threatening allergic reaction). Pregnant women and those with diabetes, autoimmune disorders, or multiple sclerosis should avoid it.
	Flaxseed (*Linum usitatissimum*)	Useful as a laxative and for hot flashes and breast pain. The oil is used for arthritis; both flaxseed and flaxseed oil have been used for cholesterol level reduction and cancer prevention.	Study results are mixed on whether flaxseed decreases hot flashes or lowers cholesterol levels.	Delays absorption of medicines, but otherwise has few side effects. Should be taken with plenty of water.
	Ginkgo (*Ginkgo biloba*)	Useful for depression, impotence, premenstrual syndrome, dementia and Alzheimer's disease, diseases of the eye, and general vascular disease.	Some promising results have been seen for Alzheimer's disease and dementia, and research continues on its ability to enhance memory and reduce the incidence of cardiovascular disease.	Gastric irritation, headache, nausea, dizziness, difficulty thinking, memory loss, and allergic reactions.
	Ginseng (*Panax ginseng*)	Affects the pituitary gland, increasing resistance to stress, affecting metabolism, aiding skin, muscle tone, and sex drive; improves concentration and muscle strength.	Studies have raised questions about appropriate dosages. Because the potency of plants varies considerably, dosage is difficult to control and side effects are fairly common.	Nervousness, insomnia, high blood pressure, headaches, chest pain, depression, and abnormal vaginal bleeding.
	Green tea (*Camellia sinensis*)	Useful for lowering cholesterol and risk of some cancers, protecting the skin from sun damage, bolstering mental alertness, and boosting heart health.	Although some studies have shown promising links between green and white tea consumption and cancer prevention, recent research questions the ability of tea to significantly reduce the risk of breast, lung, or prostate cancer.	Insomnia, liver problems, anxiety, irritability, upset stomach, nausea, diarrhea, or frequent urination.

Sources: National Center for Complementary and Alternative Medicine, "Herbs at a Glance," April 2011, http://nccam.nih.gov/health/herbsataglance.htm; Office of Dietary Supplements, National Institutes of Health, "Dietary Supplement Fact Sheets," 2011, http://ods.od.nih.gov/factsheets/list-all/; Web MD, "Experts Explain Green Tea's Potential Benefits for Everything from Fighting Cancer to Helping Your Heart," Julie Edgar, reviewed by Jonathan L Gelfand, MD, www.webmd.com/food-recipes/features/health-benefits-of-green-tea.

the Internet may have varying levels of the active ingredient or may contain additives to which the consumer may have an adverse reaction.

As a result of such concerns, pressure has mounted to establish an approval process for dietary supplements similar to the process the FDA uses for drugs. In the meantime, if you're considering purchasing a dietary supplement, look for the USP Verified Mark on the label (Figure 18.6). The USP (United States Pharmacopeia) is a nonprofit, scientific organization. It does not regulate or determine the safety of medications, foods, or dietary supplements, but it does offer verification services to manufacturers of dietary supplement products.

Dietary supplement products must meet stringent quality and manufacturing criteria to earn the USP Verified Mark.[29]

Health Insurance

Whether you're visiting your regular doctor, consulting a specialist, or preparing for a hospital stay, chances are that you'll be using some form of health insurance to pay for your care. Insurance typically allows you, the consumer, to pay into a pool of funds and then bill the insurance carrier for health care charges you incur. The fundamental principle of

TABLE
18.3 Common Nonherbal Supplements: Benefits, Research, and Risks

Supplement	Claims	Research Findings	Potential Risks
Dehydroepiandrosterone (DHEA) (hormone)	Fights aging, boosts immunity, strengthens bones, and improves brain functioning.	No proven antiaging benefits.	Could increase cancer risk and lead to liver damage, even when taken briefly.
Vitamin E	Reduces risk of heart disease; better chance of survival after heart attack.	Prevention of heart disease research results are mixed. Some researchers are now testing if it is protective for young, healthy people against eventual heart disease.	High doses cause bleeding when taken with blood thinners.
Glucosamine (biological substance that helps the body grow cartilage)	Useful for arthritis and related degenerative joint diseases; relieves swelling and decreases pain.	Early research shows it reduces mild to moderate joint pain when taken with chondroitin sulfate.	Few side effects noted.
L-Carnitine (amino acid derivative)	Improves athletic performance, increases fat-burning enzymes, combats fatigue and aging.	No consistent evidence it improves performance in healthy athletes. Some evidence it enhances mental function in older adults with mild cognitive impairment.	Interacts with some drugs. Nausea, vomiting, abdominal cramps, diarrhea, "fishy" body odor; more rarely, muscle weakness, seizures in patients with seizure disorders.
Melatonin (hormone)	Useful in regulating circadian rhythms and sleep patterns and treating insomnia; claims of antiaging benefits.	Some evidence supports its usefulness in regulating sleep patterns. No scientific support for antiaging claims.	Nausea, headaches, dizziness, blood vessel constriction; possibly a danger for people with high blood pressure or other cardiovascular problems.
SAMe (pronounced "sammy") (biological compound that aids over 40 functions in the body)	Useful in treatment of mild to moderate depression and in treatment of arthritis pain.	Studies have supported its usefulness in treating depression and arthritis pain.	Fewer side effects than prescription antidepressants, but questions remain over correct dosage, form, and long-term side effects.
Zinc (mineral)	Supports immune system; used to lessen duration and severity of cold symptoms; aids wound healing.	Research results are mixed, possibly due to the wide variety of cold viruses and differences of formulations and dosages in zinc lozenges.	Excessive intake associated with reduced immune function, reduced levels of high-density lipoproteins ("good" cholesterol).

Source: Office of Dietary Supplements, National Institutes of Health, "Dietary Supplement Fact Sheets," Modified August 2010, http://ods.od.nih.gov/Health_Information/Information_About_Individual_Dietary_Supplements.aspx.

insurance underwriting is that the cost of health care can be predicted for large populations. This is how health care **premiums,** payments made by the policyholders and/or their employer to the insurance company, are calculated. Policyholders pay premiums into a pool of funds, from which insurance companies pay claims. When you are sick or injured, the insurance company pays your care provider out of the pool regardless of your total contribution. Depending on circumstances, you may never pay for what your medical care costs, or you may pay much more for insurance than your medical bills ever total. The idea is that you pay

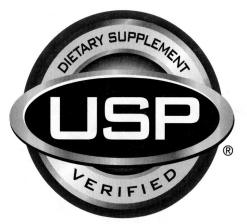

FIGURE 18.6 **The U.S. Pharmocopeia Verified Mark**

Source: Used with permission of The United States Pharmacopeial Convention. www.uspverified.org

affordable premiums so that you never have

premium Payment made to an insurance carrier, usually in monthly installments, that covers the cost of an insurance policy.

to face catastrophic bills. In profit-oriented systems, insurers prefer to have healthy people in their plans who pour money into risk pools without taking money out.

Insurance Coverage by the Numbers

In 2010, the average family's annual health insurance premium was more than $13,000.[30] For workers employed in organizations that offer health care insurance, most of this cost is hidden: The worker pays 15 percent to 25 percent of the full premium, usually as a deduction from his or her paycheck, and earns lower wages in return for the remaining cost of the coverage. However, people who are self-employed or work in companies that do not provide group health insurance must pay their premiums independently, and millions of employed but uninsured Americans do not find them affordable. In total, over 48 million Americans—16 percent—are uninsured; that is, they have no private health insurance and are not eligible for Medicare, Medicaid, or other government health programs.[31] Of these uninsured, 75 percent are workers or the dependents of workers. Almost 12 percent of all the uninsured are children under age 18.[32]

Lack of health insurance has been associated with delayed health care and increased mortality. *Underinsurance* (i.e., the inability to pay out-of-pocket expenses despite having insurance) also may result in adverse health consequences. The number of underinsured is not tracked by the government, but a 2008 study estimated that 25 million Americans between the ages of 19 and 64 are underinsured (at risk for spending more than 10% of their income on medical care because their insurance is inadequate).[33]

Among young adults ages 18 to 24, 31 percent do not have health insurance coverage.[34] However, for young adults who are college students, the statistics are different. In a 2011 national survey of college students, 7 percent of respondents said they did not have health insurance.[35] However, those who are covered only under their school's health care plan—almost 15 percent according to the same survey—may not realize that such plans are usually short term and have a low upper limit of benefits, which would be problematic if the student were to have a severe illness or injury. Few students buy higher-level catastrophic plans, however.

Racial and ethnic minorities are overly represented in the number of uninsured Americans. Almost a third of all Hispanic Americans are uninsured compared to 18.7 percent of African Americans and 11.5 percent of whites.[36] Issues such as citizenship and language barriers contribute to some of the disparities in access to health insurance for many in our country.

Why should all Americans be concerned about those who are uninsured and underinsured? People without adequate health care coverage are less likely than other Americans to have their children immunized, seek early prenatal care, obtain annual blood pressure checks and other screenings, and seek attention for symptoms of health problems. Experts believe that this ultimately leads to higher system costs because their conditions go undetected at their earliest, most treatable stage, deteriorating to a more debilitating and costly stage before they are forced to seek help, often in an emergency room. Because emergency care is far more expensive than clinic care, uninsured and underinsured patients are often unable to pay, and the cost is absorbed by "the system" in the form of higher hospital costs, insurance premiums, and taxes.

See It! Videos

Should conventional doctors incorporate CAM therapies into their treatments? Watch **Holistic Health Care** at www.pearsonhighered.com/donatelle.

what do you think?

Why is it important that private insurance cover preventive or lower-level care as well as hospitalization and high-technology interventions?

● What kinds of incentives would cause you to seek care early rather than delay care?

People without insurance can't gain access to preventive care, so they seek care only in an emergency or crisis. Because emergency care is extraordinarily expensive, they often are unable to pay, and the cost is absorbed by those who can pay—the insured or taxpayers.

Private Health Insurance

Originally, health insurance consisted solely of coverage for hospital costs (it was called *major medical*), but gradually it was extended to cover routine physicians' treatment and other services, such as dental and vision care and pharmaceuticals. These payment mechanisms laid the groundwork for today's steadily rising health care costs. Hospitals were reimbursed for the costs of providing care plus an amount for profit. This system provided no incentive to contain costs, limit the number of procedures, or curtail capital investment in redundant equipment and facilities. Physicians were reimbursed on a fee-for-service (indemnity) basis determined by "usual, customary, and reasonable"

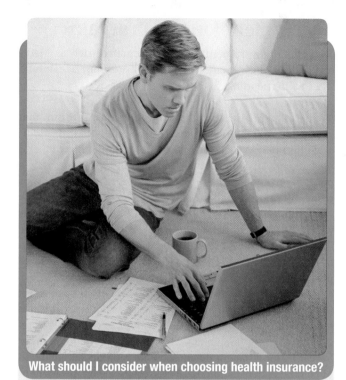

What should I consider when choosing health insurance?

Choosing a health insurance plan can be confusing. Some things to think about include how comprehensive your coverage needs to be, how convenient your care must be, how much you are willing to spend on premiums and co-payments, what the overall cost will be, and whether the services of the plan meet your needs.

fees. This system encouraged physicians to charge high fees, raise them often, and perform as many procedures as possible. Until the mid to late twentieth century, most insurance did not cover routine or preventive services, and consumers generally waited until illness developed to see a doctor instead of seeking preventive care. Consumers were also free to choose any provider or service they wished, including even inappropriate—and often very expensive—levels of care.

To limit potential losses, private insurance companies began increasingly employing several mechanisms: cost sharing (in the form of deductibles, co-payments, and coinsurance), waiting periods, exclusions, "preexisting condition" clauses, and upper limits on payments:

- **Deductibles** are payments (commonly $250 to $1,000) you make for health care before insurance coverage kicks in to pay for eligible services.
- **Co-payments** are set amounts that you pay per service or product received, regardless of the total cost (e.g., $20 per doctor visit or per prescription filled).
- **Coinsurance** is the percentage of costs that you must pay based on the terms of the policy (e.g., 20% of the total bill).
- Some plans specify a *waiting period* (e.g., 6 months) before they will provide coverage.
- All insurers set some limits on the types of *covered services* (e.g., most exclude cosmetic surgery, private rooms, and experimental procedures).

- **Preexisting condition clauses** limited the insurance company's liability for medical conditions that a consumer had before obtaining coverage. For example, if a person applying for insurance had cancer, the insurer could deny the application entirely, or agree to cover the applicant but only for conditions unrelated to the cancer. Under the 2010 Patient Protection and Affordable Care Act (ACA), starting in 2014, no one can be discriminated against due to a preexisting condition.
- Some insurance plans also imposed an *annual upper limit* or *lifetime limit,* after which coverage would end. The ACA makes this practice illegal as of 2014.

We discuss the ACA and its provisions in more detail shortly.

Managed Care

Managed care describes a health care delivery system consisting of the following elements:

- A network of physicians, hospitals, and other providers and facilities linked contractually to deliver comprehensive health benefits within a predetermined budget, sharing economic risk for any budget deficit or surplus
- A budget based on an estimate of the annual cost of delivering health care for a given population
- An established set of administrative rules requiring patients to follow the advice of participating health care providers in order to have their health care paid for under the terms of the health plan

Types of managed care plans include health maintenance organizations (HMOs), preferred provider organizations (PPOs), and point of service (POS). Approximately 66 million Americans are enrolled in HMOs, the most common type.[37]

Many managed care plans pay their contracted health care providers through **capitation,** that is, prepayment of a fixed monthly amount for each patient without regard for the type or number of health services provided. Some plans pay health care providers a salary, and some are still fee-for-service plans. As with other insurance plans, enrollees are members of a risk pool, and it is expected that some persons will use no services, some will use a modest amount, and others will have high-cost usage over a given year. Doctors have the incentive to keep their patient pool healthy and avoid catastrophic ailments that are preventable; usually such incentives come back in terms of increased salaries, bonuses, and other benefits. As such, prevention and health education to reduce risk and intervene early to avoid major problems are often capstone components of such plans.

Managed care plans have grown steadily over the past decade with a proportionate decline of enrollment in traditional indemnity insurance plans. The reason for this shift is that indemnity insurance, which pays providers and hospitals on a fee-for-service basis with no built-in incentives to

managed care Cost-control procedures used by health insurers to coordinate treatment.

capitation Prepayment of a fixed monthly amount for each patient without regard to the type or number of services provided.

45%

of Americans report taking at least one prescription drug in the past month; 18% report taking three or more such drugs.

control costs, has become unaffordable or unavailable for most Americans.

Health Maintenance Organizations

Health maintenance organizations (HMOs) provide a wide range of covered health benefits (e.g., physician visits, laboratory tests, surgery, and usually a prescription drug benefit) for a fixed amount prepaid by the patient, the employer, Medicaid, or Medicare (discussed later). Usually, HMO premiums are the least expensive form of managed care (saving between 10% and 40% more than other plans), but they are also the most restrictive (offering little or no choice in doctors and certain services). These premiums are 8 to 10 percent lower than for traditional plans, there are low or no deductibles or coinsurance payments, and co-payments are modest.

The downside of HMOs is that patients are typically required to use the plan's doctors and hospitals. Within an HMO, the PCP serves as a "gatekeeper," coordinating the patient's care and providing referrals to specialists and other services. As more and more people enroll in HMOs, concerns have arisen about care allocation and access to services, profit-motivated medical decision making, and the degree of focus on prevention and intervention.

Medicare A federal health insurance program that covers people age 65 and older, the permanently disabled, and people with end-stage kidney disease.

Medicaid A federal–state matching funds program that provides health insurance to low-income people.

Preferred Provider Organizations

Preferred provider organizations (PPOs) are networks of independent doctors and hospitals that contract to provide care at discounted rates. Although they offer greater choices in doctors than HMOs do, they are less likely to coordinate a patient's care. Members may choose to see doctors who are not on the preferred list, but this choice may involve having to pay a higher percentage of the cost of care.

Point of Service

Point of service (POS) plans—a hybrid of HMO and PPO plans—provide a more familiar form of managed care for people used to traditional indemnity insurance, which may explain why it is among the fastest growing of managed care plans. Under POS plans, members select an in-network PCP, but they can go to nonnetwork providers for care without a referral and must pay the extra cost.

No matter what type of plan you're in, a special savings account for health-related expenses could save you money. How do such accounts work, and are they right for you? See the **Money & Health** box and find out.

Government-Funded Programs

The federal government, through programs such as Medicare and Medicaid, currently funds 45 percent of the total U.S. health spending.[38]

Medicare

Medicare is a federal insurance program that covers a broad range of services except long-term care. Medicare covers 99 percent of Americans over age 65, all totally and permanently disabled people (after a waiting period), and all people with end-stage kidney failure—together, these groups comprise over 45 million people, or 1 in 7 Americans.[39] By 2030, it is estimated that 1 in 5—or 77 million—Americans will be insured by Medicare. As the costs of medical care have continued to increase, Medicare has placed limits on the amount of reimbursement to providers. As a result, some providers no longer accept Medicare patients.

To control hospital costs, in 1983 the federal government set up a prospective payment system based on *diagnosis-related groups (DRGs)* for Medicare. Nearly 500 groupings were created to establish how much a hospital would be reimbursed for caring for a patient diagnosed with a particular condition or combination of conditions. DRGs are based on the assumption that patients with similar health status and conditions will require a similar amount of hospital resources. If the costs of treating a patient are less than the predetermined amount, the hospital can keep the difference. However, if a patient's care costs more than the set amount, the hospital must absorb the difference (with a few exceptions that must be reviewed by a panel). This system motivates hospitals to discharge patients quickly, to provide more ambulatory care, and to admit patients classified into the most favorable (profitable) DRGs. Many private health insurance companies have also adopted reimbursement rates based on DRGs. In 1998, the federal Health Care Financing Administration (HCFA) expanded the prospective payment system to include payments for outpatient surgery and skilled nursing care.

In its continuing effort to control rising costs, HCFA, now known as the Centers for Medicare and Medicaid Services (CMS), has encouraged the growth of HMO plans for Medicare-eligible persons. Under this system, commercial managed care insurance plans receive a fixed per capita premium from CMS and then offer more preventive services with lower out-of-pocket co-payments. These managed care plans encourage providers and patients to utilize health care resources under administrative rules similar to commercial HMO plans.

Medicaid

In contrast to Medicare, **Medicaid**, covering approximately 58 million people, is a federal–state matching funds program that provides health insurance for people defined as low-income, including many who are blind, disabled, elderly, pregnant, or eligible for Temporary Assistance for Needy Families (TANF). Medicaid relies on funds provided by both federal and state sources. Because each state determines income eligibility, covered services, and payments to providers, there are vast differences in the way Medicaid operates from state to state. Beginning in 2014, the ACA will

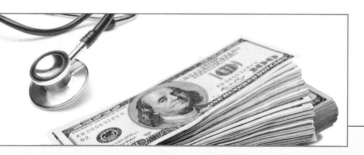

Money&Health

HEALTH CARE SPENDING ACCOUNTS

A Flexible Spending Account (FSA) for health care and a Health Savings Account (HSA) are savings plans that give you the opportunity to save money tax free to be used toward qualified health care expenses. As long as you're not claimed as a dependent on someone else's tax return, you can open one, either an FSA through your employer or an HSA through your bank.

If you're an employee, upon enrollment you identify the amount you want diverted from your paycheck into your FSA before taxes are withheld. The maximum you can contribute varies with different employers and health plans. One drawback to the FSA is that any funds still in the account at the end of the plan year are forfeited. This is known as the "use it or lose it" rule. Therefore, you need to estimate carefully what your out-of-pocket health expenses will be during the plan year.

With an HSA, there is no time limit on when the funds have to be used. Contributions to the account can be made from your paycheck by your employer as pre-tax deductions, or you can make them yourself, in which case you can claim them as an "above-the-line" deduction (a deduction from your gross income) when you file your tax return.

What expenses can you pay for with the money in your account? Deductibles, co-payments, eyeglasses, contact lenses, and prescription drugs are all allowed. Visits to approved health care providers, including dentists and optometrists, also are payable from your account if you have no health insurance coverage for them. You can even use the funds to pay for OTC drugs such as pain relievers or allergy medications as long as you have a written statement from your care provider that the OTC item is being purchased for a specific medical condition.

Does a health care spending account make sense for you? If you currently pay out-of-pocket for more than one or two health care visits a year, a few prescriptions, contact lenses, etc., and the money you use for these expenses comes from taxable income, then a health care savings plan might be worth a closer look. Contact your employee benefits specialist, your tax preparer, or a customer service provider at your bank.

---

provide generous federal subsidies to states that expand Medicaid coverage to all Americans living below 133 percent of the federal poverty level (in 2012, the poverty level was $19,090 for a three-person household). Although states would be responsible for only a small percentage of the funding, some have refused any expansion to their Medicaid programs.

The Children's Health Insurance Program (CHIP) was created in 1997 and reauthorized through new legislation in 2009. It provides health insurance coverage to more than 5 million uninsured children. Like Medicaid, it is jointly funded by federal and state funds and is administered by state governments.

Issues Facing Today's Health Care System

In recent decades, the number of Americans without health insurance rose dramatically as people with preexisting conditions, the self-employed, and low-wage workers in businesses that don't offer group plans found themselves unable to obtain or afford coverage. In 2010, Congress passed the Patient Protection and Affordable Care Act (ACA) to provide a means for these and all Americans to obtain affordable heath care. In addition to increasing access to care, the

ACA is expected to address America's high cost of care and to improve the overall quality of care. Here, we examine these three key issues, as well as the potential impact of the ACA.

See the **Be Healthy, Be Green** box on the following page for a discussion of another concern about the health care system: the amount of waste it produces and its impact on the environment.

Access

Access to health care is determined by numerous factors, the most significant of which are the supply and proximity of providers and facilities and insurance coverage.

Access to Providers, Facilities, and Treatments

In 2012, there were almost 700,000 physicians in the United States.[40] However, there is an oversupply of higher-paid specialists and a shortage of lower-paid primary care physicians (family practitioners, internists, pediatricians, etc.). Inner cities and some rural areas face constant shortages of physicians. Similarly, of the nearly 5,000 non-federal hospitals in the United States, over 60 percent serve urban areas, leaving many rural communities without readily accessible care.[41]

Managed care health plans determine access on the basis of participating providers, health plan benefits, and administrative rules. Often this means that consumers do not have

BE HEALTHY, BE GREEN

THE PERILS OF MEDICAL WASTE

MEDICAL WASTE

Legitimate concerns about the spread of infectious diseases, especially in hospital and clinic settings, have caused providers to rely on one-time-use items such as latex gloves, needles, bandages, and much more. All these items contribute substantially to medical waste.

Some estimate that the volume of hospital-generated medical waste is as much as 2 million tons each year. Approximately 15 percent of potentially infectious medical waste is combined with medical waste that is not deemed infectious and then disposed of in landfills. As water percolates through solid-waste disposal sites such as landfills, it collects contaminants and forms a substance called *leachate*. This can contaminate groundwater and surface water. Pollution in the ocean is also a major problem, as it directly affects all sea life and indirectly affects human health. In 1988, the Environmental Protection Agency banned dumping waste into the ocean, but the ban wasn't enforced until January 1992. Most of the waste that was dumped in the 1980s and early 1990s is still there today.

Currently, the vast majority—over 90 percent—of potentially infectious medical waste in the United States and around the world is incinerated, resulting in carbon emissions and other pollution such as particulate matter. Alternatives to incineration of medical waste include thermal treatment, such as microwave technologies; steam sterilization, such as autoclaving; and chemical mechanical systems that break down organic and inorganic wastes without polluting.

PHARMACEUTICAL WASTE

In addition to medical waste, hospitals generate a substantial amount of pharmaceutical waste—both hazardous and nonhazardous—that requires proper disposal. The primary culprit is medications that have been dispensed but not completely used. Consumers also generate pharmaceutical waste. Studies have shown

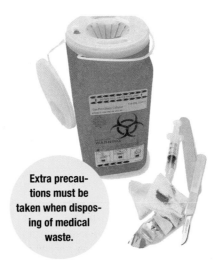

Extra precautions must be taken when disposing of medical waste.

that nearly 54 percent of consumers put unwanted medications in the trash, and 35 percent flush them down the toilet.

Prescription drug waste can contaminate our water supply through a number of avenues. First, medicines disposed of down the toilet or drain can easily be incorporated into groundwater, lakes, rivers, and streams. This may harm fish and wildlife that live in lakes, rivers, and the ocean. In addition, these drugs can end up back in our drinking water supply. This leads to elevated levels of chemicals that many water treatment facilities are not equipped to filter. Pharmaceutical drugs have been detected in the drinking water supplies of major metropolitan areas all across the United States. To date, the federal government has not set limits on the amount of these drugs that can be present in drinking water and does not require any testing for their presence.

Prescription drugs that are thrown away add to our growing landfills and can contribute to the toxicity of leachate. Moreover, medications thrown away in household trash can cause harm if they are retrieved by others. Here are some recommended ways to dispose of unused medications:

✴ Send your medicine to those in need. Some organizations collect unused, unexpired medicine to send to other countries

where prescription drugs are harder to get. Many states have passed legislation for recycling unused medications in nursing homes or other locations, but implementation has proven difficult. Nonprofits, such as the Iowa Prescription Drug Corporation (www.iowapdc .org), have developed and administered statewide drug-donation programs.

✴ Take your drugs back to the pharmacy. Many community pharmacies are starting take-back programs for unused or unneeded prescriptions. The pharmacy then disposes of these drugs safely. In some cases, pharmacies return unused pharmaceuticals to manufacturers for processing; in other cases, unused prescription medications are destroyed safely.

✴ If there is no take-back program in your community, pour the medication whole (do not crush tablets or capsules) into used coffee grounds, sawdust, cat litter, or another unpalatable substance, seal it in a plastic trash bag, and dispose of the bag.

✴ A few medications can be harmful or even fatal if consumed by someone other than the patient for whom the drug was prescribed. These medications are typically packaged with special instructions indicating that, if they cannot be brought to a take-back program, they should be disposed of by flushing. To find out if your medication is recommended for disposal by flushing, check with your pharmacist or visit the National Institutes of Health's Daily Med site at http://dailymed.nlm.nih.gov/ dailymed.

Sources: Environmental Protection Agency, "Medical Waste Frequent Questions," 2010, www.epa.gov/ wastes/nonhaz/industrial/medical/mwfaqs.htm; National Conference of State Legislatures, "State Prescription Drug Return, Reuse, and Recycling Laws," 2010, www.ncsl.org/default.aspx?tabid=14425; U.S. Food and Drug Administration, "Disposal of Unused Medicines: What You Should Know," 2012, January, www.fda.gov/drugs/resourcesforyou/consumers/ buyingusingmedicinesafely/ensuringsafeuseof medicine/safedisposalofmedicines/ucm186187.htm.

the freedom to choose specialists, facilities, or treatment options beyond those contracted with the health plan and recommended by their primary care provider.

Access to Quality Health Insurance Even if care providers and facilities are only a few miles away, not all Americans have equal access to them. A key disparity is the quality of the patient's health insurance plan. Otis W. Brawley, Chief Medical Officer for the American Cancer Society, uses the term "wallet biopsy" to describe the assessment a physician makes of a patient's—or his or her insurance company's—ability to pay for prescribed tests and procedures. Patients with excellent insurance coverage may then be encouraged to undergo expensive tests and treatments (a practice that can lead to useless or even harmful overtreatment, which we address shortly), whereas patients with poor insurance may not be informed of the full variety of diagnostic and treatment options.[42]

Key provisions in the ACA aim to increase access to quality health insurance among Americans. These include the following:

- Insurers are now required to cover several preventive services, such as health screenings for cancer, blood glucose, and blood pressure.
- Insurers are required to cover young adults on a parent's plan through age 26.
- As of 2014, Americans with preexisting conditions cannot be denied coverage.
- Both annual and lifetime limits on benefits will be phased out by 2014.
- As of 2014, Affordable Insurance Exchanges (AIEs) will facilitate consumer shopping and enrollment in plans with the same kinds of choices that members of Congress have. For example, five New England states are currently working to create an AIE intended to use its buying power to increase access to affordable coverage to New England residents.
- Small businesses, which typically paid as much as 18 percent more than large businesses for health insurance coverage for their employees, now qualify for special tax credits to help fund insurance plans.

Even before passage of the ACA, Congress provided assistance with insurance coverage for employees who change jobs. Under the Consolidated Omnibus Budget Reconciliation Act (COBRA) passed in 1986, Congress provided for former employees, retirees, spouses, and dependents to continue their insurance for up to 18 months at group rates. People who enroll in COBRA pay a higher amount than they did when they were employed, as they're covering both the personal premium and the amount previously covered by the employer.

See It! Videos

Do you benefit from health care reform? Watch **What Health Care Reform Means to You** at www.pearsonhighered.com/donatelle.

Cost

Both per capita and as a percentage of gross domestic product (GDP), we spend more on health care than any other nation. In 2011, our national health expenditures reached $2.7 trillion, over $8,600 for every man, woman, and child. This translates into 17.9 percent of our GDP.[43] Does this sound like a lot? Consider that health care expenditures are projected to grow by 6.2 percent each year, reaching over $4.7 trillion annually by 2021—nearly 20 percent of our projected GDP.[44]

Why are America's health care costs so high? Many factors are involved: duplication of services; an aging population; growing rates of obesity, inactivity, and related health problems; demand for new diagnostic and treatment technologies; an emphasis on crisis-oriented care instead of prevention; physician overtreatment, whether to avoid malpractice suits or to increase income; and inappropriate use of services by consumers, including use of emergency services for routine care, and family demands for futile and expensive procedures for patients who are dying.

Our insurance system is also to blame. Currently, more than 2,000 companies provide health insurance in the United States, each with different coverage structures and administrative requirements. This lack of uniformity prevents our system from achieving the *economies of scale* (bulk purchasing at a reduced cost) and administrative efficiency realized in countries where there is a single-payer delivery system. According to the Health Insurance Association of America, commercial insurance companies commonly experience administrative costs greater than 10 percent of the total health care insurance premium, whereas the administrative cost of the government's Medicare program is less than 4 percent. These administrative expenses contribute to the high cost of health care and force companies to require employees to share more of the costs, cut back on benefits, and drop some benefits altogether. These costs are largely passed on to consumers in the form of higher prices for goods and services. See **Figure 18.7** on the following page for a breakdown of how health care dollars are spent.

The ACA's provision for Affordable Insurance Exchanges would increase bulk purchasing and reduce administrative costs, thus achieving some savings. Moreover, the ACA mandates the following cost-control measures:

- Insurance companies that spend less than 80 percent of premium dollars on medical care in a given year now have to send enrollees a rebate.
- All insurance companies now have to publicly justify their actions if they plan to raise rates by 10 percent or more.
- Tougher screening procedures and penalties are helping to reduce health care fraud.

what do you think?

Do you believe prospective patients should have access to information about practitioners' and facilities' malpractice records?
- How about their success and failure rates or outcomes of various procedures?

Total expenditures = $2.2 trillion

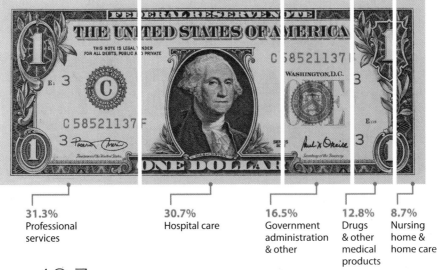

31.3%
Professional
services

30.7%
Hospital care

16.5%
Government
administration
& other

12.8%
Drugs
& other
medical
products

8.7%
Nursing
home &
home care

FIGURE 18.7 **Where Do We Spend Our Health Care Dollars?**

Source: Data are from National Center for Health Statistics, *Health, United States, 2010, with Special Feature on Medical Technology* (Hyattsville, MD: National Center for Health Statistics, 2011).

Quality

The United States has several mechanisms for ensuring quality services: Providers are assessed according to education, licensure, certification/registration, accreditation, peer review, and the legal system of malpractice litigation. Over-the-counter and prescription medications, as well as medical devices, must be approved by the Food and Drug Administration. Insurance companies and government pay-ers may also require a higher level of quality by linking payment to whether a practitioner is board certified, a facility is accredited, or a treatment is an approved therapy. In addition, most insurance plans now require prior authorization and/or second opinions, not only to reduce costs but also to improve quality of care.

Nevertheless, although our health care spending far exceeds that of any other nation, we rank far below many other nations in key indicators of quality. For example, in 2011, life expectancy in the United States, at 78.49 years, was lower than that of 49 other nations of the world.[45] And our infant mortality rate, at 5.98 deaths per every 1,000 live births, is higher than that of 48 other nations.[46] The ACA is intended to improve the quality of health care in the United States. As a first step, in 2011, the Department of Health and Human Services released to Congress a National Strategy for Quality Improvement in Health Care. Its priorities include a new emphasis on promoting the safest, most preventive, and most effective care, increased communication and coordination among providers, and ensuring that patients and families are engaged as partners in their care.[47]

Despite these provisions, many health experts feel that the ACA does not begin to go far enough in addressing the unequal access, high cost, and poor quality of our health care system. They assert that our system has failed, and an entirely new system must be put in its place. See the **Points of View** box on the following page for a discussion of the pros and cons of a system of national health insurance that advocates believe would address these key concerns.

On a personal level, perhaps the most important measurement is how you and your loved ones experience the health care provided.

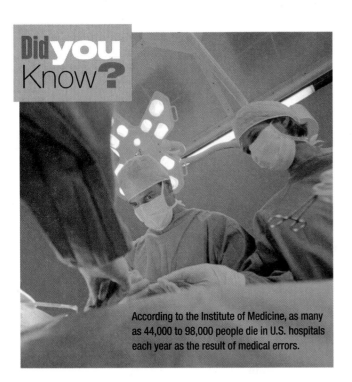

Did you Know?

According to the Institute of Medicine, as many as 44,000 to 98,000 people die in U.S. hospitals each year as the result of medical errors.

National Health Care:

IS IT A GOVERNMENT RESPONSIBILITY?

Whether universal health care coverage will—or should—be achieved in the United States and through what mechanism remain hotly debated topics. Proponents of reform argue that health care is a basic human right and should be available and affordable for everyone. They point to other Western countries, such as Canada, the United Kingdom, and France, that currently provide health care to all citizens through a national service funded through taxes. Opponents of health care reform feel that health care is not a right, but a commodity. They contend that the high cost of changing the system is more than the United States can afford and that the government should not interfere in what has been largely a free-market industry. In addition, lobbying efforts by the insurance industry, pharmaceutical manufacturers, the medical community, and special interest groups have all played a role in thwarting comprehensive reform.

In 2010, Congress passed the Patient Protection and Affordable Care Act (ACA). This act does not provide for a system of national health care but is merely a set of initial steps toward increasing the number of insured Americans. Still, it has been subjected to intense and often rancorous debate. The reforms mandated by the ACA are currently being implemented, and their actual effects are uncertain.

Arguments for National Health Insurance

◯ Health care is a human right. The United Nations Universal Declaration of Human Rights states that "everyone has the right to a standard of living adequate for the health and well-being of oneself and one's family, including . . . medical care."

◯ Americans would be more likely to engage in preventive health behaviors and clinicians would be encouraged to practice preventive medicine; people without insurance often avoid preventive care checkups and inquiring early about suspected symptoms due to cost concerns.

◯ Medical professionals could concentrate on the care of patients rather than on insurance procedures, malpractice liability, and other administrative distractions.

◯ Taxes already pay for a substantial amount of our health care expenditures.

◯ Providing all citizens the right to health care is good for economic productivity because it allows them to live longer and healthier lives, thus contributing to society for a longer time.

Arguments against National Health Insurance

◯ Health care is not a right, because it is not in the Bill of Rights in the U.S. Constitution, which lists rights that the government cannot infringe upon, not services or goods that the government must ensure for the people. Amending the U.S. Constitution to acknowledge a right to health care would be bad for economic productivity.

◯ It is the individual's responsibility, not the government's, to ensure personal health. Diseases and health problems can often be prevented by individuals choosing to live healthier lifestyles.

◯ Expenses for health care would have to be paid for with higher taxes or spending cuts in other areas such as defense and education.

◯ Profit motives, competition, and individual ingenuity have always led to greater cost control and effectiveness. These concepts should be brought to health care reform.

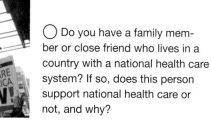

Where Do You Stand?

◯ Do you think that all Americans should have the right to health care?

◯ Is health insurance a personal responsibility?

◯ Do you currently have health insurance? If you don't, what are the barriers that prevent you from having health insurance?

◯ If you do have health insurance, are you currently paying for it? If you are not paying for it, who is?

◯ Do you have a family member or close friend who lives in a country with a national health care system? If so, does this person support national health care or not, and why?

Sources: Right to Health Care ProCon.org, "Should All Americans Have the Right (Be Entitled) to Health Care?" Updated October 2010, http://healthcare.procon.org; The White House, "Health Care Reform: The Affordable Care Act," 2010, www.whitehouse.gov/healthreform/healthcare-overview.

Are You a Smart Health Care Consumer?

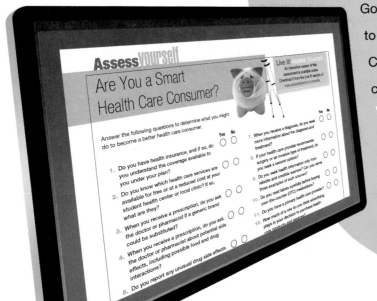

Go online to www.pearsonhighered.com/donatelle to fill out the "Are You a Smart Health Care Consumer?"* If you need to make some changes, follow the strategies outlined in the **YOUR PLAN FOR CHANGE** box.

*If your instructor so chooses, Assess Yourself Activities are available as a printed supplement or as assignable homework online at www.pearsonhighered.com/myhealth.

MyHealthLab®

YOUR PLAN FOR CHANGE

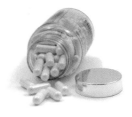

Once you have considered your responses to the **Assess yourself** questions, you may want to change or improve certain behaviors in order to get the best treatment from your health care provider and the health care system.

Today, you can:

○ Research your insurance plan. Find out which health care providers and hospitals you can visit, the amounts of co-payments and premiums you are responsible for, and the drug coverage of your plan.

○ Update your medicine cabinet. Dispose properly of any expired prescriptions or OTC medications. Keep on hand a supply of basic items, such as pain relievers, antiseptic cream, bandages, cough suppressants, and throat lozenges.

Within the next 2 weeks, you can:

○ Find a regular health care provider if you do not already have one and make an appointment for a general checkup.

○ Check with your insurance provider and see what CAM practitioners and therapies are covered.

○ Find out what alternative therapies your college's health clinic offers.

By the end of the semester, you can:

○ Become an advocate for others' health. Write to your congressperson or state legislature to express your interest in health care reform.

○ Make relaxation and mind–body stress-reducing techniques a part of your everyday life. This can simply mean practicing meditation, deep breathing, or even taking long walks in nature. You don't need to visit a CAM practitioner or follow a specific therapeutic practice to benefit from methods of relaxation, meditation, and spiritual awakening.

Summary

* Self-care and individual responsibility are key factors in reducing rising health care costs and improving health status. Advance planning can help you navigate health care treatment in unfamiliar situations or emergencies. Assess health professionals by considering their qualifications, their record of treating similar problems, and their ability to work with you.

* In theory, conventional Western (allopathic) medicine is based on scientifically validated methods and procedures. Medical doctors, specialists of various kinds, nurses, physician assistants, and other health care professionals practice allopathic medicine.

* Throughout the world people are using complementary and alternative medicine (CAM) in increasing numbers. Alternative medical systems include traditional Chinese medicine (TCM), ayurveda, homeopathy, and naturopathy. CAM also includes manipulative and body-based practices, energy medicine, mind–body medicine, and natural products.

* Consumers need to understand that the FDA does not study and approve dietary supplements before they are brought to market. Thus there is no guarantee of their safety or effectiveness. However, the USP Verified Mark does indicate that a supplement has met certain criteria for product purity and manufacturing standards.

* Health insurance is based on the concept of spreading risk. Insurance is provided by private insurance companies (which charge premiums) and the government Medicare and Medicaid programs (which are funded by taxes). Managed care (in the form of HMOs, PPOs, and POS plans) attempts to control costs by streamlining administrative procedures and promoting preventive care, among other initiatives.

* Concerns about the U.S. health care system include access, cost, and quality. The Patient Protection and Affordable Care Act was passed by Congress in 2010 to address these issues. Its provisions are currently being implemented, but many public health experts feel that it does not go far enough in addressing the fundamental flaws in the system.

Pop Quiz

1. Of the following conditions, which would be appropriately managed by self-care?
   a. A persistent temperature of 104°F or higher
   b. Sudden weight loss of more than a few pounds without changes in diet or exercise patterns
   c. A sore throat, runny nose, and cough that persist for several days
   d. Yellowing of the skin or the whites of the eyes

2. What medical practice is based on procedures whose objective is to heal by countering the patient's symptoms?
   a. Allopathic medicine
   b. Homeopathic medicine
   c. Ayurvedic medicine
   d. Chiropractic medicine

3. What mechanism used by private insurance companies requires that the subscriber pay a certain amount for health care before the insurance company will begin paying for services?
   a. Coinsurance
   b. Cost sharing
   c. Co-payments
   d. Deductibles

4. Deborah, 28, is a single parent who is unemployed. Her medical bills are paid by a federal health insurance program for the poor. This agency is
   a. an HMO.
   b. Social Security.
   c. Medicaid.
   d. Medicare.

5. CAM therapies focus on treating the mind and the whole body, which makes them part of a
   a. natural approach.
   b. psychological approach.
   c. holistic approach.
   d. gentle approach.

6. What type of medicine addresses imbalances of *qi*?
   a. Chiropractic medicine
   b. Ayurvedic medicine
   c. Traditional Chinese medicine
   d. Homeopathic medicine

7. The population group with the largest percentage of uninsured individuals is
   a. Americans over age 65.
   b. college students.
   c. African Americans.
   d. Hispanic Americans.

8. Which of the following is a form of energy medicine?
   a. Alexander technique
   b. Psychoneuroimmunology
   c. Reiki
   d. Shiatsu

9. Which of the following health care providers holds a medical degree?
   a. Doctor of science in nursing
   b. Ophthalmologist
   c. Osteopath
   d. Naturopathic physician

10. The USP Verified Mark indicates that a supplement
    a. meets quality and manufacturing standards.
    b. is effective.
    c. is FDA approved.
    d. is safe for children.

Answers to these questions can be found on page A-1.

Think about It!

1. List several conditions (resulting from illness or accident) for which you wouldn't need to seek medical help. When would you consider each condition to be bad enough to require medical attention? How would you decide where to go for treatment?

2. Describe your rights as a patient. Have you ever received treatment that violated these rights? If so, what action, if any, did you take?

3. Discuss how medical and pharmaceutical waste has a negative impact on the environment. What are two ways in which you personally can reduce such waste?

4. What are some of the potential benefits and risks of CAM? Why do you think these practices and products are becoming so popular?

5. What can you do to ensure that you are receiving accurate information regarding CAM treatments or medicines? Which federal agency oversees CAM in the United States?

Accessing Your Health on the Internet

The following websites explore further topics and issues related to personal health. For links to the websites below, visit the Companion Website for *Access to Health,* 13th Edition, at www.pearsonhighered.com/donatelle.

1. *Agency for Healthcare Research and Quality (AHRQ).* AHRQ's website is a gateway to consumer health information. It provides links to sites that can address health care concerns and provide information on what questions to ask, what to look for, and what you should know when making critical decisions about personal care. www.ahrq.gov

2. *Food and Drug Administration (FDA).* The FDA provides news on the latest government-approved home health tests and other health-related products. www.fda.gov

3. *The Leapfrog Group.* A nationwide coalition of more than 150 public and private organizations, the Leapfrog Group focuses on identifying and devising solutions for problems in the U.S. hospital system that can lead to medical errors. www.leapfroggroup.org

4. *National Committee for Quality Assurance (NCQA).* The NCQA assesses and reports on the quality of managed care plans, including HMOs. www.ncqa.org

5. *HealthCare.Gov.* This site provides up-to-date information regarding the 2010 Patient Protection and Affordable Care Act, which mandates health insurance for previously uninsured Americans. www.healthcare.gov

6. *National Center for Complementary and Alternative Medicine (NCCAM).* A division of the National Institutes of Health, NCCAM is dedicated to providing the latest information and research on complementary and alternative practices. http://nccam.nih.gov

7. *National Institutes of Health, Office of Dietary Supplements.* This excellent resource includes access to a database of federally funded research projects pertaining to dietary supplements. http://ods.od.nih.gov

References

1. Gebhardt, M.C., "Communication Matters," *American Academy of Orthopaedic Surgeons AAOS Now,* May 2011, www.aaos.org/news/aaosnow/may11/managing5.asp.

2. D. Merenstein et al., "Use and Costs of Nonrecommended Tests during Routine Preventive Health Exams," *American Journal of Preventive Medicine* 30, no. 6 (2006): 521–27; Thomson Reuters, "Waste in the U.S. Healthcare System Pegged at $700 Billion in Report from Thomson Reuters," October 26, 2009, http://thomsonreuters.com/content/press_room/tsh/waste_US_healthcare_system.

3. N. Kwon, "Patient Rights," 2006, www.emedicinehealth.com/patient_rights/article_em.htm.

4. American College Health Association, *American College Health Association–National College Health Assessment (ACHA-NCHA): Reference Group Data Report Spring 2008* (Baltimore: American College Health Association, 2008), www.achancha.org/reports_ACHA-NCHAoriginal.html.

5. U.S. Food and Drug Administration, "The Possible Dangers of Buying Medicine over the Internet," 2010, www.fda.gov/ForConsumers/ConsumerUpdates/ucm048396.htm.

6. Mayo Clinic Staff, "Complementary and Alternative Medicine: What Is It?" Mayo Clinic, October 2009, www.mayoclinic.com/health/alternative-medicine/PN00001.

7. National Center for Complementary and Alternative Medicine, "The Use of Complementary and Alternative Medicine in the United States," Updated December 2008, http://nccam.nih.gov/news/camstats/2007/camsurvey_fs1.htm.

8. National Center for Complementary and Alternative Medicine, "Health Topics A to Z," 2012, http://nccam.nih.gov/health/atoz.htm.

9. National Center for Complementary and Alternative Medicine, "Ayurvedic Medicine: An Introduction," NCCAM Publication no. D287, Updated July 2009, http://nccam.nih.gov/health/ayurveda/introduction.htm.

10. American Institute of Homeopathy, "Homeopathy: Efficacy and Evidence Base," 2007, http://homeopathyusa.org/homeopathy-now.html; Health Alternatives Online, "Homeopathy," 2008, www.healthalternativesonline.com/homeopathy.html.

11. National Center for Complementary and Alternative Medicine, "Chiropractic: An Introduction," NCCAM Publication no. D403, Modified February 2012, http://nccam.nih.gov/health/chiropractic/introduction.htm.

12. Bureau of Labor Statistics, U.S. Department of Labor, "Chiropractors," *Occupational Outlook Handbook, 2012–2013 Edition,* March 29, 2012, www.bls.gov/ooh/Healthcare/Chiropractors.htm.

13. National Center for Complementary and Alternative Medicine, "Massage Therapy: An Introduction," NCCAM Publication no. D327, Updated August 2010, http://nccam.nih.gov/health/massage/massageintroduction.htm.

14. Ibid.

15. Bureau of Labor Statistics, U.S. Department of Labor, "Massage Therapists,"

Occupational Outlook Handbook, 2012–2013 Edition, Modified March 29, 2012, www.bls.gov/ooh/Healthcare/Massage-therapists.htm.

16. National Center for Complementary and Alternative Medicine, "What Is CAM?" Updated July 2011, http://nccam.nih.gov/health/whatiscam; U.S. Trager Association, "The Trager Approach," 2010, www.trager-us.org/trager-approach.html.

17. National Center for Complementary and Alternative Medicine, "What Is CAM?" 2010.

18. Agency for Healthcare Research and Quality, U.S. Department of Health and Human Services, "Complementary and Alternative Therapies for Back Pain II," Evidence Report/Technology Assessment 194 (October 2010), AHRQ Publication No. 10(11)-E007, www.ahrq.gov/downloads/pub/evidence/pdf/backpaincam/backcam2.pdf.

19. National Center for Complementary and Alternative Medicine, "Acupuncture: An Introduction," NCCAM Publication no. D404, 2011, http://nccam.nih.gov/health/acupuncture/introduction.htm.

20. Psychoneuroimmunology Research Society, "Mission Statement," November 17, 2010, www.pnirs.org/society/index.cfm.

21. E. Broadbent and H. E. Koschwanez, "The Psychology of Wound Healing," *Current Opinions in Psychiatry* 25, no 2 (2012): 135–40.

22. M. R. Irwin and R. Olmstead, "Mitigating Cellular Inflammation in Older Adults: A Randomized Controlled Trial of Tai Chi," *American Journal of Geriatric Psychiatry,* September 19, 2011 [E-pub ahead of print].

23. J. J. Mao et al., "Complementary and Alternative Medicine Use among Cancer Survivors: A Population-Based Study," *Journal of Cancer Survivorship: Research and Practice* 5, no. 1 (2011): 8–17.

24. Academy of Nutrition and Dietetics, "Functional Foods," *Journal of the American Dietetic Association* 109, no. 4 (2009): 735–46.

25. M. G. Shrime et al., *Journal of Nutrition* 141, no 11 (2011): 1982–88.

26. Office of Dietary Supplements, National Institutes of Health, "Dietary Supplements: Background Information," Updated June 2011, http://ods.od.nih.gov/factsheets/dietarysupplements.asp.

27. National Center for Complementary and Alternative Medicine, "Kava," June 2008, http://nccam.nih.gov/health/kava/ataglance.htm.

28. Mayo Clinic Staff, "Herbal Supplements: What to Know before You Buy," Updated November 17, 2011, www.mayoclinic.com/health/herbal-supplements/SA00044.

29. U.S. Pharmacopeial Convention, "USP & Patients/Consumers," 2012, www.usp.org/usp-consumers.

30. National Conference of State Legislators, "Health Insurance: Premiums and Increases," August 2011, www.ncsl.org/issues-research/health/health-insurance-premiums.aspx

31. U.S. Centers for Disease Control and Prevention/National Center for Health Statistics, "Health Insurance Coverage: Early Release of Estimates from the 2010 National Health Interview Survey," 2011, www.cdc.gov/nchs/nhis/released201106.htm.

32. Ibid.

33. C. Schoen et al., "How Many Are Underinsured? Trends among U.S. Adults, 2003 and 2007," *Health Affairs* Web Exclusive, June 10, 2008: w298–w309.

34. U.S. Centers for Disease Control and Prevention/National Center for Health Statistics, "Health Insurance Coverage," 2011.

35. American College Health Association. *American College Health Association-National College Health Assessment II: Reference Group Executive Summary Fall 2011* (Baltimore, MD: American College Health Association; 2012).

36. U.S. Centers for Disease Control and Prevention/National Center for Health Statistics, "Health Insurance Coverage," 2011.

37. Kaiser Family Foundation, "Total HMO Enrollment, July 2010," 2011, www.statehealthfacts.org/comparecat.jsp?cat=7&rgn=6&rgn=1.

38. Centers for Medicare & Medicaid Services, "National Health Expenditure Projections 2010–2020: Forecast Summary," 2012, www.cms.gov/Research-Statistics-Data-and-Systems/Statistics-Trends-and-Reports/NationalHealthExpendData/Downloads/proj2010.pdf.

39. Centers for Medicare and Medicaid Services, "Medicare Enrollment: National Trends 1966–2008," 2009, www.cms.hhs.gov/MedicareEnRpts/Downloads/HISMI08.pdf.

40. Bureau of Labor Statistics, U.S. Department of Labor, "Physicians and Surgeons," *Occupational Outlook Handbook, 2012–2013,* Modified March 2012, www.bls.gov/oco/ocos074.htm.

41. American Hospital Association, "Fast Facts on U.S. Hospitals. www.aha.org/research/rc/stat-studies/fast-facts.shtml.

42. O. W. Brawley, *How We Do Harm: A Doctor Breaks Ranks about Being Sick in America* (New York: St. Martin's Press, 2011).

43. Centers for Medicare and Medicaid Services, *National Health Expenditure Projections 2011–2021,* 2012, www.cms.gov/Research-Statistics-Data-and-Systems/Statistics-Trends-and-Reports/NationalHealthExpendData/Downloads/Proj2011PDF. pdf.

44. Ibid.

45. Central Intelligence Agency, "Country Comparison: Life Expectancy at Birth. CIA World Factbook," 2012, www.cia.gov/library/publications/the-world-factbook/rankorder/2102rank.html.

46. Central Intelligence Agency, "Country Comparison: Infant Mortality Rate. CIA Factbook," 2012, www.cia.gov/library/publications/the-world-factbook/rankorder/2091rank.html.

47. Department of Health and Human Services, "Report to Congress: National Strategy for Quality Improvement in Health Care," 2011, www.healthcare.gov/law/resources/reports/nationalqualitystrategy032011.pdf.

10 Preventing Violence and Abuse

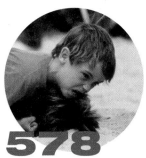

578
What makes some people act out their anger with violence?

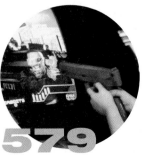

579
Does violence in the media cause violence in real life?

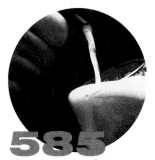

585
What does *acquaintance rape* mean?

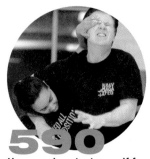

590
How can I protect myself from becoming a victim of violence?

OBJECTIVES

✳ Differentiate between intentional and unintentional injuries and discuss societal and personal factors that contribute to violence in American society.

✳ Discuss factors that contribute to homicide, domestic violence, intimate partner violence, sexual victimization, and other intentional acts of violence.

✳ Describe strategies to prevent intentional injuries and reduce their risk of occurrence.

✳ Explain potential risks to students on campus and potential strategies that campus leaders, law enforcement officials, and individuals can develop to prevent students from becoming victims.

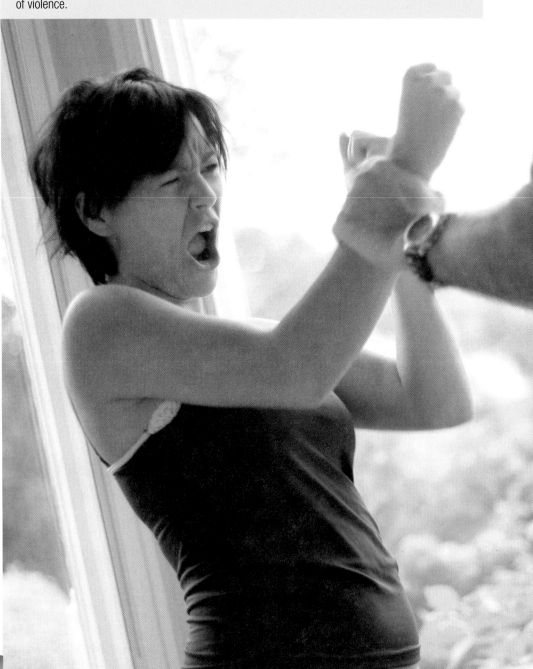

Fear follows crime, and is its punishment.
—Voltaire, 1694–1778

Acts of hatred and brutality have always played a major role in human history as humans struggle to dominate one another. Today, violence is pervasive and takes many forms; news reports seem to depict a never-ending story of murder and mayhem. In the wake of such reports, many people live in fear, even though they may not have experienced violence personally. Are our fears justified? Is violence in the United States worse than ever? And to which kinds of violence are college students particularly vulnerable?

Before we can discuss the extent and nature of violence, it's important to understand what the word *violence* means. The World Health Organization (WHO) defines **violence** as "the intentional use of physical force or power, threatened or actual, against oneself, another person, or a group or community that results in or has a high likelihood of resulting in injury, death, psychological harm, maldevelopment or deprivation."[1] Today, most experts realize that emotional and psychological forms of violence can be as devastating as physical blows to the body.

The U.S. Public Health Service historically categorized violence resulting in injuries as either intentional or unintentional, based on the intent to cause harm. Today, experts recognize that intent is not always completely clear and that distinguishing cause and intent can be difficult. Typically, **intentional injuries**—those committed with intent to harm—include assaults, homicides, self-inflicted injuries, and suicides. **Unintentional injuries** are those committed without apparent intent to harm, such as motor vehicle crashes and other types of accidents.[2] (Unintentional injuries are discussed in detail in Focus On: Reducing Your Risk of Unintentional Injury.)

Why do we focus attention on violence in an introductory health text? The answer is simple: Young adults are disproportionately affected by violence and injury. In fact, homicide and suicide are the second and third leading causes of death of young adults.[3] Intimate partner violence, assaults, harassment, and psychological abuse are possible threats to student health. These intentional injuries can harm emotional health, leading to depression, drug abuse, poor grades, dropping out, or even suicide.

Violence in the United States

Violence has been a part of the American landscape since colonial times. However, it wasn't until the 1980s that the U.S. Public Health Service identified violence as a leading cause of death and disability and gave it chronic disease status, indicating that it was a pervasive threat to society. Statistics from the Federal Bureau of Investigation (FBI) have shown that, after steadily increasing from 1973 to 2006, the rates of overall crime and certain types of violent crime have decreased over the past few years.[4] Violent crimes involve force or threat of force, and include four offenses: *murder and nonnegligent manslaughter, forcible rape, robbery,* and *aggravated assault.* In 2011, reported crimes were at historically low levels, with incidence of events in all four of the violent crime categories declining by several percentage points. Overall, the nation experienced a 4 percent decrease in violent crimes and a 0.8 percent decline in property crimes[5] (Figure 19.1).

Why be concerned about violence if violent crime rates are decreasing? The answer is that there are no reliable statistics for many forms of violence, and most violence is underreported. See Figure 19.2 on the next page for the frequency of several types of violent crimes. Also, while total crime rates may be down, there are huge disparities in crime rates based on race, sex, age, socioeconomic status, geography, and

violence Aggressive behaviors that produce injuries and can result in death.

intentional injuries Injury, death, or psychological harm inflicted with the intent to harm.

unintentional injuries Injury, death, or psychological harm caused unintentionally or without premeditation.

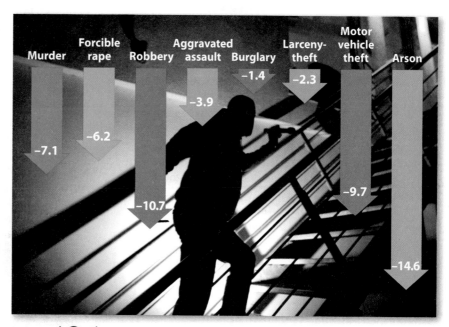

FIGURE 19.1 **Declining Crime Rates**

According to the FBI's *Preliminary Semiannual Uniform Crime Report,* violent crime in the nation dropped 6.2 percent and property crime declined 2.8 percent during the first 6 months of 2010, compared to the same period in 2009.

Source: Data from Federal Bureau of Investigation, *Crime in the United States, Preliminary Semiannual Uniform Crime Report,* January through December 2010, Table 3, www.fbi.gov/about-us/cjis/ucr/crime-in-the-u.s/2010/preliminary-crime-in-the-us-2009/prelimiucrjan-jun_10_excels/table-3.

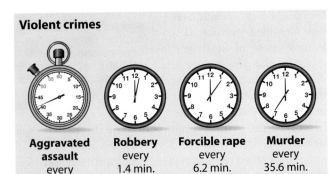

Violent crimes

Aggravated assault every 40.5 sec.

Robbery every 1.4 min.

Forcible rape every 6.2 min.

Murder every 35.6 min.

FIGURE 19.2 **Crime Clock**
The Crime Clock represents the annual ratio of crime to fixed time intervals. The Crime Clock should not be taken to imply a regularity in the commission of crime.
Source: Adapted from Federal Bureau of Investigation, "Crime in the United States, 2010," 2011, www.fbi.gov/about-us/cjis/ucr/crime-in-the-u.s/2010/crime-in-the-u.s.-2010/offenses-known-to-law-enforcement/crime-clock.

other factors. Finally, there were still an estimated 4.3 million violent crimes against U.S. residents aged 12 and older in 2009.[6] Even if we have never been victimized personally, we all are victimized by violent acts that cause us to be fearful, restrict our liberty, and damage the reputation of our campus, city, or nation. If you don't go out for a walk or run at night because you are worried about being attacked, you are a victim of societal violence.

Violence on U.S. Campuses

On April 16, 2007, a deadly mass shooting took place at Virginia Tech, taking the lives of 32 people and wounding 17 more. The tragedy sparked dialogue and action on campuses across the nation and throughout the world. In 2008, another shooting occurred at Northern Illinois University, and increased priority was placed on campus security and student and faculty safety. On April 2, 2012, a former student at Oikos University in Northern California shot and killed 7 people before surrendering to police. Today, it would be hard to find a campus without a safety plan in place to prevent and respond to violent crime. Campuses have stepped up to protect their students and their images, but many forms of campus violence continue to be a problem.

93%

of crimes against college students occur at off-campus locations.

Relationship violence is one of the most prevalent problems on campus. In the most recent American College Health Association survey, 11.1 percent of women and 6.6 percent of men reported being emotionally abused in the past 12 months by a significant other. Almost 7 percent of women and 3.8 percent of men reported being stalked, and 2.4 percent of women and 2 percent of men and women reported being involved in a physically abusive relationship. Nearly 1 percent of men and over 2 percent of women reported being in a sexually abusive relationship.[7]

The statistics on reported campus violence represent only a glimpse of the big picture. It is believed that fewer than 25 percent of campus crimes in general are reported to *any* authority. Even though as many as 20 to 25 percent of college women will be raped or sexually assaulted before they graduate, 95 percent of these women never report these crimes.[8] Why would students fail to report crimes? Typical reasons include concerns over privacy, fear of retaliation, embarrassment or shame, lack of support, perception that the crime was too minor, or uncertainty that it was a crime. This is particularly true in the case of crimes such as acquaintance rape, stalking, and hazing. See the **Student Health Today** boxes on pages 577 and 578 for further exploration of these issues.

Factors Contributing to Violence

Several factors increase the likelihood of violent acts, as discussed in the following list:[9]

- **Poverty.** Low socioeconomic status can create an environment of hopelessness in which some people view violence as the only way of obtaining what they want. Children raised in lower-income homes have higher rates of violence than those in higher-income homes.[10]
- **Unemployment.** Financial strain, losing or fear of losing a job, economic downturns, and living in economically depressed areas can increase rates and severity of violence.[11]
- **Parental influence.** Children raised in environments in which shouting, hitting, emotional abuse, antisocial behavior, and other forms of violence are commonplace are more apt to act out these behaviors as adults.[12]
- **Cultural beliefs.** Cultures that objectify women and empower men to be tough and aggressive show higher rates of violence in the home.[13]
- **Discrimination or oppression.** Whenever one group is oppressed or perceives that its members are oppressed by those of another group, violence against others is more likely.
- **Religious beliefs and differences.** Extreme religious beliefs can lead people to think that violence against others is justified.

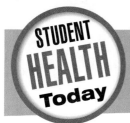

SEXUAL ASSAULT: A CULTURE OF SILENCE?

How many students do you think are sexually assaulted during a typical year on campus? Would it surprise you to know that most schools indicate that there were zero rapes or sexual assaults on their campuses during the past year? A crime prevention program at one major university had over 46 sexual assault clients in a recent academic year, yet none of these reports showed up in the university's annual security report. Likewise, a counseling program at a large Midwestern university served 62 students, faculty, and staff who reported being raped or almost raped in the previous year. Those assaults didn't show up on university reports either. How can this be?

A federal law known as the Clery Act requires colleges and universities to solicit information about crime from women's centers, student health centers, residence hall directors, coaches, and the like and to report this information. But Clery statistics are "official statistics," meaning that a victim must report an assault to campus security for the crime to be listed. If victims talk only with campus counselors and not to security officers, confidentiality issues prevent counselors from reporting these cases. Thus, for a variety of reasons, the Clery Act isn't working as intended.

Why are victims so unwilling to report crimes? The reasons include the following:

✳ Victims often blame themselves for getting into a dangerous situation.

✳ Drinking too much is often cited as a contributing factor, and many feel that if they hadn't had so much to drink, the assault might not have happened.

✳ Often there are no witnesses, and the difficulty of proving that a sexual assault occurred in a "he said, she said" situation is more than victims can manage.

✳ Conflicting lines of authority among local police, campus police, and university officials can block swift action. Rape is a felony, so some question whether hearings and other disciplinary actions should be conducted on campus or whether police should handle such matters exclusively.

✳ Lengthy university hearings and investigations can impose a heavy burden on victims and their families, leading many to drop charges.

✳ Victims fear retaliation or being labeled as promiscuous or a troublemaker.

Efforts are underway to change campus culture by educating students about their options, informing counselors and support staff of their legal responsibilities, and improving reporting protocols. However, the process is slow. Schools fear

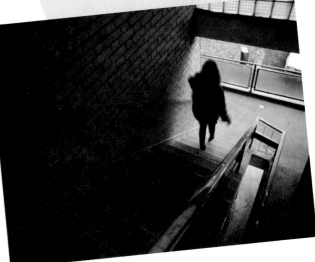

The reluctance to report sexual assault on campus and the difficulty of pursuing criminal proceedings in the campus environment can create turmoil in victims' lives while too rarely leading to punishment of offenders.

negative publicity from reports of rape and sexual assault. A school's image could be tarnished, possibly affecting enrollment and fund-raising efforts.

Sources: Center for Public Integrity, "Sexual Assault on Campus: A Frustrating Search for Justice," Updated February 2010, www.publicintegrity.org/investigations/campus_assault; Center for Public Integrity, "Barriers Curb Reporting on Campus Sexual Assault," 2009, www.publicintegrity.org/investigations/campus_assault/articles/entry/1822.

● **Political differences.** Civil unrest and differences in political party affiliations and beliefs have historically been triggers for violent acts.

● **Breakdowns in the criminal justice system.** Overcrowded prisons, lenient sentences, early releases from prison, and inadequate treatment and training in prison encourage repeat offenses and future violence.

● **Stress.** People who are in crisis or under stress are more apt to be highly reactive, striking out at others or acting irrationally.[14]

● **Heavy substance use.** Alcohol and drug abuse are often catalysts for violence and risk factors for domestic violence and other crimes.[15]

What Makes Some People Prone to Violence?

In addition to the broad, societal-based factors that contribute to crime, personal factors also can increase risks for violence. Emerging evidence suggests that the family and home environment in general may be the greatest contributor to eventual violent behavior among family members.[16] The following are several other predictors of aggressive behavior.[17]

Anger People who anger quickly often have a low tolerance for frustration. The cause may be genetic or physiological; there is evidence that some people are born with

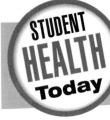

Hazing: Over the Top and Dangerous for Many

We've all seen instances of hazing—those silly, humiliating things sorority or fraternity initiates, rookie team members, or new club recruits are asked to do. However, with the death of Robert Cameron, a 26-year-old drum major at Florida A&M in 2011, the issue of hazing became headline news. Injuries, deaths, and the potential for lawsuits against those who participate all have hazing in the national spotlight. Currently, hazing is considered a crime in 44 states. Most institutions have policies against hazing, but few students ever report it, and only when high-profile cases make it into the media do most of us pay attention.

Just what is hazing? Essentially it is "any activity expected of someone joining or participating in a group that humiliates, degrades, abuses, or endangers them regardless of a person's willingness to participate." Typically, it involves forcing students to consume excessive alcohol; dress in humiliating garb; undergo forced sleep deprivation; endure verbal abuse from group members; or physical abuse in the form of beatings, heat or cold exposure, or forced sexual acts. These activities can range from practical jokes to situations where life and limb are endangered. For those who are victimized and don't find their forced hazing humorous, psychological and physical damage can be serious.

According to a recent national study, 55 percent of college students involved in clubs, teams, and organizations experience hazing, and 47 percent of students come to college already having experienced hazing. Yet many students are unaware of its dangers or legal implications, and 9 out of 10 students who experience hazing in college do not realize they've been hazed.

In 95 percent of cases in which students identified their experience as hazing, they did not report the events to campus officials. There may be several reasons for this underreporting, but one reason seems to be that more students perceive positive rather than negative outcomes of hazing, for example, feeling a sense of accomplishment or belonging. Students also report that school administrators do little to prevent hazing beyond maintaining a "hazing is not tolerated" stance. If schools are to have an impact on the prevalence of hazing on their campuses, they need to implement broader prevention and intervention efforts and work to educate their campus community on the physical and legal perils of hazing.

Source: Adapted from E. Allan and M. Madden, *Hazing in View: College Students at Risk* (Orono, ME: National Collaborative for Hazing Research and Prevention, 2008), www.hazingstudy.org. Reprinted by permission of Elizabeth Allan.

---

primary aggression Goal-directed, hostile self-assertion that is destructive in nature.

reactive aggression Hostile emotional reaction brought about by frustrating life experiences.

strong tendencies toward being angry. Family background may be the most important factor. Typically, anger-prone people come from families that are disruptive, chaotic, and unskilled in emotional expression.[18] Also, people who are taught not to express anger in public do not know how to handle it when it reaches a level they can no longer hide.[19]

Aggressive behavior is often a key aspect of violent interactions. **Primary aggression** is goal-directed, hostile self-assertion that is destructive in nature. **Reactive aggression** is more often part of an emotional reaction brought about by frustrating life experiences. Whether aggression is reactive or primary, it is most likely to flare up in times of acute stress.

Substance Abuse Substance abuse and violence are closely linked, even though research has yet to show that substance abuse actually causes violence. Consider the following:[20]

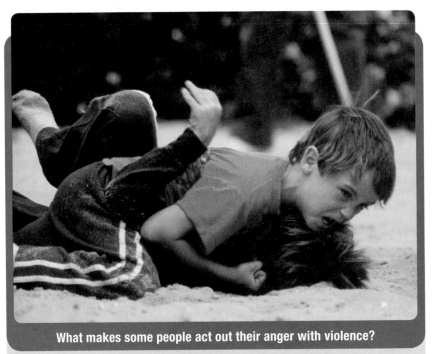

What makes some people act out their anger with violence?

If you are like most people, you probably acted out your anger more as a child than you do today. With age and maturity, most people learn to control outbursts of anger in a socially acceptable and rational manner. However, some people go through life acting out their aggressive tendencies in much the same way they did as children—with anger and violence that are a form of self-assertion or a response to frustration.

- Consumption of alcohol—by perpetrators of the crime, the victim, or both—immediately precedes over half of all violent crimes, including murder.
  - Criminals using illegal drugs commit robberies and assaults more frequently than criminals who do not use them, and do so especially during periods of heavy drug use.
  - In domestic assault cases, more than 86 percent of the assailants and 42 percent of victims reported using alcohol at the time of the attack.
- Alcohol abuse, particularly binge drinking, is associated with physical victimization among males and sexual victimization (particularly rape) among females on campuses.
- Numbers of suicide attempts and completions are highly correlated to drug and alcohol intake.

Crime Victimization Survey, the violent crime rate declined by 41 percent and the property crime rate fell by 32 percent over the 10-year period from 1999 to 2010. In 2010, the rate of violent crime declined by another 13 percent and property crime declined by another 6 percent—reaching all-time historic lows.[23] Some researchers even argue that playing violent video games or watching violent movies is actually cathartic and that people who engage in these activities report relieved stress afterward.[24]

Just because a connection between the media and violence has not been established, however, that does not mean it's healthy to consume an excessive amount of it. Concern has been raised that people who spend too much time in front of the TV or online may miss the important communication lessons that come from talking with people in person and learning to get along with others. In addition, debate continues over whether a person who sees so much violence enacted in the media becomes *desensitized* to violence.

what do you think?

Do you think the media influence your behavior? If so, in what ways?
- Could that influence lead to your becoming violent? Why or why not?
- Are there instances in which curtailing violent viewing or restricting the nature and extent of violence and sex in the media is warranted? If so, under what circumstances?

How Much Impact Do the Media Have?

Although the media are blamed for having a major role in the escalation of violence, this association is not as clear as you might suspect. Several early studies seemed to support a link between exposure to violent media and subsequent violent behavior. However, much of this research has been called into question. Analyses of earlier studies indicate that many of them used inappropriate measures of violence, had methodological problems, were inherently biased, or otherwise did not support an association between media violence and criminal aggression.[21]

Critics of previous studies point out that today's young people are exposed to more media violence—on the Internet and TV, and in movies and video games—than any previous generation, without any measurable impact on crime rates. Rates of violent crime and victimization among teens age 10 to 17 have fallen to the lowest rates ever recorded.[22] According to the National

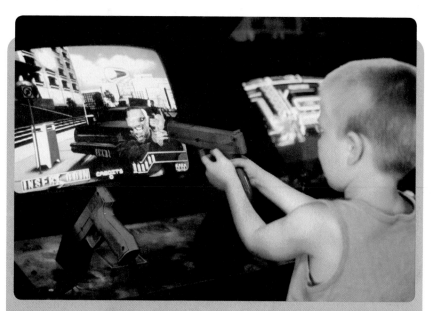

Does violence in the media cause violence in real life?

Evidence of the real-world effects of violence in the media is inconclusive. Arguably, Americans today—especially children—are exposed to more depictions of violence in the news, movies, music, and games than ever before, but research has not shown a clear link between a person's exposure to violent media and his or her propensity to engage in violent acts. Regardless, many people are concerned that children today are exposed to more violence than they have the emotional or cognitive maturity to handle.

Interpersonal Violence

Intentional injury can be categorized into three major types: *interpersonal violence, collective violence,* and *self-directed violence,* although there is some degree of overlap among these groups.[25] Interpersonal violence and collective violence are discussed below. Self-directed violence, including suicide and self-mutilation, is discussed in **Chapter 2. Interpersonal violence** includes violence inflicted against one individual by another or by a small group of others. Homicide, hate crimes, domestic violence, child abuse, elder abuse, and sexual victimization all fit into this category.

interpersonal violence Violence inflicted against one individual by another or by a small group of others.

homicide Death that results from intent to injure or kill.

hate crime Crime targeted against a particular societal group and motivated by bias against that group.

ethnoviolence Violence directed at persons affiliated with a particular ethnic group.

Homicide

Homicide, defined as murder or nonnegligent manslaughter (killing another human), is the fifteenth leading cause of death in the United States, but the second leading cause of death for persons aged 15 to 24. It accounts for 18,000 premature deaths in the United States annually, the majority of which are caused by firearms.[26] Over half of all homicides occur among people who know one another. In two thirds of these cases, the perpetrator and the victim are friends or acquaintances; in one third, they belong to the same family.[27]

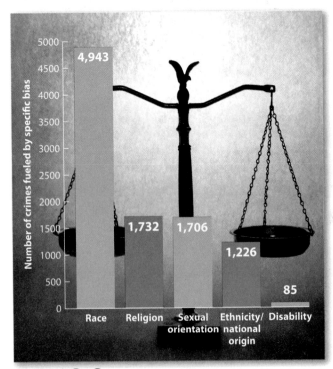

FIGURE 19.3 Bias-Motivated Crimes, 2009
Source: Data from Federal Bureau of Investigation, "Hate Crime Statistics, 2009," 2010, www.fbi.gov/ucr/hc2009.

Rank	Country	Homicide Rate
1	Colombia	0.617847 per 1,000 people
2	South Africa	0.496008 per 1,000 people
5	Russia	0.201534 per 1,000 people
6	Mexico	0.130213 per 1,000 people
16	Zimbabwe	0.0749938 per 1,000 people
24	United States	0.042802 per 1,000 people
26	India	0.0344083 per 1,000 people
40	France	0.0173272 per 1,000 people
43	Australia	0.0150324 per 1,000 people
44	Canada	0.0149063 per 1,000 people
55	Ireland	0.00946215 per 1,000 people
60	Japan	0.00499933 per 1,000 people
61	Saudi Arabia	0.00397456 per 1,000 people

TABLE 19.1 Per Capita Homicide Rates in Selected Nations

Source: Nationmaster, "Crime Statistics: Murders (per capita) (most recent) by Country," www.nationmaster.com, Accessed March 2010. Used with permission.

Homicide rates reveal clear differences across races and ages. Whereas overall homicide rates in the United States have fluctuated minimally and have even decreased in some populations, those involving young victims and perpetrators, particularly young black males, have surged. From 2002 to 2007, the number of homicides involving black male victims age 15 to 24 rose by 31 percent, and those involving them as perpetrators increased by 41 percent.[28] How do homicide rates compare by race in general? Overall, in 2008 in the United States, population-based rates of homicide were 3.3 per 100,000 for whites, 20.6 per 100,000 for blacks, and 6.1 per 100,000 for all other races combined.[29]

The rates of homicide in the United States are higher than in many other developed nations, as shown in Table 19.1. See the **Health Headlines** box for a discussion of guns and violence.

Hate and Bias-Motivated Crimes

A **hate crime** is a crime committed against a person, property, or group of people that is motivated by the offender's bias against a race, religion, disability, sexual orientation, or ethnicity. As a result of national efforts to promote understanding and appreciation of diversity, reports of hate crimes have declined since 2008. According to the FBI's most recent *Hate Crime Statistics* report, there were 8,336 reported victims of hate crimes in 2009[30] (Figure 19.3). Over 62 percent of the persons who committed these crimes were white, 18.5 percent were black, and the remaining offenders' race was listed as "various" or "unknown."

Bias-related crime, both on campus and in the community, is sometimes referred to as **ethnoviolence,** which refers to violence among ethnic groups in the larger society that

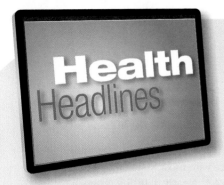

BRINGING THE GUN DEBATE TO CAMPUS

On average, each year in the United States 100,000 people are shot. Over 31,000 of them die, and of those who survive, many experience significant physical and emotional repercussions. Some facts about guns and gun violence include the following:

✳ Firearm homicide is a leading cause of death for people age 15 to 24, second only to motor vehicle crashes. The rate of firearm deaths for this age group is 42.7 times higher in the United States than it is in 22 other high-income countries with stricter gun laws and fewer guns.

✳ Handguns are consistently responsible for more murders than any other type of weapon (see the chart).

✳ Today, 35 percent of American homes have a gun on the premises, with nearly 300 million privately owned guns registered—and millions more that are unregistered and/or illegal.

✳ The presence of a gun in the home triples the risk of a homicide in that location and increases suicide risk more than five times.

What factors contribute to gun deaths in the United States? Gun critics argue that large numbers of guns in the United States as well as relatively lax gun-control laws are the culprits. However, gun-rights advocates say that the problem lies not with guns, but with the people who own them, and point to countries such as Canada, with similar numbers of guns as in the United States, but with much lower gun-related crime rates.

High-profile shootings at schools and other public places have brought

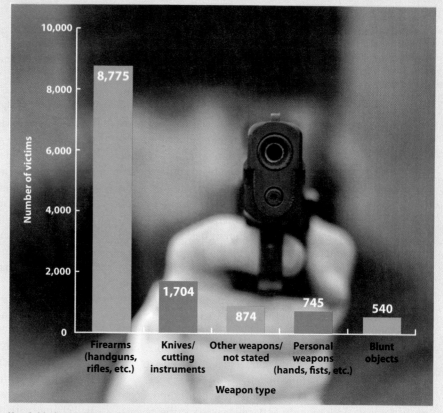

Homicide in the United States by Weapon Type, 2010
Sixty-seven percent of murders in the United States are committed using firearms, far outweighing all other weapons combined.

Source: Data from U.S. Department of Justice, Federal Bureau of Investigation, *Crime in the United States, 2010, Expanded Homicide Data*, Table 8, www.fbi.gov/about-us/cjis/ucr/crime-in-the-u.s/22010/crime-in-the-u.s.-2010/tables/10shrtbl08.xls.

the gun debate to campuses. Although many states have passed laws prohibiting or restricting guns on campuses, Utah, Florida, Texas, Arizona, and others have legislation pending or passed to allow licensed gun owners (faculty, staff, and students) to carry concealed weapons on campus. Proponents argue that there is no evidence that legally allowing guns on campus would increase the risk of campus violence. What do you think?

✳ How would you feel about students in your classes having guns? Would it make you feel more or less safe? What about bringing a gun to a sporting event, party on campus, or other venue?

✳ Do you think making guns illegal on campus would prevent students from bringing guns to school? Why or why not?

✳ What factors should be taken into consideration as states vote on guns on campus?

Sources: J. Fox and M. Zawitz, *Homicide Trends in the United States*, U.S. Department of Justice, Office of Justice Programs, Bureau of Justice Statistics, Revised 2009, www.ojp.usdoj.gov/bjs/homicide/homtrnd.htm; Brady Campaign to Prevent Gun Violence, "Facts: Gun Violence," Revised 2010, www.bradycampaign.org/facts/gunviolence; Brady Campaign to Prevent Gun Violence, "Guns in Colleges and Schools," Revised 2009, www.bradycampaign.org/stateleg/publicplaces/gunsoncampus; S. Lewis, "Concealed Carry on Campus—Guns on Campus—College Campus Carry," CNN Report, 2011, www.campuscarry.com; National Center for Injury Prevention and Control, "WISQARS Injury Mortality Reports 1999–2007," Accessed May 9, 2011, http://webapp.cdc.gov/sasweb/ncipc/mortrate.html; National Center for Injury Prevention and Control, "WISQARS Nonfatal Injury Reports 2001–2009," www.cdc.gov/injury/wisqars/nonfatal.html; M. Miller and D. Hemenway, "Guns and Suicide in the United States," *New England Journal of Medicine* 359 (2008): 989–91.

prejudice A negative evaluation of an entire group of people that is typically based on unfavorable and often wrong ideas about the group.

discrimination Actions that deny equal treatment or opportunities to a group, often based on prejudice.

domestic violence The use of force to control and maintain power over another person in the home environment, including both actual harm and the threat of harm.

intimate partner violence (IPV) Violent behavior that occurs between people in an intimate relationship (current or former spouses or dating partners).

is based on prejudice and discrimination. **Prejudice** is an irrational attitude of hostility directed against an individual, group, or race or the supposed characteristics of an individual, group, or race. **Discrimination** constitutes actions that deny equal treatment or opportunities to a group of people, often based on prejudice. Often prejudice and discrimination stem from a fear of change and a desire to blame others when forces such as the economy and crime seem to be out of control. Teaching tolerance, understanding, and respect for people from different backgrounds can reduce the risks of terrorism.

Common reasons given to explain bias-related and hate crimes include (1) *thrill seeking* by multiple offenders through a group attack; (2) *feeling threatened* that others will take their jobs or property or best them in some way; (3) *retaliating* for some real or perceived insult or slight; and (4) *fearing the unknown or differences*. For other people, hate crimes are a part of their mission in life, either due to religious zeal or distorted moral beliefs.

Nearly 12 percent of all bias-related and hate crimes occur on campuses, and schools and colleges have the fastest-growing risks for such crimes.[31] Campuses have responded to reports of hate crimes by offering courses that emphasize diversity, zero tolerance for violations, training faculty appropriately, and developing policies that enforce punishment for hate crimes. Sadly, many assaults are not reported because the victims fear retaliation.

Domestic Violence

Domestic violence refers to the use of force to control and maintain power over another person in the home environment. It can occur between parent and child, between spouses or intimate partners, or between siblings or other family members. The violence may involve emotional abuse, verbal abuse, threats of physical harm, and physical violence ranging from slapping and shoving to beatings, rape, and homicide.

Intimate Partner Violence and Women

Intimate partner violence (IPV) occurs when two people in an intimate relationship (current and former spouses or dating partners) engage in violence. Women are more likely than men to become victims of intimate partner violence.

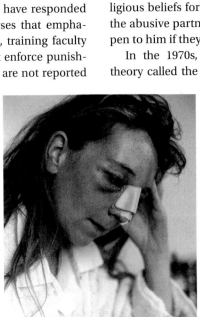

People who stay with their abusers may do so because they are dependent on the abuser, because they fear the abuser, or even because they love the abuser. In some cultures, women may not be free to leave an abusive relationship because of restrictive laws, religious beliefs, or social mores.

70%

of all hate crimes are committed against a person or persons; the rest are crimes against property.

Each year, over 12 million adults in America are victims of intimate partner violence with most cases of rape or severe IPV occurring before age 24.[32] Nearly 1 in 5 women have been raped in their lifetime compared to 1 in 71 men. The vast majority of these assaults are perpetrated by men—either men on women, or men on men.[33] Homicide committed by a current or former intimate partner is the leading cause of death of pregnant women in the United States.[34] In addition, 74 percent of all murder-suicides in the United States involve an intimate partner. Ninety-four percent of those murders were females killed by a male partner—most often in the bedroom.[35]

The Cycle of IPV Have you ever heard of a woman who is repeatedly beaten by her partner and wondered, "Why doesn't she just leave him?" There are many reasons some women find it difficult to break their ties with their abusers. Some women, particularly those with small children, are financially dependent on their partners. Others fear retaliation against themselves or their children. Some hope the situation will change with time, and others stay because cultural or religious beliefs forbid divorce. Finally, some women still love the abusive partner and are concerned about what will happen to him if they leave.

In the 1970s, psychologist Lenore Walker developed a theory called the *cycle of violence* that explained predictable, repetitive patterns of psychological and/or physical abuse that seemed to occur in abusive relationships.[36] Walker's initial work was criticized by some for its lack of scientific rigor. In her most recent book, *The Battered Woman Syndrome,* Walker's conclusions were based on improved quantitative analysis, reviews of recent research, and an extensive list of experts in the field of violence.[37]

Today, the cycle of violence continues to be important to understanding why people stay in otherwise unhealthy relationships. The cycle consists of three major phases:

1. Tension building. This phase typically occurs prior to the overtly abusive act and includes breakdowns in communication, anger, psychological aggression and violent language, growing tension, and fear.

2. Incident of acute battering. At this stage, the batterer usually is trying to "teach her a lesson," and when he feels he has inflicted enough pain, he'll stop. When the acute attack is over, he may respond with shock and denial about his own behavior or blame her for "making him" do it.

3. Remorse/reconciliation. During this "honeymoon" period, the batterer may be kind, loving, and apologetic, swearing that he will work to change his behavior. However, when the same things that triggered past abuse begin to resurface, the cycle starts over again.

For a woman who gets caught in this cycle, it is often very hard to summon the resolution to extricate herself. Most need effective outside intervention.

Causes of Domestic Violence and IPV There is no single reason to explain abuse in relationships. Alcohol abuse is often associated with such violence, and marital dissatisfaction is also a predictor. Numerous studies also point to differences in communication patterns between abusive and nonabusive relationships. Many experts believe that men who engage in severe violence are more likely than other men to suffer from personality disorders.[38]

Intimate Partner Violence: Men As Victims We may think that intimate partner violence happens only to women, but every year in the United States men experience nearly 3 million physical assaults by an intimate partner, male or female. In fact, gay men appear to be just as susceptible to male-perpetrated violence as are women in heterosexual relationships, and abuse of heterosexual men by their female partners is likely more common than statistics show. Several studies indicate that between 20 and 24 percent of men have experienced physical, sexual, or psychological intimate partner violence during their lifetime.[39]

Why don't men report abuse? Reasons include the following:

● A sense of humiliation and/or fear that no one will believe them
● Abuse that has reached the point that they believe they deserve bad treatment
● Belief that not hitting back is a sign of honor, strength, or masculinity
● Lack of awareness and support services for men in abusive relationships

Recognizing that a problem exists, communities across the nation are responding with education and awareness programs and resources such as support groups and counseling to help male victims protect themselves and make positive changes in their lives.

Child Abuse and Neglect

Children living in families in which domestic violence or sexual abuse occurs are at great risk for damage to personal health and well-being. **Child maltreatment** is defined as any act or series of acts of commission or omission by a parent or caregiver that results in harm, potential for harm, or threat of harm to a child.[40] **Child abuse** refers to *acts of commission,* which are deliberate or intentional words or actions that cause harm, potential harm, or threat of harm to a child. The abuse may be sexual, psychological, physical, or any combination of these. **Neglect** is an *act of omission,* meaning a failure to provide for a child's basic physical, emotional, or education needs or to protect a child from harm or potential harm. Failure to provide food, shelter, clothing, medical care, or supervision, or exposing a child to unnecessary environmental violence or threat are examples of neglect. Although exact figures for child abuse are difficult to obtain, in 2011 an estimated 3.3 million cases of child abuse were reported, involving the alleged maltreatment of approximately 6 million children. The United States has the worst record in the industrialized nations that report these statistics, losing 5 children every day to abuse.[41] Figure 19.4 shows the rates of abuse among children in different age groups.

child maltreatment Any act or series of acts of commission or omission by a parent or caregiver that results in harm, potential for harm, or threat of harm to a child.

child abuse Deliberate, intentional words or actions that cause harm, potential for harm, or threat of harm to a child.

neglect Failure to provide a child's basic needs such as food, clothing, shelter, and medical care.

There is no single profile of a child abuser. The most common perpetrators in child maltreatment cases are biological parents. Frequently, the perpetrator is a young adult in his or her midtwenties without a high school diploma, living at or below the poverty level, depressed, socially isolated, with a poor self-image, and having difficulty coping with stressful situations. In many instances, the perpetrator has experienced violence and is frustrated by life.

It is important to remember that child abuse occurs at every socioeconomic level, across ethnic and cultural lines, within all religions, and at all levels of education. Not all violence against children is physical. Health

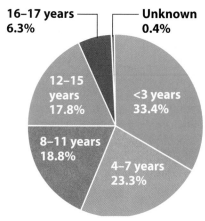

16–17 years 6.3%
Unknown 0.4%
12–15 years 17.8%
<3 years 33.4%
8–11 years 18.8%
4–7 years 23.3%

FIGURE 19.4 Child Abuse and Neglect Victims by Age, 2009

Source: U.S. Department of Health and Human Services, Administration on Children, Youth and Families, *Child Maltreatment 2009* (Washington, DC: U.S. Government Printing Office, 2010), www .acf.hhs.gov/programs/cb/pubs/cm09.

can be severely affected by psychological violence—assaults on personality, character, competence, independence, or general dignity as a human being. Negative consequences of this kind of victimization can include depression, low self-esteem, and a pervasive fear of offending the abuser.

Elder Abuse

By 2030, the number of people in the United States over the age of 65 will exceed 71 million—nearly double their number in 2000. Elder abuse is a problem for many of today's seniors and is perhaps one of the most under-studied violence topics. Those who are socially isolated are more likely to suffer abuse. Statistics are scarce, but estimates indicate that between 700,000 and 3.5 million older Americans may be abused, neglected, or exploited each year.[42] Many victims fail to report because they are embarrassed or because they don't want the abuser to get in trouble or retaliate by putting them in a nursing home or escalating the abuse. Some do not report due to feeling guilty because someone has to take care of them. Others suffer from dementia and may not be aware of the abuse. A variety of social services focus on protecting our seniors, just as we endeavor to protect other vulnerable populations.

Sexual Victimization

The term *sexual victimization* refers to any situation in which an individual is coerced or forced to comply with or endure another's sexual acts or overtures. It can run the gamut from harassment to stalking to assault and rape. As with all forms of violence, both men and women are susceptible to sexual victimization. Young people are especially vulnerable; 60 percent of female victims of sexual violence and 69 percent of male victims were first raped before the age of 18.[43] Sexual victimization and violence can have devastating and far-reaching effects on people of any age. Depression, suicide risk, drug and alcohol abuse, traumatic stress disorders, self-harm, and a host of interpersonal problems often increase among women and men who have been victimized sexually.[44]

sexual assault Any act in which one person is sexually intimate with another without that person's consent.

rape Sexual penetration without the victim's consent.

aggravated rape Rape that involves one or multiple attackers, strangers, weapons, or physical beating.

simple rape Rape by one person, usually known to the victim, that does not involve physical beating or use of a weapon.

acquaintance rape Any rape in which the rapist is known to the victim (replaces the formerly used term *date rape*).

Sexual Assault and Rape

Sexual assault is any act in which one person is sexually intimate with another person without that person's consent. This may range from simple touching to forceful penetration and may include, for example, ignoring indications that intimacy is not wanted, threatening force or other negative consequences, and actually using force.

Considered the most extreme form of sexual assault, **rape** is defined as "penetration without the victim's consent."[45] Incidents of rape generally fall into one of two types—aggravated or simple. An **aggravated rape** is any rape involving one or multiple attackers, strangers, weapons, or physical beatings. A **simple rape** is a rape perpetrated by one person, whom the victim knows, and does not involve a physical beating or use of a weapon. Most rapes are classified as simple rape, but that terminology should not be taken to mean that a simple rape is any less violent or criminal. The FBI ranks rape as the second most violent crime, trailing only murder.[46]

According to the National Center for Injury Prevention and Control, 1 in 6 women and 1 in 33 men reported experiencing an attempted or completed rape at some time in their lives.[47] An estimated 63 percent of all sexual assaults reported by women victims were committed by someone the victim knew.[48] Men can also be victims of rape and sexual assault, and a growing number have come forward to report their abusers. Over 41 percent of male victims were first raped before the age of 12, and 28 percent were first raped between the ages of 12 and 17. The vast majority of these rapes were committed by someone the victim knew.[49]

By most indicators, reported cases of rape appear to have declined in the United States since the early 1990s, even as reports of other forms of sexual assault have increased. This decline is thought to be due to shifts in public awareness and attitudes about rape, combined with tougher crime policies, major educational campaigns, and media attention. These changes enforce the idea that rape is a violent crime and should be treated as such. However, studies indicate that only 16 percent of all rapes are actually reported to law enforcement.[50]

What's Working for You?

Maybe you already practice some strategies to stay safe in social situations. Which of these are you already incorporating into your life?

- [ ] When I go to parties, I go with a friend and we look out for each other.
- [ ] I decide before I go how much I am going to drink.
- [ ] I don't leave bars alone with people I've just met.

Acquaintance Rape

The terms *date rape* and *acquaintance rape* have been used interchangeably in the past. However, most experts now believe that the term *date rape* is inappropriate because it implies a consensual interaction in an arranged setting and may, in fact, minimize the crime of rape when it occurs. Today, **acquaintance rape** refers to any rape in which the rapist is known to the victim. Acquaintance rape is more common when drugs or alcohol have been consumed by the offender or victim. Most acquaintance rapes happen to women age 15 to 24, and the most likely victim is an 18-year-old new college student.[51]

Rape on U.S. Campuses An estimated 673,000 (about 12%) of the nearly 6 million women currently attending college in the United States have been raped, many by forcible means that resulted in injury.[52] By some estimates, as many as 25 percent of college women have experienced an attempted or completed rape in college.[53] More than 80 percent of these rapes were committed by an attacker the victim knew, most occurred on campus, and alcohol was often involved, as were the two most common rape-facilitating drugs, Rohypnol and gamma-hydroxybutyrate (GHB).[54]

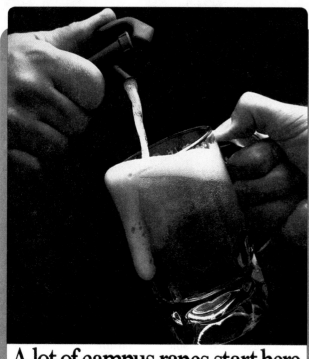

A lot of campus rapes start here.

Whenever there's drinking or drugs, things can get out of hand. So it's no surprise that many campus rapes involve alcohol.

But you should know that under any circumstances, sex without the other person's consent is considered rape. A felony, punishable by prison. And drinking is no excuse.

That's why, when you party, it's good to know what your limits are. You see, a little sobering thought now can save you from a big problem later.

What does *acquaintance rape* mean?

The term *date rape* was formerly used to describe a sexual assault that occurred in the context of a dating relationship. The term has fallen out of favor because the word *date* implies something reciprocal or arranged, thus minimizing the crime. The term *acquaintance rape* is now more commonly used, referring to any rape in which the rapist is known to the victim, even if only minimally. Acquaintance rape is particularly common on college campuses, where alcohol and drug use can impair young people's judgment and self-control.

84%

of sexual assaults on college campuses are acquaintance rapes.

In 1992, Congress passed the Campus Sexual Assault Victim's Bill of Rights, known as the *Ramstad Act*. The act gives victims the right to call in off-campus authorities to investigate serious campus crimes. In addition, it requires universities to set up educational programs and notify students of available counseling. More recent provisions of the act specify notification procedures and options for victims, rights of victims and accused perpetrators, and consequences if schools do not comply. It also requires the Department of Education to publish campus crime statistics annually.

Video Tutor: Acquaintance Rape on Campus

Marital Rape Although its legal definition varies within the United States, *marital rape* can be any unwanted intercourse or penetration (vaginal, anal, or oral) obtained by force, threat of force, or when the spouse is unable to consent.[55] This problem has undoubtedly existed since the origin of marriage as a social institution, and it is noteworthy that marital rape did not become a crime in all 50 states until 1993. Even more noteworthy is the fact that 30 states still allow exemptions from marital rape prosecution, meaning that the judicial system may treat it as a lesser crime.[56]

Although research in this area is scarce, it has been estimated that 10–14 percent of married women are raped by their husbands in the United States. About one third of women report having had "unwanted sex" with their partner.[57] In general, women under the age of 25 and those from lower socioeconomic groups are at highest risk of marital rape. Internationally, women raised in cultures where male dominance is the norm and women are treated as property tend to have higher rates of forced sex within the confines of marriage. Women who are pregnant, ill, or separated or divorced have higher rates, as do women from homes where other forms of domestic violence are common and where there is a high rate of alcoholism or substance abuse.

Child Sexual Abuse Sexual abuse of children by adults or older children includes sexually suggestive conversations; inappropriate kissing; touching; petting; oral, anal, or vaginal intercourse; and other kinds of sexual interaction. Recent studies indicate that the rates of sexual abuse in children range from 3 to 32.2 percent of all children, with girls being at greater risk than young boys, even though young boys are abused in significant numbers.[58]

Most experts believe that as high as these numbers are, the shroud of secrecy surrounding this problem makes it likely the number of actual cases are grossly underestimated. Unfortunately, the programs taught in schools today may give children the false impression that they are more likely to be assaulted by a stranger. In reality, 90 percent of child sexual abuse victims know their perpetrator, with nearly 70 percent of children abused by family members, usually an adult male.[59]

People who were abused as children bear spiritual, psychological, and/or physical scars. Studies have shown that child sexual abuse has an impact on later life: Children who experience sexual abuse are at increased risk for anxiety disorders, depression, eating disorders, post-traumatic stress disorder (PTSD), and suicide attempts.[60] Youth who have been sexually abused are 25 percent more likely to experience teen pregnancy, 30 percent more likely to abuse their own children, and are much more likely to have problems with alcohol abuse or drug addiction.[61]

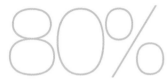

of college students who have experienced sexual harassment report being harassed by another student or former student.

Sexual Harassment

Sexual harassment is defined as unwelcome sexual conduct that is related to any condition of employment or evaluation of student performance. Unwelcome sexual advances, requests for sexual favors, and other verbal or physical conduct of a sexual nature constitute sexual harassment when:

- Submission to such conduct is made either explicitly or implicitly a term or condition of an individual's employment or education;
- Submission to or rejection of such conduct by an individual is used as the basis for employment or education-related decisions affecting such an individual; or
- Such conduct is sufficiently severe or pervasive that it has the effect, intended or unintended, of unreasonably interfering with an individual's work or academic performance because it has created an intimidating, hostile, or offensive environment and would have such an effect on a reasonable person of that individual's status.[62]

Commonly, people think of harassment as involving only faculty members or persons in power, where sex is used to exhibit control of a situation. However, peers can harass one another too. Sexual harassment may include unwanted touching; unwarranted sex-related comments or subtle pressure for sexual favors; deliberate or repeated humiliation or intimidation based on sex; and gratuitous comments, jokes, questions, or remarks about clothing or bodies, sexuality, or past sexual relationships.

sexual harassment Any form of unwanted sexual attention related to any condition of employment, education, or performance evaluation.

stalking Willful, repeated, and malicious following, harassing, or threatening of another person.

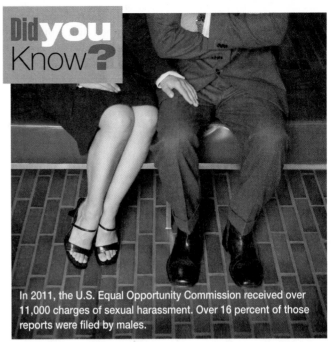

In 2011, the U.S. Equal Opportunity Commission received over 11,000 charges of sexual harassment. Over 16 percent of those reports were filed by males.

Source: Data are from U.S. Equal Employment Opportunity Commission, "Sexual Harassment Charges," 2011, www.eeoc.gov/eeoc/statistics/enforcement/sexual_harassment.cfm, Accessed July 2012.

Most schools and companies have sexual harassment policies in place, as well as procedures for dealing with harassment problems. If you feel you are being harassed, the most important thing you can do is be assertive:

- **Tell the harasser to stop.** Be clear and direct. Tell the person if it continues that you will report it. If the harassing is via phone or Internet, block the person.
- **Document the harassment.** Make a record of each incident. If the harassment becomes intolerable, a record of exactly what occurred (and when and where) will help make your case. Save copies of all communication from the harasser.
- **Try to make sure you aren't alone in the harasser's presence.** Witnesses to harassment can ensure appropriate validation of the event.
- **Complain to a higher authority.** Talk to legal authorities or your instructor, adviser, or counseling center psychologist about what happened.
- **Remember that you have not done anything wrong.** You will likely feel awful after being harassed (especially if you have to complain to superiors). However, feel proud that you are not keeping silent.

Stalking

Stalking can be defined as a course of conduct directed at a specific person that would cause a reasonable person to feel fear. This may include repeated visual or physical proximity, nonconsensual written or verbal communication, and implied or explicit threats.[63] Stalking can even occur online (see the **Tech & Health** box on page 587 for information on staying safe when using social networking sites).[64]

One in six women has experienced stalking victimization in her lifetime, during which she felt very fearful or believed

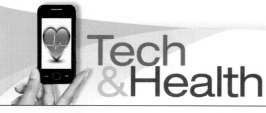

Tech &Health   SOCIAL NETWORKING SAFETY

At any given time, millions of people are chatting online with friends, family, and strangers, and posting photos and personal information that may be available to people they barely know or don't know at all. Social networking sites raise important concerns about potential risks—from stalking and identity theft, to gossip and slander, to embarrassment and defamation. For example, see the following:

* A first-year student at Virginia Commonwealth University was murdered by someone she met on MySpace.
* A student at the University of Kansas learned the consequences of revealing too much information on Facebook when she was stalked by a man who found her class schedule online.
* In Britain, 4.5 million Web users between the ages of 14 and 21 were vulnerable to identity fraud because of information provided on their social networking sites when security measures were hacked.
* Hiring and firing decisions have been influenced by information employees and job applicants made publicly available on Facebook and Twitter.
* Underage users may pose as adults, leading to claims of inappropriate sexual contact with minors and other criminal offenses on the part of people interacting with them online.

Very real threats to health, reputation, financial security, and future employment lie in wait for those who post indiscriminately and unwisely to the Web. To safely enjoy the benefits and avoid the risks of social networking sites, you'll need to be savvy and

use common sense. The following tips will help you remain safe and protect your identity when you express yourself online:

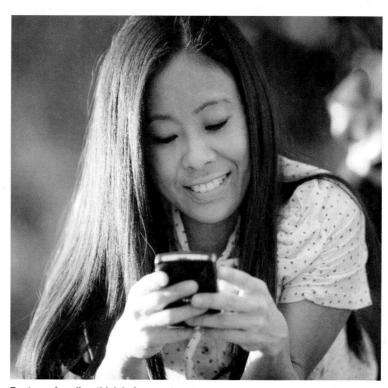

To stay safe online, think before you tweet.

* Don't post anything on the Web that you wouldn't want someone to pick out of your trash and read. Your address, phone numbers, banking information, calendar, family secrets, and other sensitive information should be kept off the sites.
* Don't post compromising pictures, videos, or other things that you wouldn't want your mother or coworkers to see.

* Never agree to meet a stranger in person whom you've met only online without bringing a trusted friend, or at the very least, notifying a close friend or family member of where you will be and when you will return. Arrange ahead of time to return home with a friend. Choose a well-established, public place and only meet during daylight hours. Don't give your address or traceable phone numbers to the person you are meeting.

that someone close to her would be harmed or killed. Much of stalking victimization is facilitated by technology. In fact, about one quarter of victims report being stalked through the use of cell phones, e-mail, text messages, sites such as Facebook, Global Positioning Systems (GPS), listening devices, and video cameras.[65] Millions of women and men are stalked annually in the United States, and the vast majority of stalkers are persons involved in relationship

breakups or are other dating acquaintances. Adults between the ages of 18 and 24 experience the highest rates of stalking. Like sexual harassment, stalking is an underreported crime. Often students do not think a stalking incident is serious enough to report, or they worry that the police will not take it seriously.

Researchers suggest several reasons for stalking: (1) Stalkers may have deficits in social skills; (2) they are young and have not yet learned how to deal with complex social relationships and situations; (3) they may not realize that their behavior constitutes stalking; (4) they have a flexible schedule and free time; and (5) they are not accountable to authority figures for their daily activities.[66] Some stalkers may not view such behaviors as criminal in nature, or they may be surprised to find out that their showing persistent interest is causing the targeted person to be anxious and fearful.

Emotional and Psychological Abuse A common and insidious form of violence between intimate partners is emotional or psychological abuse. Emotional abuse can occur in any intimate relationship but is particularly prevalent in romantic and sexual relationships. This abuse can take the form of constant criticism, verbal attacks, displays of explosive anger meant to intimidate, and controlling behavior. Psychological abusers seek to intimidate and debase their partners, thereby gaining control over the partner and the relationship. Often this form of abuse can lead to or accompany physical abuse and sexual coercion. If you observe that a friend's intimate partner is verbally or emotionally abusive or controlling, encourage him or her to seek counseling before the situation escalates.

collective violence Violence perpetrated by groups against other groups.

Social Contributors to Sexual Violence Sexual violence and intimate partner violence share common factors that increase the likelihood of their occurrence. Certain societal assumptions and traditions can promote sexual violence, including the following:[67]

● **Minimization.** Many people assume that sexual assault is rare because official crime statistics are low. However, rape is the most underreported of all serious crimes; 1 out of every 6 women in the United States has been a victim of sexual assault.

● **Trivialization.** Many people think that rape committed by a husband or intimate partner doesn't count as rape.

● **Blaming the victim.** In spite of efforts to combat this type of thinking, there is still the belief that a scantily clad woman "asks" for sexual advances.

● **Pressure to be macho.** Males are taught from a young age that showing emotions is a sign of weakness. This portrayal often depicts men as aggressive and predatory and females as passive targets.

● **Male socialization.** Many still believe that "sowing wild oats" and "boys will be boys" are merely a normal part of male development. Women are often *objectified* (treated as sexual objects) in the media, which contributes to the idea that it's natural for men to be predatory.

● **Male misperceptions.** With media implying that sex is the focus of life, it's not surprising that some men believe that when a woman says no, she is really asking to be seduced. Later, these same men may be surprised when the woman says she was raped.

● **Situational factors.** Dates in which the male makes all the decisions, pays for everything, and generally controls the entire situation are more likely to end in an aggressive sexual scenario. Alcohol and other drugs increase the risk and severity of assaults.

Collective Violence

Collective violence is violence perpetrated by groups against other groups and includes violent acts related to political, governmental, religious, cultural, or social clashes. Gang violence and terrorism are two forms of collective violence that have become major threats in recent years.

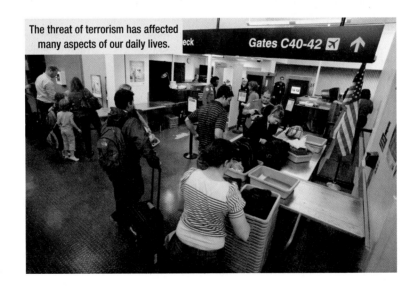

The threat of terrorism has affected many aspects of our daily lives.

Gang Violence

Gang violence includes drug trafficking, sex trafficking, shootings, beatings, thefts, carjackings, and the killing of innocent victims caught in the crossfire of gang shootouts. Once thought to occur only in urban areas, gang violence now is a growing threat in rural and suburban communities as well.[68]

Why do young people join gangs? Although the reasons are complex, gangs seem to meet many of the personal needs of young people. Often, gangs give members a sense of self-worth, companionship, security, and excitement. In other cases, gangs provide economic security through drug sales, prostitution, and other types of criminal activity. The age range of gang members is typically 12 to 22. Risk factors include low self-esteem, academic problems, low socioeconomic status, alienation from family and society, a history of family violence, and living in gang-controlled neighborhoods.[69] Once young people become involved in gang subculture, it is difficult for them to leave. Threats of violence or fear of not making it on their own discourage even those who are seriously trying to get out.

Terrorism

Numerous terrorist attacks around the world reveal the vulnerability of all nations to domestic and international threats. Today, threats against our airlines, mass transportation systems, cities, national monuments, and our population fuel our fears of looming terrorist attacks. Effects on our economy, travel restrictions, additional security measures, and military buildups are but a few of the examples of how terrorist threats have affected our lives. As defined in the U.S. Code of Federal Regulations, **terrorism** is the "unlawful use of force or violence against persons or property to intimidate or coerce a government, the civilian population, or any segment thereof in furtherance of political or social objectives."[70]

Over the past decade, the Centers for Disease Control and Prevention (CDC) established the Emergency Preparedness and Response Division. This group monitors potential public health problems, such as bioterrorism, chemical emergencies, radiation emergencies, mass casualties, national disaster and severe weather; develops plans for mobilizing communities in the case of emergency; and provides information about terrorist threats. In addition, the Department of Homeland Security works to prevent future attacks, and the FBI and other government agencies work to ensure citizens' health and safety.

How to Avoid Becoming a Victim of Violence

It is far better to prevent a violent act than to recover from it. Both individuals and communities can play important roles in preventing violence and intentional injuries.

Self-Defense against Personal Assault and Rape

Assault can occur no matter what preventive actions you take, but commonsense self-defense tactics can lower the risk. Self-defense is a process that includes increasing your awareness, developing self-protective skills, taking reasonable precautions, and having the judgment necessary to respond quickly to changing situations. It is important to know ways to avoid and extract yourself from potentially dangerous situations. The **Skills for Behavior Change** box identifies practical tips for preventing dating violence.

terrorism Unlawful use of force or violence against persons or property to intimidate or coerce a government, civilian population, or any segment thereof in furtherance of political or social objectives.

Most attacks by unknown assailants are planned in advance. Many rapists use certain ploys to initiate their attacks. Examples include asking for help, offering help, staging a deliberate "accident" such as bumping into you, or posing as a police officer or other authority figure. Sexual assault frequently begins with a casual, friendly conversation.

Trust your intuition. Be assertive and direct to someone who is getting out of line or becoming threatening—this may convince a would-be attacker to back off. Don't try to be nice,

Skills for Behavior Change

Reducing Your Risk of Dating Violence

❯ Prior to your date, think about your values and set personal boundaries.

❯ Watch your alcohol consumption. Drinking can get you into situations you'd otherwise avoid.

❯ Do not accept beverages or open-container drinks from anyone you do not know well and trust. At a bar or a club, accept drinks only from the bartender or server.

❯ Never leave a drink or food unattended. If you get up to dance, have someone you trust watch your drink or take it with you.

❯ Go out with several couples or in groups when dating someone new.

❯ Stick with your friends. Agree to keep an eye out for one another at parties, and agree to leave together and check in with one another. Never leave a bar or party alone with a stranger.

❯ Pay attention to your date's actions. If someone seems to be controlling or pushy and attempts to make every decision for you, it may mean trouble. Trust your intuition.

❯ Practice what you will say if things go in an uncomfortable direction. You have the right to express your feelings, and it is okay to be assertive. Do not be swayed by arguments such as "What about my feelings?" or "You were leading me on."

and don't fear making a scene. Use the following tips to let a potential assailant know that you are prepared to defend yourself:

- **Speak in a strong voice.** Use commands such as, "Leave me alone!" rather than questions such as, "Will you please leave me alone?" Sound like you mean it.
- **Maintain eye contact.** This keeps you aware of the person's movements and conveys an aura of strength and confidence.
- **Stand up straight, act confident, and remain alert.** Walk as though you own the sidewalk.

If you are attacked, act immediately. Draw attention to yourself and your assailant. Scream "Fire!" as loudly as you can. Research has shown that passersby are much more likely to help if they hear the word *fire* rather than just a scream.

What to Do if Rape Occurs

If you are a rape victim, report the attack. This gives you a sense of control. Follow these steps:

- Call 9-1-1 (if a phone is available).
- Do not bathe, shower, douche, clean up, or touch anything the attacker may have touched.
- Save the clothes you were wearing, and do not launder them. They will be needed as evidence. Bring a clean change of clothes to the clinic or hospital.
- Contact the rape assistance hotline in your area, and ask for advice on counseling if you need additional help.

If a friend is raped, here's how you can help:

- Believe her. Don't ask questions that may appear to implicate her in the assault.
- Recognize that rape is a violent act and that the victim was not looking for this to happen.
- Encourage your friend to see a doctor immediately, because she may have medical needs but feel too embarrassed to seek help on her own. Offer to go with her.
- Encourage her to report the crime.
- Be understanding, and let her know you will be there for her.
- Recognize that this is an emotional recovery, and it may take time for her to bounce back.
- Encourage your friend to seek counseling.

Campuswide Responses to Violence

Increasingly, campuses have become microcosms of the greater society, complete with the risks, hazards, and dangers that people face in the world. Many college administrators have been proactive in establishing violence-prevention

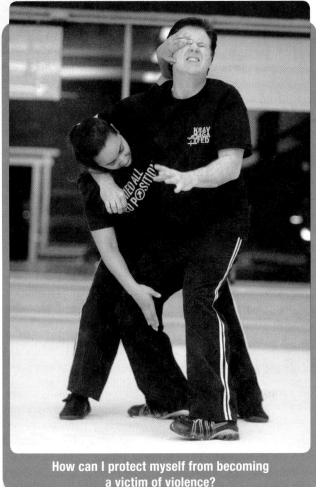

How can I protect myself from becoming a victim of violence?

One of the best ways to protect yourself from violence is to avoid situations or circumstances that could lead to it. Another way to protect yourself is to learn self-defense techniques. College campuses often offer safety workshops and self-defense classes to arm students with the physical and mental skills that may help them repel or deter an assailant.

policies, programs, and services. They have also begun to examine the aspects of campus culture that promote and tolerate violent acts.[71]

Prevention and Early Response Efforts

The Virginia Tech and Northern Illinois tragedies of 2007 and 2008 prompted vast restructuring of existing policies and strategies for prevention, risk notification, and emergency response drills. Campuses are reviewing the effectiveness of emergency messaging systems. E-mail alerts can only reach those who are at their computers or who receive e-mail updates on mobile devices, so campuses are implementing cell phone alert systems. The REVERSE 9-1-1 system uses database and geographic information system (GIS) mapping technologies to notify campus police and community members in the event of problems, and other systems allow administrators to send out alerts in text, voice, e-mail, or instant message format. Some schools program the phone numbers, photographs, and basic student information for all incoming first-year students into a university security system so that in the event of a threat, students need only hit a button on their phones, whereupon campus police will be notified and tracking devices will pinpoint their location.

Changes in the Campus Environment

There are many changes that can be made to the campus environment to improve safety. Campus lighting, parking lot security, emergency call boxes, removal of overgrown shrubbery, and stepped-up security are increasingly on the radar of campus safety personnel. Buildings can be designed with better lighting and enhanced security features, and security cameras can been installed in hallways, classrooms, and public places. Safe rides are provided for students who have consumed too much alcohol, and health promotion programs have stepped up their violence prevention efforts through seminars on acquaintance rape, sexual assault, harassment, and other topics.

Campus Law Enforcement

Campus law enforcement has changed over the years by increasing both its numbers and its authority to prosecute student offenders. Campus police are responsible for emergency responses, and they have the power to enforce laws with students in the same way infractions are handled in the general community. In fact, many campuses now hire state troopers or local law enforcement officers to deal with campus issues rather than maintain a separate police staff.

Coping in the Event of Campus Violence

Although schools have worked tirelessly to prevent violence, it can still occur. In its aftermath, some may find it difficult to remain on campus as it represents a place of violation and lack of safety; others may experience problems with concentration, studying, and other daily activities. Although there is no easy "fix" for these traumatic events, several strategies can be helpful. First, members of the campus community should

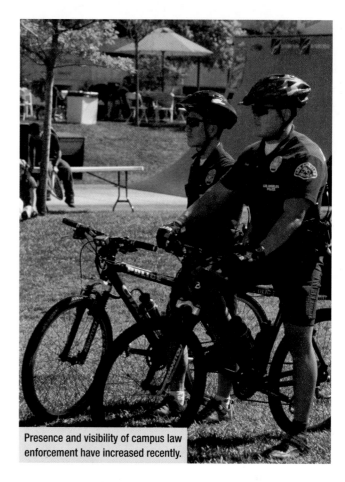

Presence and visibility of campus law enforcement have increased recently.

be allowed to mourn. Memorial services and acknowledgment of grief, fear, anger, and other emotions are critical to healing. Second, students, faculty, and staff should be involved in planning to prevent future problems—it can help to impart a feeling of control. Third, students should seek out support groups, therapists who specialize in treating PTSD, and trusted family members or friends if they need to talk and work through their feelings. Journaling or writing about feelings can also help.

Community Strategies for Preventing Violence

There are many steps you can take to ensure your personal safety (see the Skills for Behavior Change box on the following page); however, it is also necessary to address the issues of violence and safety at a community level. Strategies recommended by the CDC's Injury Response initiatives include the following:

● Inoculate children against violence in the home. Teaching youth principles of respect and responsibility are fundamental to the health and well-being of future generations.

● Develop policies and laws that prevent violence.

Stay Safe on All Fronts

Follow these tips to protect yourself from assault.

OUTSIDE ALONE

❭ Carry a cell phone and keep it turned on, but don't use it. Be aware of what is happening around you.

❭ If you are being followed, don't go home. Head for a location where there are other people. If you decide to run, run fast and scream loudly to attract attention.

❭ Vary your routes. Stay close to other people.

❭ Park in lighted areas; avoid dark areas where someone could hide.

❭ Carry pepper spray or other deterrents. Consider using your campus escort service.

❭ Tell others where you are going and when you expect to be back.

IN YOUR CAR

❭ Lock your doors. Do not open your doors or windows to strangers.

❭ If someone hits your car, drive to the nearest gas station or other public place if you are able. Call the police or road service for help, and stay in your car until help arrives.

❭ If a car appears to be following you, do not drive home. Drive to the nearest police station.

IN YOUR HOME

❭ Install dead bolts on all doors and locks on all windows. Make sure the locks work, and don't leave a spare key outside. Consider installing an alarm system.

❭ Lock doors when at home, even during the day. Close blinds and drapes whenever you are away and in the evening when you are home.

❭ Rent apartments that require a security code or clearance to gain entry, and avoid easily accessible apartments, such as first-floor units. When you move into a new residence, pay a locksmith to change the keys and locks.

❭ Don't let repair people in without asking for identification, and have someone else with you when repairs are being made.

❭ Keep a cell phone near your bed and program it to dial 9-1-1.

❭ If you return home to find your residence has been broken into, don't enter. Call the police. If you encounter an intruder, it is better to give up money or valuables than to resist.

● Develop skills-based educational programs that teach the basics of interpersonal communication, elements of healthy relationships, anger management, conflict resolution, appropriate assertiveness, stress management, and other health-based behaviors.

● Involve families, schools, community programs, athletics, music, faith-based organizations, and other community groups in providing experiences that help young people to develop self-esteem and self-efficacy.

● Promote tolerance and acceptance and establish and enforce policies that forbid discrimination.

● Improve community services focused on family planning, mental health services, day care and respite care, and alcohol and substance abuse prevention.

● Make sure walking trails, parking lots, and other public areas are well lit, unobstructed, and patrolled regularly to reduce threats.

● Improve community-based support and treatment for victims and ensure that individuals have choices available when trying to stop violence in their lives.

Are You at Risk for Violence?

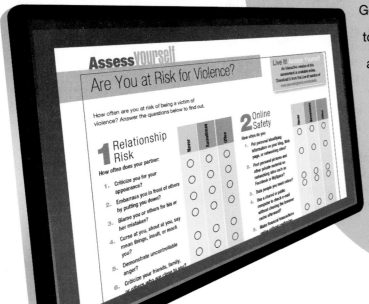

Go online to www.pearsonhighered.com/donatelle to fill out the "Are You at Risk for Violence?" assessment.* If you need to make some changes, follow the strategies outlined in the **YOUR PLAN FOR CHANGE** box.

*If your instructor so chooses, Assess Yourself Activities are available as a printed supplement or as assignable homework online at www.pearsonhighered.com/myhealth.

MyHealthLab®

YOUR PLAN FOR CHANGE

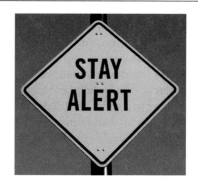

The **Assess** yourself activity gave you the chance to consider symptoms of abuse in your relationships and signs of unsafe behavior in other realms of your life. Now that you are aware of these signs and symptoms, you can work on changing behaviors to reduce your risk.

Today, you can:

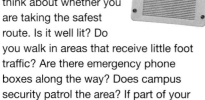

○ Pay attention as you walk your normal route around campus, and think about whether you are taking the safest route. Is it well lit? Do you walk in areas that receive little foot traffic? Are there emergency phone boxes along the way? Does campus security patrol the area? If part of your route seems unsafe, look around for alternate routes. Vary your route when possible.

○ Look at your residence's safety features. Is there a secure lock, dead bolt, or keycard entry system on all outer doors? Can windows be closed and locked? Are the outside areas well lit? If you notice any potential safety hazards, report them to your landlord or campus residential life administrator right away.

Within the next 2 weeks, you can:

○ If you are worried about potentially abusive behavior in a partner or a friend's partner, visit the campus counseling center and ask about resources on campus or in your community that can be of help. Consider talking to a counselor about your concerns or sitting in on a support group.

○ The next time you attend a party, set limits for yourself in order to remain in control of your behavior and to avoid putting yourself in a dangerous or compro-

mising position. Decide ahead of time on the number of drinks you will have, arrange with a friend to monitor each other's behavior, and be sure you have a reliable, safe way of getting home.

By the end of the semester, you can:

○ Sign up for a self-defense or violence prevention class or workshop.

○ Get involved in an on-campus or community group dedicated to promoting safety. You might want to attend a meeting of an antiviolence group, join in a Take Back the Night rally, or volunteer at a local rape crisis center or battered women's shelter.

Summary

* Violence affects everyone in society—from the direct victims, to children and families who witness it, and those who modify their behaviors because they are fearful.

* Factors that lead to violence include poverty or economic difficulties, unemployment, parental and family influences, cultural beliefs, discrimination or oppression, religious or political differences, breakdowns in the criminal justice system, and stress. Anger and substance abuse can contribute to violence and aggression.

* Interpersonal violence includes homicide, domestic violence, child abuse, elder abuse, and sexual victimization. Each of these causes significant emotional, social, and physical risks to health.

* Forms of collective violence, including gang violence and terrorism, result in fear, anxiety, and issues of discrimination.

* Proven strategies to reduce the risk of becoming a victim of violence include: Recognize how to protect yourself and your friends, know where to turn for help, and have honest, straightforward dialogue about sexual matters in dating situations. Alcohol moderation is another key factor in reducing your risks.

* Shootings and extreme acts of violence on campuses have resulted in a groundswell of activities designed to protect students and ensure their safety. Preventing violence is a public health priority that involves community activism, prioritizing mental and emotional health, and providing skills training in anger management, stress management, conflict resolution, and other key coping skills.

Pop Quiz

1. _____ is an example of an *intentional injury*.
   a. A car accident
   b. Murder
   c. Accidental drowning
   d. Road rage

2. Emotional reaction brought about by frustrating life experience is called
   a. reactive aggression.
   b. primary aggression.
   c. secondary aggression.
   d. tertiary aggression.

3. When Jane began a new job with all male coworkers, her supervisor told her that he enjoyed having an attractive woman in the workplace, and he winked at her. His comment constitutes
   a. acquaintance rape.
   b. sexual assault.
   c. sexual harassment.
   d. sexual battering.

4. Psychologist Lenore Walker developed a theory known as the
   a. aggression cycle.
   b. sexual harassment cycle.
   c. cycle of child abuse.
   d. cycle of violence.

5. What is the single greatest cause of injury to women?
   a. Rape
   b. Mugging
   c. Auto accidents
   d. Domestic violence

6. In a sociology class, some students were discussing sexual assault. One student commented that some women dress too provocatively. The assumption this student made is
   a. minimization.
   b. trivialization.
   c. blaming the victim.
   d. "boys will be boys."

7. Rape by a person the victim knows and that does not involve a physical beating or use of a weapon is called
   a. simple rape.
   b. sexual assault.
   c. simple assault.
   d. aggravated rape.

8. Which of the following is *not* a contributor to violence?
   a. Cultural beliefs
   b. Poverty
   c. Physical appearance
   d. Unemployment

9. Which of the following is an example of stalking?
   a. Making intimate and sexually implied comments to another person
   b. Repeated visual, physical, or virtual seeking out of another person
   c. Unwelcome sexual conduct by the perpetrator
   d. Sexual abuse of a child

10. Jack beats his wife Melissa "to teach her a lesson." Afterward, he denies attacking her. This illustrates which phase of the cycle of violence?
    a. Acute battering
    b. Fear/depression
    c. Remorse/reconciliation
    d. Tension building

Answers to these questions can be found on page A-1.

Think about It!

1. What forms of violence do you think are most significant or prevalent in the United States today? Why?

2. What type of violence is most common on your campus? How do you think campus violence affects students at your school? Are there differences in how men and women respond to news that there has

been a rape or violent assault on campus? If so, why?

3. Have you known anyone personally who has been sexually assaulted on campus? What actions were taken to help him or her cope with the assault? What campus services, if any, were used?

4. Why do some people develop into violent or abusive adults and others become pacifists or peaceful adults? What key factors influence violent offenders to be violent?

5. What actions need to be taken to stem the tide of violence in the United States at the individual level? At the community level? In schools? On college campuses? Nationally?

Accessing Your Health on the Internet

The following websites explore further topics and issues related to personal health. For links to the websites below, visit the Companion Website for *Access to Health,* 13th Edition, at www.pearsonhighered.com/donatelle.

1. *Communities against Violence Network.* This site provides an extensive, searchable database for information about violence against women, with articles about everything from domestic violence to legal information and statistics. www.cavnet.blogspot.com

2. *Men Can Stop Rape.* Practical suggestions for men interested in helping to protect women from sexual predators and assault are provided on this site. www.mencanstoprape.org

3. *National Center for Injury Prevention and Control.* The Web-based Injury Statistics Query and Reporting System (WISQARS) database of this CDC section provides statistics and information on fatal and nonfatal injuries, both intentional and unintentional. www.cdc.gov/injury

4. *National Center for Victims of Crime.* Information and resources for victims of crimes ranging from

hate crimes to sexual assault are available here. www.ncvc.org

5. *National Sexual Violence Resource Center.* This is an excellent resource for victims of sexual violence. www.nsvrc.org

6. *CyberAngels.* On this site you will find information on online safety, as well as help and advice for victims of cyberstalking, identity theft, and related personal invasions via technology. www.cyberangels.org

References

1. World Health Organization, *World Report on Violence and Health* (Geneva: World Health Organization, 2002), www.who.int/violence_injury_prevention/violence/world_report/en.

2. World Health Organization, "Training for the Health Sector: Children's Health and the Environment," 2010.

3. Society of Public Health Educators (SOPHE) Unintentional Injury and Violence Prevention, "Injury 101: Violence/Intentional Injury," 2009, www.sophe.org/ui/injury-violence.shtml.

4. U.S. Department of Justice, Federal Bureau of Investigation, "Crime in the United States, Preliminary Semiannual Uniform Crime Report for 2011," July 2012, www.fbi.gov/news/pressrel/press-releases/fbi-releases-preliminary-annual-crime-statistics-for-2011.

5. Ibid.

6. Bureau of Justice Statistics. "Criminal Victimization," 2009, Accessed 2010, http://bjs.ojp.usdoj.gov/index.cfm?ty=pbdetail&iid=2217.

7. American College Health Association, *American College Health Association—National College Health Assessment II: Reference Group Data Report Fall 2011* (Baltimore: American College Health Association, 2012), www.acha-ncha.org/reports_ACHA-NCHAII.html.

8. Center for Public Integrity, "Sexual Assault on Campus: A Frustrating Search for Justice," Updated February 2010, www.publicintegrity.org/investigations/campus_assault.

9. World Health Organization Violence Prevention Alliance, "The Ecological Framework," 2010, www.who.int/violenceprevention/approach/ecology/en/index.html; Centers for Disease Control and Prevention, National Center for Injury Prevention and Control, "Understanding Youth Violence," 2009, Available

at www.cdc.gov/violenceprevention/youthviolence.

10. Substance Abuse and Mental Health Services Administration, "The NSDUH Report: Violent Behaviors and Family Income among Adolescents," August 19, 2010, Newsletter, www.oas.samhsa.gov/2k10/189/ViolentBehaviorsHTML.pdf; Q. Li, R. Kirby, R. Sigler, et al. "A Multilevel Analysis of Individual, Household, and Neighborhood Correlates of Intimate Partner Violence among Low-Income Pregnant Women in Jefferson County, Alabama," *American Journal of Public Health,* March 2010; 100(3): 531–39; L. Kiss, L. Glima-Schraiber, L. Heise, et al. "Gender-Based Violence and Socioeconomic Inequalities: Does Living in More Deprived Neighborhoods Increase Women's Risk of Intimate Partner Violence?" *Social Science & Medicine* 74, no. 8, 1172–79.

11. U.S. Department of Justice, National Institute of Justice, "Economic Distress and Intimate Partner Violence," 2009, www.ojp.usdoj.gov/nij/topics/crime/intimate-partner-violence/economic-distress.htm.

12. J. H. Derzon, "The Correspondence of Family Features with Problem, Aggressive, Criminal and Violent Behaviors: A Meta-Analysis," *Journal of Experimental Criminology* 6, no. 3 (2010): 263–92, DOI: 10.1007/s11292-010-9098-0; C. Ferguson, C. San Miguel, and R. Hartley, "A Multivariate Analysis of Youth Violence and Aggression: The Influences of Family, Peers, Depression, and Media Violence," *Journal of Pediatrics* 155, no. 6 (2009): 904–08.

13. M. Flood and B. Pease, "Factors Influencing Attitudes to Violence against Women," *Trauma, Violence and Abuse* 10, no. 2 (2009): 125–42.

14. Centers for Disease Control and Prevention, "Understanding Intimate Partner Violence," Fact Sheet, 2012, www.cdc.gov/ViolencePrevention/pdf/IPV_Factsheet-a.pdf.

15. G. Stuart et al., "Examining the Interface between Substance Misuse and Intimate Partner Violence," *Substance Abuse Research and Treatment* 3 (2009): 25–29.

16. T. Frisell et al., "Violent Crime Runs in Families: A Total Population Study of 12.5 Million Individuals," *Psychological Medicine* 41, no. 1 (2010): 97–105, DOI: 10.1017S0023329170000462.

17. J. H. Derzon, "The Correspondence of Family Features with Problem, Aggressive, Criminal and Violent Behaviors: A Meta-Analysis," *Journal of Experimental Criminology* 6, no. 3 (2010): 263–92, DOI: 10.1007/s11292-010-9098-0; C. Cook,

et al., "Predictors of Bullying and Victimization in Childhood and Adolescence: A Meta-Analytic Investigation," *School Psychology Quarterly* 25, no. 2 (2010): 65–83.

18. R. Kendra, K. Bell, and J. Guimond. "The Impact of Child Abuse History, PTSD and Anger Arousal on Dating Violence Perpetrators Among College Women," *Journal of Family Violence* 27, no. 3 (2012): 165–75.

19. D. Matsumoto, S. Yoo, and J. Chung, "The Expression of Anger across Culture," in *International Handbook of Anger*, eds. M. Potegal et al. (New York: Springer, 2010).

20. M. Randolph et al., "Alcohol Use and Sexual Risk Behavior among College Students: Understanding Gender and Ethnic Differences," *American Journal of Drug & Alcohol Abuse* 35, no. 2 (2009): 80–84; E. Reed, H. Amaro, A. Matsumoto, and D. Kaysen, "The Relation between Interpersonal Violence and Substance Use among a Sample of University Students: Examination of the Role of Victim and Perpetrator Substance Use," *Addictive Behaviors* 34, no. 3 (2009): 316–18; T. Messman-Moore, R. Ward, and A. Brown, "Substance Use and PTSD Symptoms Impact the Likelihood of Rape and Revictimization in College Women," *Journal of Interpersonal Violence* 24, no. 3 (2009): 499–521; J. McCauley, K. Calhoun, and C. Gidycz, "Binge Drinking and Rape: A Prospective Examination of College Women with a History of Previous Sexual Victimization," *Journal of Interpersonal Violence* 25, no. 9 (2010): 1655–68.

21. Ferguson and J. Kilburn, "The Public Health Risks of Media Violence: A Meta-Analytic Review," *The Journal of Pediatrics* 154, no. 5 (2009): 759–63, www.jpeds.com/article/S0022-3476(08)01037-8/fulltext; C. Ferguson et al., "Personality and Media Influences on Violence and Depression in a Cross National Sample of Young Adults: Data from Mexican Americans, English and Croatians," *Computers in Human Behavior* 27, no. 3 (2011): 1195–1200, DOI:10.1016/j.chb.2010.12.015; J. Savage and C. Yancey, "The Effects of Media Violence Exposure on Criminal Aggression: A Meta-Analysis," *Criminal Justice and Behavior* 35, no. 6 (2008): 772–91.

22. C. Ferguson et al., "Personality, Parental and Media Influences on Aggressive Personality and Violent Crime in Youth," *Journal of Aggression, Maltreatment and Trauma* 17, no. 4 (2008): 395–414; B. Wilson, "Media and Children's Aggression, Fear, and Altruism," *The Future of Children* 18, no. 1 (2008): 1550–54; L. Price and V. Maholmes, "Understanding the Nature and Consequences of Children's Exposure to Violence: Research Perspectives,"

Clinical Child and Family Psychology Review 12, no. 2 (2009): 65–70.

23. U.S. Department of Justice, Office of Justice Programs, Bureau of Justice Statistics, *National Crime Victimization Survey: Criminal Victimization*, 2009 (Washington, DC: Bureau of Justice Statistics, 2010); U.S. Department of Justice, Bureau of Justice Statistics, Crime Victimization, 2010, updated 2011, http://bjs.ojp.usdoj.gov/index.cfm?ty=pbdetail&iid=2224.

24. C. Ferguson, *Violent Crime: Clinical and Social Implications* (Thousand Oaks, CA: Sage, 2010).

25. World Health Organization, *World Report on Violence and Health*, 2002.

26. A. M. Miniño, J. Xu, and K. D. Kochanek, Centers for Disease Control and Prevention, National Center for Health Statistics, "Deaths: Preliminary Data for 2008," *National Vital Statistics Reports* 59, no. 2 (2010): 31, 55, www.cdc.gov/nchs/data/nvsr/nvsr59/nvsr59_02.pdf.

27. U.S. Department of Justice, Federal Bureau of Investigation, *Crime in the United States 2009*, 2010, www2.fbi.gov/ucr/cius2009.

28. J. Fox and M. Swatt, *The Recent Surge in Homicides Involving Young Black Males and Guns: Time to Reinvest in Prevention and Crime Control* (Alexandria, VA: American Statistical Association, 2008), Available at www.ncjrs.gov/App/publications/abstract.aspx?ID=248092.

29. Centers for Disease Control and Prevention, "FastStats: Assault or Homicide," 2009, www.cdc.gov/nchs/FASTATS/homicide.htm.

30. Federal Bureau of Investigation, "Hate Crime Statistics, 2009," February 2011, www.fbi.gov/ucr/hc2009/index.html.

31. Ibid.

32. Centers for Disease Control, "National Intimate Partner and Sexual Violence Survey Fact Sheet, Highlights of 2010 Findings," updated June 2012, http://www.cdc.gov/ViolencePrevention/pdf/NISVS_FactSheet-a.pdf.

33. Ibid.

34. P. Lin and J. Gill, "Homicides of Pregnant Women," *Journal of Forensic Medicine and Pathology*, March 5, 2010, DOI: 10-1097/PAF.obo13e3181d3dc3b.

35. Violence Policy Center, *American Roulette: Murder-Suicide in the United States*. 4th. (Washington, DC): Violence Policy Center, 2012, Available at http://www.vpc.org/studies/amroul2012.pdf.

36. L. Walker, *The Battered Woman* (New York: Harper and Row, 1979).

37. L. Walker, *The Battered Woman Syndrome*. 3rd ed. (New York: Springer, 2009).

38. L. Rosen and J. Fontaine, *Compendium of Research on Violence against Women*,

1993–Present (Washington, DC: National Institute of Justice, 2009), DOJ (US) NCJ223572, Available at www.ojp.usdoj.gov/nij/pubs-sum/vaw-compendium.htm.

39. Centers for Disease Control and Prevention, National Center for Injury Prevention and Control, "Understanding Intimate Partner Violence Fact Sheet," 2009, www.cdc.gov/violenceprevention/pdf/IPV_factsheet-a.pdf; National Domestic Violence Hotline, "Abuse in America," www.ndvh.org/get-educated/abuse-in-america.

40. U.S. Department of Health and Human Services, Administration for Children and Families, "Definition of Child Abuse and Neglect: Summary of State Laws," 2009, www.childwelfare.gov/systemwide/laws_policies/statutes/define.cfm.

41. Childhelp, National Child Abuse Statistics, "Child Abuse in America," 2012, www.childhelp.org/pages/statistics.

42. C. Cooper, A. Selwood, and G. Livingston, "The Prevalence of Elder Abuse and Neglect: A Systematic Review," *Age and Ageing* 37, no. 2 (2008): 151–60; U.S. Department of Health and Human Services, National Institute on Aging, "Elder Abuse," 2011; United States Department of Health and Human Services, National Institute on Aging, "Elder Abuse," 2011, www.nia.nih.gov/health/publication/elder-abuse; U.S. Department of Justice, Elder Abuse and Mistreatment Fact Sheet, November,2011, www.ojp.gov/newsroom/factsheets/ojpfs_elderabuse.html.

43. Centers for Disease Control and Prevention, National Center for Injury Prevention and Control, "Sexual Violence: Facts at a Glance," 2008, Available at www.cdc.gov/violenceprevention/sexualviolence/index.html.

44. D. Kilpatrick et al., "Drug-Facilitated, Incapacitated, and Forcible Rape: A National Study," National Crime Victims Research and Treatment Center, February 1, 2007, www.ncjrs.gov/pdffiles1/nij/grants/219181.pdf.

45. Centers for Disease Control and Prevention, "Sexual Violence: Facts at a Glance," 2008.

46. M. Rand, *National Crime Victimization Survey: Criminal Victimization, 2008* (Washington, DC: Bureau of Justice Statistics, 2009), NCJ 227777, Available at http://bjs.ojp.usdoj.gov/index.cfm?ty=pbdetail&iid=1975.

47. Centers for Disease Control and Prevention, National Center for Injury Prevention and Control, "Understanding Sexual Violence Fact Sheet," 2009, www.cdc.gov/violenceprevention/sexualviolence/index.html.

48. M. Rand, *National Crime Victimization Survey*, 2009.

49. Centers for Disease Control and Prevention, "Sexual Violence: Facts at a Glance," 2008; L. Schneider, L. Mori, P. Lambert, and A. Wong, "The Role of Gender and Ethnicity in Perceptions of Rape and Its Aftereffects," *Sex Roles* 60, no. 5/6 (2009): 410–21.

50. D. Kilpatrick et al., "Drug-Facilitated, Incapacitated, and Forcible Rape," 2007.

51. J. Carr, *American College Health Association Campus Violence White Paper*, (Baltimore: American College Health Association, 2005), Available at www.acha.org/Publications/Guidelines_WhitePapers.cfm.

52. D. Kilpatrick et al., "Drug-Facilitated, Incapacitated, and Forcible Rape," 2007.

53. Centers for Disease Control and Prevention, "Understanding Sexual Violence Fact Sheet," 2009.

54. University of Illinois at Chicago, "Most Sexual Assaults Drug Facilitated, Study Claims," *ScienceDaily* (May 13, 2006), Accessed May 18, 2008, www.sciencedaily.com/releases/2006/05/060513122928.htm.

55. R. Bergen and E. Barnhill, "Marital Rape: New Research and Directions," National Online Resource Center on Violence against Women, 2006, http://new.vawnet.org/category/Main_Doc.php?docid=248.

56. R. Bergen and E. Barnhill, National Online Resource Center on Violence Against Women, "Summary: Marital Rape: New Research and Directions," 2011.

57. Ibid.

58. L. P. Chen et al., "Sexual Abuse and Lifetime Diagnosis of Psychiatric Disorders: Systematic Review and Meta-Analysis," *Mayo Clinic Proceedings* 85, no. 7 (2010): 618–29.

59. Childhelp, National Child Abuse Statistics, May 6, 2011, www.childhelp.org/pages/statistics#stats-sources.

60. L. P. Chen et al., "Sexual Abuse and Lifetime Diagnosis of Psychiatric Disorders" 2010; R. Gilbert, et al., "Burden and Consequences of Child Maltreatment in High-Income Countries," *Lancet* 373, no. 3 (2009): 68–81; T. Hilberg, C. Hamilton-Giachrtsis, and L. Dixon, "Review of Meta-Analyses on the Association between Child Sexual Abuse and Adult Mental Health Difficulties: A Systematic Approach." *Trauma, Violence, Abuse* 12, no. 1 (2011): 38–49.

61. Childhelp, National Child Abuse Statistics, Accessed June 2012.

62. Oregon State University, Sexual Harassment Policy, Accessed May 6, 2011, http://oregonstate.edu/affact/sexual-harassment-policy-0.

63. Centers for Disease Control, "Sexual Violence, Stalking, and Intimate Partner Violence Widespread in the US," NISVS 2010 Summary Report, Press Release, December 2011.

64. Ibid.

65. Ibid.

66. Ibid.

67. Centers for Disease Control and Prevention Injury Center, "Preventing Intimate Partner Violence, Sexual Violence and Child Maltreatment," 2006, www.cdc.gov/ncipc/pub-res/research_agenda/07_violence.htm; P. York, "Traditional Gender Role Attitudes and Violence against Women: A Test of Feminist Theory," Paper presented at the annual meeting of the American Society of Criminology (November 13, 2007), Accessed June 2008, www.allacademic.com/meta/p200649_index.html.

68. U.S. Department of Justice, National Drug Intelligence Center, *National Gang Threat Assessment 2009* (Washington, DC: National Drug Intelligence Center, 2009), 2009-M0335-001, Available at www.justice.gov/ndic/pubs32/32146/index.htm.

69. National Youth Violence Prevention Resource Center, "Youth Gangs and Violence," updated January 4, 2008, www.safeyouth.org/scripts/faq/youthgang.asp.

70. U.S. Code of Federal Regulations, Title 28CFR0.85.

71. J. Carr, *American College Health Association Campus Violence White Paper*, 2005.

Reducing Your Risk of Unintentional Injury

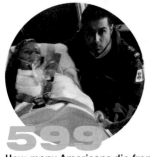

How many Americans die from unintentional injuries each year?

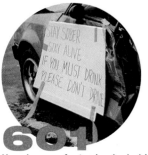

How large a factor is alcohol in motor vehicle crashes?

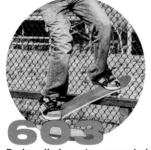

Do I really have to wear a helmet while I'm skateboarding?

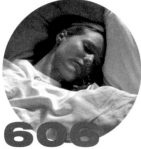

What's the top cause of fire-related deaths?

When Matt planned his birthday trip for spring break, he never thought he'd be spending part of the day in a hospital room. After drinking for several hours at the cantina on the beach, he and his friends started back to their hotel to continue the party by the swimming pool. They had all been drinking heavily, and they were in a celebratory mood when two of Matt's friends picked him up and threw him into the water, shouting, "Happy Birthday!" When he hit the water, Matt started thrashing, but he was too drunk to understand what was happening or figure out what to do. All he knew was an all-consuming panic as

he inhaled the water. Then he passed out. Fortunately, another hotel patron sitting by the pool recognized what his friends were too intoxicated to realize: Matt was drowning. She jumped into the water and pulled Matt's limp body to the edge, screaming to his friends, "Dial 9-1-1!" Then she started cardiopulmonary resuscitation (CPR). As the ambulance arrived, Matt regained consciousness, but even hours later, in his hospital room, he had no memory of what had really happened to him.

Drowning is just one of many unintentional injuries in which alcohol commonly plays a role. Alcohol reduces your ability to stay alert, to maintain an

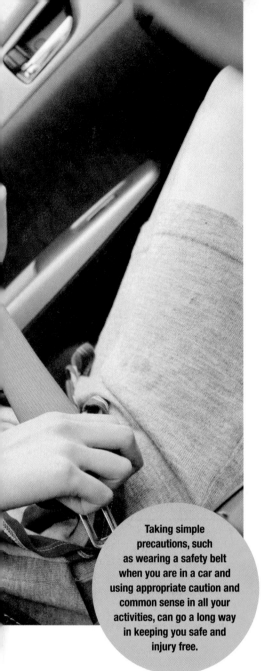

Taking simple precautions, such as wearing a safety belt when you are in a car and using appropriate caution and common sense in all your activities, can go a long way in keeping you safe and injury free.

by cell phone use or another activity, or impaired by substance abuse, sleep deprivation, or other circumstances.

How big a problem is unintentional injury? For Americans age 15 to 44, unintentional injuries are the leading cause of death, killing approximately 40,000 people in the prime of life.[1] In fact, unintentional injuries are responsible for about 28 percent of all deaths in this age group.[2] As you might expect, motor vehicle accidents are responsible for the greatest percentage of unintentional injury deaths. However, many other mechanisms are responsible for significant mortality each year, most notably poisonings, falls, chokings, drownings, and fires.[3]

In this text, we'll discuss the most common unintentional injuries, beginning with motor vehicle crashes, which are the leading cause of death of young adults.[4] For each injury type, we'll identify steps you can take to reduce your risk as well as strategies for managing an injury situation should one occur.

awareness of your surroundings, and to make good decisions. Other factors—such as drowsiness, distraction, and failing to take sensible precautions—increase your risk for injury for similar reasons. In fact, although the term **unintentional injury** might sound academic, most health professionals shy away from the more familiar term *accidental injury* because it implies that these injuries occur without individuals having any control over their situation. As we saw with Matt's near-drowning, "accidents" often occur as a consequence of people's poor choices. Car "accidents," for example, often occur because the driver was distracted

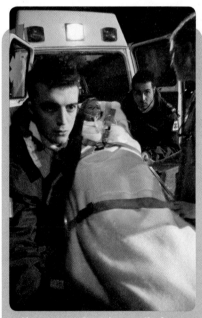

How many Americans die from unintentional injuries each year?

Unintentional injuries killed over 118,000 Americans in 2010. That's over 320 people per day. Most strategies for preventing unintentional injuries focus on changing something about the person, the environment, or the circumstances that put people in harm's way.

See It! Videos

For true stories of the tragic effects of traumatic brain injuries, watch **Driven Mad** at www.pearsonhighered.com/donatelle.

Are You at Risk on the Road?

In 2010, over 35,000 people died in motor vehicle accidents (MVAs).[5] That's nearly 100 Americans every day. What factors contribute to MVAs? And how can you reduce your risk?

Five Factors Affect Motor Vehicle Safety

In the blink of an eye, your actions could transform your vehicle from a pleasant mode of *transportation* into a deadly weapon. Five factors—distracted driving, impaired driving, speeding, vehicle safety issues, and driver age—contribute to the majority of MVAs.[6] As you read about each of these, notice that most are within your personal control.

Distracted Driving Four types of activities constitute distracted driving: looking at something other than the road; hearing something not related to driving; manipulating something other than the steering wheel; and thinking about something other than driving.[7] In 2010, 3,092 Americans died in over a million distraction-affected crashes.[8]

Although there's no conclusive evidence identifying the forms of distraction most likely to contribute to MVAs, the behaviors of greatest concern are texting and talking on a cell phone. Overall, 9 percent of all U.S. drivers and 25 percent of drivers age 18 to 29 report texting "regularly or fairly often" while driving, and 25 percent of all U.S. drivers, and 40 percent of drivers age 18 to 29 report that they talk on their cell phone "regularly or fairly often" while driving.[9] How do these behaviors contribute to MVAs? The

unintentional injury Any injury committed or sustained without intent of harm.

Banning Phone Use While Driving:
GOOD IDEA OR GOING TOO FAR?

A whopping 75 percent of U.S. drivers in their teens and twenties have reported answering a text or chatting on the phone while driving in the past month. The problem is that as of 2009, the most recent year for which statistics are available, the proportion of drivers reportedly distracted at the time of a fatal crash reached 11 percent. That same year, nearly 1,000 deaths and 24,000 injuries were due to distracted driving specifically involving use of a cell phone.

Thirty-seven states now ban texting while driving, and ten states ban all handheld phone use. No state bans all cell phone use for all drivers, but 31 states ban all use—including hands-free phone use—for novice drivers. Are these laws necessary to protect American drivers, passengers, cyclists, and pedestrians, or do they go too far?

Arguments in Favor of Banning Cell Phone Use While Driving

○ Laws against driving under the influence of alcohol or other drugs and laws mandating seat belt use have saved millions of lives. Cell phone bans could do the same.

○ Statistics have shown that drivers who use handheld devices are four times as likely to get into crashes resulting in injury than are drivers who don't use them.

Arguments Opposing Banning Cell Phone Use While Driving

○ Talking with passengers, eating, working a GPS device, putting on makeup, and changing the radio station are also shown to greatly increase the chance of accidents. Why ban cell phone use without banning the other activities?

○ These laws are difficult to enforce and spend tax dollars that might be better spent improving traffic safety in other ways.

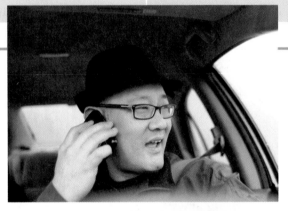

Where Do You Stand?

○ What are your own state's laws regarding cell phone use? If it is against the law in your state, do you obey the rules?

○ Do you think texting while driving should be banned? What about use of a handheld cell phone? What about use of a hands-free cell phone? Why?

○ Do you agree with state laws banning all cell phone use for novice drivers?

○ Do you personally think that other driving distractions are as dangerous as cell phone use? Is it possible to avoid getting distracted while driving?

Sources: National Highway Traffic Safety Administration, Traffic Safety Facts: Distracted Driving, 2009, (Washington, DC: US Department of Transportation, National Highway Traffic Safety Administration, September 2010), DOT-HS-811-379, www.distraction.gov; Governors Highway Safety Association, "Cell Phone and Texting Laws," Updated April 2012, www.ghsa.org/html/stateinfo/laws/cellphone_laws.html; M. Reardon, "Study: Distractions, Not Pones, Cause Care Crashes," in CNET.com Signal Strength, January 29, 2010, http://news.cnet.com/8301-30686_3-1044717-266.html.

National Safety Council estimates that about every 24 seconds, somewhere in the United States an MVA occurs because drivers are texting or talking on a cell phone.[10] Given these statistics, it's no wonder that laws regulating cell phone use while driving have been passed in several states, and 37 states now ban text-messaging for all drivers.[11] See the **Points of View** box for more on laws banning phone use while driving.

Other common distractions for drivers include manipulating handheld music and Internet devices, adjusting CD players or the radio, looking in the mirror, calling out the window, and eating. Nearly 8 out of 10 MVAs happen within just 3 seconds of a driver becoming distracted.[12] The next time you're tempted to text, make a call, or even swat an insect while driving, don't do it. Pull over. Handle the distraction. Then rejoin the traffic when you're ready to give it your full attention.

Impaired Driving Every day, 32 people in the United States die in MVAs that involve an alcohol-impaired driver.

This amounts to nearly 12,000 deaths, or 1 death every 45 minutes. Viewed another way, nearly 32 percent of all MVA fatalities are due to alcohol impairment.[13] If you think these deaths occur mainly among older adults, think again: 67 percent of alcohol-impaired drivers involved in fatal crashes are between the ages of 21 and 34.[14]

Although alcohol is the primary cause of impairment while driving, other substances and situations are also responsible. For example, use of drugs other than alcohol, including marijuana, cocaine, and prescription medications, is an increasing problem among young adult drivers and is a significant cause of MVA injury and death.[15] In one study of nighttime drivers, over 11 percent tested positive for illicit drugs.[16] Drowsiness can impair driving, too; many researchers contend that driving while sleep deprived is as dangerous as driving drunk. In 2009, an estimated 30,000 MVAs involved drowsy drivers. These resulted in 832 deaths.[17]

Both public health and law enforcement agencies are cooperating on several measures to keep impaired drivers off the road. These include the following:

● Promotion of designated driver programs, including measures such as public funding of "safe rides" for people who have been drinking and provision of nonalcoholic beverages free of charge to designated drivers.
● Strict enforcement of existing laws defining impaired driving and the legal drinking age
● Implementation of measures to prevent repeat offenses by anyone previously convicted of driving while impaired:
  • Mandatory alcohol or other drug abuse treatment
  • Installation of ignition interlock systems that prevent vehicle operation by anyone with a blood alcohol

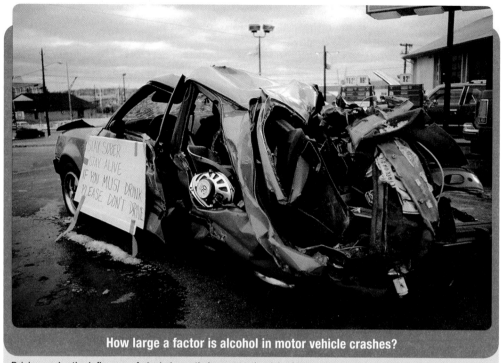

How large a factor is alcohol in motor vehicle crashes?
Driving under the influence of alcohol greatly increases the risk of being involved in a motor vehicle crash. Of all drivers between the ages of 21 and 24 involved in fatal crashes, more than 1 out of 3 were legally drunk.

concentration above a specified safe level
  • Revoking the driver's license
● Stricter testing for and punishment of those who abuse prescription medicines and/or drive when sleep impaired.

Speeding Speeding is a factor in 1 out of every 3 fatal crashes. Driver surveys suggest that many people speed because they don't perceive it as dangerous—they believe that traffic laws are overly restrictive and don't apply to them! Unfortunately, such attitudes lead to more than 13,000 deaths each year.[18]

Vehicle Safety Issues Wearing a safety belt cuts your risk of death or serious injury in a crash by almost half.[19] In 2009, 53 percent of drivers and passengers killed in MVAs were not wearing safety belts,[20] so buckle up and insist any passengers do the same. If you're transporting an infant or child in your vehicle, follow state laws governing use and location of age-appropriate safety seats.

Vehicles can include many safety features, from air bags to stability con-

trol. Unfortunately, people who don't have the financial resources to drive vehicles with all of the state-of-the-art features—and that group often includes college students—are at increased risk during MVAs. Still, the next time you're planning to purchase a car, new or used, look for the following features recommended by the Insurance Institute for Highway Safety:

1. Does the car have front air bags? Side air bags? Remember, air bags do not eliminate the need for everyone to wear safety belts.
2. Does the car have antilock brakes? Traction and electronic stability control? Each of these features can mean the difference between life, injury, or death.
3. Does the car have impact-absorbing crumple zones?
4. Are there strengthened passenger compartment side walls?
5. Is there a strong roof support? (The center doorpost on four-door models gives you an extra roof pillar.)

Another factor in MVA safety is the size of the vehicles involved. All cars sold in the United States must meet U.S. Department of Transportation standards for crash worthiness, no matter their size. However, in crashes involving multiple vehicles, the death rate in 2007 for people in minicars was almost twice the rate for people in very large cars.[21] Many college students drive minicars because they are more affordable and use less gas, but the laws of physics make such cars more dangerous, especially in frontal collisions with larger cars.

What about motorcycles? Per vehicle mile traveled, motorcyclists are about 25 times more likely than passenger car occupants to die in an MVA, and 5 times more likely to be injured. In 2009, this translated into 4,462 motorcyclist deaths and 90,000 injuries.[22]

95%

of college students surveyed reported that they mostly or always wear a seat belt when driving or riding in a car.

Many motorcyclists involved in MVAs have avoided severe injuries because they were wearing a helmet. In 2009, for every 100 motorcyclists killed in crashes while not wearing a helmet, 37 could have been saved by helmet use. Although the benefits of helmets and protective clothing are well established, only 20 states have full helmet requirements for anyone riding a motorcycle.[23] To find out what your state requirements are, go to www.iihs.org/laws/helmetusecurrent.aspx.

Driver Age Many of us assume that seniors are the age group most often involved in MVAs. Sensory impairments and slowed reflexes can increase accident rates among people 65 and older, but rates are at their peak among teen drivers, especially the first year that a teen has a license. Overall, teen drivers are four times more likely than older drivers to be involved a crash.[24] Graduated driver licensing (GDL) programs, which have been implemented

Minimizing the Chance of Injury During A Car Accident

If a car accident is unavoidable, you can still behave in a way that lessens the chance of serious injury. Some tips include the following:

❱ Generally, it's safer to veer right rather than left.
❱ Steer, don't skid, off the road to avoid rolling your vehicle.
❱ If you have to hit a vehicle, better to sideswipe one moving in your direction than to hit one in the oncoming lane.
❱ Avoid hitting pedestrians, motorcyclists, and bicyclists at all costs.

in many states, have been shown to reduce MVA fatalities in crashes involving teens by nearly 20 percent.[25] They are also thought to reduce the risk of all MVAs involving teen drivers by 20 to 40 percent.[26] Typically, GDL programs involve several stages for teens to complete before becoming fully licensed.

Practice Risk-Management Driving Techniques

Although you can't control what other drivers are doing, you can reduce your risk of injury in an MVA by practicing risk-management driving techniques. These include the following:

● Don't manipulate electronic devices while driving. Avoid talking on a cell phone while driving, even if the phone is hands free.
● Don't drink and drive. If you plan to party with friends, designate a sober driver or arrange in advance for a taxi or "safe ride," or plan to spend the night where you are.
● Don't drive when tired or when in a highly emotional or stressed state.
● Surround your car with a safety "bubble." The rear bumper of the car ahead of you should be at least 3 seconds away.
● Scan the road ahead of you and to both sides.
● Drive with your low-beam headlights on, *day and night,* to make your car more visible to other drivers.

● Anticipate the actions of other drivers as much as you can, and be on the alert for unsignaled lane changes, sudden braking, or other unexpected maneuvers.
● Obey all traffic laws.
● Whether you are the driver or a passenger, always wear a seat belt.

Even the most careful drivers may find themselves having to avoid an accident at some time in their lives. See the **Skills for Behavior Change** box for tips on how to manage your risk.

Can You Play It Safe and Still Have Fun?

Recreational activities among young people that commonly involve injury include biking, skateboarding, snow sports, swimming and boating, and using fireworks. By following some basic guidelines while doing these activities, you can have fun and be safe.

Follow Bike Safety Rules

Currently, over 63 million Americans of all ages ride bicycles for transportation, recreation, and fitness. The National Highway Traffic Safety Administration (NHTSA) reports about 700 to 750 deaths per year from cycling accidents. The great majority of cycling deaths

(87%) involve cyclists age 16 and older.[27] Most fatal collisions are due to cyclists' errors, usually failure to yield at intersections. However, alcohol also plays a significant role in bicycle deaths and injuries: In 2009, nearly one fourth (24%) of cyclists killed were legally drunk, and in one third of all fatal accidents between motor vehicles and bicycles, either the driver or the cyclist was drunk.[28]

All cyclists should wear a properly fitted bicycle helmet every time they ride (Figure 1). In spite of this, fewer than one third of all college students report "mostly or always" wearing a helmet while biking.[29] The NHTSA reports that a helmet is the single most effective way to prevent head injury resulting from a bicycle crash. Moreover, bear in mind that cyclists are considered vehicle operators; they are required to obey the same rules of the road as do drivers.

Cyclists should consider the following suggestions:

● Wear a helmet approved by the American National Standards Institute (ANSI) or the Snell Memorial Foundation.
● Watch the road and listen for traffic sounds! Never listen to an MP3 player or talk on a cell phone, even hands free, while cycling.
● Don't drink and ride.
● Follow all traffic laws, signs, and signals.

● Ride with the flow of traffic.
● Wear light or brightly colored, reflective clothing that is easily seen at dawn, dusk, and during full daylight.
● Avoid riding after dark. If you must ride at night, use a front light and a red reflector or flashing rear light, as well as reflective tape or other markings on your bike and clothing.
● Know and use proper hand signals.
● Keep your bicycle in good condition.
● Use bike paths whenever possible.
● Stop at stop signs and traffic lights.

Stay Safe on Your Board

According to the U.S. Consumer Product Safety Commission (CPSC), approximately 26,000 people are treated in hospital emergency rooms each year with skateboard-related injuries. These injuries are most commonly due to falls or collisions, and some are fatal. Three factors commonly contribute to skateboard injury: lack of protective equipment, poor board maintenance, and irregular riding surfaces. Both inexperience and overconfidence also play a role: One third of all injuries happen to people who have been skateboarding for less than a week, but the majority of injuries occur among people who have been skating for more than a year, typically when they are attempting difficult stunts.[30]

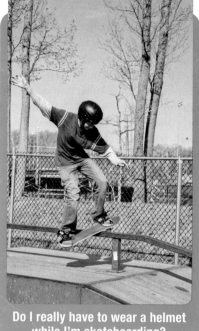

Do I really have to wear a helmet while I'm skateboarding?

Many skateboarding injuries occur among people who have been practicing the sport for more than a year, often when they attempt a stunt beyond their level of skill. Wearing a helmet, no matter how experienced a skateboarder you are, will help protect you in case of a fall.

Skateboard safety tips from the CPSC include the following:[31]

● Wear an approved helmet designed for skateboarding, with a hard shell and foam interior.
● Wear skateboarding gloves, wrist guards, and knee and elbow pads. Wear flat-soled shoes.
● Maintain your board. Between uses, check it for loose, broken, sharp, or cracked parts. Tighten screws or have the board professionally repaired if necessary.
● Examine the surface where you'll be riding for holes, bumps, and debris.
● Never skateboard in the street, and never hitch a ride from a car, bicycle, or other vehicle.
● Practice complicated stunts in specially designed areas, wearing lots of protective padding.
● Practice safe falling: If you start to lose your balance, crouch down; if you fall, try to "relax and roll."
● Don't ride alone.
● Don't drink and ride.

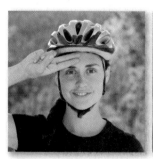 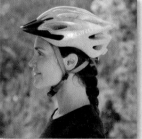 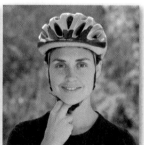

❶ The helmet should sit level on your head and low on your forehead—one or two finger-widths above your eyebrows.

❷ The sliders on the side straps should be adjusted to form a "V" shape under, and slightly in front of, your ears. Lock the sliders if possible.

❸ The chin strap buckle should be centered under your chin. Tighten the strap until it is snug, so that no more than two fingers fit under the strap.

FIGURE 1 Fitting a Bicycle Helmet

When your helmet is fitted correctly, opening your mouth wide in a yawn should cause the helmet to pull down on your head. Also, you should not be able to rock the helmet back more than the width of two fingers above the eyebrows or forward into your eyes.

Video Tutor: Biking Safety

Stay Safe in the Snow

The National Ski Areas Association (NSAA) reports that a skiing or snowboarding fatality occurs at the rate of 3.8 per 1 million participants per year.[32] That translates into about 40 fatalities on the slopes in an average year. Severe nonfatal injuries, such as head trauma and spinal cord injury, also occur, but at a similarly low rate. This makes snow sports much safer, overall, than bicycling, swimming, and many others. More good news is that the rate of injury has been declining for decades, largely because of the use of shorter skis, improved safety features on equipment, and increased safety efforts at resorts, such as having more monitors on the slopes, setting aside special family skiing areas, and encouraging helmet use.

These safety measures are critical because when collisions and other accidents occur on the slopes, they can be fatal or leave the victim permanently paralyzed. One of the most important ways to protect yourself while skiing or snowboarding is to wear an approved helmet. The NSAA reports that helmet use reduces the risk of any head injury by 30 to 50 percent. It's also important to keep skis and snowboards in good condition and to ski according to your ability. Pay attention to the locations of other skiers, and if you stop, move to the side of the trail. Finally, observe all posted signs and warnings.

Stay Safe in the Water

Drowning is the sixth leading cause of unintentional injury death among Americans of all ages, with 1 in 5 of those deaths occurring in children age 14 and younger. Males are nearly four times more likely than females to die from unintentional drowning.[33] As we saw with Matt at the beginning of this chapter, alcohol plays a significant role in many drownings: About half of all fatal drownings among adolescents and adults involve alcohol.[34]

personal flotation device A device worn to provide buoyancy and keep the wearer, conscious or unconscious, afloat with the nose and mouth out of the water; also known as a life jacket.

Swimming The American Red Cross reports that almost half of adults surveyed say they've had an experience in which they nearly drowned.[35] Most drownings occur during water recreation—swimming, diving, or just simply having fun—in unorganized or unsupervised areas, such as ponds or pools without lifeguards present. Many drowning victims were strong swimmers, so all swimmers should take the following precautions:

- Don't drink alcohol before or while swimming.
- Don't enter the water without a lifejacket unless you can swim at least 50 feet unassisted.
- Know your limitations; get out of the water when you start to feel even slightly fatigued.
- Never swim alone, even if you are a skilled swimmer. You never know what might happen.
- Never leave a child unattended, even in extremely shallow water.
- Before entering the water, check the depth. Most neck and back injuries result from diving into water that is too shallow.
- Never swim in a river with currents too swift for easy, relaxed swimming.
- Never swim in muddy or dirty water that obstructs your view of the bottom. Water that is discolored and choppy or foamy may indicate a rip current.
- If you are caught in a rip current, swim parallel to the shore. Once you are free of the current, swim toward the shore.
- Learn cardiopulmonary resuscitation (CPR). In the event of an emergency, in the time it might take for paramedics to arrive, your CPR skills could make a difference

in someone's life. CPR performed by bystanders has been shown to improve outcomes in drowning victims.[36]

Boating In 2010, the U.S. Coast Guard received reports of 3,153 injured boaters and 672 deaths.[37] About 70 percent of boating fatalities are drownings, and among those who drown, 9 out of 10 are not wearing a **personal flotation device**—that is, a lifejacket. Other boating fatalities are due to trauma, hypothermia, carbon monoxide poisoning, and other causes.[38]

Alcohol sharply raises the death risk for boaters: About one third of all boating fatalities involve alcohol. In fact, the effects of alcohol can be more pronounced during boating than they are during driving. This is due to boat and engine noise, vibration, wind, sun, glare, temperature, and wave action. When boat operators are drinking, both collisions with other boats and falls overboard are much more likely. If someone who has been drinking does fall overboard, he or she is more likely to drown or to die of hypothermia. Unfortunately, the "designated driver" concept does not apply to boating because intoxicated passengers often cause or directly contribute to boating accidents. The U.S. Coast Guard and every state have

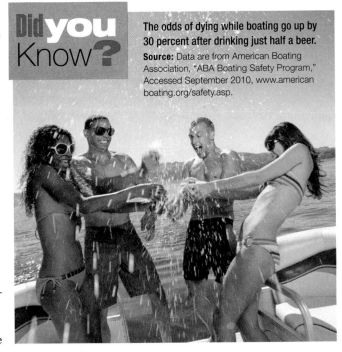

Did you Know?

The odds of dying while boating go up by 30 percent after drinking just half a beer.

Source: Data are from American Boating Association, "ABA Boating Safety Program," Accessed September 2010, www.americanboating.org/safety.asp.

"Boating Under the Influence" (BUI) laws that carry stringent penalties for violation, including fines, license revocation, and even jail time.[39]

The following boating safety tips are from the American Boating Association:[40]

- Share your plans for your outing. Before leaving home, let others know where you are going, who will be with you, and when you expect to return.
- Check the weather. Listen to boating advisories regarding high winds, storms, and other environmental factors.
- Make sure your boat is seaworthy. Even if you are just going for a short trip, make sure the vessel doesn't leak, has enough fuel (if powered), and has the proper safety equipment.
- Make sure you have enough life jackets for all who are on board and that they are easily accessible.
- Carry an emergency radio and cell phone.
- Don't drink alcohol before you leave, and don't bring any aboard.

In addition, the U.S. Coast Guard recommends that before setting out, you put on your life jacket. Most modern life jackets are thin and flexible and can be worn comfortably all day. Children must wear a life jacket once the vessel is under way, unless they are below deck. Even if you and your companions decide not to put on life jackets initially, a life jacket must be immediately available for every person aboard. Bear in mind that you need to wear a life jacket not only when sailing or motorboating, but also when canoeing, kayaking, and rafting!

Have Fun with Fireworks—Safely

It's the Fourth of July, and you're celebrating with friends and family. Your cousin has fished out of his basement a box of old fireworks and invites you to help him shoot them off. Should you do it? Each year, fireworks cause an estimated 7,000 injuries in the United States, often the loss of fingers or hands. And using improperly stored fireworks is a risk factor. Here are some safety tips for fireworks use from the National Council on Fireworks Safety:[41]

- Only use fireworks outdoors in an open area, at least 50 feet from spectators, buildings, dry grasses, and the like.
- Have plenty of water handy—either a hose or a bucket.
- When lighting fireworks, crouch down and reach out. Never bend over them. Don't hold onto them or throw them: Light the fuse and step away.
- Use only commercial fireworks, never homemade ones: They can kill you.
- Never tamper with fireworks, for example, trying to combine the powders. Use them only as intended.
- Never try to relight a "dud" firework. It could explode in your hand. Set it aside for 20 minutes, then soak it in a bucket of water.
- Alcohol and fireworks don't mix. Anyone who has been drinking should keep away from fireworks.

Before using any type of fireworks, check your state laws. You can find a state-by-state directory of fireworks-related laws at www.fireworksafety.com.

How Can You Avoid Injuries at Home?

Injuries within the home typically occur in the form of poisonings, falls, or burns. Some populations, such as the elderly, are particularly vulnerable. However, older adults are not the only victims; each year, hundreds of young adults, teens, and children are brought to hospital emergency rooms for treatment of home-based injuries.

Prevent Poisoning

A **poison** is any substance that is harmful to your body when ingested, inhaled, injected, or absorbed through the skin. Any substance can be poisonous if too much is taken. On an average day in the United States, 87 people die as a result of unintentional poisoning.[42] This makes poisonings second only to MVAs as a cause of unintentional injury deaths. Moreover, in 2010, over 830,000 people were treated in emergency departments for unintentional poisoning.

Tips to Prevent Poisonings
The safety tips below were adapted from the American Association of Poison Control Centers:

- Read and follow all usage and warning labels before taking medications or working with chemicals, including household products.
- Never share or sell your prescription drugs.
- Never mix household products together, as combinations of products can give off toxic fumes.
- When working with chemicals, wear a protective mask and make sure the area in which you are working is well ventilated. Wear gloves and other protective clothing if there is any possibility of skin contact, and eyeglasses or an eye guard if splashing could occur.
- Be especially careful with medications, dietary supplements, and alcohol around children. Keep such items out of sight, preferably in a locked cabinet, and never refer to medication as "candy."
- Program the national poison control number, 1-800-222-1222, into your cell phone. The line is open 24 hours a day, 7 days a week.

What to Do in Case of Poisoning
If you suspect you have ingested or inhaled a poison, or you are with someone who has collapsed, dial 9-1-1. If you are with someone who is not breathing and you are trained in CPR, provide CPR until paramedics arrive. If the victim is awake and alert, dial the poison control hot line (1-800-222-1222). Follow the instructions you are given: If you are told to take the person to a hospital emergency room, bring along the suspected poison, if possible.

---

poison Any substance harmful to the body when ingested, inhaled, injected, or absorbed through the skin.

Avoid Falls

Falls are the third most common cause of death from unintentional injury, and a very common source of injury in the home. About 20 to 30 percent of people who fall suffer moderate to severe injury such as bruises, a fracture, a dislocation, or a head injury. In fact, falls are the most common cause of traumatic brain injury.[43] Although falls are most common among older adults, people of all ages experience them, and many are preventable.

Observe the following measures to reduce your risk of falls:

- Leave nothing lying around on the floor and nothing on the stairs.
- Avoid using small scatter rugs and mats, which can slide out from under your feet. Use rubberized liners or strips to secure large rugs to the floor.
- Train your pets to stay away from your feet.
- Install slip-proof mats, treads, or decals in showers and tubs and on the stairs.
- If you need to reach something in a high cupboard or closet, or to change a ceiling light, use an appropriate step stool or short ladder. Don't try to balance on a ledge or on any piece of furniture not designed to bear and balance body weight.
- When using a ladder, make sure it's stable before climbing.
- Wear supportive shoes. Flip-flops and shoes without laces can trip you up.

Reduce Your Risk of Fire

In 2010, more than 2,600 Americans—not including firefighters—died in a fire.[44] On an average day, nine college campuses in the United States will experience a fire in a residential structure. The three main causes of fires in campus housing are cooking, careless smoking, and arson. However, a variety of other factors typically contribute to injuries from dormitory fires:[45]

1. **Alcohol is often a key factor.** In more than 50 percent of fire fatalities, victims were intoxicated at the time of the fire.

2. **Student apathy.** Many students do not believe that fire is a risk to them and ignore both fire drills and actual fire alarms.

3. **Lack of preparation.** Building evacuations are delayed because of inadequate fire drills, inability to recall exit routes, and so on.

4. **Failure of early detection.** Smoke alarms and fire alarm systems have not been maintained in working order or have been vandalized and not repaired.

5. **Delayed response.** Students fail to properly notify the fire department using the 9-1-1 system.

Fire Prevention Tips to prevent fires include the following:

- Extinguish all cigarettes in ashtrays before bed, and never smoke in bed!
- Set lamps away from drapes, linens, and paper.
- In the kitchen, keep hot pads and kitchen cloths away from stove burners, avoid reaching over hot pans. Use caution when lighting barbecue grills.
- Keep candles under control and away from combustibles. Never leave candles unattended or burning while you sleep.
- Avoid overloading electrical circuits with appliances and cords. Older buildings are at particular risk for fire from such overloads.
- Have the proper fire extinguishers ready in case of fire, and replace batteries in smoke alarms and test them periodically.

What to Do in a Fire If a fire breaks out in your dorm or apartment, your priority is to get out. Don't take time to phone before leaving. Don't gather up your stuff. First, feel the door handle: If it's hot, don't open the door! Go to a window, open it as fully as possible, and call for help. Hang a sheet from the window to let rescuers know where you are. If no one is outside,

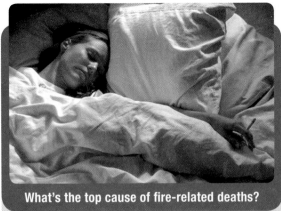

What's the top cause of fire-related deaths?

Smoking is the number one cause of fire-related deaths. If you fall asleep with a lit cigarette, bedding and clothing can quickly ignite. If you can't quit, take it outside.

call 9-1-1. If smoke is entering your room, seal the cracks in the door with blankets or towels. Then stay low until you're rescued—there is less smoke close to the floor.

If the door handle is not hot, open the door cautiously. If the hallway is clear to the exit, get out, yelling, "Fire!" and knocking on doors as you leave. If you encounter smoke, stay low to the floor—crawl if necessary—to make your way out. If you pass a fire alarm on your way out, pull it. Always use the stairs, never an elevator. Once you're outside, dial 9-1-1.

The same tips apply when you're staying in a hotel or motel. Always bring a flashlight with you when traveling, and study the evacuation plan posted in your room. Before going to bed, locate the two exits nearest your room and the fire alarms on your floor.

Learn First Aid and CPR

If you were to encounter someone who is injured, would you offer assistance? Many bystanders don't because they lack training and are afraid their efforts will do more harm than good. However, one simple action can help any injury victim: Dial 9-1-1. As soon as your call is answered, describe the situation, then follow the advice you're given. (First aid measures are provided in **Appendix B,** "Providing Emergency Care.")

If you witness someone who has collapsed and you cannot detect a pulse, the American Heart Association advises that you call 9-1-1 and then begin chest compressions.[46] This technique simply requires you to push down in the middle of the victim's chest hard and fast (about 100 compressions per minute). Traditional **cardiopulmonary resuscitation (CPR)**, which includes mouth-to-mouth resuscitation as well as chest compression, is preferable for victims of near-drowning and other forms of respiratory collapse. Everyone is encouraged to get training in CPR, and the course is offered on most college campuses.

Limit Your Exposure to Loud Noise

Our modern society is too often filled with excessive noise. Take a look at **Figure 2**, which shows the decibel (dB) levels of various common sounds. In general, noise levels above 85 dB (about as loud as a diesel truck) increase risks for hearing loss. When you consider the many such noises people are exposed to every day, it should be no surprise that hearing loss is becoming increasingly common. In fact, more than 36 million U.S. adults have hearing loss. Although you might think hearing loss is only a problem for the very old, 26 million Americans between the ages of 20 and 69 have hearing loss due to exposure to loud sounds either at

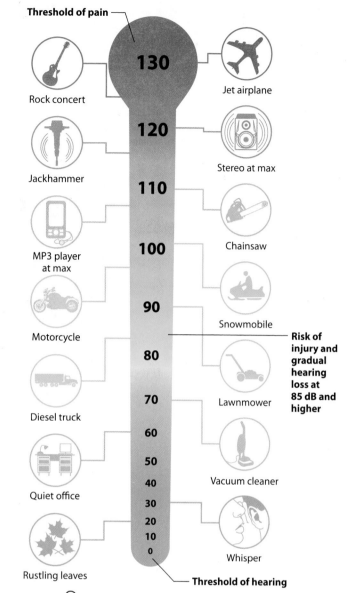

Threshold of pain

130 — Rock concert / Jet airplane

120 — Jackhammer / Stereo at max

110 — /

100 — MP3 player at max / Chainsaw

90 — Motorcycle / Snowmobile

80 — / Lawnmower

70 — Diesel truck /

60 — /

50 — / Vacuum cleaner

40 — Quiet office /

30 — /

20 — /

10 — / Whisper

0 — Rustling leaves

Threshold of hearing

Risk of injury and gradual hearing loss at 85 dB and higher

FIGURE 2 **Noise Levels of Various Sounds (dB)**
Decibels increase logarithmically, so each increase of 10 db represents a tenfold increase in loudness.

Source: Adapted from National Institute on Deafness and Other Communication Disorders, "How Loud Is Too Loud? Bookmark," Updated June 2010, www.nidcd .nih.gov/health/hearing/ruler.asp.

work or in leisure activities.[47] In fact, according to the Bureau of Labor Statistics, occupational hearing loss is the most commonly recorded occupational illness in manufacturing, accounting for 1 in 9 reportable illnesses.[48] These numbers may be just the tip of the iceberg, as a person's hearing loss must be determined to be work-related and severe enough to cause hearing impairment in order to be recordable by the Occu-

pational Safety and Health Administration (OSHA). Many more workers are likely to have measurable occupational hearing loss, though they have not yet become hearing impaired.

Noise-induced hearing loss results when exposure to high-decibel noise,

cardiopulmonary resuscitation (CPR) Emergency technique to provide lifesaving chest compression and mouth-to-mouth resuscitation when an individual has stopped breathing and has no pulse.

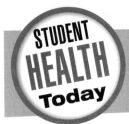

TURNING DOWN THE TUNES

Increasingly, children and young adults experience hearing loss due to use of portable music devices such as MP3 players. High frequency, duration of use. and high volume all make hearing loss a high-risk side effect when using earphones. Any sound above 90 decibels (dB) can cause hearing loss if the exposure is prolonged, and many people listen to music at volumes higher than this throughout the day, every day.

What can you do to avoid hearing loss while still enjoying your music? The most important step is to keep the volume at or below 80 dB—or at a level at which you can still comfortably carry on a conversation. If you do that, you won't need to limit

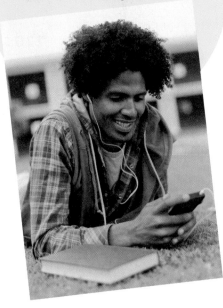

Hearing loss is becoming more frequent as music lovers increase the frequency, duration, and volume of their listening time.

the amount of time you spend listening to music. Another way to tell if your volume is set too loud is to ask people nearby if they can hear your music. If they can, it's definitely too loud. Finally, debate continues over the relative safety of over-the-ear earphones versus in-the-ear ear buds; however, experts agree that earphones are probably safer.

Sources: American Academy of Audiology, "turn it to the left!", 2011, www.turnittotheleft.com/news/keymessagesandfacts.htm; H. Keppler et al., "Short-Term Auditory Effects of Listening to an MP3 Player," *Archives of Otolaryngology—Head & Neck Surgery* 136, no. 6 (2010): 538–48.

usually over extended periods of time, damages sensory receptors in the cochlea, or inner ear. Hearing loss can be temporary or permanent, and in general worsens with age. One of the highest rates of sudden noise-induced hearing loss is among adults age 20 to 29. A recent study of college students who reported having normal hearing revealed that, when tested, 12 percent showed at least moderate hearing loss.[49] The study authors identified a correlation between use of a personal music player and increased risk for hearing loss. Several other studies have also linked hearing loss in young adults to the use of portable listening devices. However, the precise decibel level, frequency, and duration of exposure that might correlate with hearing loss is currently under investigation.[50] Check out the **Student Health Today** box for more details and tips for protecting your hearing while enjoying your tunes.

Another source of hearing impairment is frequent concert attendance. Most rock musicians use earplugs when performing or rehearsing, and their audiences would be wise to do the same. Hearing loss may result from one evening in front of huge speakers at a rock concert. If you can't hear the person standing next to you at a concert, then you should put in earplugs or look for a quieter spot. In addition, you should rest your ears between nights out partying or attending concerts or loud sporting events.

How Can You Avoid Injury While Working?

American adults spend most of their waking hours on the job. Although most job situations are pleasant and

productive, others pose hazards. Over 4,500 fatal work injuries occurred in the United States in 2010. Transportation incidents made up the largest number of fatal work injuries (nearly 40%). In addition, workers in material moving, construction, and extraction (mining) and those in the service industry are at high risk of fatal injuries. Farmers, fishing workers, and loggers are also at high risk.[51]

Although on-the-job deaths capture media attention, workers may also be seriously injured or disabled at their jobs. Common work injuries include cuts and lacerations, chemical burns, fractures, sprains and strains (often of the back), and repetitive motion disorders. Because so many work injuries are due to overexertion, poor body mechanics, or repetitive motion, they are largely preventable. We discuss these problems and share some prevention strategies here.

Protect Your Back

Low back pain (LBP), usually as a result of injury, is epidemic throughout the world and is the major cause of disability for people age 20 to 45 in the United States, who suffer more frequently and severely from this problem than older people do.[52] It is one of the most commonly experienced chronic ailments among college students. In a recent survey, nearly 13 percent of college students reported having seen their doctor in the previous year because of back pain.[53]

Because most injuries to the back are in the lumbar spine area (lower back), strengthening core muscle groups and stretching muscles to avoid cramping and spasms are key strategies to reduce risks. Frequently, sports injuries, stress on spinal bones and tissues, the sudden jolt of a car accident, or other obvious causes are the culprits. Other times, sitting too long in the same position or hunching over your computer while you're pulling an all-nighter can leave you with pain so severe that you can't stand up or walk comfortably. Carrying heavy backpacks between classes is another frequent source of LBP.

You can avoid typical risks by using common sense and thinking "safety" when engaging in activities that could injure your back. Getting up and stretching after long hours in a static position is another great strategy to avoid problems. Maintaining good posture can also reduce back problems.

Other measures you can take to reduce the risk of back pain include the following:

- Invest in a high-quality, supportive mattress.
- Avoid high-heeled shoes, which tilt the pelvis forward.
- Control your weight. Extra weight puts increased strain on your knees, hips, and back.
- Warm up and stretch before exercising or lifting heavy objects.
- When lifting something heavy, use your leg muscles and use proper form (Figure 3). Do not bend from the waist or take the weight load on your back.
- Buy a desk chair with good lumbar support.
- Move your car seat forward so your knees are elevated slightly.
- Engage in exercise regularly, particularly in core exercises that strengthen the abdominal muscles and stretch the back muscles.
- Downsize your backpack.

Maintain Alignment while Sitting

How many hours have you sat glued to a workstation, laptop, netbook, tablet computer, pocket computer, mobile device, or an ordinary book today? Were you slouching, hunched over, or sitting up straight? Your answers are probably reflected in the degree of aching and stiffness you may be feeling right now. So how can you maintain a healthy alignment while you sit and work? Try these strategies:

1. Sit comfortably with your feet flat on the floor or on a footrest, and your knees level with your hips. Raise or lower your chair, or move to a different chair, to achieve this position.

2. Your middle back should be firmly against the back of the chair. The small of your back should be supported, too. If you can't feel the chair back supporting your lumbar region, try placing a small cushion or even a rolled towel behind the curve of your lower back.

3. Keep your shoulders relaxed and straight, not rolled or hunched forward.

4. The angle of your elbows should be 90 degrees to your upper arms. Change your position or the position of your device to achieve this angle.

5. Ideally, you should be looking straight ahead, not peering down at the device's screen.

Avoid Repetitive Motion Disorders

It's the end of the term, and you have finished the last of several papers. After hours of nonstop typing, your hands are numb and you feel an intense, burning pain that makes the thought of typing one more word almost unbearable. If this happens, you may be suffering from one of several **repetitive motion disorders (RMDs)**, sometimes called *overuse syndrome, cumulative trauma disorders,* or *repetitive stress injuries.* These refer to a family of painful soft tissue injuries that begin with inflammation and gradually become disabling.

Repetitive motion disorders include carpal tunnel syndrome, bursitis, tendonitis, and ganglion cysts, among

repetitive motion disorder (RMD) An injury to soft tissue, tendons, muscles, nerves, or joints due to the physical stress of repeated motions.

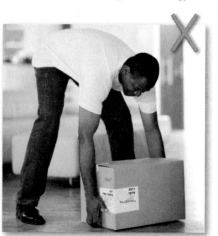

ⓐ Attempting to lift a heavy object by bending at your waist is a common cause of back injury.

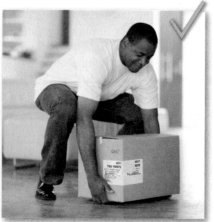

ⓑ Start as close to the object as possible, with it positioned between your knees as you squat down. Keep your feet parallel, or stagger one foot in front of the other. Keep the object close to your body as you stand, using your legs, not your back, to lift.

FIGURE 3 **Lifting a Heavy Object**

others.[54] Twisting of the arm or wrist, overexertion, and incorrect posture or position are usually contributors. The areas most likely to be affected are the hands, wrists, elbows, and shoulders, but the neck, back, hips, knees, feet, ankles, and legs can be affected, too. Over time, RMDs can cause permanent damage to nerves, soft tissue, and joints. Usually, RMDs are associated with repeating the same task in an occupational setting and gradually irritating the area in question. However, certain sports (tennis, golf, and others), gripping the wheel while driving, keyboarding or texting, and a number of newer technology-driven activities can also result in RMDs.

Because many of these injuries occur in everyday work, play, and athletics, they are often not reported to national agencies that keep track of injury statistics. Many people just pop over-the-counter pain remedies and continue working until the pain becomes unbearable. Nevertheless, reports of increasing numbers of cases of disorders like "BlackBerry thumb," carpal tunnel syndrome, and other maladies are widespread.

25%

of all emergency room hospital visits could be avoided if people knew basic first aid and CPR.

One of the most common RMDs is **carpal tunnel syndrome (CTS)**, an

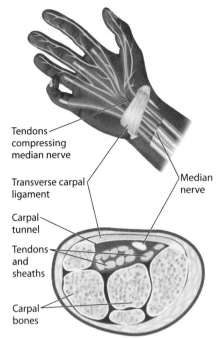

Tendons compressing median nerve

Transverse carpal ligament

Median nerve

Carpal tunnel

Tendons and sheaths

Carpal bones

Cross-section through wrist

FIGURE 4 Carpal Tunnel Syndrome
The carpal tunnel is a space beneath the transverse carpal ligament and above the carpal bones of the wrist. The median nerve and the tendons that allow you to flex your fingers run through this tunnel. Carpal tunnel syndrome occurs when repetitive use prompts inflammation of the tissues and fluids of the tunnel. This in turn compresses the median nerve.

inflammation of the soft tissues within the "tunnel" through the carpal bones of the wrist (Figure 4). This puts pressure on the median nerve, which runs down the forearm through the tunnel to innervate the hand. Symptoms include numbness, tingling, and pain in the fingers and hands. Carpal tunnel syndrome typically results from spending hours typing at the computer keyboard, flipping groceries through computerized scanners, or manipulating other objects in jobs "made simpler" by technology. The risk for CTS can be reduced by proper design of workstations, protective

wrist pads, and worker training. Physical and occupational therapy is an important part of treatment and recovery.

Are You Prepared for Environmental Events?

A **natural disaster** is any extreme environmental event that causes widespread destruction of land and/or property, injuries, and sometimes deaths. Some, such as hurricanes and volcanic eruptions, may be predictable, whereas others, like earthquakes and many tornadoes, can occur without warning. If a natural disaster were to strike without warning in your region, would you be prepared?

The first step in preparedness is to learn what types of natural disasters typically affect the area where you live. If you've relocated from New England to the Midwest to attend school, for example, you may want to learn about tornado preparedness. If you attend school in the Southeast, hurricanes would also be a key concern. To learn more about specific types of disasters, log on to the Centers for Disease Control and Prevention (CDC) website at www .cdc.gov and search the event name. For instance, the CDC's hurricane page provides key facts; basic steps to prepare yourself, your residence, and even your pets; a list of emergency supplies you'd need; information on how to evacuate safely; and steps to take to get through the storm safely if you're ordered *not* to evacuate. You can always find advisories and other information about weather-related events in your area—from blizzards to gales to flash floods—by visiting the National Weather Service website at www.weather.gov.

Are You at Risk for a Motor Vehicle Accident?

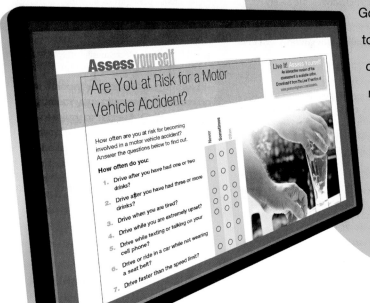

Go online to www.pearsonhighered.com/donatelle to fill out the "Are You at Risk for a Motor Vehicle Accident?" assessment.* If you need to make some changes, follow the strategies outlined in the **YOUR PLAN FOR CHANGE** box.

*If your instructor so chooses, Assess Yourself Activities are available as a printed supplement or as assignable homework online at www.pearsonhighered.com/myhealth.

MyHealthLab®

YOUR PLAN FOR CHANGE

The **Assess** yourself activity helped you identify the ways you take risks on the road. Depending on your responses, you might choose to make some of the following changes.

Today, you can:
○ Fasten your seat belt before you turn the ignition key, and ask everyone in your vehicle to do the same.

○ Commit to turning off your cell phone and other handheld devices before you drive.

○ Drive within the posted speed limit.

Within the next 2 weeks, you can:
○ Offer to be the designated driver the next time you go out with friends.

○ Get 7 to 8 hours of sleep before setting out on a long drive.

By the end of the semester, you can:
○ Bring your car in for a tune-up, and have the mechanic check that the seat belts and air bags are functioning properly.

References

1. S. L. Murphy, J. Q. Xu, and K. D. Kochanek, "Deaths: Preliminary Data for 2010," *National Vital Statistics Reports* 60, no. 4 (2012), www.cdc.gov/nchs/data/nvsr/nvsr60/nvsr60_04.pdf.
2. S. L. Murphy, J. Q. Xu, and K. D. Kochanek, "Deaths: Preliminary Data for 2010," 2012.
3. National Safety Council, "Safety at Home," 2012, www.nsc.org/safety_home/Pages/safety_at_hom.aspx.
4. National Safety Council, "Defensive Driving," 2010, www.nsc.org/safety_road/DefensiveDriving/Pages/defensive_driving.aspx.
5. S. L. Murphy, J. Q. Xu, and K. D. Kochanek, "Deaths: Preliminary Data for 2010," 2012.
6. National Safety Council, "Driver Safety," 2010, www.nsc.org/safety_road/DriverSafety/Pages/driver_safety.aspx.
7. Governors Highway Safety Association, *Distracted Driving: What Research Shows and What States Can Do*, Executive Summary, 2011, www.ghsa.org/html/publications/pdf/sfdist11execsum.pdf.
8. National Safety Council, "Distracted Driving: Research and Statistics," 2012, www.nsc.org/safety_road/Distracted_Driving/Pages/DistractedDrivingResearchandStatistics.aspx.
9. U.S. Centers for Disease Control and Prevention, "Distracted Driving," 2011, www.cdc.gov/Motorvehiclesafety/Distracted_Driving/.
10. National Safety Council, "Distracted Driving: Research and Statistics," 2012.
11. Governors Highway Safety Association, "Cell Phone and Texting Laws," Updated April 2012, www.ghsa.org/html/stateinfo/laws/cellphone_laws.html.
12. Centers for Disease Control and Prevention, "Parents Are the Key: Eight Danger Zones," Updated October 2009, www.cdc.gov/parentsarethekey/danger/index.html.
13. National Highway Traffic Safety Administration, *Traffic Safety Facts 2010 Motor Vehicle Crashes: Overview* (Washington, DC: NHTSA's National Center for Statistics and Analysis, February, 2012), DOT HS 811 552, www-nrd.nhtsa.dot.gov/Pubs/811552.pdf.
14. National Highway Traffic Safety Administration, *Traffic Safety Facts 2009 Data: Alcohol-Impaired Driving* (Washington, DC: NHTSA's National Center for Statistics and Analysis, 2010), DOT HS 811 385, www-nrd.nhtsa.dot.gov/Pubs/811385.pdf.
15. National Institute on Drug Abuse, "NIDA InfoFacts: Drugged Driving," Revised December 2010, http://drugabuse.gov/infofacts/driving.html.
16. Ibid.
17. National Highway Traffic Safety Administration, "Traffic Safety Facts: Drowsy Driving," 2011, DOT HS 811 449, www-nrd.nhtsa.dot.gov/Pubs/811449.pdf.
18. National Safety Council, "Speeding," 2010, www.nsc.org/safety_road/DriverSafety/Pages/speeding.aspx.
19. Centers for Disease Control and Prevention, "Policy Impact: Seat Belts," Updated January, 2012, www.cdc.gov/Motorvehiclesafety/seatbeltbrief.
20. Ibid.
21. Insurance Institute for Highway Safety, "New Crash Tests Demonstrate the Influence of Vehicle Size and Weight on Safety in Crashes; Results Are Relevant to Fuel Economy Policies," April 2009, www.iihs.org/news/rss/pr041409.html.
22. National Highway Traffic Safety Administration, *Traffic Safety Facts 2009 Data: Motorcycles* (Washington, DC: NHTSA's National Center for Statistics and Analysis, 2011), DOT HS 811 389, www-nrd.nhtsa.dot.gov/Pubs/811389.pdf.
23. Ibid.
24. Centers for Disease Control and Prevention, "Parents Are the Key," 2009.
25. A. Williams and R. Shults, "Graduated Driver Licensing Research, 2007–Present: A Review and Commentary," *Journal of Safety Research* 41, no. 2 (2010): 77–84.
26. National Safety Council, "Graduated Driver Licensing," 2010, www.nsc.org/safety_road/TeenDriving/GDL/Pages/GraduatedDriverLicensing.aspx.
27. National Highway Traffic Safety Administration, *Traffic Safety Facts 2009 Data: Bicyclists and Other Cyclists* (Washington, DC: NHTSA's National Center for Statistics and Analysis, 2011), DOT HS 811 386, www.nrd.nhtsa.dot.gov/cats/listpublications.aspx?Id=A&ShowBy=DocType.
28. Ibid.
29. American College Health Association, *American College Health Association—National College Health Assessment (ACHA-NCHA): Reference Group Executive Summary Fall 2011*, (Baltimore: American College Health Association, 2011), www.achancha.org/docs/ACHA-NCHA_Reference_Group_ExecutiveSummary_Fall2011.pdf.
30. Consumer Product Safety Commission, "Fact Sheet: Skateboards," 2009, www.cpsc.gov/cpscpub/pubs/rec_sfy.html.
31. Consumer Product Safety Commission. "CPSC Fact Sheet: Skateboarding Safety," December 2011, www.cpsc.gov/CPSCPUB/PUBS/093.pdf.
32. National Ski Areas Association, "Facts about Skiing/Snowboarding Safety," Updated November 2010, www.nsaa.org/nsaa/press/facts-ski-snbd-safety.asp.
33. Centers for Disease Control and Prevention, "Unintentional Drowning: Fact Sheet," May 2011, www.cdc.gov/HomeandRecreationalSafety/Water-Safety/waterinjuries-factsheet.html.
34. Ibid.
35. American Red Cross, "Summer Water Safety Guide," March 2009, http://american.redcross.org/site/DocServer/watersafety0609.pdf?docID=735.
36. Centers for Disease Control and Prevention, "Unintentional Drowning," 2011.
37. U. S. Coast Guard, "Coast Guard News: Recreational Boating Fatalities Reach Record Low," June 2011, http://coastguardnews.com/recreational-boating-fatalities-reach-record-low/2011/06/15/.
38. Centers for Disease Control and Prevention, "Unintentional Drowning," 2011.
39. U. S. Coast Guard, "Boating Safety Resource Center: Boating Under the Influence Initiatives," October 2011, www.uscgboating.org/safety/boating_under_the_influence_initiatives.aspx.
40. American Boating Association, "Boating Safety—It Could Mean Your Life," 2010, www.americanboating.org/safety.asp.
41. National Council on Fireworks Safety, "Key Fireworks Safety Information," 2010, www.fireworksafety.com.
42. Centers for Disease Control and Prevention, "Poisoning in the United States: Fact Sheet," 2010, www.cdc.gov/HomeandRecreationalSafety/Poisoning/poisoning-factsheet.htm.
43. Centers for Disease Control and Prevention, "Falls Among Older Adults: An Overview," September 2011, www.cdc.gov/HomeandRecreationalSafety/Falls/adultfalls.html.
44. Centers for Disease Control and Prevention, "Fire Deaths and Injuries: Fact Sheet," October 2011, www.cdc.gov/HomeandRecreationalSafety/Fire-Prevention/fires-factsheet.html.
45. U.S. Fire Administration, "Fire Safety 101: Colleges and Universities," 2006, www.usfa.fema.gov/citizens/college/101.shtm.
46. American Heart Association, "Hands-Only CPR," February 2011, http://handsonlycpr.org/.
47. National Institute on Deafness and Other Communication Disorders, "Quick Statistics," 2010, www.nidcd.nih.gov/health/statistics/quick.htm.
48. National Institute for Occupational Safety and Health, "Occupationally Induced Hearing Loss," 2010, www.cdc.gov/niosh/docs/2010-136.

49. C. G. LePrell, et al., "Evidence of Hearing Loss in a 'Normally-Hearing' College Student Population," *International Journal of Audiology* 50, Suppl 1 (2011): S21-1.

50. F. Zhao, V. K. Manchalah, D. French, and S. M. Price, "Music Exposure and Hearing Disorders: An Overview," *International Journal of Audiology* 49, no. 1 (2010): 54–64.

51. U.S. Bureau of Labor Statistics, "Census of Fatal Occupational Injuries Summary, 2010," August 2011, www.bls.gov/news .release/cfoi.nr0.htm.

52. National Institute of Neurological Disorders and Stroke, "Low Back Pain Fact Sheet," June 2010, www.ninds.nih.gov/ disorders/backpain/detail_backpain .htm.

53. American College Health Association, *ACHA-NCHA Reference Group Executive Summary Fall 2011*, 2011.

54. National Institute of Neurological Disorders and Stroke, "NINDS Repetitive Motion Disorders Information Page," October, 2011, www.ninds.nih.gov/ disorders/repetitive_motion/ repetitive_motion.htm.

20 Preserving and Protecting Your Environment

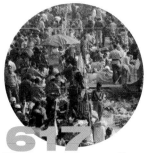

617

Why is population growth an environmental issue?

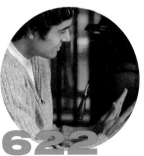

622

How can air pollution be a problem indoors?

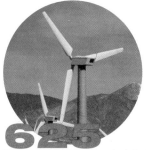

625

How can I help prevent global warming?

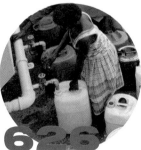

626

How large a concern is water scarcity?

OBJECTIVES

✳ Explain the environmental impact associated with global population growth.

✳ Describe major causes of air pollution and the consequences of greenhouse gas accumulation and ozone depletion.

✳ Identify sources of pollution and chemical contaminants often found in water.

✳ Distinguish municipal solid waste from hazardous waste and list strategies for reducing land pollution.

✳ Discuss the health concerns associated with ionizing and nonionizing radiation.

✳ Describe the physiological consequences of noise pollution and how to prevent or reduce its effects.

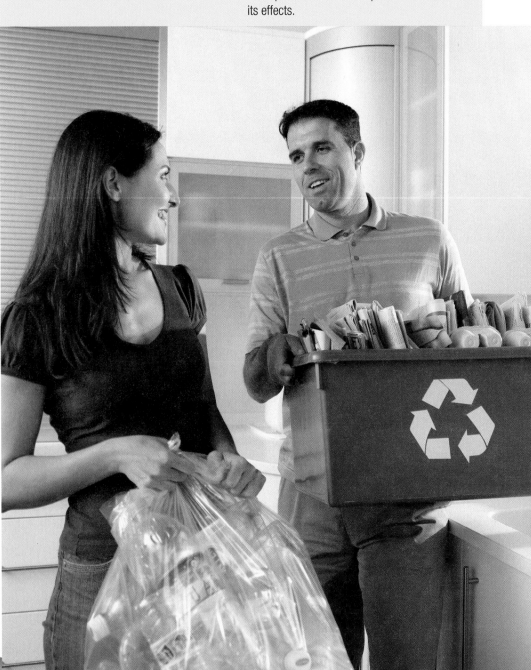

The threat from climate change is serious, it is urgent, and it is growing. Our generation's response to this challenge will be judged by history, for if we fail to meet it—boldly, swiftly, and together—we risk consigning future generations to an irreversible catastrophe.
—*President Barack Obama, United Nations Summit on Climate Change, September 22, 2009*

We live in an especially dangerous time. The global population has grown more in the past 50 years than at any other time in human history. More people pose a potentially devastating threat to the water we drink, the air we breathe, the food we eat, and our capacity to survive. Polar ice caps and glaciers are melting at rates that surpass even the most dire predictions of a decade ago, and threats of rising sea levels loom large. One in four species of mammals in the world is now threatened with extinction as humans destroy habitat, exacerbate drought and flooding through climate change, and pollute the environment. Clean water is becoming scarce, fossil fuels are being depleted, and the amount of solid and hazardous waste is growing.

This chapter provides an overview of the factors contributing to the global environmental crisis. It also provides a blueprint for action—by individuals, communities, policymakers, and governments. Staying informed and becoming involved in the process are key things you can do to help.

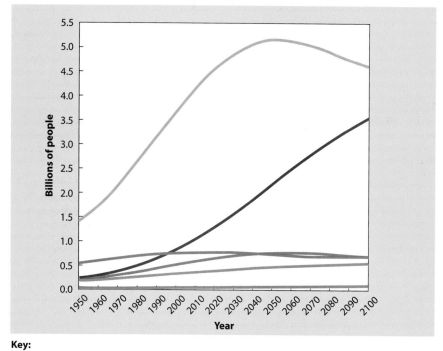

Key:
- Asia
- Africa
- Latin America and the Caribbean
- Europe
- Northern America
- Oceania

FIGURE 20.1 **Projected World Population Growth, 1950–2100**

Source: United Nations, Department of Economic and Social Affairs, Population Division. World Population Prospects: The 2010 Revision. http://esa.un.org © 2011. Reprinted by permission.

The Threat of Overpopulation

As anthropologist Margaret Mead put it, "Every human society is faced with not one population problem but two: how to beget and rear enough children and how not to beget and rear too many." The United Nations projects that the world population will grow from its current 7 billion in 2012 to 9.3 billion by 2050 and to 10.1 billion by 2100.[1] Newer reports increase the population growth in 2050 to over 10.5 billion, indicating that recent increases in fertility rates in the United States and Europe will increase all previous estimates.[2] (See Figure 20.1.) Population experts believe that slowing world population growth is the most critical environmental challenge today.[3]

Measuring the Impact of People

While many people question *when* we will reach the "tipping point" at which we will be unable to restore the balance between humans and nature, others argue that it may already be too late. The global demand for natural resources has doubled since 1996. It now takes 1.5 years to regenerate the renewable resources used in 1 year by humans. By 2030, one report indicates that it will take the equivalent of two planets to meet the demand for resources. Simply put, we are running out of the natural resources necessary to sustain us, and the problem is growing at an unprecedented rate.[4] In addition, our impact on other aspects of life on Earth is evident in many areas. For example, consider the following:

● **Impact on other species.** Changes in the **ecosystem** are resulting in extinctions. Twelve percent of all birds are threatened, with seabirds taking the greatest hit (over 38% are threatened). More than 100 species of mammals are already extinct, with others, such as tigers, already having populations decline by 95 percent in the last century. About a third of amphibians (frogs, toads, and salamanders) are already gone, and many of those that survive have chemically induced ailments or genetic mutations that will hasten their demise. Along with mammals, rapid declines in plant species are reasons for concern.[5]

● **Impact on the food supply.** We are currently fishing the oceans at rates that are 250 percent more than they can regenerate, and scientists project a global collapse of all fish species by 2050.[6]

Aquatic ecosystems continue to be heavily contaminated by chemical and human waste. Drought and erosion and natural disasters make growing food increasingly difficult, and food shortages and famine are occurring in many regions of the world with increasing frequency.

● **Land degradation and contamination of drinking water.** The per capita availability of freshwater is declining rapidly, and contaminated water remains the greatest single environmental cause of human illness. Unsustainable land use and climate change are increasing land degradation, including erosion, nutrient depletion, deforestation, and other problems that will inevitably affect human life.

● **Energy consumption.** "Use it *and* lose it" is an apt saying for our use of nonrenewable energy sources in the form of **fossil fuels** (oil, coal, natural gas). Although we are seeing a shift toward renewable energy sources, such as hydropower, solar and wind power, and biomass power, the predominant energy sources are still fossil fuels. Currently, the United States is the largest consumer of liquid fossil fuels, the largest consumer of natural gas, and among the top three to four consumers of nuclear power, coal, and hydroelectric power.[7] In many developing regions of the world, demand for fossil fuels is growing at unprecedented rates. (See **Figure 20.2**.)

Factors That Affect Population Growth A number of factors have led to the world population's increase. Key among them are changes in fertility and mortality rates.

Fertility rate refers to the average number of births per woman in a specific country or region. Today, the U.S. fertility rate is just over 2 births per woman, compared to nearly 3.5 births per woman during the baby boom years following World War II.[8] In India and in many Asian, Latin American, and African countries,

ecosystem Collection of physical (nonliving) and biological (living) components of an environment and the relationships between them.

fossil fuels Carbon-based material used for energy; includes oil, coal, and natural gas.

fertility rate Average number of births a female in a certain population has during her reproductive years.

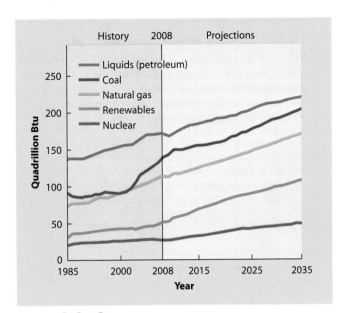

FIGURE 20.2 World Energy Consumption by Fuel, 1990–2035 (Quadrillion Btu)
Liquid fuels include petroleum. The last year with real data is 2008; years thereafter projected estimates.

Source: U.S. Energy Information Administration, *International Energy Outlook 2011*, Figure 2, Page 2, Available at http://205.254.135.7/forecasts/ieo/pdf/0484(2011).pdf.

birth rates can range from 5 to nearly 8 per woman, which leads to rapid population increases in many poorer nations (see **Table 20.1**).[9] In countries where women have little say over reproductive choices and where birth control is either not

TABLE 20.1 Selected Total Fertility Rates Worldwide, 2012

Country	Number of Children Born per Woman*	Rank
Niger	7.5	1
Uganda	6.65	2
Afghanistan	5.64	9
India	2.58	80
Mexico	2.27	98
Saudi Arabia	2.26	100
United States	2.06	122
Australia	1.77	159
Canada	1.59	176
China	1.55	180
Russia	1.43	195
Japan	1.39	203

*Indicates average number of children that would be born per woman if all women lived to the end of their childbearing years and bore children according to a given fertility rate at each age.

Source: "Total Fertility Rate (Children Born/Woman) 2012 Country Ranks, by Rank 2012." Data from *CIA World Fact Book*, www.photius.com/rankings/population/total_fertility_rate_2012_0.html.

available or frowned upon, pregnancy rates continue to rise. Mortality rates from chronic and infectious diseases have declined in both developed and developing regions as a result of improved public health infrastructure, increased availability of drugs and vaccines, better disaster preparedness, and other factors. Consequently, people are living longer and consuming more resources over the course of their lifetimes.

Differing Growth Rates

The country projected to have the largest increase in population in coming decades is India, which is expected to add another 600 million people by 2050, surpassing China as the most populous nation.[10] High infant mortality rates, the traditional view of children as "social security" (working to assist families in daily survival and supporting parents when they grow too old to work), the low educational and economic status of women, lack of reproductive choices, and a preference for sons, which keeps parents of girls trying for a boy, are all factors that favor large families in developing nations.

The population sizes in wealthier nations are static or declining, with one notable exception—the United States. With a population of over 314 million, the United States leads most other industrialized nations, with a growth rate of nearly 1 percent in 2012. Each day, the United States adds 8,000 people, or about 3 million people per year. It is also among the five countries of the world with the biggest "ecological footprint," exerting a greater impact on many of the planet's resources than any other nation.[11] Overall, we are among the leading users of fossil fuels and other energy sources, we are among the largest emitters of greenhouse gases, the largest forest-product consumers, and the generators of the most municipal solid waste per person.[12]

Zero Population Growth

Recognizing that population control will be essential in the decades ahead, many countries have already enacted strict population control measures or have encouraged their citizens to limit the size of their families. Proponents of *zero population growth (ZPG)* believe that each couple should produce only two offspring. When the parents die, these two children are their replacements, allowing the population to stabilize. Currently, there are over 20 countries in the world with zero or negative population growth, meaning that deaths surpass births or there are an equal number of births and deaths. Education may be the single biggest contributor to zero population growth. As education levels of women increase and women achieve equality in pay, job status, and social status, fertility rates decline. Also, as women gain choices in birth control, access to health care, and information about family planning, they tend to marry later and have fewer children.[13]

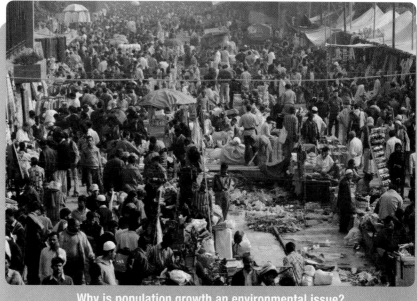

Why is population growth an environmental issue?

Every year the global population grows by 90 million, but Earth's resources are not expanding. Population increases are believed to be responsible for most of the current environmental stress.

"Why Should I Care?"

Imagine waking up in the morning to find you have no water for a shower, the electricity stops working throughout the day, gas stations have no fuel for sale, and basic necessities are either unavailable or unaffordable. Such scenarios are not science fiction. Major difficulties loom unless we take action to change our current rate of population growth and our consumption of natural resources and unless the global community acts to enforce policies to check rampant population growth.

what do you think?

Should individuals get tax breaks for having fewer children?
● How would such policies compare to our current policies?
● Can you think of other policies that might be effective in encouraging population control and resource conservation in the United States?

Air Pollution

The term *air pollution* refers to the presence, in varying degrees, of substances (suspended particles and vapors) not found in clean air.[14] From the beginning

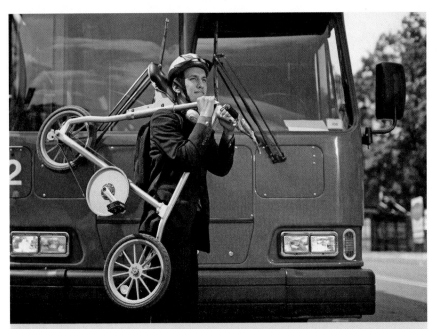

Reducing our individual carbon footprint is a key goal in combating air pollution, global warming, and climate change. Making small changes such as driving less, riding your bike more, taking public transportation or carpooling, turning off lights, recycling, and composting can all help to reduce your carbon footprint.

made. The act established standards for six of the most widespread air pollutants that seriously affect health: sulfur dioxide, particulates, carbon monoxide, nitrogen dioxide, ground-level ozone, and lead. Other common air pollutants include carbon dioxide and hydrocarbons. There have been major decreases in these six criteria pollutants, even as populations have increased in the United States. Today, however, ozone and particulate matter continue to be present at significant.[17] See Table 20.2 on page 619 for an overview of the sources and effects of these pollutants.

Photochemical Smog

Smog is a brownish haze produced by the photochemical reaction of sunlight with hydrocarbons, nitrogen compounds, and other gases in vehicle exhaust. It is sometimes called *ozone pollution* because ozone is a main component of smog. Smog tends to form in areas that experience a **temperature inversion**, in which a cool layer of air is trapped under a layer of warmer air, preventing the air from circulating. Smog is more likely to occur in valley areas surrounded by hills or mountains, such as Los Angeles. The most noticeable adverse effects of smog are difficulty breathing, burning eyes, headaches, and nausea. Long-term exposure poses serious health risks, particularly for children, older adults, pregnant women, and people with chronic respiratory disorders.

Air Quality Index The Air Quality Index (AQI) is a measure of how clean or polluted the air is on a given day if there are any health concerns related to air quality. The AQI focuses on health effects that can happen within a few hours or days after breathing polluted air.

The AQI scale is from 0 to 500: The higher the AQI value, the greater the level of air pollution and associated health risks. An AQI value of 100 generally corresponds to the national air quality standard for the pollutant, which is the level the EPA has set to protect public health. AQI values below 100 are generally considered satisfactory. When AQI values rise above 100, air quality is considered unhealthy at certain levels for specific groups of people and at higher levels for everyone. As shown in Figure 20.3 on the following page, the EPA has divided the AQI scale into six categories with corresponding color codes. National and local weather reports generally include information on the day's AQI.

of time, natural events, living creatures, and toxic by-products have been polluting the environment. As such, air pollution is not a new phenomenon. What is new is the vast array of **pollutants** that exist today and their potential interactive effects.

Air pollutants are either *naturally occurring* or *anthropogenic* (caused by humans). Naturally occurring air pollutants include particulate matter, such as ash from volcanic eruptions. Anthropogenic sources include those caused by *stationary sources* (e.g., power plants, factories, and refineries) and *mobile sources,* such as vehicles. Mobile sources are *on-road* vehicles (cars, trucks, and buses) or *off-road* sources (such as construction equipment). Planes, trains, and watercraft are considered *non-road* sources.[15] According to Environmental Protection Agency estimates, mobile sources are the major contributors of key air pollutants, such as carbon monoxide (CO), sulfur oxides (SO_x), and nitrogen oxides (NO_x). Motor vehicles alone contribute about 60 percent of all CO emissions, and non-road sources contribute another 22 percent.[16]

pollutant Substance that contaminates some aspect of the environment and causes potential harm to living organisms.

smog Brownish haze that is a form of pollution produced by the photochemical reaction of sunlight with hydrocarbons, nitrogen compounds, and other gases in vehicle exhaust.

temperature inversion Weather condition that occurs when a layer of cool air is trapped under a layer of warmer air.

acid deposition Acidification process that occurs when pollutants are deposited by precipitation, clouds, or directly on the land.

Components of Air Pollution

Concern about air quality prompted Congress to pass the *Clean Air Act* in 1970 and to amend it in 1977 and again in 1990. Since then, several minor amendments have been

Acid Deposition and Acid Rain

Acid deposition is replacing the term *acid rain* in scientific circles; it refers to the deposition of *wet* (rain, snow, sleet, fog, cloud water, and dew) and *dry* (acidifying particles and gases) acidic components that fall to the earth in dust or

20.2 Sources, Health Effects, and Environmental Impacts of Six Major Air Pollutants

Pollutant	Description	Sources	Health Effects	Welfare Effects
Carbon monoxide (CO)	Colorless, odorless gas	Motor vehicle exhaust; indoor sources include kerosene and wood-burning stoves	Headaches, reduced mental alertness, heart attack, cardiovascular diseases, impaired fetal development, death	Contributes to the formation of smog
Sulfur dioxide (SO_2)	Colorless gas that dissolves in water vapor to form acid and interacts with other gases and particles in the air	Coal-fired power plants, petroleum refineries, manufacture of sulfuric acid, and smelting of ores containing sulfur	Eye irritation, wheezing, chest tightness, shortness of breath, lung damage	Contributes to the formation of acid rain, visibility impairment, plant and water damage, aesthetic damage
Nitrogen dioxide (NO_2)	Reddish brown, highly reactive gas	Motor vehicles, electric utilities, and other industrial, commercial, and residential sources that burn fuels	Susceptibility to respiratory infections, irritation of the lungs and respiratory symptoms (e.g., cough, chest pain, difficulty breathing)	Contributes to the formation of smog, acid rain, water quality deterioration, global warming, and visibility impairment
Ozone (O_3)	Gaseous pollutant when formed in the stratosphere	Vehicle exhaust and certain other fumes; formed from other air pollutants in the presence of sunlight	Eye and throat irritation, coughing, respiratory tract problems, asthma, lung damage	Plant and ecosystem damage, global warming
Lead (Pb)	Metallic element	Metal refineries, lead smelters, battery manufacturers, iron and steel producers	Anemia, high blood pressure, brain and kidney damage, neurological disorders, cancer, lowered IQ	Affects animals, plants, and the aquatic ecosystem
Particulate matter (PM)	Very small particles of soot, dust, or other matter, including tiny droplets of liquids	Diesel engines, power plants, industries, windblown dust, wood stoves	Eye irritation, asthma, bronchitis, lung damage, cancer, heavy metal poisoning, cardiovascular effects	Visibility impairment, atmospheric deposition, aesthetic damage

Source: U.S. Environmental Protection Agency, "Air and Radiation: Air Pollutants," 2012, www.epa.gov/air/urbanair/ and www.epa.gov/air/airpollutants.html.

smoke.[18] Sulfur dioxides (SO_2) and nitrogen oxides (NO_x) are the key culprits in much of the damage, causing damage to plants, aquatic animals, forests, and humans over time. In the United States, roughly two thirds of all sulfur dioxide and one fourth of all nitrogen oxides come from electric power generation that relies on burning fossil fuels such as coal.[19] When coal-powered plants, oil refineries, and other facilities burn these fuels, sulfur and nitrogen in the emissions combine with oxygen and sunlight to become sulfur dioxide and nitrogen oxide. Small acid particles are carried by the wind and combine with moisture to produce acidic rain or snow.[20]

Although there have been substantial reductions in SO_2 and NO_x emissions from power plants that use the fossil fuels coal, gas, and oil in the last decade, full recovery is still years away. Calls for increased production of coal and more refineries in the United States may result in significant increases in emissions in the next decades unless policies mandating "cleaner" coal technology are put into effect and monitored. Currently, China leads the world in coal production and usage at nearly 76 quadrillion Btu, projected to rise to over 114 quadrillion Btu by 2035. The United States is the second biggest user, with current usage of 20 quadrillion Btu, projected to increase to over 25 quadrillion Btu by 2035. Global pressure to reduce use and invest in technology to dramatically reduce emissions from coal production and burning is a key aspect of 2012 global environmental meetings in Rio de Janeiro and in other parts of the world. Although coal is "cleaner" than it was a decade ago from a production standpoint, the idea of "clean coal" is far from reality.[21]

When the AQI is in this range:	... air quality conditions are	... as symbolized by this color:
0 to 50	Good	Green
51 to 100	Moderate	Yellow
101 to 150	Unhealthy for sensitive groups	Orange
151 to 200	Unhealthy	Red
201 to 300	Very unhealthy	Purple
301 to 500	Hazardous	Maroon

FIGURE 20.3 Air Quality Index

The EPA provides individual air quality indexes (AQIs) for ground-level ozone, particle pollution, carbon monoxide, sulfur dioxide, and nitrogen dioxide. All of the AQIs are presented using the general values, categories, and colors of this figure.

Source: U.S. Environmental Protection Agency, "Air Quality Index: A Guide to Air Quality and Your Health," Updated July 2010, www.airnow.gov/index.cfm?action=aqibasics.aqi.

18,6 million

barrels of oil are consumed each day in the U.S.

Acid deposition gradually acidifies ponds, lakes, and other bodies of water. Once the acid content of the water reaches a certain level, plant and animal life cannot survive.[22] Ironically, acidified lakes and ponds become a crystal-clear deep blue, giving the illusion of beauty and health even as they wreak destruction. Every year, acid deposition destroys millions of trees in Europe and North America. Sugar maples and other trees in the northeastern United States appear to be the newest victims of acid deposition as they are having difficulty regenerating seedlings destroyed by these deposits. Scientists have concluded that much of the world's forestlands are now experiencing damaging levels of acid deposition.[23]

Acid deposition aggravates and may even cause bronchitis, asthma, and other respiratory problems, and people with emphysema or heart disease may suffer from exposure.[24] It may also be hazardous to fetuses. Acid deposition can cause metals such as aluminum, cadmium, lead, and mercury to **leach**

leach To dissolve and filter through soil.

out of the soil. If these metals make their way into water or food supplies, they can cause cancer in humans.

Indoor Air Pollution

A growing body of scientific evidence indicates that the air within homes and other buildings can be 10 to 40 times more hazardous than outdoor air, even in the most industrialized cities. Potentially dangerous chemical compounds can increase risks of cancer, contribute to respiratory problems, reduce the immune system's ability to fight disease, and increase problems with allergies and allergic reactions: The higher the dose of these pollutants and the more airtight the house, the greater the risk. In fact, according to a spokesperson for the EPA, "Indoor air pollution causes 50 percent of illnesses globally. That's more than all cancers and heart diseases combined."[25]

Indoor air pollution comes primarily from woodstoves, furnaces, passive cigarette smoke exposure, mold, asbestos, formaldehyde, radon, and lead. That "new car" smell we like is often related to potentially harmful chemicals found in interior fabrics, upholstery, and glues. Today, more and more manufacturers are offering green building products and furnishings, such as natural fiber fabrics, untreated wood for furniture and floors, low-VOC paints, and many other products, in an attempt to reduce potential pollutants. See the **Skills for Behavior Change** box for ideas on how to become a more environmentally conscious consumer.

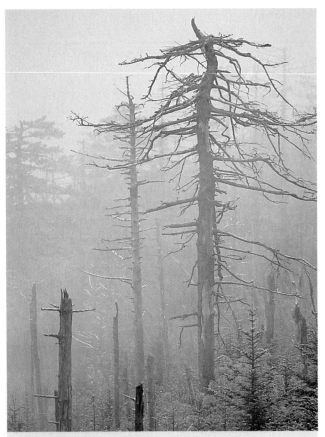

Acid deposition has many harmful effects on the environment. Because its toxins seep into groundwater and enter the food chain, it also poses health hazards to humans.

Skills for Behavior Change

Shopping to Save the Planet

❯ Look for products with less packaging or with refillable, reusable, or recyclable containers.
❯ Bring your own reusable cloth grocery bags to the store. Be sure to wash them after transporting uncooked meat, fish, or poultry.
❯ Buy foods that are produced sustainably.
❯ Purchase organic foods or foods produced with fewer chemicals and pesticides.
❯ Do not buy plastic bottles of water. Purchase a hard plastic or stainless steel reusable water bottle and fill it from a filtered source.
❯ Do not use caustic cleaning products. Simple vinegar is usually just as effective and less harsh on your home and the environment, and many natural products are available.
❯ Buy laundry products that are free of dyes, fragrances, and sulfates.
❯ Purchase appliances with the Energy Star logo.
❯ Use reusable cups, mugs, plates, and utensils rather than disposable products.
❯ Buy recycled paper products.
❯ Purchase bed linens and bath towels that are made from bamboo, hemp, or organic cotton.

Pollutant	Sources	Health Effects
Asbestos	Deteriorating or damaged insulation; fireproofing, acoustical materials, and floor tiles	Long-term risk of chest and abdominal cancers and lung diseases. Smokers are at higher risk of developing asbestos-induced lung cancer.
Lead	Lead-based paint, contaminated soil, dust, and drinking water	At or above 80 µg/dL of blood (high levels) it can cause convulsions, coma, and death. Lower levels can cause central nervous system, kidney, and blood disorders. Blood lead levels as low as 10 µg/dL can impair mental and physical development.
Radon	Uranium in the soil or rock on which homes are built can lead to air exposure inside. Well water also can be a source.	A major nontobacco cause of lung cancer from air and drinking water exposure; it also has a synergistic effect with smoking exposure.
Environmental tobacco smoke	Smoke from the burning end of cigarettes, pipes, or cigars or smoke exhaled by a smoker; consists of a complex mixture of 4,000+ compounds	Over 40 compounds linked to increased risk of lung cancer; asthma, lower respiratory infections; sudden infant death syndrome (SIDS) and heart disease
Biological contaminants (molds, mildew, viruses, animal dander, cat saliva, dust mites, cockroaches, and pollen)	Improper ventilation and moisture buildup, lack of cleanliness/sanitation, contaminated heating systems, faulty construction, household pets, rodents, insects, damp carpets	Allergic reactions, including hypersensitivity, rhinitis, asthma, infectious illnesses, sneezing, watering eyes, coughing, shortness of breath, dizziness, lethargy, fever, digestive problems
Combustion products	Unvented kerosene heaters, woodstoves, fireplaces, gas stoves	Carbon monoxide causes headaches, dizziness, weakness, nausea, confusion and disorientation, chest pain, death. Nitrogen dioxide causes irritation of nose and eyes, respiratory distress. Particles cause lung damage and irritation.
Benzene	Paint, new carpet, new drapes, upholstery, fast-drying glues, caulks	Headaches, eye/skin irritation, fatigue, cancer
Formaldehyde	Tobacco smoke, plywood, cabinets, furniture, particleboard, new carpet and drapes, wallpaper, ceiling tile, paneling	Headaches, eye/skin irritation, drowsiness, fatigue, respiratory problems, memory loss, depression, gynecological problems, cancer
Chloroform	Paint, new drapes, new carpet, upholstery	Headaches, asthma attacks, dizziness, eye/skin irritations
Toluene	All paper products, most finished wood products	Headaches, eye/skin irritation, sinus problems, dizziness, cancer
Hydrocarbons	Tobacco smoke, gas burners and furnaces	Headaches, fatigue, nausea, dizziness, breathing difficulty
Ammonia	Tobacco smoke, cleaning supplies, animal urine	Eye/skin irritation, headaches, nosebleeds, sinus problems
Trichloroethylene	Paints, glues, caulking, vinyl coatings, wallpaper	Headaches, eye/skin irritation, upper respiratory irritation

Source: U.S. Environmental Protection Agency, "The Inside Story: A Guide to Indoor Air Quality," Updated April 2010, www.epa.gov/iaq/pubs/insidest.html.

Multiple factors, including age, individual sensitivity, preexisting medical conditions, liver function, and the condition of the immune and respiratory systems, contribute to a person's risk for being affected by indoor air pollution.[26] Those with allergies may be particularly vulnerable, as may those living in newer airtight, energy-efficient homes. Health effects may develop over years of exposure or may occur in response to toxic levels of pollutants. Room temperature and humidity also play a role. Table 20.3 lists major sources of indoor air pollution and possible health effects.

Preventing indoor air pollution should focus on three main areas: *source control* (eliminating or reducing individual contaminants), *ventilation improvements* (increasing the amount of outdoor air coming indoors), and *air cleaners* (removing particulates from the air).[27]

Environmental Tobacco Smoke

Perhaps the greatest source of indoor air pollution is *environmental tobacco smoke (ETS)*, also known as secondhand smoke, which contains carbon monoxide and cancer-causing particulates. The level of carbon monoxide in cigarette smoke in enclosed spaces has been found to be 4,000 times higher than that allowed in the clean air standard established by the EPA. Moreover, the Surgeon General has reported that there are more than

50 carcinogens in environmental tobacco smoke. Ten to 15 percent of nonsmokers are extremely sensitive to tobacco smoke, experiencing itchy eyes, breathing difficulties, headaches, nausea, and dizziness in response to very small amounts of smoke. The only truly effective way to eliminate ETS in public places is to enact strict no-smoking policies; ventilation and separate smoking areas are not sufficient. The CDC estimates that every U.S. state will have some form of smoking ban by 2020. Many major U.S. cities have banned smoking in public buildings and certain workplaces. As of 2011, Maine, Louisiana, California, Arkansas, and counties in several other states have also banned smoking in automobiles where children are present.

20–100

potentially dangerous chemical compounds can be found in the air of the average U.S. home.

Home Heating Woodstoves emit significant levels of particulates and carbon monoxide in addition to other pollutants, such as sulfur dioxide. If you rely on wood for heating, make sure that your stove is properly installed, vented, and maintained. Burning properly seasoned wood reduces particulates. People who rely on oil- or gas-fired furnaces also need to make sure that these appliances are properly installed, ventilated, and maintained. Inexpensive monitors are available to detect high carbon monoxide levels in the home.

Asbestos The mineral compound **asbestos** was once commonly used in insulating materials and also found its way into vinyl flooring, shingles/roofing materials, heating pipe coverings, and many other products in buildings constructed before 1970. When bonded to other materials, asbestos is relatively harmless, but if its tiny fibers become loosened and airborne, they can embed themselves in the lungs. Their presence leads to cancer of the lungs, stomach, and chest lining and other life-threatening lung diseases called *mesothelioma* and *asbestosis*. If asbestos is detected in the home, it must be removed or sealed off by a professional.

Formaldehyde **Formaldehyde** is a colorless, strong-smelling gas present in some carpets, draperies, furniture, particleboard, plywood, wood paneling, countertops, and many adhesives. It is released into the air in a process called *outgassing*. Outgassing is highest in new products, but the process can continue for many years. Exposure to formaldehyde can cause respiratory problems, dizziness, fatigue, nausea, and rashes. Long-term exposure can lead to central nervous system disorders and cancer. Ask about the formaldehyde content of products you are considering for your home, and avoid those that contain it.

Radon **Radon** is an odorless, colorless gas penetrates homes through cracks, pipes, or sump pits, and other openings in the basement or foundation. The U.S. Surgeon General warns that radon is the second leading cause of lung cancer, after smoking, each year.[28] The EPA estimates that as many as 8.1 million homes (1 out of every 15) have elevated levels of radon.[29] Since 1988, the EPA and the Office of the Surgeon General have recommended that homes be tested for radon below the third floor and that Americans test their homes every 2 years or when they move into a new home. Low-cost radon test kits are available online, in hardware stores, and through other retail outlets.

Lead This metal pollutant is sometimes found in paint, batteries, drinking water, pipes, dishes with lead-based glazes, dirt, soldered cans, and some candies made in Mexico. In recent years, toys produced in China and other regions of the world have been recalled due to unsafe levels of lead in their paint. Lead affects the circulatory, reproductive, urinary, and nervous systems and can accumulate in bone and other tissues. It is particularly detrimental to children and fetuses and can cause birth defects, learning problems, behavioral abnormalities, and other health problems. By some estimates, as many as 25 percent of U.S. homes still have lead-based paint hazards, and an estimated 250,000 American children

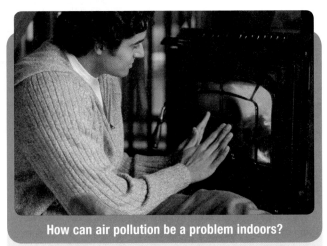

How can air pollution be a problem indoors?

Inside air can be 10 to 40 times more hazardous than outside air. Indoor air pollution comes from woodstoves, furnaces, tobacco smoke, asbestos, formaldehyde, radon, lead, mold, and household chemicals.

ages 1 to 5 have unsafe blood lead levels.[30] To reduce unsafe exposure, keep areas where children play clean and dust free, regularly wash the child's hands and toys, leave lead-based paint undisturbed if it is in good condition, and if lead paint must be removed, hire a professional contractor.

Mold Molds are fungi that live both indoors and outdoors in most regions of the country. They produce tiny reproductive spores, which waft through the indoor and outdoor air. When they land on a damp spot indoors, they may begin growing and digesting whatever they are on, including wood, paper, carpet, and food. In general, molds are harmless; however, some people are sensitive or allergic to them. In such people, exposure to molds may lead to nasal stuffiness, eye irritation, wheezing, or skin irritation. For those who are very sensitive, molds may cause fever or shortness of breath.[31] For ways to reduce your exposure to mold, see the **Skills for Behavior Change** box.

Sick Building Syndrome **Sick building syndrome (SBS)** is said to exist when 80 percent of a building's occupants report air pollution-related problems. Poor ventilation is a primary cause, along with faulty furnaces, pet dander, mold, and dust. Volatile compounds from products such as hair spray, cleaners, and adhesives can cause problems, as can heavy metals such as lead, particularly in older buildings. Symptoms include eye irritation, sore throat, queasiness, and worsening of asthma.

Indoor air pollution and SBS are increasing concerns in the classroom and workplace. Many people complain of maladies that lessen or vanish when they leave their workplace. Studies show that significant numbers of U.S. schools have unsatisfactory indoor air quality, often due to poor ventilation, construction techniques that block outside air, and the use of synthetic materials.[32] Poor air quality can trigger allergies, asthma, and other health problems among students.[33]

Ozone Layer Depletion

The ozone layer forms a protective stratum in the stratosphere—the highest level of Earth's atmosphere, located 12 to 30 miles above the surface. The ozone layer protects our planet and its inhabitants from ultraviolet B (UVB) radiation, a primary cause of skin cancer. Such radiation damages DNA and weakens human and animal immune systems (radiation in general is discussed later in this text).

In the 1970s, scientists began to warn of a breakdown in the ozone layer. Instruments developed to test atmospheric contents indicated that certain chemicals, especially **chlorofluorocarbons (CFCs)**, were contributing to the ozone layer's rapid depletion. Chlorofluorocarbons were used as refrigerants, aerosol propellants, and cleaning solvents, and were also used in medical sterilizers, rigid foam insulation, and Styrofoam. When released into the air through spraying or outgassing, CFCs migrate into the ozone layer, where they decompose and release chlorine atoms. These atoms cause ozone molecules to break apart and levels to be depleted.

The U.S. government banned the use of aerosol sprays containing CFCs in the 1970s. The discovery of an ozone "hole" over Antarctica led to the 1987 Montreal Protocol treaty, whereby the United States and other nations agreed to further reduce the use of CFCs and other ozone-depleting chemicals. The treaty was amended in 1995 to ban CFC production in developed countries. Today, more than 190 countries have signed the treaty as the international community strives to preserve the ozone layer.[34] Although the ban on CFCs is believed to be responsible for slowing the depletion of the ozone layer, some CFC replacements may also be damaging because they contribute to the enhanced greenhouse effect.

Global Warming

More than 100 years ago, scientists theorized that carbon dioxide emissions from the burning of fossil fuels would create a buildup of **greenhouse gases** (gases that trap heat in the atmosphere), which contribute to warming of the earth's surface.[35] In recent years,

See It! Videos

How did Earth Day start? Watch **Going Green** at www.pearsonhighered.com/donatelle.

sick building syndrome (SBS) Problem that exists when 80 percent of a building's occupants report maladies that tend to lessen or vanish when they leave the building.

chlorofluorocarbons (CFCs) Chemicals that contribute to the depletion of the atmospheric ozone layer.

greenhouse gases Gases that accumulate in the atmosphere where they contribute to global warming by trapping heat near the earth's surface.

these predictions have been supported by reports from leading international scientists in the field and accounts in the popular media, such as the documentary *An Inconvenient Truth,* all detailing indicators of a planet in trouble.

The *greenhouse effect* is a natural phenomenon in which greenhouse gases such as **carbon dioxide (CO_2)** form a layer in the atmosphere, allowing solar heat to pass through and trapping some of the heat close to the surface, where it warms the planet (Figure 20.4). Human activities such as burning fossil fuels and land clearing have increased greenhouse gases in the atmosphere, resulting in the **enhanced greenhouse effect**, in which excess solar heat is trapped, raising the planet's temperature. According to data from the National Oceanic and Atmospheric Administration (NOAA) and the National Aeronautics and Space Administration (NASA), Earth's surface temperature has risen about 1.2° to 1.4°F since 1900,[36] with each of the last 35 years of data indicating significantly higher rates. In fact, 2011 tied 1997 as the warmest year globally since records were first collected in 1880.[37] Furthermore, the consensus is that temperatures will continue to rise, perhaps by as much as 5° to 10° in the next 100 years, unless immediate steps are taken to reverse the trend. Results of such a temperature increase—which might include rising sea levels (potentially flooding entire regions), glacier retreat, arctic shrinkage at the poles, altered patterns of agriculture (including changes in growing seasons and alterations of climatic zones), deforestation, drought, extreme weather events, increases in tropical diseases, changes in disease trends and patterns, loss of biological species (over 100 species of mammals are already extinct), and economic devastation—would be catastrophic.

Greenhouse gases include carbon dioxide, nitrous oxide, methane, CFCs, and hydrocarbons. The most predominant is carbon dioxide, which accounts for 49 percent of all greenhouse gases. The United States is the greatest producer of greenhouse gases, responsible for over 22 percent of all output, and this output is expected to increase 43 percent by 2025.[38] Rapid deforestation of the tropical rain forests of Central and South America, Africa, and southeast Asia also contributes to the rapid rise in greenhouse gases. Trees take in carbon dioxide, transform it, store the carbon for food,

carbon dioxide (CO_2) Gas created by the combustion of fossil fuels and is exhaled by animals; used by plants for photosynthesis; the primary greenhouse gas in the atmosphere.

enhanced greenhouse effect Warming of the earth's surface as a direct result of human activities that release greenhouse gases into the atmosphere, trapping more of the sun's radiation than is normal.

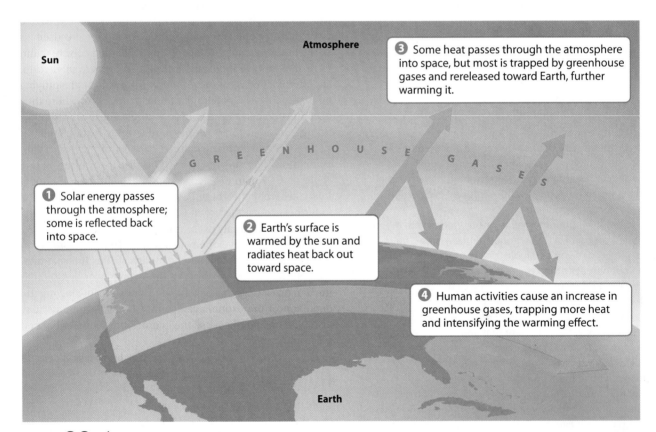

Sun

Atmosphere

❸ Some heat passes through the atmosphere into space, but most is trapped by greenhouse gases and rereleased toward Earth, further warming it.

GREENHOUSE GASES

❶ Solar energy passes through the atmosphere; some is reflected back into space.

❷ Earth's surface is warmed by the sun and radiates heat back out toward space.

❹ Human activities cause an increase in greenhouse gases, trapping more heat and intensifying the warming effect.

Earth

FIGURE 20.4 **The Enhanced Greenhouse Effect**
The natural greenhouse effect is responsible for making Earth habitable; it keeps the planet 33°C (60°F) warmer than it would otherwise be. An increase in greenhouse gases resulting from human activity is creating the enhanced greenhouse effect, trapping more heat and causing dangerous global climate change.

Video Tutor: Enhanced Greenhouse Effect

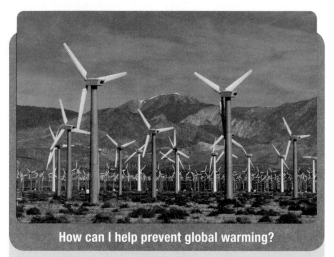

How can I help prevent global warming?

Global warming is a global problem. We need to work with other nations to ensure that all do their part. By reducing your use of fossil fuels, using high-efficiency vehicles, and supporting increased use of renewable resources such as solar, wind, and water power, you can help combat global warming.

and release oxygen into the air. As we lose forests at the rate of hundreds of acres per hour, we lose the capacity to dissipate carbon dioxide.

A 1997 United Nations treaty, the Kyoto Protocol, outlined an international plan to reduce the manmade emissions responsible for climate change. It went into effect in 2005 and required participating countries to reduce their emissions between 2008 and 2012 by at least 5 percent below 1990 levels.[39] More than 160 countries signed on to the Kyoto Protocol, including more than 30 industrialized countries.[40] The United States opted out of this proposal, ostensibly because of concerns that major developing nations, including India and China, were not required to reduce emissions under the treaty. A follow-up summit in Copenhagen in 2009 sought to restrict global temperatures to a rise of 2°C by 2050. These talks stalled with disagreements between the West and developing countries. A major United Nations Conference on Sustainable Development and Environmental concerns (RIO+20) took place in 2012 in Rio de Janeiro. However, leaders of many nations, including the United States, France, Germany, and the United Kingdom opted not to attend, and the resulting paper generated by the conference contained only nonbinding objectives.

Reducing Air Pollution and the Threat of Global Warming

Air pollution and climate change problems are rooted in our energy, transportation, and industrial practices. Clearly, we must develop comprehensive national strategies that encourage the use of renewable resources such as solar, wind, and water power. Because industrial production is a key contributor to fossil fuel emissions, clean energy, green factories,

improved technology, and governmental regulation are necessary for preventing climate change.

Most experts agree that reducing consumption of fossil fuels, shifting to alternative energy sources, improving gas mileage, and using mass transportation are crucial to air pollution reduction. Many cities have taken steps in this direction by setting high parking fees and road-usage tolls in congested areas. Although stricter laws on vehicular carbon emissions and the development of cars that operate on electricity, hydrogen, biodiesel, ethanol, or other alternative energy sources are promising, we have a long way to go to reduce fossil-fuel consumption.

Meanwhile, many communities have created bicycle lanes and hold "bike to work" days. Scooters and other low-energy modes of transportation are becoming increasingly popular. Some college campuses have enacted policies allowing skateboard and Rollerblade use on campus. Other campuses provide scooter and bike garages to protect them from theft and vandalism and to encourage students to use energy-efficient transportation. You can participate in this effort by finding ways to reduce your own **carbon footprint**, or the amount of CO_2 emissions you contribute to the atmosphere in your daily life.

carbon footprint Amount of greenhouse gases produced, usually expressed in equivalent tons of carbon dioxide emissions.

Water Pollution and Shortages

Seventy-five percent of Earth is covered with water in the form of oceans, seas, lakes, rivers, streams, and wetlands. Underneath the surface are reservoirs of groundwater. We draw our drinking water from this underground source and from freshwater on the surface. However, just 1 percent of the entire water supply is available for human use; the rest is too salty, too polluted, or locked away in polar ice caps.[41]

We cannot take the safety of our water supply for granted. Over half the global population faces a shortage of clean water. More than 2.6 billion people, about 40 percent of the planet's population, have no access to basic sanitation or adequate toilet facilities. More than 1 billion have no access to clean water, and more than 4,500 children die every day from illnesses caused by lack of safe water and sanitation.[42] Many regions of the world are already experiencing severe freshwater shortages due to poor sanitation; overuse by agriculture, industry, and consumers; and dwindling supplies at a time when populations are growing. Between now and 2040, severe increases in global demand will affect economic growth and population health. Annual global water requirements will reach 6,900 billion cubic meters in 2030, 40 percent above current sustainable water supplies.[43]

Considering how little water is available to meet the world's agricultural, manufacturing, community, personal, and sanitation needs, it is no wonder that clean water is a precious commodity that must not be wasted. Although the United States makes up just over 5 percent of the world's population, it is the third largest consumer of water after the much more populated countries of China and India. While

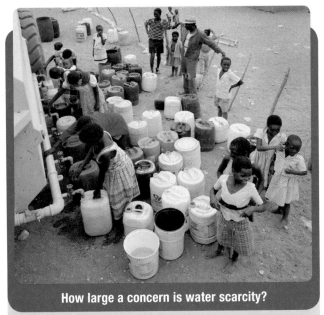

How large a concern is water scarcity?

The lack of clean water and sanitation is a major global problem. *Closed basins* are defined as regions where existing water cannot meet the agricultural, industrial, municipal, and environmental needs. The Stockholm International Water Institute estimates that 1.4 billion people live in a closed basin, and the problem is worsening; the Food and Agriculture Organization estimates that number will increase to 1.8 billion by 2025.

Skills for Behavior Change

Waste Less Water!

IN THE KITCHEN

❯ Turn off the tap while washing dishes. Use only half a sink, and don't run rinse water until you need it. Shut it off after a quick rinse.
❯ Repair leaky pipes and faucets. More than 3,000 gallons of water each year are lost to leaks.
❯ Equip faucets with aerators to reduce water use by 4 percent.
❯ Run dishwashers only when they are full, and use the energy-saving mode.

IN THE LAUNDRY ROOM

❯ Wash only full loads or use a washing machine that adjusts to allow a reduced water level for smaller loads. Use cold water whenever possible to save energy. Upgrade to a high-efficiency washer to use 30 percent less water per load.
❯ Limit the use of the dryer and line dry clothing when possible.
❯ Buy soaps that are dye free, fragrance free, and biodegradable whenever possible.

IN THE BATHROOM

❯ Detect and fix leaks. A leaky toilet can waste about 200 gallons of water per day.
❯ Replace old toilets with a high-efficiency models that use 60 to 80 percent less water per flush.
❯ Take showers instead of baths, and limit showers to the time it takes to lather up and rinse off. Ideally, get wet, shut off water, lather up, and turn on water to rinse.
❯ Replace old showerheads with efficient models that use 60 percent less water per minute.
❯ Turn off the tap while brushing your teeth to save up to 8 gallons of water per day.

---

point source pollutant Pollutant that enters waterways at a specific location.

the average person uses about 100 to 150 gallons of water for household use, the per capita freshwater usage is over 750,000 gallons a day! Why so high? Because this usage figure considers total water usage, of which agriculture makes up 92 percent of the total. Grain, meat, and dairy production are the biggest agricultural users, followed by industrial use, power plant cooling, and other high-use activities.[44] The Skills for Behavior Change box presents simple conservation measures that you can adopt to save water where you live.

Water Contamination

Any substance that gets into the soil can potentially enter the water supply. Industrial pollutants and pesticides eventually work their way into the soil, then into groundwater. Underground storage tanks for gasoline may leak. U.S. Geological Survey researchers discovered the presence of low levels of many chemical compounds in a network of 139 targeted streams across the United States. Steroids, pharmaceuticals, personal care products, hormones, insect repellent, and wastewater compounds were all detected.[45]

Tap water in the United States is among the safest in the world. The Safe Drinking Water Act (SDWA) is the main federal law that ensures the quality of Americans' drinking water. Under the SDWA, the EPA sets standards for drinking water quality and oversees the states, localities, and water suppliers who implement those standards. Cities and municipalities have strict policies and procedures governing water treatment, filtration, and disinfection to screen out pathogens and microorganisms. However, their ability to filter out increasing amounts of chemical by-products and other substances is in question. According to a recent Associated Press inquiry, a "vast array of pharmaceuticals—including antibiotics, anticonvulsants, mood stabilizers, and sex hormones—have been found in the drinking water supplies of at least 41 million Americans."[46]

Congress has coined two terms that describe general sources of water pollution. **Point source pollutants** enter a waterway at a specific location through a pipe, ditch, culvert, or other conduit. The major sources of point source pollution are sewage treatment plants and industrial facilities.

Nonpoint source pollutants—commonly known as *run-off* and *sedimentation*—drain or seep into waterways from broad areas of land. Nonpoint source pollution results from a variety of land use practices, including soil erosion and sedimentation, construction and engineering project wastes, pesticide and fertilizer runoff, urban street runoff, acid mine drainage, septic tank leakage, and sewage sludge (Figure 20.5).

Pollutants causing the greatest potential harm are the following:

● **Gasoline and petroleum products.** There are more than 2 million underground storage tanks for gasoline and petroleum products in the United States, most located at gasoline filling stations. The EPA indicates that many sites are in compliance with cleanup and leak-monitoring protocols. However, many underground storage tanks that are yet unidentified or are either out of compliance or currently unmonitored are thought to be leaking after years of corrosion.[47]

● **Chemical contaminants.** *Organic solvents* are chemicals designed to dissolve grease and oil. These extremely toxic substances are used to clean clothing, painting equipment, plastics, and metal parts. Many household products (e.g., stain removers, degreasers, drain cleaners, septic system cleaners, and paint removers) also contain these toxic chemicals. Organic solvents enter the water supply in different ways. Consumers often dump leftover products into the toilet or into street drains. Industries pour leftovers into barrels, which are then buried. Eventually the chemicals eat through the barrels and leach into groundwater. For a description of one energy-harnessing process that poses groundwater risks, see the **Points of View** box on fracking on the following page.

● **Polychlorinated biphenyls.** Fire resistant and stable at high temperatures, **polychlorinated biphenyls (PCBs)** were used for many years as insulating materials in high-voltage electrical equipment, such as transformers and older fluorescent lights. The human body does not excrete ingested PCBs but rather stores them in the liver and fatty tissues. PCB exposure is associated with birth defects, cancer, and various skin problems. As of 1977, PCBs are no longer manufactured in the United States, but approximately 500 million pounds have been dumped into landfills and waterways, where they continue to pose an environmental threat.[48]

● **Dioxins.** **Dioxins** are chlorinated hydrocarbons found in herbicides (chemicals used to kill vegetation) and are produced during certain industrial processes. Dioxins have the ability to accumulate in the body and are much more toxic than PCBs. Long-term effects include possible immune system damage and increased risk of infections and cancer. Exposure to high concentrations of PCBs or dioxins for a short period of time can also have severe consequences, including nausea, vomiting, diarrhea, painful rashes and sores, and chloracne, an ailment in which the skin develops hard, black, painful pimples that may never heal.

● **Pesticides.** **Pesticides** are chemicals designed to kill insects, rodents, plants, and fungi. More than 1,055 active ingredients are sold as pesticides in thousands of products.[49] Americans use more than 1.2 billion of pounds of pesticides each year, but only 10 percent actually reach the targeted organisms. The other 90 percent settle on the land and in our air and water. Pesticides evaporate readily and are often dispersed by winds over a large area or carried out to sea. In tropical regions, many farmers use pesticides heavily, and the climate promotes their rapid release into the atmosphere. Pesticide residues cling to fruits and vegetables and can accumulate in the body. Potential hazards associated with exposure to pesticides include birth defects, liver and kidney damage, and nervous system disorders.

● **Lead.** **Lead** can leach into tap water from lead pipes or water lines, usually in older homes. The EPA has issued updated standards to dramatically reduce the levels of lead in drinking water, stipulating that lead values must not exceed 15 parts per billion (ppb). (The previous standard allowed up to 50 ppb.) If lead is present in your water supply, you can reduce your risk by running the tap for several minutes before using the water for drinking or cooking. This flushes out water that has been standing in lead-contaminated lines. The EPA also recommends using filtration systems that attach to faucets and remove lead and other particles from water.[50]

nonpoint source pollutant Pollutant that runs off or seeps into waterways from broad areas of land.

polychlorinated biphenyls (PCBs) Toxic chemicals that were once used as insulating materials in high-voltage electrical equipment.

dioxins Highly toxic chlorinated hydrocarbons contained in herbicides and produced during certain industrial processes.

pesticides Chemicals that kill pests such as insects or rodents.

lead Highly toxic metal found in emissions from lead smelters and processing plants; also sometimes found in pipes or paint in older buildings.

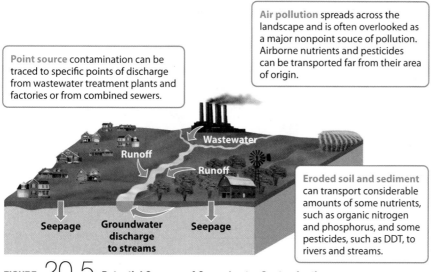

Point source contamination can be traced to specific points of discharge from wastewater treatment plants and factories or from combined sewers.

Air pollution spreads across the landscape and is often overlooked as a major nonpoint souce of pollution. Airborne nutrients and pesticides can be transported far from their area of origin.

Eroded soil and sediment can transport considerable amounts of some nutrients, such as organic nitrogen and phosphorus, and some pesticides, such as DDT, to rivers and streams.

Wastewater

Runoff

Runoff

Seepage

Groundwater discharge to streams

Seepage

FIGURE 20.5 **Potential Sources of Groundwater Contamination**

Source: Adapted from U.S. Geological Survey, Wisconsin Water Science Center, "Learn More about Groundwater," 2008, http://wi.water.usgs.gov/gwcomp/learn.

Fracking: ENVIRONMENTAL THREAT OR ROAD TO ENERGY INDEPENDENCE?

Hydraulic fracturing, more commonly known as *fracking,* is a relatively new method of extracting natural gas from the ground that has recently grown popular. North America has vast reserves of natural gas, but most of them are trapped in shale beds that have long been inaccessible to cost-effective tapping. According to some experts, these deposits could provide the United States with enough natural gas to power the country for a century, helping us to become energy independent in the years ahead. But the process also has many people concerned about the environmental risks that go with it.

In fracking, underground rock and dense soil are cracked open by pumping highly pressurized fluids into them. This creates fissures that allow oil or gas to flow to the surface for extraction. Much of the fracking liquid, a mixture of water, sand, ceramic beads, and other chemicals, comes up with the gas or oil and is stored in chemical pools for delivery to treatment plants. However, some scientists and members of the public are concerned that a portion of this toxic, chemical-laden sludge can seep down and contaminate aquifers that supply drinking water to many regions of the country. In addition to potential groundwater contamination, the EPA has noted that fracking causes airborne pollution from methane, sulfur oxide, benzene, and other pollutants, each of which pose significant risks to human health and the environment. At present, fewer regulations exist to control the safe collection of harmful gases from fracking compared with other energy technologies. In the last year, a rash of earthquakes in regions of the country where shale gas is being extracted by fracking sparked speculation that changing the internal pressures of the earth's surface may pose risks that have yet to be explored. To date, the science supporting fracking as a harmless process or a highly risky process is lacking. In the meantime, the fracking industry is growing rapidly, with sand-mining production escalating daily in the upper Midwest in anticipation of a fracking boom that extends well beyond any underground rumbling.

Arguments for Fracking

○ Increased U.S. energy production and energy independence are important to the health of the economy.

○ The process provides jobs to spur economic growth and reduce unemployment.

○ Accessing these reserves provides profits for land owners, mineral rights owners, and large gas, oil, and supplying companies.

○ Local business increases in communities where fracking operations occur.

○ Fracking costs less than extraction of natural gas by other methods

Arguments against Fracking

○ Contamination of underground wells, surface waters, and aquifers pose risks to health.

○ Clean up of this sort of groundwater contamination is difficult, if not impossible, with current technology.

○ Illegal, unregulated dumping of waste from fracking process occurs.

○ Regulation and oversight continue to be "in progress" rather than clearly defined.

○ There is a possibility for far-reaching effects, such as earthquakes, due to fracking.

○ Air pollution problems risk health.

Where Do You Stand?

○ How would you prioritize the competing needs of jobs, energy production (that may cause pollution), and environmental destruction or danger?

○ What criteria should be used to set rules for when or how fracking should take place?

Sources: EPA, "Natural Gas Extraction: Hydraulic Fracturing," 2012, www.epa.gov/hydraulicfracture/; U.S. Energy Information Administration (EIA), "What Is Shale Gas and Why Is It Important?" 2012, www.eia.gov/energy_in_brief/about_shale_gas.cfm.

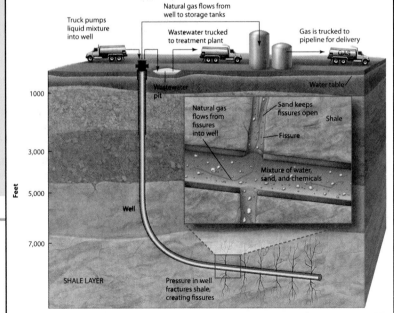

Hydraulic Fracturing (Fracking)

Source: Adapted from schematic found in "EPA Study of Hydraulic Fracturing and Drinking Water Safety; Initial Recommendations by Science Advisory Board," U.S. Environmental Protection Agency, 2010.

Land Pollution

Much of the waste that ends up polluting water starts out polluting the land. Growing population creates more pressure on the land to accommodate increasing amounts of refuse, much of which is nonbiodegradable and some of which is directly harmful to living organisms.

Solid Waste

Each day, every person in the United States generates more than 4.4 pounds of **municipal solid waste (MSW)**, more commonly known as trash or garbage, totaling about 250 million tons of trash each year, with organic materials making up the largest share. Paperboard accounts for 29 percent and yard trimmings and food scraps account for another 27 percent (Figure 20.6).[51]

Increasing amounts of electronic waste (known as "E-waste") is generated each year; however, the vast majority of E-waste (nearly 83%) ends up in landfills; recycling rates are just shy of 18 percent.[52] There are several options for reducing electronic waste, including recycling, participating in electronic reuse programs, and donating your consumer electronics. Find more information on electronic waste recycling in your state and ways to reduce electronic waste at www.greenergadgets.org and www.ecyclingcentral.com.

Americans generate about 250 million tons of waste per year. The good news is that these numbers are down from historic highs in the 1990s. The bad news is that we recycle only slightly over one third of the waste we generate. Experts

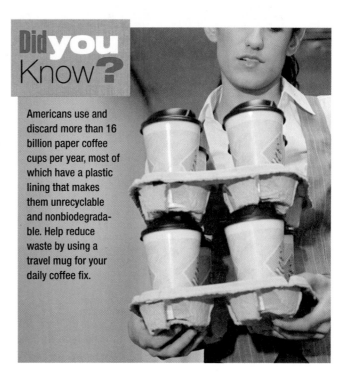

believe we could recycle up to 90 percent of trash (Figure 20.7). Currently, 34.8 percent of all MSW in the United States is recycled or composted, over 14 percent is burned at combustion facilities, and the remaining 54 percent is disposed of in landfills.[53]

The number of U.S. landfills has actually decreased in the past decade, but their sheer mass has increased. Many people worry that we are rapidly losing our ability to dispose of all of the waste we create. As communities run out of landfill space, it is becoming common to haul garbage to other states or to dump it illegally in woods, waterways, or oceans, where it contaminates ecosystems, or to ship it to landfills in developing countries, where it becomes someone else's problem. In today's throwaway society, we need to become aware of the amount of waste we generate and to look for ways to recycle, reuse, and—most desirable of all—reduce what we consume.

Communities, businesses, and individuals can adopt several strategies to reduce MSW:

- *Source reduction* (*waste prevention*) involves altering the design, manufacture, or use of products and materials to reduce the amount and toxicity of waste. The most effective waste-reducing strategy is to prevent waste from being generated in the first place. One key area is packaging. Do we

municipal solid waste (MSW) Solid waste such as durable and nondurable goods, containers and packaging, food waste, yard waste, and miscellaneous waste from residential, commercial, institutional, and industrial sources.

what do you think?

Do you know people who throw away recyclable items rather than recycling them?

● What do you think motivates their behavior?

● How might you encourage them to recycle more than they do now?

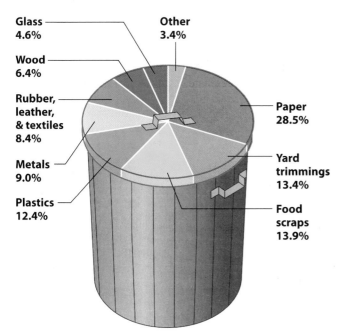

- Glass 4.6%
- Other 3.4%
- Wood 6.4%
- Rubber, leather, & textiles 8.4%
- Metals 9.0%
- Plastics 12.4%
- Paper 28.5%
- Yard trimmings 13.4%
- Food scraps 13.9%

FIGURE 20.6 What's in Our Trash?

Source: Data are from U.S. Environmental Protection Agency, *Municipal Solid Waste Generation, Recycling, and Disposal in the United States: Facts and Figures for 2010*, EPA-530-F-11-005, December 2011, www.epa.gov/wastes/nonhaz/municipal/pubs/msw_2010_rev_factsheet.pdf.

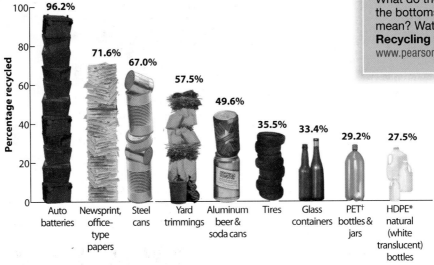

†High-density polyethylene
*Polyethylene terephthalate

FIGURE 20.7 **How Much Do We Recycle?**

Source: Data are from U.S. Environmental Protection Agency, *Municipal Solid Waste Generation, Recycling, and Disposal in the United States: Facts and Figures for 2010*, EPA-530-F-11-005, December 2011, www.epa.gov/wastes/nonhaz/municipal/pubs/msw_2010_rev_factsheet.pdf.

really need to buy products that have three outer shells of plastic and take lawn shears to break into? Consumers can help by boycotting such packaging strategies. See the **Money & Health** box on plastic bag bans and use taxes on the following page.

● *Recycling* involves sorting, collecting, and processing materials to be reused in manufacturing new products. This process diverts items such as paper, cardboard, glass, plastic, and metals from the waste stream. Be responsible and recycle everything that is recyclable, particularly E-waste and paper.

● *Composting* involves collecting organic waste, such as food scraps and yard trimmings, and allowing it to decompose with the help of microorganisms (mainly bacteria and fungi). This process produces a nutrient-rich substance used to fertilize gardens and for soil enhancement. Many communities now have yard carts that allow you to mix your food scraps in with yard trimmings. Find out what options are available in your area.

● *Combustion with energy recovery* typically involves the use of boilers and industrial furnaces to incinerate waste and use the burning process to generate energy.

Hazardous Waste

Hazardous waste is defined as waste with properties that make it capable of harming human health or the environment. In 1980, the Comprehensive Environmental Response, Compensation and Liability Act, known as the **Superfund**, was enacted to provide funds for cleaning up hazardous waste dump sites. This Superfund is financed through taxes on the chemical and petroleum industries (87%) and through federal tax revenues (13%). To date, 32,500 potentially hazardous waste sites have been identified, and 90 percent of these have been cleared or "recovered."[54] Currently, there are 66 priority sites being actively cleared, with thousands more sites, costing billions of dollars, possible for future clean up. Newer technologies are being investigated, including nanotechnologies that could reduce costs by as much as 75 percent.

The large number of U.S. hazardous waste dump sites indicates the severity of our toxic chemical problem. American manufacturers generate more than 1 ton of chemical waste per person per year (275 million tons annually). Many wastes are now banned from land disposal or are being treated to reduce their toxicity before they become part of land disposal sites. The EPA has developed protective requirements for land disposal facilities, such as double liners, detection systems for substances that may leach into groundwater, and groundwater monitoring systems.

hazardous waste Toxic waste that poses a hazard to humans or to the environment.

Superfund Fund established under the Comprehensive Environmental Response, Compensation, and Liability Act to be used for cleaning up toxic waste dumps.

What's Working for You?

Our individual choices can make a huge difference in the amount of resources used and the amount of waste generated each day. Maybe you have already begun to take action. Which of the following behaviors do you engage in?

☐ I buy local foods to avoid excess transportation costs and to obtain fresh food.

☐ When there are choices in packaging, I opt for packages with less plastic and unnecessary waste.

☐ I turn off lights when I leave a room and unplug my computer and other electronics when I'm not using them for extended periods.

☐ I shut off the faucet when brushing my teeth and take shorter showers.

☐ I only run full loads in the dishwasher.

Money&Health

PLASTIC BAG BANS AND TAXES: WHAT ARE THE COSTS AND BENEFITS?

In the past few years, San Francisco; Los Angeles; Seattle; Portland, Oregon; Austin, Texas; Washington, DC; and most of Hawaii are just a few of the places that have enacted taxes or bans on plastic bags at the checkout counter. Proponents of the bans and taxes say plastic bags are bad for the environment because they are made from nonbiodegradeable petroleum, are infrequently recycled, and are commonly littered, ending up in waterways where they become a wildlife hazard.

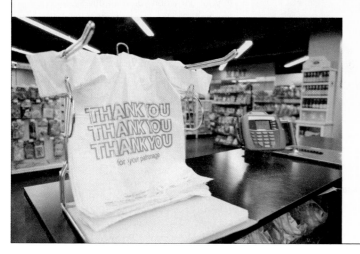

When thrown away as trash, they sit in landfills for decades. But how do bag bans and taxes impact our wallets?

Many locations with bag taxes require stores to charge customers a nominal fee, often a nickel per single-use plastic bag. By contrast, reuseable cloth bags are usually sold for several dollars apiece. Of course, the upfront costs of the reuseable bags are recouped over time.

How much tax revenue is collected by communities with bag taxes varies widely. In Washington, DC, a 5-cent disposable bag tax at grocery, convenience, and liquor stores instituted in 2010 was expected to add $3.6 million dollars to government revenues, most of which was earmarked for clean-up efforts on a local river. However, the District of Columbia reported the tax only netted $2 million that year. But what wasn't so good for the tax coffers appeared to pay off for the environment: One survey of DC residents indicated 75 percent reduced plastic bag usage after the tax was imposed, and, likewise, local businesses reported that bag use was down about 50 percent.

Sources: "D.C. Bag Tax Nets $2 Million," Associated Press, January 5, 2011; "Public Perceptions and Willingness to Address Litter in the District of Columbia," a research report by the Alice Ferguson Foundation, funded by Washington's District Department of Environment (DDOE), 2011, www .fergusonfoundation.org/trash_initiative/AFF_DC_%20ResearchMemo021511.pdf.

52%

of all waste produced in Switzerland is recycled, compared to only 31.5% of all U.S. waste.

Radiation

Radiation is energy that travels in waves or particles. There are many different types of radiation, ranging from radio waves to gamma rays, all making up the electromagnetic spectrum. Exposure to radiation is an inescapable part of life on this planet, and only some of it poses a threat to human health.

Nonionizing Radiation

Nonionizing radiation is radiation at the lower end of the electromagnetic spectrum. This radiation moves in relatively long wavelengths and has enough energy to move atoms around or cause them to vibrate but not enough to remove electrons or alter molecular structure. Examples of nonionizing radiation are radio waves, TV signals, microwaves, infrared waves, and visible light. Concerns have been raised about the safety of radio frequency waves generated by cell phones (see the **Tech & Health** box on the following page).

nonionizing radiation Electromagnetic waves having relatively long wavelengths and enough energy to move atoms around or cause them to vibrate.

ionizing radiation Electromagnetic waves and particles having short wavelengths and energy high enough to ionize atoms.

radiation absorbed dose (rad) Unit of measure of radiation exposure.

Ionizing Radiation

Ionizing radiation is caused by the release of particles and electromagnetic rays from atomic nuclei during the normal process of disintegration. This type of radiation has enough energy to remove electrons from the atoms it passes through. Some naturally occurring elements, such as uranium, emit ionizing radiation. The sun is another source of ionizing radiation, in the form of high-frequency ultraviolet rays—those against which the ozone layer protects us.

Radiation exposure is measured in **radiation absorbed doses** or **rads** (also called *roentgens).* Radiation can cause

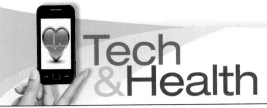

Tech & Health

ARE CELL PHONES HAZARDOUS TO YOUR HEALTH?

Cell phones are used by billions of people around the globe. But cell phones also emit radio frequency (RF) energy when turned on. Depending on how close the phone is to your head, as much as 60 percent of the energy penetrates the skull, neck, and upper torso, some of it reaching as far as 1.5 inches into the brain. Could this harm you?

At high power levels, RF energy damages the body. But in the United States, safety standards for cell phone radiation are set by the Federal Communications Commission, which looks at research to determine a threshold at which RF energy emissions begin to be harmful. Currently, cell phones must emit levels no higher than less than half the safety threshold.

The U.S. Food and Drug Administration, the World Health Organization, and other major health agencies agree that, so far, research finds no link between cell phones and cancer or other disorders. However, they also point to the need for more research, since cell phones are relatively new technology and no long-term studies exist. Three large studies com-

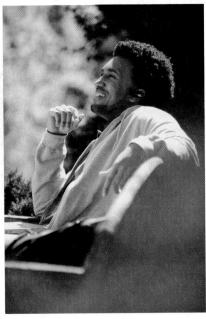

A hands-free device lets you keep your phone—and any radio-frequency energy it may emit—away from your head.

pared cellphone use among brain cancer patients and individuals free of brain cancer, finding no correlation between phone use and tumors. Yet preliminary results

from smaller, well-designed studies have continued to raise questions.

If you are concerned about risk from cell phone usage, a few small changes in behavior can greatly reduce on the amount of RF energy your body absorbs. First, limit the amount of time you spend talking on the phone. When you do make calls, use a hands-free device that keeps the phone away from your head. However, a caveat—wireless earpieces also emit energy, so only keep them turned on and in your ear when you are actively engaged in a call. Finally, you can opt to buy a phone that emits lowers RF energy than others. Information on phone emissions is available from manufacturers in the form of specific absorption rate (SAR) charts, which are readily available on the Internet.

Sources: National Research Council, *Identification of Research Needs Relating to Potential Biological or Adverse Health Effects of Wireless Communications Devices* (Washington, DC: National Academies Press, 2008); American Cancer Society, "Cellular Phones," 2008, www.cancer.org/docroot/PED/content/PED_1_3X_Cellular_Phones.asp; National Cancer Institute, "Cell Phones and Cancer Risk," 2011, www.cancer.gov/cancertopics/factsheet/Risk/cellphones.

---

damage at dosages as low as 100 to 200 rads. At this level, signs of radiation sickness include nausea, diarrhea, fatigue, anemia, sore throat, and hair loss. At 350 to 500 rads, these symptoms become more severe, and death may result because the radiation hinders bone marrow production of the white blood cells we need to protect us from disease. Dosages above 600 to 700 rads are fatal.

Recommended maximum "safe" exposure ranges from 0.5 to 5 rads per year.[55] Approximately 50 percent of the radiation to which we are exposed comes from background sources, including natural and human-made sources. Natural sources include radon gas in the air and cosmic radiation. Human-made sources include certain building materials. Another 45 percent comes from medical and dental X rays. The remaining 5 percent is nonionizing radiation that comes from such sources as computer monitors, microwave ovens, televisions, and radar screens.[56] Most of us are exposed to far less radiation than the safe maximum dosage per year. The effects of long-term exposure to relatively low levels of radiation are unknown. Some scientists believe that such

exposure can cause lung cancer, leukemia, skin cancer, bone cancer, and skeletal deformities.

Nuclear Power Plants

Currently, nuclear power plants account for less than 1 percent of the total radiation to which we are exposed; however, the number of U.S. plants may increase in the next decade, so that percentage may increase. Proponents of nuclear energy believe that it is a safe and efficient way to generate electricity. Initial costs of building nuclear power plants are high, but actual power generation is relatively inexpensive. A 1,000-megawatt reactor produces enough energy for 650,000 homes and saves 420 million gallons of fossil fuels each year. In some areas where nuclear power plants were decommissioned, electricity bills tripled when power companies turned to hydroelectric or fossil fuel sources to generate electricity. Nuclear reactors discharge fewer carbon oxides into the air than do fossil fuel–powered generators. Advocates believe that converting to nuclear power could help slow global warming.

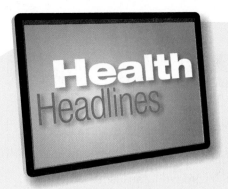

THE NUCLEAR EMERGENCY AFTER THE JAPANESE TSUNAMI

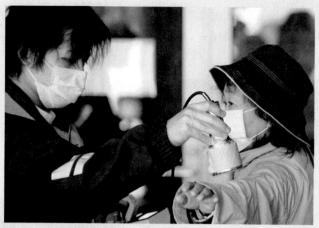

Testing a resident for radiation in Fukushima, Japan.

On March 11, 2011, an earthquake registering 9.0 on the Richter scale occurred off the coast of Japan. The earthquake, the largest to strike Japan in recorded history, initiated a devastating tsunami that leveled cities and washed over farmlands in northern Japan. The combined damaging effects of the earthquake and tsunami also triggered the worst nuclear emergency since Chernobyl. The Fukushima Daiichi Nuclear Power Station, positioned in the region hardest hit by the tsunami, suffered several explosions, multiple fires, radioactive gas leaks, and a partial meltdown in three of its reactors. Despite continued exposure to toxic radioactive material and risk to their lives, nuclear plant workers labored for weeks to stave off a full-scale meltdown and to minimize the destruction to the public and surrounding region by attempting to cool and repair the damaged reactors.

There continues to be significant concern for public safety due to exposure to radioactive materials through the air, food, and water supplies. Of all the hundreds of dangerous radioactive chemicals released during the Fukushima Daiichi nuclear emergency, scientists expressed the most concern about the levels of iodine, plutonium, cesium, and strontium in the atmosphere, water, and food supplies. According to reports of tests on food and drinking water samples made in late March 2011, iodine and cesium were detected, but the majority of measurements remained below regulation values.

Additionally, small amounts of plutonium were also found in the soil outside the plant, though not enough to pose a significant health risk. Long-term health outcomes associated with the Fukushima Daiichi nuclear emergency will be closely monitored by Japanese officials as well as by officials globally. This emergency has spurred Japan and other nations to reconsider the safety of nuclear power plants and the policies necessary to protect the environment and public health.

Sources: "Japan's Nuclear Emergency," *Washington Post*, 2011, www.washingtonpost.com/wp-srv/special/world/japan-nuclear-reactors-and-seismic-activity/; "Earthquake, Tsunami, and Nuclear Crisis," *New York Times*, 2011, http://topics.nytimes.com/top/news/international/countriesandterritories/japan/index.html.

The advantages of nuclear energy must be weighed against the disadvantages. Disposal of nuclear waste is extremely problematic. In addition, a reactor core meltdown could pose serious threats to the immediate environment and to the world in general. A **nuclear meltdown** occurs when the temperature in the core of a nuclear reactor increases enough to melt the nuclear fuel and breach the containment vessel. Most modern facilities seal the reactors and containment vessels in concrete buildings with pools of cold water on the bottom. If a meltdown occurs, the building and the pool are supposed to prevent radiation from escaping.

The International Atomic Energy Agency ranks nuclear and radiological accidents and incidents by severity on a scale of 1 to 7. To date, we have had two major nuclear disasters that resulted in a 7, the highest severity rating, meaning that there was a major release of radioactive material with widespread health and environmental consequences. The first was the 1986 reactor core fire and explosion at the Chernobyl nuclear power plant in Russia, which has led to conservative estimates of from 2,000 to as many as 724,000 deaths. Many regions surrounding the area may be uninhabitable for decades.[57] The damage to the Fukushima Daiichi Nuclear Power Station in northern Japan caused by the March 2011 earthquake and tsunami was also listed as a level 7 nuclear disaster, the worst since Chernobyl, and has awakened the worldwide fears about nuclear power. Even so, the use of nuclear power worldwide is expected to double in the next 20 to 25 years.[58] Some research suggests that there may be as many as 400,000 additional cancer patients and over 40,000 deaths from thyroid cancer alone among those within 200 kilometers of the Fukushima Daiichi plant; however, exact information is difficult to obtain.[59] See the **Health Headlines** box for a look at recent events surrounding nuclear energy.

nuclear meltdown Accident that results when the temperature in the core of a nuclear reactor increases enough to melt the nuclear fuel and breach the containment vessel.

Are You Doing All You Can to Protect the Environment?

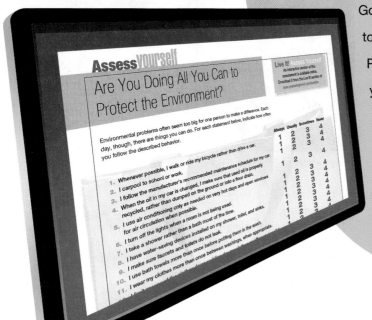

Go online to www.pearsonhighered.com/donatelle to fill out the "Are You Doing All You Can to Protect the Environment?" assessment.* If you need to make some changes, follow the strategies outlined in the **YOUR PLAN FOR CHANGE** box.

*If your instructor so chooses, Assess Yourself Activities are available as a printed supplement or as assignable homework online at www.pearsonhighered.com/myhealthlab.

MyHealthLab®

YOUR PLAN FOR **CHANGE**

Now that you have considered your results from the **Assess** yourself activity, you can take steps to become more environmentally responsible.

Today, you can:

○ Find out how much energy you are using. Visit www.carbonfund.org, www.carbonoffsets.org, or www.greatestplanet.org to find out what your carbon footprint is and to learn about projects you can

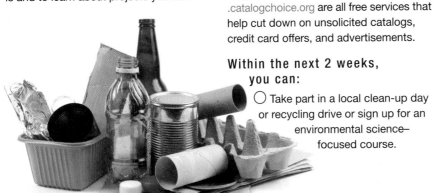

support to offset your own emissions and energy usage.

○ Reduce paper waste in your mailbox. The Direct Marketing Association's Mail Preference Service site (www.dmachoice.org), 1-888-5-OPT-OUT, and www.catalogchoice.org are all free services that help cut down on unsolicited catalogs, credit card offers, and advertisements.

Within the next 2 weeks, you can:

○ Take part in a local clean-up day or recycling drive or sign up for an environmental science–focused course.

By the end of the semester, you can:

○ Check if your campus dining hall composts. If they don't, ask them to start.

○ Make a habit of recycling everything you can, from bottles to batteries.

○ Take part in an environmental activism group on campus or in your community. Let your legislators know how you feel about environmental issues and vote for candidates with pro-environment records.

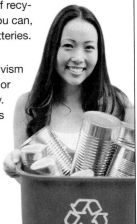

Summary

* Population growth is the single largest factor affecting the environment. Demand for more food, water, and energy—as well as places to dispose of waste—puts great strain on the earth's resources.
* The primary constituents of air pollution are sulfur dioxide, particulate matter, carbon monoxide, nitrogen dioxide, ozone, lead, carbon dioxide, and hydrocarbons. Indoor air pollution is caused primarily by tobacco smoke, woodstove smoke, furnace emissions, asbestos, formaldehyde, radon, lead, and mold.
* Air pollution is depleting Earth's protective ozone layer and contributing to global warming by enhancing the greenhouse effect.
* Water pollution can be caused by either point sources (direct entry) or nonpoint sources (runoff or seepage). Major contributors to water pollution include petroleum products, organic solvents, polychlorinated biphenyls (PCBs), dioxins, pesticides, and lead.
* Municipal solid waste (MSW) includes household trash, plastics, glass, metals, and paper. Many of these items can be recycled. Limited landfill space creates problems in dealing with growing volumes of MSW. Hazardous waste is toxic; improper disposal creates health hazards for people in surrounding communities.
* Nonionizing radiation comes from electromagnetic fields, such as those around power lines. Ionizing radiation results from the erosion of atomic nuclei. The disposal and storage of radioactive waste from nuclear power plants pose potential public health problems.

Pop Quiz

1. The United States is responsible for what percentage of total global resource consumption?
   a. 10 percent
   b. 25 percent
   c. 50 percent
   d. 70 percent

2. Which of the following statements about fertility rates are *correct*?
   a. The United States has shown increases in fertility rates in recent years.
   b. As education levels of women increase and women achieve more equal pay and social status with men, fertility rates typically go down.
   c. Many regions of the world are showing declining fertility rates.
   d. All of the above are correct.

3. One source of indoor air pollution is a gas present in some carpets and home furnishings known as
   a. lead.
   b. asbestos.
   c. radon.
   d. formaldehyde.

4. Which substance separates into stringy fibers that can become embedded in the lungs and cause disease?
   a. Asbestos
   b. Particulate matter
   c. Radon
   d. Formaldehyde

5. The terms *point source* and *nonpoint source* are used to describe the two general sources of
   a. water pollution.
   b. air pollution.
   c. noise pollution.
   d. ozone depletion.

6. The air pollutant that originates primarily from motor vehicle emissions is
   a. particulates.
   b. nitrogen dioxide.
   c. sulfur dioxide.
   d. carbon monoxide.

7. Which gas can potentially become cancer causing when it seeps into a home?
   a. Carbon monoxide
   b. Radon
   c. Hydrogen sulfide
   d. Ozone

8. The barrier that protects us from the sun's harmful ultraviolet rays is
   a. photochemical smog.
   b. the ozone layer.
   c. gray air smog.
   d. the greenhouse effect.

9. A DVD you recently purchased had less packaging than those you had bought previously. This change in packaging design is an example of reducing municipal solid waste by
   a. source reduction.
   b. recycling.
   c. composting.
   d. incineration.

10. Some herbicides contain toxic substances known as
    a. THMs.
    b. PCPs.
    c. dioxins.
    d. PCBs.

Answers to these questions can be found on page A-1.

Think about It!

1. How are the rapid increases in global population and consumption of resources related? Is population control the best solution? Why or why not?
2. What are the primary sources of air pollution? What can be done to reduce air pollution?
3. What are the causes and consequences of global warming? What can individuals do to reduce the threat of global warming?
4. What are point and nonpoint sources of water pollution? What can be done to reduce or prevent water pollution?

5. How do you think communities and governments could encourage recycling efforts? Or, should industry be forced to reduce packaging and waste? Which do you think would have the biggest impact? Why?

Accessing Your Health on the Internet

The following websites explore further topics and issues related to personal health. For links to the websites below, visit the Companion Website for *Access to Health,* 13th Edition, at www.pearsonhighered.com/donatelle.

1. *Environmental Literacy Council.* This website is an excellent source of information about environmental issues in general. Topics range from how the ozone layer works to why the rain forests are important ecosystems. www.enviroliteracy.org

2. *Environmental Protection Agency (EPA).* The EPA is the U.S. government agency responsible for overseeing environmental regulation and protection issues. www.epa.gov

3. *National Center for Environmental Health (NCEH).* This site provides information on a wide variety of environmental health issues and includes a series of helpful fact sheets. www.cdc.gov/nceh

4. *National Environmental Health Association (NEHA).* This organization provides educational resources and opportunities for environmental health professionals. www.neha.org

5. *Environmental Working Group (EWG).* This organization provides resources for consumers, such as a guide to fruits and vegetables ranking the best to worst in terms of pesticide contaminants. They also work for national policy change. www.ewg.org

References

1. United Nations, "World Population to Reach 10 Billion by 2100 if Fertility in All Countries Converges to Replacement Level," 2011, http://esa.un.org/unpd/wpp/index.htm.

2. Worldwatch Institute, "U.N. Raises 'Low' Population Projections for 2050," May 12, 2012, www.worlwatch.org.node/6038.

3. United Nations, *Global Environment Outlook: Environment for Development* (GEO-5): Summary for Policy Makers, 2012, www.uncsd2012.org/rio20/content/documents/280GEO5_SPM_English.pdf.

4. World Wildlife Report, *Living Planet Report 2012,* www.worldwildlife.org/science/2012%20Living%20Planet%20Report/index.html; United Nations, *Global Environmental Outlook,* 2012.

5. United Nations, *Global Environment Outlook,* 2012.

6. United Nations Environmental Program (UNEP), *Green Economy Report,* 2010, www.unep.org/greeneconomy/greeneconomyreport/tabid/29846/default.aspx.

7. U.S. Energy Information Administration, "Independent Statistics and Analysis," 2012, www.eia.gov/oiaf/aeo/tablebrowser/#release=IEO2011&subject=1-IEO2011&table=9-IEO2011&region=0-0&cases=Reference-0504a_1630.

8. N. Eberstadt, "Born in the USA," American Enterprise Institute for Public Policy Research, 2007, www.aei.org/article/25988.

9. "Total Fertility Rate (Children Born/Woman) 2012 Country Ranks, by Rank 2012," *CIA World Fact Book,* www.photius.com/rankings/population/total_fertility_rate_2012_0.html.

10. U.S. Census Bureau, Population Division, "International Data Base Country Rankings," 2010, http://sasweb.ssd.census.gov/idb/ranks.html.

11. U.S. Census Bureau, U.S. and World Population Clocks, "U.S. POPClock Projection," May 19, 2012, www.census.gov/population/www/popclockus.html.

12. World Wildlife Federation, *Living Planet Full Report,* 2012.

13. U.S. Department of Health and Human Services, Healthy People 2010. 2nd ed., vol. 1, *Objectives for Improving Health: Focus Area 9 Family Planning* (Washington, DC: U.S. Government Printing Office, 2000), Available at www.healthypeople.gov/document/HTML/volume1/09Family.htm; Women Deliver, "Women Deliver 2010: Ministers' Forum Statement," 2010, www.womendeliver.org/updates/entry/women-deliver-2010-ministers-forum-statement/.

14. R. H. Friis, *Essentials of Environmental Health* (Boston: Jones and Bartlett, 2007), 232.

15. U.S. Environmental Protection Agency, "Air Pollution Control Orientation Course: Criteria Pollutants," Updated January 2010, www.epa.gov/apti/course422/ap5.html.

16. Ibid.

17. Environmental Protection Agency, "Our Nation's Air: Status and Trends Through 2010," February 2012; American Lung Association, "Health Effects of Ozone and Particle Pollution," in *State of the Air 2010* (Washington, DC: American Lung Association, 2010), Available at www.stateoftheair.org/2010/health-risks.

18. A. Soos, "Acid Rain Change," Environmental News Network, 2012, www.enn.com/enn_news/article/43885.

19. Ibid.; American Lung Association, "Health Effects of Ozone," 2010.

20. U.S. Environmental Protection Agency, "Acid Rain–Reducing Acid Rain," www.epa.gov/aciderain/reducing/index.html.

21. U.S. Energy Information Administration, "Independent Statistics and Analysis," 2012.

22. U.S. Environmental Protection Agency, "Acid Rain: Effects of Acid Rain—Surface Waters and Aquatic Animals," www.epa.gov/acidrain/effects/surface_water.html.

23. Ibid.; A. Soos, "Acid Rain Change," 2012.

24. U.S. Environmental Protection Agency, "Acid Rain: Effects of Acid Rain—Human Health," www.epa.gov/acidrain/effects/health.html.

25. S. McMahon, et al., "Common Toxins in our Homes, Schools and Workplaces," Global Indoor Health Network, 2012, http://globalindoorhealthnetwork.com/files/GIHN_position_statement.pdf.

26. U.S. Environmental Protection Agency, "An Introduction to Indoor Air Quality," Updated April 2010, www.epa.gov/iaq/ia-intro.html.

27. Ibid.

28. U.S. Environmental Protection Agency, "Indoor Air Quality: Radon: Health Risks," Updated March 2010, www.epa.gov/radon/healthrisks.html.

29. U.S. Environmental Protection Agency, "U.S. Homes above EPA's Radon Action Level," Updated June 2010, http://cfpub.epa.gov/eroe/index.cfm?fuseaction=detail.viewInd&lv=list.listByAlpha&r=201747.

30. Centers for Disease Control and Prevention, "Lead," Updated July 2010, www.cdc.gov/nceh/lead.

31. National Center for Environmental Health, "Mold: Basic Facts," 2010, www.cdc.gov/mold/faqs.htm#affect.

32. North Carolina Department of Health and Human Services, Epidemiology, "Indoor Air Quality: Schools," Updated July 2010, www.epi.state.nc.us/epi/air/schools.html.

33. U.S. Environmental Protection Agency, "IAQ Tools for Schools: Improved Academic

Performance: Evidence from Scientific Literature," Updated May 2010, www.epa.gov/iaq/schools/student_performance/evidence.html.

34. U.S. Environmental Protection Agency, "Ozone Layer Depletion: Ozone Science: Brief Questions and Answers on Ozone Depletion," Updated February 2010, www.epa.gov/ozone/science/q_a.html.

35. S. Arrhenius, "On the Influence of Carbonic Acid in the Air Upon the Temperature of the Ground," *Philosophical Magazine and Journal of Science* 5, 41 (1896): 237–75.

36. U.S. Environmental Protection Agency, "Climate Change: Basic Information," 2011, http://epa.gov/climatechange/basicinfo.html.

37. NOAA, State of the Climate Global Analysis, 2011, www.ncdc.noaa.gov/satc/global/2011/2011/13.

38. U.S. Government Accountability Office, *Climate Change: Trends in Greenhouse Gas Emissions and Emissions Intensity in the United States and Other High-Emitting Nations*, (Washington, DC: Government Printing Office, 2012).

39. United Nations Framework Convention on Climate Change, "Kyoto Protocol," 2010, http://unfccc.int/kyoto_protocol/items/2830.php.

40. D. Malakoff and E. M. Williams, "Q & A: An Examination of the Kyoto Protocol," 2007, www.npr.org/templates/story/story.php?storyId=5042766.

41. U.S. Geological Survey, "Water Science for Schools: Where Is Earth's Water Located?" Modified July 2010, http://ga.water.usgs.gov/edu/earthwherewater.html.

42. Department of National Intelligence, "Global Water Security," ICA 2012-08, 2012, www.dni.gov/nic/ICA_Global%20Water%20Security.pdf.

43. Department of National Intelligence, "Global Water Security," ICA 2012-08, 2012, www.dni.gov/NIC/ICA_Global%20Water%20Security.pdf.

44. A. Hekstra and M. Mekonnen, "The Water Footprint of Humanity, *Proceedings of the National Academy of Sciences* 109, no. 9 (2012): 3232–37.

45. U.S. Geological Survey, "Emerging Contaminants in the Environment," 2011, http://toxics.usgs.gov/regional/emc/; U.S. Environmental Protection Agency, "Pharmaceuticals and Personal Care Products (PPCPs)," 2010, www.epa.gov/ppcp/faq.html.

46. J. Donn et al., "AP Probe Finds Drugs in Drinking Water," Associated Press, March 8, 2008.

47. Environmental Protection Agency, Office of Underground Storage Tanks, "FY 2010 Annual Report on the Underground Storage Tank Program," 2010, www.epa.gov/oust.

48. Agency for Toxic Substances and Disease Registry (ATSDR), "Toxic Substances Portal: Polychlorinated Biphenyls (PCBs)," Updated April 2010, www.atsdr.cdc.gov/substances/toxsubstance.asp?toxid=26.

49. U.S. Environmental Protection Agency, "Pesticides: Topical and Chemical Fact Sheets: Assessing Health Risks from Pesticides," Updated September 2009, www.epa.gov/pesticides/factsheets/riskassess.htm.

50. Environmental Protection Agency, "Filters/Home Water Treatment Units (HWTUs)," Updated May 2012, http://safewater.supportportal.com/link/portal/23002/23015/ArticleFolder/1774/Filters-Home-Water-Treatment-Units-HWTUs.

51. U.S. Environmental Protection Agency, *Municipal Solid Waste Generation, Recycling, and Disposal in the United States: Facts and Figures for 2010*, EPA-530-F-11-005 (Washington, DC: U.S. Environmental Protection Agency, 2011), www.epa.gov/osw/nonhaz/municipal/pubs/msw_2010_rcv_factsheet.pdf.

52. EPA Office of Solid Waste, *Municipal Solid Waste in the United States, Facts and Figures for 2010*, EPA-530-F-11-005, 2011, www.epa.gov/osw/nonhaz/municipal/pubs/msw_2010_rev_factsheet.pdf.

53. Ibid.

54. U.S. Environmental Protection Agency, "Superfund: Superfund National Accomplishments Summary, Fiscal Year 2009," Updated May 2010, www.epa.gov/superfund/accomp/numbers09.html.

55. U.S. Nuclear Regulatory Commission, "Radiation Basics," 2011, http://nrc.gov/about-nrc/radiation/health-effects/radiation-basics.html.

56. National Council on Radiation Protection and Measurements, "NCRP Report No. 160 Section 1 Pie Chart," 2010, www.ncrponline.org/Publications/160_Pie_charts.html.

57. R. Balmforth, "Factbox: Key Facts on Chernobyl Nuclear Accident," Reuters, March 15, 2011.

58. U.S. Energy Information Administration, "Independent Statistics and Analysis," 2012.

59. M. Penny and M. Selden. "The Severity of the Fukushima Daiichi Nuclear Disaster: Comparing Chernobyl and Fukushima," Global Research, 2011, www.globalresearch.ca/PrintArticle.php?articleId=24949.

21 Preparing for Aging, Death, and Dying

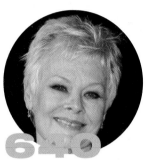

640

Is it really possible to "age gracefully"?

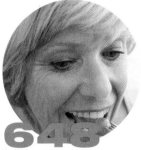

644

Is memory loss an inevitable part of aging?

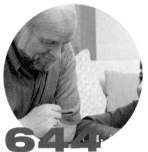

648

Is there any way to slow down the aging process?

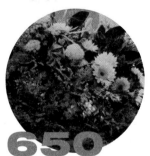

650

How can I help a friend who has just experienced a loss?

OBJECTIVES

✶ Define *aging* and the concepts of biological, psychological, social, legal, and functional age.

✶ List the characteristics of successful aging.

✶ Explain how the growing population of older adults will affect society, including considerations of economics, health care, living arrangements, and ethical and moral issues.

✶ Explain the biological and psychosocial theories of aging and summarize major physiological changes that occur as a result of the normal aging process.

✶ Describe unique health challenges faced by older adults and strategies for successful and healthy aging that can begin during young adulthood.

✶ Discuss death, the stages of the grieving process, and strategies for coping with death.

✶ Explain the ethical concerns that arise from the concepts of the right to die and rational suicide.

✶ Review the decisions that need to be made when someone is dying or has died, including hospice care, funeral arrangements, wills, and organ donation.

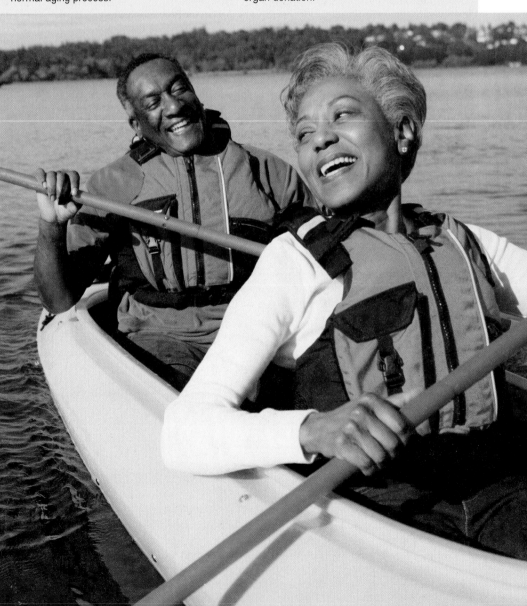

In a society that seems to worship youth, researchers have begun to offer good—even revolutionary—news about the aging process. Growing older doesn't have to mean a slow slide into declining physical and mental health. Health promotion, disease prevention, and wellness-oriented activities can prolong vigor and productivity, even among those who haven't always led model lifestyles or made healthful habits a priority. Numerous research studies show that people who make even modest lifestyle changes can reap significant health benefits. In fact, getting older can mean getting better in many ways—particularly socially, psychologically, spiritually, and intellectually.

Aging has traditionally been described as the patterns of life changes that occur in members of all species as they grow older. Some believe that aging begins at the moment of conception. Others contend that it starts at birth. Still others believe that true aging does not begin until we reach our forties. The study of individual and collective aging processes, known as **gerontology**, explores the reasons for aging and the ways in which people cope with and adapt to this process. Chronological age has traditionally been used to assign people to particular stages of life. However, definitions of aging that consider only years lived rather than quality of life warrant reexamination.

Redefining Aging

Gerontologists have identified several age-related characteristics that define where a person is in terms of biological, psychological, social, legal, and functional life-stage development:[1]

- **Biological age** refers to the relative age or condition of a person's organs and body systems. Research shows that healthy lifestyle behaviors such as being active, eating a healthy diet, and not smoking are the most influential factors on how your body ages.[2]
- **Psychological age** refers to a person's adaptive capacities, such as coping abilities and intelligence, and to the awareness of individual capabilities, self-efficacy, and general ability to adapt to new situations. Research demonstrates that many older adults maintain a positive attitude and successfully cope with the physical and cognitive changes associated with aging.[3]
- **Social age** refers to a person's habits and roles relative to society's expectations.
- **Legal age** is probably the most common definition of age in the United States. Based on chronological years, legal age is used as a factor in determining voting rights, driving privileges, drinking rights, eligibility for Social Security payments, and other rights and obligations.
- **Functional age** refers to a person's status in terms of physical and mental performance.

Hear It! Podcasts

Want a study podcast for this chapter? Download the podcast **Life's Transitions: The Aging Process** at www.pearsonhighered.com/donatelle.

What Is Successful Aging?

Many of today's "elderly" individuals lead active, productive lives. For instance, nearly 21.7 percent of Americans age 65 or over have completed bachelor's through doctoral or professional degrees.[4] The majority of adults over 65 continue to work, care for and help others, engage in social and leisure activities, and remain otherwise active.[5]

Typically, people who age successfully have the following characteristics:

- They stay active, through leisure activities and regular exercise.
- They maintain a normal weight range.
- They eat a healthy diet containing low levels of saturated fats, with plenty of fruits, vegetables, and whole grains.
- They participate in meaningful activities, such as volunteering and other social activities.
- They don't smoke, and they consume alcohol in moderation.[6]

The question is not how many years someone has lived, but how much life the person has packed into those years. This quality-of-life index, combined with the chronological process, appears to be the best indicator of "aging gracefully." Most experts agree that the best way to experience a productive, full, and satisfying old age is to lead a productive, full, and satisfying life prior to old age.

aging Patterns of life changes that occur in members of all species as they grow older.

gerontology The study of individual and collective aging processes.

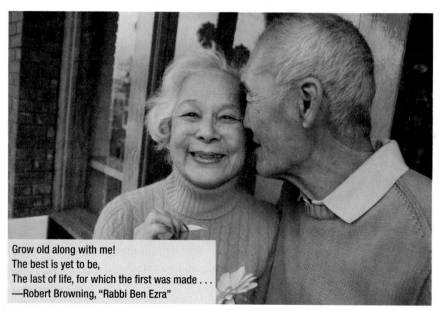

Grow old along with me!
The best is yet to be,
The last of life, for which the first was made . . .
—Robert Browning, "Rabbi Ben Ezra"

Older Adults: A Growing Population

The United States and much of the developed world are on the brink of a *longevity revolution,* one that will affect society in ways that we have not yet begun to understand. According to the latest statistics, life expectancy for a child born in 2012 is 78.49 years, more than 30 years longer than for a child born in 1900.[7] Today there are 40.4 million people age 65 or older in the United States, making up over 13 percent of the total population.[8] By 2030, the older population is expected to be twice as large as in 2000, growing to 72.1 million and representing 19.3 percent of the population. In comparison, a mere 3 million people were age 65 and older in 1900 (Figure 21.1).[9] Other nations report a similar trend. The Population Reference Bureau predicts that by 2050, the percentage of adults over 60 years old will double to 22 percent.[10]

Within the United States, the population of those over 65 will increase substantially over the next two decades, due to the aging "baby boomer" generation and medical advances that prolong life beyond anything imaginable in previous generations. Baby boomers, people born between 1946 and 1964, started turning 65 in 2011. With this aging boom will come a generation of Americans who are better educated, more racially diverse, and more health savvy than past generations. Having come of age as the driving force behind the growth and economic power of the late 20th century, their expectations for health care will be high. Their impact on the economy, housing market, health care system, and Social Security will be profound.

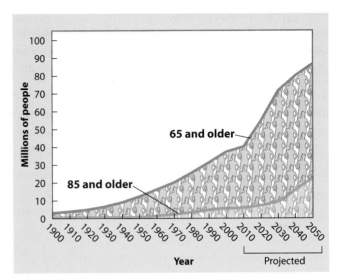

FIGURE 21.1 **Number of Americans 65 and Older (in millions), Years 1900–2008, and Projected 2010–2050**
Source: Data from U.S. Census Bureau, Decennial Census, Population Estimates and Projections. Available at www.census.gov.
Note: Data for 2010–2050 are projections of the population.

Health Issues for an Aging Society

Meeting an older population's financial and medical needs, providing health care and adequate housing, and addressing end-of-life ethical considerations are all of concern in an aging society. You may have heard various political and media debates about the potential bankruptcy of the Social Security system and heavy increases in out-of-pocket expenses for Medicare recipients. Many fear that the combination of fewer younger workers paying into the system and more older people drawing benefits for longer periods will result in tremendous shortfalls.

Health Care Costs Older Americans averaged $4,843 in out-of-pocket medical expenses in 2010, an increase of 49 percent since 2000.[11] These costs included $3,085 (65%) for insurance; $821 (17%) for drugs; $795 (18%) for medical services; and $158 (3%) for medical supplies.[12] As people live longer, the chances of developing a costly chronic disease increase, and as technology improves, chronic illnesses that once were quickly fatal may now be treated successfully for years. Most older adults have at least one chronic condition, and many have multiple conditions. It is estimated that 34 percent of older adults have hypertension, 50 percent have been diagnosed with arthritis, 32 percent with heart disease, 23 percent with cancer, and 19 percent with diabetes.[13] Among people turning 65 today, nearly 69 percent will need some form of long-term care, whether in the community or in a residential care facility.[14]

Is it really possible to "age gracefully"?

The people we often think of as aging gracefully—such as actress Dame Judi Dench—are those who continue to be active and productive; who are not frightened or ashamed of growing older; who adapt to the changing circumstances of their lives; and who strive to be healthy, vibrant, and alive at any age.

90%

of older adults live independently in the community.

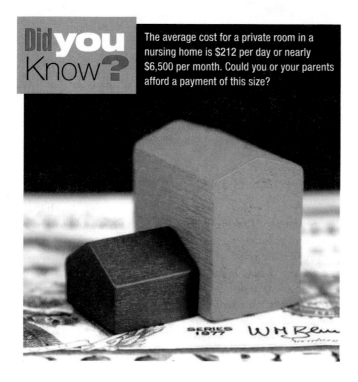

If you have the money, the sky's the limit in terms of superb care for your later years. However, tremendous income-based disparities exist in caring for the elderly. Those without means are more likely to be shut out of all but the most meager care situations.

Ethical and Moral Considerations Difficult ethical questions arise when we consider the implications of an already overburdened health care system. Questions have already surfaced regarding the efficacy of hooking up a terminally ill older person to costly machines that prolong life for a few weeks or months, but overtax health care resources, or performing costly surgeries such as hip replacements on people in their eighties and nineties. Is the prolonging of life at all costs a moral imperative, or will future generations devise a set of criteria for deciding who will be helped and who will not? Such debates leave much room for careful thought and discussion.

Housing and Living Arrangements Most older adults never live in a nursing home. Many live with a spouse, while others live alone or with relatives or friends (Figure 21.2). Increasing numbers of people spend their later years in communities that offer various levels of assistance. Some of these communities allow individuals to purchase their own homes and live fairly independently, sometimes with electronically monitored devices that allow some form of supervision. Other communities and facilities include 24/7 monitoring of unique needs, such as Alzheimer's or other disabilities. Newer, technologically advanced housing includes physiological monitoring that records heart rate and other life indicators to ensure prompt emergency services in case of problems.

Theories of Aging

Social gerontologists, behaviorists, biologists, geneticists, and physiologists continue to explore various potential explanations for why the body breaks down over time. One explanation for the biological cause of aging is the *wear-and-tear theory*, which states that, like everything else in the world, the human body wears out. Inherent in this theory is the idea that the more you abuse your body, the faster it will wear out. Another theory, the *cellular theory*, proposes that at birth we have only a certain number of usable cells, which are genetically programmed to reproduce a limited number of times. Once cells reach the end of their reproductive cycle, they die, and the organs they make up begin to deteriorate.

According to the *genetic mutation theory*, the number of body cells exhibiting unusual or different characteristics increases with age. Proponents of this theory believe that aging is related to the amount of mutational damage within the genes. The more mutation there is, the greater the chance that cells will not function properly.

Finally, the *autoimmune theory* attributes aging to the decline of the body's immunological system. Studies indicate that as we age, the ability to produce necessary antibodies declines, and our immune systems become less effective in fighting disease. At the same time, the white blood cells active in the immune response become less able to recognize foreign invaders and more likely to mistakenly attack the body's own proteins.

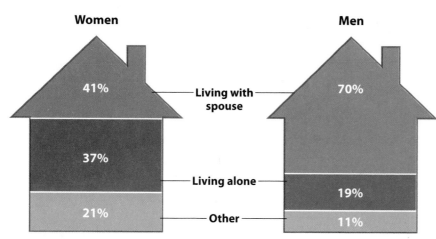

Women   **Men**

41% — Living with spouse — 70%

37% — Living alone — 19%

21% — Other — 11%

FIGURE 21.2 **Living Arrangements of Americans Age 65 and Older** Percentages may not total 100% due to rounding.

Source: Administration on Aging, U.S. Dept. of Health and Human Services, "A Profile of Older Americans: Living Arrangements, 2011," 2012, www.aoa.gov/AoARoot/Aging_Statistics/Profile/2011/6.aspx.

Physical and Mental Changes of Aging

Although the physiological consequences of aging can differ in severity and timing, certain standard changes occur as a result of the aging process. Many of these changes are physical (see Figure 21.3), whereas others are mental or psychosocial.

The Skin

As a normal part of aging, the skin becomes thinner and loses elasticity, particularly in the outer surfaces. Fat deposits, which add to the soft lines and shape of the skin, diminish. Because of the loss of body fat, thinning of the epithelium, and diminished glandular activity, older adults experience greater difficulty regulating body temperature. This limits their ability to withstand extreme cold or heat, which increases the risks of hypothermia, heatstroke, and heat exhaustion.

Starting at about age 30, lines develop on the forehead as a result of smiling, squinting, and other facial expressions. During the forties, these lines become more pronounced, with added "crow's feet" around the eyes. In a person's fifties and sixties, the skin begins to sag and lose color, which leads to pallor in the seventies. Body fat in underlying layers of skin continues to be redistributed away from the limbs and extremities into the body's trunk region. Age spots become more numerous because of excessive pigment accumulation under the skin, particularly in areas of the skin exposed to heavy sun.

osteoporosis Degenerative bone disorder characterized by increasingly porous bones.

Bones and Joints

Throughout the life span, bones are continually changing because of the accumulation and loss of minerals. By the third or fourth decade of life, mineral loss from bones becomes more prevalent than mineral accumulation, which results in a weakening and porosity (diminishing density) of bony tissue. **Osteoporosis** is a disease characterized by low bone density and structural deterioration of bone tissue. These porous, fragile bones are susceptible to fracture and may lead to crippling malformation of the spine characteristic of the dowager's hump seen in stooped individuals.

Many people think osteoporosis is a disease affecting only older women, but it can occur at any age and affects men, as

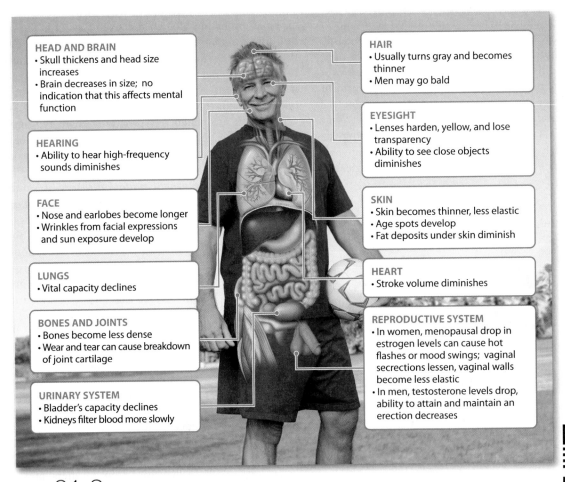

HEAD AND BRAIN
• Skull thickens and head size increases
• Brain decreases in size; no indication that this affects mental function

HEARING
• Ability to hear high-frequency sounds diminishes

FACE
• Nose and earlobes become longer
• Wrinkles from facial expressions and sun exposure develop

LUNGS
• Vital capacity declines

BONES AND JOINTS
• Bones become less dense
• Wear and tear can cause breakdown of joint cartilage

URINARY SYSTEM
• Bladder's capacity declines
• Kidneys filter blood more slowly

HAIR
• Usually turns gray and becomes thinner
• Men may go bald

EYESIGHT
• Lenses harden, yellow, and lose transparency
• Ability to see close objects diminishes

SKIN
• Skin becomes thinner, less elastic
• Age spots develop
• Fat deposits under skin diminish

HEART
• Stroke volume diminishes

REPRODUCTIVE SYSTEM
• In women, menopausal drop in estrogen levels can cause hot flashes or mood swings; vaginal secrections lessen, vaginal walls become less elastic
• In men, testosterone levels drop, ability to attain and maintain an erection decreases

FIGURE 21.3 **Normal Effects of Aging on the Body**

Video Tutor: Effects of Aging on Body

well. More than 44 million Americans have osteoporosis, including 14 million men. Each year, about half of all women over 50—and up to 1 in 4 men—will break a bone because of osteoporosis.[15] Bone density scans using dual-energy X-ray absorptiometry can screen for osteoporosis. With early detection, steps can be taken to reverse bone loss and prevent fractures.

Some of the factors that predispose a person to developing osteoporosis are intrinsic and cannot be controlled, including gender, age, body size, ethnicity, and family history. You cannot modify these factors, but there *are* things you can do to prevent the disease. During your lifetime, bone is constantly being added (formation) and being broken down and removed (reabsorption). At around age 30, a person reaches *peak bone mass*. After this point, a slow and steady decline occurs. Individuals who develop strong, dense, healthy bones through proper diet and exercise can minimize this decline and reduce their risk for osteoporosis.

Adequate calcium intake is important, as is vitamin D, which helps the body absorb and use calcium more efficiently. Bone is a living tissue that grows stronger with exercise and weight-bearing activity; therefore, bone loss can be slowed or prevented with regular weight-bearing exercise, such as walking, jogging, and dancing, as well as through strength training. Unhealthy behaviors that contribute to bone loss include smoking, excessive alcohol consumption, and anorexia nervosa.

Another bone condition that afflicts almost 27 million Americans is *osteoarthritis,* a progressive breakdown of joint cartilage that becomes more common with age and is a major cause of disability in the United States.[16]

Head and Face

With age, features of the head enlarge and become more noticeable. Increased cartilage and fatty tissue cause the nose to grow a half inch wider and another half inch longer. Earlobes get fatter and grow longer. As the skull becomes thicker with age, the overall head circumference increases one quarter of an inch per decade, even though the brain itself shrinks.

50%

of older adults in long-term care facilities experience urinary incontinence.

Urinary Tract

At age 70, the kidneys can filter waste from the blood only half as fast as they could at age 30. The need to urinate more frequently occurs because the bladder's capacity declines from 2 cups of urine at age 30 to 1 cup at age 70.

One problem sometimes associated with aging is **urinary incontinence,** which ranges from passing a few drops of urine while laughing or sneezing to having no control over urination. Urinary incontinence affects more than half of all persons in long-term care facilities, and it is the second leading cause of institutionalization.[17]

Incontinence can pose major social, physical, and emotional problems. Embarrassment and fear of wetting oneself may cause an older person to become isolated and avoid social functions. Caregivers may become frustrated with incontinent patients. Prolonged wetness and the inability to properly care for oneself can lead to tissue irritation, infections, and other problems. However, incontinence is not an inevitable part of aging. Most cases are caused by persistent infections, medications, treatable neurological problems that affect the central nervous system, weakness in the pelvic wall, and so on. When the problem is treated, the incontinence is usually resolved.[18]

Heart and Lungs

Resting heart rate stays about the same over the course of a person's life, but the stroke volume (the amount of blood the heart pushes out per beat) diminishes as heart muscle deteriorates. Vital capacity, or the amount of air that moves when you inhale and exhale at maximum effort, also declines with age. Exercise can do a great deal to preserve heart and lung function. Not smoking and avoiding smoke-filled environments are important ways of reducing risks.

The Senses

With aging, the senses (vision, hearing, touch, taste, and smell) become less acute. By age 30, the lens of the eye begins to harden, which can cause problems by the early forties. The lens begins to yellow and lose transparency, and the pupil shrinks, allowing less light to penetrate. By age 60, depth perception declines, and farsightedness often develops. **Cataracts** (clouding of the lens) and **glaucoma** (elevated pressure within the eyeball) become more likely. Eventually, a tendency toward color blindness may develop, especially for shades of blue and green. **Macular degeneration** is the breakdown

urinary incontinence Inability to control urination.

cataracts Clouding of the lens that interrupts the focusing of light on the retina, resulting in blurred vision or eventual blindness.

glaucoma Elevation of pressure within the eyeball, leading to hardening of the eyeball, impaired vision, and possible blindness.

macular degeneration Breakdown of the macula, the light-sensitive part of the retina responsible for sharp, direct vision.

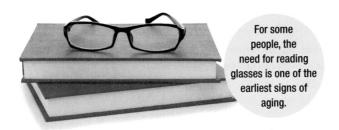

For some people, the need for reading glasses is one of the earliest signs of aging.

of the light-sensitive area of the retina responsible for the sharp, direct vision needed to read or drive. Its effects can be devastating to independent older adults; the causes are still being investigated.

With age, the ear structure also experiences changes and often deteriorates. The eardrum thickens, and the inner ear bones are affected. The inner ear is the portion that controls balance (equilibrium). As a result, it often becomes difficult for a person to maintain balance. Studies have shown that exercises including resistance/strength training, yoga, and tai chi can improve balance in older adults.[19] The ability to hear high-frequency consonants (e.g., *s*, *t*, and *z*) also diminishes with age. Much of the actual hearing loss lies in the inability to distinguish extreme ranges of sound rather than an inability to distinguish normal conversational tones.

Many studies have indicated that with age, there is a reduced or changed sensation of pain, vibration, cold, heat, pressure, and touch. Some of these changes may be caused by decreased blood flow to the touch receptors or to the brain and spinal cord.[20] It may become difficult, for example, to tell the difference between cool and cold. Decreased temperature sensitivity increases the risk of injuries such as hypothermia and frostbite.

The senses of taste and smell are closely connected. The number of taste buds decreases starting at about age 40 in women and age 50 in men. Each remaining taste bud also begins to atrophy (lose mass). The sense of smell may diminish, especially after age 70. This may be related to loss of nerve endings in the nose. Studies on the cause of decreased sense of taste and smell have conflicting results. Some studies have indicated that normal aging produces very little change in taste and smell.[21] Therefore, changes may be related to chronic diseases, smoking, and environmental exposures over a lifetime.

Sexual Function

As men age, they experience noticeable alterations in sexual function. Although the degree and rate of change vary greatly from man to man, several changes generally occur, including a slowed ability to obtain an erection, diminished ability to maintain an erection, and a decline in angle of the erection. Men may also experience a longer refractory period between orgasms and shortened duration of orgasm.

Women also experience several changes in sexual function as they age. Menopause usually occurs between the ages of 45 and 55. Women may experience hot flashes, mood swings, weight gain, development of facial hair, or other hormone-related symptoms. The walls of the vagina become less elastic, and the epithelium thins, possibly making intercourse painful. Vaginal secretions, particularly during sexual activity, diminish. The breasts become less firm, and loss of fat in various areas leads to fewer curves, with a decrease in the soft lines of body contours.

Although these physiological changes may sound discouraging, sex is still an essential component in the lives of those in their mid-fifties and older, and many people remain sexually active throughout their entire adult lives. According to studies, the proportion of elderly couples (couples between their mid-50s and age 70) who engaged in sexual activity is approximately 50 percent.[22] In addition, approximately 20 to 30 percent of both men and women remain sexually active well into their eighties. With the advent of drugs such as Viagra and medical interventions designed to treat sexual dysfunction, many older adults are able to be sexually active. However, adults over the age of 61 reported the lowest percentages of condom use, with 5.1 percent for men and 7.4 percent for women, signifying a need for education with this population.

Mental Function and Memory

Given an appropriate length of time, older people learn and develop skills in a manner similar to younger people. Researchers have also determined that what many older adults lack in speed of learning they make up for in practical knowledge—that is, the "wisdom of age." Memory loss is

See It! Videos
Why do some seniors prefer work over retirement? Watch **Seniors Say No to Retirement** at www.pearsonhighered.com/donatelle.

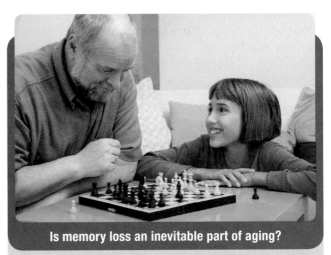

Is memory loss an inevitable part of aging?

No. In fact, all of us have periods when remembering things seems more difficult than during other times due to stress, illness, grief, task overload, injury or trauma, relationship problems, or other challenges. Certain physiological conditions or diseases may cause older people to experience memory loss, but in general the knowledge and memories gained through a lifetime remain intact.

not necessarily a normal part of aging; however, as a person ages, drug interactions, vascular deficiencies, hormonal or biochemical imbalances, and other physiological changes can make memory lapses occur more frequently. Although short-term memory may fluctuate on a daily basis, in the absence of disease, the ability to remember events from past decades seems to remain largely unchanged.

What can you do to help improve memory and overall mental functioning as you age? Generally, those who maintain their memory in old age have exercised and kept their cardiovascular system and other body systems healthy over the years. Another key to maintaining memory is keeping your mind active as well. Those who foster their creative side and engage their minds by reading books, solving puzzles (crossword, Sudoku), playing musical instruments, volunteering, and, in general, sharpening their brains seem to fare much better in the memory department. As with the physical aspects of the body, "use it or lose it" applies to your brain acuity.

Depression

Most older adults lead healthy, fulfilling lives. However, while research indicates that depression is the most common psychological problem affecting this population, the rate of major depression is actually lower among older people than it is among younger adults. Regardless of age, people who have a poor perception of their health, have multiple chronic illnesses, take a lot of medications, abuse alcohol or other drugs, lack social support, and do not exercise face more challenges to their emotional resilience.

Dementias and Alzheimer's Disease

Memory failure, errors in judgment, disorientation, or erratic behavior can occur at any age and for various reasons, including nutrient deficiency (such as vitamin B deficiency), alcohol abuse, medication interactions, vascular problems, tumors, hormonal or metabolic imbalances, or any number of problems. Often, when the underlying issues are corrected, the memory loss and disorientation also improve. The terms *dementing diseases,* or **dementias,** are used to describe either reversible symptoms or progressive forms of brain malfunctioning.

Although there are many types of dementia, one of the most common forms is **Alzheimer's disease (AD).** Affecting an estimated 5.4 million Americans, this disease is one of the most painful and devastating conditions that families can endure.[23] It kills its victims twice: first through a slow loss of personhood (memory loss, disorientation, personality changes, and eventual loss of independent functioning), and then through the deterioration of body systems as they gradually succumb to the powerful impact of neurological problems.

The number of individuals with AD has significantly increased in the United States. Because of the increase in the number of people over 65 in the United States, the annual total number of new cases of Alzheimer's and other dementias is projected to double by 2050. An estimated 15 million family members and friends cared for a person with Alzheimer's disease or another dementia in 2011.[24] Patients with AD live for an average of 4 to 6 years after diagnosis, although the disease can last for up to 20 years.[25] Caring for a person with AD can be a heavy financial burden; the average cost of nursing care is between $79,110 and almost $87,235 each year.[26] Most people associate the disease with the aged, but AD has been diagnosed in people in their late forties.

Alzheimer's disease is a degenerative illness that involves areas of the brain developing "tangles" that impair the way nerve cells communicate, eventually causing them to die. This degeneration occurs in the sections of the brain that affect memory, speech, and personality, leaving the parts that control other functions, such as heartbeat and breathing, functioning at near-normal levels. Thus, the mind begins to go while the body lives on.

This disease characteristically progresses in stages, each of which is marked by increasingly impaired memory and judgment. In later stages of the disease, these symptoms can be accompanied by agitation and restlessness (especially at night), loss of sensory perceptions, muscle twitching, and repetitive actions. Many patients become depressed, combative, and aggressive. In the final stage, disorientation is often complete. The person becomes dependent on others for eating, dressing, and other activities. Identity loss and speech problems are common. Eventually, control of bodily functions may be lost.

Researchers are investigating several possible causes of AD, including genetic predisposition, immune system malfunction, a slow-acting virus, chromosomal or genetic defects, chronic inflammation, uncontrolled hypertension, and neurotransmitter imbalance. There is no treatment that can stop the progression of AD, but there are medications that can prevent some symptoms from progressing for a short period of time or relieve symptoms such as sleeplessness, anxiety, and depression. Some researchers are looking at anti-inflammatory drugs, theorizing that AD may develop in response to an inflammatory ailment. Others are focusing on studying deposits of protein called plaques and their role in damaging and killing nerve cells.[27]

dementias Progressive brain impairments that interfere with memory and normal intellectual functioning.

Alzheimer's disease (AD) Chronic condition involving changes in nerve fibers of the brain that results in mental deterioration.

4%

of Alzheimer's cases occur before age 65.

Alcohol and Drug Use and Abuse

Those who are prone to alcoholism in their younger years are likely to continue drinking later in life. Alcohol abuse is more common among older men than it is among older women. Yet, those age 65 and older have the lowest rates of drinking among any age group. Those who do drink do so less than younger persons.[28]

If recent studies are accurate, the reason there aren't many heavy drinkers among older adults may be that very heavy drinkers tend to either die of alcoholic complications before they grow old or because they are afraid of combining alcohol with their prescription drugs. Most older adults who consume alcohol are not alcoholics but rather social drinkers.

Older people rarely use illicit drugs, but some do overuse or misuse prescription drugs. *Polypharmacy,* or polydrug use (the simultaneous use of multiple medications), is common in older adults. It is estimated that 88 percent of adults age 60 years and older take at least one prescription drug, compared to 48 percent of adults age 20 to 59 years. Furthermore, 37 percent of adults age 65 years and over reported taking five or more prescribed drugs. Anyone who combines different drugs runs the risk of dangerous drug interactions.[29]

People also must be aware of the possible effects of medications they take, alone or in combination. It is estimated that almost 100,000 Americans are hospitalized for adverse drug reactions each year, with most of these events linked to drugs for treatment of diabetes or to blood thinners.[30] Nearly two thirds of the hospitalizations were due to unintentional overdoses. The risks of adverse effects are even greater for people with impaired circulation and declining kidney and liver function.

Currently, there is no one system that tracks all of a patient's prescriptions. To avoid drug interactions and other problems, older adults should use the same pharmacy consistently, ask questions about medicines, dosages, and possible drug interactions, and read the directions carefully.

Strategies for Healthy Aging

As you know from reading this book, you can do many things to prolong and improve the quality of your life. To provide for healthy older years, make each of the following part of your younger years.

Improve Fitness

Just about any moderate-intensity exercise that gets your heart beating faster and increases strength and/or flexibility will maximize your physical health and functional years. One of the physical changes that the body undergoes is *sarcopenia,* age-associated loss of muscle mass. The less muscle

TABLE 21.1 Exercise Recommendations for Adults over Age 65		
Option 1:	**Option 2:**	**Option 3:**
Moderate-intensity aerobic activity (e.g., brisk walking) at least 2 hours and 30 minutes every week **and** muscle-strengthening activity, working all major muscle groups, on 2 or more days a week	Vigorous-intensity aerobic activity (e.g., jogging or running) at least 1 hour and 15 minutes every week **and** muscle-strengthening activity, working all major muscle groups, on 2 or more days a week	An equal mix of moderate- and vigorous-intensity aerobic activity **and** muscle-strengthening activity on 2 or more days a week

Source: Centers for Disease Control, "How Much Physical Activity Do Older Adults Need?" 2011, www.cdc.gov/physicalactivity/everyone/guidelines/olderadults.html.

you have, the less energy you will burn even while resting. The lower your metabolic rate, the more likely you will gain weight. With regular strength training, you can increase your muscle mass, boost your metabolism, strengthen your bones, prevent osteoporosis, and feel better and function more efficiently.

Both aerobic and muscle-strengthening activities are critical for healthy aging. Table 21.1 lists basic recommendations for aerobic and strength-training exercises for older adults. In addition to these, the Centers for Disease Control and Prevention recommends that people who are at risk of falling perform regular balance exercises.[31] It is also recommended that older adults or individuals with chronic conditions develop an activity plan with a health professional to manage risks and take therapeutic needs into account. This will maximize the benefits of physical activity and ensure your safety. The **Health in a Diverse World** box on the following page describes more of the benefits of physical activity.

Eat for Longevity

Certain nutrients are especially essential for healthy aging:

- **Calcium.** Bone loss tends to increase in women, particularly in the hip region, shortly before menopause. During perimenopause and menopause, this bone loss accelerates rapidly, with an average of about 3 percent skeletal mass lost per year over a 5-year period. The result is an increased risk for fracture and disability. Adequate consumption of calcium throughout one's life can help prevent bone loss.
- **Vitamin D.** Vitamin D is necessary for adequate calcium absorption, yet as people age, particularly in their fifties and sixties, they do not absorb vitamin D from foods as readily as before. If vitamin D is unavailable, calcium levels are also likely to be lower.

See It! Videos

What can you do to increase your chances of living until age 100? Watch **Vitality Project** at www.pearsonhighered.com/donatelle.

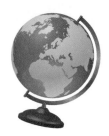

KEEPING FIT AS WE AGE

Physical activity is the key for maintaining health and independence as people age, but regular physical activity is not widespread among older adults. According to the National Institutes of Health, regular physical activity is reported by only 30 percent of Americans age 45 to 64, 25 percent of those age 65 to 74, and 11 percent of those age 85 and older.

The Centers for Disease Control and Prevention identifies regular physical activity as one of the most important things that can be done to maintain your health as you age. The benefits include:

✳ Maintenance and improvement of physical strength and fitness
✳ Improvement of balance
✳ Better management of diseases such as diabetes, heart disease, and osteoporosis
✳ Reduction in feelings of depression and improved mood and overall well-being

Recent studies have found that older adults who keep active may reduce their

Many forms of activity can improve physical fitness.

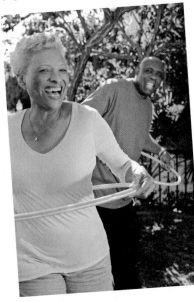

odds of losing their mental abilities. "If we want to become a healthy and fit

nation, we need to increase the number of Americans who are healthy at every stage of life," U.S. Surgeon General Dr. Regina Benjamin stated.

A new program called Go4Life (http://go4life.nia.nih.gov) is meant to encourage people 50 and older to become and stay active to improve their health. Go4Life provides older adults with resources to be physically active, such as sample exercise programs and videos. Go4Life is based on studies demonstrating the benefits of exercise and physical activity for older people, including those with chronic health conditions. This program shows them that, even with physical limitations, it is possible to exercise safely. Programs like Go4Life are also important because they are able to reach out to older adults who have traditionally not been physically active.

Source: National Institute on Aging, "New Go4Life Campaign Focuses on Fitness for Older Adults," October 2011, www.nia.nih.gov/newsroom/2011/10/new-go4life-campaign-focuses-fitness-older-adults.

● **Protein.** As some older adults become concerned about cholesterol and fatty foods and others face a limited food budget, they often cut back on protein. Meat and seafood products cost more and have the "fat" stigma associated with animal products. Yet protein is necessary for muscle mass, and protein insufficiencies can spell trouble.

Other nutrients, including vitamin E, folic acid (folate), iron, potassium, CoQ10, and vitamin B_{12} (cobalamin), are important to the aging process, and most of these are readily available in any diet that follows the U.S. Department of Agriculture's (USDA) MyPlate recommendations (www.choosemyplate.gov).

Develop and Maintain Healthy Relationships

Social bonds lend vigor and energy to life. Be willing to give to others, and seek variety in your relationships rather than befriending only people who agree with you. By interacting

with diverse people and considering different points of view, we gain a new perspective on life.

Enrich the Spiritual Side of Life

Although we often take the spiritual side of life for granted, cultivating a relationship with nature, the environment, a higher being, and yourself is a key factor in personal growth and development. Take time for thought and quiet contemplation, and enjoy the sunsets, sounds, and energy of life. Setting aside time for quiet, meaningful moments will leave you invigorated and refreshed—better able to cope with life's ups and downs.

What's Working for You?

Maybe you're already on the path to aging well. Which of these are you already incorporating into your life?

☐ I exercise on a regular basis and eat a healthy diet most of the time.

☐ I stay engaged in work, school, and/or volunteer activities that have meaning for me.

☐ I keep in touch with family and old friends and have a strong support network.

☐ I get out socially on a regular basis.

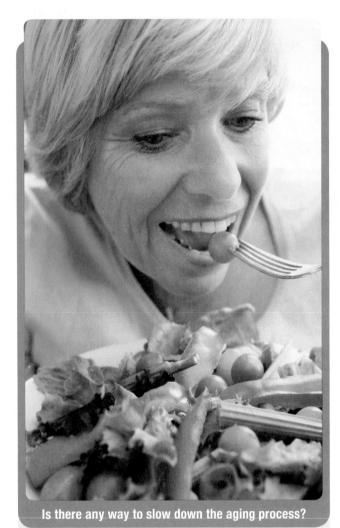

Is there any way to slow down the aging process?

Aging is inevitable, but if you take good care of your body, mind, and spirit, you can prevent disease and delay the deterioration of abilities that can lead to disability or a poor quality of life in old age. Participating in regular physical activity and following a healthy diet are two of the most important things you can do to stay active and thrive throughout all the years of your life.

Understanding the Final Transitions: Dying and Death

Throughout history, humans have attempted to determine the nature and meaning of death. Individuals' feelings about death vary widely, depending on many factors, including age, religious beliefs, family orientation, health, personal experience with death, and the circumstances of the death itself. To cope effectively with dying, we must address the individual needs of those involved.

death The permanent ending of all vital functions.

brain death Irreversible cessation of all functions of the entire brainstem.

dying Process of decline in body functions that results in the death of an organism.

Defining Death

According to the *Merriam Webster Dictionary*, **death** can be defined as the "a permanent cessation of all vital functions: the end of life."[32] This definition has become more significant as medical advances make it increasingly possible to postpone death. Legal and ethical issues led to the Uniform Determination of Death Act in 1981. This act, which several states have adopted, reads as follows: "An individual who has sustained either (1) irreversible cessation of circulatory and respiratory functions, or (2) irreversible cessation of all functions of the entire brain, including the brainstem, is dead. A determination of death must be made in accordance with accepted medical standards."[33]

The concept of **brain death,** defined as the irreversible cessation of all functions of the entire brainstem, has gained increasing credence. As defined by the Ad Hoc Committee of the Harvard Medical School, brain death occurs when the following criteria are met:[34]

- Unreceptivity and unresponsiveness—that is, no response even to painful stimuli
- No movement for a continuous hour after observation by a physician, and no breathing after 3 minutes off a respirator
- No reflexes, including brainstem reflexes; fixed and dilated pupils
- A "flat" electroencephalogram (EEG, which monitors electrical activity of the brain) for at least 10 minutes
- All of these tests repeated at least 24 hours later with no change
- Certainty that hypothermia (extreme loss of body heat) or depression of the central nervous system caused by use of drugs such as barbiturates are not responsible for these conditions

The Harvard report provides useful guidelines; however, the definition of death and all its ramifications continues to concern us.

what do you think?

Why is there so much concern over the definition of *death*?
- How does modern technology complicate the understanding of when death occurs?

The Dying Process

Dying is the process of decline in body functions that results in the death of an organism. It is a complex process that includes physical, intellectual, social, spiritual, and emotional dimensions. Now that we have examined the physical indicators of death, we must consider the emotional aspects of dying and "social death."

Coping Emotionally with Death

Science and medicine have enabled us to understand many changes throughout the life span, but they have not fully explained the nature of death. This may explain why the transition from life to death evokes so much mystery and emotion. Although emotional reactions to dying vary, many people share similar experiences during this process.

Kübler-Ross and the Stages of Dying Much of our knowledge about reactions to dying is based on the work of Elisabeth Kübler-Ross, a pioneer in **thanatology,** the study of death and dying. In 1969, Kübler-Ross published *On Death and Dying,* a sensitive analysis of the reactions of terminally ill patients. This pioneering work encouraged the development of death education as a discipline and prompted efforts to improve the care of dying patients. Kübler-Ross identified five psychological stages (Figure 21.4) that people coping with death often experience.[35]

1. Denial. ("Not me, there must be a mistake.") A person intellectually accepts the impending death but rejects it emotionally and feels a sense of shock and disbelief. The patient is too confused and stunned to comprehend "not being" and thus rejects the idea.

2. Anger. ("Why me?") The person becomes angry at having to face death when others, including loved ones, are healthy and not threatened. The dying person perceives the situation as unfair or senseless and may be hostile to friends, family, physicians, or the world in general.

3. Bargaining. ("If I'm allowed to live, I promise . . .") The dying person may resolve to be a better person in return for an extension of life or may secretly pray for a short postponement of death to experience a special event, such as a family wedding or birth.

4. Depression. ("It's really going to happen, and I can't do anything about it.") Depression eventually sets in as vitality diminishes and the person begins to experience symptoms with increasing frequency. The person's deteriorating condition becomes impossible for him or her to deny. Common feelings experienced during this stage include doom, loss, worthlessness, and guilt over the emotional suffering of loved ones and arduous but seemingly futile efforts of caregivers.

5. Acceptance. ("I'm ready.") This is often the final stage. The patient stops battling with emotions and becomes tired and weak. With acceptance, the person does not "give up" and become sullen or resentfully resigned to death, but rather becomes passive.

Some of Kübler-Ross's contemporaries consider her stage theory too neat and orderly. Subsequent research has indicated that the experiences of dying people do not fit easily into specific stages, and patterns vary from person to person. Some people never go through this process and instead remain emotionally calm; others may shift back and forth between various stages. Even if it is not accurate in all its particulars, Kübler-Ross's theory does offer valuable insights for those seeking to understand or deal with the process of dying.

Corr's Coping Approach Charles Corr developed an alternative model based on the idea that there are unique challenges and responses for the dying person and those who love him or her.[36] He suggests four dimensions of coping with loss: *physical*—doing everything possible to make oneself comfortable and minimize pain; *psychological*—living to the fullest, focusing on life accomplishments, and seeking satisfaction in daily activities; *social*—nurturing relationships, keeping loved ones involved, and sharing emotions; and *spiritual*—identifying what matters in life and reaffirming meaningful experiences.

thanatology The study of death and dying.

social death A seemingly irreversible situation in which a person is not treated like an active member of society.

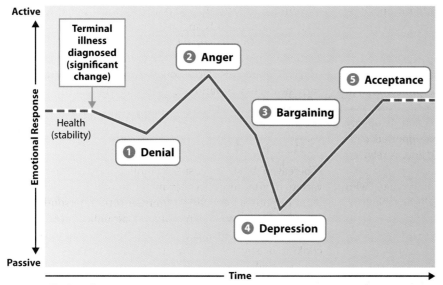

FIGURE 21.4 **Kübler-Ross's Stages of Dying**
Kübler-Ross developed this model while working with terminally ill patients. She later expanded the model to apply to people experiencing grief or significant loss of any kind.

Social Death

The need for recognition and appreciation within a social group is nearly universal. Loss of being valued or appreciated by others can lead to **social death,** a situation in which a person is not treated like an active member of society. Numerous studies indicate that people are treated differently when they are dying, leading them to feel more isolated and unable to talk about their feelings: The dying person may be excluded from conversations or referred to as if he or she were already dead.[37] Dying patients are often moved to terminal wards and may be given minimal care; medical personnel may make degrading or impersonal comments about dying patients in their presence. In addition, inadequate pain control may contribute to patient suffering and anger or hostility, making caregiver assistance more difficult.

A decrease in meaningful social interaction often strips dying and bereaved people of their identity as valued members of society at a time when being able to talk, share, and make important decisions or say important things is critical.

Coping with Loss

Coping with the loss of a loved one is extremely difficult. The dying person, as well as close family and friends, frequently suffers emotionally and physically from the loss of critical relationships and roles.

Bereavement is generally defined as the loss or deprivation that a survivor experiences when a loved one dies. The death of a parent, spouse, sibling, child, friend, or pet will result in different kinds of feelings for different people. We should not make assumptions about the value a person places on his or her relationship with the deceased or the nature of his or her feelings about the loss. For example, often people fail to recognize the importance a pet can have, especially in single people's lives; for some, the loss of a pet may be as significant as the loss of a child. The loss of a loved one leaves "holes" and inevitable changes. Loneliness and despair may envelop the survivors. Understanding these normal reactions, along with time, patience, and support from loved ones can do much to help the bereaved heal and move on, even though they will not forget.

Grief occurs in reaction to significant loss, including one's own impending death, the death of a loved one, or a *quasi-death* experience (a significant loss such as the end of a relationship or job, which involves separation, rejection, or a change in personal identity). Grief may be experienced as a mental, physical, social, or emotional reaction and often includes changes in patterns of eating, sleeping, working, and even thinking.

When a person experiences a loss that cannot be openly acknowledged, publicly mourned, or socially supported, coping may be much more difficult. This type of grief is referred to as *disenfranchised grief*. It may occur among people who experience a miscarriage, who are developmentally disabled, or who are close friends rather than blood relatives of the deceased. It may also include relationships that are not socially approved, such as extramarital affairs or homosexual relationships.

Symptoms of grief vary in severity and duration, depending on the situation and the individual. However, the bereaved person can benefit from emotional and social support from family, friends, clergy, employers, and traditional support organizations. The larger and stronger the support system, the easier readjustment is likely to be. See the **Skills for Behavior Change** box to learn how you can best help a grieving friend.

The term *mourning* is often incorrectly equated with the term *grief*. As we have noted, *grief* refers to a wide variety of feelings and actions that occur in response to bereavement. **Mourning,** in contrast, refers to culturally prescribed and accepted time periods and behavior patterns for the expression of grief. In Judaism, for example, *sitting shivah* is a designated mourning period of 7 days that involves prescribed rituals and prayers. Depending on a person's relationship with the deceased, various other rituals may continue for up to a year.

What Is "Typical" Grief?

A bereaved person may suffer emotional pain and exhibit a variety of grief responses for many months after the death. Grief responses vary widely from person to person but frequently include such symptoms as periodic waves of prolonged physical distress, a feeling of tightness in the throat, choking or shortness of breath, sighing, feelings of emptiness, muscular weakness, or intense anxiety that is described as actually painful.

Other common symptoms of grief include insomnia, memory lapses, loss of appetite, difficulty concentrating, a tendency to engage in repetitive or purposeless behavior, a feeling of being removed from reality, difficulty making

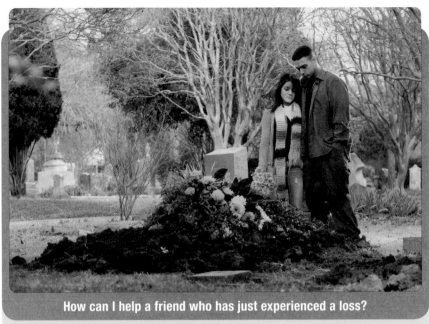

How can I help a friend who has just experienced a loss?

The most important thing you can do for a grieving friend is offer emotional support and a caring presence. Knowing what to say is less important than knowing how to listen. Acknowledge the loss, let your friend know you care, and be there when he or she needs to talk or express grief.

bereavement Loss or deprivation experienced by a survivor when a loved one dies.

grief An individual's reaction to significant loss, including one's own impending death, the death of a loved one, or a quasi-death experience; grief can involve mental, physical, social, or emotional responses.

mourning Culturally prescribed behavior patterns for the expression of grief.

decisions, lack of organization, excessive talking, social withdrawal or hostility, guilty feelings, and preoccupation with the image of the deceased. Susceptibility to disease increases with grief and may even be life threatening in severe and enduring cases.

The rate of the healing process depends on the amount and quality of grief work that a person does. **Grief work** is the process of integrating the reality of the loss into everyday life and learning to feel better. Often, a bereaved person must deliberately and systematically work at reducing denial and coping with the pain that comes from remembering the deceased.

Grief and Trauma

Disasters, war, and other events can leave many people suddenly bereaved of spouses, children, parents, close friends, and coworkers. In the immediate aftermath of the event, some bereaved survivors feel numb or unable to accept the loss. Many feel shocked, lost, anxious, and depressed. For many, the pain from their loss can be intense and unrelenting. These emotional and bodily reactions may be very strong and can themselves be traumatizing, especially if they are unfamiliar and unexpected. This secondary reaction can further amplify the pain caused by the loss.

> **grief work** Process of accepting the reality of a person's death and coping with memories of the deceased.

It is important to realize that intense and unfamiliar emotionality is entirely normal and does not necessarily have implications for long-term emotional stability or health. However, if the symptoms linger and become increasingly debilitating, the condition turns into what is now being referred to as unresolved, traumatic, or complicated grief, which has features of both depression and post-traumatic stress disorder (PTSD). The most characteristic symptoms are intrusive thoughts and images of the deceased person and a painful yearning for his or her presence. Other complications are denial of the death, imagining that the dead person is alive, desperate loneliness and helplessness, anger and bitterness, and wanting to die. Treatment requires professional therapy and can include a promising new treatment called traumatic grief therapy, which uses cognitive behavioral methods for traumatic symptoms and stress relief, along with interpersonal techniques to encourage reengagement with the world.

Worden's Model of Grieving Tasks

William Worden, a researcher into the death process, developed an active grieving model that suggests four developmental tasks that a grieving person must complete in the grief work process:[38]

1. **Accept the reality of the loss.** This task requires acknowledging and realizing that the person is dead. Traditional rituals, such as the funeral, help many bereaved people move toward acceptance.

2. **Work through the pain of grief.** It is necessary to acknowledge and work through the pain associated with loss, or it will manifest itself through other symptoms or behaviors.

3. **Adjust to an environment in which the deceased is missing.** The bereaved may feel lonely and uncertain about a new identity without the person who has died. This loss confronts them with the challenge of adjusting their own sense of self.

4. **Emotionally relocate the deceased and move on with life.** Individuals never lose memories of a significant relationship. They may need help in letting go of the emotional energy that used to be invested in the person who has died, and they may need help in finding an appropriate place for the deceased in their emotional lives. See the **Skills for Behavior Change** box on the following page for more suggestions on living with grief.

Children and Death

Children are highly valued in our society, and their deaths are considered major tragedies. No matter what the cause of death—miscarriage, fatal birth defects, childhood illness,

Talking to Friends When Someone Dies

DO . . .

) Let your genuine concern and caring show; say you are sorry about their loss and pain.

) Be available to listen, run errands, help with children, or whatever else seems needed at the time.

) Allow them to express as much grief as they are feeling at the moment and are willing to share.

) Encourage them to be patient with themselves and not worry about things they should be doing.

) Allow them to talk about the person who has died as much and as often as they want to.

) Reassure them that they did everything they could, that the medical care given was the best, or whatever else you know to be true and positive about the care given.

DON'T . . .

) Let your own sense of helplessness keep you from reaching out to those who are bereaved.

) Avoid them because you are uncomfortable.

) Say you know how they feel (unless you've suffered a similar loss, you probably don't).

) Say, "You ought to be feeling better by now" or anything else that implies judgment about their feelings or what they should be doing.

) Change the subject when they mention the person who has died.

accident, suicide, homicide, natural disaster, neglect, or war injuries—the grief experienced when a child dies may be overwhelming.

Siblings of a deceased child may have a particularly hard time with grief work. Because so much attention and energy are devoted to the deceased child, the surviving children may feel emotionally abandoned by their parents. They may feel uncomfortable talking about death, and they may also receive less social support and sympathy than their parents do.

Bereaved children usually have limited experience with death and therefore have not yet learned how to deal with major loss. Often, when children suffer a loss, they will continue to behave "normally" to the adult observer. When it comes to complex emotional issues, children do not always show their feelings as openly as adults. Children tend to experience more prolonged grieving periods. They worry about whether they caused the death and whether they will die or will lose someone else they love, and they worry about what will happen to them and to the person who died. It can be helpful for family members to involve children in the dying process and to talk

> ## what do you think?
>
> **If you have experienced a death among your family or friends, how did you grieve?**
> ● Did you accomplish Worden's tasks?
> ● Did any of the models discussed match your experience?

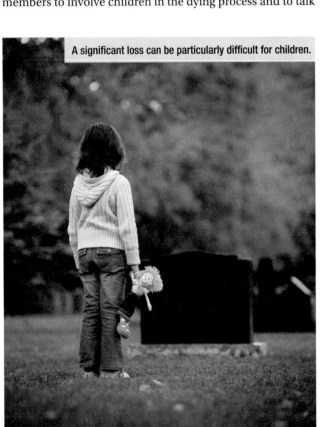

A significant loss can be particularly difficult for children.

with them about the death while reassuring them of their safety. A professional counselor may also be of help in assisting children who are coping with loss.

Life-and-Death Decision Making

When a loved one is dying, many complex and emotional—and often expensive—life-and-death decisions must be made during a highly distressing period.

The Right to Die

Few people would object to the right to a dignified death. Going beyond that concept, however, many people today believe that they should be allowed to die if their condition is terminal and their existence depends on mechanical life-support devices or artificial feeding or hydration systems. Artificial life-support techniques that may be legally refused by competent patients include electrical or mechanical heart resuscitation, mechanical respiration by machine, nasogastric tube feedings, intravenous nutrition, gastrostomy (tube feeding directly into the stomach), and medications to treat life-threatening infections.

As long as a person is conscious and competent, he or she has the legal right to refuse treatment, even if this decision will hasten death. However, when a person is in a coma or otherwise incapable of speaking on his or her own behalf, medical personnel, family members, and administrative policy will dictate treatment. This issue has evolved into a battle involving personal freedom, legal rulings, health care administration policy, and physician responsibility. The living will and other **advance directives** were developed to assist in solving these conflicts.

Even young, apparently healthy people need a **living will.** Consider Terri Schiavo, who collapsed at age 26 from heart failure that led to irreversible brain damage. Schiavo, unable to survive without life support, never left any written guidelines about her wishes should she become incapacitated. After a 15-year legal battle between her parents, who wanted her to be kept alive, and her husband, who felt she should be allowed to die, the courts sided with her husband, and she was removed from life support. There are examples of living wills online, including at http://estate.findlaw.com/living-will/sample-living-will-form.html.

Many legal experts suggest that you take the following steps to ensure that your wishes are carried out.[39]

- **Be specific.** Complete an advance directive that permits you to make very specific choices about a variety of procedures, including cardiopulmonary resuscitation (CPR); being placed on a ventilator; being given food, water, or medication through tubes; being given pain medication; and organ donation.
- **Get an agent.** You may want to appoint a family member or friend to act as your agent, or *proxy,* by completing a form known as either a *durable power of attorney for health care* or a *health care proxy.*
- **Discuss your wishes.** Discuss your preferences in detail with your proxy and your doctor.
- **Deliver the directive.** Distribute several copies, not only to your doctor and your agent, but also to your lawyer and to immediate family members or a close friend. Make sure *someone* knows to bring a copy to the hospital in the event you are hospitalized.

One alternative to the traditional advance directive or living will is a document called *Five Wishes* that is written in uncomplicated language and meets the legal requirements for advance directive statutes in most states. This document differs from most other living wills because it addresses personal, emotional, and spiritual needs, as well as medical needs.[40] It is available at low cost online at www.agingwithdignity.org.

Rational Suicide and Euthanasia

Although exact numbers are not known, estimates are that thousands of terminally ill people every year decide to kill themselves rather than endure constant pain and slow decay. This alternative to the extended dying process is known as **rational suicide.** To these people, the prospect of an undignified death is unacceptable. This issue has been complicated by advances in death prevention techniques that allow terminally ill patients to exist in an irreversible disease state for extended periods of time.

According to public opinion polls, most Americans believe that suicide is morally wrong but are divided on whether physician-assisted suicide is morally acceptable. Roughly 70 percent of Americans believe doctors should be allowed to help end an incurably ill patient's life painlessly at the patient's request.[41]

Physician-assisted suicide is not a new phenomenon. It has been practiced in many societies throughout history and currently is legal in some European countries, such as Belgium and the Netherlands. Legalization of assisted suicide has been debated in many U.S. states. Currently, more than 30 states have statutes explicitly prohibiting assisted suicide and only three states—Oregon, Washington, and Montana—have laws allowing for physician-assisted suicide under certain circumstances.[42] See the **Points of View** box on the following page for a discussion of this topic.

Euthanasia is often referred to as "mercy killing." The term **active euthanasia** refers to ending the life of a person (or animal) who is suffering greatly and has no chance of recovery. An example might be a physician-prescribed lethal injection, as in physician-assisted suicide. **Passive euthanasia** refers to the intentional withholding of treatment that would prolong life. Deciding not to place a person with massive brain trauma on life support is an example of passive euthanasia. Advance directives, such as "do not resuscitate" orders, can provide legal justification for various forms of passive euthanasia.

advance directive Document that stipulates an individual's wishes about medical care; used to make treatment decisions when an individual becomes physically unable to voice his or her preferences.

living will Type of advance directive.

rational suicide The decision to kill oneself rather than endure constant pain and slow decay.

active euthanasia "Mercy killing" in which a person or organization knowingly acts to end the life of a terminally ill person.

passive euthanasia Intentional withholding of treatment that would prolong life.

palliative care Any form of medical care focused on relieving the pain, symptoms, and stress of serious illness to improve the quality of life for patients and their families.

Making Final Arrangements

Caring for a dying person and his or her loved ones involves a wide variety of psychological, legal, social, spiritual, economic, and interpersonal issues.

Hospice Care: Positive Alternatives

Since the mid-1970s, hospice programs in the United States have grown from a mere handful to more than 5,100 and are available in nearly every community.[43] These programs are a form of **palliative care** that focus on reducing pain and suffering while attending to the emotional and spiritual needs of dying individuals and their caregivers. Hospice care may help the survivors cope better with the death experience.

Physician-Assisted Suicide:
SHOULD IT BE LEGALIZED?

Physician-assisted suicide (also known as *physician aid-in-dying*) refers to a practice in which the physician provides, at a terminally ill patient's request, a lethal dose of medication that the patient intends to use to end his or her own life. Currently, more than 30 states have statutes explicitly prohibiting assisted suicide. Only Oregon, Montana, and Washington allow physician-assisted suicide under certain circumstances. Oregon's Death with Dignity Act states that a person must be 18 years or older, a resident of Oregon, competent to make health decisions, and diagnosed with a terminal illness that will lead to death within 6 months. The physician must determine that all of these factors have been met. The arguments for and against the legalization of physician-assisted suicide within individual states continue to be debated. Below are some of the major points from both sides of the issue.

Arguments in Favor of Legalization of Physician-Assisted Suicide

○ Decisions about time and circumstances regarding death are personal, and a competent person with a terminal illness should have the right to choose death.

○ For some patients, treatment refusal does not lead to death quickly enough; therefore, their only option is to commit suicide. Justice requires that patients should be allowed to choose death.

○ Many terminal conditions are accompanied by tremendous suffering and pain. Physician-assisted suicide is a compassionate response to unbearable suffering.

○ Physician-assisted suicide already occurs, but behind closed doors and in secret. Legalization of physician-assisted suicide would promote open discussion of existing practices.

○ Physician-assisted suicide is not a new phenomenon. It has been practiced in many societies throughout history and currently is legal in some European countries, such as Belgium and the Netherlands.

Arguments against Legalization of Physician-Assisted Suicide

○ It is unethical to take a human life, and historical, ethical traditions of medicine strongly oppose taking life. The Hippocratic Oath states, "I will not administer poison to anyone where asked," and "Be of benefit, or at least do no harm."

○ There is an important difference between passively letting someone die and actively killing. Treatment refusal or withholding treatment equates to letting a patient die (passive) and is justifiable, whereas physician-assisted suicide equates to killing (active) and is not morally justifiable.

○ Certain groups of terminally ill people, lacking access to care and support, may be pushed into assisted suicide. Physician-assisted suicide may become a cost-containment strategy. Burdened family members and health care providers may encourage the option of assisted suicide.

○ There may be uncertainty in the diagnosis and prognosis of the terminal illness. There may be errors in diagnosis and treatment of depression, or inadequate treatment of pain.

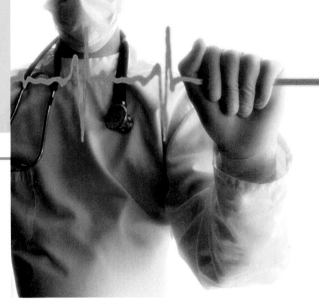

Where Do You Stand?

○ Do you think physician-assisted suicide should be legalized in your state?

○ What criteria do you think should be used to monitor physician-assisted suicide if it were widely legalized?

○ What are your feelings on physician-assisted suicide in general? Is it an appropriate option for patients diagnosed with devastating terminal illnesses?

Sources: C. H. Braddock III and M. R. Tonelli, University of Washington, School of Medicine, "Physician Aid-in-Dying," Revised 2012, http://depts.washington.edu/bioethx/topics/pad.html; Oregon Department of Human Services, "FAQ's about the Death with Dignity Act," Updated 2012, http://public.health.oregon.gov/ProviderPartnerResources/EvaluationResearch/DeathwithDignityAct/Pages/faqs.aspx; International Task Force on Euthanasia and Assisted Suicide, "Assisted Suicide Laws," Updated February 2012, www.patientsrightscouncil.org/site/assisted-suicide-state-laws.

Making Funeral Arrangements

Anthropological evidence indicates that all cultures throughout human history have developed some sort of funeral ritual. For this reason, social scientists agree that funerals assist survivors in coping with their loss. In the United States, with its diversity of religious, regional, and ethnic customs, funeral practices vary. (See the **Be Healthy, Be Green** box on the following page to learn how environmental responsibility is influencing today's funeral, burial, and memorial practices.) In some faiths, the deceased may be displayed to formalize last respects and increase social support of the bereaved. This part of the funeral ritual is referred to as a *wake* or *viewing*. The funeral service may be held in a church, a funeral chapel, or at the burial site. Some people choose to replace the funeral service with a simple memorial service held within a few days of the burial. Social interaction that is part of funeral and memorial services is valuable in helping survivors cope.

In addition to details related to the type of funeral or memorial service and the method of burial or body disposition, loved ones must also consider the cost of funeral and memorial options. They usually have to contact friends and relatives, plan for the arrival of guests, choose markers, submit obituary information to newspapers, and deal with many other details. Even though funeral directors are available to facilitate decision making, the bereaved may experience undue stress, especially if the death is sudden and unexpected. People who make their own funeral arrangements ahead of time can save their loved ones the difficulty of having to make these decisions during a very stressful time.

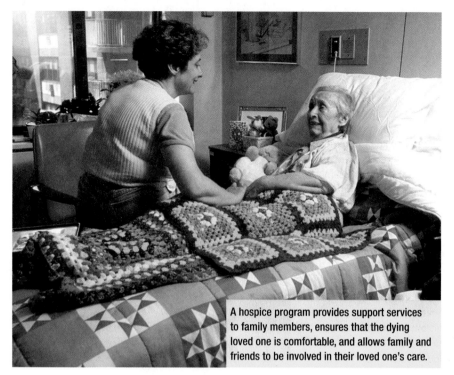

A hospice program provides support services to family members, ensures that the dying loved one is comfortable, and allows family and friends to be involved in their loved one's care.

Hospice volunteers provide much needed "respite" care for caregivers who often face emotional and physical challenges in caring for dying loved ones.

The primary goals of **hospice** programs are to relieve the dying person's pain; offer emotional support to the dying person and loved ones; and restore a sense of control to the dying person, family, and friends. Hospice programs usually include the following characteristics:

- There is overall medical direction of the program, with all health care provided under the direction of a qualified physician. Emphasis is placed on symptom control, primarily the alleviation of pain.
- Services are provided by an interdisciplinary team.
- Coverage is provided 24 hours a day, 7 days a week, with emphasis on the availability of medical and nursing skills.
- Carefully selected and extensively trained volunteers who augment but do not replace staff service are an integral part of the health care team.
- Care of the family extends through the bereavement period.
- Patients are accepted on the basis of their health needs, not their ability to pay.

Despite the growing number of individuals and families who consider hospice facilities, some people prefer to die in a hospital, and others choose to die at home. In some communities, hospice services are available as in-home care. Individuals and families should decide as early as possible what type of terminal care is most desirable and feasible to allow time for the necessary emotional, physical, and financial preparations.

Wills

The issue of inheritance is controversial in some families and should be resolved before a person dies to reduce both conflict and needless expense. Unfortunately, many people are so intimidated by the thought of making a will that they never do so and die **intestate** (without a will). This is tragic, especially because the procedure for establishing a legal will is relatively simple and inexpensive. In addition, if you don't make a will before you die, the courts (as directed by state laws) will make a will for you. Legal issues, rather than your wishes, will preside. Furthermore, settling an estate takes longer when a person dies without a will.

hospice Type of end-of-life care designed to maximize quality of life and help dying people have peace, comfort, and dignity.

intestate Dying without a will.

GREEN GOODBYES

Worldwide, more than 56 million people die each year. Nearly all of those people are given some form of burial, funeral, or cremation, and yet traditional practices can have significant and negative environmental impacts. With growing awareness of these impacts has come an increased interest in ways to "go green" in funeral, burial, and cremation practices.

Each year, more than 20,000 cemeteries in the United States bury millions of feet of hardwood; tens of thousands of tons of steel, copper, and bronze; and more than a million tons of reinforced concrete. In addition, it is estimated that more than 1 million gallons of embalming fluid are buried in the United States every year. These chemicals (including formaldehyde, glutaraldehyde, phenol, methanol, antibiotics, dyes, and more) eventually make their way into the soil and can potentially contaminate water supplies.

Instead of traditional cemetery and burial sites, you can opt for a green burial site that prohibits the use of formaldehyde-based embalming fluids, metal caskets, and concrete burial vaults. Typically, these sites are located in nature preserves that eschew the manicured expanses of lawn present in modern cemeteries. They have restrictions on the density of burials allowed, as well as strict guidelines aimed at conservation and preservation of the ecosystem. To find locations of natural cemeteries, start by checking out www.naturalburial.coop or www.greenburialcouncil.org.

Many green cemeteries and other burial sites choose to plant living markers instead of erecting tombstones. Traditional grave markers are made of stone, a nonrenewable resource, and most leave a carbon footprint, as both the mining and shipping of them produce excess carbon. In contrast, a living marker is a tree, bush, plant, or flowers planted in memory of the deceased loved one. This not only reduces waste and negative environmental impact, but also contributes to the development of green landscape.

Green coffins are also available as an alternative to traditional coffins made of metal, plastic, endangered hardwood, or particleboard with formaldehyde glues. Greener options include coffins made of oak, pine, cardboard, willow, seagrass, wicker, fair-trade bamboo, and other natural materials that are more sustainable, biodegradable, and renewable. In addition, some burial sites allow one to forgo the coffin altogether and bury loved ones in natural-cloth shrouds.

Cremation has historically been viewed as a more ecofriendly option because the environmental footprint is much less than that of traditional burials. Although cremation does not involve the land use that burial does, it takes a lot of energy, approximately the same amount required to power an average car for a distance of 4,800 miles, and the burning process releases carbon and particulate emissions into the air. However, these emissions are relatively low in comparison to others in our society. Some fast-food restaurants release 0.46 pound of carbon an hour, whereas the human cremation process emits only 0.08 pound an hour. Environmental monitoring agencies have imposed emission standards on crematoriums that help to keep the levels down. Furthermore, some crematoriums are installing additional filters to catch smaller particulate matter.

Another alternative to traditional burial is the controversial and relatively new process of "promession," or freeze-drying.

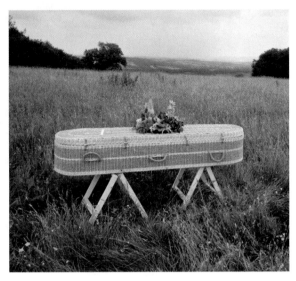

Ecofriendly burial options include coffins made of biodegradable materials, such as this wicker model.

This technique, developed by Swedish biologist Susanne Wiigh-Mäsak, was patented in 1999 and first introduced to the public in May 2001. Currently, there are a few facilities in Europe that perform promession. The first step in promession involves freezing the body in a vat of liquid nitrogen, a process that makes the body very brittle. Next, the body is gently broken apart with ultrasonic vibration. This creates a damp powder that is then dried and packaged in a small biodegradable coffin that can be buried alongside a living memorial plant. As the "promains" become wet from rain and watering, they naturally decompose, composting the soil and providing nourishment to the living memorial.

Sources: S. Grover, "How to Go Green: Funerals," Planet Green, 2010, http://planetgreen .discovery.com/go-green/funerals/funerals-basics .html; Green Burial Council, "Frequently Asked Questions," 2012, www.greenburialcouncil.org/ faqs-fiction/.

Trusts

Trusts are estate-planning tools that can help you manage property during your life if you are disabled by accident or illness and ensure a smooth transition of affairs after your death. While a trust sounds appealing, there are some aspects to be aware of. A living trust is more expensive to set up than a typical will because it must be actively managed after it is created. Most importantly, however, a living trust is useless unless it is funded, and it can only control those assets that have been placed into it. If your assets have not been transferred or if you die without funding the trust, the trust will be of no benefit: Your estate will still be subject to probate, and there may be significant estate tax issues.[45]

Organ Donation

Organ donation takes healthy organs and tissues from one person for transplantation into another. Experts say that the organs from one donor can save or help as many as 50 people. You can donate internal organs (kidneys, heart, liver, pancreas, intestines, lungs); skin; bone and bone marrow; and corneas. Most organ and tissue donations occur after the donor has died, but some organs and tissues can be donated while the donor is alive.[44]

Organ donation saves lives: Approximately 79 people receive organ transplants every day. However, an average of 18 people die each day waiting for transplants because of the shortage of donated organs.[45] The number of patients waiting for organs continues to significantly outnumber the donor organs available, and the gap is increasing (Figure 21.5).

People of all ages and background can be organ donors. It's especially important to consider becoming an organ donor if you are African American, Asian or Pacific Islander, Native American, or Hispanic. Members of these groups have a higher prevalence of certain chronic conditions that affect the kidney, heart, lung, pancreas, and liver, all of which can be treated with organ transplantation. Matching blood type is necessary for transplants, and because certain blood types are more common in particular ethnic groups, the need for minority donor organs is especially high.[46]

If you want to be an organ donor, the most important thing to do is to enroll in your state's donor registry. Go to www .organdonor.gov to sign up under your state. It is also a good idea to indicate your decision on your driver's license, tell your family about your donation decision, tell your physician, and include the donation in your will and living will. Uniform donor cards are available through the U.S. Department of

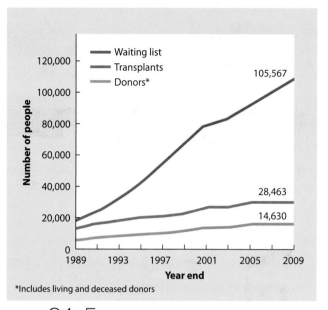

FIGURE 21.5 **Organ Donors and Patients Needing and Receiving Transplants, 1989–2009**

Source: U.S. Department of Health and Human Services, "The Need Is Real: Data," 2011, www.organdonor.gov/about/data.html.

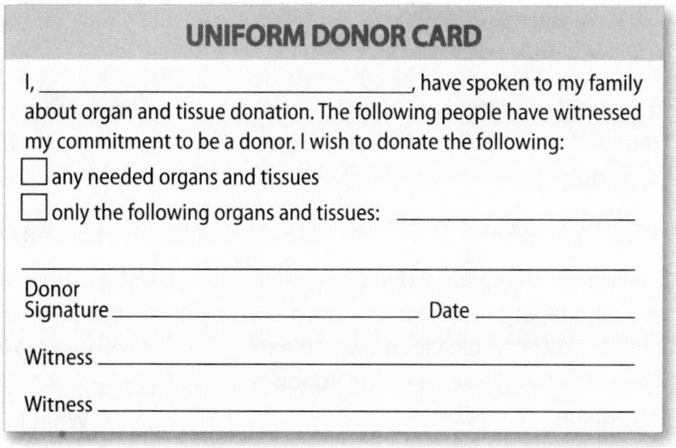

Health and Human Services and through many health care foundations and nonprofit organizations (Figure 21.6).

Although some people are opposed to organ transplants and tissue donation, others experience personal fulfillment from knowing that their organs may extend and improve someone else's life after their own death.

UNIFORM DONOR CARD

I, _____, have spoken to my family about organ and tissue donation. The following people have witnessed my commitment to be a donor. I wish to donate the following:

☐ any needed organs and tissues

☐ only the following organs and tissues: _____

_____

Donor
Signature _____ Date _____

Witness _____

Witness _____

FIGURE 21.6 **Organ Donor Card**
Each organ and tissue donor can save or improve the lives of as many as 50 people.

Are You Afraid of Death?

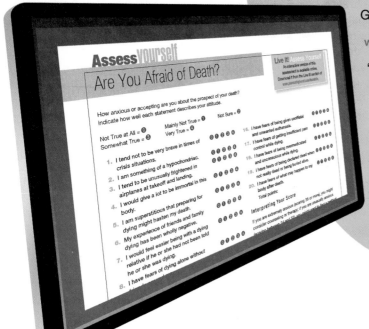

Assess Yourself
Are You Afraid of Death?

Go online to the **Live It!** section of www.pearsonhighered.com/donatelle to take the "Are You Afraid of Death?" assessment.* Use the strategies outlined in the **YOUR PLAN FOR CHANGE** box to take steps to lessen your fears about death and dying.

*If your instructor so chooses, Assess Yourself Activities are available as a printed supplement or as assignable homework online at www.pearsonhighered.com/myhealthlab.

MyHealthLab®

YOUR PLAN FOR CHANGE

After completing the "Are You Afraid of Death?" **Assess yourself** activity, you can begin to change beliefs that may be causing you anxiety on the subject of death and dying.

Today, you can:

◯ Learn about advance directives. Visit a low-cost legal clinic for information and a sample. You can also locate samples online, including the *Five Wishes* document, which is available at www.agingwithdignity.org.

◯ Fill out an organ donation card. Knowing that you may be able to prolong another person's life after your death can help you feel more at peace with your mortality.

Within the next 2 weeks, you can:

◯ Write down a list of goals you want to attain by ages 30, 40, and 50. Think about the steps you need to take to attain these goals.

◯ Talk to family members about their life goals. What have they achieved, and what do they wish they had done differently? What can you learn from their experiences?

By the end of the semester, you can:

◯ Consider how you feel about various medical techniques that might be used in the event you become incapacitated. Do you feel comfortable being kept alive by a machine? Make your wishes on these matters known to family members and friends, and put them in writing.

◯ Talk to your parents or grandparents about the arrangements they prefer in the event of their death. Do they want a burial or cremation? A full funeral or a small service? Making these decisions now will save you and your loved ones stress later.

Summary

* Aging can be defined in terms of biological age, psychological age, social age, legal age, or functional age. The growing number of older adults (age 65 and older) has an increasing impact on society in terms of the economy, health care, housing, and ethical considerations.

* Biological explanations of aging include the wear-and-tear theory, the cellular theory, the genetic mutation theory, and the auto-immune theory. Psychosocial theories center on adaptation and adjustments related to self-development.

* Aging changes the body and mind in many ways. Physical changes occur in the skin, bones and joints, head, urinary tract, heart and lungs, senses, sexual function, and temperature regulation. Major physical concerns are osteoporosis, urinary incontinence, and changes in eyesight and hearing. Most older people maintain a high level of mental functioning and memory. Potential mental problems include depression and Alzheimer's disease.

* Lifestyle choices we make today will affect health status later in life. Choosing to exercise, eat a healthy diet, foster lasting relationships, engage in spiritual development, and avoid unhealthy habits such as smoking will contribute to healthy aging.

* *Death* can be defined biologically in terms of brain death or the ces-sation of vital functions. Dying is a multifaceted emotional process, and individuals may experience emotional stages such as denial, anger, bargaining, depression, and acceptance. Social death results when a person is no longer treated as an active member of society.

* Grief is the state of distress felt after loss. People differ in their responses to grief. Children need to be helped through the process of grieving.

* Hospice services are available to provide care for the terminally ill and their caregivers. The right to die by rational suicide involves ethical, moral, and legal issues.

* After death, funeral arrangements must be made quickly and customs vary by family, region, religious affiliation, and cultural background.

* Decisions made in advance of ill-ness and death through advance directives, wills, trusts, and organ donation cards make the process easier for survivors.

Pop Quiz

1. Which biological theory of aging supports the concept that body cells are able to reproduce only so many times throughout life?
   a. Wear-and-tear theory
   b. Cellular theory
   c. Autoimmune theory
   d. Genetic mutation theory

2. The progressive breakdown of joint cartilage is known as
   a. osteoporosis.
   b. osteoarthritis.
   c. calcium loss.
   d. vitamin D deficiency.

3. Martha's ophthalmologist tells her she has a condition that involves the breakdown of the light-sensitive area of the retina that is affecting her sharp, direct vision. What is this condition?
   a. Cataracts
   b. Glaucoma
   c. Macular degeneration
   d. Nearsightedness

4. What is the most common form of dementia in older adults?
   a. Alzheimer's disease
   b. Incontinence
   c. Depression
   d. Psychosis

5. The keys to successful aging include
   a. being physically active.
   b. eating a healthy diet.
   c. not smoking.
   d. All of the above

6. The study of death and dying is known as
   a. thanatology.
   b. gerontology.
   c. biology.
   d. geriatrics.

7. The Kübler-Ross stage of dying in which the individual rejects death emotionally and feels a sense of shock and disbelief is known as
   a. acceptance.
   b. bargaining.
   c. denial.
   d. anger.

8. A culturally prescribed and accepted period of grief for some-one who has died is known as
   a. bereavement.
   b. grief work.
   c. coping with loss.
   d. mourning.

9. Grief work is
   a. the process of integrating the reality of a loss with everyday life and learning to feel better.
   b. the total acceptance that a loved one has died.
   c. assigning feelings to the loss of a loved one.
   d. completing the cultural rituals required to express one's grief.

10. Kerri's elderly grandmother is ter-minally ill and wants to die without medical intervention. Her family has agreed to withhold treatment that may prolong her life. This is called
    a. rational suicide.
    b. health care proxy.
    c. passive euthanasia.
    d. active euthanasia.

Answers to these questions can be found on page A-1.

Think about It!

1. Discuss when you think people should start deciding whether to have an advance directive. What are some important considerations when preparing an advance directive?
2. As the older population grows, how will it affect your life? Would you be willing to pay higher taxes to support government programs for older adults? Why or why not?
3. List the major physical and mental changes that occur with aging. Which of these, if any, can you change? Discuss actions you can start taking now to ensure a healthier aging process.
4. Explain why so many of us deny death. How could death become a more acceptable topic to discuss?
5. Debate whether rational suicide should be legalized for the terminally ill. What restrictions would you include in a law?

Accessing Your Health on the Internet

The following websites explore further topics and issues related to personal health. For links to the websites below, visit the Companion Website for *Access to Health*, 13th Edition, at www.pearsonhighered.com/donatelle.

1. *AARP.* This site includes comprehensive information on issues related to aging, including longevity and caregiving. www.aarp.org
2. *Administration on Aging.* This U.S. Department of Health and Human Services link is dedicated to addressing the health needs of older adults. www.aoa.gov
3. *Alzheimer's Association.* This site includes media releases, position statements, fact sheets, and research on Alzheimer's disease. www.alz.org
4. *Grieving.com.* This forum site addresses all aspects of grief and loss, including terminal illness, non-death losses, and caregiving. http://forums.grieving.com
5. *National Hospice and Palliative Care Organization.* This site offers information on hospice care, including resources for finding a hospice, end-of-life issues, and advance directives. www.nhpco.org
6. *National Institute on Aging.* A site that provides information and research updates on aging-related issues. www.nia.nih.gov
7. *Organ Donation and Transplant Association of America.* This site provides information related to organ donation. http://odtaa.org

References

1. J. C. Cavanaugh and F. Blanchard-Fields, *Adult Development and Aging*, 6th ed. (Belmont, CA: Wadsworth, Cengage Learning, 2011); S. Hillier and G. Barrow, *Aging, the Individual, and Society*, 9th ed. (Belmont, CA: Wadsworth, Cengage Learning, 2011).
2. Centers for Disease Control and Prevention and the Merck Company Foundation, *The State of Aging and Health in America 2007* (Whitehouse Station, NJ: The Merck Company Foundation, 2007), Updated 2009. Available at www.cdc.gov/aging/data/stateofaging.htm.
3. Ibid.
4. Administration on Aging, U.S. Department of Health and Human Services, "A Profile of Older Americans: 2010, Education," 2011, Available from www.aoa.gov/AoAroot.
5. Federal Interagency Forum on Aging Related Statistics, "Older Americans 2010: Key Indicators of Well-Being," (Washington, DC: U.S. Government Printing Office, 2011), Available at www.agingstats.gov/agingstatsdotnet/main_site/default.aspx.
6. National Institute on Aging, "Healthy Aging: Lessons from the Baltimore Longitudinal Study of Aging," 2010. Available at www.nia.nih.gov/health/publication/healthy-aging-lessons-baltimore-longitudinal-study-aging.
7. Central Intelligence Agency, "The World Factbook. Country Comparisons: Life Expectancy at Birth," 2012. Available at www.cia.gov/library/publications/the-world-factbook/rankorder/2102rank.html.
8. Administration on Aging, U.S. Department of Health and Human Services, "A Profile of Older Americans: 2011, Education," 2012, Available at www.aoa.gov/aoaroot/aging_statistics/Profile/.
9. Federal Interagency Forum on Aging Related Statistics, "Older Americans 2010: Key Indicators of Well-Being," 2011.
10. Population Reference Bureau, "America's Aging Population," *Population Bulletin* 66, no. 1 (2011); "Networks of Cities Tackle Age-Old Problem," *Bulletin of the World Health Organization* 88 (2010): 406–407.
11. Administration on Aging, "A Profile of Older Americans: 2011," 2012, www.aoa.gov/aoaroot/aging_statistics/Profile/2011/9.aspx.
12. Administration on Aging, "A Profile of Older Americans: 2011, Health and Health Care," 2012, Available at www.aoa.gov/aoaroot/aging_statistics/Profile/.
13. Ibid.
14. Florida Health Care Association, "Facts about Long-term Health Care in Florida," 2010. www.fhca.org/media_center/long_term_health_care_facts/.
15. Osteoporosis and Related Bone Diseases—National Resource Center, "Fast Facts about Osteoporosis," 2011, www.niams.nih.gov/bone/hi/ff_osteoporosis.htm; National Institute of Arthritis and Musculoskeletal Disease, "Osteoporosis," Reviewed May 2009, www.niams.nih.gov/Health_Info/Bone?Osteoporosis/default.asp; National Osteoporosis Foundation, "Bone Health Basics," 2011, www.nof.org/aboutosteoporosis/bonebasics/whybonehealth.
16. Centers for Disease Control and Prevention, "Osteoarthritis," 2011, www.cdc.gov/arthritis/basics/osteoarthritis.htm.
17. National Association for Continence, "Statistics," 2012, www.nafc.org.
18. Ibid.
19. T. E. Howe, et. al., "Exercise for Improving Balance in Older People," *Cochrane Database of Systematic Reviews*, 2011, www.summaries.cochrane.org/CD004963/exercise-for-improving-balance-in-older-people.
20. Medline Plus, "Aging Changes in the Senses," 2012, www.nlm.nih.gov/medlineplus/ency/article/004013.html.
21. B. J. Cowart, "Smell and Taste in Aging," 2011, *Perfumer and Flavorist* 36, no. 1 (2011): 34–36.
22. L. Fisher, Sex, *Romance, and Relationships: AARP Survey of Midlife and Older Adults* (Washington, DC: AARP, 2010); V. Schick, et al., "Sexual Behaviors, Condom Use, and Sexual Health of Americans over 50: Implications for Sexual Health Promotion for Older Adults," *The Journal of Sexual Medicine* 7 (2010):

315–29; Center for Sexual Health Promotion, National Survey of Sexual Health and Behavior, 2010. Available at www.nationalsexstudy.indiana.edu.

23. Alzheimer's Association, *2012 Alzheimer's Disease Facts and Figures* (Chicago: Alzheimer's Association, 2012).

24. Ibid.

25. Ibid.

26. Ibid.

27. Alzheimer's Association, "What Is Alzheimer's?" 2011, www.alz.org/alzheimers_disease_what_is_alzheimers.asp.

28. National Center for Health Statistics, *Health, United States, 2010* (Hyattsville, MD: National Center for Health Statistics, 2011), Table 64, "Lifetime Alcohol Drinking Status among Adults," Available at www.cdc.gov/nchs/hus.htm; National Institute on Aging, "AgePage: Alcohol Use in Older People," Updated April 2012, www.nia.nih.gov/HealthInformation/Publications/alcohol.htm.

29. Centers for Disease Control and Prevention, "Prescriptive Drug Use Continues to Increase," *NCHS Data Brief* 42, September 2010.

30. D.S. Budnitz, et al., "Emergency Hospitalizations for Adverse Drug Events in Older Americans," *The New England Journal of Medicine* 365 (2011): 2002–2012.

31. Centers for Disease Control and Prevention, "Making Physical Activity a Part of an Older Adult's Life," 2011. Available at www.cdc.gov/physicalactivity/everyone/getactive/olderadults.html.

32. Merriam-Webster, "Death," *Merriam-Webster's Collegiate® Dictionary*. 11th ed. 2011, Merriam-Webster, Inc., www.merriam-webster.com. Used by permission.

33. President's Commission on the Uniform Determination of Death, *Defining Death: Medical, Ethical and Legal Issues in the Determination of Death* (Washington, DC: U.S. Government Printing Office, 1981).

34. Ad Hoc Committee of the Harvard Medical School to Examine the Definition of Brain Death, "A Definition of Irreversible Coma," *Journal of the American Medical Association* 205 (1968): 377.

35. Elisabeth Kübler-Ross and David Kessler, "The Five Stages of Grief," 2011, www.grief.com/the-five-stages-of-grief.

36. C. Corr, C. Nabe, and D. Corr, *Death and Dying, Life and Living*. 6th ed. (Belmont, CA: Wadsworth, 2009).

37. Victorian Government Health Information, "Death and Dying," 2011, www.health.vic.gov.au/dementia/index.htm.

38. Behavior Neuropathy Clinic, "Grief and the Grieving Process," 2010, www.adhd.com.au/grief.htm.

39. American Bar Association, Commission on Law and Aging, *Consumer's Tool Kit for Health Care Advance Planning*, 2d ed. (Washington, DC: American Bar Association, 2012), Available at www.abanet.org/aging/toolkit/home.html.

40. Aging with Dignity, "Five Wishes," 2012, www.agingwithdignity.org/five-wishes.php.

41. Public Agenda, "Right to Die," 2011, www.publicagenda.org/articles/right-die.

42. Oregon Department of Human Services, "FAQs about the Death with Dignity Act," Updated 2011, www.public.health.oregon.gov/ProviderPartner Resources/EvaluationResearch/DeathwithDignityAct/Pages/faqs.aspx#similar; International Task Force on Euthanasia and Assisted Suicide, "Assisted Suicide Laws," Updated February 2012, www.internationaltaskforce.org/assisted_suicide_laws.htm.

43. National Hospice, and Palliative Care Organization, *NHPCO Facts and Figures: Hospice Care in America, 2011 Ed.* (Alexandria, VA: National Hospice and Palliative Care Organization, 2012), 460.

44. U.S. National Library of Medicine, " Organ Donation" 2012, www.nlm.nih.gov/medlineplus/organdonation.html.

45. U.S. Department of Health and Human Services, "The Need Is Real," 2012, www.organdonor.gov/about/data.html.

46. Mayo Clinic, "Organ Donation: Don't Let These Myths Confuse You," 2011, www.mayoclinic.com/health/organ-donation/FL00077.

Answers to Chapter Review Questions, Appendix A

Chapter 1
1. b; 2. d; 3. b; 4. a; 5. d;
6. a; 7. a; 8. a; 9. a; 10. c

Chapter 2
1. a; 2. b; 3. a; 4. b; 5. c; 6. a;
7. b; 8. b; 9. c; 10. b

Chapter 3
1. c; 2. c; 3. d; 4. d; 5. c; 6. d;
7. c; 8. c; 9. c; 10. b

Chapter 4
1. b; 2. b; 3. c; 4. c; 5. a; 6. c;
7. a; 8. d; 9. a; 10. d

Chapter 5
1. a; 2. d; 3. c; 4. a; 5. a; 6. b;
7. b; 8. b; 9. b; 10. a

Chapter 6
1. b; 2. b; 3. a; 4. c; 5. b; 6. a;
7. c; 8. d; 9. c; 10. a

Chapter 7
1. d; 2. a; 3. a; 4. b; 5. b;
6. a; 7. b; 8. b; 9. b; 10. c

Chapter 8
1. c; 2. c; 3. b; 4. b; 5. c; 6. b;
7. a; 8. a; 9. d; 10. a

Chapter 9
1. c; 2. d; 3. c; 4. b; 5. a; 6. c;
7. d; 8. c; 9. b; 10. a

Chapter 10
1. d; 2. d; 3. b; 4. c; 5. d;
6. b; 7. d; 8. b; 9. b; 10. a

Chapter 11
1. c; 2. d; 3. d; 4. d; 5. b;
6. b; 7. c; 8. d; 9. c; 10. a

Chapter 12
1. b; 2. b; 3. c; 4. b; 5. d;
6. c; 7. d; 8. d; 9. b; 10. a

Chapter 13
1. c; 2. c; 3. b; 4. b; 5. c; 6. c;
7. a; 8. d; 9. c; 10. b

Chapter 14
1. a; 2. c; 3. c; 4. d; 5. a; 6. d;
7. c; 8. b; 9. c; 10. a

Chapter 15
1. c; 2. b; 3. a; 4. d; 5. c; 6. d;
7. b; 8. d; 9. a; 10. c

Chapter 16
1. b; 2. d; 3. a; 4. a; 5. c; 6. d;
7. a; 8. d; 9. a; 10. c

Chapter 17
1. c; 2. b; 3. c; 4. d; 5. c; 6. a;
7. b; 8. c; 9. b; 10. a

Chapter 18
1. c; 2. a; 3. d; 4. c; 5. c; 6. c;
7. d; 8. c; 9. b; 10. a

Chapter 19
1. b; 2. a; 3. c; 4. d; 5. d; 6. c;
7. a; 8. c; 9. b; 10. a

Chapter 20
1. b; 2. d; 3. d; 4. a; 5. a;
6. a; 7. b; 8. b; 9. a; 10. c

Chapter 21
1. b; 2. b; 3. c; 4. a; 5. d; 6. a;
7. c; 8. d; 9. a; 10. d

Providing Emergency Care

Ideally, first-aid procedures should be performed only by someone who has received formal training from the American Red Cross or another reputable institution. (There are numerous classes and opportunities in most communities for updating your skills in these areas. Check for such classes at your university or local community college.) If you do not have such training, contact a physician or call your local emergency medical service (EMS) by dialing 9-1-1 or your local emergency number. In life-threatening situations, however, you may need to begin first aid immediately and continue until help arrives. This section contains basic information for various emergency situations. Simply reading these directions, however, may not prepare you fully to handle these situations. For this reason, you may want to enroll in a first-aid course.

Calling for Emergency Assistance

When calling for emergency assistance, be prepared to give exact details. Be clear and thorough, and do not panic. Never hang up until the dispatcher has informed you that he or she has all the information needed. Be ready to answer the following questions:

- Where are you and the victim located? (This is the most important information that the EMS will need.)
- What is your phone number and name?
- What has happened? Was there an accident, or is the victim ill?
- How many people need help?
- What is the nature of the emergency? What is the victim's apparent condition?
- Are there any life-threatening situations that the EMS should know about (for example, fires, explosions, or fallen electrical lines)?
- Is the victim wearing a medic-alert tag (a tag indicating a specific medical condition such as diabetes)?

Administering First Aid

According to the laws in most states, you are not required to administer first aid unless you have a special obligation to the victim. For example, parents must provide first aid for their children, and a lifeguard must provide aid to a swimmer.

Before administering first aid, you should obtain the victim's consent. If the victim refuses aid, you must respect that person's rights. However, you should make every reasonable effort to persuade the victim to accept your help. In emergency situations, consent is *implied* if the victim is unconscious. Once you begin to administer first aid, you are required by law to continue. You must remain with the victim until someone of equal or greater competence takes over.

Can you be held liable if you fail to provide adequate care or if the victim is further injured? To protect people who render first aid, most states have Good Samaritan laws, which grant immunity (protection from civil liability) if you act in good faith to provide care to the best of your ability, according to your level of training. Because these laws vary, you should become familiar with the Good Samaritan laws in your state.

First-Aid Supplies

Every home, car, and boat should be supplied with a basic first-aid kit, which should be stored in a convenient place but kept out of the reach of children. Following is a list of supplies that should be included:

- Bandages, including triangular bandages (36 inches by 6 inches), butterfly bandages, a roller bandage, rolled white gauze bandages (2- and 3-inch widths), adhesive bandages
- Sterile gauze pads and absorbent pads
- Adhesive tape (2- and 3-inch widths)
- Cotton-tip applicators
- Scissors
- Thermometer
- Antibiotic ointment
- Aspirin
- Calamine lotion
- Antiseptic cream or petroleum jelly
- Safety pins
- Tweezers
- Latex gloves
- Flashlight
- Paper cups
- Blanket

You cannot be prepared for every medical emergency, but these essential tools and a knowledge of basic first aid will help you cope with many emergency situations, including the ones discussed below.

Cessation of Breathing

If someone has stopped breathing, you should perform mouth-to-mouth resuscitation. This involves the following steps:

1. Check for responsiveness by gently tapping or shaking the victim. Ask loudly, "Are you okay?"

2. Call the local EMS for help (usually 9-1-1).

3. Gently roll the victim onto his or her back.

4. Open the airway by tilting the victim's head back—place your hand nearest the victim's head on the victim's forehead, and apply backward pressure to tilt the head back and lift the chin.

5. Check for breathing (3 to 5 seconds): look, listen, and feel for breathing.

6. Give two slow breaths.
- Keep the victim's head tilted back.
- Pinch the victim's nose shut.
- Seal your lips tightly around the victim's mouth.
- Give two slow breaths, each lasting 1.5 to 2 seconds.
- Watch for the chest to rise and fall.

7. Check for pulse at side of neck; feel for pulse for 5 to 10 seconds.

8. Begin rescue breathing.
- Keep the victim's head tilted back.
- Pinch the victim's nose shut.
- Give one breath about every 5 seconds (12 breaths per minute).
- Look, listen, and feel for breathing between breaths.

9. Recheck pulse every minute.
- Keep the victim's head tilted back.
- Feel for pulse for 5 to 10 seconds.
- If the victim has a pulse but is not breathing, continue rescue breathing. If there is no pulse, begin CPR (see below).

There are some variations when performing this procedure on infants and children. For infants, at step 8, you should give one slow breath every 3 seconds. You should not pinch the nose. Instead, seal your lips tightly around the infant's nose and mouth. For children aged 1 to 8, at step 8, give one slow breath every 4 seconds.

Sudden Collapse

If an adult has a sudden cardiac arrest, his or her survival depends largely on being given immediate cardiopulmonary resuscitation (CPR). People are often afraid to offer aid for fear of doing something wrong or making matters worse. In addition, some people are squeamish about performing the artificial respiration that is part of traditional CPR. However, studies have shown that simply providing hands-only CPR to an adult who has collapsed can double that person's chance of survival. The American Heart Association now recommends that anyone, trained or untrained, who witnesses an adult's sudden collapse should call 9-1-1 and then immediately begin hands-only CPR. That means uninterrupted chest compressions—pushing hard in the center of the victim's chest—at a rate of about 100 per minute until the EMS arrives.

Conventional CPR, a technique that involves a combination of artificial respiration and chest compressions, is still recommended for infants or children, drowning victims, drug overdose, or other respiratory problems, and on adult victims who are found already unconscious and not breathing normally. The American Red Cross, the American Heart Association, and other organizations offer courses in mouth-to-mouth resuscitation and CPR as well as general first aid. If you have taken a CPR course in the past, you should be aware that certain changes have been made in the procedure. Consider taking a refresher course.

Choking

Choking occurs when an object obstructs the trachea (windpipe), thus preventing normal breathing. Failure to expel the object and restore breathing can lead to death within 6 minutes. The universal signal of distress related to choking is the clasping of the throat with one or both hands. Other signs of choking include not being able to talk and/or noisy and difficult breathing. If a victim can cough or speak, do not interfere. The most effective method for assisting choking victims is the Heimlich maneuver (Figure 1), which involves the application of pressure to the victim's abdominal area to expel the foreign object, as described below.

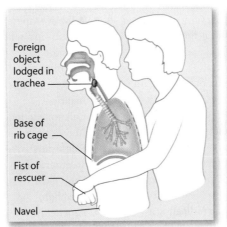

Foreign object lodged in trachea

Base of rib cage

Fist of rescuer

Navel

a Standing behind the victim, place a fist thumb-side in just above the victim's navel and cover it with your other hand.

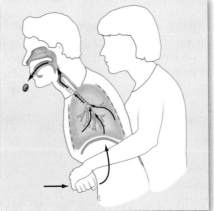

b Press sharply upward and inward, using enough force to push the diaphragm and lungs up and create air pressure that will expel the object.

FIGURE 1 **Heimlich Maneuver**

The Heimlich maneuver can be used to dislodge an object that is blocking a person's airway, causing him or her to choke. The technique shown here is appropriate for use on a person who is either sitting or standing.

Source: Adapted from Johnson, Michael D., *Human Biology: Concepts And Current Issues*, 5th, © 2010. Printed and Electronically reproduced by permission of Pearson Education, Inc., Upper Saddle River, New Jersey.

If the Choking Victim Is Standing or Seated

1. Recognize that the victim is choking. Without startling him or her, approach from behind.

2. Wrap your arms around the victim's waist, making a fist with one hand.

3. Place the thumb side of the fist on the middle of the victim's abdomen, just above the navel and well below the tip of the sternum.

4. Cover your fist with your other hand.

5. Press fist into victim's abdomen, with up to five quick upward thrusts.

6. After every five abdominal thrusts, check the victim and your technique.

7. If the victim becomes unconscious, gently lower him or her to the ground.

8. Try to clear the airway by using your finger to sweep the object from the victim's mouth or throat.

9. Give two rescue breaths. If the passage is still blocked and air will not go in, repeat the Heimlich maneuver.

If the Choking Victim Is Lying Down

1. Facing the person, kneel with your legs astride the victim's hips. Place the heel of one hand against the abdomen, slightly above the navel and well below the tip of the sternum. Put the other hand on top of the first hand.

2. Press inward and upward using both hands with up to five quick abdominal thrusts.

3. Repeat the following steps in this sequence until the airway becomes clear or the EMS arrives:
- Finger sweep.
- Give two rescue breaths.
- Do up to five abdominal thrusts.

Alcohol Poisoning

Alcohol overdose is considered a medical emergency when an irregular heartbeat or coma occurs. The two immediate causes of death in such cases are cardiac arrhythmia and respiratory depression. If a person is seriously uncoordinated and has possibly also taken a depressant, the risk of respiratory failure is serious enough that a physician should be contacted. When dealing with someone who is drunk, remember these points:

1. Stay calm. Assess the situation.

2. Keep your distance. Before approaching or touching the person, explain what you intend to do.

3. Speak in a clear, firm, reassuring manner.

4. Keep the person still and comfortable.

5. Stay with the person if she or he is vomiting. When helping him or her to lie down, turn the head to the side to prevent it from falling back. This helps to keep the person from choking on vomit.

6. Monitor the person's breathing.

Seizures

If you are with someone experiencing a seizure, there are several steps you can take to help ensure his or her safety during and after the episode:

1. Note the length of the attack. Seizures in which a person remains unconscious for long periods of time should be monitored closely. If medical help arrives, be sure to tell them how long the person has been unconscious.

2. Remove obstacles that could harm the victim. Because seizure victims may lose motor control during a convulsion, they inadvertently thrash around. To reduce the chances of serious injury, clear away any objects that could pose a threat.

3. Loosen clothing, and turn the victim's head to the side. This will help ensure that the person can breathe freely and will allow fluids or vomit to drain from the mouth.

4. Do not force objects into the victim's mouth. Although seizure victims may bite their tongues, causing possible damage, they will not swallow them. If the victim's mouth is clamped shut, forcing objects into the mouth may break teeth or cause more harm than doing nothing.

5. Get help. After you have completed steps 1 through 4, get help or send someone for help. This is particularly important if the victim does not regain consciousness within a few minutes.

6. Reassure the victim. Too often, the seizure victim regains consciousness only to face a crowd of staring people. When administering first aid, try to dissuade curious bystanders from hanging around. Calmly reassure the victim that everything is okay.

7. Allow the person to rest. After a seizure, many people will be exhausted. Allow them to sleep if possible.

Bleeding

External Bleeding   Control of external bleeding is an important part of emergency care. Survival is threatened by the loss of 1 quart of blood or more. There are three major procedures for the control of external bleeding:

- **Direct pressure.** The best method is to apply firm pressure by covering the wound with a sterile dressing, bandage, or clean cloth. Wearing disposable latex gloves or an equally protective barrier, apply pressure for 5 to 10 minutes to stop bleeding.
- **Elevation.** Elevate the wounded section of the body to slow the bleeding. For example, a wounded arm or leg should be raised above the level of the victim's heart.
- **Pressure points.** Pressure points are sites where an artery that is close to the body's surface lies directly over a bone (Figure 2). Pressing the artery against the bone can limit the flow of blood to the injury. This technique should be used only as a last resort when direct pressure and elevation have failed to stop bleeding.

For serious wounds, seek medical attention immediately.

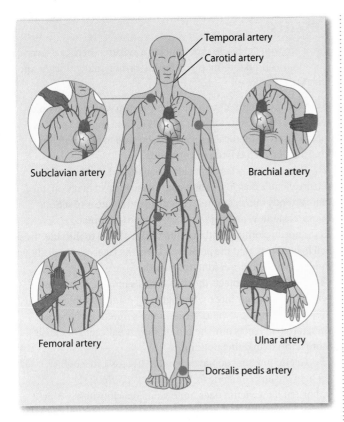

FIGURE 2 **Pressure Points**
Pressure can be applied to these points to stop bleeding. However, unless absolutely necessary, avoid applying pressure to the carotid arteries, which supply blood to the brain. Never apply pressure to both carotid arteries at the same time.

Internal Bleeding Although internal bleeding may not be immediately obvious, you should be aware of the following signs and symptoms:

- Symptoms of shock (discussed below)
- Coughing up or vomiting blood
- Bruises or contusions of the skin
- Bruises on chest or fractured ribs
- Black, tarlike stools
- Abdominal discomfort or pain (rigidity or spasms)

In some cases, a person who has suffered an injury (such as a blow to the head, chest, or abdomen) that does not cause external bleeding may bleed internally. If you suspect internal bleeding, follow these steps:

1. Have the person lie on his or her back on a flat surface with knees bent.
2. Treat for shock. Keep the victim warm. Cover the person with a blanket, if possible.
3. Expect vomiting. If this occurs, keep the victim on his or her side for drainage, to prevent inhalation of vomit, and to prevent expulsion of vomit from the stomach.
4. Do *not* give the victim any medications or fluids.
5. Send someone to call for emergency medical help immediately.

Nosebleeds

1. Have the victim sit down and lean slightly forward to prevent blood from running into the throat. If you do not suspect a fracture, pinch the person's nose firmly closed using the thumb and forefinger. Keep the nose pinched for at least 5 minutes.
2. While the nose is pinched, apply a cold compress to the surrounding area.
3. If pinching does not work, gently pack the nostril with gauze or a clean strip of cloth. Do not use absorbent cotton, which will stick. Be sure that the ends of the gauze or cloth hang out so that it can be easily removed later. Once the nose is packed with gauze, pinch it closed again for another 5 minutes.
4. If the bleeding persists, seek medical attention.

Shock

Shock is a condition in which the cardiovascular system fails to provide sufficient blood circulation to all parts of the body. Victims of shock display some or all of the following symptoms:

- Dilated pupils
- Cool, moist skin
- Weak, rapid pulse
- Vomiting
- Delayed or unrelated responses to questions

All injuries result in some degree of shock. Therefore, treatment for shock should be given after every major injury. The following are basic steps for treating shock:

1. Have the victim lie flat with his or her feet elevated approximately 8 to 12 inches. (In the case of chest injuries, difficulty breathing, or severe pain, the victim's head should be slightly elevated if there is no sign of spinal injury.)
2. Keep the victim warm. If possible, wrap him or her in blankets or other material. Keep the victim calm and reassured.
3. Seek medical help.

Treatment for Burns

Minor Burns For minor burns caused by fire or scalding water, apply running cold water or cold compresses for 20 to 30 minutes. Never put butter, grease, salt water, aloe vera, or topical burn ointments or sprays on burned skin. If the burned area is dirty, gently wash it with soap and water, and blot it dry with a sterile dressing.

Major Burns For major burn injuries, call for help immediately. Wrap the victim in a clean, dry sheet. Do not clean the burns or try to remove any clothing attached to burned skin. Remove jewelry near the burned skin immediately, if possible. Keep the victim lying down and calm.

Chemical Burns Remove clothing surrounding the burn. Wash skin that has been burned by chemicals by flushing with water for at least 20 minutes. Seek medical assistance as soon as possible.

Electrical Shock

Do not touch a victim of electrical shock until the power source has been turned off. Approach the scene carefully, avoiding any live wires or electrical power lines. Pay attention to the following:

1. If the victim is holding onto the live electrical wire, do not remove it unless the power has been shut off at the plug, circuit breaker, or fuse box.

2. Check the victim's breathing and pulse. Electrical current can paralyze the nerves and muscles that control breathing and heartbeat. If necessary, give mouth-to-mouth resuscitation. If there is no pulse, CPR might be necessary. (Remember that only trained people should perform CPR.)

3. Keep the victim warm and treat for shock. Once the person is breathing and stable, seek medical help or send someone else for help.

Poisoning

Among adults, almost all poisonings are caused by an overdose of a prescription drug, most commonly an opioid pain medication, or an illegal drug, such as cocaine or heroin. Among children, the majority of poisonings are caused by household products.

You should keep emergency telephone numbers for the poison control center and the local EMS close at hand. Many people keep these numbers on labels on their telephones. Check the front of your telephone book for these numbers. Be prepared to answer the following questions and to give the following information when calling for help:

- What was ingested? Have the container of the product and the remaining contents ready so you can describe it. Bring the container with you to the emergency room.
- When was the substance taken?
- How much was taken?
- Has vomiting occurred? If the person has vomited, save a sample to take to the hospital.
- Are there any other symptoms?
- How long will it take to get to the nearest emergency room?

When caring for a person who has ingested poison, keep these basic principles in mind:

1. Maintain an open airway. Make sure the person is breathing.

2. Call the local poison control center. Follow their advice for neutralizing the poison.

3. If the poison control center or another medical authority advises you to induce vomiting, then do so.

4. If a corrosive or caustic (that is, acid or alkali) substance was swallowed, immediately dilute it by having the victim drink at least one or two 8-ounce glasses of cold water or milk.

5. Place the victim on his or her left side. This position will delay advancement of the poison into the small intestine, where absorption into the victim's circulatory system is faster.

Injuries of Joints, Muscles, and Bones

Sprains   Sprains result when ligaments and other tissues around a joint are stretched or torn. The following steps should be taken to treat sprains:

1. Elevate the injured joint to a comfortable position.

2. Apply an ice pack or cold compress to reduce pain and swelling.

3. Wrap the joint firmly with a roller bandage.

4. Check the fingers or toes periodically to ensure that blood circulation has not been obstructed. If the bandage is too tight, loosen it.

5. Keep the injured area elevated, and continue ice treatment for 24 hours.

6. Apply heat to the injury after 48 hours if there is no further swelling.

7. If pain and swelling continue or if a fracture is suspected, seek medical attention.

Fractures   Any deformity of an injured body part usually indicates a fracture. A fracture is any break in a bone, including chips, cracks, splinters, and complete breaks. Minor fractures (e.g., hairline cracks) might be difficult to detect and might be confused with sprains. If there is doubt, treat the injury as a fracture until X rays have been taken.

Do not move the victim if a fracture of the neck or back is suspected, because this could result in a spinal cord injury. If the victim must be moved, splints should be applied to immobilize the fracture in order to prevent further damage and to decrease pain. Following are some basic steps for treating fractures and applying splints to broken limbs:

1. If the person is bleeding, apply direct pressure above the site of the wound.

2. If a broken bone is exposed, do not try to move it back into the wound. This can cause contamination and further injury.

3. Do not try to straighten out a broken limb. Splint the limb as it lies.

4. The following materials are needed for splinting:
   - *Splint:* wooden board, pillow, or rolled up magazines and newspapers
   - *Padding:* towels, blankets, socks, or cloth
   - *Ties:* cloth, rope, or tape

5. Place splints and padding above and below the joint. Never put padding directly over the break. Padding should protect bony areas and the soft tissue of the limb.

6. Tie splints and padding into place.

7. Check the tightness of the splints periodically. Pay attention to the skin color, temperature, and pulse below the fracture to make sure the blood flow is adequate.

8. Elevate the fracture and apply ice packs to prevent swelling and reduce pain.

Head Injuries

All head injuries can potentially lead to brain damage, which may result in a cessation of breathing and pulse.

Minor Head Injuries

1. For a minor bump on the head resulting in a bruise without bleeding, apply ice to decrease the swelling.

2. If there is bleeding, apply even, moderate pressure. Do not use excessive pressure because the skull may be fractured.

3. Observe the victim for a change in consciousness. Observe the size of pupils, including whether both pupils are dilated to the same degree, and note signs of inability to think clearly. Check for any signs of numbness or paralysis. Allow the victim to sleep, but wake him or her periodically to check for awareness.

Severe Head Injuries

1. If the victim is unconscious, check the airway for breathing. If necessary, perform mouth-to-mouth resuscitation.

2. If the victim is breathing, check the pulse. If it is less than 55 or more than 125 beats per minute, the victim may be in danger.

3. Check for bleeding. If fluid is flowing from the ears or nose, do not stop it.

4. Do not remove any objects embedded in the victim's skull.

5. Cover the victim with blankets to maintain body temperature, but guard against overheating.

6. Seek medical help as soon as possible.

Temperature-Related Emergencies

Frostbite   Frostbite is damage to body tissues caused by intense cold, generally occurring at temperatures below 32°F. When skin is exposed to the cold, ice crystals form beneath the skin. Avoid rubbing frostbitten tissue, because the ice crystals can scrape and break blood vessels. The body parts most likely to suffer frostbite are the toes, ears, fingers, nose, and cheeks. To treat frostbite, follow these steps:

1. Bring the victim to a medical facility as soon as possible.

2. Cover and protect the frostbitten area. If possible, apply a steady source of external warmth, such as a warm compress. Avoid walking if the feet are frostbitten.

3. If the victim cannot be transported, warm the body part by immersing it in warm water (100°F to 105°F). Continue to warm until the frostbitten area is warm to the touch when removed from the bath. Do not allow the body part to touch the sides or bottom of the water container. After warming, dry gently and wrap the body part in bandages to protect from refreezing.

Hypothermia   Hypothermia is a condition of generalized cooling of the body, resulting from exposure to cold temperatures or immersion in cold water. It can occur at any temperature below 65°F and can be made more severe by wind chill and moisture. The following are key symptoms of hypothermia:

- Shivering
- Vague, slow, slurred speech
- Poor judgment
- A cool abdomen
- Lethargy, or extreme exhaustion
- Slowed breathing and heartbeat
- Numbness and loss of feeling in extremities

After contacting the EMS, take the following steps:

1. Get the victim out of the cold.

2. Keep the victim in a flat position. Do not raise the legs.

3. Squeeze as much water as possible from wet clothing, and layer dry clothing over wet clothing. Removal of clothing may jostle the victim and lead to other problems.

4. Give the victim warm drinks only if he or she is able to swallow. Do not give the victim alcohol or caffeinated beverages, and do not allow the victim to smoke.

5. Do not allow the victim to exercise.

Heatstroke   Heatstroke, the most serious heat-related disorder, results from the failure of the brain's heat-regulating mechanism (the hypothalamus) to cool the body. The following are signs and symptoms of heatstroke:

- Rapid pulse
- Hot, dry, flushed skin (absence of sweating)
- Disorientation leading to unconsciousness
- High body temperature

Body temperature should be reduced as quickly as possible. Immerse the victim in a cool bath, lake, or stream. If there is no water nearby, loosen clothing and use a fan to help lower the victim's body temperature.

Heat Exhaustion   Heat exhaustion results from excessive loss of salt and water. The onset is gradual, with the following symptoms:

- Fatigue and weakness
- Anxiety
- Nausea
- Profuse sweating and clammy skin
- Normal body temperature

Move the victim to a cool place and have him or her lie down flat, with feet elevated 8 to 12 inches. Replace lost fluids slowly and steadily. Sponge or fan the victim.

Heat Cramps   Heat cramps result from excessive sweating, resulting in an excessive loss of salt and water. Although heat cramps are the least serious heat-related emergency, they are the most painful. The symptoms include muscle cramps, usually starting in the arms and legs. To relieve symptoms, the victim should drink electrolyte-rich beverages or a light saltwater solution or eat salty foods.

Nutritive Value of Selected Foods and Fast Foods

This section presents nutritional information about a wide array of foods, including many fast foods. Values are given for calories, protein, carbohydrates, fiber, fat, saturated fat, and cholesterol for common foods and serving sizes. Use this information to assess your diet and make improvements. This is only a sampling of the most common foods. See the MyDietAnalysis database for a more extensive list of foods.

MDA Code	Food Name	Amt	Wt (g)	Ener (kcal)	Prot (g)	Carb (g)	Fiber (g)	Fat (g)	Sat (g)	Chol (g)
Beverages										
Alcoholic Beverages										
22831	Beer	12 fl. oz	360	157	1	13		0	0	0
34053	Beer, light	12 fl. oz	353	105	1	5	0	0	0	0
22606	Beer, nonalcoholic	12 fl. oz	353	73	1	14	0	0	0	0
22884	Wine, red	1 fl. oz	29	24	0	1		0	0	
22861	Wine, white	1 fl. oz	29	24	0	1		0	0	
22514	Gin, 80 proof	1 fl. oz	28	64	0	0	0	0	0	0
22593	Rum, 80 proof	1 fl. oz	28	64	0	0	0	0	0	0
22515	Tequila, 80 proof	1 fl. oz	28	64	0	0	0	0	0	0
22594	Vodka, 80 proof	1 fl. oz	28	64	0	0	0	0	0	0
22670	Whiskey, 80 proof	1 fl. oz	28	64	0	0	0	0	0	0
Coffee, Tea, and Dairy Drink Mixes										
20012	Coffee, brewed	1 cup	237	2	0	0	0	0	0	0
20686	Coffee, decaffeinated, brewed	1 cup	237	0	0	0	0	0	0	0
20439	Coffee, espresso	1 cup	237	5	0	0	0	0	0.2	0
20402	Coffee, from mix, French vanilla, sugar & fat free	1 ea	7	25	0	5	0	0	0.1	0
85	Chocolate milk, prepared w/ syrup	1 cup	282	254	9	36	1	8	4.7	25
46	Hot cocoa, w/ aspartame, sodium, vitamin A, prepared w/ water	1 cup	256	74	3	14	2	1	0.4	0
48	Hot cocoa, prep from dry mix w/ water	1 cup	275	151	3	32	1	2	0.9	0
166	Hot cocoa, w/ marshmallows, from dry packet	1 ea	28	112	1	21	1	4	4.2	0
39	Chocolate flavor, dry mix, prepared w/ milk	1 cup	266	226	9	32	1	9	4.9	24
41	Strawberry flavor, dry mix, prepared w/ milk	1 cup	266	234	8	33	0	8	5.1	32
20014	Tea, brewed	1 cup	237	2	0	1	0	0	0	0
20036	Tea, herbal (not chamomile) brewed	1 cup	237	2	0	0	0	0	0	0
Fruit and Vegetable Beverages and Juices										
71080	Apple juice, canned or bottled, unsweetened	1 ea	262	121	0	30	1	0	0.1	0
20277	Capri Sun All Natural Juice Drink, Fruit Punch	1 ea	210	99	0	26	0	0	0	0
5226	Carrot juice, canned	1 cup	236	94	2	22	2	0	0.1	0
3042	Cranberry juice cocktail	1 cup	253	137	0	34	0	0	0	0
20024	Fruit punch, canned	1 cup	248	117	0	30	0	0	0	0
20035	Fruit punch, from frozen concentrate	1 cup	247	114	0	29	0	0	0	0
20101	Grape drink, canned	1 cup	250	152	0	39	0	0	0	0
3053	Grapefruit juice, from frozen concentrate, unsweetened	1 cup	247	101	1	24	0	0	0	0
20045	Lemonade flavor drink, from dry mix	1 cup	266	72	0	18	0	0	0	0
20047	Lemonade w/ aspartame, low kcal, from dry mix	1 cup	237	7	0	2	0	0	0	0
20070	Orange drink, canned	1 cup	248	122	0	31	0	0	0	0
20004	Orange flavor drink, from dry mix	1 cup	248	122	0	31	0	0	0	0
71108	Orange juice, canned, unsweetened	1 ea	263	124	2	29	1	0	0	0
3090	Orange juice, fresh	1 cup	248	112	2	26	0	0	0.1	0
3091	Orange juice, from frozen concentrate, unsweetened	1 cup	249	112	2	27	0	0	0	0
5397	Tomato juice, canned w/o salt	1 cup	243	41	2	10	1	0	0	0
20849	Vegetable and fruit, mixed juice drink	4 oz	113	33	0	8	0	0	0	0
20080	Vegetable juice cocktail, canned	1 cup	242	46	2	11	2	0	0	0

Ener = energy (kilocalories); **Prot** = protein; **Carb** = carbohydrate; **Fiber** = dietary fiber; **Fat** = total fat; **Sat** = saturated fat; **Chol** = cholesterol.

MDA Code	Food Name	Amt	Wt (g)	Ener (kcal)	Prot (g)	Carb (g)	Fiber (g)	Fat (g)	Sat (g)	Chol (g)
Soft Drinks										
20006	Club soda	1 cup	237	0	0	0	0	0	0	0
20685	Low-calorie cola, w/ aspartame, caffeine free	12 fl. oz	355	4	0	1	0	0	0	0
20843	Cola, w/ higher caffeine	12 fl. oz	370	152	0	39	0	0	0	0
20008	Ginger ale	1 cup	244	83	0	21	0	0	0	0
20032	Lemon-lime soft drink	1 cup	246	98	0	25	0	0	0	0
20027	Pepper-type soft drink	1 cup	246	101	0	26	0	0	0.2	0
20009	Root beer	1 cup	246	101	0	26	0	0	0	0
Other										
20033	Soy milk	1 cup	245	132	8	15	1	4	0.5	0
20041	Water, tap	1 cup	237	0	0	0	0	0	0	0
Breakfast Cereals										
40095	All-Bran/Kellogg	0.5 cup	30	78	4	22	9	1	0.2	0
40032	Cap'n Crunch/Quaker	0.75 cup	27	109	1	23	1	2	1.1	0
40297	Cheerios/Gen Mills	1 cup	30	110	3	22	3	2	0.3	0
40126	Cinnamon Toast Crunch/Gen Mills	0.75 cup	30	130	2	24	1	3	0.4	0
40195	Corn Flakes/Kellogg	1 cup	28	101	2	24	1	0	0	0
40089	Corn Grits, instant, plain, prepared/Quaker	1 pkg	137	104	2	22	2	1	0.1	
40206	Corn Pops/Kellogg	1 cup	31	117	1	28	0	0	0.1	0
40179	Cream of Rice, prepared w/ salt	1 cup	244	127	2	28	0	0	0	0
40182	Cream of Wheat, instant, prepared w/ salt	1 cup	241	149	4	32	1	1	0.1	0
40104	Crispix/Kellogg	1 cup	29	109	2	25	0	0	0.1	0
40218	Froot Loops/Kellogg	1 cup	30	112	2	26	3	1	0.6	0
40217	Frosted Flakes/Kellogg	0.75 cup	31	114	1	28	1	0	0	0
11916	Frosted Mini-Wheats, bite size/Kellogg	1 cup	55	189	6	45	6	1	0.2	0
40209	Raisin Bran/Kellogg	1 cup	61	196	5	47	7	1	0.2	0
40210	Rice Krispies/Kellogg	1.25 cup	33	128	2	28	0	0	0.1	0
60887	Shredded wheat, large biscuit	2 ea	38	127	4	30	5	1	0.2	0
40211	Special K/Kellogg	1 cup	31	117	7	22	1	0	0.1	0
Dairy and Cheese										
500	Cream, half & half	2 Tbs	30	39	1	1	0	3	2.1	11
11	Milk, condensed, sweetened, canned	2 Tbs	38	123	3	21	0	3	2.1	13
19	Milk, lowfat, 1% fat, chocolate	1 cup	250	158	8	26	1	2	1.5	8
218	Milk, 2%, w/ added vitamins A & D	1 cup	245	130	8	13	0	5	3	20
6	Milk, nonfat/skim, w/ added vitamin A	1 cup	245	83	8	12	0	0	0.1	5
1	Milk, whole, 3.25%	1 cup	244	149	8	12	0	8	4.6	24
20	Milk, whole, chocolate	1 cup	250	208	8	26	2	8	5.3	30
72088	Yogurt, fruit variety, nonfat	1 cup	245	233	11	47	0	0	0.3	5
1287	American cheese, nonfat slices	1 pce	21	32	5	2	0	0	0.1	3
13349	Cheez Whiz cheese sauce/Kraft	2 Tbs	33	91	4	3	0	7	4.3	25
1014	Cottage cheese, 2% fat	0.5 cup	113	97	13	4	0	3	1.1	11
1015	Cream cheese	2 Tbs	29	99	2	1	0	10	5.6	32
1452	Cream cheese, fat free	2 Tbs	29	30	5	2	0	0	0.2	3
1016	Feta, crumbled	0.25 cup	38	99	5	2	0	8	5.6	33
47887	Mozzarella, whole milk, slice	1 ea	34	102	8	1	0	8	4.5	27
1075	Parmesan, grated	1 Tbs	5	22	2	0	0	1	0.9	4
1024	Ricotta, part skim	0.25 cup	62	86	7	3	0	5	3.1	19
1064	Ricotta, whole milk	0.25 cup	62	108	7	2	0	8	5.1	32
Eggs and Egg Substitutes										
19525	Egg substitute, liquid	0.25 cup	63	53	8	0	0	2	0.4	1
19506	Egg, white, raw	1 ea	33	16	4	0	0	0	0	0
19509	Egg, whole, fried	1 ea	46	90	6	0	0	7	2	210
19515	Egg, whole, hard boiled	1 ea	37	57	5	0	0	4	1.2	157
19521	Egg, whole, poached	1 ea	37	53	5	0	0	4	1.1	156
19516	Egg, whole, scrambled	1 ea	61	102	7	1	0	7	2.2	215
19508	Egg, yolk, raw, fresh	1 ea	17	53	3	1	0	4	1.6	205

MDA Code	Food Name	Amt	Wt (g)	Ener (kcal)	Prot (g)	Carb (g)	Fiber (g)	Fat (g)	Sat (g)	Chol (g)
Fruit										
72101	Apricots, canned, heavy syrup, drained	1 cup	182	151	1	39	5	0	0	0
3164	Fruit cocktail canned in juice	1 cup	237	109	1	28	2	0	0	0
71079	Apple w/ skin, raw	1 cup	125	65	0	17	3	0	0	0
3331	Applesauce w/ added vitamin C	0.5 cup	128	97	0	25	2	0	0	0
3657	Apricot, raw	1 cup	165	79	2	18	3	1	0	0
3210	Avocado, California, peeled, raw	1 ea	173	289	3	15	12	27	3.7	0
71082	Banana, peeled, raw	1 ea	81	72	1	19	2	0	0.1	0
71976	Grapefruit, fresh	0.5 ea	154	60	1	16	6	0	0	0
3055	Grapes, Thompson seedless, fresh	0.5 cup	80	55	1	14	1	0	0	0
3642	Melon, fresh, wedge	1 pce	69	23	1	6	1	0	0	0
3168	Mixed fruit (prune, apricot, & pear) dried	1 oz	28	69	1	18	2	0	0	0
3216	Nectarine, raw	1 cup	138	61	1	15	2	0	0	0
3726	Peach, peeled, raw	1 ea	79	31	1	8	1	0	0	0
3106	Pear, raw	1 ea	209	121	1	32	6	0	0	0
3766	Raisins, seedless	50 ea	26	78	1	21	1	0	0	0
72113	Pineapple, fresh, slice	1 pce	84	38	0	10		0		
3085	Orange, fresh	1 ea	184	86	2	22	4	0	0	0
3135	Strawberries, halves/slices, raw	1 cup	166	53	1	13	3	0	0	0
Grain Products										
Breads, Rolls, and Bread Crumbs										
71170	Bagel, cinnamon-raisin	1 ea	26	71	3	14	1	0	0.1	0
71167	Bagel, egg	1 ea	26	72	3	14	1	1	0.1	6
71152	Bagel, plain/onion/poppy/sesame, enriched	1 ea	26	67	3	13	1	0	0.1	0
42433	Biscuit, w/ butter	1 ea	82	273	5	28	1	16	3.9	1
71192	Biscuit, plain or buttermilk, refrig dough, baked, reduced fat	1 ea	21	63	2	12	0	1	0.3	0
42004	Bread crumbs, dry, plain, grated	1 Tbs	7	27	1	5	0	0	0.1	0
49144	Bread, crusty Italian w/ garlic	1 pce	50	186	4	21		10	2.4	6
70964	Bread, garlic, frozen/Campione	1 pce	28	101	2	12	1	5	0.8	
42069	Bread, oat bran	1 pce	30	71	3	12	1	1	0.2	0
42095	Bread, wheat, reduced kcal	1 pce	23	46	2	10	3	1	0.1	0
71247	Bread, white, commercially prepared, crumbs/cubes/slices	1 pce	9	24	1	5	0	0	0.1	0
42084	Bread, white, reduced kcal	1 pce	23	48	2	10	2	1	0.1	0
26561	Buns, hamburger, Wonder	1 ea	43	117	3	22	1	2	0.4	
42021	Hamburger/hot dog bun, plain	1 ea	43	120	4	21	1	2	0.5	0
42115	Cornbread, prepared from dry mix	1 pce	60	188	4	29	1	6	1.6	37
71227	Pita bread, white, enriched	1 ea	28	77	3	16	1	0	0	0
71228	Pita bread, whole wheat	1 ea	28	74	3	15	2	1	0.1	0
71368	Roll, dinner, plain, homemade w/ reduced fat (2%) milk	1 ea	43	136	4	23	1	3	0.8	15
42161	Roll, French	1 ea	38	105	3	19	1	2	0.4	0
71056	Roll, hard/kaiser	1 ea	57	167	6	30	1	2	0.3	0
42297	Tortilla, corn, w/o salt, ready to cook	1 ea	26	58	1	12	1	1	0.1	0
90645	Taco shell, baked	1 ea	5	23	0	3	0	1	0.3	0
Crackers										
71451	Cheez-its/Goldfish crackers, low sodium	55 pce	33	166	3	19	1	8	3.2	4
43507	Oyster/soda/soup crackers	1 cup	45	189	4	33	1	4	0.9	0
70963	Ritz crackers/Nabisco	5 ea	16	79	1	10	0	4	0.9	
43587	Saltine crackers, original premium/Nabisco	5 ea	14	56	1	10	0	1	0	0
43545	Sandwich crackers, cheese filled	4 ea	28	134	3	17	1	6	1.7	1
43546	Sandwich crackers, peanut butter filled	4 ea	28	138	3	16	1	7	1.4	0
44677	Snackwell Wheat Cracker/Nabisco	1 ea	15	62	1	12	1	2		
43581	Wheat Thins, baked/Nabisco	16 ea	29	140	3	20	1	6	0.9	0
43508	Whole wheat cracker	4 ea	32	137	3	22	3	5	0.7	0

MDA Code	Food Name	Amt	Wt (g)	Ener (kcal)	Prot (g)	Carb (g)	Fiber (g)	Fat (g)	Sat (g)	Chol (g)
Muffins and Baked Goods										
42723	English muffin, plain	1 ea	57	132	5	26		1	0.2	
62916	Muffin, blueberry, commercially prepared	1 ea	11	43	1	5	0	2	0.4	4
44521	Muffin, corn, commercially prepared	1 ea	57	174	3	29	2	5	0.8	15
44514	Muffin, oatbran	1 ea	57	154	4	28	3	4	0.6	0
44518	Toaster muffin, blueberry	1 ea	33	103	2	18	1	3	0.5	2
Noodles and Pasta										
38048	Chow mein noodles, dry	1 cup	45	237	4	26	2	14	2	0
38047	Egg noodles, enriched, cooked	0.5 cup	80	110	4	20	1	2	0.3	23
38060	Spaghetti, whole wheat, cooked	1 cup	140	174	7	37	6	1	0.1	0
38251	Egg noodles, enriched, cooked w/ salt	0.5 cup	80	110	4	20	1	2		23
38102	Macaroni noodles, enriched, cooked	1 cup	140	221	8	43	3	1	0.2	0
38118	Spaghetti noodles, enriched, cooked	0.5 cup	70	111	4	22	1	1	0.1	0
Grains										
38076	Couscous, cooked	0.5 cup	78	88	3	18	1	0	0	0
38080	Oats	0.25 cup	39	152	7	26	4	3	0.5	0
38010	Rice, brown, long grain, cooked	1 cup	195	216	5	45	4	2	0.4	0
38256	Rice, white, long grain, enriched, cooked w/ salt	1 cup	158	205	4	45	1	0	0.1	0
38019	Rice, white, long grain, instant, enriched, cooked	1 cup	165	193	4	41	1	1	0	0
Pancakes, French Toast, and Waffles										
42156	French toast, homemade, w/reduced fat (2%) milk	1 pce	65	149	5	16		7	1.8	75
45192	Pancake/waffle, buttermilk/Eggo/Kellogg	1 ea	42	99	3	16	0	3	0.6	5
45117	Pancakes, plain, homemade	1 ea	77	175	5	22	1	7	1.6	45
45193	Waffle, lowfat, homestyle, frozen	1 ea	35	83	2	15	0	1	0.3	9
Meat and Meat Substitutes										
Beef										
10093	Beef, average of all cuts, lean & fat (1/4" trim), cooked	3 oz	85	260	22	0	0	18	7.3	75
10705	Beef, average of all cuts, lean (1/4" trim), cooked	3 oz	85	184	25	0	0	8	3.2	73
10133	Beef, whole rib, roasted, 1/4" trim	3 oz	85	305	19	0	0	25	10	71
58129	Ground beef (hamburger), 25% fat, cooked, pan-browned	3 oz	85	236	22	0	0	15	6	76
58119	Ground beef (hamburger), 15% fat, cooked, pan-browned	3 oz	85	218	24	0	0	13	5	77
58109	Ground beef (hamburger), 5% fat, cooked, pan-browned	3 oz	85	164	25	0	0	6	2.9	76
10791	Porterhouse steak, lean & fat (1/4" trim), broiled	3 oz	85	280	19	0	0	22	8.7	61
58257	Rib eye steak, small end (ribs 10–12), 0" trim, broiled	3 oz	85	210	23	0	0	13	4.9	94
58094	Skirt steak, trimmed to 0" fat, broiled	3 oz	85	187	22	0	0	10	4	51
58328	Strip steak, top loin, 1/8" trim, broiled	3 oz	85	171	25	0	0	7	2.7	67
10805	T-Bone steak, lean & fat (1/4" trim), broiled	3 oz	85	260	20	0	0	19	7.6	55
11531	Veal, average of all cuts, cooked	3 oz	85	197	26	0	0	10	3.6	97
Chicken										
15057	Chicken breast, w/o skin, fried	3 oz	85	159	28	0	0	4	1.1	77
15080	Chicken, dark meat, w/ skin, roasted	3 oz	85	215	22	0	0	13	3.7	77
15026	Chicken, dark meat, w/o skin, fried	3 oz	85	203	25	2	0	10	2.7	82
15042	Chicken drumstick, w/o skin, fried	3 oz	85	166	24	0	0	7	1.8	80
15048	Chicken, wing, w/o skin, fried	3 oz	85	180	26	0	0	8	2.1	71
15059	Chicken, wing, w/o skin, roasted	3 oz	85	173	26	0	0	7	1.9	72
Turkey										
51151	Turkey bacon, cooked	1 oz	28	108	8	1	0	8	2.4	28
*51098	Turkey patty, breaded, fried	1 ea	42	119	6	7	0	8	2	32
16110	Turkey breast w/ skin, roasted	3 oz	85	130	25	0	0	3	0.7	77
16038	Turkey breast, no skin, roasted	3 oz	85	115	26	0	0	1	0.2	71
16101	Turkey, dark meat w/ skin, roasted	3 oz	85	155	24	0	0	6	1.8	100
16003	Turkey, ground, cooked	1 ea	82	193	22	0	0	11	2.8	84
Lamb										
13604	Lamb, average of all cuts (1/4" trim), cooked	3 oz	85	250	21	0	0	18	7.5	83
13616	Lamb, average of all cuts, lean (1/4" trim), cooked	3 oz	85	175	24	0	0	8	2.9	78

MDA Code	Food Name	Amt	Wt (g)	Ener (kcal)	Prot (g)	Carb (g)	Fiber (g)	Fat (g)	Sat (g)	Chol (g)
Pork										
12000	Bacon, broiled, pan-fried, or roasted	3 pcs	19	103	7	0	0	8	2.6	21
28143	Canadian bacon	1 pce	56	68	9	1		3	1	27
12211	Ham, cured, boneless, regular fat (11% fat), roasted	1 cup	140	249	32	0	0	13	4.4	83
12309	Pork, average of retail cuts, cooked	3 oz	85	203	22	0	0	12	4.2	75
12097	Pork, ribs, backribs, roasted	3 oz	85	315	21	0	0	25	9.4	100
12099	Pork, ground, cooked	3 oz	85	253	22	0	0	18	6.6	80
Lunchmeats										
13000	Beef, thin slices	1 oz	28	33	5	1	0	1	0.3	14
58275	Bologna, beef and pork, low fat	1 ea	14	32	2	0	0	3	1	5
13157	Chicken breast, oven roasted deluxe	1 oz	28	29	5	1	0	1	0.2	14
13306	Corned beef, cooked, chopped, pressed	1 ea	71	101	14	1	0	5	2	46
13264	Ham, slices, regular (11% fat)	1 cup	135	220	22	5	2	12	4	77
13101	Pastrami, beef, cured	1 oz	28	42	6	0	0	2	0.8	19
13215	Salami, beef, cotto	1 oz	28	59	4	1	0	4	1.9	24
16160	Turkey breast slice	1 pce	21	22	4	1	0	0	0.1	9
58279	Turkey ham, sliced, extra lean, prepackaged or deli-sliced	1 cup	138	171	27	4	0	5	1.5	92
Sausage										
13070	Chorizo, pork & beef	1 ea	60	273	14	1	0	23	8.6	53
57877	Frankfurter, beef	1 ea	45	148	5	2	0	13	5.3	24
13012	Frankfurter, turkey	1 ea	45	100	6	2	0	8	1.8	35
57890	Italian sausage, pork, cooked	1 ea	83	286	16	4	0	23	8	47
13021	Pepperoni sausage	1 pce	6	27	1	0	0	2	0.8	6
13185	Pork sausage links, cooked	2 ea	48	165	8	0	0	15	5.1	37
58227	Sausage, pork, precooked	3 oz	85	321	12	0	0	30	9.9	63
58007	Turkey sausage, breakfast links, mild	2 ea	56	132	9	1	0	10	2.1	90
Meat Substitutes										
7509	Bacon substitute, vegetarian, strips	3 ea	15	46	2	1	0	4	0.7	0
7722	Garden patties, frozen/Worthington, Morningstar	1 ea	67	118	12	9	3	4	0.5	1
7674	Harvest burger, original flavor, vegetable protein patty	1 ea	90	138	18	7	6	4	1	0
90626	Sausage, vegetarian, meatless	1 ea	28	72	5	3	1	5	0.8	0
7726	Spicy black bean burger/Worthington, Morningstar	1 ea	78	133	13	15	5	4	0.6	1
Nuts										
4519	Cashews, dry roasted w/ salt	0.25 cup	34	196	5	11	1	16	3.1	0
4728	Macadamia nuts, dry roasted, unsalted	1 cup	134	962	10	18	11	102	16	0
4592	Mixed nuts, w/ peanuts, dry roasted, salted	0.25 cup	34	203	6	9	3	18	2.4	0
4626	Peanut butter, chunky w/ salt	2 Tbs	32	188	8	7	3	16	2.6	0
4756	Peanuts, dry roasted w/o salt	30 ea	30	176	7	6	2	15	2.1	0
4696	Peanuts, raw	0.25 cup	36	207	9	6	3	18	2.5	0
4540	Pistachio nuts, dry roasted, salted	0.25 cup	32	182	7	9	3	15	1.8	0
Seafood										
17029	Bass, freshwater, cooked w/ dry heat	3 oz	85	124	21	0	0	4	0.9	74
17037	Cod, Atlantic, baked/broiled (dry heat)	3 oz	85	89	19	0	0	1	0.1	47
19036	Crab, Alaskan King, boiled/steamed	3 oz	85	83	16	0	0	1	0.1	45
17090	Haddock, baked or broiled (dry heat)	3 oz	85	95	21	0	0	1	0.1	63
17291	Halibut, Atlantic & Pacific, baked or broiled (dry heat)	3 oz	85	119	23	0	0	3	0.4	35
17181	Salmon, Atlantic, farmed, cooked w/ dry heat	3 oz	85	175	19	0	0	11	2.1	54
17099	Salmon, Sockeye, baked or broiled (dry heat)	3 oz	85	184	23	0	0	9	1.6	74
71707	Squid, fried	3 oz	85	149	15	7	0	6	1.6	221
17066	Swordfish, baked or broiled (dry heat)	3 oz	85	132	22	0	0	4	1.2	43
56007	Tuna salad, lunchmeat spread	2 Tbs	26	48	4	2	0	2	0.4	3
17151	White tuna, canned in water, drained	3 oz	85	109	20	0	0	3	0.7	36
17083	White tuna, canned in oil, drained	3 oz	85	158	23	0	0	7	1.1	26

MDA Code	Food Name	Amt	Wt (g)	Ener (kcal)	Prot (g)	Carb (g)	Fiber (g)	Fat (g)	Sat (g)	Chol (g)
Vegetables and Legumes										
Beans										
7038	Baked beans, plain or vegetarian, canned	1 cup	254	239	12	54	10	1	0.2	0
5197	Bean sprouts, mung, canned, drained	1 cup	125	15	2	3	1	0	0	0
7012	Black beans, boiled w/o salt	1 cup	172	227	15	41	15	1	0.2	0
5862	Beets, boiled w/ salt, drained	0.5 cup	85	37	1	8	2	0	0	0
90018	Cowpeas, cooked w/ salt	1 cup	171	198	13	35	11	1	0.2	0
7081	Hummus, garbanzo or chickpea spread, homemade	1 Tbs	15	27	1	3	1	1	0.2	0
7087	Kidney beans, canned	1 cup	256	215	13	37	14	2	0.3	0
7006	Lentils, boiled w/o salt	1 cup	198	230	18	40	16	1	0.1	0
7051	Pinto beans, canned	1 cup	240	206	12	37	11	2	0.4	0
6748	Snap green beans, raw	10 ea	55	17	1	4	1	0	0	0
5320	Snap yellow beans, raw	0.5 cup	55	17	1	4	2	0	0	0
90026	Split peas, boiled w/ salt	0.5 cup	98	114	8	20	8	0	0.1	0
7054	White beans, canned	1 cup	262	299	19	56	13	1	0.2	0
Fresh Vegetables										
9577	Artichokes (globe or French) boiled w/ salt, drained	1 ea	20	11	1	2	2	0	0	0
6033	Arugula/roquette, raw	1 cup	20	5	1	1	0	0	0	0
90406	Asparagus, raw	10 ea	35	7	1	1	1	0	0	0
5558	Broccoli stalks, raw	1 ea	114	32	3	6	3	0	0.1	0
5036	Cabbage, raw	1 cup	70	18	1	4	2	0	0	0
90605	Carrots, baby, raw	1 ea	15	5	0	1	0	0	0	0
5049	Cauliflower, raw	0.5 cup	50	12	1	2	1	0	0	0
90436	Celery, raw	1 ea	17	3	0	1	0	0	0	0
7202	Corn, white, sweet, ears, raw	1 ea	73	63	2	14	2	1	0.1	0
5900	Corn, yellow, sweet, boiled w/ salt, drained	0.5 cup	82	79	3	17	2	1	0.2	0
5908	Eggplant (brinjal) boiled w/ salt, drained	1 cup	99	33	1	8	2	0	0	0
5087	Lettuce, looseleaf, raw	2 pcs	20	3	0	1	0	0	0	0
51069	Mushrooms, brown, Italian, or crimini, raw	2 ea	28	6	1	1	0	0	0	0
90472	Onions, chopped, raw	1 ea	70	28	1	7	1	0	0	0
5116	Peas, green, raw	1 cup	145	117	8	21	7	1	0.1	0
7932	Peppers, jalapeno, raw	1 cup	90	27	1	5	2	1	0.1	0
90493	Peppers, sweet green, chopped/sliced, raw	10 pcs	27	5	0	1	0	0	0	0
6990	Pepper, sweet red, raw	1 ea	10	3	0	1	0	0	0	0
9251	Potatoes, red, flesh and skin, baked	1 ea	138	123	3	27	2	0	0	0
9245	Potatoes, russet, flesh and skin, baked	1 ea	138	134	4	30	3	0	0	0
5146	Spinach, raw	1 cup	30	7	1	1	1	0	0	0
90525	Squash, zucchini w/ skin, slices, raw	1 ea	118	20	1	4	1	0	0.1	0
6924	Sweet potato, baked in skin w/ salt	0.5 cup	100	92	2	21	3	0	0.1	0
5180	Tomato sauce, canned	0.5 cup	123	30	2	7	2	0	0	0
90532	Tomato, red, ripe, whole, raw	1 pce	15	3	0	1	0	0	0	0
5306	Yam, peeled, raw	0.5 cup	75	88	1	21	3	0	0	0
Soy and Soy Products										
7564	Tempeh	0.5 cup	83	160	15	8		9	1.8	0
7015	Soybeans, cooked	1 cup	172	298	29	17	10	15	2.2	0
7542	Tofu, firm, silken, 1" slice	3 oz	85	53	6	2	0	2	0.3	0
Meals and Dishes										
92216	Tortellini with cheese filling	1 cup	108	332	15	51	2	8	3.9	45
57658	Chili con carne w/ beans, canned entree	1 cup	222	269	16	25	9	12	3.9	29
57703	Chili, vegetarian chili w/ beans, canned entree/Hormel	1 cup	247	205	12	38	10	1	0.1	0
57068	Macaroni and cheese, unprepared/Kraft	1 ea	70	260	9	48	1	4	2	15
70958	Stir fry, rice & vegetables, w/ soy sauce/Hanover	1 cup	137	130	5	27	2	0		
70943	Beef & bean burrito/Las Campanas	1 ea	114	296	9	38	1	12	4.2	13
16195	Chicken & vegetables/Lean Cuisine	1 ea	297	232	20	26	4	5	1.9	30
70917	Hot Pockets, beef & cheddar, frozen	1 ea	142	403	16	39		20	8.8	53
70918	Hot Pockets, croissant pocket w/ chicken, broccoli, & cheddar, frozen	1 ea	128	301	11	39	1	11	3.4	37

MDA Code	Food Name	Amt	Wt (g)	Ener (kcal)	Prot (g)	Carb (g)	Fiber (g)	Fat (g)	Sat (g)	Chol (g)
56757	Lasagna w/ meat sauce/Stouffer's	1 ea	215	249	17	27	2	8	4.1	28
11029	Macaroni & beef in tomato sauce/Lean Cuisine	1 ea	283	326	21	40	3	9	3.7	32
5587	Mashed potatoes, from granules w/ milk, prep w/ water & margarine	0.5 cup	105	122	2	17	1	5	1.2	2
70898	Pizza, pepperoni, frozen	1 ea	146	432	16	42	3	22	7	22
56703	Spaghetti w/ meat sauce/Lean Cuisine	1 ea	326	284	14	49	5	4	1.1	13
Snack Foods										
10051	Beef jerky	1 pce	20	81	7	2	0	5	2.1	10
63331	Breakfast bars, oats, sugar, raisins, coconut	1 ea	43	200	4	29	1	8	5.5	0
61251	Cheese puffs and twists, corn based, low fat	1 oz	28	123	2	21	3	3	0.6	0
44032	Chex snack mix	1 cup	42	180	4	32	2	4	0.6	
23059	Granola bar, hard, plain	1 ea	24	115	2	16	1	5	0.6	0
23104	Granola bar, soft, plain	1 ea	28	126	2	19	1	5	2.1	0
44012	Popcorn, air-popped	1 cup	8	31	1	6	1	0	0	0
44076	Potato chips, plain, no salt	1 oz	28	152	2	15	1	10	3.1	0
5437	Potato chips, sour cream & onion	1 oz	28	151	2	15	1	10	2.5	2
44015	Pretzels, hard	5 pcs	30	114	3	24	1	1	0.1	0
44021	Rice cake, brown rice, plain, salted	1 ea	9	35	1	7	0	0	0.1	0
44058	Trail mix, regular	0.25 cup	38	173	5	17		11	2.1	0
Soups										
50398	Beef barley, canned/Progresso Healthy Classics	1 cup	241	142	11	20	3	2	0.7	19
50081	Chicken noodle, chunky, canned	1 cup	240	89	8	10	1	2	1	12
50085	Chicken rice, chunky, ready to eat, canned	1 cup	240	127	12	13	1	3	1	12
50088	Chicken vegetable, chunky, canned	1 cup	240	166	12	19		5	1.4	17
90238	Chicken, chunky, canned	1 cup	240	170	12	17	1	6	1.9	29
50697	Cup of Noodles, ramen, chicken flavor, dry/Nissin	1 ea	64	296	6	37		14	6.3	
50009	Minestrone, canned, made w/ water	1 cup	241	82	4	11	1	3	0.6	2
92163	Ramen noodle, any flavor, dehydrated, dry	0.5 cup	38	166	4	24	1	6	2.9	0
50043	Tomato vegetable, from dry mix, made w/ water	1 cup	253	56	2	10	1	1	0.4	0
50028	Tomato, canned, made w/ water	1 cup	244	73	2	16	1	1	0.2	0
50014	Vegetable beef, canned, made w/ water	1 cup	244	76	5	10	2	2	0.8	5
50013	Vegetarian vegetable, canned, made w/ water	1 cup	241	67	2	12	1	2	0.3	0
Desserts										
62904	Brownie, commercially prepared, square, lrg, 2-3/4" × 7/8"	1 ea	56	227	3	36	1	9	2.4	10
46062	Cake, chocolate, homemade, w/o icing	1 pce	95	352	5	51	2	14	5.2	55
46091	Cake, yellow, homemade, w/o icing	1 pce	68	245	4	36	0	10	2.7	37
71337	Doughnut, cake, w/ chocolate icing, lrg, 3 1/2"	1 ea	57	258	3	29	1	14	7.7	11
45525	Doughnut, cake, glazed/sugared, med, 3"	1 ea	45	192	2	23	1	10	2.7	14
47026	Animal crackers/Arrowroot/Tea Biscuits	10 ea	12	56	1	9	0	2	0.4	0
90636	Chocolate chip cookie, commercially prepared 3.5" to 4"	1 ea	40	190	2	26	1	9	4	0
47006	Chocolate sandwich cookie, creme filled	3 ea	30	141	2	21	1	6	1.9	0
62905	Fig bar, 2 oz	1 ea	57	197	2	40	3	4	0.6	0
90640	Oatmeal cookie, commercially prepared, 3-1/2" to 4"	1 ea	25	112	2	17	1	5	1.1	0
47010	Peanut butter cookie, homemade, 3"	1 ea	20	95	2	12		5	0.9	6
62907	Sugar cookie, refrigerated dough, baked	1 ea	23	111	1	15	0	5	1.4	7
57894	Pudding, chocolate, ready to eat	1 ea	113	160	2	26	0	5	1.4	1
2612	Pudding, vanilla, ready to eat	1 ea	113	147	2	26	0	4	1.1	1
2651	Rice pudding, ready to eat	1 ea	142	168	5	28	1	4	2.5	26
57902	Tapioca pudding, ready to eat	1 ea	113	147	2	25	0	4	1.1	1
71819	Frozen yogurts, chocolate, nonfat	1 cup	186	199	8	37	4	1	0.9	7
72124	Frozen yogurts, flavors other than chocolate	1 cup	174	221	5	38	0	6	4	23
2010	Ice cream, light, vanilla, soft serve	0.5 cup	88	111	4	19	0	2	1.4	11
90723	Ice popsicle	1 ea	59	47	0	11	0	0	0	0
42264	Cinnamon rolls w/ icing, refrigerated dough/Pillsbury	1 ea	44	145	2	23	0	5	1.5	0
71299	Croissant, butter	1 ea	67	272	5	31	2	14	7.8	45
45572	Danish, cheese	1 ea	71	266	6	26	1	16	4.8	16
45593	Toaster pastry, Pop Tart, apple-cinnamon/Kellogg	1 ea	52	205	2	37	1	5	0.9	0

MDA Code	Food Name	Amt	Wt (g)	Ener (kcal)	Prot (g)	Carb (g)	Fiber (g)	Fat (g)	Sat (g)	Chol (g)
23014	Chocolate syrup, fudge-type	2 Tbs	38	133	2	24	1	3	1.5	0
510	Whipped cream topping, pressurized	2 Tbs	8	19	0	1	0	2	1	6
54387	Whipped topping, frozen, low fat	2 Tbs	9	21	0	2	0	1	1.1	0

Fats, Oils, and Condiments

MDA Code	Food Name	Amt	Wt (g)	Ener (kcal)	Prot (g)	Carb (g)	Fiber (g)	Fat (g)	Sat (g)	Chol (g)
90210	Butter, unsalted	1 Tbs	14	100	0	0	0	11	7.2	30
8084	Oil, vegetable, canola	1 Tbs	14	124	0	0	0	14	1	0
8008	Oil, olive, salad or cooking	1 Tbs	14	119	0	0	0	14	1.9	0
8111	Oil, safflower, salad or cooking, greater than 70% oleic	1 Tbs	14	120	0	0	0	14	0.8	0
44483	Shortening, household	1 Tbs	13	113	0	0	0	13	3.2	0
1708	Barbecue sauce, original	2 Tbs	36	63	0	15		0		
27001	Ketchup	1 ea	6	6	0	2	0	0	0	0
53523	Cheese sauce, ready to eat	0.25 cup	63	110	4	4	0	8	3.8	18
54388	Cream substitute, powdered, light	1 Tbs	6	25	0	4	0	1	0.2	0
50939	Gravy, brown, homestyle, canned	0.25 cup	60	25	1	3		1	0.3	2
23003	Jelly	1 Tbs	19	51	0	13	0	0	0	0
25002	Maple syrup	1 Tbs	20	52	0	13	0	0	0	0
44476	Margarine, regular, 80% fat, with salt	1 Tbs	14	101	0	0	0	11	2	0
8145	Mayonnaise, safflower/soybean oil	1 Tbs	14	99	0	0	0	11	1.2	8
8502	Miracle Whip, light/Kraft	1 Tbs	16	37	0	2	0	3	0.5	4
435	Mustard, yellow	1 tsp	5	3	0	0	0	0	0	0
23042	Pancake syrup	1 Tbs	20	47	0	12	0	0	0	0
23172	Pancake syrup, reduced kcal	1 Tbs	15	25	0	7	0	0	0	0
53524	Pasta sauce, spaghetti/marinara	0.5 cup	125	109	2	17	3	3	0.9	2
53646	Salsa picante, mild	2 Tbs	30	8	0	1	0	0		0
504	Sour cream, cultured	2 Tbs	29	56	1	1	0	6	3.3	15
53063	Soy sauce	1 Tbs	18	11	2	1	0	0	0	0
53652	Taco sauce, red, mild	1 Tbs	16	7	0	1	0	0		0
53004	Teriyaki sauce	1 Tbs	18	16	1	3	0	0	0	0
8024	Thousand Island, regular	1 Tbs	16	58	0	2	0	5	0.8	4
8013	Blue/Roquefort cheese, regular	2 Tbs	31	146	0	1	0	16	2.5	9
90232	French, regular	1 Tbs	12	56	0	2	0	6	0.7	0
44498	Italian, fat-free	1 Tbs	14	7	0	1	0	0	0	0
44696	Ranch, reduced fat	1 Tbs	15	29	0	3	0	2	0.2	2
8035	Vinegar & oil, homemade	2 Tbs	31	140	0	1	0	16	2.8	0

Fast Food

MDA Code	Food Name	Amt	Wt (g)	Ener (kcal)	Prot (g)	Carb (g)	Fiber (g)	Fat (g)	Sat (g)	Chol (g)
6177	Baked potato, topped w/ cheese sauce	1 ea	296	474	15	47		29	10.6	18
56629	Burrito w/ beans & cheese	1 ea	93	189	8	27		6	3.4	14
66023	Burrito w/ beans, cheese, & beef	1 ea	102	166	7	20		7	3.6	62
66024	Burrito w/ beef	1 ea	110	262	13	29		10	5.2	32
56600	Biscuit w/ egg sandwich	1 ea	136	373	12	32	1	22	4.7	245
66029	Biscuit w/ egg, cheese, & bacon sandwich	1 ea	144	433	17	35	0	25	8.5	239
66013	Cheeseburger, double, condiments & vegetables	1 ea	166	417	21	35		21	8.7	60
56649	Cheeseburger, large, one meat patty w/ condiments & vegetables	1 ea	219	451	25	37	3	23	8.5	74
15063	Chicken, breaded, fried, dark meat (drumstick or thigh)	3 oz	85	248	17	9		15	4.1	95
15064	Chicken, breaded, fried, light meat (breast or wing)	3 oz	85	258	19	10		15	4.1	77
56000	Chicken filet, plain	1 ea	182	515	24	39		29	8.5	60
56635	Chimichanga w/ beef & cheese	1 ea	183	443	20	39		23	11.2	51
5461	Cole slaw	0.75 cup	99	151	1	15	2	10	1.6	4
56606	Croissant w/ egg & cheese sandwich	1 ea	127	368	13	24		25	14.1	216
56607	Croissant w/ egg, cheese, & bacon sandwich	1 ea	129	413	16	24		28	15.4	215
66021	Enchilada w/ cheese	1 ea	163	319	10	29		19	10.6	44
66020	Enchirito w/ cheese, beef, & beans	1 ea	193	344	18	34		16	7.9	50
66031	English muffin w/ cheese & sausage sandwich	1 ea	115	389	15	29	1	24	9.4	49
66010	Fish sandwich w/ tartar sauce	1 ea	158	431	17	41		23	5.2	55
90736	French fries fried in vegetable oil, medium	1 ea	134	427	5	50	5	23	5.3	0
56638	Frijoles (beans) w/ cheese	0.5 cup	84	113	6	14		4	2	18

MDA Code	Food Name	Amt	Wt (g)	Ener (kcal)	Prot (g)	Carb (g)	Fiber (g)	Fat (g)	Sat (g)	Chol (g)
56664	Ham & cheese sandwich	1 ea	146	352	21	33		15	6.4	58
56662	Hamburger, large, double, w/ condiments & vegetables	1 ea	226	540	34	40		27	10.5	122
56659	Hamburger, one patty w/ condiments & vegetables	1 ea	110	279	13	27		13	4.1	26
66007	Hamburger, plain	1 ea	90	266	13	30	1	10	3.2	30
5463	Hash browns	0.5 cup	72	235	2	23	2	16	3.6	0
66004	Hot dog, plain	1 ea	98	242	10	18		15	5.1	44
2032	Ice cream sundae, hot fudge	1 ea	158	284	6	48	0	9	5	21
6185	Mashed potatoes	0.5 cup	121	100	3	20		1	0.6	2
56639	Nachos w/ cheese	7 pcs	113	346	9	36		19	7.8	18
6176	Onion rings, breaded, fried	8 pcs	78	259	3	29		15	6.5	13
6173	Potato salad	0.33 cup	95	108	1	13		6	1	57
56619	Pizza w/ pepperoni 12" or 1/8	1 pce	108	275	15	30		11	3.4	22
66003	Roast beef sandwich, plain	1 ea	139	346	22	33		14	3.6	51
56671	Submarine sandwich, cold cuts	1 ea	228	456	22	51		19	6.8	36
57531	Taco	1 ea	171	371	21	27		21	11.4	56
71129	Shake, chocolate, 12 fl. oz	1 ea	250	318	8	51	5	9	5.8	32
71132	Shake, vanilla, 12 fl. oz	1 ea	250	370	8	49	2	16	9.9	58

Source: This food composition table has been prepared for Pearson Education, Inc., and is copyrighted by ESHA Research in Salem, Oregon, the developer of the MyDietAnalysis software program.

Glossary

% Daily Values (%DVs) Percentages listed as "% DV" on food and supplement labels; identify how much of each listed nutrient a serving of food contributes to a 2,000 calorie/day diet.

5-year survival rates The percentage of people in a study or treatment group who are alive 5 years after they were diagnosed with or treated for a disease such as cancer.

abortion Termination of a pregnancy by expulsion or removal of an embryo or fetus from the uterus.

abstinence Refraining from a behavior.

accountability Accepting responsibility for personal decisions, choices, and actions.

acid deposition Acidification process that occurs when pollutants are deposited by precipitation, clouds, or directly on the land.

acquaintance rape Any rape in which the rapist is known to the victim (replaces the formerly used term *date rape*).

acquired immunodeficiency syndrome (AIDS) A disease caused by a retrovirus, the human immunodeficiency virus (HIV), that attacks the immune system, reducing the number of helper T cells and leaving the victim vulnerable to infections, malignancies, and neurological disorders.

active euthanasia "Mercy killing" in which a person or organization knowingly acts to end the life of a terminally ill person.

acupressure Branch of traditional Chinese medicine related to acupuncture. Uses application of pressure to selected body points to balance energy.

acupuncture Branch of traditional Chinese medicine that uses the insertion of long, thin needles to affect flow of energy (*qi*) along pathways (meridians) within the body.

acute stress The short-term physiological response to an immediate perceived threat.

adaptive response Form of adjustment in which the body attempts to restore homeostasis.

adaptive thermogenesis Theoretical mechanism by which the brain regulates metabolic activity according to caloric intake.

addiction Persistent, compulsive dependence on a behavior or substance, including mood-altering behaviors or activities, despite ongoing negative consequences.

advance directive Document that stipulates an individual's wishes about medical care; used to make treatment decisions when an individual becomes physically unable to voice his or her preferences.

aerobic capacity (or power) The functional status of the cardiorespiratory system; refers specifically to the volume of oxygen the muscles consume during exercise.

aerobic exercise Any type of exercise that increases heart rate.

aggravated rape Rape that involves one or multiple attackers, strangers, weapons, or physical beating.

aging Patterns of life changes that occur in members of all species as they grow older.

alcohol abuse Use of alcohol in a way that interferes with work, school, or personal relationships or that entails violations of the law.

alcohol poisoning Potentially lethal blood alcohol concentration that inhibits the brain's ability to control consciousness, respiration, and heart rate; usually occurs as a result of drinking a large amount of alcohol in a short period of time. Also known as *acute alcohol intoxication.*

alcoholic hepatitis Condition resulting from prolonged use of alcohol in which the liver is inflamed; can be fatal.

Alcoholics Anonymous (AA) Organization whose goal is to help alcoholics stop drinking; includes auxiliary branches such as Al-Anon and Alateen.

alcoholism (alcohol dependence) Condition in which personal and health problems related to alcohol use are severe, and stopping alcohol use results in withdrawal symptoms.

alleles One of potentially several variants of the same gene.

allergen An antigen that induces a hypersensitive immune response.

allergies Hypersensitivity reactions in which the body produces antibodies to a normally harmless substance in the environment.

allergy Hypersensitive reaction to a specific antigen in which the body produces antibodies to a normally harmless substance.

allopathic medicine Conventional, Western medical practice; in theory, based on scientifically validated methods and procedures.

allostatic load Wear and tear on the body caused by prolonged or excessive stress responses.

alternative insemination Fertilization procedure accomplished by depositing semen from a partner or donor into a woman's vagina via a thin tube.

alternative (whole) medical systems Complete systems of theory and practice that involve several CAM domains.

alternative medicine Treatment used in place of conventional medicine.

altruism Giving of oneself out of genuine concern for others.

altruism Giving of oneself out of genuine concern for others.

alveoli Tiny air sacs of the lungs where gas exchange occurs (oxygen enters the body and carbon dioxide is removed).

Alzheimer's disease (AD) Chronic condition involving changes in nerve fibers of the brain that results in mental deterioration.

amino acids The nitrogen-containing building blocks of protein.

amniocentesis Medical test in which a small amount of fluid is drawn from the amniotic sac to test for Down syndrome and other genetic abnormalities.

amniotic sac Protective pouch surrounding the fetus.

amphetamines A large and varied group of synthetic agents that stimulate the central nervous system.

anabolic steroids Artificial forms of the hormone testosterone that promote muscle growth and strength.

anal intercourse Insertion of the penis into the anus.

androgyny Combination of traditional masculine and feminine traits in a single person.

anemia Condition that results from the body's inability to produce adequate hemoglobin.

aneurysm A weakened blood vessel that may bulge under pressure and, in severe cases, burst.

angina pectoris Chest pain occurring as a result of reduced oxygen flow to the heart.

angiography A technique for examining blockages in heart arteries.

angioplasty A technique in which a catheter with a balloon at the tip is inserted into a clogged artery; the balloon is inflated to flatten fatty deposits against artery walls, and a stent is typically inserted to keep the artery open.

anorexia nervosa Eating disorder characterized by excessive preoccupation with food, self-starvation, or extreme exercising to achieve weight loss.

antagonism A drug interaction in which two drugs compete for the same available receptors, potentially blocking each other's actions.

antibiotic resistance The ability of bacteria or other microbes to withstand the effects of an antibiotic.

antibiotics Medicines used to kill microorganisms, such as bacteria.

antibodies Substances produced by the body that are individually matched to specific antigens.

antigen Substance capable of triggering an immune response.

antioxidants Substances believed to protect against oxidative stress and resultant tissue damage.

anxiety disorders Mental illness characterized by persistent feelings of threat and worry in coping with everyday problems.

appetite The desire to eat; normally accompanies hunger but is more psychological than physiological.

appraisal The interpretation and evaluation of information provided to the brain by the senses.

arrhythmia An irregularity in heartbeat.

arteries Vessels that carry blood away from the heart to other regions of the body.

arterioles Branches of the arteries.

arthritis Painful inflammatory disease of the joints.

asbestos Mineral compound that separates into stringy fibers and lodges in the lungs, where it can cause disease.

asthma A chronic respiratory disease characterized by attacks of wheezing, shortness of breath, and coughing spasms.

atherosclerosis Condition characterized by deposits of fatty substances (plaque) on the inner lining of an artery.

atria (singular: *atrium*) The heart's two upper chambers, which receive blood.

autoerotic behaviors Sexual self-stimulation.

autoimmune disease Disease caused by an overactive immune response against the body's own cells.

autoinoculate Transmit a pathogen from one part of your body to another part.

autonomic nervous system (ANS) The portion of the central nervous system regulating body functions that a person does not normally consciously control.

autosomal dominant disorder Single-gene disorder that occurs in individuals who have inherited at least one copy of an autosome with the affected dominant allele.

autosomal recessive disorder Single-gene disorder that occurs in individuals who have inherited two copies of an autosome with the affected recessive allele.

ayurveda (ayurvedic medicine) A comprehensive system of medicine, derived largely from ancient India, that places equal emphasis on the body, mind, and spirit, and strives to restore the body's innate harmony through diet, exercise, meditation, herbs, massage, exposure to sunlight, and controlled breathing.

background distressors Environmental stressors of which people are often unaware.

bacteria (singular: *bacterium*) Simple, single-celled microscopic organisms; about 100 known species of bacteria cause disease in humans.

barbiturates Drugs that depress the central nervous system and have sedating, hypnotic, and anesthetic effects.

barrier method Contraceptive methods that block the meeting of egg and sperm by means of a physical barrier (such as condom, diaphragm, or cervical cap);a chemical barrier (such as spermicide); or both.

basal body temperature The lowest temperature the body reaches, usually during sleep.

basal metabolic rate (BMR) The rate of energy expenditure by a body at complete rest in a neutral-environment.

behavioral genetics The science that studies the role of inheritance in human behavior.

belief Appraisal of the relationship between some object, action, or idea and some attribute of that object, action, or idea.

benign Harmless; refers to a noncancerous tumor.

benzodiazepines A class of central nervous system depressant drugs with sedative, hypnotic, and muscle relaxant effects.

bereavement Loss or deprivation experienced by a survivor when a loved one dies.

bidis Hand-rolled flavored cigarettes.

binge drinking A pattern of drinking alcohol that brings blood alcohol concentration (BAC) to 0.08 gram-percent or above; corresponds to consuming five or more drinks (adult male) or four or more drinks (adult female) in 2 hours.

binge-eating disorder A type of eating disorder characterized by binge eating once a week or more, but not typically followed by a purge.

biofeedback A technique using a machine to self-monitor physical responses to stress.

biopsy Removal and examination of a tissue sample to determine if a cancer is present.

biopsychosocial model of addiction Theory of the relationship between an addict's biological (genetic) nature and psychological and environmental influences.

bipolar disorder Form of mood disorder characterized by alternating mania and depression; also called *manic depression.*

bisexual Experiencing attraction to and preference for sexual activity with people of both sexes.

blood alcohol concentration (BAC) The ratio of alcohol to total blood volume; the factor used to measure the physiological and behavioral effects of alcohol.

body composition Describes the relative proportions of fat and lean (muscle, bone, water, organs) tissues in the body.

body image Most fundamentally, what you believe about your overall body and how you feel subjectively about your body, including shape, weight, and how you picture yourself in your mind.

body mass index (BMI) A number calculated from a person's weight and height that is used to assess risk for possible present or future health problems.

brain death Irreversible cessation of all functions of the entire brainstem.

bronchitis Inflammation of the lining of the bronchial tubes.

bulimia nervosa Eating disorder characterized by binge eating followed by inappropriate measures, such as vomiting, to prevent weight gain.

calorie A unit of measure that indicates the amount of energy obtained from a particular food.

cancer staging A classification system that describes how far a person's disease has advanced.

cancer A large group of diseases characterized by the uncontrolled growth and spread of abnormal cells.

candidiasis Yeastlike fungal infection often transmitted sexually; also called *moniliasis* or *yeast infection.*

capillaries Minute blood vessels that branch out from the arterioles and venules; their thin walls permit exchange of oxygen, carbon dioxide, nutrients, and waste products among body cells.

capitation Prepayment of a fixed monthly amount for each patient without regard to the type or number of services provided.

carbohydrates Basic nutrients that supply the body with glucose, the energy form most commonly used to sustain normal activity.

carbon dioxide (CO_2) Gas created by the combustion of fossil fuels and is exhaled by animals; used by plants for photosynthesis; the primary greenhouse gas in the atmosphere.

carbon footprint Amount of greenhouse gases produced, usually expressed in equivalent tons of carbon dioxide emissions.

carbon monoxide Gas found in cigarette smoke that reduces the ability of blood to carry oxygen.

carcinogens Cancer-causing agents.

cardiometabolic risks Physical and biochemical changes that are risk factors for the development of cardiovascular disease and type 2 diabetes.

cardiopulmonary resuscitation (CPR) Emergency technique to provide lifesaving chest compression and mouth-to-mouth resuscitation when an individual has stopped breathing and has no pulse.

cardiorespiratory fitness The ability of the heart, lungs, and blood vessels to supply oxygen to skeletal muscles during sustained physical activity.

cardiovascular disease (CVD) Diseases of the heart and blood vessels.

cardiovascular system Organ system, consisting of the heart and blood vessels, that transports nutrients, oxygen, hormones, metabolic wastes, and enzymes throughout the body.

carotenoids Fat-soluble plant pigments with antioxidant properties.

carpal tunnel syndrome A common occupational injury in which the median nerve in the wrist becomes irritated, causing numbness, tingling, and pain in the fingers and hands.

carrier Individual who has one copy of an autosome with a recessive allele for a particular trait, but is unaffected by it.

cataracts Clouding of the lens that interrupts the focusing of light on the retina, resulting in blurred vision or eventual blindness.

celiac disease An inherited autoimmune disorder causing malabsorption of nutrients from the small intestine and triggered by the consumption of gluten.

celibacy State of not engaging in sexual activity.

cell-mediated immunity Aspect of immunity that is mediated by specialized white blood cells that attack pathogens and antigens directly.

cervical caps Small cup made of latex or silicone that is designed to fit snugly over the entire cervix; should always be used with spermicide.

cervix Lower end of the uterus that opens into the vagina.

cesarean section (C-section) Surgical birthing procedure in which a baby is removed through an incision made in the mother's abdominal wall and uterus.

chancre Sore often found at the site of syphilis infection.

chemotherapy The use of drugs to kill cancerous cells.

chewing tobacco Stringy form of tobacco that is placed in the mouth and then sucked or chewed.

chickenpox A highly infectious disease caused by the herpes varicella zoster virus.

child abuse Deliberate, intentional words or actions that cause harm, potential for harm, or threat of harm to a child.

child maltreatment Any act or series of acts of commission or omission by a parent or caregiver that results in harm, potential for harm, or threat of harm to a child.

chiropractic medicine Manipulation of the spine to allow proper energy flow.

chlamydia Bacterially caused STI of the urogenital tract.

chlorofluorocarbons (CFCs) Chemicals that contribute to the depletion of the atmospheric ozone layer.

cholesterol A lipid found in foods and synthesized by the body. Although essential to functioning, cholesterol circulating in the blood can accumulate on the inner walls of blood vessels.

chorionic villus sampling (CVS) Prenatal test that involves snipping tissue from the fetal sac to be analyzed for genetic defects.

chromosome disorder A disorder arising from a missing or extra chromosome or damage to part of a chromosome.

chromosome Discrete bundle of DNA, 46 of which are present in the nucleus of almost all cells of the human body.

chronic disease A disease that typically begins slowly, progresses, and persists, with a variety of signs and symptoms that can be treated but not cured by medication.

chronic lower respiratory disease (CLRD)

chronic mood disorder Experience of persistent emotional states, such as sadness, despair, and hopelessness.

chronic obstructive pulmonary disease (COPD) The chronic lung diseases of emphysema and chronic bronchitis.

chronic stress An ongoing state of physiological arousal in response to ongoing or numerous perceived threats.

cirrhosis The last stage of liver disease associated with chronic heavy alcohol use, during which liver cells die and damage becomes permanent.

clitoris Pea-sized nodule of tissue located at the top of the labia minora; central to sexual arousal in women.

club drugs Synthetic analogs (drugs that produce similar effects) of existing illicit drugs.

codependence A self-defeating relationship pattern in which a person is controlled by an addict's addictive behavior.

cognitive restructuring The modification of thoughts, ideas, and beliefs that contribute to stress.

cohabitation Intimate partners living together without being married.

collateral circulation Adaptation of the heart to partial damage accomplished by rerouting needed blood through unused or underused blood vessels while the damaged heart muscle heals.

collective violence Violence perpetrated by groups against other groups.

colonization The process of bacteria or some other infectious organisms establishing themselves in a host without causing infection.

common-law marriage Cohabitation lasting a designated period of time (usually 7 years) that is considered legally binding in some states.

comorbidities The presence of one or more diseases at the same time.

complementary medicine Treatment used in conjunction with conventional medicine.

complete proteins Proteins that contain all nine of the essential amino acids.

complex carbohydrates A carbohydrate consisting of long chains of sugar molecules; also called a polysaccharide.

compulsion Preoccupation with a behavior and an overwhelming need to perform it.

compulsive exercise Disorder characterized by a compulsion to engage in excessive amounts of exercise and feelings of guilt and anxiety if the level of exercise is perceived as inadequate.

compulsive shoppers People who are preoccupied with shopping and spending.

computerized axial tomography (CAT) scan A scan by a machine that uses radiation to view internal organs not normally visible in X rays.

conception Fertilization of an ovum by a sperm.

conflict resolution Concerted effort by all parties to constructively resolve points of contention.

conflict Emotional state that arises when opinions differ or the behavior of one person interferes with the behavior of another.

congeners Forms of alcohol that are metabolized more slowly than ethanol and produce toxic by-products.

congenital cardiovascular defect Cardiovascular problem that is present at birth.

congestive heart failure (CHF) or heart failure (HF) An abnormal cardiovascular condition that reflects impaired cardiac pumping and blood flow; pooling blood leads to congestion in body tissues.

consummate love A combination of intimacy, compassion, and commitment.

contemplation Practice of concentrating the mind on a spiritual or ethical question or subject, a view of the natural world, or an icon or other image representative of divinity.

contraception (birth control) Methods of preventing conception.

contraceptive sponge Contraceptive device, made of polyurethane foam and containing nonoxynol-9, that fits over the cervix to create a barrier against sperm.

coping Managing events or conditions to lessen the physical or psychological effects of excess stress.

coronary artery disease (CAD) A narrowing or blockage of coronary arteries, usually caused by atherosclerotic plaque buildup.

coronary bypass surgery A surgical technique whereby a blood vessel taken from another part of the body is implanted to bypass a clogged coronary artery.

coronary heart disease (CHD) A narrowing of the small blood vessels that supply blood to the heart.

coronary heart disease (CHD) A narrowing of the small blood vessels that supply blood to the heart.

coronary thrombosis A blood clot occurring in a coronary artery.

coronary thrombosis A blood clot occurring in a coronary artery.

corpus luteum Cells that form from the remains of the graafian follicle following ovulation; it secretes estrogen and progesterone during the second half of the menstrual cycle.

cortisol Hormone released by the adrenal glands that makes stored nutrients more readily available to meet energy demands.

countering Substituting a desired behavior for an undesirable one.

Cowper's glands Glands that secrete a preejaculate fluid that lubricates the urethra and neutralizes any acid remaining in the urethra after urination.

Crohn's disease An autoimmune inflammatory disease of the gastrointestinal tract characterized by cramping and diarrhea.

cross-tolerance Development of a physiological tolerance to one drug that reduces the effects of another, similar drug.

cunnilingus Oral stimulation of a woman's genitals.

death The permanent ending of all vital functions.

defensive medicine The use of medical practices designed to avert the possibility of malpractice suits in the future.

dehydration Loss of water from body tissues.

dehydration Abnormal depletion of body fluids; a result of lack of water.

delayed ejaculation Persistent difficulty in reaching orgasm despite normal desire and stimulation.

delirium tremens (DTs) State of confusion, delusions, and agitation brought on by withdrawal from alcohol.

dementias Progressive brain impairments that interfere with memory and normal intellectual functioning.

denial Inability to perceive or accurately interpret the self-destructive effects of the addictive behavior.

dentist Specialist who diagnoses and treats diseases of the teeth, gums, and oral cavity.

Depo-Provera Injectable method of birth control that lasts for 3 months.

depressants Drugs that slow down the activity of the central nervous system.

determinants of health The range of personal, social, economic, and environmental factors that influence health status.

detoxification The early abstinence period during which an addict adjusts physically and cognitively to being free from the substance's influence.

detoxification The early abstinence period during which an addict adjusts physically and cognitively to being free from the influences of the addiction.

diabetes mellitus A group of diseases characterized by elevated blood glucose levels.

diaphragm Latex, cup-shaped device designed to cover the cervix and block access to the uterus; should always be used with spermicide.

diastolic pressure The lower number in the fraction that measures blood pressure, indicating pressure on arterial walls during the relaxation phase of heart activity.

dietary supplements Products taken by mouth and containing dietary ingredients such as vitamins and minerals that are intended to supplement existing diets.

digestive process The process by which the body breaks down foods and either absorbs or excretes them.

dilation and evacuation (D&E) Abortion technique that uses a combination of instruments and vacuum aspiration; fetal tissue is both sucked and scraped out of the uterus.

dioxins Highly toxic chlorinated hydrocarbons contained in herbicides and produced during certain industrial processes.

dipping Placing a small amount of chewing tobacco between the lower lip and teeth for rapid nicotine absorption.

disaccharides Combinations of two monosaccharides.

discrimination Actions that deny equal treatment or opportunities to a group, often based on prejudice.

disease prevention Actions or behaviors designed to keep people from getting sick.

disordered eating A pattern of atypical eating behaviors that is used to achieve or maintain a lower body weight.

disordered gambling Compulsive gambling that cannot be controlled.

distillation Process in which alcohol vapors are condensed and mixed with water to make hard liquor.

distress Stress that can have a detrimental effect on health; negative stress.

DNA (deoxyribonucleic acid) Compound residing in the nucleus of body cells that stores in its sequence of chemical subunits the instructions for assembling body proteins.

domestic violence The use of force to control and maintain power over another person in the home environment, including both actual harm and the threat of harm.

dominant Term describing an allele that is expressed even if there is only one copy in the pair.

Down syndrome Syndrome caused by the presence of an extra chromosome that results in mental retardation and distinctive physical characteristics.

drug abuse Excessive use of a drug.

drug misuse Use of a drug for a purpose for which it was not intended.

dying Process of decline in body functions that results in the death of an organism.

dysfunctional families Families in which there is violence; physical, emotional, or sexual abuse; parental discord; or other negative family interactions.

dysmenorrhea Condition of pain or discomfort in the lower abdomen just before or during menstruation.

dyspareunia Pain experienced by women during intercourse.

dyspnea Shortness of breath, usually associated with disease of the heart or lungs.

dysthymic disorder (dysthymia) Type of depression that is milder and harder to recognize than major depression; chronic; and often characterized by fatigue, pessimism, or a short temper.

eating disorder A psychiatric disorder characterized by severe disturbances in body image and eating behaviors.

eating disorders not otherwise specified (EDNOS) Eating disorders that are a true psychiatric illness but that do not fit the strict diagnostic criteria for anorexia nervosa, bulimia nervosa, or binge-eating disorder.

ecological or public health model A view of health in which diseases and other negative health events are seen as a result of an individual's interaction with his or her social and physical environment.

ecosystem Collection of physical (nonliving) and biological (living) components of an environment and the relationships between them.

ectopic pregnancy Dangerous condition that results from the implantation of a fertilized egg outside the uterus, usually in a fallopian tube.

ejaculation Propulsion of semen from the penis.

ejaculatory duct Tube formed by the junction of the seminal vesicle and the vas deferens that carries semen to the urethra.

electrocardiogram (ECG) A record of the electrical activity of the heart; may be measured during a stress test.

embolus A blood clot that becomes dislodged from a blood vessel wall and moves through the circulatory system.

embryo Fertilized egg from conception through the eighth week of development.

emergency contraceptive pills (ECPs) Drugs taken within 3 to 5 days after unprotected intercourse to prevent fertilization or implantation.

emotional health The feeling part of psychological health; includes your emotional reactions to life.

emotional intelligence Ability to identify, monitor, and manage one's own emotions and to understand those of others; includes the ability to use the information to guide one's thinking and actions The ability to identify, use, understand and manage your emotions in positive and constructive ways.

emotions Intensified feelings or complex patterns of feelings.

emphysema A respiratory disease in which the alveoli become distended or ruptured and are no longer functional.

emphysema Chronic lung disease in which the tiny air sacs in the lungs are destroyed, making breathing difficult.

enablers People who knowingly or unknowingly protect addicts from the natural consequences of their behavior.

endemic Describing a disease that is always present to some degree.

endometriosis Disorder in which endometrial tissue establishes itself outside the uterus.

endometrium Soft, spongy matter that makes up the uterine lining.

endorphins Opioid-like hormones that are manufactured in the human body and contribute to natural feelings of wellbeing.

energy medicine Therapies using energy fields, such as magnetic fields or biofields.

enhanced greenhouse effect Warming of the earth's surface as a direct result of human activities that release greenhouse gases into the atmosphere, trapping more of the sun's radiation than is normal.

environmental stewardship Responsibility for environmental quality shared by all those whose actions affect the environment.

environmental tobacco smoke (ETS) Smoke from tobacco products, including secondhand and mainstream smoke.

epidemic Disease outbreak that affects many people in a community or region at the same time.

epididymis Duct system atop the testis where sperm mature.

epilepsy A neurological disorder caused by abnormal electrical brain activity; can be accompanied by altered consciousness or convulsions.

epinephrine Also called *adrenaline*, a hormone that stimulates body systems in response to stress.

erectile dysfunction (ED) Difficulty in achieving or maintaining an erection sufficient for intercourse.

ergogenic drug Substance believed to enhance athletic performance.

erogenous zones Areas of the body that, when touched, lead to sexual arousal.

essential amino acids Nine of the basic nitrogen-containing building blocks of human proteins, which must be obtained from foods

estrogens Hormones secreted by the ovaries that control the menstrual cycle.

ethnoviolence Violence directed at persons affiliated with a particular ethnic group.

ethyl alcohol (ethanol) Addictive drug produced by fermentation that is the intoxicating substance in alcoholic beverages.

eustress Stress that presents opportunities for personal growth; positive stress.

evidence-based practice Decisions regarding patient care based on clinical expertise, patient values, and current best scientific evidence.

exercise addicts People who exercise compulsively to try to meet needs of nurturance, intimacy, self-esteem, and self-competency.

exercise metabolic rate (EMR) The energy expenditure that occurs during exercise.

exercise Planned, structured, and repetitive bodily movement done to improve or maintain one or more components of physical fitness.

extensively drug-resistant TB (XDR-TB) Form of TB that is resistant to nearly all existing antibiotics.

fallopian tubes Tubes that extend from near the ovaries to the uterus; site of fertilization and passageway for fertilized eggs.

family of origin People present in the household during a child's first years of life—usually parents and siblings.

fats Essential nutrients needed for energy, cell function, insulation of body organs, maintenance of body temperature, and healthy skin and hair.

fellatio Oral stimulation of a man's genitals.

female athlete triad A syndrome of three interrelated health problems seen in some female athletes: disordered eating, amenorrhea, and poor bone density.

female condom Single-use polyurethane sheath for internal use during vaginal or anal intercourse to catch semen upon ejaculation.

female orgasmic disorder A woman's inability to achieve orgasm.

fermentation Process in which yeast organisms break down plant sugars to yield ethanol.

fertility awareness methods (FAMs) Several types of birth control that require alteration of sexual behavior rather than chemical or physical intervention in the reproductive process.

fertility rate Average number of births a female in a certain population has during her reproductive years.

fertility A person's ability to reproduce.

fetal alcohol syndrome (FAS) Birth defect involving physical and mental impairment that results from the mother's alcohol consumption during pregnancy.

fetal alcohol syndrome (FAS) Pattern of birth defects, learning, and behavioral problems in a child caused by the mother's alcohol consumption during pregnancy.

fetus Developing human from the ninth week until birth.

fiber The indigestible portion of plant foods that helps move food through the digestive system and softens stools by absorbing water.

fibrillation A sporadic, quivering pattern of heartbeat that results in extreme inefficiency in moving blood through the cardiovascular system.

fight-or-flight response Physiological arousal response in which the body prepares to combat or escape a real or perceived threat.

FITT Acronym for **F**requency, **I**ntensity, **T**ime, and **T**ype; the terms that describe the recommended levels of exercise to improve a health-related component of physical fitness.

flexibility The range of motion, or the amount of movement possible, at a particular joint or series of joints.

food allergy An immune response against a specific food that the majority of people can eat without problem.

food allergy Overreaction by the immune system to normally harmless proteins, which are perceived as allergens. In response, the body produces antibodies, triggering allergic symptoms.

food intolerance Difficulty or inability to digest certain foods due to problems with the physical, hormonal, or biochemical systems in your digestive tract. Dairy (lactose) and gluten (wheat protein) are common food intolerances.

food intolerance Adverse effects that result when people who lack the digestive chemicals needed to break down certain substances eat those substances.

food irradiation Exposing foods to low doses of radiation to kill microorganisms or keep them from reproducing.

formaldehyde Colorless, strong-smelling gas released through outgassing; causes respiratory and other health problems.

fossil fuels Carbon-based material used for energy; includes oil, coal, and natural gas.

frequency As part of the FITT prescription, refers to how many days per week a person should exercise.

functional foods Foods believed to have specific health benefits and/or to prevent disease.

fungi A group of multicellular and unicellular organisms that obtain their food by infiltrating the bodies of other organisms, both living and dead; several microscopic varieties are pathogenic.

gastroesophageal reflux disease (GERD) Chronic condition in which stomach acid backflows into the esophagus, causing heartburn and potential damage to the esophagus.

gay Sexual orientation involving primary attraction to people of the same sex.

gender identity Personal sense or awareness of being masculine or feminine, a male or a female.

gender roles Expression of maleness or femaleness in everyday life.

gender-role stereotypes Generalizations concerning how men and women should express themselves and the characteristics each possesses.

gender Characteristics and actions associated with being feminine or masculine as defined by the society in which one lives.

gene Discrete segment of DNA in a chromosome that stores the code for assembling a particular body protein.

general adaptation syndrome (GAS) The pattern followed in the physiological response to stress, consisting of the alarm, resistance, and exhaustion phases.

generalized anxiety disorder (GAD) A constant sense of worry that may cause restlessness, difficulty in concentrating, tension, and other symptoms.

generic drugs Medications marketed by chemical names rather than brand names.

genetically modified (GM) foods Foods derived from organisms whose DNA has been altered using genetic engineering techniques.

genital herpes STI caused by the herpes simplex virus.

genital warts Warts that appear in the genital area or the anus; caused by the human papillomavirus (HPV).

genome All of the genetic information an organism possesses.

gerontology The study of individual and collective aging processes.

gestational diabetes Form of diabetes mellitus in which women who have never had diabetes have high blood sugar (glucose) levels during pregnancy.

glaucoma Elevation of pressure within the eyeball, leading to hardening of the eyeball, impaired vision, and possible blindness.

glycogen The polysaccharide form in which glucose is stored in the liver and, to a lesser extent, in muscles.

gonads Reproductive organs that produce germ cells and sex hormones. In males, the testes, and in females, the ovaries).

gonorrhea Second most common bacterial STI in the United States; if untreated, may cause sterility.

graafian follicle Mature ovarian follicle that contains a fully developed egg (ovum).

greenhouse gases Gases that accumulate in the atmosphere where they contribute to global warming by trapping heat near the earth's surface.

grief work Process of accepting the reality of a person's death and coping with memories of the deceased.

grief An individual's reaction to significant loss, including one's own impending death, the death of a loved one, or a quasi-death experience; grief can involve mental, physical, social, or emotional responses.

habit A repeated behavior in which the repetition may be unconscious.

hallucinogens Substances capable of creating auditory or visual distortions and heightened states.

hangover Physiological reaction to excessive drinking, including headache, upset stomach, anxiety, depression, diarrhea, and thirst.

hate crime Crime targeted against a particular societal group and motivated by bias against that group.

hay fever A chronic allergy-related respiratory disorder that is most prevalent when ragweed and flowers bloom.

hazardous waste Toxic waste that poses a hazard to humans or to the environment.

health belief model (HBM) Model for explaining how beliefs may influence behaviors.

health disparities Differences in the incidence, prevalence, mortality, and burden of diseases and other health conditions among specific population groups.

health promotion The combined educational, organizational, procedural, environmental, social, and financial supports that help individuals and groups reduce negative health behaviors and promote positive change.

health-related quality of life Assessment of impact of health status—including elements of physical, mental, emotional, and social function—on overall quality of life.

health The ever-changing process of achieving individual potential in the physical, social, emotional, mental, spiritual, and environmental dimensions.

healthy life expectancy Expected number of years of full health remaining at a given age, such as at birth.

heat cramps Involuntary and forcible muscle contractions that occur during or following exercise in hot and/or humid weather.

heat exhaustion A heat stress illness caused by significant dehydration resulting from exercise in hot and/or humid conditions.

heatstroke A deadly heat stress illness resulting from dehydration and overexertion in hot and/or humid conditions.

hepatitis A viral disease in which the liver becomes inflamed, producing symptoms such as fever, headache, and possibly jaundice.

herpes gladiatorum A skin infection caused by the herpes simplex type 1 virus and seen among athletes participating in contact sports.

heterosexual Experiencing primary attraction to and preference for sexual activity with people of the opposite sex.

high-density lipoproteins (HDLs) Compounds that facilitate the transport of cholesterol in the blood to the liver for metabolism and elimination from the body.

high-density lipoproteins (HDLs) Compounds that facilitate the transport of cholesterol in the blood to the liver for metabolism and elimination from the body.

histamine Chemical substance that dilates blood vessels, increases mucous secretions, and produces other symptoms of allergies.

histamine Chemical substance that dilates blood vessels, increases mucus secretions, and triggers other allergy symptoms.

holistic Relating to or concerned with the whole body and the interactions of systems, rather than treatment of individual parts.

homeopathic medicine Unconventional Western system of medicine based on the principle that "like cures like."

homeostasis A balanced physiological state in which all the body's systems function smoothly.

homicide Death that results from intent to injure or kill.

homosexual Experiencing primary attraction to and preference for sexual activity with people of the same sex.

hormonal methods Contraceptive methods that introduce synthetic hormones into a woman's system to prevent ovulation, thicken cervical mucus, or prevent a fertilized egg from implanting.

hormone replacement therapy (menopausal hormone therapy) Use of synthetic estrogens and progesterone to compensate for hormonal changes in a woman's body during menopause.

hospice Type of end-of-life care designed to maximize quality of life and help dying people have peace, comfort, and dignity.

hostility The cognitive, affective, and behavioral tendencies toward anger and cynicism.

human chorionic gonadotropin (HCG) Hormone detectable in blood or urine samples of a mother within the first few weeks of pregnancy.

human immunodeficiency virus (HIV) The virus that causes AIDS by infecting helper T cells.

human papillomavirus (HPV) A group of viruses, many of which are transmitted sexually; some types of HPV can cause genital warts or cervical cancer.

humoral immunity Aspect of immunity that is mediated by antibodies secreted by white blood cells.

hunger The physiological impulse to seek food, prompted by the lack or shortage of basic foods needed to provide the energy and nutrients that support health.

hymen In some women, a thin tissue covering the vaginal opening.

hyperglycemia Elevated blood glucose level.

hyperplasia A condition characterized by an excessive number of fat cells.

hypertension Sustained elevated blood pressure.

hypertrophy The act of swelling or increasing in size, as with cells.

hypnosis A trancelike state that allows people to become unusually responsive to suggestion.

hyponatremia or water intoxication Overconsumption of water, which leads to a dilution of sodium concentration in the blood with potentially fatal results.

hypothalamus A structure in the brain that controls the sympathetic nervous system and directs the stress response.

hypothalamus Area of the brain located near the pituitary gland; works in conjunction with the pituitary gland to control reproductive functions.

hypothermia Potentially fatal condition caused by abnormally low body core temperature.

hysterectomy Surgical removal of the uterus.

hysterotomy Surgical removal of the fetus from the uterus.

idiopathic Of unknown cause.

imagined rehearsal Practicing, through mental imagery, to become better able to perform an event in actuality.

immunocompetence The ability of the immune system to respond to attack.

immunocompromised Having an immune system that is impaired.

immunotherapy Treatment strategies based on the concept of regulating the immune system by administering antibodies or desensitizing shots of allergens.

immunotherapy Treatment strategies based on the concept of regulating the immune system, as by administering antibodies or desensitization shots of allergens.

in vitro fertilization (IVF) Fertilization of an egg in a nutrient medium and subsequent transfer back to the mother's body.

incomplete proteins Proteins that lack one or more of the essential amino acids.

incubation period The time between exposure to a disease and the appearance of symptoms.

induction abortions Abortion technique in which chemicals are injected into the uterus through the uterine wall; labor begins, and the woman delivers a dead fetus.

infection The state of pathogens being established in or on a host and causing disease.

infertility Inability to conceive after a year or more of trying.

inflammatory bowel disease (IBD) A group of disorders in which the intestines become inflamed.

influenza A common viral disease of the respiratory tract.

inhalants Products that are sniffed or inhaled in order to produce highs.

inhalation The introduction of drugs through breathing into the lungs.

inheritance Process by which physical and biological characteristics—called traits—are transmitted from parents to their offspring.

inhibited sexual desire Lack of sexual appetite or lack of interest and pleasure in sexual activity.

inhibition A drug interaction in which the effects of one drug are eliminated or reduced by the presence of another drug at the same receptor site.

injection The introduction of drugs into the body via a hypodermic needle.

insulin resistance State in which body cells fail to respond to the effects of insulin; obesity increases the risk that cells will become insulin resistant.

insulin Hormone secreted by the pancreas and required by body cells for the uptake and storage of glucose.

intact dilation and extraction (D&X) Late-term abortion procedure in which the body of the fetus is extracted up to the head and then the contents of the cranium are aspirated.

intensity As part of the FITT prescription, refers to how hard or how much effort is needed when a person exercises.

intentional injuries Injury, death, or psychological harm inflicted with the intent to harm.

Internet addiction Compulsive use of the computer, PDA, cell phone, or other forms of technology to access the Internet for activities such as e-mail, games, shopping, social networking, or blogging.

interpersonal violence Violence inflicted against one individual by another or by a small group of others.

intersexuality Not exhibiting exclusively male or female sex characteristics.

intervention A planned confrontation with an alcoholic led by a professional counselor in which family members and/or friends try to get the alcoholic to face the reality of his or her problem and to seek help.

intervention A planned process of confronting an addict; carried out by close family, friends, and significant others.

intestate Dying without a will.

intimate partner violence (IPV) Violent behavior that occurs between people in an intimate relationship (current or former spouses or dating partners).

intimate relationships Relationships with family members, friends, and romantic partners, characterized by behavioral interdependence, need fulfillment, emotional attachment, and emotional availability.

intolerance A drug interaction in which the combination of two or more drugs in the body produces extremely uncomfortable symptoms.

intrauterine device (IUD) A device, often T-shaped, that is implanted in the uterus to prevent pregnancy.

ionizing radiation Electromagnetic waves and particles having short wavelengths and energy high enough to ionize atoms.

irritable bowel syndrome (IBS) Nausea, pain, gas, or diarrhea caused by certain foods or stress.

ischemia Reduced oxygen supply to a body part or organ.

jealousy Aversive reaction evoked by a real or imagined relationship involving a person's partner and a third person.

labia majora "Outer lips," or folds of tissue covering the female sexual organs.

labia minora "Inner lips," or folds of tissue just inside the labia majora.

leach To dissolve and filter through soil.

lead Highly toxic metal found in emissions from lead smelters and processing plants; also sometimes found in pipes or paint in older buildings.

learned behavioral tolerance The ability of heavy drinkers to modify behavior so they appear to be sober even when they have high BAC levels.

learned helplessness Pattern of responding to situations by giving up because of repeated failure in the past.

learned optimism Teaching oneself to think positively.

lesbian Sexual orientation involving attraction of women to other women.

leukoplakia Condition characterized by leathery white patches inside the mouth, which is produced by contact with irritants in tobacco juice.

libido Sexual drive or desire.

life expectancy Expected number of years of life remaining at a given age, such as at birth.

living will Type of advance directive.

locavore A person who primarily eats food grown or produced locally.

locus of control The location, *external* (outside oneself) or *internal* (within oneself), that an individual perceives as the source and underlying cause of events in his or her life.

loss of control Inability to reliably predict whether a particular instance of involvement with the addictive substance or behavior will be healthy or damaging.

low back pain (LBP) Pain or discomfort in the lumbosacral region of the back.

low sperm count Sperm count below 20 million sperm per milliliter of semen.

low-density lipoproteins (LDLs) Compounds that facilitate the transport of cholesterol in the blood to the body's cells and cause the cholesterol to build up on artery walls.

low-density lipoproteins (LDLs) Compounds that transport cholesterol in the blood to the body's cells.

lymphocyte A type of white blood cell involved in the immune response.

macrophage A type of white blood cell that ingests foreign material.

macular degeneration Breakdown of the macula, the light-sensitive part of the retina responsible for sharp, direct vision.

magnetic resonance imaging (MRI) A device that uses magnetic fields, radio waves, and computers to generate an image of internal tissues of the body for diagnostic purposes without the use of radiation.

mainstream smoke Smoke that is drawn through tobacco while inhaling.

major depression Severe depressive disorder with physical effects such as sleep disturbance and exhaustion, and mental effects such as the inability to concentrate; also called *clinical depression.*

male condom Single-use sheath of thin latex or other material designed to fit over an erect penis and to catch semen upon ejaculation.

malignant melanoma A virulent cancer of the melanocytes (pigment-producing cells) of the skin.

malignant Very dangerous or harmful; refers to a cancerous tumor.

managed care Cost-control procedures used by health insurers to coordinate treatment.

manipulative and body-based practices Treatments involving manipulation or movement of one or more body parts.

marijuana Chopped leaves and flowers of *Cannabis indica* or *Cannabis sativa* plants (hemp); a psychoactive stimulant.

masturbation Self-stimulation of genitals.

measles A viral disease that produces symptoms such as an itchy rash and a high fever.

Medicaid A federal-state matching funds program that provides health insurance to low-income people.

medical abortion Termination of a pregnancy during the first 9 weeks using hormonal medications that cause the embryo to be expelled from the uterus.

medical model A view of health in which health status focuses primarily on the individual and a biological or diseased organ perspective.

Medicare A federal health insurance program that covers people age 65 and older, the permanently disabled, and people with end-stage kidney disease.

meditation A relaxation technique that involves deep breathing and concentration.

meditation Practice of emptying the mind of thought.

menarche The first menstrual period.

meningitis An infection of the meninges, the membranes that surround the brain and spinal cord.

menopause Permanent cessation of menstruation, generally occurs between the ages of 45 and 55.

mental health The thinking part of psychological health; includes your values, attitudes, and beliefs.

mental illnesses Disorders that disrupt thinking, feeling, moods, and behaviors, and that impair daily functioning.

metabolic syndrome (MetS) A group of metabolic conditions occurring together that increase a person's risk of heart disease, stroke, and diabetes.

metastasis Process by which cancer spreads from one area to different areas of the body.

methicillin-resistant *Staphylococcus aureus* (MRSA) Highly resistant form of staph infection that is growing in international prevalence.

migraine A condition characterized by localized headaches that possibly result from alternating dilation and constriction of blood vessels.

mind–body medicine Techniques designed to enhance the mind's ability to affect bodily functions and symptoms.

mindfulness Practice of purposeful, nonjudgmental observation in which we are fully present in the moment.

minerals Inorganic, indestructible elements that aid physiological processes.

miscarriage Loss of the fetus before it is viable; also called *spontaneous abortion.*

modeling Learning specific behaviors by watching others perform them.

monogamy Exclusive sexual involvement with one partner.

mononucleosis A viral disease that causes pervasive fatigue and other long-lasting symptoms.

monosaccharides Simple sugars that contain only one molecule of sugar.

mons pubis Fatty tissue covering the pubic bone in females; in physically mature women, the mons is covered with coarse hair.

morbidly obese Having a body weight 100 percent or more above healthy recommended levels; in an adult, having a BMI of 40 or more.

mortality The proportion of deaths to population.

motivation A social, cognitive, and emotional force that directs human behavior.

mourning Culturally prescribed behavior patterns for the expression of grief.

multidrug-resistant TB (MDR-TB) Form of TB that is resistant to at least two of the best antibiotics available.

multifactorial disease Disease caused by interactions of several factors.

multifactorial disorder A disorder attributable to more than one of a variety of factors.

mumps A once common viral disease that is controllable by vaccination.

municipal solid waste (MSW) Solid waste such as durable and nondurable goods, containers and packaging, food waste, yard waste, and miscellaneous waste from residential, commercial, institutional, and industrial sources.

muscle dysmorphia Body image disorder in which men believe that their body is insufficiently lean or muscular.

muscular endurance A muscle's ability to exert force repeatedly without fatiguing or the ability to sustain a muscular contraction for a length of time.

muscular strength The amount of force that a muscle is capable of exerting in one contraction.

mutant cells Cells that differ in form, quality, or function from normal cells.

myocardial infarction (MI) or heart attack A blockage of normal blood supply to an area in the heart.

natural disaster Any extreme environmental event that causes widespread destruction of land and/or property, injuries, and sometimes deaths.

naturopathic medicine System of medicine originating from Europe that views disease as a manifestation of alterations in the body's natural self-healing processes and that emphasizes health restoration as well as disease treatment.

negative consequences Severe problems associated with addiction, such as physical damage, legal trouble, financial problems, academic failure, or family dissolution.

neglect Failure to provide a child's basic needs such as food, clothing, shelter, and medical care.

neoplasm A new growth of tissue that serves no physiological function and results from uncontrolled, abnormal cellular development.

neurotransmitter One of many chemical substances, such as acetylcholine or dopamine, that transmits nerve impulses between nerve fibers.

neurotransmitters Biochemical messengers that bind to specific receptor sites on nerve cells.

nicotine poisoning Symptoms often experienced by beginning smokers, including dizziness, diarrhea, lightheadedness, rapid and erratic pulse, clammy skin, nausea, and vomiting.

nicotine withdrawal Symptoms including nausea, headaches, irritability, and intense tobacco cravings suffered by nicotine-addicted individuals who stop using tobacco.

nicotine Primary stimulant chemical in tobacco products that is highly addictive.

nonionizing radiation Electromagnetic waves having relatively long wavelengths and enough energy to move atoms around or cause them to vibrate.

nonpoint source pollutant Pollutant that runs off or seeps into waterways from broad areas of land.

nonverbal communication Unwritten and unspoken messages, both intentional and unintentional.

nuclear meltdown Accident that results when the temperature in the core of a nuclear reactor increases enough to melt the nuclear fuel and breach the containment vessel.

nurse practitioner (NP) Professional nurse with advanced training obtained through either a master's degree program or a specialized nurse practitioner program.

nurse Health professional who provides many services for patients and who may work in a variety of settings.

nutraceuticals Term often used interchangeably with *functional foods;* refers to the combined nutritional and pharmaceutical benefit derived through use of foods or food supplements.

nutrients The constituents of food that sustain humans physiologically: water, proteins, carbohydrates, fats, vitamins, and minerals.

nutrition The science that investigates the relationship between physiological function and the essential elements of foods eaten.

NuvaRing Soft, flexible ring inserted into the vagina that releases hormones, preventing pregnancy.

obesity A body weight more than 20 percent above healthy recommended levels; in an adult, a BMI of 30 or more.

obesogenic Characterized by environments that promote increased food intake, nonhealthful foods, and physical inactivity; refers to conditions that lead people to become excessively fat.

obsession Excessive preoccupation with an addictive object or behavior.

obsessive-compulsive disorder (OCD) Form of anxiety disorder characterized by recurrent, unwanted thoughts and repetitive behaviors.

oncogenes Suspected cancer-causing genes present on chromosomes.

one repetition maximum (1 RM) The amount of weight or resistance that can be lifted or moved only once.

open relationship Relationship in which partners agree that sexual involvement can occur outside the relationship.

ophthalmologist Physician who specializes in the medical and surgical care of the eyes, including prescriptions for glasses.

opioids Drugs that induce sleep and relieve pain, including derivatives of opium and synthetics with similar chemical properties; also called *narcotics.*

opium The parent drug of the opioids; made from the seedpod resin of the opium poppy.

opportunistic infections Infections that occur when the immune system is weakened or compromised.

optometrist Eye specialist whose practice is limited to prescribing and fitting lenses.

oral contraceptives Pills containing synthetic hormones that prevent ovulation by regulating hormones.

oral ingestion Intake of drugs through the mouth.

organic Grown without use of toxic and persistent pesticides, chemicals, or hormones.

Ortho Evra Patch that releases hormones similar to those in oral contraceptives; each patch is worn for 1 week.

osteoarthritis (OA) Progressive deterioration of bones and joints that has been associated with the wear-and-tear theory of aging.

osteopath General practitioner who receives training similar to a medical doctor's but with an emphasis on the skeletal and muscular systems; often uses spinal manipulation as part of treatment.

osteoporosis Degenerative bone disorder characterized by increasingly porous bones.

ovarian follicles Areas within the ovary in which individual eggs develop.

ovaries Almond-sized organs that house developing eggs and produce hormones.

overload A condition in which a person feels overly pressured by demands.

overuse injuries Injuries that result from the cumulative effects of day-after-day stresses placed on tendons, muscles, and joints.

overweight Having a body weight more than 10 percent above healthy recommended levels; in an adult, having a BMI of 25 to 29.

ovulation The point of the menstrual cycle at which a mature egg ruptures through the ovarian wall.

ovum Single mature egg cell.

palliative care Any form of medical care focused on relieving the pain, symptoms, and stress of serious illness to improve the quality of life for patients and their families.

palliative treatment Those treatments designed to treat or ease symptoms but not cure the disease.

pancreas Organ that secretes digestive enzymes into the small intestine and hormones, including insulin, into the bloodstream.

pandemic Global epidemic of a disease.

panic attack Severe anxiety reaction in which a particular situation, often for unknown reasons, causes terror.

Pap test A procedure in which cells taken from the cervical region are examined for abnormal cellular activity.

parasitic worms The largest of the pathogens, most of which are more a nuisance than they are a threat.

parasympathetic nervous system Branch of the autonomic nervous system responsible for slowing systems stimulated by the stress response.

passive euthanasia Intentional withholding of treatment that would prolong life.

pathogen A disease-causing agent.

pelvic inflammatory disease (PID) Inflammation of the female genital tract that may cause scarring or blockage of the fallopian tubes, resulting in infertility.

pelvic inflammatory disease (PID) Term used to describe various infections of the female reproductive tract.

penis Male sexual organ that releases sperm into the vagina.

perfect-use failure rate The number of pregnancies (per 100 users) likely to occur in the first year of use of a particular birth control method if the method is used consistently and correctly.

perineum Tissue that forms the "floor" of the pelvic region.

peripheral artery disease (PAD) Atherosclerosis occurring in the lower extremities, such as in the feet, calves, or legs, or in the arms.

personal flotation device A device worn to provide buoyancy and keep the wearer, conscious or unconscious, afloat with the nose and mouth out of the water; also known as a life jacket.

personality disorder Mental disorder characterized by inflexible patterns of thought and beliefs that lead to socially distressing behavior.

pesticides Chemicals that kill pests such as insects or rodents.

phobia Deep and persistent fear of a specific object, activity, or situation that results in a compelling desire to avoid the source of the fear.

physical activity Refers to all body movements produced by skeletal muscles resulting in substantial increases in energy expenditure.

physical fitness A balance of health-related attributes that allow you to perform moderate to vigorous physical activities on a regular basis and complete daily physical tasks without undue fatigue.

physician assistant (PA) A midlevel practitioner trained to handle most standard cases of care under the supervision of a physician.

physiological dependence The adaptive state that occurs with regular addictive behavior and results in withdrawal syndrome.

pituitary gland Endocrine gland that controls the release of hormones from the gonads.

placenta Network of blood vessels connected to the umbilical cord that transports oxygen and nutrients to a developing fetus and carries away fetal wastes.

plant sterols Essential components of plant membranes that, when consumed in the diet, appear to help lower cholesterol levels.

plaque Buildup of deposits in the arteries.

platelet adhesiveness Stickiness of red blood cells associated with blood clots.

pneumonia Inflammatory disease of the lungs characterized by chronic cough, chest pain, chills, high fever, and fluid accumulation; may be caused by bacteria, viruses, fungi, chemicals, or other substances.

point source pollutant Pollutant that enters waterways at a specific location.

poison Any substance harmful to the body when ingested, inhaled, injected, or absorbed through the skin.

pollutant Substance that contaminates some aspect of the environment and causes potential harm to living organisms.

polychlorinated biphenyls (PCBs) Toxic chemicals that were once used as insulating materials in high-voltage electrical equipment.

polydrug use Taking several medications, vitamins, recreational drugs, or illegal drugs simultaneously.

pornography Visual or literary depictions of sexual activity intended to be sexually arousing.

positive reinforcement Presenting something positive following a behavior that is being reinforced.

post-traumatic stress disorder (PTSD) Collection of symptoms that may occur as a delayed response to a traumatic event or series of events.

postpartum depression Mood disorder experienced by women who have given birth; involves depression, fatigue, and other symptoms and may last for weeks or months.

power Ability to make and implement decisions.

prayer Communication with a transcendent Presence.

prayer Communication with a transcendent Presence.

pre-diabetes Condition in which blood glucose levels are higher than normal, but not high enough to be classified as diabetes.

pre-gaming Drinking heavily at home before going out to an event or other location.

preconception care Medical care received prior to becoming pregnant that helps a woman assess and address potential health issues.

preeclampsia Pregnancy complication characterized by high blood pressure, protein in the urine, and edema.

prejudice A negative evaluation of an entire group of people that is typically based on unfavorable and often wrong ideas about the group.

premature ejaculation Ejaculation that occurs prior to or almost immediately following penile penetration of the vagina; also known as *early ejaculation*.

premenstrual dysphoric disorder (PMDD) Group of symptoms similar to but more severe than PMS, including severe mood disturbances.

premenstrual syndrome (PMS) Mood changes and physical symptoms that occur in some women 1 to 2 weeks prior to menstruation.

premium Payment made to an insurance carrier, usually in monthly installments, that covers the cost of an insurance policy.

primary aggression Goal-directed, hostile self-assertion that is destructive in nature.

primary care practitioner (PCP) A medical practitioner who treats routine ailments, advises on preventive care, gives general medical advice, and makes appropriate referrals when necessary.

prion A recently identified self-replicating protein-based pathogen.

process addictions Behaviors such as disordered gambling, compulsive buying, compulsive Internet or technology use, work addiction, compulsive exercise, and sexual addiction that are known to be addictive because they are mood altering.

procrastinate To intentionally put off doing something.

progesterone Hormone secreted by the ovaries; helps the endometrium develop and helps maintain pregnancy.

proof Measure of the percentage of alcohol in a beverage; the proof is double the percentage of alcohol in the drink.

prostate gland Gland that secretes nutrients and neutralizing fluids into the semen.

prostate-specific antigen (PSA) An antigen found in prostate cancer patients.

prostitution Practice of engaging in sexual acts for money.

proteins Large molecules made up of chains of amino acids; essential constituents of all body cells.

protozoans Microscopic single-celled organisms that can be pathogenic.

psychoactive drugs Drugs that have the potential to alter mood or behavior.

psychological hardiness A personality trait characterized by control, commitment, and the embrace of challenge.

psychological health The mental, emotional, social, and spiritual dimensions of health.

psychological resilience The process of adapting well in the face of adversity, trauma, tragedy, threats, or significant sources of stress, such as family and relationship problems, serious health problems, or workplace and financial stressors.

psychoneuroimmunology (PNI) The study of the interactions of behavioral, neural, and endocrine functions and the functioning of the body's immune system.

puberty Period of sexual maturation.

pubic lice Parasitic insects that can inhabit various body areas, especially the genitals.

rabies A viral disease of the central nervous system; often transmitted through animal bites.

radiation absorbed dose (rad) Unit of measure of radiation exposure.

radiotherapy The use of radiation to kill cancerous cells.

radon Naturally occurring radioactive gas resulting from the decay of certain radioactive elements.

rape Sexual penetration without the victim's consent.

rational suicide The decision to kill oneself rather than endure constant pain and slow decay.

reactive aggression Hostile emotional reaction brought about by frustrating life experiences.

receptor sites Specialized areas of cells and organs where chemicals, enzymes, and other substances interact.

recessive Term describing an allele that is expressed only in the absence of a dominant allele, that is, if both alleles are recessive or if the recessive gene is on the X chromosome of the twenty-third pair.

relapse The tendency to return to the addictive behavior after a period of abstinence.

religion System of beliefs, practices, rituals, and symbols designed to facilitate closeness to the sacred or transcendent.

repetitive motion disorder (RMD) An injury to soft tissue, tendons, muscles, nerves, or joints due to the physical stress of repeated motions.

resting metabolic rate (RMR) The energy expenditure of the body under BMR conditions plus other daily sedentary activities.

Rh factor Antigen present in the red blood cells of 85% of people; those with the Rh factor are known as Rh positive (Rh^+); those without it are Rh negative (Rh^-).

rheumatic heart disease A heart disease caused by untreated streptococcal infection of the throat.

rheumatoid arthritis An autoimmune inflammatory joint disease.

RICE Acronym for the standard first aid treatment for virtually all traumatic and overuse injuries: **r**est, **i**ce, **c**ompression, and **e**levation.

rickettsia A small form of bacteria that live inside other living cells.

risk behaviors Actions that increase susceptibility to negative health outcomes.

rubella (German measles) A milder form of measles that causes a rash and mild fever in children and may damage a fetus or a newborn baby.

satiety The feeling of fullness or satisfaction at the end of a meal.

saturated fats Fats that are unable to hold any more hydrogen in their chemical structure; derived mostly from animal sources; solid at room temperature.

schizophrenia Mental illness with biological origins characterized by irrational behavior, severe alterations of the senses, and often an inability to function in society.

scrotum External sac of tissue that encloses the testes.

seasonal affective disorder (SAD) Type of depression that occurs in the winter months, when sunlight levels are low.

secondary sex characteristics Characteristics associated with sex but not directly related to reproduction, such as vocal pitch, body hair, and location of fat deposits.

self-disclosure Sharing personal feelings or information with others.

self-efficacy Belief in one's ability to perform a task successfully.

self-efficacy Describes a person's belief about whether he or she can successfully engage in and execute a specific behavior.

self-esteem Refers to one's realistic sense of self-respect or self-worth.

self-injury Intentionally causing injury to one's own body in an attempt to cope with overwhelming negative emotions; also called *self-mutilation, self-harm,* or *nonsuicidal self-injury* (NSSI).

self-nurturance Developing individual potential through a balanced and realistic appreciation of self-worth and ability.

self-talk The customary manner of thinking and talking to yourself, which can affect your self-image.

semen Fluid containing sperm and nutrients that increase sperm viability and neutralize vaginal acid.

seminal vesicles Glandular ducts that secrete nutrients for the semen.

serial monogamy Series of monogamous sexual relationships.

set point theory Theory that a form of internal thermostat controls our weight and fights to maintain this weight around a narrowly set range.

sexual addiction Compulsive involvement in sexual activity.

sexual assault Any act in which one person is sexually intimate with another without that person's consent.

sexual aversion disorder Desire dysfunction characterized by sexual phobias and anxiety about sexual contact.

sexual dysfunction Problems associated with achieving sexual satisfaction.

sexual fantasies Sexually arousing thoughts and dreams.

sexual harassment Any form of unwanted sexual attention related to any condition of employment, education, or performance evaluation.

sexual identity Recognition of oneself as a sexual being; a composite of biological sex characteristics, gender identity, gender roles, and sexual orientation.

sexual orientation A person's enduring emotional, romantic, or sexual attraction to other persons.

sexual performance anxiety Sexual difficulties caused by anticipating some sort of problem with the sex act.

sexual prejudice Negative attitudes and hostile actions directed at those with a different sexual orientation.

sexuality Thoughts, feelings, and behaviors associated with being male or female, experiencing attraction, being in love, and being in relationships that include sexual intimacy.

sexually transmitted infections (STIs) Infectious diseases caused by pathogens transmitted through some form of sexual contact.

shaping Using a series of small steps to gradually achieve a particular goal.

shingles A disease characterized by a painful rash that occurs when the chickenpox virus is reactivated.

sick building syndrome (SBS) Problem that exists when 80 percent of a building's occupants report maladies that tend to lessen or vanish when they leave the building.

sidestream smoke Cigarette, pipe, or cigar smoke breathed by nonsmokers, commonly called *secondhand smoke.*

simple carbohydrates A carbohydrate made up of only one sugar molecule, or of two sugar molecules bonded together; also called *simple sugars.*

simple rape Rape by one person, usually known to the victim, that does not involve physical beating or use of a weapon.

single-gene disorder A disorder characterized by structural and/or functional impairments resulting from a defect involving only one gene.

sinoatrial node (SA node) Cluster of electric pulse-generating cells that serves as a natural pacemaker for the heart.

situational inducement Attempt to influence a behavior through situations and occasions that are structured to exert control over that behavior.

smog Brownish haze that is a form of pollution produced by the photochemical reaction of sunlight with hydrocarbons, nitrogen compounds, and other gases in vehicle exhaust.

snuff Powdered form of tobacco that is sniffed or absorbed through the mucous membranes in the nose or placed inside the cheek and sucked.

social bonds Degree and nature of interpersonal contacts.

social cognitive model Model of behavior change emphasizing the role of social factors and thought processes (cognition) in behavior change.

social death A seemingly irreversible situation in which a person is not treated like an active member of society.

social health Aspect of psychological health that includes interactions with others, ability to use social supports, and ability to adapt to various situations.

social learning theory Theory that people learn behaviors by watching role models—parents, caregivers, and significant others.

social phobia Phobia characterized by fear and avoidance of social situations; also called *social anxiety disorder.*

social physique anxiety (SPA) A desire to look good that has a destructive effect on a person's ability to function well in social interactions and relationships.

social support Network of people and services with whom you share ties and from whom you get support.

socialization Process by which a society communicates behavioral expectations to its members.

spermatogenesis The development of sperm.

spermicide Substance designed to kill sperm.

spiritual health Aspect of psychological health that relates to having a sense of meaning and purpose to one's life, as well as a feeling of connection with others and with nature.

spiritual intelligence (SI) The ability to access higher meanings, values, abiding purposes, and unconscious aspects of the self, a characteristic that helps us find a moral and ethical path to guide us through life.

spirituality An individual's sense of peace, purpose, and connection to others and beliefs about the meaning of life.

stalking Willful, repeated, and malicious following, harassing, or threatening of another person.

standard drink Amount of any beverage that contains about 14 grams of pure alcohol.

staphylococci A group of round bacteria, usually found in clusters, that cause a variety of diseases in humans and other animals.

starch Polysaccharide that is the storage form of glucose in plants.

static stretching Stretching techniques that slowly and gradually lengthen a muscle or group of muscles and their tendons.

stent A stainless steel, mesh-like tube that is inserted to prop open the artery.

sterilization Permanent fertility control achieved through surgical procedures.

stigma Negative perception about a group of people or a certain situation or condition.

stillbirth Fetus that is dead at birth.

stimulants Drugs that increase activity of the central nervous system.

Streptococcus A round bacterium, usually found in chain formation.

stress inoculation Stress-management technique in which a person consciously tries to prepare ahead of time for potential stressors.

stress A series of physiological responses and adaptations in response to a real or imagined threat to one's well-being.

stressor A physical, social, or psychological event or condition that upsets homeostasis and produces a stress response.

stroke A condition occurring when the brain is damaged by disrupted blood supply; also called *cerebrovascular accident.*

subjective well-being An uplifting feeling of inner peace.

suction curettage Abortion technique that uses gentle suction to remove fetal tissue from the uterus.

sudden cardiac death Death that occurs as a result of abrupt, profound loss of heart function.

sudden infant death syndrome (SIDS) Sudden death of an infant under 1 year of age for no apparent reason.

suicidal ideation A desire to die and thoughts about suicide.

Superfund Fund established under the Comprehensive Environmental Response, Compensation, and Liability Act to be used for cleaning up toxic waste dumps.

suppositories Mixtures of drugs and a waxy medium (designed to melt at body temperature) that are inserted into the anus or vagina.

survivorship Physical, psychological, emotional, and economic issues of cancer from diagnosis until the end of life.

sympathetic nervous system Branch of the autonomic nervous system responsible for stress arousal.

sympathomimetics Food substances that can produce stresslike physiological responses.

synergism The interaction of two or more drugs that produces more profound effects than would be expected if the drugs were taken separately; also called *potentiation.*

syphilis One of the most widespread bacterial STIs; characterized by distinct phases and potentially serious results.

systolic pressure The upper number in the fraction that measures blood pressure, indicating pressure on arterial walls when the heart contracts.

tar Thick, brownish sludge condensed from particulate matter in smoked tobacco.

target heart rate The heart rate range of aerobic exercise that leads to improved cardiorespiratory fitness (i.e., 64% to 95% of maximal heart rate).

temperature inversion Weather condition that occurs when a layer of cool air is trapped under a layer of warmer air.

teratogenic Causing birth defects; may refer to drugs, environmental chemicals, radiation, or diseases.

terrorism Unlawful use of force or violence against persons or property to intimidate or coerce a government, civilian population, or any segment thereof in furtherance of political or social objectives.

testes Male sex organs that manufacture sperm and produce hormones.

testosterone Male sex hormone manufactured in the testes.

tetrahydrocannabinol (THC) The chemical name for the active ingredient in marijuana.

thanatology The study of death and dying.

thrombolysis Injection of an agent to dissolve clots and restore some blood flow, thereby reducing the amount of tissue that dies from ischemia.

thrombus Blood clot attached to a blood vessel's wall.

time As part of the FITT prescription, refers to how long a person needs to exercise each time.

tolerance Phenomenon in which progressively larger doses of a drug or more intense involvement in a behavior is needed to produce the desired effects.

toxic shock syndrome (TSS) Potentially life-threatening disease that occurs when specific bacterial toxins multiply and spread to the bloodstream, most commonly through improper use of tampons or diaphragms.

toxins Poisonous substances produced by certain microorganisms that cause various diseases.

toxoplasmosis Disease caused by an organism found in cat feces that, when contracted by a pregnant woman, may result in stillbirth or birth defects.

traditional Chinese medicine (TCM) Ancient comprehensive system of healing that uses herbs, acupuncture, and massage to bring the body into balance and to remove blockages of vital energy flow that lead to disease.

trans fats (trans fatty acids) Fatty acids that are produced when polyunsaturated oils are hydrogenated to make them more solid.

transdermal The introduction of drugs through the skin.

transgendered Having a gender identity that does not match one's biological sex.

transient ischemic attack (TIA) Brief interruption of the blood supply to the brain that causes only temporary impairment; often an indicator of impending major stroke.

transsexual Person who is psychologically of one sex but physically of the other.

transtheoretical model Model of behavior change that identifies six distinct stages people go through in altering behavior patterns; also called the *stages of change model.*

traumatic injuries Injuries that are accidental and occur suddenly and violently.

trichomoniasis Protozoan STI characterized by foamy, yellowish discharge and unpleasant odor.

triglycerides The most common form of lipid in the body; excess calories are converted into triglycerides and stored as body fat.

triglycerides The most common form of fat in foods and in the body; made up of a molecule called glycerol and three fatty acid chains.

trimesters A 3-month segment of pregnancy.

triple marker screen (TMS) Common maternal blood test that can be used to identify fetuses with certain birth defects and genetic abnormalities.

tubal ligation Sterilization of a woman that involves cutting and tying off or cauterizing the fallopian tubes.

tuberculosis (TB) A disease caused by bacterial infiltration of the respiratory system.

tumor A neoplasmic mass that grows more rapidly than surrounding tissue.

type 1 diabetes Form of diabetes mellitus in which the pancreas is not able to make insulin, and therefore blood glucose cannot enter the cells to be used for energy.

type 2 diabetes Form of diabetes mellitus in which the pancreas does not make enough insulin or the body is unable to use insulin correctly.

type As part of the FITT prescription, refers to what kind of exercises a person should do.

typical-use failure rate The number of pregnancies (per 100 users) likely to occur in the first year of use of a particular birth control method if the method's use is not consistent or always correct.

ulcerative colitis (UC) An inflammatory disorder that affects the mucous membranes of the large intestine, producing bloody diarrhea.

ultrasonography (ultrasound) Common prenatal test that uses sound waves to create a visual image of a developing fetus.

underweight Having a body weight more than 10 percent below healthy recommended levels; in an adult, having a BMI below 18.5.

unintentional injuries Injury, death, or psychological harm caused unintentionally or without premeditation.

unintentional injury Any injury committed or sustained without intent of harm.

unsaturated fats Fats with one or more chemical bonds that exclude hydrogen; derived mostly from plants; liquid at room temperature.

urethral opening Opening through which urine is expelled.

urinary incontinence Inability to control urination.

urinary tract infection (UTI) Infection, more common among women than men, of the urinary tract; causes include untreated STIs.

uterus (womb) Hollow, pear-shaped muscular organ whose function is to contain a developing fetus.

vaccination Inoculation with killed or weakened pathogens or similar, less dangerous antigens to prevent or lessen the effects of some disease.

vaginal intercourse Insertion of the penis into the vagina.

vagina Muscular, tube-shaped organ in females that serves as a passageway connecting the vulva to the uterus.

vaginismus State in which the vaginal muscles contract so forcefully that penetration cannot occur.

values Principles that influence our thoughts and emotions and guide the choices we make in our lives.

variant sexual behavior A sexual behavior that is not commonly practiced.

vas deferens Tube that transports sperm from the epididymis to the ejaculatory duct.

vasectomy Male sterilization procedure that involves cutting and tying off the vasa deferentia.

vasocongestion Engorgement of the genital organs with blood.

vegetarian A person who follows a diet that excludes some or all animal products.

veins Vessels that transport waste and carry blood back to the heart from other regions of the body.

ventricles The heart's two lower chambers, which pump blood through the blood vessels.

venules Branches of the veins.

very-low-calorie diets (VLCDs) Diets with a daily caloric value of 400 to 700 calories.

violence Aggressive behaviors that produce injuries and can result in death.

virulent Strong enough to overcome host resistance and cause disease.

viruses Pathogens that invade and inject their own DNA or RNA into a host cell, take it over, and force it to make copies of themselves.

visualization The creation of mental images to promote relaxation.

vitamins Essential organic compounds that promote metabolism, growth, and reproduction and help maintain life and health.

vulva External female genitalia.

waist-to-hip ratio Waist circumference divided by hip circumference; a high ratio indicates increased health risks due to unhealthy fat distribution.

wellness The achievement of the highest level of health possible in each of several dimensions.

whole grains Grains that are milled in their complete form and thus include the bran, germ, and endosperm, with only the husk removed.

withdrawal Contraceptive method that involves withdrawing the penis from the vagina before ejaculation; also called *coitus interruptus.*

withdrawal A series of temporary physical and biopsychosocial symptoms that occurs when an addict abruptly abstains from an addictive chemical or behavior.

work addiction The compulsive use of work and the work persona to fulfill needs for intimacy, power, and success.

X-linked dominant disorder Single-gene disorder that occurs in individuals who have inherited at least one copy of an X chromosome with the affected dominant allele.

X-linked recessive disorder Single-gene disorder that occurs in males who have inherited one copy of an X chromosome with the affected recessive allele and in females who have inherited two copies.

yo-yo diets Cycles in which people diet and regain weight.

yoga System of physical and mental training involving controlled breathing, physical postures *(asanas),* meditation, chanting, and other practices believed to cultivate unity with the *Atman,* or Absolute.

zoonotic diseases Diseases of animals that may be transmitted to humans.

Photo Credits

Stock Photo, Inc.; May/Photo Researchers, Inc.; Phanie/Photo Researchers, Inc.; Life Measurement, Inc.; p. 252 top: Image Source/Getty Images; p. 252 bottom: EPF/Alamy; p. 254: Murat Giray Kaya/iStockphoto; p. 255: UpperCut Images/Alamy; p. 260: Dennis MacDonald/PhotoEdit

FOCUS ON Enhancing Your Body Image Opener: Yellowj/Shutterstock; p. 266 top to bottom: Pictorial Press Ltd/Alamy; Trinity Mirror/Mirrorpix/Alamy; LatitudeStock/Alamy; itanistock/Alamy; Pascal Broze/Getty Images; p. 268 left: Custom Medical Stock Photo/Alamy; p. 268 right: Sakala/Shutterstock; p. 269 top left: Pictorial Press Ltd/Alamy; p. 269 top right: Trinity Mirror/Mirrorpix/Alamy; p. 269 bottom: Brand X Pictures/Jupiter Images; p. 270: LatitudeStock/Alamy; p. 271 left: Brand X Pictures/Jupiter Images; p. 271 right: Gollykim/iStockphoto; p. 272: itanistock/Alamy; p. 273: Chistopher LaMarca/Redux Pictures; p. 274: moodboard/Corbis; p. 275 top: Pascal Broze/Getty Images; p. 275 bottom: Sharon Dominick/iStockphoto; p. 276 top: Loretta Hostettler/iStockphoto; p. 276 bottom: Photodisc/Thinkstock; p. 277: Lucas Allen White/Shutterstock

Chapter 9 Opener: jazavac/Fotolia; p. 280 top to bottom: Exactostock/SuperStock; Rolf Adlercreutz/Alamy; Goodshoot/Jupiter Images; Dennis Welsh/AGE Fotostock America, Inc.; p. 281: Dylan Ellis/Corbis; p. 282: Miroslav Georgijevic/iStockphoto; p. 283: John Fryer/Alamy; p. 285 top: Sharon Dominick/iStockphoto; p. 285 bottom left to right: Teo Lannie/Getty Images; Elena Dorfman, Pearson Science Photodisc/Getty Images; Exactostock/SuperStock Anton Gvozdikov/iStockphoto; p. 286 top: Exactostock/SuperStock; p. 286 bottom: George Doyle/Getty Images; p. 288: Masterfile Corporation; p. 289 top left to right: Walter Cruz/MCT/Newscom; Craig Veltri/iStockphoto; Paul Maguire/iStockphoto Tatuasha/Shutterstock; Stephen VanHorn/Alamy; Graca Victoria/Shutterstock; Rod Ferris/Shutterstock; p. 289 bottom left to right: zimmytws/Shutterstock; KJ Pargeter Images/iStockphoto; Enderbirer/iStockphoto; Ali Ender Birer/Shutterstock; Dandanian/iStockphoto; p. 290: Rolf Adlercreutz/Alamy; p. 291 left to right: Dan Dalton/Getty Images; MIXA/Getty Images Daniel Grill/Alamy; p. 292 top left: Creative Digital Visions; p. 292 top right: Karl Weatherly/Getty Images; p. 292 bottom: Ammentorp Photography/Alamy; p. 293 Kathy Willens/AP Images; p. 294 left to right: Radu Razvan/Shutterstock; Pearson Education Pearson Education; p. 295 all: Pearson Education; p. 296: Masterfile Corporation; p. 297: Goodshoot/Jupiter Images; p. 298: michaeljung/Shutterstock; p. 299: Thomas Smith Photography/Alamy Images; p. 301: Dennis Welsh/AGE Fotostock America, Inc; p. 302: Ingram Publishing/Getty Images; p. 303: Radius Images/Getty Images; p. 304: © Morgan Lane Studios/iStockphoto; p. 305: Jacqueline Perez/iStockphoto

Chapter 10 Opener: Monkey Business Images/Shutterstock; p. 310 top to bottom: Hill Creek Pictures/Alamy Images; Juice Images/AGE Fotostock America, Inc.; Cassiede Alain/Shutterstock; UpperCut Images/Alamy Images; p. 311: MATT DUNHAM/AP Images; p. 312: Hill Creek Pictures/Alamy Images; p. 313: Juice Images/AGE Fotostock America, Inc.; p. 314: sumnersgraphicsine/iStockphoto; p. 315 top: Cassiede Alain/Shutterstock; p. 315 bottom: RubberBall/Alamy Images; p. 317: John Howard/Getty Images; p. 318: Alamy Images; p. 319: Denis Pepin/iStockphoto; p. 321 top: amana images inc./Alamy; p. 321 bottom: UpperCut Images/Alamy Images; p. 323: Image Source/AGE Fotostock America, Inc.; p. 324: Blend Images/Alamy Images

Chapter 11 Opener: Monkey Business Images/Fotolia; p. 328 top to bottom: Goodshoot/Jupiter Images; Image Source/Getty Images; Stockbyte/Getty Images; Roger Allyn Lee/SuperStock; p. 330: Goodshoot/Jupiter Images; p. 331: INSADCO Photography/Alamy; p. 333: I Love Images/Getty Images; p. 334: Image Source/Getty Images; p. 335: Murat Giray Kaya/iStockphoto; p. 336 left: CNRI/SPL/Photo Researchers, Inc.; p. 336 right: Martin M. Rotker/Photo Researchers, Inc.; p. 337: Bill Roth/AP Images; p. 339: Stockbyte/Getty Images; p. 340: Rafael Laguillo/iStockphoto; p. 341: Roy McMahon/Corbis; p. 344 top: Roger Allyn Lee/Superstock; p. 344 bottom: Thinkstock/Getty Images; p. 346: vario images GmbH & Co.KG/Alamy; p. 347: Jiang Jin/Superstock, Inc.

Chapter 12 Opener: LanaK/Fotolia; p. 354 top to bottom: Kristin Piljay Rayman/Getty Images; Oral Health America; Image Source/Alamy Images; p. 356: Kristin Piljay; p. 359: Elizabeth Weinberg/Getty Images; p. 360: Elvele Images Ltd/Alamy Images; p. 361 all: James Steveson/Photo Researchers, Inc.; p. 362 top: Rayman/Getty Images; p. 362 bottom: Image 100/Alamy Images; p. 363: Oral Health America; p. 364 top: TPH/allOver Photography/Alamy Images; p. 364 bottom: Liaison/Getty Images; p. 365: Sharon Dominick/iStockphoto; p. 367: Image Source/Alamy Images; p. 369: Comstock Images/Getty Images; p. 372: Tatiana Popova/Getty Images; p. 373 top to bottom: Josh Sher/Photo Researchers, Inc.; Bloomberg via Getty Images; Michael Newman/PhotoEdit Inc. Gustoimages/Photo Researchers, Inc. Jane Stockman/Dorling Kindersley Limited Eric; Nelson/Custom Medical Stock Photo, Inc.; ICP/Alamy Images; p. 374 fStop/Alamy Images

Chapter 13 Opener: SW Production/Getty Images; p. 380 top to bottom: AF archive/Alamy; David Hoffman/Alamy Images; Manchan/Getty Images; Jupiterimages/Getty Images; p. 382 top: Image Source/Getty Images; p. 382

bottom: Craig Wactor/Shutterstock; p. 383: Science Photo Library/Alamy Images; p. 384 top: Lori Sparkla/Shutterstock; p. 384 bottom: sumnersgraphicsine/iStockphoto; p. 385: AF archive/Alamy; p. 386: Thomas M Perkins/Shutterstock; p. 388: Image Source/Getty Images; p. 390: Banana stock/Getty Images; p. 391 all: Faces of Meth Program; p. 393 top: Karen Mower/iStockphoto; p. 393 bottom: © Bubbles Photolibrary/Alamy; p. 395: Park Street/PhotoEdit, Inc.; p. 396: Gregor Buir/Shutterstock; p. 397: David Hoffman/Alamy Images; p. 398 top: PeerPoint/Alamy; p. 398 bottom: Bob Cheung/Shutterstock; p. 399 top: Martyn Vickery/Alamy; p. 399 bottom: Janine Wiedel Photolibrary/Alamy; p. 400 epa european pressphoto agency b.v./Alamy; p. 401: Manchan/Getty Images; p. 404 top: Jupiterimages/Getty Images; p. 404 bottom: Arresting Images; p. 405: TommL/iStockphoto

Chapter 14 Opener: Chepko Danil Vitalevich/Shutterstock; p. 410 top to bottom: PhotoAlto/SuperStock; Peter Llewellyn(L)/Alamy Peter Bernik/Shutterstock; SHASHANK BENGALI/MCT/Newscom; p. 414: Alamy Images; p. 415: Michael Krinke/iStockphoto; p. 417 top: Murat Giray Kaya/iStockphoto; p. 417 bottom: PhotoAlto/SuperStock; p. 419: Science Photo Library/Getty Images; p. 420 left to right: Gary Gaugler/Photo Researchers, Inc.; Dr. Linda Stannard, UCT/Photo Researchers, Inc.; Steve Gschmeissner/Photo Researchers, Inc.; Eye of Science/Photo Researchers, Inc.; Mediscan/Alamy; p. 421: Exactostock/SuperStock; p. 423: Lev Ezhov/iStockphoto; p. 424: yZUMA Press/Newscom; p. 425: Sidea Revuz/Photo Researchers, Inc.; p. 426: Alexei Zaycev/iStockphoto; p. 427: Peter Llewellyn(L)/Alamy; p. 428: Sharon Dominick/iStockphoto; p. 429: Peter Bernik/Shutterstock; p. 430 left: Western Ophthalmic Hospital/Photo Researchers, Inc.; p. 430 right: Centers for Disease Control & Prevention; p. 432 top to bottom: SPL/Photo Researchers, Inc.; Martin M. Rotker/Photo Researchers, Inc.; Photo Researchers, Inc.; p. 433 left: NMSB/Custom Medical Stock Photo, Inc.; p. 433 right: Dr. Herrmann/Centers for Disease Control and Prevention (CDC); p. 434 left: Dr.; p. Marazzi/Photo Researchers, Inc.; p. 434 right: Centers for Disease Control and Prevention (CDC); p. 435: © Pixtal/SuperStock/Glow Images; p. 436 top: Meckes/Ottawa/Photo Researchers, Inc.; p. 436 bottom: SHASHANK BENGALI/MCT/Newscom; p. 438: Kevin Foy/Alamy; p. 439: Nick Ut/AP Wide World Photos; p. 440: Caro/Alamy; p. 442: Brandon Brown/iStockphoto

FOCUS ON Understanding Your Health Inheritance Opener: Kzenon/Fotolia; p. 446 top to bottom: Scott Bauer/Photo Researchers, Inc.; Adam Hart-Davis/Photo Researchers, Inc.; Christina Kennedy/Alamy Leila Cutler/Alamy Images; p. 447: sumnersgraphicsine/iStockphoto; p. 448: Ingram Publishing/Getty Images; p. 449 top: Scott Bauer/Photo Researchers, Inc.; p. 449 bottom: Addenbrookes Hospital/Photo Researchers, Inc.; p. 450: Schultheiss Selection GmbH & CoKG/Getty Images; p. 451 top: Friedrich Stark/Alamy Images; p. 451 bottom: Adam Hart-Davis/Photo Researchers, Inc.; p. 452: Exactostock/Superstock; p. 453: Christina Kennedy/Alamy; p. 454 top: Marcel Jancovic/Shutterstock; p. 454 bottom: Leila Cutler/Alamy Images

Chapter 15 Opener: Brocreative/Shutterstock; p. 458 top to bottom: MBI/Alamy moodboard/Alamy; Thinkstock/Jupiter Images; Red Images, LLC/Alamy; p. 466 top: HA Photos/Alamy; p. 466 bottom: Sharon Dominick/iStockphoto; p. 468: MBI/Alamy; p. 470 top: Radius Images/Alamy; p. 470 bottom: moodboard/Alamy; p. 473: Ariusz Nawrocki/iStockphoto; p. 474 top: Julien Bastide/Shutterstock; p. 474 bottom: Moodboard/Getty Images; p. 475 top: Tish1/Shutterstock; p. 475 bottom: Thinkstock/Jupiter Images; p. 476: Michael Ventura/Alamy; p. 477 top: Red Images, LLC/Alamy; p. 477 bottom: DK Images

FOCUS ON Minimizing Your Risk for Diabetes Opener: Philippe Garo/Science Source/Photo Researchers, Inc.; p. 482 top to bottom: John Giustina/Getty Images; Terry Vine/Corbis Stockxpert/Thinkstock; JERILEE BENNET/KRT/Newscom; p. 483: Bochkarev Photography/iStockphoto; p. 486 top: Kamdyn R Switzer/Cal Sport Media/Newscom; p. 486 bottom: Murat Giray Kaya/iStockphoto; p. 487 top: moodboard/Superstock; p. 487 bottom: John Giustina/Getty Images; p. 488: Elfina Photo Art/iStockphoto; p. 489 top: Terry Vine/Corbis; p. 489 bottom left: SHOUT/Alamy; p. 489 bottom right: Paul Parker/Photo Researchers Inc.; p. 491: Stockxpert/Thinkstock; p. 492: JERILEE BENNET/KRT/Newscom

Chapter 16 Opener: Purestock/Getty Images; p. 496 top to bottom: Philippe Psaila/Photo Researchers, Inc.; Blend Images/Alamy Images; BSIP SA/Alamy Images; Exactostock/SuperStock; p. 498: Philippe Psaila/Photo Researchers, Inc.; p. 500 top: Getty Images; p. 500 bottom: Sharon Dominick/iStockphoto; p. 501: Dawn Poland/iStockphoto; p. 502: Gord Horne/iStockphoto; p. 503: Blend Images/Alamy Images; p. 505: BSIP SA/Alamy Images; p. 506: Garo/Photo Researchers, Inc.; p. 507: Sharon Dominick/iStockphoto; p. 508: Exactostock/SuperStock; p. 509 left to right: James Stevenson/SPL/Photo Researchers, Inc.; Dr. p. Marazzi/SPL/Photo Researchers, Inc.; Dr. p. Marazzi/SPL/Photo Researchers, Inc.; p. 510: David Sacks/Getty Images; p. 511: .shock/Shutterstock; p. 513: PCN Photography/Alamy; p. 514: Science Photo Library/Photo Researchers, Inc.; p. 516: Blend Images/Alamy; p. 517: W. G. Murray/Alamy; p. 518: mark wragg/iStockphoto

Chapter 17   Opener: Sam Edwards/AGE Fotostock America, Inc.; p. 522 top to bottom: Custom Medical Stock Photo/Alamy Images; Science Photo Library/ Alamy Images; Gladskikh Tatiana/Shutterstock; Chassenet/Alamy; p. 523: allOver Photography/Alamy Images; p. 524: Andrew Aitchison/Alamy; p. 525: Robert Matton AB/Alamy; p. 526: Custom Medical Stock Photo/Alamy Images; p. 527: PhotoAlto/Alamy Images; p. 529: Science Photo Library/Alamy; p. 530: Vanja Gavric/Alamy; p. 532: Corbis RF/Alamy; p. 533: Gladskikh Tatiana/Shutterstock; p. 536: Jack Sullivan/Alamy; p. 537: Gautier Willaume/Shutterstock; p. 538: Chassenet/Alamy; p. 539: Alexander Tsiaras/Photo Researchers, Inc.

Chapter 18   Opener: AVAVA/Fotolia; p. 544 top to bottom: Jiang Jin/Superstock; Thomas Boehm/Alamy; Michael Newman/PhotoEdit Inc.; Tetra Images/Alamy; p. 545: OJO Images Ltd/Alamy; p. 547: Jiang Jin/SuperStock; p. 548: Tatiana Popova/Shutterstock; p. 500: IIene MacDonald/Alamy; p. 553: Thomas Boehm/ Alamy; p. 555: Murat Giray Kaya/iStockphoto; p. 556: Bananastock/Jupiter Images; p. 558: Rayman/Getty Images; p. 559: Michael Newman/PhotoEdit; p. 560 top to bottom: Elena Elisseeva/Shutterstock Shapiso/Shutterstock Joanna Wnuk/ Shutterstock; WEKWEK/iStockphoto eAlisa/Shutterstock; p. 562:; Jochen Tack/ Alamy; p. 563: Tetra Images/Alamy; p. 566: Comstock Images/Thinkstock; p. 568 top: David Mager/Pearson Learning Photo Studio; p. 568 bottom: Pixland/Getty Images; p. 569: Frances Roberts/Alamy; p. 570: jo unruh/iStockphoto

Chapter 19   Opener: Chris Rout/Alamy; p. 574 top to bottom: Catherine Ursillo/ Photo Researchers, Inc.; D. Hurst/Alamy Images; Bill Aron/Photo Edit Inc.; Tariq Zehawi/Newscom; p. 575: Jochen Tack/Alamy; p. 577: David White/Alamy Images; p. 578: Catherine Ursillo/Photo Researchers, Inc.; p. 579 top: Sharon Dominick/iStockphoto; p. 579 bottom: D. Hurst/Alamy Images; p. 580: Think-stock; p. 581: Dean Millar/iStockphoto; p. 582: Janine Wiedel Photolibrary/Alamy; p. 584: Sharon Dominick/iStockphoto; p. 585: Bill Aron/PhotoEdit Inc.; p. 586: Roy McMahon/Glow Images; p. 587: reddroomstudios/iStockphoto; p. 588: Michael Dwyer/Alamy; p. 590 Tariq Zehawi/Newscom; p. 591: A. Ramey/PhotoEdit; p. 593 left: Eric Ferguson/iStockphoto; p. 593 right: Daniel Deitschel/iStockphoto

FOCUS ON Reducing Your Risk of Unintentional Injury   Opener: payless-images/Fotolia; p. 598 top to bottom: Radius Images/Alamy; Paul Conklin/ PhotoEdit inc.; Stephen Bonk/Shutterstock; Jeff Greenberg/PhotoEdit Inc.; p. 599: Radius Images/Alamy Images; p. 600: Peter Kim/Shutterstock; p. 601: Paul Conklin/PhotoEdit Inc.; p. 603 top: Stephen Bonk/Shutterstock; p. 603 bottom: Kristin Piljay/Pearson Education; p. 604: PNC/Getty Images; p. 606: Jeff Greenberg/ PhotoEdit Inc.; p. 607: sumnersgraphicsine/iStockphoto; p. 608: Hybrid Images/ AGE Fotostock America, Inc.; p. 609 left: Science Photo Library/Alamy Images; p. 609 right: Science Photo Libarary/Alamy

Chapter 20   Opener: Dev Carr/AGE Fotostock America, Inc.; p. 614 top to bot-tom: brianindia/Alamy; Real World People/Alamy; David King/Dorling Kindesley Ltd. qaphotos.com/Alamy; p. 617 top: brianindia/Alamy; p. 617 bottom: Murat Giray Kaya/iStockphoto; p. 618: Masterfile Corporation; p. 620: Will and Demi McIntyre/Photo Researchers, Inc.; p. 622: Real World People/Alamy; p. 625: David King/Dorling Kindersley; p. 626: qaphotos.com/Alamy; p. 629: Image Source/Corbis; p. 631: Patrick Lane/Somos Images/Corbis/Glow Images; p. 632: Blend Images/Alamy; p. 633: CHINE NOUVELLE/SIPA/Newscom; p. 634 left: iStockphoto; p. 634 right: Jupier Images/Thinkstock

Chapter 21   Opener: Andersen Ross/Blend Images; p. 638 top to bottom: Newscom Fancy/Alamy; Monkey Business Images/Shutterstock; Dream Pictures/ Corbis; p. 639: Ronnie Kaufman/Blend Images/Getty Images; p. 640: Newscom; p. 641: Markos Dolopikos/Alamy; p. 642: Moodboard/Corbis; p. 643: Sharon Dominick/iStockphoto; p. 644 top: Elnur/Shutterstock; p. 644 bottom: Fancy/ Alamy; p. 647: Thinkstock/Getty Images; p. 648: Monkey Business Images/ Shutterstock; p. 650: DreamPictures/Corbis; p. 652: Matthew Plexman/Masterfile; p. 654: Pascal Broze/Photo Researchers, Inc.; p. 655: Richard Hutchings/ PhotoEdit Inc.; p. 656: Apex News and Pictures Agency/Alamy; p. 658: Daniel Cardiff/iStockphoto

Index